ONCOLOGY NURSING

Second Edition

Shirley E. Otto,
MSN, RN, OCN, CRNI

Oncology Clinical Nurse Specialist
St. Francis Regional Medical Center
Wichita, Kansas

*with **189** illustrations*

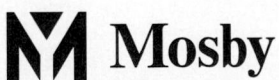 Mosby

St. Louis Baltimore Boston Chicago London Madrid Philadelphia Sydney Toronto

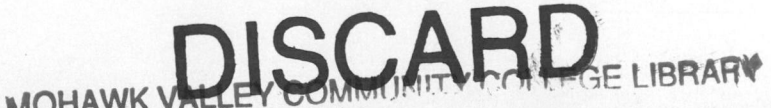

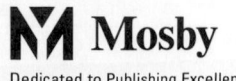

Mosby
Dedicated to Publishing Excellence

Editor: Don Ladig
Developmental Editor: Jolynn Gower
Project Manager: Linda Clarke
Production Editor: Allan S. Kleinberg
Cover Designer: John Grizzell
Manufacturing Supervisor: Kathy Grone

SECOND EDITION

Printed in the United States of America
Composition by Graphic World, Inc.
Printing/binding by Maple-Vail Book Mfg. Group

Mosby–Year Book, Inc.
11830 Westline Industrial Drive
St. Louis, Missouri 63146

Library of Congress Cataloging-in-Publication Data
Oncology nursing / [edited by] Shirley E. Otto. — 2nd ed.
        p.   cm.
    Includes bibliographical references and index.
    ISBN 0-8016-7816-1
    1. Cancer—Nursing.   I. Otto, Shirley E.
    [DNLM: 1. Neoplasms—nursing.   2. Neoplasms—therapy.
 3. Oncologic Nursing.   WY 156 05748 1993]
 RC266.053   1993
 610.73'698—dc20
 DNLM/DLC
 for Library of Congress   93-28963
                                                               CIP

94 95 96 97 98 / 9 8 7 6 5 4 3 2 1

ONCOLOGY NURSING

DISCARD

To those who knew me best
and loved me most,
my mother,

Esther Blaney,

and my daughters,

Carla Jo and Carmen Joy Otto

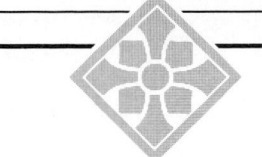

Contributors

Joyce Alexander MSN, RN, OCN **(Chapter 4)**

Oncology Clinical Nurse Specialist
Emory University Hospital
Atlanta, Georgia

Cynthia Brogden, MSN, RN, OCN **(Chapter 13)**

Clinical Nurse Specialist
University of Kansas Medical Center
Kansas City, Kansas
Kansas City Free Health Clinic
Kansas City, Missouri

Stephanie Chang, MN, RN, OCN **(Chapter 5)**

Oncology Clinical Nurse Specialist
University of California at Los Angeles
Assistant Professor of Nursing
University of California at Los Angeles School of Nursing
Los Angeles, California

Jane C. Clark, MN, RN, OCN **(Chapters 11 and 17)**

Clinical Nurse Specialist
Assistant Professor
Emory University Hospital
Atlanta, Georgia

Frances Cornelius, MSN, RN **(Chapter 26)**

Instructor
University of Pittsburgh School of Nursing
Department of Health and Community Systems
Pittsburgh, Pennsylvania

Rebecca Crane, MN, RN, OCN **(Chapter 7)**

Assistant Clinical Professor
UCLA School of Nursing
Oncology/Breast Clinical Nurse Specialist
Harbour UCLA Medical Center
Torrence, California

Betty Thomas Daniel, MS, RN, OCN **(Chapter 9)**

Clinical Nurse Specialist GI Oncology/Endocrinology
The University of Texas M.D. Anderson Cancer Center
Houston, Texas

Marilyn Davis, MS, RN **(Chapter 10)**

Project Manager, Oncology/Biotech
Schering Laboratories
Washington, DC

Mary Gullatte, MN, RN, OCN **(Chapter 3)**

Head Nurse-Medical Oncology
Emory University Hospital
Atlanta, Georgia
Director/Consultant
Staff Development & Health Education
Marietta, Georgia

Ryan Iwamoto, ARNP, MN **(Chapter 21)**

Clinical Nurse Specialist
Section of Radiation Therapy Oncology
Virginia Mason Clinic
Seattle, Washington

Noella Devolder McCray, MN, RN, OCN **(Chapter 30)**

Oncology Program Director
Independence Regional Health Center
Kansas City, Missouri

Linda Meili, BSN, RN, OCN **(Chapters 2, 14, and 25)**

Case Manager, Breast Cancer Clinic
Vincent T. Lombardi Cancer Center
Georgetown University Hospital
Washington, DC

Jill Grodecki Moore, MSN, RN **(Chapters 16 and 24)**

Clinical Nurse Specialist
Harper Hospital
Detroit, Michigan

Mary E. Murphy, MS, RN, OCN **(Chapters 6 and 8)**

Instructor, Sinclair Community College
Education Coordinator, Hospice of Dayton
Dayton, Ohio

Shirley E. Otto, MSN, RN, OCN, CRNI **(Chapters 18 and 22 and Appendices)**

Oncology Clinical Nurse Specialist
St. Francis Regional Medical Center
Wichita, Kansas

Jeanne Parzuchowski, MS, RN, OCN **(Chapter 12)**

Urologic Oncology Program Coordinator
Detroit Medical Center Oncology Program
Detroit, Michigan

Karen Pfeifer, MSN, RN, CNA, OCN **(Chapters 1 and 20)**

Director of Nursing Resources
Zale Lipshy University Hospital
  at Southwestern Medical Center
Dallas, Texas

Paula Trahan Rieger, MSN, RN, OCN **(Chapter 23)**

Clinical Nurse Specialist
Immunology/ChemoPharmacology
The University of Texas M.D. Anderson Cancer Center
Houston, Texas

Sandra Lee Schafer, MN, RN, OCN **(Chapter 19)**

Clinical Nurse Specialist in Cancer Care
Shadyside Hospital
Pittsburgh, Pennsylvania

Susan L. Penny Schmidt, MS, RN, OCN **(Chapter 15)**

Oncology Clinical Nurse Specialist
New Hanover Regional Medical Center
Wilmington, North Carolina

Lisa Schulmiester, MN, RN, CS, OCN **(Chapter 27)**

Clinical Instructor
Louisiana State University Medical Center
New Orleans, Louisiana

Suzanne Shaffer, MN, RN, OCN **(Chapter 29)**

Hematology Clinical Nurse Specialist
Nursing Services
University of Kansas Medical Center
Kansas City, Kansas

Judith A. Shell, MS, RN, OCN **(Chapters 15 and 31)**

Oncology Clinical Nurse Specialist
Butterworth Hospital
Grand Rapids, Michigan

Carol J. Swenson, MS, RN, OCN **(Chapter 28)**

Oncology Clinical Nurse Specialist
Swedish American Hospital
Rockford, Illinois

Sandra Szekely, BSN, RN **(Chapter 24)**

Assistant Administrative Manager
Bone Marrow Transplant
Harper Hospital
Detroit, Michigan

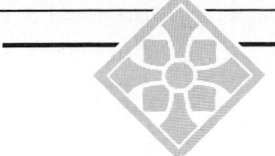

Consultants

Patricia J. Bluml, BSN, RN, OCN

Bone Marrow Transplant Clinical Nurse Specialist
St. Francis Regional Medical Center
Wichita, Kansas

Margaret Barton Burke, MS, RN, OCN

Oncology Consultant
West Roxbury, Massachusetts

Patricia C. Cloud, MSN, RN, OCNS

Doctoral Candidate
Oncology Clinical Nurse Specialist
Texas Woman's University
Houston, Texas

Ruth V. Cook, RN, MSN

Oncology Clinical Nurse Specialist
Magee Women's Hospital
Pittsburgh, Pennsylvania

Jeanne Held, MSN, RN, CS

Medical Oncology Clinical Nurse Specialist
Albert Einstein Medical Center
Philadelphia, Pennsylvania

Barbara Carlile Holmes, RN, MSN, OCN, C/PhD

Oncology Nursing Consultant
San Antonio, Texas

Patricia P. Lillis, DSN

Associate Professor and Chair
Department of Adult Nursing
The Medical College of Georgia
Augusta, Georgia

Lynn W. Nichols, MSN, RN

Associate Professor
Department of Nursing
State University of New York College at Plattsburgh
Plattsburgh, New York

Janet S. Nussbaum, EdD, RNC, OCN

Assistant Professor
College of Nursing
University of South Carolina
Columbia, South Carolina

Elizabeth Outlaw, RN, MA

Per Diem Oncology Staff Nurse
Stamford Hospital
Stamford, Connecticut

Jacqueline A. Rohaly, MSN, RN, OCN

Clinical Nurse Specialist
Oncology/Hematology
Medical Nursing Service
Hines VA Hospital
Hines, Illinois

Kathrine Roth, RN, MSN, OCN

Clinical Nurse Specialist
Oncology, Hematology, and Bone Marrow Transplant
University of Wisconsin Hospital and Clinics
Madison, Wisconsin

Barbara J. Schroeder, MS, RN

Oncology Clinical Nurse Specialist
Mayo Clinic
Rochester, Minnesota

Denice Sheehan, RN, MSN, OCN

Nursing Supervisor
Hospice of the Western Reserve
Mentor, Ohio

Kathleen M. Shuey, MS, RN, OCN

Clinical Nurse Specialist, Thoracic
M.D. Anderson Cancer Center
Houston, Texas

Nancy Short, MSN

Clinical Nurse Specialist
Duke University Medical Center
Durham, North Carolina

Patricia A. Stuckey, MSN, RN, OCN

Assistant Professor, Retired
School of Nursing
Virginia Commonwealth University
Medical College of Virginia
Richmond, Virginia

Linda Tenenbaum, RN, MSN, OCN

Professor of Nursing
Broward Community College
Ft. Lauderdale, Florida

Lindsey Trammell, RN, MSN

Oncology Clinical Nurse Specialist
University of Alabama in Birmingham
Comprehensive Cancer Center
Birmingham, Alabama

Claudette Varricchio, DSN, RN, OCN, FAAN

Nurse Consultant, Program Director
Department of Health and Human Services
National Institute of Health
National Cancer Institute
Bethesda, Maryland

Sally P. Weinrich, PhD, RN

Associate Professor
College of Nursing
University of South Carolina
Columbia, South Carolina

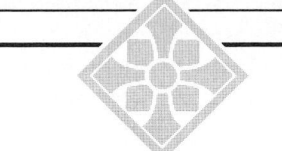

Preface

Oncology Nursing's first edition was designed to provide the most current and relevant information needed for nursing care of patients with cancer. The book's strong clinical focus made it a valuable resource for nurses in a variety of settings, including major cancer centers, local hospitals, clinics, physicians' offices, and patients' homes. Based on the many excellent comments and compliments received, the book met the varied nursing practice needs:

"Someone wrote an oncology book with the staff nurse in mind. I can read, interpret, and incorporate the concepts into my nursing practice."

"It was the book of *choice* to prepare/review for the oncology nursing certification exam."

"The book is an excellent resource for the clinical nurse specialist preparing informal/formal clinical educational programs."

Other health care professionals stated that they found the book to be an excellent resource enabling them to become more knowledgeable in cancer care.

This second edition of *Oncology Nursing* combines several excellent suggestions to provide an enhanced and more comprehensive text. The original format has stayed the same, but the book has been expanded with more disease, treatment, and supportive care chapters, and a 200 word glossary has been added. Each chapter received major revisions, and new features such as geriatric considerations, patient teaching priorities, disease and treatment related complications, and future directions and advances in therapy were incorporated throughout all the chapters.

Unit I opens with a chapter on cancer pathophysiology that gives a fundamental explanation of carcinogenesis, neoplastic classification systems, cell cycle properties, and the metastatic process. Chapters covering epidemiology; prevention, screening, and detection; and diagnosis and staging complete the unit. The most recent National Cancer Institute and American Cancer Society guidelines, recommenda-

tions, and statistics are incorporated throughout the book. New information regarding chemoprevention trials for prevention of breast and prostate cancer, environmental issues, and socioeconomic factors of poor and underserved Americans will be of interest to many nurses.

The chapters in Unit II cover clinical management of the most common cancers (bone, brain/CNS, breast, colorectal, gastrointestinal, genitourinary, gynecologic, head and neck, HIV-related cancers, leukemia, lung, lymphoma, myeloma, and skin cancers) and oncologic complications. The disease chapters examine the epidemiology, etiology, prevention, screening, and detection of the particular type of cancer being discussed. Information on how the disease is classified, diagnosed, and staged, its clinical features, and the metastatic process precedes sections that explain the most prevalent treatments and prognosis for each type of cancer. Nursing diagnosis and interventions are presented in nursing management sections incorporated in each chapter. Additional features include geriatric considerations, patient teaching priorities, and disease/treatment related complications. The chapter on oncologic complications defines the major complications that may occur as a result of cancer or its treatment. Etiology, incidence and risk factors, pathophysiology, clinical features, diagnostic evaluation, treatment modalities, and nursing management are covered for each of the following complications: disseminated intravascular coagulation, hypercalcemia, malignant pleural effusion, neoplastic cardiac tamponade, septic shock, spinal cord compression, superior vena cava syndrome, and syndrome of inappropriate antidiuretic hormone secretion. Algorithms for decision tree assessment and management of the varied oncologic complications have been added.

Unit III, which discusses cancer treatment modalities, includes chapters on surgery, radiation therapy, chemotherapy, biotherapy, bone marrow transplant, and cancer clinical trials. These chapters examine the principles and roles of each therapy. The surgery chapter explores pre-, peri-, and post-operative nursing assessment and interventions. Radiation therapy issues such as whole body, fractionated dose schedules, hyperthermia, and intraoperative therapies are included. The chapters on biotherapy and chemotherapy detail what the agents are and how they work, provide administration guidelines, and explain safe handling, storage, and disposal. The bone marrow transplantation chapter provides pretransplant and posttransplant conditioning, intervention, and follow-up medical/nursing treatment protocols. All the chapters explain how to monitor for and manage side effects. Additional information includes ambulatory care setting and home care considerations and future directions and advances in all these therapies.

Unit IV, which features chapters on home care and cancer resources, nutrition, pain management, protective mechanisms, and psychosocial and sexuality issues, is intended to equip the nurse to better support and care for the patient and family regardless of the type of cancer or method of treatment. The home care/cancer resources chapter provides many resources and guidelines to assist the nurse in discharging the patient from the acute care, ambulatory care, and/or extended care setting to the patient's home. Checklists for caregiver and home care/extended care assessment are provided. Multiple professional and public national and local resources are profiled. The nutrition chapter addresses the impact of cancer on nutritional status; assessment parameters are identified, and interventions for oral, enteral, and parenteral nutrition are suggested. Additional features include geriatric and ethical considerations. The chapter on pain management discusses analgesic, nonanalgesics, and nonsteroidal drugs as well as drug administration principles specific to route, dose titration, schedule, and side effects. Noninvasive pain management strategies are presented. Invasive pain management modalities are defined, rationales for the procedures are given, and potential outcomes are discussed. New pain management guidelines from the American Pain Society have been incorporated throughout the chapter; multiple professional and patient pain management resources are listed. Protective mechanisms, such as skin, mucous membrane, and bone marrow, are defined and parameters of nursing assessment with effective interventions are provided.

The sexuality chapter discusses the impact of cancer and its therapy on sexuality. Many sensitive issues are explored, and strategies intended to help the patient enhance self and sexual images are provided. The internal and external factors that have an impact on the patient and family with cancer are explored in the psychological chapter. These include advanced directives, quality of life, disability information, hospice care, survivorship, and the well-being of the professional and lay caregiver.

About one in three, or 85 million Americans, will eventually develop cancer. The vast majority of nurses in all practice settings feel the impact of the disease personally or professionally at some time during their careers. Because we believe the nurse is vital in providing high-quality care for patients with cancer, the nurse's role is interwoven throughout each chapter and then focused in nursing management sections. These sections include nursing diagnosis and interventions to provide the nurse with concrete guidelines to assure the best quality care throughout the course of the disease. Compassionate, competent, and conscientious nursing care is the right of the patient and family with cancer. What we say and do can *make a difference* in the quality of life for these individuals.

ACKNOWLEDGMENTS

I wish to express my sincere appreciation to the many people who made this publication possible: the contributing authors, Karen, Linda, Mary G., Joyce, Stephanie, Mary M., Becky, Betty, Marilyn, Jane, Jeanne, Cynthia, Susan, Judy, Jill, Sandy L.S., Ryan, Paula, Sandy S., Fran, Lisa, Carol, Suzanne, and Noella; and all the Mosby staff; to Ann Healy, St. Francis Regional Medical Center; and to all my oncology peers who have encouraged me. Thank you.

Shirley E. Otto

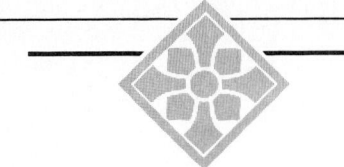

Contents in Brief

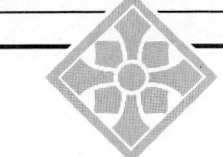

Contents

UNIT I

CLINICAL ASPECTS OF THE CANCER DIAGNOSIS

CHAPTER 1

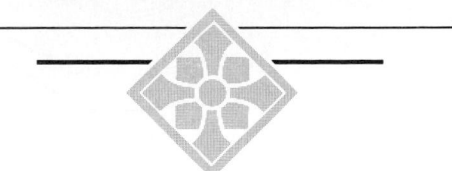

Pathophysiology

Karen A. Pfeifer

Cancer, the second most common cause of death in the United States, kills approximately 526,000 persons each year. Cancer is the primary cause of death from disease in children between the ages of 1 and 14 years, and approximately 60% of all cancer deaths occur among those individuals older than 65 years of age.[1,40]

Medical researchers have identified approximately 100 different types of cancers. Each cancer cell within these various diseases has an altered morphology and biochemistry from the normal cell. Cancer is not a disorderly growth of immature cells, but rather, a logical coordinated process in which a normal cell undergoes changes and acquires special capabilities.[24]

THE NORMAL CELL

The basic unit of structure and function in all living things is the *cell*. Approximately 60,000 billion cells are in the adult human body, and, although there are many different types of cells, all of them have certain common characteristics. For example, all cells need nourishment to maintain life, and all cells use almost identical nutrients. All cells use oxygen (O_2); the O_2 combines with fat, protein, or carbohydrates (CHO) to release the energy needed for cells to function. The mechanisms for changing nutrients into energy are generally the same in all cells, and all cells deliver their end-products of chemical reactions into nearby fluids. Most cells have the ability to reproduce. Whenever cells are destroyed, the remaining cells of the same type reproduce until the correct number has been replenished. This orderly replacement of cells is governed by a control mechanism that stops when the loss or damage has been corrected. Dynamic, active, and orderly, the healthy cell is a small powerhouse, laboratory, factory, and duplicating machine—perfectly copying itself over and over.[18,29] Fig-

ure 1-1 shows the phases and characteristics of *mitosis* (cell division).

PROLIFERATIVE GROWTH PATTERNS

Cancer cells are not subject to the usual restrictions placed by the host on cell proliferation. Proliferation is not always indicative of cancer, however. Abnormal cellular growth is classified as *nonneoplastic* and *neoplastic growth*.[11,18,30,38,41]

Nonneoplastic Growth Patterns

The four common nonneoplastic growth patterns are hypertrophy, hyperplasia, metaplasia, and dysplasia.[11,18,30,38,41]

Hypertrophy is an increase in cell size. It commonly results from increased workload, hormonal stimulation, or compensation directly related to the functional loss of other tissue.[41]

Hyperplasia is a reversible increase in the number of cells of a certain tissue type, resulting in increased tissue mass. Hyperplasia commonly occurs as a normal physiologic response at times of rapid growth and development (e.g., pregnancy and adolescence). It is abnormal when the volume of cells produced exceeds the normal physiologic demand.[11,18,38,41]

In *metaplasia*, one adult cell type is substituted for another type not usually found in the involved tissue (e.g., glandular for squamous). The process is reversible if the stimulus is removed, or metaplasia may progress to dysplasia if the stimulus persists. Metaplasia can be induced by inflammation, vitamin deficiencies, irritation, and various chemical agents. A common area for metaplasia to occur is the uterine cervix.[11,18,38,41]

Dysplasia is characterized by alterations in normal adult cells in which the cell varies from its normal

Interphase
- Cell grows in size
- Chromosomes elongate
- DNA replicates

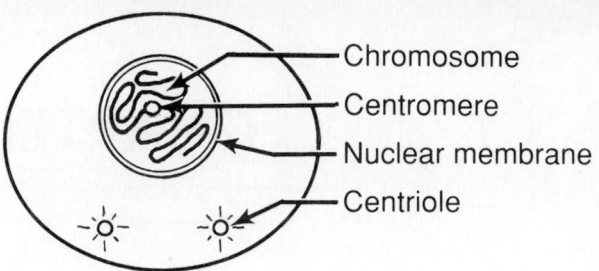

Chromosome
Centromere
Nuclear membrane
Centriole

Prophase
- DNA coils
- Centrioles move to opposite poles

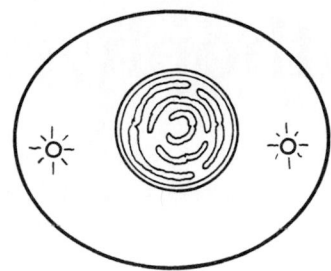

Metaphase
- Chromosomes align across cell equator
- Nucleoli and nuclear membrane disappear

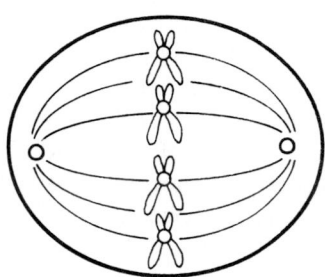

Anaphase
- Chromosomes divide
- Chromosomes move to opposite poles

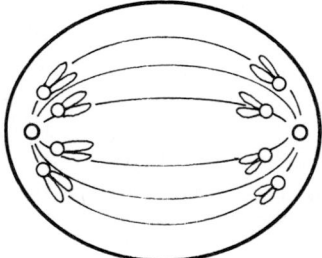

Telophase
- Chromosomes elongate
- Nuclear membranes reappear and enclose chromosomes
- Cytokinesis occurs
- Centrioles replicate

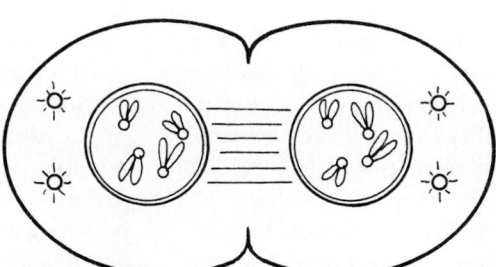

Figure 1–1   Mitosis: phases and characteristics. (From Griffiths M, Murray K, and Russo P: Oncology nursing: pathophysiology, assessment, and intervention, New York, 1984, Macmillan Publishing Co.)

size, shape, or organization, or one mature cell type is replaced with a less mature cell type. The common stimulus creating a dysplasia is usually an external one (e.g., radiation, inflammation, toxic chemicals, or chronic irritation). Dysplasia is possibly reversible if the stimulus is removed.[18,38,41]

Hyperplasia, metaplasia, and dysplasia are not neoplastic conditions but may precede the development of cancer.[41]

Neoplastic Growth Patterns

Anaplasia means "without form" and is an irreversible change where the structures of adult cells regress to more primitive levels. It is a hallmark of cancer. Anaplastic cells lose the capacity for specialized functions and are positionally and cytologically disorganized.*

Neoplasm means "new growth" and describes an abnormal tissue mass that extends beyond the boundaries of normal tissue, failing to fulfill the normal function of cells in that tissue. Neoplasms are characterized by uncontrolled functioning, unregulated division and growth, and abnormal motility. Some neoplasms are potentially harmful to the host, because they occupy space and compete for essential nutrients. Neoplastic growths are referred to as *benign neoplasms* or *malignant neoplasms*. Benign neoplasms include papillomas or warts. Malignant neoplasms include solid tumors and leukemia; these have the ability to destroy the host. *Cancer* is the common term for all malignant neoplasms.† Table 1-1 summarizes the differences between benign and malignant growths.

CHARACTERISTICS OF CANCER CELLS
Microscopic Properties

Microscopic examination of cancer cells shows certain structural changes that are described in pathologic terms. These changes are:

- *Pleomorphism.* Cancer cells vary in size and shape. Some are unusually large, while others are too small. Multiple nuclei may be seen.
- *Hyperchromatism.* Nuclear *chromatin*, the major component of genes, is more pronounced upon staining.
- *Polymorphism.* The nucleus is larger and varies in shape.
- *Aneuploidy.* Unusual numbers of chromosomes are seen.
- *Abnormal chromosome arrangements.* A variety of possibilities exist including *translocations*, the exchange of material between chromosomes, *deletions*, loss of chromosome sections, *additions*, ex-

*References 17, 18, 25, 32, 38, 41.
†References 11, 18, 20, 25, 40, 41.

Table 1–1 Comparison of Benign and Malignant Growths

Characteristic	Malignant Tumor	Benign Tumor
Encapsulated	Rarely	Usually
Differentiated	Poorly	Partially
Metastasis	Frequently present	Absent
Recurrence	Frequent	Rare
Vascularity	Moderate to marked	Slight
Mode of growth	Infiltrative and expansive	Expansive
Cell characteristics	Cells abnormal and become more unlike parent cells	Fairly normal and similar to parent cells

From Bender CM and Yasko JM: Problems with abnormal cell growth. In Lewis SM and Collier IC, editors: Medical-surgical nursing: assessment and management of clinical problems, ed 3, St Louis, 1992, Mosby.

tra chromosomes, and *fragile sites*, weak sections on chromosomes.[25,41,44]

Kinetic Properties

Cancer cells possess certain kinetic characteristics:

- *Loss of proliferative control.* All cancer cells possess this characteristic. The need for cell renewal or replacement is the usual stimulus for cell proliferation. Cell production stops when the stimulus is gone, producing a balance between cell production and cell loss. In cancer, proliferation continues once the stimulus initiates the process, and cancer cells progress in continued, uncontrolled growth. The host's normal control mechanisms fail to stop this proliferation.[11,18]
- *Loss of capacity to differentiate. Differentiation* is the process by which cells diversify and acquire specific structural and functional characteristics. In cancer, *differentiation* refers to the extent to which cancer cells resemble comparable normal cells. Cancer cells vary in their ability to retain the original tissue's morphologic and functional traits. Cells that closely resemble the normal cell but form slow-growing, usually encapsulated tumors are *well differentiated*. These cells have recognizable specialized structures and functions. Cells that grow rapidly and do not have the original tissue's morphologic characteristics and specialized cell functions are call *undifferentiated*. These cells have lost the capacity for specialized functions. The process by which cells lose characteristics of normal cells is called *dedifferentiation*. The more undifferentiated a malignant cell, the more virulent it is thought to be. It is possible to cause cells at one level of differentiation to transform

Table 1–2 Paraneoplastic Syndromes

Clinical Syndrome	Underlying Cancers	Causal Substance
Cushing's syndrome	Bronchogenic (small cell) carcinoma Pancreatic carcinoma Neural tumors	Adrenocorticotropic hormone (ACTH) or ACTH-like substance
Hyponatremia	Bronchogenic carcinoma Intracranial neoplasms	Antidiuretic hormone (ADH) or ADH-like substance
Hypercalcemia	Bronchogenic squamous cell carcinoma Breast carcinoma Renal carcinoma Adult T-cell lymphoma	(?) Parathyroid hormone-like substance Transforming growth factor (TGF)-α
Hyperthyroidism	Blood dyscrasias Bronchogenic carcinoma Prostatic carcinoma	Thyroid-stimulating hormone (TSH) or TSH-like substance
Hypoglycemia	Fibrosarcoma Other mesenchymal sarcomas Hepatocellular carcinoma	Insulin or insulin-like substance
Carcinoid syndrome	Bronchial adenoma (carcinoid) Pancreatic carcinoma Gastric carcinoma	Serotonin, bradykinin, (?) histamine
Polycythemia	Renal carcinoma Cerebellar hemangioma Hepatocellular carcinoma	Erythropoietin
Venous thrombosis	Pancreatic carcinoma Bronchogenic carcinoma Other cancers	(?) Hypercoagulability

From Volker DL: Pathophysiology of cancer. In Clark JC and McGee RF, editors: Core curriculum for oncology nursing, Philadelphia, 1992, WB Saunders Co. Modified from Cotran RS, Kumar V, and Robbins SL: Robbins pathologic basis of disease, ed 4, Philadelphia, 1989, WB Saunders Co.

into less well-differentiated cells by exposing them to cancer-causing agents.[11,18,25,38,41]

- *Altered biochemical properties.* Because of the cancer cell's loss of the capacity to differentiate, certain biochemical properties may be missing because of the cell's new immature state, or cells may acquire new properties because of enzyme pattern changes or alterations in DNA. Examples of these *altered biochemical properties* include production of tumor-associated antigens marking the cancer cell as "non-self"; continued reproduction despite diminished concentrations of growth hormones; higher rates of anaerobic glycolysis, making the cell less dependent on O_2; loss of cell-to-cell cohesiveness and adhesiveness; and abnormal production of hormones or hormone-like substances that induce paraneoplastic syndromes. In the latter, cancer cells may inappropriately secrete hormones in an organ or tissue that does not normally produce or release those hormones, resulting in signs and symptoms not directly related to the local effects of the tumor.

For example, in bronchogenic carcinoma, antidiuretic hormone (ADH) is produced, resulting in hyponatremia.[5,11,25,41] See Table 1-2.

- *Chromosomal instability.* Cancer cells are less genetically stable than normal cells owing to the development of abnormal chromosome arrangements. Chromosomal instability results in new, increasingly malignant mutants as cancer cells proliferate. These mutant cells can create a surviving subpopulation of advanced neoplasms with unique biologic and cytogenetic characteristics that are highly resistant to therapy.*

- *Capacity to metastasize. Metastasis,* the spread of cancer cells from a *primary* (parent) site to distant secondary sites, is aided by the production of enzymes on the surface of the cancer cell. Cancer cells become increasingly malignant with each mutation, and there is an association between a cell's degree of malignancy and its ability to metastasize.[11,18,26,41]

---

*References 10, 11, 14, 19, 41, 44.

CELLULAR KINETICS

The field of *cellular kinetics* is the study of the quantitative growth and division of cells.[11,35,41]

Cell Cycle

The *cell cycle* is the sequence of events involved in replication and distribution of DNA to the daughter cells produced by cell division. All cells, nonmalignant and malignant, progress through the five phases of the cell cycle. These *five phases* are G_0, G_1, S, G_2, and M (see Figure 1-2).[3,11,18,41]

G_0 PHASE (POSTMITOTIC RESTING PHASE). The G_0 phase encompasses that period of the cell cycle when normal renewable tissue is not actively proliferating. In this phase, cells perform all functions except those related to proliferation. This category includes nondividing cells and resting cells. Normal cells in the G_0 phase are activated to reenter the reproductive cycle only by certain stimuli (e.g., the death of a cell of the same type).*

G_1 PHASE (GROWTH OR POSTMITOTIC/PRESYNTHESIS PERIOD). The G_1 phase, which lasts from 12 to 14 hours, extends from the completion of the previous cell division to the beginning of chromosome replication. This is a period of decreased metabolic activity. Cells carry out their designated physiologic functions, synthesizing proteins needed in the formation of ribonucleic acid (RNA). The G_1 phase is primarily a stage of readiness, as cells prepare for entry into the S phase.*

S PHASE (SYNTHESIS). In the S phase, which lasts approximately 7 to 20 hours, RNA is synthesized, which is essential for the synthesis of deoxyribonucleic acid (DNA). DNA synthesis is limited exclusively to this phase. *Histones*, the basic protein of chromatin, are also synthesized in the S phase. Cells are most vulnerable to damage during the S phase.*

G_2 PHASE (POSTSYNTHETIC/PREMITOTIC PHASE). The G_2 phase, which lasts from 1 to 4 hours, is one of relative hypoactivity, as the cells await entry into the mitotic phase. This phase encompasses the interval from the termination of DNA synthesis to the beginning of cell division. Some additional protein synthesis occurs in G_2, but it is mostly synthesis of structural proteins versus enzymes. Some additional RNA synthesis occurs also.[3,11,18,38,41]

M PHASE (MITOSIS). In the M phase, which lasts from 40 minutes to 2 hours, mitosis and cell division occur. Protein synthesis continues but is drastically reduced. Duplication of DNA must be complete before cells enter the mitotic cycle. This phase is further subdivided into four stages: *prophase, metaphase, anaphase*, and *telophase* (review Figure 1-1). It is important to note that *interphase* encompasses all events before

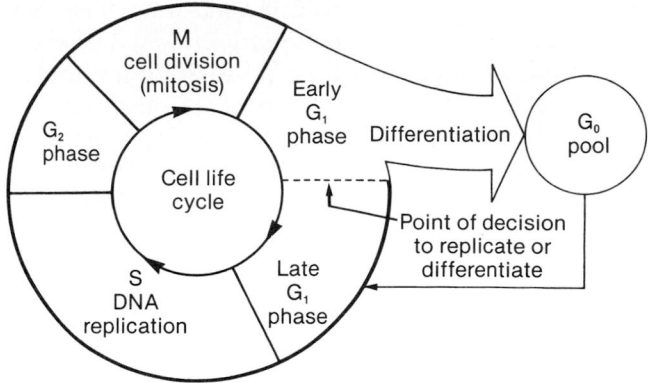

Figure 1–2 Cell generation cycle. (Courtesy Adria Laboratories, Columbus, Ohio.)

mitosis (i.e., G_1, S, and G_2). After mitosis, the daughter cells either return to the G_0 phase and stop dividing or, if a stimulus for cell division exists, enter the G_1 phase and begin the cell reproductive cycle again.*

Cancer cells are able to complete the cell cycle quicker by decreasing the length of time spent in the G_1 phase. They are also much less likely to enter or remain in the G_0 phase of the cell cycle than are normal cells; thus, they divide continuously.[3,11,24,38]

The number of cells in the body "in cycle" is only a small fraction of the total number of cells, and this is true of cancer cells as well. The duration of the M, G_2, and S phases is relatively constant, whereas the time a cell spends in G_1 varies from a few hours to several days. This determines the overall length of the cell cycle. The *cell cycle time* (T_c) is the sum of M, G_1, S, and G_2:

$$T_c = TM + TG_1 + TS + TG_2$$

Those cells in the late G_1 or early S phase of the cell cycle are the most vulnerable to dedifferentiation.[3,11,18,25,41]

TUMOR GROWTH

In normal cell proliferation, cell birth approximates cell death. The body's demand for an increase in the number of cells and for cell replacement is initiated by loss of cells of the same type or by extra tissue function demands. All elements of normal tissue growth are found in cancer cell growth and reproduction. However, progressive failure of intrinsic normal growth mechanisms produces the growth common to cancer.[28,30,38]

A common misconception is that cancer is a population of cells that reproduces much faster than normal cells. In fact, many cancers are rather slow-growing when compared to some normal cells (e.g., cells

---

*References 3, 11, 18, 25, 38, 41.

*References 3, 11, 18, 25, 38, 41.

of the epithelial lining and bone marrow cells). Not all cancer cells can proliferate indefinitely, but every neoplasm contains cells that fail to abide by the restraints placed on proliferation. This results in cell growth beyond normal margins and pressure on other organs and may contribute to the tendency of cancer cells to invade neighboring tissues and structures.[25]

Tumor Growth Properties

In general, cancer cells possess the following properties[20,34]:

- *Immortality of transformed cells.* Cancer cells are capable of passing through an infinite number of population doublings if sufficient nutrition and growth factors are available.[20]
- *Decreased contact inhibition of movement.* Normal cells adjust to the proximity of neighboring cells by halting growth. They arrest movement when another cell is encountered and symmetrically arrange themselves around each other. Cancer cells invade others without respect to these constraints.[20,25]
- *Decreased contact inhibition of cell division.* Normal cells stop dividing because of full contact with other cells, not because nutrients become depleted or because of accumulated wastes. When normal cells are surrounded, they simply stop dividing. Cancer cells lack or exhibit decreased contact inhibition of growth, continuing to divide; even piling atop one another.[20,25]
- *Decreased adhesiveness.* Cancer cells are less adhesive, resulting in increased cell mobility. This is possibly due to the loss of extracellular *fibronectin.* Fibronectin, a *large external transformation-sensitive* glycoprotein (LETS), facilitates intercellular adhesion by collagen and elastin links.[20,21,25,41]
- *Loss of anchorage dependence.* Cancer cells do not need a surface on which to attach and proliferate. This property affects cells shape and adhesiveness because the cell assumes a more rotund shape.[20]
- *Loss of restrictive point control.* In the normal cell, several environmental growth conditions (e.g., high cell density or depletion of essential amino acids, glucose, and lipids) cause the cell to be blocked in G_1. This is called the *restriction point of* G_1 or the point where the cell is blocked from continuing the cell cycle. Cancer cells lose this stringent restriction point control and continue to proliferate in spite of suboptimal nutrition and high cell density.[20]

Tumor Growth Concepts

Normal cells are divided into three major categories of cell growth: *static* (nondividing), *expanding* (rest-ing), and *renewing* (continuously dividing). Static cells do not continue to divide after the postembryonic period. If these cells are damaged or destroyed, they cannot be replaced. Examples are nerve and brain cells. Expanding cells temporarily stop reproduction on reaching normal size, but they can reenter the cell cycle and divide during times of physiologic need. Examples are liver, kidney, and endocrine gland cells. Renewing cells have the highest level of reproductive activity. These cells have a finite lifespan and continuously replicate to replace dying cells. Examples are germ cells, epithelial cells of the gastrointestinal mucosa, and blood cells. Likewise, not all cancer cells participate in active proliferation. Tumors are composed of mixtures of nondividing, resting, and continuously dividing cells.[11,18]

In the simplest model for cell growth, a cell divides to produce two daughter cells, each of which then divides, producing four cells, eight cells, and so on. Thus, cell numbers increase in powers of two *(exponential growth).*[35,41]

The growth rate of tumors is expressed in doubling time. *Tumor volume-doubling time* (DT) is the time needed for a tumor mass to double its volume. Tumor cells undergo a series of doublings as the tumor increases in size. The average DT of most primary solid tumors is approximately 2 to 3 months, with a range of 11 to 90 weeks. In general, a tumor must progress through approximately 30 doublings before becoming palpable. The minimum clinically detectable body burden of tumor *(tumor volume)* is 10 billion cells (1 g). Tumor masses are usually 100 billion cells or 10 g at detection. Death of the host usually occurs when the body burden of tumor equals or exceeds 1 trillion cells or 1 kg of tumor. This growth from 1 g to 1 kg of tumor requires only 10 more doublings.[11,18,28,35,41]

Because not all tumor cells divide simultaneously, *growth fraction* (GF) is an important concept in the determination of DT. GF is the ratio of the total number of cells to the number of proliferating cells. Tumors with larger GFs increase their tumor mass more quickly.[11,25,41] As tumor volume increases, GF decreases. In the latter stages of tumor growth, the tumor usually has only a small proportion of actively proliferating cells. The tumor loses cells by differentiation, death, or desquamation. Cell growth usually continues only at the periphery of the tumor with the center becoming increasingly dormant and eventually turning necrotic. Finally, the tumor reaches a point where cell death approximates cell birth, and a plateau is reached. The rapid proliferation of tumor cells followed by this continuous, but slowed, proliferation is called the *Gompertz function.* The Gompertz function can be expressed by the *Gompertz growth curve* (see Figure 1-3). The growth curve illustrates the initial exponential growth of cancer cells, followed by the steady and progressive decrease in the GF due to a

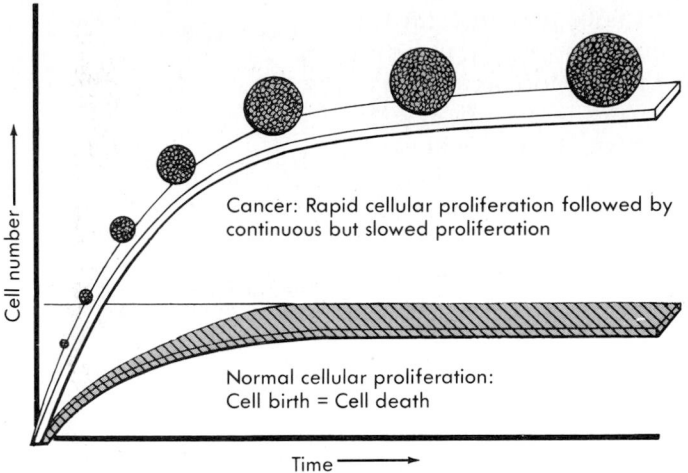

Figure 1–3   Gompertz function as viewed by growth curve. (From Goodman M: Cancer: chemotherapy and care, part I, 1990, Bristol Laboratories, Division of Bristol-Myers Co., Evansville, Ind.)

decrease in the fraction of proliferating cells and an increase in the rate of cell death.*

CARCINOGENESIS

Carcinogenesis is the process by which normal cells are transformed into cancer cells. Although numerous theories have been proposed to explain it, no single unifying hypothesis has been offered or accepted. The exact cause of most human cancers is still unknown today.[11,41,43]

An understanding of the following terms is necessary before theories of carcinogenesis can be discussed:

- *Initiating agent* (carcinogen). An initiating agent is a chemical, biologic, or physical agent capable of permanently, directly, and irreversibly changing the molecular structure of the genetic component (DNA) of a cell. This predisposes the cell to transformation when exposed to a prolonged or continuous promoting agent. An initiating agent may cause: (1) complete division of the DNA chain in one or more places; (2) elimination of one of the component parts of the DNA chain (e.g., sugars or bases); or (3) errors in DNA repair. It may act at the initial point of contact, in the organ where carcinogens have accumulated, or at the site of metabolism or excretion. *Viral, environmental or life-style,* and *genetic factors* have all been identified as initiators of carcinogenesis.[36,38,41]

- *Promoting agent* (cocarcinogen). A promoting agent alters the expression of genetic information of the cell, thereby enhancing cellular transformation. Examples include hormones, plant products, and drugs. Promoting agents do not directly

react with a cell's genetic material and cannot mutate DNA by themselves. Although they work in conjunction with initiating agents to promote neoplastic change, promoting agents do not themselves cause cancer. The effects of promoting agents are temporary and reversible.[11,38,41]

- *Complete carcinogen.* A complete carcinogen possesses both initiating and promoting properties and is capable of inducing cancer on its own. The ability to act as a complete carcinogen may be dose related. Radiation is an example of a dose-related complete carcinogen.[11,24,36,43]

- *Reversing agent.* A reversing agent inhibits the effects of promoting agents by stimulating metabolic pathways in the cell that destroy carcinogens or altering the initiating potency of chemical carcinogens. Examples include drugs, enzymes, and vitamins.[41,43]

- *Oncogene.* An oncogene is a gene that has evolved to control growth and repair of tissues. It is the genetic code that functions as the "off" and "on" signals that cells send and receive to control reproduction. Oncogenes include *proto-oncogenes,* the portion of DNA that regulates normal cell proliferation and repair, and *antioncogenes,* the portion of DNA that stops cell division. Oncogenes are the targets of carcinogens, producing mutations that may leave protooncogenes permanently in the "on" position and prevent antioncogenes from exerting the "off" signal at the appropriate time.[41,43]

- *Progression.* As tumor cells proliferate, they undergo changes in their microscopic structures. This is referred to as *progression,* or the change in a tumor from a preneoplastic state, or low degree of malignancy, to a rapidly growing, virulent tumor. Tumor progression may be characterized by

*References 11, 18, 27, 28, 35, 38, 41.

changes in growth rate, invasive potential, metastatic frequency, morphologic traits, and responsiveness to therapy. Progression occurs as a result of a cell type that grows more rapidly or metabolizes at a faster rate than other cells in the tumor mass. This cell then becomes the dominant cell type. Also, cytotoxic treatments may enhance tumor progression by their mutagenic effects, hastening the appearance of increasingly malignant variants.[11]

- *Heterogeneity.* The concept of heterogeneity is closely related to progression. It refers to differences among individual cells within a tumor. As mentioned earlier, cancer cells have a higher frequency of random mutation because of their genetic instability. These mutations produce clones whose acquired genetic variability results in heterogeneity within a tumor. Cells within a tumor can be heterogeneous with respect to ability to invade surrounding tissue, genetic composition, growth rate, metastatic potential, hormone receptors, and susceptibility to antineoplastic therapy. The degree of heterogeneity increases as the tumor increases in size.[10,11,13,19]

- *Transformation.* Transformation is a multistep process by which cells become progressively dedifferentiated after exposure to an initiating agent. There is probably more than one way to transform a cell. Transformation, however, generally results from a genetic alteration in the cell, which deregulates the control of cell proliferation. The controversy centers around the question of what stimuli induce the needed transformation in a cell's DNA. Many authorities feel that as much as 80% of known human cancers are the direct result of an individual's exposure to environmental carcinogens.[11,41,43]

Theories of Carcinogenesis

Carcinogenesis is believed to involve two or more steps. The *Berenblum theory,* first proposed in 1947, states that cancer occurs as the result of two distinct events: *initiation* and *promotion.* Initiation occurs first and is usually believed to be rapid and mutational. The change is brought about by an initiating agent (e.g., a chemical substance). The second event involves a promoting agent, and its effect is generally believed to include changes in cell growth, transport, and metabolism. Without promotion, initiation will not result in a truly transformed cell. Promotion may occur shortly after initiation or much later in an individual's life. Initiation produces a change in the cell, but cancer will not develop until the cell is affected by one or several promoting agents (see Figure 1-4).[4]

Over the years, Berenblum's theory has evolved into the *three-stage theory of carcinogenesis.* This theory

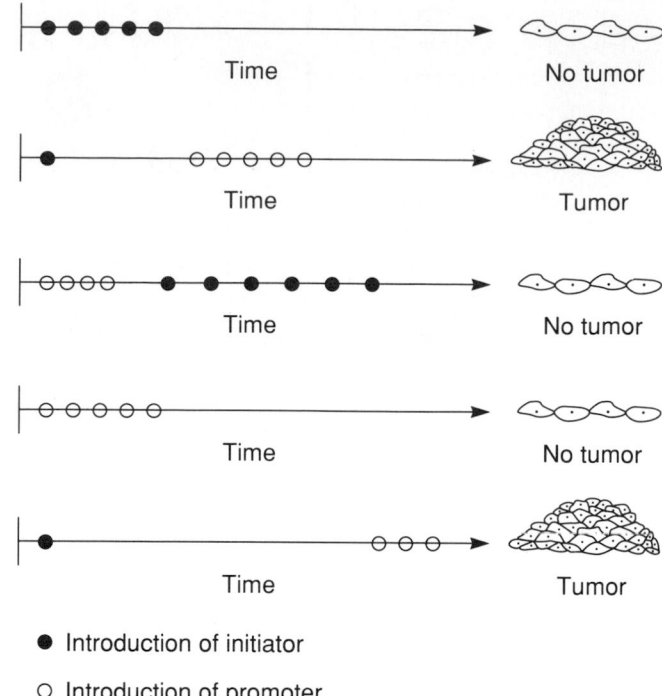

● Introduction of initiator

○ Introduction of promoter

Figure 1-4   The interactions of initiation and promotion.

proposes that the process of transforming a normal cell into a cancer cell consists of three distinct phases with several substages, all of which occur in the cell's DNA.

In the first stage, *initiation,* a carcinogen damages DNA by altering a specific gene. This gene either (1) undergoes repair and no cancer results, (2) permanently changes but causes no cancer unless subsequently exposed to the action of a cocarcinogen at a later date, or (3) transforms and produces a cancer cell if the initiator is a complete carcinogen.[41,43]

In the second stage, *promotion,* cocarcinogens are subsequently introduced, resulting in either reversible or irreversible damage to the proliferating mechanism of the cell. Irreversible damage results in cancer cell transformation. Cocarcinogens' effects may be inhibited by cancer-reversing agents (e.g., Vitamin C; certain host characteristics, such as an effective immune system; or limited time or dose exposure to the cocarcinogen).[41,43]

In the final stage, *progression,* both mutagenic and nonmutagenic events occur, leading to morphologic changes within the cell and increased grades of malignant behavior (e.g., invasion, metastasis, and drug resistance). This process is irreversible.[41,43]

Carcinogenesis is a process that can occupy the better part of a person's life. Obviously, in humans, carcinogenesis is more complex than any researcher-induced laboratory model. The distinction between the three stages is often blurred and complicated by the presence of a *latent period* between the initial exposure to a carcinogen and the actual development of a clinically detectable malignancy. This latent period is not characterized by particular clinical or subjective signs or symptoms, nor have any tests been developed to detect latent transformed cells. It is therefore impossible to predict whether certain segments of a population are at risk for developing cancer. Tumors might not appear for 20, 30, or 40 years in these risk grops. Also, for most persons diagnosed with cancer, there is no obvious history of exposure to a carcinogen. This phenomenon, known as the *multiple factor effect*, plays a significant role in human carcinogenesis.[41,43]

Medical researchers have not been able to prove definitively that the initial event in carcinogenesis is a mutation. Whatever causes cancer, the final result is an irreversible change in the cellular genetic code. This leads to cell clones that eventually give rise to clinically detectable cancer.[24,41,43]

Hormonal Carcinogenesis

Changes in a person's hormonal environment most likely result from an overproduction of endogenous hormones or an excessive administration of exogenous hormones. Four main types of human cancer (i.e., cancer of the prostate, brain, breast, and en-dometrium) occur in hormone-responsive tissues *(target tissues)*. Although target tissues require hormones for normal growth and function, there is little evidence that hormones produce any direct carcinogenic effects. Hormones do not interact with or exert an effect on nucleic acid. Rather, hormones promote the carcinogenic process by sensitizing a cell to the carcinogenic insult or modifying the growth of an established tumor.[18,22]

Chemical Carcinogenesis

Many chemical compounds are known carcinogens. Chemical carcinogens include compounds or elements that alter DNA. The relationship between chemical carcinogens and neoplasia has been documented for several centuries, beginning with the high incidence of scrotal cancer observed among chimneysweeps. However, chemical carcinogens are not confined solely to the occupational arena. Environmental chemical carcinogens range from food preservatives to atmospheric pollution. The list of known human chemical carcinogens is short; the list of suspected human chemical carcinogens is longer and grows yearly. Examples of known or suspected chemicals and mixtures that act as carcinogens are listed in Table 1-3.[24,33,41,43]

Table 1–3 Chemicals and Mixtures that are Carcinogenic or Probably Carcinogenic in Humans

Agent	Site
LIFE-STYLE/PERSONAL-CHOICE EXPOSURE	
Tobacco	Lung, pancreas, oral cavity and pharynx, larynx, urinary tract
Tobacco quids and betel nut	Oral mucosa
Ethanol with smoking	Esophagus
INDUSTRIAL EXPOSURE	
Arsenic compounds	Skin, lungs
p-Biphenylamine and *o*-nitrobiphenyl	Urinary bladder
Asbestos	Pleura, peritoneum, lung
Asbestos with cigarette smoking	Synergistic increase in lung
Benzidine (4,4'-diaminobiphenyl)	Urinary bladder
Bis(chloromethyl) ether	Lung
Bis(2-chloroethyl) sulfide	Respiratory tract
Chromium compounds	Lung
2(or β)-Naphthylamine	Urinary bladder
Nickel compounds	Lungs, nasal sinuses
Soots, tars, oils	Skin, lungs
Vinyl chloride	Liver mesenchyme
Radon gas (radiation)	Lung
Radon gas with cigarette smoking	Synergistic increase in lung
DRUGS AND THERAPEUTIC EXPOSURE	
N,N-Bis(2-chloroethyl)-2-naphthylamine (Chlornaphazine)	Urinary bladder
Cancer chemotherapy regimens (alkylating agents)	Leukemias, lymphomas, solid tumors
Diethylstilbestrol	Vagina
Estrogen	Breast, uterus
Phenacetin	Renal pelvis
Psoralen with ultraviolet radiation	Skin

From Lieberman MW and Lebovitz RM: Neoplasia. In Kissane JM, editor: Anderson's pathology, ed 9, St Louis, 1990, Mosby.

Different chemical carcinogens show no similarities in their chemical structures, except for the property of *electrophilicity* (electron-loving or seeking). All chemical carcinogens are initially electrophilic or become so as a result of the host's metabolism. These carcinogenic molecules tend to be highly reactive and search for other biologic molecules that have excess electrons or are electron-donating, primarily DNA, RNA, and proteins.[41,43]

Chemical carcinogens may be divided into two categories regardless of origin. The first category, *direct-acting chemical carcinogens*, acts directly on nucleic acids and proteins. These carcinogens form reactive ions that mutate DNA and do not require metabolic activation by the host. Examples include busulfan and nitrogen mustard. The second category involves *procarcinogens*, which are not directly effective as carcinogens but can mutate DNA after metabolic activation. These must be activated by carcinogen-activating enzymes attached to cells. Most chemical carcinogens are procarcinogens. Examples include soot, coal tar products, and cigarette smoke. Once metabolized, procarcinogens become *ultimate carcinogens*.[18,41,43]

In summary, most chemical carcinogens are mutagens and must be biochemically changed to reveal their potential mutagenicity. However, some chemical carcinogens may be active in their original form. Their main mechanism of action appears to be interference with nuclear DNA.[18]

Viral Carcinogenesis

Although evidence of viral carcinogenesis in animals has existed for many years, the connection between viruses and human cancers has been a fairly recent development. Viruses are thought to contribute to human carcinogenesis by infecting the host DNA, resulting in proto-oncogenic changes and cell mutation. Viral carcinogens may be *slow-acting* (adenoviruses, herpes viruses) or *fast-acting* (human T-cell lymphomaleukemia virus or HTLV) and are *tissue specific*, infecting tissue selectively. Age and immunocompetence are believed to interact with and affect a person's vulnerability to viral carcinogens.[11,38,41,43]

The link between the Epstein-Barr virus (EBV) and Burkitt's lymphoma and nasopharyngeal cancer as well as that of hepatitis B virus (HBV) to hepatocellular cancer has been firmly established. The herpes simplex 2 virus is believed to be linked to the development of cervical cancer, but the evidence for this is not conclusive. Cytomegaloviruses (CMVs) have been linked to Kaposi's sarcoma and are found in the tissues of persons with different cancers. See Table 1-4 for additional information on oncogenic viruses.[18,24,38]

Time-space clusters of persons with leukemia and Hodgkin's disease suggest an infectious etiology. However, other environmental factors may be equally significant in both of these conditions. In the past, the importance of viruses in carcinogenesis was con-

Table 1-4   Oncogenic Viruses

Family	Virus	Associated Tumors	Other Risk Factors
DNA VIRUSES			
Hepadenovirus	Hepatitis B group (HBV)	Liver cancer	Alcohol Smoking Fungal toxins Other viruses
Papovavirus	Human papilloma virus (HPV)	Genital, laryngeal, and skin warts	
		Skin cancers in clients with epidermodysplasia verruciformis	Sunlight Genetic disorders possibly affecting immunity
		In situ and invasive cancers of the vulva and uterine cervix	
Herpesvirus	Epstein-Barr virus (EBV)	Burkitt's lymphoma Immunoblastic lymphoma Nasopharyngeal carcinoma	Malaria Immune deficiency Histocompatibility antigen genotype
	Herpes simplex type 2 (HSV-2)	Cancer of uterine cervix	
	Cytomegalovirus (CMV)	Kaposi's sarcoma	Immune deficiency Histocompatibility antigen genotype
RNA VIRUSES			
Type D	Human T-cell leukemia virus-1 (HTLV-1)	Adult T-cell leukemia/lymphoma	

From Fernoglio-Preiser CM et al: New concepts in neoplasia as applied to diagnostic pathology, Baltimore, 1986, Williams & Wilkins.

sidered minimal; however, as more information is uncovered about these relationships, this is changing.[18,24]

Radiation Carcinogenesis

Radiation is a carcinogen and has the potential to be a complete carcinogen. Damage to the cell by this source may give rise to cancer when damage affects proto-oncogenes or antioncogenes. The first documented evidence of radiation carcinogenesis was shown when skin cancer occurred as a result of chronic exposure to radioactive chemicals, x-rays, and other radioactive materials (e.g., paints). Radiation appears to initiate carcinogenesis by damaging susceptible DNA, producing changes in the DNA structure. These changes may be single- and double-strand breaks or cross-linking of spiral changes. Cell death may result, or the cells may become permanently altered and escape normal control mechanisms.[11,18,24,41]

Both *ionizing* and *electromagnetic radiation* have been known to cause cancer in animals and humans. Sources of ionizing radiation exposure include: radioactive ground minerals, diagnostic or therapeutic x-rays, and synthetic radioactive materials (e.g., radioisotopes). Factors that apparently influence the risk of carcinogenesis by ionizing radiation include the following:

- Host characteristics—among these are level of tissue oxygenation, genetic make-up, age, and degree of stress
- Cell cycle phase—cells in G_2 are more sensitive than cells in S or G_1
- Degree of differentiation—immature cells are most vulnerable
- Cellular proliferation rate—cells with high mitotic rates are most vulnerable
- Tissue type—gastrointestinal and hematopoietic tissues are extremely sensitive to radiation
- Rate of dose and total dose—the higher the dose rate and total dose, the greater is the chance for mutation to occur

Less than 3% of human cancers have been related to ionizing radiation.[11,24,38,41]

Sources of ultraviolet radiation (UVL) include the sun and certain industrial sources (e.g., welding arcs and germicidal lights). The risk of developing skin cancer from sunlight is well documented. Sunlight is responsible for the majority of cases of squamous and basal cell carcinomas of the skin. UVL from the sun has little ability to penetrate body tissues, leaving the skin most vulnerable to its effects. The longer and more intense the exposure to the sun, the greater is the chance of developing skin cancer. Persons at greatest risk are fair-skinned white individuals (Irish, Scotch, Welsh, albinos, those with xeroderma pigmentosum) and those who work outdoors. UVL increases the risk of basal cell epithelioma and melanoma.[18,24,38,41]

The long latency period between exposure and tumor growth has hindered the evaluation of radiation as a carcinogen, but several types of human cancers have been associated with previous exposure to radiation. Leukemia, particularly acute myelogenous leukemia (AML) and chronic myelogenous leukemia (CML), lymphoma, skin cancer, osteosarcoma, and cancers of the lung, thyroid, and breast have all been shown to occur at varying lengths of time after radiation exposure.[9,41]

Immune System in Carcinogenesis

The immune system normally controls the proliferation of potential cancer cells. Potentially cancerous cells constantly arise within the human body but are continuously screened by the immune system and eliminated before a tumor can be established. Human immunity to malignant disease is a function of *humoral factors* (tumor-specific antibodies) and *cellular factors* (sensitized lymphocytes and macrophages). Cancer cells often possess antigens that differ from the person's own antigens and, therefore, are recognized as foreign cells by the immune system and are destroyed.[38]

Cancer should arise only when the immune system is overwhelmed, as in malnutrition, chronic disease, advancing age, and stress. Support for this theory comes from the recognition that immunosuppressed or immunodeficient persons have a much higher chance of developing cancer than persons with normal immune system function. When evaluated at the time of initial diagnosis, persons with cancer often have abnormal immune function. However, not all types of cancer are increased by immunodeficiency.[38]

TUMOR NOMENCLATURE
Histogenetic Classification System

Tumors are grouped according to the tissue from which they originate and are described by the *histogenetic classification system*. In this classification system, tumors are described by Latin and Greek terms (see Table 1-5).[29]

Benign tumors usually end in the suffix *oma*, the Greek root for *tumor*. When the suffix *oma* follows a prefix designating a specific tissue, a benign tumor can be identified. For example, fibromas and adenomas are benign tumors of fibrous and glandular tissue, respectively. Exceptions to this rule include hepatomas and melanomas. By name, these cancers should be benign. However, melanomas are malignant neoplasia of melanocytes, and hepatomas are malignant neoplasia of the liver.[17,25,37,41]

Malignant tumors also use the suffix *oma* to designate the presence of a tumor. However, malignant

Table 1–5   Classification of Tumors

Site	Benign	Malignant
EPITHELIAL TISSUE TUMORS*	**-OMA**	**-CARCINOMA**
Surface epithelium	Papilloma	Carcinoma
Glandular epithelium	Adenoma	Adenocarcinoma
CONNECTIVE TISSUE TUMORS†	**-OMA**	**-SARCOMA**
Fibrous tissue	Fibroma	Fibrosarcoma
Cartilage	Chondroma	Chondrosarcoma
Striated muscle	Rhabdomyoma	Rhabdomyosarcoma
Bone	Osteoma	Osteosarcoma
NERVOUS TISSUE TUMORS‡	**-OMA**	**-OMA**
Meninges	Meningioma	Meningeal sarcoma
Nerve cells	Ganglioneuroma	Neuroblastoma
HEMATOPOIETIC TISSUE TUMORS		
Lymphoid tissue	—	Hodgkin's disease, malignant lymphoma
Plasma cells		Multiple myeloma
Bone marrow		Lymphocytic and myelogenous leukemia

*Body surfaces, lining of body cavities, and glandular structures.
†Supporting tissue, fibrotic tissues, and blood vessels.
‡Brain nerves and retina.
From Bender CM and Yasko JM: Problems with abnormal cell growth. In Lewis SM and Collier IC, editors: Medical-surgical nursing: assessment and management of clinical problems, ed 3, St Louis, 1992, Mosby.

tumors of epithelial origin are designated by the root *sarc* (flesh) and those of connective tissue origin are designated by the root *carcin* (crablike).[37,41] *Sarcomas* comprise about 10% of human cancers. Prefixes that describe specific connective tissue sarcomas include the following[18,25,29,37,41]:

Osteo—sarcomas arising in the bone
Chondro—sarcomas arising from cartilage
Lipo—sarcomas arising from fat
Rhabdo—sarcomas arising from skeletal muscle
Leiomyo—sarcomas arising from smooth muscle
Carcinomas comprise about 80% of human cancers. Certain prefixes are used to describe the type of epithelial tissue from which carcinomas originate. For example, *adeno* describes tumors originating from glandular (columnar) epithelium. *Squamous* describes tumors arising from squamous epithelial tissue.[25,37,41]

Blastoma is a suffix used for neoplasms with histologic features suggesting origin in embryonal tissue. Examples include neuroblastoma, hepatoblastoma, nephroblastoma, and retinoblastoma (i.e., tumors that arise in the adrenal gland, liver, kidney, and retina, respectively). *Mixed tumors* contain more than one neoplastic cell type. *Teratomas* are a special type of mixed tumor and may be benign or malignant. These tumors arise from totipotential (germ) cells and may be composed of several differentiated tissue types. Teratomas arise from three germ layers: endoderm, ectoderm, and mesoderm.[17,25,41]

Hematologic Malignancies

Leukemia is a cancer of the hematologic system and is a diffuse rather than a solid tumor. This disease is characterized by the abnormal proliferation and release of leukocyte (white blood cell) precursors. Leukemia is classified as either *lymphoid* or *myeloid* according to the predominant cell type and as *acute* or *chronic* according to the level of maturity shown by the predominant cell. Acute leukemia is characterized by the proliferation of primitive white blood cells; chronic leukemia is characterized by the proliferation of mature cells. The prefix *lympho* describes a leukemia of lymphoid (lymphatic system) origin. The prefix *myelo* or *granulo* describes a leukemia of myeloid (bone marrow) origin. The suffix *blastic* describes immature white blood cells, while the suffix *cystic* describes the presence of more mature cells. For example, acute lymphoblastic leukemia describes a white blood cell disease that involves immature cells of lymphoid origin.[38,41] For additional information on leukemia, see Chapter 14.

Malignant lymphoma is a cancer of the lymphoid tissue. Both *non-Hodgkin's lymphoma* and *Hodgkin's disease* are classified according to four primary features: cell type, degree of differentiation, type of reaction elicited by tumor cells, and growth patterns. If a nodular growth pattern is observed, the term *nodular* is used after the cell type. If no mention of growth pattern is made, the lymphoma is of a *diffuse* type.[38,41]

For additional information on lymphoma, see Chapter 16.

Multiple myeloma is a cancerous proliferation of plasma cells (B lymphocytes). It is characterized by bone marrow involvement, bone destruction, and the presence of a homogeneous immunoglobulin in the urine or serum.[9,41] For additional information on multiple myeloma, see Chapter 17.

ROUTES OF TUMOR SPREAD

Cancer may remain a locally invasive process, or it may spread to nonadjacent areas by hematogenous or lymphatic channels. Some tumors exhibit an orderly pattern of progression. Initially, they grow locally, and, as tumor growth continues, tumor cells spread to and colonize regional nodes. Finally, distant metastases occur. Other tumors metastasize to distant organs before or with their spread to regional nodes. Because there are different patterns of tumor spread, it is important to determine the extent of disease in the cancer patient.[19]

The spread of cancer depends on a series of events that occur at the surface of the tumor cell and in the vascular bed of the person with cancer. The spread of cancer cells from a primary tumor occurs by two major processes: *direct spread* to contiguous areas or *metastatic spread* to nonadjacent tissues. Dissemination of cancer cells may not be limited to only one process, because spread by one route may permit entry into another.[11,15,42]

Direct Spread

Direct invasion is the ability of a tumor to penetrate and destroy adjoining tissue. Factors believed to enhance this process include the following[11,26,41]:

- *Tumor angiogenesis factor.* This substance, when secreted by cancer cells, stimulates new capillary formation. Once a tumor becomes vascularized, its growth rate increases, and its ability to invade local tissue is enhanced.[11,15]
- *Mechanical pressure and rate of tumor growth.* Rapid tumor growth creates an intratumor pressure that forces fingerlike projections of cancer cells into adjacent tissues. Uncontrolled replication produces densely packed and expanding tumor masses that exert pressure on adjacent tissues. Tumors extend into normal tissue along natural fracture lines that part in response to mechanical pressure.[11,25]
- *Cell motility and loss of cellular adhesiveness.* Cancer cells have a propensity for locomotion, and this, coupled with the slippery nature of cancer cells, promotes tumor cell dispersion.[18]
- *Tumor-secreted enzymes.* Recent research documents a strong association between the invasive potential of some tumor cells and the intracellular levels of specific enzymes (e.g., *plasminogen activator*). These enzymes may play a role in the destruction of normal tissue barriers, allowing invasion of cancer cells.[26]

Direct spread of tumor cells also occurs by *serosal seeding*. After tumor cells spread locally into tissue and penetrate body cavities, these cells can embolize, attaching to the serosal surfaces of organs within the cavity. Serosal seeding commonly occurs with lung and ovarian tumors. Although tumor cells implant on the surface of organs in the pleural and peritoneal cavities, tumor cell infiltration into the parenchyma of the organ is uncommon.[11]

Surgical instrumentation also provides a direct pathway for the spread of cancer cells. Contamination of normal tissue can occur during the course of surgical procedures (e.g., diagnostic biopsy and paracentesis). Tumor cells may be seeded by needles as they are removed, or manipulation of the tumor during surgery may release cells into the circulation.[11]

Metastatic Spread

Metastasis is derived from the Greek prefix *meta*, indicating a change. This process permits the release of cells from the primary site and subsequent spread and attachment to structures in distant sites (see Figure 1-5). The ability of a cancer cell to invade adjacent tissues and metastasize to distant sites is its most virulent property. This is an important characteristic of cancer. Benign tumors do not metastasize. Up to 75% of those persons who die with cancer have metastatic lesions in the liver, and it is estimated that liver failure is the direct cause of death in 40% of persons with liver involvement. Anorexia and cachexia secondary to metastatic disease are also frequent causes of death.[11,18,38,42]

The sequence of events in the metastatic process by *hematogenous channels* (dissemination of tumor cells through veins or arteries) is as follows:

- *Growth and progression of the primary tumor.* The first requirement for metastasis is rapid growth of the primary tumor. Most tumors must reach 10 billion cells or 1 cm in size before metastasis is possible.[15,18]
- *Angiogenesis at the primary site.* As in direct invasion, release of tumor angiogenesis factor stimulates new capillary formation. An avascular tumor is rarely metastatic. It has been shown experimentally that tumor cells do not enter the bloodstream until after the primary tumor has been vascularized.[2,15]
- *Detachment.* Cancer cells are more motile than normal cells. The period of least cellular adhesiveness is during mitosis; a tumor with a high

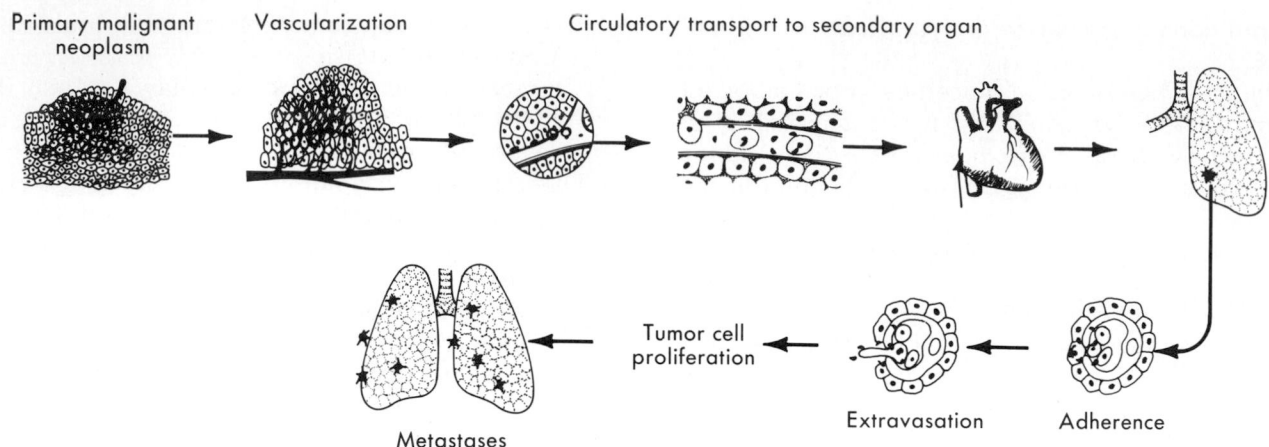

Figure 1–5   Lymphatic-hematogenic spread. (From Beare P and Meyers J: Principles and practice of adult health nursing, ed 1, St Louis, 1990, Mosby.)

mitotic index might be able to detach more cells than normal tissue. In the advancing tips of a tumor's capillaries, wide gaps exist between these endothelial cells, and there is no basement membrane in the foremost part of the capillaries. This may explain the apparent ease with which tumor cells can enter the bloodstream from a vascularized tumor.[2,15]

- *Circulation of tumor cells.* Tumor cells have been found in the bloodstream of both patients and animals with vascularized tumors. In some animal tumors, cancer cells are shed into the circulation continuously, as many as 1 million cells per day. However, most of these cells usually die. Only about 1% or less survive to become a viable metastatic lesion. It seems that the circulatory system itself is cytotoxic. The longer tumor cells circulate in the bloodstream, the higher their death rate. Factors that inhibit coagulation also keep tumor cells circulating and reduce the number of tumor emboli that attach to the vascular bed. Other causes of cell death have been proposed (i.e., immunologic destruction of circulating tumor cells).[6,8,15,18]
- *Arrest of tumor cells on vascular endothelium.* After entering the bloodstream, tumor cells aggregate with lymphocytes, platelets, or other tumor cells and form a fibrin-platelet clot. This protects the tumor cells from the hostile environment and promotes metastasis by enhancing their ability to adhere to the capillary walls of the target organ.[11]
- *Site predilection.* Site predilection does not depend on the anatomy of the circulation as previously believed. Tumor cells flow through the circulatory system based on venous drainage from the primary tumor. However, the site and survival of disseminated tumor cells depend on the *qualities and properties unique to the tumor cell* itself. Certain

tumor cells possess an affinity for specific organs. The metastatic process is not random.[12,15,18,23,31]
- *Escape from the circulation.* Once implanted into the vessel wall of the chosen organ, tumor cells must exit the organ's circulation and penetrate its tissue in order to proliferate (*extravasation*). This process is complex. Arrested tumor cells appear to damage the intact endothelium of the blood vessel by compression. Once the endothelium is damaged, tumor cells escape through the vessel wall and invade the organ tissue itself (see Figure 1-6).[7,11,15]
- *Angiogenesis of metastatic implant.* Once tumor cells arrive in the extravascular tissue, they continue to grow as a small cluster up to about 10 million cells. Continued growth, however, requires the induction of new capillaries. Without an adequate blood supply, tumor cells remain dormant and harmless, receiving only enough diffused nutrition to maintain viability. New blood vessels, induced again by the tumor's release of tumor angiogenesis factor, are needed for the continued growth of the new metastatic lesion.[11,15,16]

Lymphatic spread occurs when the cancer cells penetrate lymphatic channels draining the affected site. Much less is known about this mechanism versus spread of cancer cells by hematogenous channels. In many cancers, the first evidence of spread of disease is a mass in the lymph nodes that drain the area or region of the body carrying the tumor. Previously, it was thought that the filtering action of lymph nodes was responsible for nodal metastasis, but recent research shows that filtration is a relatively minor factor. Perhaps the physiochemical changes on the cancer cell's surface and lymph node interaction is also important in determining whether and where cancer cells become lodged in lymph nodes. Conventional thinking has also been that lymph nodes become pos-

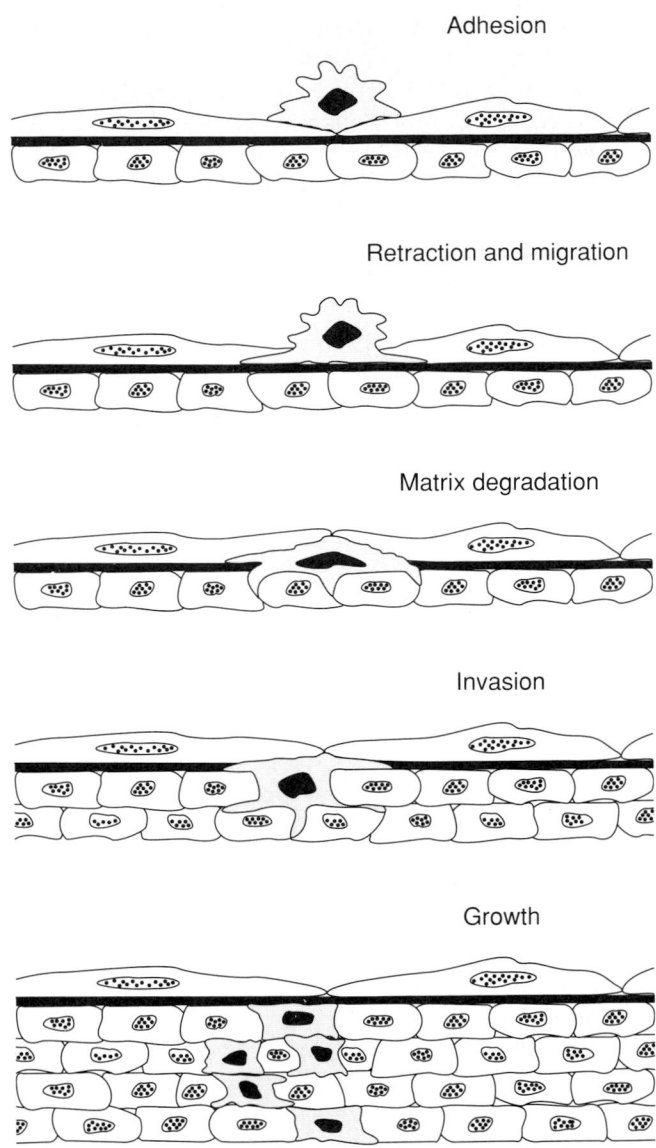

Adhesion

Retraction and migration

Matrix degradation

Invasion

Growth

Figure 1–6 Cancer cells exit from the bloodstream.

itive primarily for anatomic reasons, because the lymph nodes that drain the primary tumor are often positive first. This is a naive assumption, however, for the same reason it is now realized that hematogenous metastases are not random or completely directed by anatomy. Indeed, in some instances, metastatic tumor cells bypass local lymph nodes and seed in more distant nodes in the lymph chain.[26,41]

Several outcomes await those cancer cells that do become lodged in lymph nodes. They may die as a result of local inflammation or the encountered environment; they can grow into a lump; or they can remain dormant for unknown reasons. A significant feature of the lymphatic system is that the main lymphatic trunk enters the venous system just before the veins enter the heart. Therefore, the lymphatic and circulatory systems are interconnected, and cancer

cells that enter the lymphatic system are able to enter the bloodstream as well.[26,41]

Carcinomatosis, the extensive dissemination of tumor cells by gravity, may also be a causal factor of metastasis. During the spread of cancer over the serous membranes of larger cavities (e.g., pleural and peritoneal), cancer cells may break away and gravitate to the lower reaches of the cavity.[25]

Host and Treatment Factors as Modifiers of Metastasis

Several factors and conditions modify the frequency of metastasis. Factors known to *increase the likelihood* of metastasis include a primary tumor of long duration; a high mitotic rate; trauma, including biopsy and tumor massage; heat; radiation; and chemotherapy. Factors known to *decrease the likelihood* of metastasis include those that reduce tumor cell adherence to endothelial cells, retard intravascular coagulation, and kill tumor cells.[25]

Although the search continues for the key cellular factors that determine metastatic potential, all that is known to date in regard to clinical application is that undifferentiated tumors are more likely to metastasize than differentiated tumors. Even with histologically similar tumors, however, individuals can exhibit different metastatic disease patterns. This suggests that host factors, such as hormonal environment and age, are important in determining how, and whether, tumors will metastasize.[25]

Other Aspects of the Metastatic Process

METASTASES FROM METASTASIS. Because a metastatic tumor is penetrated by new blood vessels in the same manner as a primary tumor, the secondary implant may itself release cells in the circulation, leading to tertiary implants. This is an important clinical concern. The decision about when, or whether, to remove metastatic lesions surgically depends partly on the threat of further metastases from a metastasis.[15,26]

INHIBITORY EFFECT OF PRIMARY TUMORS. There is remarkable evidence that a primary tumor can inhibit the growth of already established metastatic lesions and, in some cases, inhibit implantation. The strength of this inhibition is directly related to tumor mass. This may explain the increased growth rate of existing metastatic lesions observed after a primary tumor is removed. It also provides further substantiation for initiating adjuvant chemotherapy after surgical resection of an advanced primary tumor instead of waiting for the first metastasis to appear.[15,26,39]

DORMANCY. Metastatic growth may appear in persons many years after apparent cure of a primary tumor. For example, in breast cancer, metastases can appear in the vertebrae 30 years after the original diagnosis. Presumably, metastatic tumor cells remain dormant for periods far beyond what would be expected based on logarithmic division of cells. Investigators do not know what causes metastatic tumor cells to go into a dormant stage and remain dormant or what causes them to eventually re-emerge. Of all aspects of metastasis, this is the least understood.[15,25,26]

CONCLUSION

The essential features of the cancer cell that distinguish it from the normal cell are its ability to reproduce uncontrollably, invade normal tissue, disseminate to distant body sites, and destroy the host. These are the essence of the transformed cell.[18]

The nurse involved in the care of cancer patients must comprehend the principles of normal and abnormal cellular physiology. These principles form the basis for defining the essential concepts related to the nursing care of the individual with cancer (e.g., teaching about health promotion and prevention, diagnosis, treatment, and follow-up) and determining implications for the professional development of the oncology nurse (e.g., use of appropriate terminology and nomenclature necessary for teaching and interdisciplinary communication; understanding rationale for treatment protocols, timing of treatment, follow-up, intensity of initial treatment protocols, current research and trends in care, and disease prognoses; initiating cancer nursing research; and enhancing participation in discussion of ethical issues related to cancer and treatment).[41]

CASE STUDY

Your patient, Mrs. H., a 68-year-old white female, is admitted for a radical vulvar excision and bilateral inguinal node dissection. The patient initially presented 2 weeks ago with a 4-year history of unremitting vulvar pruritis and the recent finding of a wart on her vulva. Initial biopsy revealed squamous cell carcinoma of the vulva. Mrs. H's pap smear results were within normal limits 6 months ago. Family history reveals a sister diagnosed with endometrial cancer 8 years ago, who is now doing well.

Discuss how you would answer this individual's questions relative to why she has developed cancer.

BIBLIOGRAPHY

1. American Cancer Society: Cancer facts and figures—1993, Atlanta, 1993, American Cancer Society.
2. Ausprunk DH and Folkman J: Migration and proliferation of endothelial cells in preformed and newly formed blood vessels during tumor angiogenesis, Microvasc Res 14:53, 1977.
3. Bender C: Implications of antineoplastic therapy for nursing. In Clark JC and McGee RF, editors: Core curriculum for oncology nursing, ed 2, Philadelphia, 1992, WB Saunders Co.
4. Berenblum I: Established principles and unresolved problems in carcinogenesis, J Natl Cancer Inst 60:723, 1978.
5. Bunn PA Jr and Ridgway EC: Paraneoplastic syndrome. In DeVita VT Jr, Hellman S, and Rosenberg SA, editors: Cancer: principles and practice of oncology, ed 3, Philadelphia, 1989, JB Lippincott Co.
6. Butler TP and Gullino PM: Quantitation of cell shedding into efferent blood of mammary adenocarcinoma, Cancer Res 35:512, 1975.
7. Chew EC, Josephson RL, and Wallace AC: Morphologic aspects of the arrest of circulating cancer cells. In Weiss L, editor: Fundamental aspects of metastasis, Amsterdam, 1975, North-Holland Publishing Co.
8. Clifton EE and Agostino D: The effects of fibrin formation and alterations in the clotting mechanism on the development of metastases, Vasc Dis 2:43, 1965.
9. Cook MB: Multiple myeloma. In Groenwald SL, Frogge MH, and Goodman M, editors: Cancer nursing: principles and practice, ed 2, Boston, 1990, Jones and Bartlett Publishers.
10. Dexter DL and Calabresi P: Intraneoplastic diversity, Biochim Biophys Acta 695:97, 1982.
11. Donehower MG: The behavior of malignancies. In Johnson BL and Gross J, editors: Handbook of oncology nursing, New York, 1985, John Wiley & Sons, Inc.
12. Fidler IJ: Selection of successive tumor lives for metastases, Nature New Biol 242:148, 1973.
13. Fidler IJ: The evolution of biological heterogeneity in metastatic neoplasms. In Nicolson GL and Miles L, editors: Cancer invasion and metastasis: biologic and therapeutic aspects, New York, 1984, Raven Press.
14. Fidler IJ and Hart IR: Biological diversity in metastatic neoplasms: origins and implications, Science 217:998, 1982.
15. Folkman J: Tumor invasion and metastasis. In Holland JF and Frei E III, editors: Cancer medicine, ed 2, Philadelphia, 1982, Lea & Febiger.
16. Folkman J and Cotran RS: Relation of vascular proliferation to tumor growth. In Richter GW and Epstein MA, editors: International review of experimental pathology, New York, 1976, Academic Press.
17. Goldfarb S: Pathology of neoplasia. In Kahn SB and others, editors: Concepts in cancer medicine, New York, 1983, Grune & Stratton, Inc.
18. Griffiths MJ, Murray KH, and Russo PC: Oncology nursing: pathophysiology, assessment, and intervention, New York, 1984, Macmillan Publishing Co.

19. Haskell CM: Introduction. In Haskell CM, editor: Cancer treatment, ed 2, Philadelphia, 1985, WB Saunders Co.
20. Holland G: Pathophysiological features of cancer: clinical knowledge for nurses. In McIntire SN and Cioppa AL, editors: Cancer nursing: a developmental approach, New York, 1984, John Wiley & Sons, Inc.
21. Hynes RO: Fibronectins, Sci Am 254:42, 1986.
22. Jordan VC: Hormones. In Kahn SB and others, editors: Concepts in cancer medicine, New York, 1983, Grune & Stratton, Inc.
23. Kinsey DL: An experimental study of preferential metastases, Cancer 13:674, 1960.
24. Kirkpatrick CS: Nurse's guide to cancer care, Totowa, NJ, 1986, Rowman Publishing Co.
25. Kupchella CE: Cellular biology of cancer. In Groenwald SL, Frogge MH, and Goodman M, editors: Cancer nursing: principles and practice, ed 2, Boston, 1990, Jones and Bartlett Publishers.
26. Kupchella CE: The spread of cancer: invasion and metastasis. In Groenwald SL, Frogge MH, and Goodman M, editors: Cancer nursing: principles and practice, ed 2, Boston, 1990, Jones and Bartlett Publishers.
27. Laishes BA: Local growth of neoplasms. In Kahn SB and others, editors: Concepts in cancer medicine, New York, 1983, Grune & Stratton, Inc.
28. LaRocca JC and Otto SE: Pocket guide to intravenous therapy, ed 2, St Louis, 1993, Mosby.
29. Luckmann J and Sorensen KC: Medical-surgical nursing: a psychophysiologic approach, ed 4, Philadelphia, 1991, WB Saunders Co.
30. Marx J: Cell growth control takes balance, Science 239:975, 1988.
31. Nicolson G: Organ specificity of tumor metastasis: role of preferential adhesion, invasion and growth of malignant cells at specific secondary sites, Cancer Metastasis Rev 7:143, 1988.
32. Potter VR: The cancer cell. In Kahn SB and others, editors: Concepts in cancer medicine, New York, 1983, Grune & Stratton, Inc.
33. Pitot HC: Principles of carcinogenesis: chemical. In DeVita VT Jr, Hellman S, and Rosenberg SA, editors: Cancer: principles and practice of oncology, ed 3, Philadelphia, 1989, JB Lippincott Co.
34. Ruddon R: Cancer biology, New York, 1981, Oxford University Press.
35. Shakney SE: Cell kinetics and cancer chemotherapy. In Calabresi P, Schein PS, and Rosenberg SA, editors: Medical oncology: basic principles and clinical management of cancer, New York, 1985, Macmillan Publishing Co.
36. Sirica AE: Pathogenesis. In Kahn SB and others, editors: Concepts in cancer medicine, New York, 1983, Grune & Stratton, Inc.
37. Sirica AE: Classification of neoplasms. In Sirica AE, editor: The pathobiology of neoplasia, New York, 1989, Plenum Press.
38. Snyder CC: Oncology nursing, Boston, 1986, Little, Brown & Co.
39. Sugarbaker EV, Thornthwaite J, and Ketcham AS: Inhibitory effect of primary tumor on metastasis. In Day SB, editor: Cancer invasion and metastasis, New York, 1977, Raven Press.
40. Thompson JM and others: Clinical nursing, ed 2, St Louis, 1989, Mosby.
41. Volker DL: Pathophysioloy of cancer. In Clark JC and McGee RF, editors: Core curriculum for oncology nursing, ed 2, Philadelphia, 1992, WB Saunders Co.
42. Wolberg WH: Metastasis. In Kahn SB and others, editors: Concepts in cancer medicine, New York, 1983, Grune & Stratton, Inc.
43. Yarbro JW: Carcinogenesis. In Groenwald SL, Frogge MH, and Goodman M, editors: Cancer nursing: principles and practice, ed 2, Boston, 1990, Jones and Bartlett Publishers.
44. Yunis JJ and Hoffman WR: Fragile sites as a mechanism in carcinogenesis, Cancer Bull 41:283, 1989.

CHAPTER 2

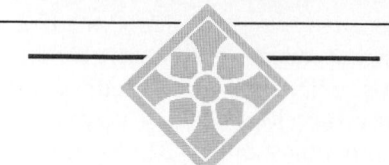

Epidemiology

Linda Meili

The science of epidemiology studies the variations in disease frequencies among human population groups and the factors influencing these variations. The goal of epidemiology is to identify the cause of disease so the causative agent may be removed, and ultimately the disease can be prevented. Unlike basic research, the emphasis of epidemiology is on humans rather than animals, and unlike clinical medicine, epidemiology studies groups or populations rather than individuals. In addition, epidemiology focuses on the events occurring before the illness, rather than the treatment after disease diagnosis. The endpoint of therapeutic research is to discover the cure for cancer: the endpoint of epidemiologic research is to prevent cancer. Epidemiology was initially associated with the study of infectious diseases. In the 1940s, however, scientists began to notice an increasing number of deaths from chronic causes, such as cancer and heart disease.

One of the earliest and best known cancer epidemiologic studies was performed by the British surgeon Percival Pott in 1775. Pott first described occupational carcinogens by noting the high incidence of scrotal cancer in chimneysweeps. The astute observation of Dr. Pott preceded the laboratory discovery of the carcinogenic properties of polycyclic hydrocarbons, such as coal and soot, by decades. Cancer epidemiology became a refined research discipline partly as a result of oncology becoming a distinct subspecialty and the beginning of the computer age.

In addition to epidemiologic principles, demography and the natural and social sciences are used to help discover causes of cancer. Examples of these fields include geographic variations in the occurrence of cancer, the relationship of cancer incidence to social habits and environmental agents, the comparison of populations with and without cancer, and results after removal of suspected cancer-causing agents.

A basic understanding of epidemiologic terminology and techniques assists oncology nurses to interpret literature about cancer causation. This knowledge allows the nurse to be an informed resource person to patients, the public, and nursing peers.

This chapter presents the terminology most frequently found in epidemiologic literature. The terms are defined, and examples of their use are illustrated. Basic information about the types of epidemiologic studies are presented. This chapter is a basis for the subsequent disease chapters of this text, which present epidemiologic information specific to that disease site.

Etiology, the cause of cancer, will be described only briefly here, since this information is presented with greater extent in the subsequent disease chapters.

TERMINOLOGY

Many terms are associated with the science of epidemiology. This chapter limits discussion to four terms that help to describe the cancer problem and are commonly used in cancer literature: incidence, prevalence, mortality, and survival.

Incidence

The number of newly diagnosed cases of cancer in a specified period of time (usually a calendar year) in a defined population is called the cancer *incidence*. For example, the incidence of breast cancer in the United States in 1993 was 183,000 newly diagnosed cases.[2] Incidence is frequently expressed in the literature as a rate per 100,000 population at risk. For example, the incidence of new breast cancer cases in Utah may be 72.3 per 100,000 population per year. The advantage of expressing incidence as a rate is that it allows comparison of rates among different populations. The statement that Utah had 750 new cases of breast cancer in 1993 and California had 18,500 new cases of breast cancer has little meaning because of their population differences. But if the rate of incidence per 100,000 population in Utah was 72.3 and in California it was 93.8, one could investigate what differences were responsible for the higher incidence rate in California. Important epidemiologic questions may arise when comparing incidence rates around the country and around the world.

Prior to 1973, cancer incidence data were collected through several periodic surveys in selected areas of the country. These surveys, coordinated by the National Cancer Institute (NCI), were conducted in 1937-1939, 1947-1948, and 1969-1971. In 1973, the NCI established and funded the Surveillance, Epidemiology, and End-Results Program (SEER), consisting of 11 population-based registries to collect data on individual cancer sites. The registries are located in Atlanta, Detroit, San Francisco/Oakland, Seattle/Puget Sound, the entire states of Connecticut, Hawaii, Iowa, New Mexico, Utah, and Puerto Rico. These registries continuously gather information on cancer incidence, mortality, and survival. These registries collect data on only about 10% of the total U.S. population, but considerable geographic and ethnic variations are represented.

In addition to SEER data, incidence information is also collected in individual hospital cancer registries. Individual tumor registries are certified by the American College of Surgeons. These registries abstract demographic and disease related information from the charts of newly diagnosed cancer patients. All patients are followed for survival data. The registries also conduct disease-specific studies as requested by the American College of Surgeons.

Incidence data collection focuses on two specific areas: demographic and medical. Demographic information extrapolates age, sex, race, marital status, and place of residence. Medical data on the same individual reports onset of illness, location of tumor, stage, histology, treatment, and survival over time. These data assist epidemiologists in describing the current cancer problem in terms of geographic distribution, age and race of patients, and increase or decrease in specific types of cancer.

Care must be exercised when deriving conclusions from incidence data. For example, there has been a slight but steady increase in the overall cancer incidence over the past decade. This information does not necessarily mean cancer is on the rise. Consider this hypothesis: more than half of all cancers are diagnosed after the age of 65; with the "graying of America," a greater portion of the population is over 65, and, therefore, this expanding aged population accounts for some of the increase in new cases. Apply this theory to these data: there were 142,900 new cases of breast cancer in 1989 compared to 183,000 in 1993. These figures would seem to indicate an increasing rate of breast cancer incidence, but, in fact, they reflect population growth because there were more women alive over the age of 50 in 1993 with the potential to develop breast cancer.

Prevalence

The measurement of all cancer cases, both old and new, at a *designated point in time,* is called cancer *prevalence.*[6] These data are not routinely collected by the SEER registries and must be determined by conducting a special survey. This is expensive and is further prohibited by the difficulty in determining who actually has been cured of the disease and should not be counted in the prevalence survey. Also consider the fact that any cancer therapy that improves survival would actually increase the prevalence of cancer.

Prevalence information is used for healthcare planning including physical facilities, manpower, and the design and implementation of screening programs.[12]

Mortality

The number of deaths attributed to cancer in a specified time period and in a defined population is the cancer *mortality.*[6] The 1993 estimated cancer mortality rate in the United States is 526,000 persons or about 1400 people a day.[1]

Unlike incidence data, mortality data have routinely been collected in the United States since 1930. The National Death Index is a centralized source for death information and can be accessed by investigators. Mortality data of comparable quality are available throughout the world and can be used for comparison of death rates. The shortcoming of mortality data, however, is accuracy. Death certificates routinely assign a single cause of death to each patient. A patient with colon cancer that metastasized to the liver may be reported to have died from liver failure rather than colon cancer.

Mortality figures are actually only a variable reflection of the cancer incidence. Therefore, when epidemiologists try to determine causes of cancer, the incidence figures are usually more helpful. Mortality data enable us to determine trends over time in the magnitude of cancer as a cause of death among members of our population.[9]

Survival

The link between incidence and mortality data is *survival analysis,* the observation over time of persons with cancer and the calculation of their probability of dying over several time periods.[12] Survival data historically have not been as available as incidence or mortality data, and it is difficult to prove how representative the existing data are.[9]

In spite of these difficulties, survival data are a useful measure of the end result of cancer treatment and can indicate improvements over time in the management of cancer. Survival data can provide a baseline for individual institutions to compare their local survival rates to national rates. Major discrepancies may indicate the need for education of community physicians regarding cancer management or more intense community education regarding early detection.[9] The disadvantage of survival data, however, is that the data are influenced by measures unrelated to treatment efficacy, such as earlier detection and changes in disease classification systems. These factors appear to lengthen survival without actually changing the natural course of the disease.[4]

The 5-year survival rate has become almost a standard term, although there is no specific biologic significance about having survived 5 years. Myers and Ries[10] studied 10-year follow-up data from the SEER program to analyze the outcome of 5-year survivors and to determine the chance of long-term survival in cancer patients. For most cancers, the chances of surviving the second 5 years are greater than surviving the first 5 years. One must consider the natural history and biology of each cancer, however. Very few pancreatic cancer patients survive the first 5 years, but those who do generally survive the following 5 years. Conversely, many breast cancer patients may survive the first 5 years after diagnosis but will not ultimately survive their cancer. The chronicity of some forms of cancer emphasizes the need for continued long-term disease follow-up beyond any arbitrary point such as 5 years.

Identification of Trends

The ultimate value of incidence, prevalence, mortality, and survival data is the identification of trends. This is the root of epidemiologic studies. A particular trend is identified that raises the question "why?" From that point, a study is designed to determine the possible cause of the trend. Why have lung cancer deaths exceeded breast cancer deaths in women? Why has the incidence of melanoma increased 1000% over the last 50 years? Why is cancer mortality higher in blacks than in whites?

The trends found in monitoring cancer incidence and mortality statistics have significant implications for cancer education and prevention. For example, the incidence of lung cancer in women increased dramatically every year this past decade. Epidemiologic studies reveal this was caused by the acceptance of and subsequent increase in women smoking after World War II. This was an impetus for education and

smoking cessation interventions targeting women. Likewise, the alarming increase in the incidence of malignant melanoma resulted in nationwide public education about the risks of sun exposure. Industry responded to both medical research and public concern by marketing more effective sunscreen products and including "sun-sense" education in their advertising campaigns.

Some examples of current trends in cancer incidence, mortality, and survival are listed in the box below.

CURRENT TRENDS IN CANCER INCIDENCE, MORTALITY, AND SURVIVAL

Incidence

There were over 1,170,000 newly diagnosed cases in the United States in 1993.

Higher rate of incidence is seen in males than females.

Overall incidence is highest in Hawaiians, lowest in American Indians.

Blacks have three times more esophageal cancer than whites.

The leading sites of incidence in males are: prostate, lung, colon.

The leading sites of incidence in females are: breast, colon, lung.

Cancers of the colon and rectum are the most frequently diagnosed malignancies.

Melanoma incidence has increased 1000% in the past 50 years.

Mortality

Over 526,000 cancer-related deaths in the United States in 1993.

Lung cancer accounts for 34% of male cancer deaths.

Lung cancer accounts for 22% of female cancer deaths.

Leading causes of male death are cancers of the lung, prostate, colon, and pancreas and leukemia.

Leading causes of female death are cancers of the lung, breast, colon, pancreas, and ovary.

Cancer is the leading cause of death in women from age 35 to 74.

For all ages, cancer is the second most common cause of death, following heart disease.

Survival

Overall 5-year survival rate for all cancers is 50%.

Large survival increases seen in Hodgkin's disease, melanoma skin cancers, and cancer of the testis, prostate, and bladder.[11]

Survival depends on extent of disease at diagnosis.

Less favorable survival rates are seen in blacks.

Five-year survival for all types of childhood cancer increased from 28% in the early 1960s to 63% in the early 1980s.[11]

Data from American Cancer Society: Cancer facts and figures—1993, Atlanta, 1993, American Cancer Society, Inc.

TYPES OF STUDIES

The epidemiologic method is composed of an orderly progression of three types of studies: descriptive, analytic, and experimental. Descriptive studies are observational in nature and record the existing patterns of disease. Identified trends generate a hypothesis as to the possible cause of the cancer trend. The intermediate step, the analytic study, tests the hypothesis and tries to identify the causal relationship. The final step, the experimental study, removes the suspected cause and evaluates the effect on the population (Figure 2-1).

Descriptive Studies

Descriptive studies form the body of data within which the hypothesis may be sought. The disease of cancer can be described many ways. One method of description might be evaluating the frequency of a cancer. This is the purpose of incidence, prevalence, and mortality data. There are specific methods available to describe the classification of the cancer: site of the tumor, morphology and grade, and the stage of the disease. This information is found in the medical record at the time of diagnosis and can be extrapolated by the epidemiologist.

Person, place, and time are classical descriptive epidemiologic variables that serve as a major source of clues to cancer etiology.

PERSON.   Age, sex, and racial differences account for fundamental differences in cancer rates.

Age. With a few exceptions, cancer becomes more prevalent in older people. Epidemiologists previously explained the increase of cancer incidence with advancing age as an increased susceptibility problem or perhaps an impaired immune system. It is now believed, however, that the increased incidence reflects the importance of duration of carcinogen exposure and of long induction periods of some cancers.[3] Indeed, more than half of all cancers are diagnosed after the age of 65.

Sex. Men tend to develop cancer more often than women, and they die more frequently from cancer than women. As women adopt roles and habits in society similar to men, the rates of non-sex–linked cancers would become similar, if indeed the current differences are related to environmental and occupational causes.[12]

Race. There are striking racial and ethnic variations in cancer incidence in this country. The male incidence of cancer is highest in blacks, followed by whites, then Hawaiians. In females, however, the exact opposite is true: Hawaiians have the highest incidence, followed by whites, then blacks.[16] There is also a significant variation in the kinds of cancer seen in different races. Compared to other races, whites have especially high rates of melanoma, Hodgkin's

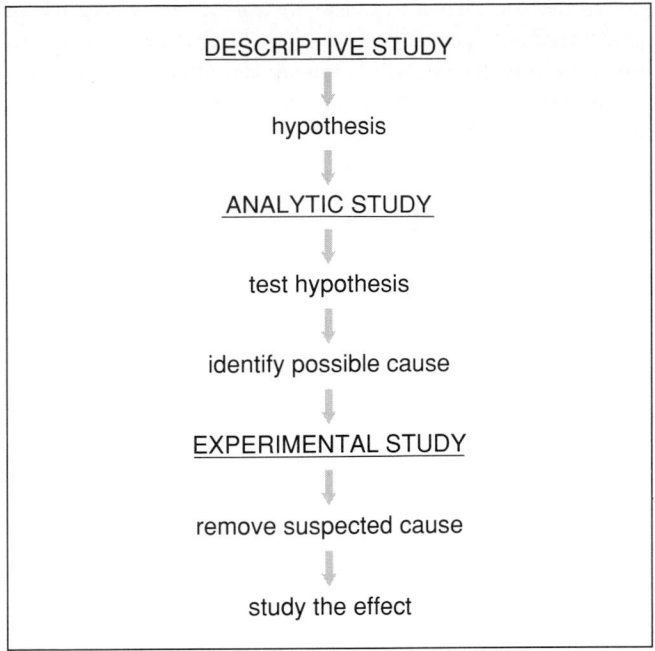

Figure 2–1 The epidemiologic method.

disease, non-Hodgkin's lymphomas, and leukemia. Blacks have elevated rates of multiple myeloma and cancers of the oral cavity, esophagus, and colon. Hispanics have especially high rates of cervical cancer, and American Indians have a remarkable prevalence of stomach cancer. Chinese people have more liver cancer diagnosed, and Japanese people have a high percentage of stomach cancers. Hawaiian women develop lung and breast cancer more frequently than others.[11] Racial and ethnic populations present unique opportunities for studying environmental and host differences.

Other Factors. Other "person" or host factors such as general health/wellness status—including nutritional status, cultural and socioeconomic variables, marital status, psychologic factors, and susceptibility factors—help to describe the cancer situation. These variables add to the body of information and may help define the hypothesis of a particular cancer cause.

PLACE.   The evaluation of incidence and mortality statistics for various geographic locales has led to the identification of major international differences in the cancer burden. Japan exemplifies a very unique cancer spectrum when compared to 24 other countries. The Japanese population has the lowest international death rate for breast cancer and the highest international mortality rate for stomach cancer.[6] Differing genetic constitutions and social habits may be possible explanations. Japanese women who migrate to Hawaii or California and adopt new habits develop cancer risks similar to American women with an increase in their breast cancer incidence and a decrease in stomach cancers.

In addition to a specific location, the category of place in descriptive studies also involves physical and biologic environmental variables such as geologic structure, water sources, flora, weather, climate, plants, and animals. "Place" descriptions also include the socioeconomic environment: urban versus rural, waste disposal systems, industrialization, pollution, and so forth. Epidemiologists may study changes in the environment that coincide with changes in cancer incidence to develop hypothesis of potential causative agent.

TIME.   Evaluating the incidence of cancer over time may indicate significant trends. The alarming increase in melanoma over the past several decades reflects societal attitudes regarding the healthy appearance of a suntan. The well-recognized time trend of mounting lung cancer deaths led to the extensive series of studies that ultimately incriminated cigarette smoking as a principal cause.

Studying descriptive data and incidence trends raises obvious questions regarding environmental, geographic, dietary, and sociocultural variables of affected populations. Sources of variability and even sources of nonvariability may serve as an element of hypothesis formulation. See the box above for factors used in descriptive epidemiologic study.

Analytic Studies

Descriptive epidemiologic studies generate possible causes of disease. These etiologic hypotheses are then tested in the second investigative phase, the analytic study. Analytic epidemiology also assists in further defining risk factors. This type of study is observational in nature and its purpose is to elucidate which type of exposure causes which kind(s) of cancer.[13] The three types of analytic studies are cross-sectional studies, case-control studies, and cohort studies. The element of time distinguishes these types of studies. A cross-sectional study occurs in the present, case-control studies are based on subjects with past exposure (retrospective), and cohort studies examine populations who have been exposed to see if they develop the disease in the future (prospective).

CROSS-SECTIONAL STUDIES.   These studies may also be called *prevalence surveys*. The purpose is to canvas a population of subjects to ascertain a relationship between the disease and variables of interest as they exist in the group at a specific time. The drawback of such a survey is that the causal nature of a relationship cannot be established because the design does not allow accounting for the time sequence of events.[15]

COHORT DESIGN.   This type of study can be thought of as a prospective investigation and may also be called a *concurrent study*. People selected for a cohort study have all had exposure to the suspected cancer-causing factor. These subjects are followed into the future to evaluate the possible development of cancer. For example, to test the hypothesis that tanning in a tanning parlor causes skin cancer, two groups of people are followed: a group that tanned in parlors and a group that did not. All subjects are followed over a period of years to determine if the exposed group had a higher incidence of skin cancer. The disease incidence or mortality rates for various levels of exposure (high, medium, low, none) are then compared. If there is a causal relationship between tanning booths and skin cancer, one would expect to see the highest incidence of skin cancer in the sample with the most frequent exposure to tanning beds.

A second type of cohort study is the *historical cohort design*, also called the *historical prospective study*. This design is frequently used in occupational studies as both the exposure and onset of cancer have already occurred. Information is collected by reviewing records of the sample under study and reconstructing the disease history.

It is important in a cohort or prospective study that the time the study begins is clearly identified, that all of the participants are free of cancer when enrolled in the study, and that all participants are followed the same way. Complete long-term follow-up of all the participants in a cohort study, using medical records, death certificates, and other available resources, is crucial. Prospective studies have the disadvantage of being very large and expensive trials that take an extended period of time to complete.

CASE-CONTROL DESIGN.   This method evaluates a case group of persons diagnosed with the cancer under study who have exposure to the suspected cancer-causing agent. This group is compared to a control group chosen from the general population. The case-control design is a retrospective study that evaluates the outcome of past events. This type of study is commonly used because it is quickly implemented and can be performed with even small numbers of cases.[13]

An example of a case-control study is the evaluation of two groups of women, one group with a diagnosis of endometrial cancer and one group without. Both groups are interviewed to determine prior use of estrogens to test the hypothesis that estrogen use causes endometrial cancer. The percentage of women with endometrial cancer who used estrogens is referred to as the "exposure frequency." If the exposure frequency is greater in the case group than the control group, then the incidence of endometrial cancer after estrogen use is greater than the incidence of endometrial cancer without estrogen use.

STUDY ANALYSIS.   The endpoint of an analytic study is the determination of risk. Risk refers to the likelihood that people who are without a disease, but who come in contact with certain factors thought to increase the disease risk, will acquire the disease.[15]

Factors associated with an increased risk of acquiring cancer are *risk factors*. Risk factors may be associated with the environment (ultraviolet radiation, toxins), personal behavior (tobacco and alcohol use, sexual practices), or personal history (genetic changes).

Risk can be calculated as either *relative* or *attributable*. Relative risk estimates how much the risk of acquiring cancer increases with exposure to a risk factor.[15] Relative risk can also be thought of as the ratio of the rate of cancer between exposed and unexposed individuals. The higher the relative risk, the stronger the association between the risk factor and the cancer. A relative risk of 1.0 means the risk is the same for both groups. Thus, a relative risk factor of 10 implies that the risk of acquiring cancer is 10 times greater for an exposed person than an unexposed person. Relative risk ratios are a useful tool for identifying factors that increase risk for developing a particular kind of cancer. Early age of sexual intercourse, multiple sexual partners, and cigarette smoking are known risk factors for developing cervical cancer; women with these behaviors show several times the rate of cervical cancer than women without these behaviors.

Attributable risk describes the expected or normal number of unexposed people who acquire cancer, such as the number of nonsmokers expected to develop lung cancer in a year. Attributable risk is calculated by simply subtracting the rate of incidence in the exposed population from the rate of incidence in the nonexposed population. If a nonsmoking population develops lung cancer at a rate of 200 per 100,000 and a smoking population develops lung cancer at a rate of 543 per 100,000, then 343 cases of lung cancer per 100,000 population were caused by smoking and could have been prevented.

Experimental Studies

An experimental study modifies host characteristics, life style changes, or uses screening to prevent disease. Experimental studies are prospective and often take the form of a randomized clinical trial. Experimental studies may also be called *intervention studies, clinical trials,* or *prophylactic studies*. An example of the experimental study design is the chemoprevention trial, in which an agent is given for the purpose of achieving regression of a precursor lesion, to prevent cancer recurrence, or to prevent the development of cancer in a high-risk population. The Breast Cancer Prevention Trial, initiated in 1992 by the National Cancer Institute and the National Surgical Adjuvant Breast and Bowel Project (NSABP) is a prospective randomized chemoprevention trial. The study will enroll 16,000 female volunteers determined to be at high risk for developing breast cancer either due to age or personal and family history. The chemopreventive agent under investigation is Tamoxifen, an antiestrogen known to be beneficial in treating both early and advanced stages of breast cancer. The objective of the study, which is double-blinded and placebo-controlled, is to determine if Tamoxifen prevents high-risk women from developing breast cancer. The population will also be assessed for lipid levels and bone density to evaluate additional potential benefits from Tamoxifen.

CAUSES OF CANCER

Because one of the primary purposes of epidemiology is to discover the causes of cancer, the concept of "cause" must be understood. *Sufficient cause* is one that produces the effect.[14] In other words, if sufficient cause existed and were removed, the event would not occur. Because cancer is a complex and multifactorial disease, there is no single sufficient cause, the removal of which will prevent the disease. What must be examined then are various components of sufficient causes. The presence of a component increases the probability of the effect, but requires other components to produce it. Components may be active or passive. Personal susceptibility factors (genetics, environment, immunity) are passive components; carcinogens are active component causes. Each of these component causes is not "complete"; blocking the action of a component cause can make an otherwise sufficient cause become insufficient to produce the effect.[14] Descriptive epidemiology factors are given in the box below.

The various theories of carcinogenesis are discussed extensively in Chapter 1. To review, initiators

---

DESCRIPTIVE EPIDEMIOLOGY FACTORS

Frequency	*Disease*	*Person*	*Place*	*Time*
Incidence	Site	Age	Physical environment	Changes in frequency patterns over specified periods of time
Prevalence	Morphology	Sex	Biologic environment	
Mortality	Grade	Race	Geographic location	
	Stage	Marital status		
		Nutritional status		
		Cultural differences		
		Socioeconomic variables		
		Psychologic factors		
		Susceptibility factors		

Table 2–1 Environmental Causes of Human Cancer

Agent	Type of Exposure	Site of Cancer
Alcoholic beverages	Drinking	Mouth, pharynx, esophagus, larynx, liver
Alkylating agents (melphalan, cyclophosphamide, chlorambucil, semustine)	Medication	Leukemia
Androgen-anabolic steroids	Medication	Liver
Aromatic amines (benzidine, 2-naphthylamine, 4-aminobiphenyl)	Manufacturing of dyes and other chemicals	Bladder
Arsenic (inorganic)	Mining and smelting of certain ores, pesticide manufacturing and use, medication, drinking water	Lung, skin, liver (angiosarcoma)
Asbestos	Manufacturing and use	Lung, pleura, peritoneum
Benzene	Leather, petroleum, and other industries	Leukemia
Bis(chloromethyl)ether	Manufacturing	Lung (small cell)
Chlornaphazine	Medication	Bladder
Chromium compounds	Manufacturing	Lung
Estrogens	Medication	
Synthetic (DES)		Cervix, vagina (adenocarcinoma)
Conjugated (Premarin)		Endometrium
Steroid contraceptives		Liver (benign)
Immunosuppressants (azathioprine, cyclosporin)	Medication	Non-Hodgkin's lymphoma, skin (squamous carcinoma and melanoma), soft tissue tumors (including Kaposi's sarcoma)
Ionizing radiation	Atomic bomb explosions, treatment and diagnosis, radium dial painting, uranium and metal mining	Most sites
Isopropyl alcohol production	Manufacturing by strong acid process	Nasal sinuses
Leather industry	Manufacturing and repair (boot and shoe)	Nasal sinuses, bladder
Mustard gas	Manufacturing	Lung, larynx, nasal sinuses
Nickel dust	Refining	Lung, nasal sinuses
Parasites	Infection	
Schistosoma haematobium		Bladder (squamous carcinoma)
Clonorchis sinensis		Liver (cholangiocarcinoma)
Phenacetin-containing analgesics	Medication	Renal pelvis
Polycyclic hydrocarbons	Coal carbonization products and some mineral oils	Lung, skin (squamous carcinoma)
Tobacco chews, including betel nut	Snuff dipping and chewing of tobacco, betel, lime	Mouth
Tobacco smoke	Smoking, especially cigarettes	Lung, larynx, mouth, pharynx, esophagus, bladder, pancreas, kidney
Ultraviolet radiation	Sunlight	Skin (including melanoma), lip
Viruses	Infection	
Epstein-Barr virus		Burkitt's lymphoma; nasopharyngeal carcinoma
Hepatitis-B virus		Hepatocellular carcinoma
Human T-lymphotrophic virus, type I		T-cell leukemia/lymphoma
Vinyl chloride	Manufacturing of polyvinyl chloride	Liver (angiosarcoma)
Wood dusts	Furniture manufacturing (hardwood)	Nasal sinuses (adenocarcinoma)

From Fraumeni JF and others: Epidemiology of cancer. In DeVita VT, Hellman S, and Rosenberg SA, editors: Cancer: principles and practice of oncology, ed 3, Philadelphia, 1989, JB Lippincott Company.

are early stage sequences of limited exposure and are irreversible, whereas promoters occur at a later stage, involve repeated exposures at frequent intervals, and are reversible. Therefore, limiting or eliminating the promoter may prevent the occurrence of cancer or reverse malignant changes. The promoter, or carcinogen, may be the active component cause. By removing this agent, sufficient cause cannot exist.

Chapter 1 also describes the various groups of carcinogens: chemicals, hormones, viruses, and radiation. In addition, specific cancer etiologies are presented in Chapter 3 and each of the disease chapters. This chapter will not repeat a discussion of these agents, but Table 2-1 lists a number of environmental causes of cancer, the type of exposure, and the kind of resulting cancer. Some of these carcinogenic agents were identified by laboratory research; others were identified by the epidemiologic methods detailed in this chapter.

An excellent historic example of an epidemiologic study is the Argonne Radium Study. In the 1920s, many people worked as "luminators" in watch factories. Their job was to apply radium paint to the numerals on watch dials. This obviously detailed work required a paintbrush with a very fine tip. This pointed tip was achieved by touching the end of the brush to the lips or tongue. This practice transferred a considerable amount of the sticky radium paint to the mouth. In a few years, a luminator may have ingested 5 mg or more of radioactive substances, which would be deposited in their bones, spleen, and liver. It would remain in these organs emitting a steady stream of radioactivity to the surrounding tissues.

By 1924, nine young women working in the same New Jersey factory died within 3 years. Other workers developed gingivitis, osteomyelitis, and anemia. The Argonne Radium Study was initiated to study the luminators as well as chemists and patients treated with radium. This became one of the largest epidemiologic studies to evaluate the health effects of ionizing radiation on humans. The Argonne Study produced an undeniable link between radiation exposure and certain forms of cancer, including osteosarcomas, paranasal sinus, and mastoid cancers.[12] Even 65 years later, this study continues as epidemiologists identify, interview, and even arrange for the exhumation of additional subjects.

A most impressive contribution of the Argonne Study is that it served as a basis for plutonium exposure guidelines during the Manhattan Project of the World War II era.

CONCLUSION

Examples of cancer-causing agents highlight the role of epidemiology in the cancer problem. Once a cancer-causing agent is identified, steps must be taken to eliminate or limit exposure. This involves public health and government agencies at the local, state, and national levels. Nurses must be knowledgeable about environmental carcinogens not only to answer patient questions, but also to take more accurate health histories and adequately assess high-risk exposures.

Nurses can use knowledge of epidemiology to increase their personal understanding of the cancer problem. Familiarity with terminology and epidemiologic methods enables the nurse to interpret medical literature more accurately; new information can be more easily understood and, therefore, integrated into the personal knowledge base. Nurses can develop a more acute awareness in their practice setting, allowing possible observations of clusters or trends. Curiosity and observation may lead to nursing research questions.

BIBLIOGRAPHY

1. American Cancer Society: Cancer facts and figures—1993, Atlanta, 1993, American Cancer Society, Inc.
2. Boring CC, Squires TS, and Tong T: Cancer statistics, 1992, Cancer 43(1):7, 1993.
3. Doll R and Peto R: The causes of cancer, J Natl Cancer Inst 66:1191, 1981.
4. Feinstein AR, Sosin DM, and Wells CK: The Will Rogers phenomenon: stage migration and new diagnostic techniques as a source of misleading statistics for survival in cancer, N Engl J Med 312:1604, 1985.
5. Fraumeni JF and others: Epidemiology of cancer. In DeVita VT, Hellman S, and Rosenberg SA, editors: Cancer: principles and practice of oncology, ed 3, Philadelphia, 1989, JB Lippincott Co.
6. Hutchison GB: The epidemiologic method. In Schottenfeld D and Fraumeni JF, editors: Cancer epidemiology and prevention, Philadelphia, 1982, WB Saunders Co.
7. Merz B: Studies illuminate hazards of ingested radiation, JAMA 258(5):584, 1987.
8. Mettlin C: Trends in years of life lost to cancer, 1970-1985, CA 39(1):33, 1989.
9. Myers MH and Hankey BF: Cancer patient survival in the United States. In Schottenfeld D and Fraumeni JF, editors: Cancer epidemiology and prevention, Philadelphia, 1982, WB Saunders Co.
10. Myers MH and Ries LG: Cancer patient survival rates: SEER Program results for 10 years of follow-up, CA 39(1):21, 1989.
11. Newell GR and others: Epidemiology of cancer. In DeVita VT, Hellman S, and Rosenberg SA, editors: Cancer: principles and practice of oncology, ed 3, Philadelphia, 1989, JB Lippincott Co.

12. Oleske D and Greenwald SL: Epidemiology of cancer. In Groenwald SL, Frogge MH, and Goodman M, editors: Cancer nursing: practice and principles, ed 2, Boston, 1990, Jones & Bartlett Publishers.

13. Oleske DM: Epidemiologic principles for nursing practice: assessing the cancer problem and planning its control. In Baird SB, McCorkle R, and Grant M, editors: Cancer nursing: a comprehensive textbook, Philadelphia, 1991, WB Saunders Co.

14. Rothman KJ: Causation and causal inference. In Schottenfeld D and Fraumeni JF, editors: Cancer epidemiology and prevention, Philadelphia, 1982, WB Saunders Co.

15. Valanis B: Epidemiology in nursing and allied health, Norwalk, Conn, 1986, Appleton-Century-Crofts.

16. Young JL and Pollack ES: The incidence of cancer in the United States. In Schottenfeld D and Fraumeni JF, editors: Cancer epidemiology and prevention, Philadelphia, 1982, WB Saunders Co.

CHAPTER 3

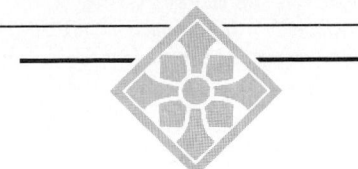

Prevention, Screening, and Detection

Mary Magee Gullatte

Approximately 76 million Americans alive today will eventually have cancer; about one in three according to present rates, striking approximately three of four families.[11] Cancer continues to be the second leading cause of death in the United States. The American Cancer Society (ACS) estimates that greater than one million new cancer cases will be diagnosed in 1992.[8]

Prevention, screening, and early detection are among the best strategies available in the quest to conquer cancer. The United States' goal in cancer control, as identified by the National Cancer Institute (NCI), is to reduce the cancer death rate by 50% for all Americans by the year 2000; saving some 230,000 lives each year.[52] These reductions are to be achieved by smoking cessation, diet modification, and early detection through screening programs, and state-of-the art cancer treatments.[23,47] Further reductions may be achieved through elimination of occupational and environmental risks and changes in lifestyle, focusing on healthy choices in diet and exercise. Early diagnosis is crucial to reducing the morbidity and mortality associated with cancer. Table 3-1 shows the positive impact of early detection on survival for the four most prevalent cancers.

Prevention of human cancers is a major focus in education and research, as America moves toward the year 2000. In spite of advances in the treatment of cancers, overall mortality statistics far exceed desired outcomes.

Neoplastic transformation is a multistep process in the development of human cancers involving three sequences of events: initiation, promotion, and progression. Goals of prevention, risk reduction, and

Table 3–1 Five-Year Survival Rates for Four Most Prevalent Cancers and Leading Causes of Cancer Deaths, Localized and Metastatic, Diagnosed between 1979 and 1984 in the United States*

Cancer	Stage at Diagnosis†	5-Year Survival Rate (%)
Female breast	Localized	90
	Distant†	17
Lung	Localized	32
	Distant	2
Colorectal	Localized	84
	Distant	6
Prostate	Localized	84
	Distant	29

From Surveillance and Operations Research Branch, National Cancer Institute. In Cancer Facts and Figures 1989, Atlanta, American Cancer Society, 1989.
*Adjusted for normal life expectancy.
†Distant stage refers to disease that has spread to other parts of the body from the primary site.

early detection are aimed at eliminating and/or modifying neoplastic transformation of human cells.

The ACS and NCI are promoting nationwide cancer education, screening, and early detection initiatives, targeting African, Hispanic, Asian-Pacific, and Native Americans and the underserved or socioeconomically disadvantaged (SED) populations. The differences in cancer incidence, mortality, and survival among minority Americans is disproportionately high for most sites when compared to nonminority Americans. Tables 3-2, 3-3, and 3-4 depict the cancer incidence, mortality, and survival rates by race/ethnic group.

Table 3–2   Cancer Incidence Rates* Per 100,000 Population by Race/Ethnic Group, 1977-1983

Cancer Site	White	Black	Chinese	Japanese	Filipino	American Indian	Mexican American	Native Hawaiian
All sites	345.1	382.8	247.6	242.5	212.4	137.6	245.1	346.5
Oral cavity	11.3	15.0	15.4	4.8	8.9	2.1	6.6	9.0
Esophagus	3.0	11.6	3.3	2.8	3.4	1.0	1.6	7.3
Stomach	7.9	14.5	10.5	26.6	7.8	15.1	15.3	27.0
Colon & rectum	50.1	50.3	40.4	48.8	30.3	9.6	26.2	31.7
Liver	1.8	3.6	9.6	3.6	5.4	2.1	3.1	5.5
Gallbladder	1.3	1.0	1.0	1.5	1.4	10.0	4.6	1.3
Pancreas	9.1	13.8	6.3	7.1	4.9	3.7	11.0	8.0
Lung	51.8	69.8	40.6	27.1	27.3	6.3	23.4	66.9
Melanoma (skin)	9.2	0.8	0.7	1.2	1.0	1.9	1.9	1.1
Breast	88.8	75.2	57.8	55.0	41.3	21.3	52.1	106.1
Cervix uteri	8.7	19.7	10.3	5.9	8.6	19.9	16.1	15.2
Corpus uteri	25.7	15.0	18.0	17.7	11.3	7.2	11.3	28.2
Ovary	13.8	10.2	9.2	8.8	9.7	7.5	11.3	14.4
Prostate	77.9	125.5	29.6	43.8	44.0	31.0	76.3	56.1
Urinary bladder	17.0	9.6	9.0	8.0	4.4	1.4	7.9	8.5
Kidney	7.1	6.8	3.5	3.6	3.1	5.7	6.4	4.2
Brain & CNS	6.1	3.4	2.4	2.4	1.9	1.2	3.7	3.0
Hodgkin's disease	3.0	1.8	0.6	0.5	1.2	0.2	2.6	1.0
Non-Hodgkin's lymphoma	10.9	7.2	8.5	7.2	8.3	2.8	6.7	8.4
Leukemia	10.6	9.1	4.8	5.7	7.1	4.6	6.9	8.2

From Cancer facts and figures for minority Americans: Atlanta, GA, p. 5, 1991, American Cancer Society.
*Age-adjusted to 1970 US standard population.

Table 3–3   Number of Cancer Deaths for Black, American Indian, Chinese, Japanese, and Hispanic Persons, United States, 1988

| Cancer Site | Black | | American Indian | Chinese | Japanese | Hispanic* |
	Males	Females				
All sites	30,321	23,647	1,151	1,388	1,012	9,602
Oral cavity	939	303	28	53	9	167
Esophagus	1,580	470	22	24	23	164
Stomach	1,316	802	48	98	130	582
Colon & rectum	2,637	3,014	102	159	153	866
Liver & other biliary	720	564	71	151	60	565
Pancreas	1,355	1,469	55	83	85	585
Lung (male)	10,112	—	197	211	127	1,218
Lung (female)	—	4,019	111	102	64	535
Breast (female)	—	4,467	66	99	62	798
Cervix uteri	—	974	29	21	8	240
Other uterus	—	953	30	31	32	231
Ovary	—	888	11	16	10	110
Prostate	4,582	—	64	26	43	482
Bladder	411	371	13	18	14	132
Kidney	501	319	30	18	19	241
Brain & CNS	358	311	22	23	14	248
Lymphomas	684	513	35	49	36	477
Leukemia	806	672	49	38	28	464
Multiple myeloma	631	716	20	15	12	179

From Cancer facts and figures for minority Americans: Atlanta, GA, p. 8, 1991, American Cancer Society.
*Persons classified as of Hispanic origin on death certificates may be of any race. Hispanic deaths are only reported for the District of Columbia and the following 26 states: Alabama, Arizona, Arkansas, California, Colorado, Georgia, Hawaii, Illinois, Indiana, Kansas, Kentucky, Maine, Mississippi, Montana, Nebraska, New Jersey, New York (including New York City), North Carolina, North Dakota, Ohio, Oregon, Rhode Island, Texas, Utah, Washington, and Wyoming. In 1980, these reporting areas accounted for about 80% of the Hispanic population in the United States. Caution should be exercised in generalizing this mortality data to the entire US Hispanic population.

Table 3—4 Five-Year Relative Survival Rates (%) by Race/Ethnic Group, 1975-1984

Cancer Site	White	Black	Chinese	Japanese	Filipino	American Indian	Mexican American	Native Hawaiian
All sites	51.9	39.6	47.5	53.1	46.1	35.4	48.4	43.2
Oral cavity	54.0	33.0	55.7	44.4	46.6	38.6	60.7	42.8
Esophagus	6.5	4.2	11.5	5.8	3.4	—	0.0	0.0
Stomach	15.3	17.5	21.6	29.8	18.8	8.9	17.8	12.9
Colon & rectum	53.2	46.7	53.1	61.7	44.8	39.7	45.0	58.4
Liver	3.8	3.1	2.0	1.5	6.7	0.0	0.0	6.6
Gallbladder	9.2	8.9	—	16.2	—	2.8	8.5	26.2
Pancreas	2.7	3.2	0.0	2.6	5.2	0.0	1.2	0.0
Lung	13.2	11.7	15.1	14.3	13.2	0.0	10.8	13.0
Melanoma (skin)	81.2	57.5	—	81.0	—	—	82.1	—
Breast	76.1	63.2	80.8	85.4	73.7	46.2	70.6	68.0
Cervix uteri	68.2	61.6	74.6	70.2	73.0	63.5	70.5	67.7
Corpus uteri	86.0	54.9	86.1	84.1	79.9	82.7	77.0	74.6
Ovary	37.6	40.9	43.3	43.5	44.7	42.9	38.7	46.8
Prostate	72.6	63.4	72.5	80.5	71.7	54.2	72.4	72.0
Urinary bladder	76.6	53.4	78.5	80.8	58.4	—	64.6	51.4
Kidney	51.9	56.3	60.7	63.1	47.0	49.7	51.4	59.0
Brain & CNS	23.3	28.5	35.9	40.6	29.6	37.6	32.2	38.9
Hodgkin's disease	74.7	71.0	—	—	43.5	—	69.0	74.1
Non-Hodgkin's lymphoma	50.2	47.9	50.3	41.1	33.8	31.1	41.1	40.2
Leukemia	35.5	28.0	19.8	26.0	22.3	21.4	25.7	21.1

From Cancer facts and figures for minority Americans: Atlanta, GA, p. 7, 1991, American Cancer Society.

The rates presented in each table depict differences in neoplastic growth that appear to be due to ethnic, cultural, environmental, economic, or hereditary differences within each group.

Cancer incidence rates are nearly twice as high or higher for African Americans as compared with whites for cancers of the esophagus, uterine, cervix, liver, stomach, prostate, and multiple myeloma.[50] Cancer mortality is higher in African Americans than in all races for several reasons, including higher rates of new disease, later stage at diagnosis, and poor survival experience.[7,12]

CANCER PREVENTION GUIDELINES

The focus of prevention of cancer in this chapter is two dimensional. *Primary prevention* aimed at measures to ensure that the cancer never develops and *secondary prevention* aimed at detecting and treating the cancer early while in its most curable stage.

The American Cancer Society estimates that 80% of all cancers may be associated with environmental exposures and are potentially preventable.[17] Smoking accounts for the highest overall health risk in the United States. Cigarette smoking is the major cause of lung cancer and is estimated to cause 83% of lung cancer deaths.[11]

Major factors placing humans at risk for developing cancer include: tobacco, diet, lifestyle, occupational and environmental exposures. Site specific guidelines related to cancer risk factors, signs and symptoms,

screening, and early detection are presented in Table 3-5. Health promotion, cancer prevention, and risk reduction guidelines of selected lifestyle, occupational, socioeconomic status (SES), and environmental factors will now be reviewed.

TOBACCO

The link between cigarette smoking and lung cancer was first suspected in the 1920s and 1930s.[14] The ACS estimates that cigarette smoking is responsible for 85% of lung cancer deaths among men and 75% among women.[11] Over the past few years the gap between the number of lung cancer deaths, caused by smoking, in men and women is narrowing. Lung cancer now exceeds breast cancer as the leading cause of cancer death in women. Passive exposure to cigarette smoke (side stream and exhaled smoke) appears to increase risk of lung cancer in nonsmokers who live with smokers.[35] Smoking is associated with cancers of the mouth, pharynx, layrnx, esophagus, pancreas, uterine cervix, kidney, and bladder.[11,37]

Racial differences in smoking habits between African Americans and whites in the United States have also been identified. African American adolescents are less likely than white adolescents to smoke; however, African American adults are more likely than white adults to begin smoking after adolescence.[12,15,19,34] Tables 3-6 and 3-7 depict differences in smoking trends by age and race. The data in these tables correlate with recent studies that indicate an

Text continued on page 37.

Table 3–5 Site Specific Cancer Risk, Screening, and Early Detection Guidelines[14,17,37]

Site	Associated Risk Factors	Signs and Symptoms	Screening and Detection
Biliary tract (Gallbladder and bile ducts)	Older Americans (age 60-70s) Female predominance Higher in white females than African American females Chronic infection with liver parasites (*Clonorchis sinensis*) Eating raw or pickled freshwater fish from Southeast Asia Chronic ulcerative colitis	Pruritis Jaundice Abdominal pain Nausea and vomiting Fever Malaise Enlarged liver Palpable mass upper right quadrant Lower extremity edema Ascites	Physical examination Ultrasound
Bladder	Occupational exposure (textile, rubber) Cigarette smoking Chronic bladder infections	Microscopic or gross hematuria Dysuria Bladder irritability Urinary urgency, frequency and/or hesitancy	Urinalysis Urine cytology Physical examination
Brain	Environmental exposures (vinyl chlorides) Epstein-Barr virus	Persistent generalized headache Vomiting Seizures Loss of fine motor control Unsteady gait Change in personality Lethargy Slurring of speech Loss of memory Impaired vision	Physical examination Prompt follow-up with onset of signs and symptoms
Breast	Previous history of cancer (colon, thyroid, endometrial, ovary, breast) Obesity High fat intake Family history of breast cancer Exposure to ionizing radiation before age 35 Early menarche Late menopause Nulliparity First pregnancy after age 30	Painless mass or thickening in breast or axilla Skin dimpling, puckering, or nipple retraction Nipple discharge or scaliness Edema (peau d'orange) Erythema, ulceration Change in size, contour, shape of breast	Consist of three modalities:[2] 1. *Breast self-examination* monthly at age 20 and older. 2. *Clinical examination* age 20–40: every 3 years over 40: every year 3. *Mammography* age 40–49: every 1–2 years age 50 & over: every year *Baseline mammogram at age 25 has been recommended for genetically predisposed women. Fine needle aspiration Ultrasound
Central nervous system	Unknown etiology Speculation related to genetic disorders	Headache Nausea/vomiting Edema Loss of fine motor coordination Unsteady gait Seizures Vision and speech problems	No effective screening measures Family history CT scan of the brain MRI Cerebrospinal fluid analysis Tumor markers Alpha-fetoprotein Beta human chorionic-gonadotropin

Table 3–5 Site Specific Cancer Risk, Screening, and Early Detection Guidelines—cont'd

Site	Associated Risk Factors	Signs and Symptoms	Screening and Detection
Cervix	Early age at first intercourse (before age 20) Multiple sex partners Smoking HPV infection (*Condyloma* or warts) Herpes simplex virus II Diet	Abnormal vaginal bleeding Persistent postcoital spotting	Pap test Pelvic examination
Colon and rectum	Colorectal polyps(s) Diets high in fat Diets low in fiber Genetic component: 　Familial polyposis 　Gardner's syndrome 　Peutz-Jeghers syndrome 　Inflammatory bowel disease 　Chron's disease 　Ulcerative colitis	Depend on the location of the tumor: *Right colon* 　Anemia 　GI bleeding 　Persistent lower abdominal pain 　Right lower quadrant mass *Left colon* 　Gross blood in the stool 　Decrease in stool caliber 　Change in bowel habits, constipation, diarrhea *Rectum* 　Hematochezia 　Tenesmus 　Feeling of incomplete evacuation 　Rectal pain (late sign) 　Prolapse of tumor	Digital rectal examination Stool occult blood testing Flexible sigmoidoscopy (see Table 3-12 for frequency of these tests/procedures)
Endometrium	Post menopause High socioeconomic status Nulliparity Obesity > 50 pounds over ideal body weight Prolonged use of exodgenous estrogen without supplemental progesterone High fat intake Diabetes Hypertension Stein-Leventhal syndrome (failure to ovulate/infertility—polycystic ovaries) Menstrual aberration	*Early sign* 　Abnormal vaginal bleeding *Late signs* 　Pain in pelvis, legs, or back 　General weakness 　Weight loss	Aspiration curettage
Esophagus	Elderly male (70–80 years old) Nitrosamines and ethanol consumption Cigarette smoking Pre-cancerous lesions Achalasia (failure of the lower esophagus to relax with swallowing) Combined smoking and drinking Barrett's esophagus (chronic gastric reflux)	*Early* 　Dysphagia 　Weight loss 　Regurgitation 　Aspiration 　Odynophagia (pain on swallowing) 　Gastroesophageal reflux *Advanced* 　Cervical adenopathy 　Chronic cough 　Choking after eating 　Massive hemoptysis 　Hematemesis 　Hoarseness	Esophagoscopy with staining techniques Brush biopsy Radioisotopes in tumor scanning

Continued.

Table 3–5 Site Specific Cancer Risk, Screening, and Early Detection Guidelines—cont'd

Site	Associated Risk Factors	Signs and Symptoms	Screening and Detection

Head and neck	Tobacco (inhaled or chewed)
	Ethyl alcohol
	Combination of tobacco and alcohol
	Poor oral hygiene
	Wood dust inhalation
	Nickel exposure
	Leukoplakia
		Mouth and oral cavity
		  Swelling
		  Ulcer that does not heal
		Nose and sinuses
		  Pain
		  Swelling
		  Bloody nasal discharge
		  Nasal obstruction
		Salivary glands
		  Painless swelling
		  Unilateral facial paralysis
		Hypopharynx
		  Dysphagia
		  Persistent earache
		  Lymphadenopathy
		Nasopharynx
		  Double vision
		  Hearing loss
		  Loss of smell
		  Hoarseness
		  Adenopathy
		Larynx
		  Hoarseness
		  Difficulty breathing
			Semiannual dental oral examination
			Awareness of signs and symptoms (cancer's seven warning signs)

HIV/AIDS related (Kaposi's sarcoma [KS])	All age groups
	Homosexual or bisexual men highest risk
	Intravenous drug users
	Unprotected sexual contact
	Multiple sex partners
		Multifocal, widespread lesions on skin (face, extremities and torso)
		Persistent intermittent fever
		Weight loss, diarrhea
		Malaise, fatigue
		Severe cellular immune deficiency
		Generalized lymphadenopathy
		Respiratory infections:
		  Pneumocystis carinii
		  Tuberculosis
		Difficulty breathing
		Oral lesions
		Enlarged liver, spleen
			High risk group
			Appearance of skin lesions
			HIV (human immunodeficiency virus) serum testing
			Oral examination

Leukemia *Acute*	Men higher risk than women Whites higher than African Americans Exposure to radiation Exposure to toxic organic chemicals (benzene) Drugs (alkylating agents, chloramphenicol)	Low grade fever Anemia, pallor Lymphadenopathy Generalized weakness Frequent infections Easy bruising Bleeding (nose, gums) Petechiae lower extremities Bone and joint pain	Complete blood count Platelet count Physical examination
Chronic	Benzene exposure High dose radiation Philadelphia chromosome	Lymphadenopathy Splenomegaly Weight loss Night sweats Malaise, weakness Recurrent infections, fever Early satiety	

Table 3–5 Site Specific Cancer Risk, Screening, and Early Detection Guidelines—cont'd

Site	Associated Risk Factors	Signs and Symptoms	Screening and Detection
Liver	Exposure to aflatoxin Environmental exposures Viral hepatitis More frequent in males Alcoholic cirrhosis Parasitic infestation Chronic venous obstruction Paraneoplastic syndromes Anabolic steroid use	*Early* Bloating Abdominal pain Fever Weight loss Decreased appetite Nausea *Advanced* Jaundice Ascites Extreme weight loss Anorexia	Annual physical examination Awareness of risk factors Ultrasound
Lung	Cigarette smoking (active and passive) Increase in age Asbestos Occupational exposure among miners Air pollution (benzopyrenes and hydrocarbons) Genetic predisposition Vitamin A deficiency	Nagging cough Dull ache in the chest Recurrent or persistent upper respiratory infection Wheezing Dyspnea Hemoptysis Change in volume, color, odor of sputum	None
Lymphoma *Hodgkins*	Epstein-Barr virus Higher socioeconomic status Small family	Persistent swelling or painless lymph nodes (neck, axilla) Recurrent fevers Night sweats Weight loss Pruritis Cough, shortness of breath Leukocytosis	Physical examination Complete blood count
Non-Hodgkins	Occupational exposure (flour and agricultural industries) Abnormalities of the immune system HIV Exposure to radiation or chemotherapy	Lymphadenopathy Fatigue Fever, chills Night sweats Decreased appetite Weight loss	
Multiple myeloma	Older Americans High levels of immunoglobulin (B-cells) African Americans at significant increased risk than whites (14 to 1)	*Early* Anemia Fatigue Bone pain (back, legs) Weakness Unexplained bleeding (nose and gums) Recurrent upper respiratory infection *Advanced* Hypercalcemia Pathologic fractures	Annual physical examination Radiologic tests
Ovary	Familial disposition Late menopause Nulliparity First pregnancy after age 30	*Early* Vague abdominal discomfort Dyspepsia Flatulence Bloating Digestive disturbance *Advanced* Abdominal distention Pain Abdominal and pelvic masses Ascites Lower extremity edema	Pelvic ultrasonography (with vaginal probe) Elevated serum markers CEA CA 125

Continued.

Table 3–5 Site Specific Cancer Risk, Screening, and Early Detection Guidelines—cont'd

Site	Associated Risk Factors	Signs and Symptoms	Screening and Detection
Pancreas	Older men Smoking Chronic pancreatitis Ethanol consumption Diabetes	*Early* 　Hypoglycemia 　Weight loss, anorexia 　Abdominal pain 　Cramping pain associated with 　　diarrhea 　Pruritis *Advanced* 　Jaundice 　Ascites 　Lower extremity edema	Blood glucose test Physical examination
Prostate	Occupational exposure Cadmium, heavy metals, chemicals Age (median age of incidence = 70 　yrs) Increased fat intake	*Early* 　Difficult starting urinary stream 　Unexplained cystitis 　Urinary bleeding 　Dribbling 　Bladder retention *Advanced* 　Bladder outlet obstruction 　Urinary retention 　Ureteral obstruction with anuria 　Azotemia 　Uremia 　Anorexia 　Hematuria 　Bone pain	Digital rectal exami- 　nation Biochemical markers Prostatic specific anti- 　gen Transrectal ultra- 　sound
Skin (Nonmel- anoma)	Fair-skinned, freckles Blonde hair, blue eyes Sun exposure Severe sunburn in childhood Familial conditions Previous skin cancers History of dysplastic nevus	Changes in a wart or mole Sore that does not heal The *ABCD*'s of skin cancer: 　*A*—Asymmetry (change in size/ 　　shape) 　*B*—Border irregularity 　*C*—Color (change in color) 　*D*—Diameter (> than 6 mm)	Extensive examination 　of the skin Mole mapping
Soft tissue sar- coma (bone or muscle)	Familial/genetic syndromes: (Von 　Recklinghausen disease) High dose radiation Toxic chemical exposure (Agent Or- 　ange)	Swelling of extremity Painless mass Fever Malaise Weight loss Occasionally hypoglycemia Functional difficulty or pain in 　joints Pathologic fractures	Annual physical ex- 　amination Awareness of cancer's 　early warning signs
Stomach	Dietary carcinogens (smoked, salt 　cured, and charcoal foods) Familial/genetic disposition Persons with Type A blood (15–20% 　increase incidence) Benign gastric ulcers	Feeling of fullness Weight loss Loss of appetite Anemia (iron deficiency) Malaise Complaints of indigestion GI bleeding Abdominal pain Persistent epigastric distress	Occult blood testing Complete blood count

Table 3-5 Site Specific Cancer Risk, Screening, and Early Detection Guidelines—cont'd

Site	Associated Risk Factors	Signs and Symptoms	Screening and Detection
Testis	Cryptorchid testes Young white males have rate four times that of African Americans	*Early* Painless mass Gynecomastia Heavy sensation in the scrotum *Advanced* Ureteral obstruction Abdominal mass Pulmonary symptoms Elevated human chorionic gonadotropin	Testicular self examination (monthly) beginning in adolescence Testicular ultrasound
Vulva	Postmenopausal History of genital warts Human papilloma virus Other sexually transmitted diseases Lower socioeconomic status Multiple sex partners Precancerous or cancerous lesions of the cervix	Lump or ulcer Itching Pain Burning bleeding Discharge	Visual and manual inspection of external genitalia Colposcopic exam in women with HPV

Table 3-6 Prevalence of Tobacco Use Among High School Students, 1990

Race/Sex	Cigarette Use*	Frequent Cigarette Use†	Smokeless Tobacco Use
White	36.4	15.9	12.6
Male	36.8	15.2	23.9
Female	36.0	16.6	1.5
Black	16.1	2.3	1.9
Male	16.8	3.0	3.1
Female	15.7	1.8	0.8
Hispanic	30.8	7.4	5.7
Male	34.7	9.6	10.9
Female	27.2	5.5	1.0

Source: Youth Risk Behavior Survey, Centers for Disease Control.
*Smoked at any time during the 30 days preceding the survey.
†Smoked on more than 25 of the 30 days preceding the survey.

Table 3-7 Trends in Smoking Prevalence, 1965-1987, Adults Ages 20 and Older[7]

Race	1965	1976	1987
African Americans	43.0%	41.2%	34.0%
Whites	40.0%	35.6%	28.8%

overall decline in cigarette smoking in the United States.[51]

One of the national health objectives for the year 2000 is to reduce the initiation of cigarette smoking among youth. Among current smokers, more than 80% started smoking before age 21 and about half started before age 18.[12] The goal is that no more than 15% of youth become regular smokers by the age of 20 years.[15,19,54,56] The following measures have been identified to achieve this goal:[15,56]

1. offer health education classes on tobacco use in schools
2. establish tobacco-free environments in schools
3. enact and enforce laws prohibiting sale and distribution of tobacco products to minors (including smokeless tobacco)
4. reduce or restrict tobacco advertising where youth are likely to be exposed
5. plan to unify all 50 states to reduce tobacco use, especially among youth.

A number of organizations offer smoking cessation programs and are reporting successes in the campaign toward a smoke-free America. Cessation of smoking reduces the risk of death from lung cancer; after 15 years, former smokers have lung cancer death rates only about two times greater than nonsmokers.[14]

DIET

Research continues into the connection between diet, cancer causation, and prevention. At this time the only consensus recommendations related to cancer, diet, and nutrition are to reduce the intake of fat, both saturated and unsaturated, and to increase the amount of daily intake of natural fiber (components that are not broken down during the digestive process) in the diet.

Specific dietary recommendations, related to macronutrients and micronutrients, chemoprevention, and sources of mutagenic and carcinogenic chemicals used to preserve, protect, or cultivate food sources, remain clouded in uncertainty. Estimates are that 30% to 60% of all cancers, in men and women respectively, are related to diet.[18,65] Foods high in fat have been associated with an increased incidence of colon, prostate, and breast cancer. Dietary fat acts as a cancer promoter. Table 3-8 depicts the median intake frequency per week for selected food, by race and sex. As much as 40% of food energy in the American diet is provided by fat.[41] Studies indicate that obesity (40% or more overweight) is a risk factor in the development of cancer of the colon, breast, endometrium, and prostate.[14,17]

Although the exact mechanism(s) of action is unknown, dietary fiber appears to offer a protective effect in relation to colon cancer. Fiber can be found in fresh fruits and vegetables, legumes, and in whole grain breads and cereals. Several functions are believed to account for the protective effect of dietary fiber. Fiber reduces the concentration of fecal bile acids, dilutes colonic content, reduces the level of fecal mutagens, and decreases transient time of fecal material in the gut.[31,49,69]

Several micronutrients have been profiled as having a protective effect in reducing cancer risk. Naturally occurring vitamin A in the form of beta-carotene, found in yellow and green vegetables and fruits, and retinol, occurring in foods of animal origin, dairy products, eggs, and liver, are associated with a protective effect against cancer. Inverse associations have been found in studies relating vitamin A precursors and cancers of the lung, larynx, esophagus, stomach, and prostate.[27,28,31]

The protective action of vitamin C hinders the formation of nitrosamines by blocking the reaction between nitrite and amines. Historical studies have shown an inverse association between vitamin C and cancers of the stomach, esophagus, larynx, and cervix.

Another micronutrient is selenium. Animal studies involving selenium indicate a protective role against chemically induced cancers. There exists a fine line between the therapeutic and toxic level of selenium, however, and the evidence does not support its use as an anticancer compound.[14,41]

The NCI estimates that dietary modifications could save 30,000 lives by the year 2000.[23,47] The NCI is currently sponsoring human chemoprevention and diet and nutrition trials in an effort to answer questions and update earlier studies related to the diet and cancer connection. The ACS, NCI, and other organizations with an interest in health promotion through dietary modifications have developed dietary guidelines to reduce cancer and other health risks. These dietary recommendations have many similarities and are summarized in the box on p. 39.

Table 3–8 Median Intake Frequency per Week for Selected Foods,* by Race and Sex

Food	White		Black		Hispanic	
	Male	*Female*	*Male*	*Female*	*Male*	*Female*
High-fiber bread or cereal	3.0	3.0	0.5	1.0	1.0	1.0
All fruit	3.0	3.9	2.5	3.2	3.4	4.2
Fruit and juice	7.5	9.0	8.0	9.0	9.1	10.2
Dried legumes, chili	0.7	0.5	1.0	0.5	2.0	1.0
Garden vegetables	4.9	5.4	5.0	5.2	6.2	7.0
Potatoes	4.0	3.0	3.0	2.7	3.2	3.0
Salad	2.0	3.0	1.0	1.2	2.0	3.0
Hamburger, beef, pork	3.3	2.5	3.2	2.7	4.0	3.2
Chicken and fish	1.6	1.7	3.0	2.9	2.3	2.0
Bacon, sausage, hot dogs, lunch meats	3.5	2.1	5.0	3.6	3.4	2.2
Beer, wine, liquors	1.9	0.2	1.3	0.0	2.6	0.1

From Cancer facts and figures for minority Americans: Atlanta, GA, p. 19, 1991, American Cancer Society.
*Estimates are weighted to reflect U.S. census population estimates for 1987.
Source: National Health Interview Survey, 1987.

**DIETARY RECOMMENDATIONS FOR
CANCER PREVENTION**

1. Reduce the amount of saturated and unsaturated fats in the diet from 40% to 30% of total daily caloric intake.
2. Increase the amount of fiber in the diet by eating fresh fruits, vegetables (especially cruciferous vegetables), and whole grain breads/cereals.
3. Drink alcoholic beverages in moderation (one or two drinks daily) or not at all.
4. Eat limited amounts of broiled, charcoaled, smoked, and salt- or nitrite-cured foods.
5. Maintain ideal body weight.

Adapted from American Cancer Society, Cancer facts and figures, 1993, Atlanta.

ALCOHOL

Excessive consumption of ethyl alcohol can lead to cancers in the head and neck, larynx, and possibly the liver and pancreas.[9,40,52,68] The synergistic effects of alcohol and tobacco can be a lethal combination. The lethal effects of alcohol and tobacco may involve the direct action of alcohol on epithelial tissues or the ability of alcohol as a solvent to increase the delivery of smoke-derived chemicals, including formaldehyde, arsenic, tar, and many others, to cause cancer.

GENETIC PREDISPOSITION

The genetic or family factor associated with cancer risk and causation is recognized but not well understood. There are two approaches in the study of familial clustering: epidemiologic and genetic. The *epidemiologic approach* examines the frequency of the disease among relatives; the *genetic approach* studies the pattern of disease expression among relatives.[1,29,44] These approaches help to provide evidence of familial aggregation but do not answer why a particular cancer expresses itself. The greatest known cancer risk exists when there is a primary relative of a patient with an autosomal dominant inherited cancer.[43-45] A thorough and complete family history can be invaluable in identifying relative risks (RR) and traits within a family aggregate.

The first report of familial aggregation of breast cancer was in Roman medical literature in 100 AD.[43] Studies in the 1930s revealed that the RR for developing breast cancer if a first-degree relative had the disease was two- to threefold. While the role of genetics is not completely clear in human oncogenesis, it is certain that the environmental carcinogens in the tissue is modified by the host-genetic make-up.[35] There is no known genetic basis to explain the major racial differences in cancer incidence and outcome.[26] Continued research into the genetic/hereditary factor in the development of human cancers represents another edge in the fight toward cancer prevention and risk reduction.

SOCIOECONOMIC FACTORS

Issues related to barriers to primary prevention and health care access have been reported as major factors in the differences in cancer incidence, delayed diagnosis, poor survival statistics, and increased mortality from cancer in minority populations. Figure 3-1 reviews the 5-year relative survival rate for all cancers diagnosed between 1981 and 1987. There is a marked difference in overall survival for African Americans and whites; the rate is 53% for whites and 38% for African Americans.[10-12,58] The estimated numbers of cancer cases and deaths for African Americans in 1991 were 112,000 and 57,000, respectively.[6,10,12]

The ACS, in collaboration with the NCI and the Centers for Disease Control (CDC), in May and June 1989 sponsored national hearings on cancer and the poor. The objective of the hearings was to determine the magnitude of unmet cancer prevention and control needs among poor and underserved Americans. The most profound findings came from the ACS's report to the nation in June of 1989. Freeman,[26] then president of the National ACS, reported five critical issues related to cancer and the poor:

1. Poor people endure greater pain and suffering from cancer than other Americans.
2. Poor people and their families must make extraordinary personal sacrifices to obtain and pay for health care.
3. Poor people face substantial obstacles in obtaining and using health insurance and often do not seek care if they cannot pay for it.
4. Current cancer education programs are culturally insensitive and irrelevant to many poor Americans.
5. Fatalism about cancer is prevalent among the poor and prevents them from seeking health care.

Freeman further reported other findings about the poor: that there are 39 million poor Americans (living below the poverty level of $11,200 a year for a family of four); two thirds of the poor are white, and nearly one third are African Americans; and a total of 37 million Americans have no health insurance.[26] Poverty is a proxy for other elements of living, including lack of education, unemployment, substandard housing, inadequate nutrition, risk-promoting behaviors and lifestyle, and limited or no access to health care.[4,10,12,26] Freeman remarked that to be poor, African American, and to have cancer is a double-jeopardy situation.[26] In large part differences in survival for African Americans and SED populations is a result of the late stage of cancer diagnosis.

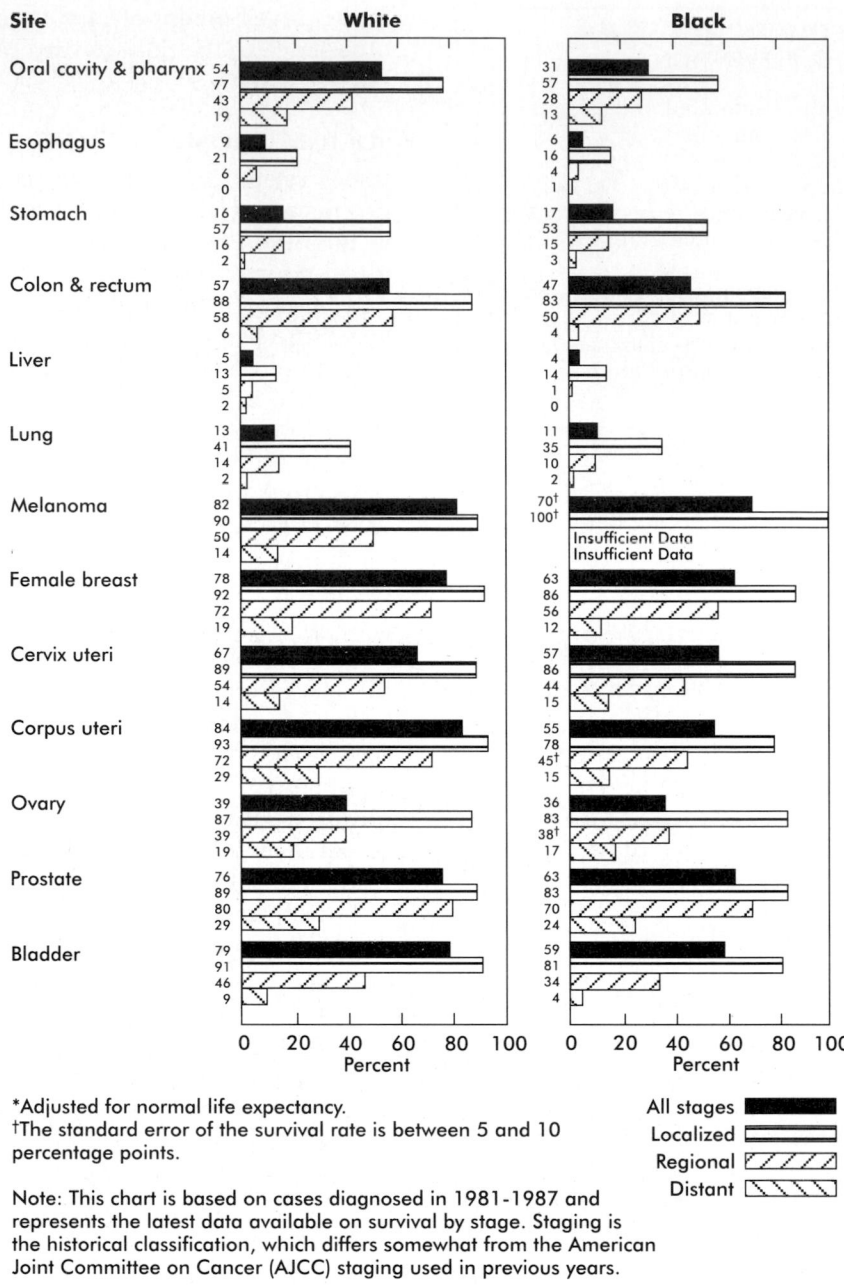

Figure 3–1 Five-year survival rates (percent)* for selected sites by race, 1981-1987. (From Boring CC, Squires TS, and Tong T: Cancer statistics, 1992, CA 42:19, 1992).

In a recent study of socioeconomic factors and cancer incidence among African Americans and whites, Baquet et al[4] found that when age-adjusted incidence data were correlated with socioeconomic status, the comparative risks changed: whites showed an elevated risk of cancer at all sites combined. These findings, presented in Table 3-9, conclude that the disproportionate distribution of African Americans at lower socioeconomic levels accounts for a large percentage of their excess cancer burden. It is therefore imperative for health care professionals to target SED and minority populations with culturally sensitive and relevant educational information on cancer prevention, risk reduction, and early detection, and to legislate for changes in health care policies to facilitate access to health care for all Americans. In the words of the great civil rights leader, the Reverend Martin Luther King, Jr., "Of all the forms of inequality, injustice in health is the most shocking and inhumane."[26]

Table 3–9 Incidence Rates* by Race, Income, and
Educational Level, Ages 25 and Over, 1978 to 1982

	White	Black
EDUCATIONAL LEVEL:		
<12 years of school	385.9	383.0
High school graduate	352.6	324.4
Some college	342.1	339.8
College graduate	338.3	270.6
Total	350.5	328.7
INCOME LEVEL (ANNUAL)		
Less than $15,000	403.2	371.7
$15,000–$24,999	352.7	341.9
$25,000–$29,999	348.1	285.8
$30,000 and over	336.8	326.6
Total	349.3	323.4

From Boring CC, Squires TS, and Heath CW. Cancer statistics for
African Americans. CA 43(1):7, 1993.
*Rates are per 100,000 and are age-adjusted to the 1970 US standard
population.

SUNLIGHT

The sun is the primary source of natural ultraviolet
(UV) light exposure that is known to cause skin cancer. The three types of skin cancers are basal cell,
squamous cell, and melanoma. Of the three types of
skin cancer, melanoma is the most potentially lethal
and is increasing in incidence at a rate of 4% per year.[11]

At highest risk for developing skin cancer are persons who work outdoors, who are fair-skinned, with
occupational exposure to coal tar, arsenic compounds,
and radium. Among African Americans the incidence
of skin cancer development is low because of heavy
skin pigmentation. Ultraviolet rays of the sun are
strongest between 10 AM and 3 PM. Sun exposure
should be limited during those hours and/or protective clothing (hats, scarves, long sleeves) should be
worn to offer some protection from the UV rays. Children should be especially protected because of the
possible link between severe sunburn in childhood
and greatly increased risk of melanoma in later life.[11]
Sunscreens should be worn when deliberate sun exposure is expected (i.e., when poolside or on the
beach). A sunscreen with a sun protection factor (SPF)
of 15 or higher should be worn on all sun exposed
skin surfaces. Sunscreens protect against a spectra of
UV rays and should be applied before sun exposure
and reapplied after being in the water. Sun tanning
parlors, which are increasing in popularity among
Americans, should be avoided.

Early detection of skin cancers is crucial to saving
lives and reducing the extent of surgical intervention.
Basal and squamous cell cancers of the skin usually
appear over areas of the body chronically exposed to
the sun including the nose, cheeks, and ears. These
cancers appear as pale, waxlike nodules or a red, scaly
patch that tends to bleed. Melanomas are small, mole-
like eruptions on the skin that can appear anywhere
on the body including the soles of the feet and palms
of the hand. Melanomas change in color, shape, and
size and can ulcerate and bleed.

A simple *ABCD* rule outlines the warning signs of
melanoma: *A* is for asymmetry; *B* is for border irregularity; *C* is for change in color or pigmentation; and
D is for diameter greater than 6 mm.[11] Adults should
practice skin self-examination and mole mapping
monthly and report any suspicious indicators to a
member of the health care team.

SEXUAL LIFE-STYLES

Sexual beliefs, attitudes, and practices are no longer
private and unassuming. The sexual mores of the
1980s and 1990s have thrust the association between
sexual activity and cancer risk from obscurity to the
front lines. The advertising slogan "sex sells" has almost prompted an attitude of "anything goes." Sexually transmitted diseases (STDs), genital cancers,
and acquired immune deficiency syndrome (AIDS)
have a documented direct relationship to sexual lifestyles and practices. The association between sex and
genital cancer has been known for over 150 years.[38]
Research indicates an association between sexual lifestyles and cancer of the cervix, vulva, vagina, and
AIDS. Risk factors common in women with cervical
cancer include: a high rate of STDs, early age at first
coitus, multiple sexual partners, and exposure to
high-risk sexual partners. Several viruses have been
implicated in the etiology of cervical neoplasia including herpes simplex virus (HSV) and human papillomavirus (HPV). Penile HPV (genital wart or condyloma) infection in a male partner places the woman
at risk of cervical cancer.

The incurable and deadly disease AIDS has cast a
shadow over the American sexual revolution/free-
dom as no other disease or health threat. Sexual behaviors considered to be high-risk factors associated
with AIDS include: unprotected vaginal or anal intercourse, internal watersports (urinating into a body
cavity such as the vagina or anus), fisting (inserting
a finger, fingers, or fist into the anus), and oral-anal
sex, also known as rimming.[38] Sharing of dirty needles
by intravenous drug users is also a high-risk factor.[36]
Male homosexuals and IV drug users are at greatest
risk for acquiring AIDS and other related neoplasms;
however, the CDC reports a growing rate of HIV and
AIDS cases among the heterosexual population.[36,63]
The mortality rate for AIDS is over 40% within the
first year of diagnosis.[38,63] Reducing the cancer risk
related to sexual lifestyles can be effected by safe sexual practices.

EARLY DETECTION AND SCREENING RECOMMENDATIONS

Americans are adopting more health conscious behaviors, which include diet modification, physical fitness, smoking cessation, and overall healthier lifestyles. Heightened awareness of health-promoting activities and early detection techniques, related to cancer, continue to be a focus of many cancer information agencies (ACS, NCI) and professional organizations like the Oncology Nursing Society and others. The ACS in 1993 updated screening and early detection guidelines (Table 3-10).

A number of socioeconomic barriers to screening and early detection exist, such as lack of health insurance, poverty, unemployment, and lack of education. Empowering people to overcome some of these barriers is key to the success of reducing cancer related deaths by the year 2000. Overall cancer survival can be increased through early detection. Regular breast, cervical, and prostate screening techniques have scientific evidence of their effectiveness in detecting cancers early. The public should be educated to individual risk factors and screening recommendations.

Table 3–10 Summary of American Cancer Society Recommendations for the Early Detection of Cancer in Asymptomatic People (Jan/Feb 1993)

Test or Procedure	Population		
	Sex	Age	Frequency
Sigmoidoscopy, preferably flexible	M & F	50 and over	Every 3 to 5 years
Fecal occult blood test	M & F	50 and over	Every year
Digital rectal examination	M & F	40 and over	Every year
Prostate examination	M	50 and over*	Every year
Pap test	F	All women who are or who have been sexually active, or have reached age 18, should have an annual Pap test and pelvic examination. After a woman has had three or more consecutive satisfactory normal annual examinations, the Pap test may be performed less frequently at the discretion of her physician.	
Pelvic examination	F	18–40	Every 1–3 years with Pap test
		Over 40	Every year
Endometrial tissue sample	F	At menopause, women at high risk§	At menopause
Breast self-examination	F	20 and over	Every month
Clinical breast examination	F	20–40	Every 3 years
		Over 40	Every year
Mammography†	F	40–49	Every 1–2 years
		50 and over	Every year
Health counseling and cancer checkup‡	M & F	Over 20	Every 3 years
	M & F	Over 40	Every year

From American Cancer Society: CA 43(1):42, 1993.
*Annual digital rectal examination and prostate-specific antigen should be performed on men age 50 and older. If either is abnormal, further evaluation should be considered.
§History of infertility, obesity, failure to ovulate, abnormal uterine bleeding, or estrogen therapy.
†Screening mammography should begin by age 40.
‡To include examination for cancers of the thyroid, testicles, prostate, ovaries, lymph nodes, oral region, and skin.

Nursing Management

Patient/family education in the prevention, screening, and early detection of cancer lays the foundation for overcoming ignorance and fear of cancer related to health beliefs, practices, and attitudes. Nurses can take active roles in sharing knowledge, skills, and expertise with those Americans with limited access to health care and who are at a higher risk for developing certain cancers. Nurses can work through neighborhood outreach groups and legislators to advocate for reduced or no cost cancer screening tests for the underserved and high-risk population. Nurses can involve at-risk youth by facilitating health education programs, conducting risk appraisals, and providing information on nutrition and lifestyle choices and changes for health promotion and disease prevention.

Overall, professional nurses can have the greatest impact on the public by "walking the talk"; i.e., by practicing good health habits, weight reduction, smoking cessation, and self-examination, and by facilitating public and professional education programs. The nurse can take a pro-active role by coordinating screening projects and participating in health fairs.

By eliciting the aid of church, social, and civic organizations, nurses can reach a large number of those individuals with limited or no access to health care and who are at greatest risk for cancer morbidity and/or mortality.[32]

NURSING DIAGNOSIS
Knowledge deficit related to prevention and early detection of site specific cancers (Table 3–5)

OUTCOME GOALS
Patient/significant other will be able to:
1. State the 7 warning signals of cancer
2. Demonstrate site related self-examination related to breast, oral, skin, vulva, penile, and testicular cancers.
3. Recognize cancer related signs and symptoms that require follow up in the health care system.
4. Identify cancer information sources (ACS, Leukemia Society, NCI).
5. Identify his/her relative risk for cancer development.

ASSESSMENTS
Assess the following:
1. Patient education level
2. Literacy level
3. Cultural/ethnic perspectives of patient/significant other
4. Beliefs and attitudes towards cancer
5. Patient/family history and relative risk of cancer development

INTERVENTIONS
1. Discuss site specific cancer risk factors.
2. Identify signs and symptoms of site specific cancer.
3. Health teaching related to diet, nutrition, and lifestyle choices.
4. Provide appropriate and culturally sensitive printed information to client.
5. Provide a list of cancer information/support agencies.
6. Instruct patient in self examination of breast, mouth, skin, cervix, vulva, penis, and testicles.
7. Review ACS screening guidelines.
8. Assist patient with access to health care issues for cancer screening and early detection.
9. Identify signs/symptoms that warrant access to the health care system.
10. Identify community resources available to help patient:
    - Stop smoking
    - Reduce stress
    - Control weight and diet
11. Identify occupational and environmental risk factors and reporting agencies: OSHA (Occupational, Safety and Health Administration), EPA (Environmental Protection Agency), NRA (Nuclear Regulatory Agency), FDA (Federal Drug Administration).
12. Provide mechanism for necessary referral and follow-up.

CONCLUSION
Cancer mortality will not be reduced without heightened public awareness and a multidisciplinary approach involving health-care professionals, epidemiologists, and researchers. Agencies such as the ACS, Leukemia Society, and the NCI play a vital role in cancer control efforts via funding and support of all aspects of cancer research and public and professional education. Additionally, these agencies and organizations must increase activity and involvement in social and political decisions influencing health care policy, cancer research, and treatment. A positive example of such efforts by the American public and support agencies is the ban on cigarette smoking on all domestic flights.

Because cancer is predominantly a disease of the elderly, many signs and symptoms can mimic the normal aging process and go ignored and undetected by the elderly and their significant others. Nurses can play a vital role in cancer prevention, screening, and risk reduction by identifying high-risk individuals, assessing lifestyle, personal and family history, and occupational or environmental exposure to carcinogens. Nurses' efforts should also include promoting follow-up and surveillance of those identified as high risk.

Underserved Americans offer the greatest challenge to nurses and other health care professionals. The underserved and SED populations make up a significant percentage of the American public and often bear the greatest burden of cancer risk and mortality. This is reflected in poorer overall survival, most frequently due to a later stage at which the cancer is detected. Millions of Americans are uninsured or underinsured, and this number is escalating with the climbing unemployment rate. Another barrier for this population is limited access to health care due to lack of health insurance, unemployment, homelessness, transportation issues, and inability to wait 6 to 8 hours in a overcrowded health care facility because of family and/or job responsibilities. Screening and early detection have little significance but to imply a death sentence to someone who has no access to health care intervention and follow up and for whom the situation seems hopeless.

To offer public health teaching and support the nurse and other health care professionals must be sensitive to social, cultural, ethnic and religious beliefs, and values and attitudes that can impact an individual's receptivity to health promotion and disease prevention strategies. Nurses can best prepare to meet the public education needs through sensitivity training sessions, developing printed materials that reflect cultural diversity, and are at an appropriate literacy level, and thorough "train the trainer" programs for volunteers. Train the trainer programs facilitate contact with previously hard to reach groups by training a volunteer from within the community or group to deliver the message of cancer prevention, risk reduction, and health promotion. Cancer prevention efforts should be aimed at improved agricultural and grain storage techniques, safe sexual practices, reducing occupational and environmental exposure to carcinogens, health promotion activities, and education.

BIBLIOGRAPHY

1. Albright LA and others: Genetic predisposition to cancer. In DeVita VT, Jr, Hellman S, and Rosenberg SA, editors: Important advances in oncology, Philadelphia, 1991, JB Lippincott.
2. American Cancer Society: Guidelines for the cancer related checkup—Update January 1992, CA 42:44, 1992.
3. Annotated bibliography of cancer—related literature on black populations, US/DHHS, Public Health Service, 1988, NIH Pub No 89-3024.
4. Baquet CR and others: Socioeconomic factors and cancer incidence among blacks and whites, J Nat Cancer Inst 83:551, 1991.
5. Bell I: Testicular self-examination, Nurs Times 86:38, 1990.
6. Black and minority health: Report of the secretary's task force, US/DHHS, Washington, DC, 1985.
7. Boring CC, Squires TS, and Heath CW: Cancer statistics for African Americans, CA 42:7, 1992.
8. Boring CC, Squires TS, and Tong T: Cancer statistics, 1992, CA 43(1):7, 1993.
9. Bridbord K: Pathogenesis and prevention of hepatocellular carcinoma, Cancer Detect Prev 14:191, 1989.
10. Cancer among blacks and other minorities: Statistical profiles, US/DHHS, Public Health Service, 1986, National Institutes of Health (NIH) Pub No 86-2785.
11. Cancer facts and figures 1993: Atlanta, Ga, 1993, American Cancer Society.
12. Cancer facts and figures for minority Americans 1991: Atlanta, GA, 1991, American Cancer Society.
13. Cancer prevention and detection: Atlanta, GA, 1989, American Cancer Society.
14. Cancer rates and risks, National Institute of Health Pub No 85-691, 1985, US Department of Health and Human Services.
15. Cigarette smoking among youth—United States, 1989: Morbidity and Mortality Weekly Report 40: 712, 1991, Centers for Disease Control, Atlanta.
16. Cook-Mozaffari P: The epidemiology of cancer of the esophagus, Nutr Cancer 1:51, 1979.
17. Croghan IT and Omoto MK: cancer prevention and risk reduction. In Baird SB, editor: A cancer source book for nurses, Atlanta, Ga, 1991, American Cancer Society.
18. Diet, nutrition and cancer prevention: a guide to food choices, US/DHHS Pub No 85-2711, 1984, National Institutes of Health.
19. Differences in age of smoking initiation between blacks and whites—United States, Morbidity and Mortality Weekly Report 40:754, 1991, Centers for Disease Control, Atlanta.
20. Dodd GD: American cancer society guidelines on screening for breast cancer: An overview, CA 42:177, 1992.
21. Drago JR: The role of new modalities's in the early detection and diagnosis of prostate cancer, CA 39:326, 1989.
22. Faulkenberry JE: Cancer in men: A case for cancer prevention and early detection, Dimen Oncol Nurs 2:17, 1988.
23. Fighting Cancer in America: Achieving the "year 2000 goal", Cancer Nurs 12:359, 1989.
24. Fink DJ: Cancer detection: The cancer related checkup guidelines. In Holleb AI, Fink DJ, and Murphy GP, editors: ACS textbook of clinical oncology, Atlanta, GA, 1991, American Cancer Society.
25. Fitzsimmons ML and others: Hereditary cancer syndromes: Nursing's role in identification and education, Oncol Nurs Forum 16:87, 1989.
26. Freeman HP: Cancer in the socioeconomically disadvantaged, CA 39:266, 1989.
27. Graham S, Mettlin C, and Marshall J: Dietary factors in the epidemiology of cancer of the larynx, Am J Epidemiol 113:675, 1981.
28. Graham S, Schotz W, and Martino P: Alimentary factors in the epidemiology of gastric cancer, Cancer 30:927, 1972.

29. Graves PL, Thomas CB, and Mead LA: Familial and psychological predictors of cancer, Cancer Detect Prev 15:59, 1991.

30. Griffiths EK and Schapira DV: Serum ferritin and stool occult blood and colon cancer screening, Cancer Detect Prev 15:303, 1991.

31. Gullatte MM: Cancer prevention and early detection in black americans: Prostate, In touch 9:4, 1988, American Cancer Society, Atlanta, GA.

32. Gullatte MM: Cancer prevention and early detection in black americans: Colon and rectum, J National Black Nurses Assoc 3:49, 1989.

33. Hahn RA and others: Prevalence of HIV infection among intravenous drug users in the United States, JAMA 261:2677, 1989.

34. Headen SW and others: Are the correlates of cigarette smoking initiation different for black and white adolescents? Am J Public Health 81:854, 1991.

35. Heath CW: Cancer prevention. In Holleb AI, Fink DJ, and Murphy GP, editors: ACS textbook of clinical oncology, Atlanta, Ga, 1991, American Cancer Society.

36. HIV—Infection prevention messages for injecting drug users: Sources of information and use of mass media—Baltimore—1989, Morbidity and Mortality Weekly Report 40:1, 1991, Centers for Disease Control, Atlanta.

37. Holleb AI, Fink DJ, and Murphy G: American cancer society textbook of clinical oncology, Atlanta, 1991, American Cancer Society.

38. Holmes BC: Sexual lifestyles and cancer risk, 1988, Atlanta, GA, American Cancer Society.

39. Increasing breast cancer screening among the medically underserved—Dade County, Florida, September 1987—March 1991, Morbidity and Mortality Weekly Report 40:261, 1991, Centers for Disease Control, Atlanta.

40. Knopp JM and Croghan IT: Screening, detection, and diagnosis. In Baird SB, editor: A cancer source book for nurses, Atlanta, Georgia, 1991, American Cancer Society.

41. Kritchewsky D: Diet and cancer. In Holleb AI, Fink DJ, and Murphy GP, editors: ACS textbook of clinical oncology, Atlanta, GA, 1991, American Cancer Society.

42. Littrup PJ, Lee F, and Mettlin C: Prostate cancer screening: current trends and future implications, CA 42:198, 1992.

43. Lynch HT: Genetics and breast cancer, New York, 1981, Van Nostrand Reinhold.

44. Lynch HT and Lynch JF: Familial factors and genetic predisposition to cancer: Population studies, Cancer Detec Prev 15:49, 1991.

45. Lynch HT: The family history and cancer control: Hereditary breast cancer, Arch Surg 125:151, 1990.

46. Miller AB: Role of early diagnosis and screening; Biomarkers, Cancer Detec Prev 15:21, 1991.

47. Phillips J: Cancer control by the year 2000: Implications for action, J Nation Black Nurses Assoc 5:42, 1991.

48. Post WJ and others: Nutrition and cancer: Educating the public through a health fair, Oncol Nurs Forum 16:115, 1989.

49. Reddy BS, Sharma C, and Simi B: Metabolic epidemiology of colon cancer: Effects of dietary fiber on fecal mutagens and bile acids in healthy subjects, Cancer Res 75:791, 1987.

50. Reis LA and others: Cancer statistics review 1973–88, National Cancer Institute, NIH Pub No 91-2789, 1991.

51. Resnicow K, Kabat G, and Wynder E: Progress in decreasing cigarette smoking. In DeVita VT, Hellman S, and Rosenberg SA, editors: Important advances in oncology, Philadelphia, 1991, JB Lippincott.

52. Rosenbaum EH, Dollinger M, and Newell GR: Risk assessment, cancer screening and prevention, Everyone's guide to cancer therapy, Kansas City, 1991, A Somerville House Book.

53. Schuman LM, Mandell JS, and Radke A: Some selected features of the epidemiology of prostate cancer: Minneapolis—St. Paul case control study 1976–79. In Magnus K, editor: Trends in cancer incidence: Causes and practical implication, Washington, DC, 1982, Hemisphere Publishing Company.

54. Smoking—attributable mortality and years of potential life lost—United States 1988, Morbidity and Mortality Weekly Report 40: 62, 1991, Centers for Disease Control, Atlanta.

55. Stromborg MF and Olsen SJ: Cancer prevention in minority populations: Cultural implications for health care professionals, St. Louis, 1993, Mosby.

56. Tobacco use among high school students—United States, 1990, Morbidity and Mortality Weekly Report 40:617, 1991.

57. Tubiana M: Trends in primary and secondary prevention, Cancer Detec Prev 15:1, 1991.

58. Underwood SM: Cancer risk reduction and early detection behaviors among black men: focus on learned helplessness, J Community Health Nurs 9:21, 1992.

59. Underwood SM: Testicular self-examination among african-american men, J Nation Black Nurses Assoc 5:18, 1991.

60. Underwood SM: African-american men: Perceptual determinants of early cancer detection and cancer risk reduction, Cancer Nurs 14:281, 1991.

61. Vainio H and Hemminki K: Use of exposure information and animal cancer data in the preven-

tion of environmental and occupational cancer, Cancer Detec Prev 15:7, 1991.

62. Vlahov D and others: Trends of HIV-1 risk reduction among initiates into intravenous drug use: 1982-1987, Am J Drug Alcohol Abuse 17:39, 1991.

63. Volker DL: Acquired immune deficiency syndrome: An overview, Dimen Oncol Nurs 2:22, 1988.

64. Watkins MC: Computerized cancer information sources, J Med Assoc Georgia 81:143, 1992.

65. White K: Diet and cancer, Med World News 52: August 1982.

66. Wholihan DJ: Incorporating cancer prevention interventions into the home health visit, Home Healthcare Nurse 9:19, 1991.

67. Willis MA and others: Inter-agency Collaboration: teaching breast self-examination to black women. Oncol Nurs Forum 16:171, 1989.

68. Wogan GN: Dietary risk factors for primary hepatocellular carcinoma, Cancer Detect Prev 14:209,1989.

69. Ziegler RG, Devesa SS, and Fravmeni JF, Jr: Epidemiologic patterns of colorectal cancer. In DeVita VT, Jr, Hellman S, and Rosenberg SA, editors: Important advances in oncology, Philadelphia, 1986, JB Lippincott.

CHAPTER 4

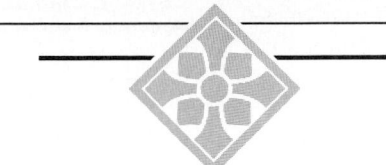

Diagnosis and Staging

Joyce Alexander

The diagnosis of cancer involves many members of the healthcare team, including the attending physician, specialists, radiologists, surgeons, oncologists, pathologists, technicians, and nurses. Treatment decisions are based upon the histology (tumor type) and the assessed extent of disease. New techniques to diagnose and stage cancers have facilitated development of sophisticated plans of treatment, which have produced improved patient survival rates as well as cures for some malignancies.

DIAGNOSIS
History and Physical Examination
A patient's past medical history and physical examination (H&P) and presenting signs and symptoms provide important data toward diagnosing a malignancy. In addition to the thorough H&P by the physician, the nurse takes a nursing history and performs a complete systems assessment, documenting variations from normal. Careful listening to the patient's experience of symptoms provides vital information. From this database, a potential diagnosis can be made and testing initiated to rule out various reasons for the patient's problem. The medical history and family history provide valuable information regarding a patient's cancer risk factors. For example, a previous diagnosis of Crohn's disease in a patient with bloody stools raises the index of suspicion that a malignancy might be present in the colon. Thorough and complete histories help guide the initial diagnostic work-up.

Physical examinations are a systematic assessment of major body sites: head, ears, nose, throat, cardiovascular system, chest, abdomen, genitourinary system, extremities, lymph nodes, and nervous system. Positive and negative findings are documented and evaluated in terms of the patient's medical history. An enlarged liver may cause the physician to suspect metastatic disease if the patient has a past history of colon or breast cancer.

A cancer diagnosis may be readily determined or difficult. The diagnostic work-up, planned from the patient's symptoms, history, and physical examination yields a presumptive malignant diagnosis. That diagnosis must be confirmed through histologic and cytologic examination. Staging completes the necessary information for planning treatment.

Diagnostic Work-up
A diagnostic work-up is initiated to determine the cause of a patient's symptoms. A wide range of diagnostic procedures may be used in the individualized work-up for each patient. Testing begins with less invasive procedures but may include highly technical innovations. After the diagnosis of malignancy is established, further diagnostic tests may be utilized to determine the stage of the cancer. Knowledge of symptoms, a high index of suspicion for malignancy, and knowledge of biologic behavior of a particular cancer are all useful in reaching a diagnosis.

RADIOLOGIC STUDIES. A work-up often begins with a basic chest x-ray. A mammogram, flat plate of the abdomen, or x-rays of the extremities may also add information. Barium studies of the gastrointestinal tract, intravenous pyelogram to evaluate the urinary tract, and myelogram evaluation of the spinal canal are added when indicated. Computed tomography (CT) combines computer technology with radiology to produce multiple cross-sectional depictions of internal structures. CT images are based on varying density of tissues. Contrast solutions containing iodine may be used to improve images. Position emission tomography (PET) is an emerging technology that will provide useful information in the future.

MAGNETIC RESONANCE IMAGING.   Magnetic resonance imaging (MRI) provides sensitive images of soft tissues, without interference from bone. Images are produced by placing the patient within a strong magnetic field, causing alignment of certain atoms within cellular molecules. Pulsed radio waves cause absorption and release of energy as the atomic nuclei change orientation. Energy differences are detected and measured by antennae and the information used by the MRI computer to produce images. MRI is superior for visualization of tissues obscured by bone in other diagnostic techniques, including the central nervous system, mediastinal, and hilar areas. MRI may also be used to visualize abnormal vascular states, edema, and other tumors.[12]

ULTRASONOGRAPHY.   High-frequency sound waves may also be used to visualize internal structures. Abdominal, pelvic, or peritoneal masses may be detected by ultrasound. This technique is also sometimes used to evaluate masses in the breast, thyroid, and prostate.

NUCLEAR MEDICINE SCANS.   Radioactive isotopes may be injected and tracked to those tissues for which the isotope has an affinity. Concentrations of the isotope in focal points indicates greater activity of cells, which may be due to disease, infection, or malignancy. Areas of decreased uptake may also be significant in tissues that normally take up an isotope. A bone scan is often done to detect areas of possible bony metastasis. Other scans, including thyroid, brain, and liver, are done to evaluate possible primary or metastatic disease in those organs. Radio-labelled monoclonal antibodies specific to tumor antigens may also be used to produce gamma camera images of tumors through a process called *immunoscintography*.[13]

VISUALIZATION.   Advances in endoscopy techniques have made visual examination of many tissues possible. Colonoscopy and flexible sigmoidoscopy are used in the diagnosis of colorectal cancer; bronchoscopy is often useful in diagnosis of cancer of bronchogenic or lung origin; gastroscopy can differentiate causes of gastric symptoms; and laparoscopy is now being used to view and biopsy abdominal tissues. These techniques are used not only to visualize the tissues but to obtain samples for pathologic examination.

LABORATORY STUDIES.   Each patient's work-up includes a battery of common laboratory procedures: complete blood count (CBC), with differential analysis of white blood cells, blood chemistries, liver function tests, renal function tests, and urinalysis. Additional laboratory studies such as serum electrophoresis, calcium and magnesium levels, and levels of tumor markers are ordered as indicated by the patient's

Table 4–1   Selected Laboratory Studies

Examination	*Detects or Assesses*
Bone marrow aspiration/ biopsy	Hematologic abnormalities Presence of metastatic disease in the marrow
Chemistry profile: bilirubin, calcium, uric acid, blood-urea-nitrogen, creatinine, electrolytes, lactic dehydrogenase, serum glutamic oxaloacetic transaminase, alkaline phosphatase, serum glutamic pyruvic transaminase, magnesium	Liver, kidney, bone abnormalities secondary to cancer, therapy, certain chronic illnesses May be used to monitor response to treatment
Complete blood count	Bone marrow abnormalities Toxicity of therapy
Creatinine clearance	Kidney function; especially important when giving nephrotoxic drugs
Hemoccult test	Presence of blood in stool; not specific for cancer
Pap smear	Cervical cancer or premalignant changes
Serum electrophoresis	Serum protein and immunoglobulin levels (multiple myeloma)
Urine catecholamines	Neuroblastoma, pheochromocytoma

symptoms. Table 4-1 lists some common laboratory studies used in a diagnostic work-up.

TUMOR MARKERS.   Tumor markers are substances that are present and measurable in the blood or tissues of patients with malignancies that are not present or are present in lesser amounts in normal individuals. The first known tumor marker, Bence-Jones protein, was discovered in 1848 in patients with multiple myeloma.[15] Tumor markers often are hormonal substances produced by specific types of cells. Chorionic gonadotropin (HCG) and alpha-fetoprotein are hormonal substances that are elevated in germ cell tumors. Antigens produced by tumor cells are also tumor markers when identified by monoclonal antibodies. Carcinoembryonic antigen (CEA) is an antigen that can be identified at increased levels in some patients with colorectal, lung, or breast cancer.[13]

CA-125 is an antigen that is elevated in the blood of patients with ovarian cancer but may be elevated in normal women as well. An antigen produced by prostate tissue, prostate specific antigen (PSA), along with acid phosphatase, is elevated in prostate cancer but may also be elevated in benign prostatic disease. Tumor markers are often elevated in nonmalignant disease. The significance of tumor marker levels may be difficult to determine and must be assessed according to the patient's symptoms and other work-

Table 4–2 Commonly Used Tumor Markers

Marker	Elevations May Indicate	Useful For
CEA (carcinoembryonic antigen)	Breast cancer, colorectal cancer, lung cancer	Monitoring or management of patients with known disease
PSA (prostate specific antigen)	Prostate cancer, benign prostate enlargement	Monitoring response of patients to treatment; arouse suspicion of prostate cancer
HCG (human chorionic gonadotropin)	Germ cell tumors (testicular, certain types ovarian, others), pregnancy	Differentiation of germ cell tumors
AFP (alpha fetal protein)	Germ cell tumors, liver cancer, benign liver disease, pregnancy	Differentiation of germ cell tumors
CA-125 (antigen)	Ovarian cancer, also elevated in some nonmalignant conditions and in some nongynecologic cancers	Monitoring response
CA-15-3 (2 antigens)	Metastatic or recurrent breast cancer	Monitoring recurrent disease
CA-19-9 (antigens)	Pancreatic cancer, colorectal cancer, gastric cancer, inflammatory bowel, biliary disease	Monitoring response to treatment

up data. Table 4-2 lists some commonly used tumor markers.[9]

Grade

Grade is a classification of tumor cells based on cellular differentiation or resemblance to normal cells in structure, function, and maturity. Actual tumor cells must be obtained and examined by the pathologist before a clinical diagnosis of cancer or a determination of the grade of the malignancy can be made. Cells may be obtained by cytologic examination techniques, biopsy, or surgical excision of a suspected mass.

CYTOLOGY.   Cytology is the examination of cells obtained from tissue scrapings, body fluids, secretions, or washings. Pap smears (named for Dr. George Papanicolaou, who developed the technique) use scrapings from the cervix to identify abnormal cervical cells. Fluids aspirated by thoracentesis, paracentesis, or lumbar puncture may yield cells for examination. Fine needle aspiration may also be used to obtain cells for evaluation. Once procured, cytology specimens must be evaluated by a skilled pathologist. False positive results are possible and negative results indicate only that no cancer cells were found in the sample.

BIOPSY.   A portion of tissue, generally obtained by surgical procedure, is examined in a biopsy specimen. Biopsy is often done as part of an endoscopic procedure or under the guidance of CT to ensure that suspicious areas are sampled. Bone marrow biopsy, which uses a special needle to aspirate bone marrow tissue, is included in the work-up for hematologic disorders, including lymphomas, and when there is suspicion of bone marrow metastasis.

EXCISION AND ANALYSIS.   Whenever a mass is surgically removed, whether or not a definitive diagnosis has been made, the tissue removed must be examined by a pathologist. The pathologist uses a number of techniques to determine the tissue type and the degree of differentiation (grade) of the tumor. Frozen section is a procedure by which a small amount of tissue is quickly frozen, sliced thinly, and stained for immediate examination. A permanent section is prepared using tissue preserved in formalin, sliced thinly, stained, and prepared for microscopic examination. The pathologist begins the examination of the tissues with an overview and measurement of the gross specimen, then proceeds to microscopic examination of prepared slides using light microscopy. Careful attention is paid to the margins of the excised specimen to determine if margins are free of malignancy.

Immunoperoxidase staining identifies specific cell types using monoclonal or polyclonal antibodies against cellular antigens.[8] PSA can be stained using a monoclonal antibody and suggests that tissue is of prostatic origin. Leukocyte common antigen can be used to identify non-Hodgkin lymphomas.[8] Electron microscopy may be used when light microscopy and special stains fail to differentiate the cell type. Genetic analysis is used to identify specific chromosomal abnormalities. Some malignancies known to have chromosomal abnormalities include chronic myelogenous leukemia, acute leukemia, peripheral neuroepithelioma, testicular cancer, and B-cell non-Hodgkin's lymphoma.[8]

In addition to determining the definitive diagnosis of cancer and the tissue of origin, the pathologist must determine the grade. Grade is a classification based on the differentiation, or maturity and resemblance to normal cells, of the malignancy. The more unlike normal tissue, and less differentiated or mature the cells, the higher the grade. Behavior of a malignancy can be predicted on the basis of grade. Table 4-3 lists grade classifications.

Table 4–3   Grades

Grade		Definition
X	Cannot be assessed	
I	Well differentiated	Mature cells resembling normal tissue
II	Moderately differentiated	Cells with some immaturity
III	Poorly differentiated	Immature cells with little resemblance to normal
IV	Undifferentiated	No resemblance to normal tissue

Table 4–4   General TNM Definitions

T	Primary tumor	Size, extent, depth of primary tumor
	TX	Primary tumor cannot be assessed
	T0	No evidence of primary tumor
	Tis	In situ
	T1–T4	Increasing size or extent of primary tumor
N	Nodal metastasis	Extent and location of involved regional lymph nodes
	NX	Regional lymph nodes cannot be assessed
	N0	No regional lymph node metastasis
	N1–N3	Increasing numbers and size of involved regional lymph nodes
M	Metastasis	Absence or presence of distant spread of disease
	MX	Distant disease cannot be assessed
	M0	No distant spread of disease
	M1	Distant spread of disease

Stage

Once a cancer diagnosis is confirmed by pathology, information from previous tests and scans is combined with additional work-up studies to determine the stage of the malignancy. Stage is a classification system based on the apparent anatomic extent of the malignancy.[1] A universal system of staging allows comparison of cancers of similar cellular origin. Classification assists in determination of a treatment plan and prognosis for the individual patient, evaluation of research, comparison of treatment results between institutions, and comparison of worldwide statistics.

A comprehensive staging system was developed by the American Joint Committee on Cancer (AJCC), a coalition sponsored by the American Cancer Society, the National Cancer Institute, the College of American Pathologists, the American College of Physicians, the American College of Radiology, and the American College of Surgeons. This group published the first staging manual in 1977. The International Union Against Cancer later joined the group and the system became international. The fourth edition, published in 1992, included recommendations of the International Federation of Gynecology and Obstetrics (FIGO) to broaden the international scope.[1]

The TNM system outlined by AJCC involves assessment of three basic components: the size of the primary tumor (T); the absence or presence of regional lymph nodes (N); and the absence or presence of distant metastatic disease (M). General definitions used throughout the system are included in Table 4-4.[1]

Information from the TNM classification is combined to define the stage. Stage classifications have been determined for most cancer sites and are published in the *Manual for Staging of Cancer*.[1] Examples for selected disease sites are included in Table 4-5 (Parts A to E). The stage is determined prior to beginning treatment, and is the basis for treatment decisions. The stage is often changed following surgery, however, when pathologic measurements more accurately define tumor size and nodal involvement.

Stage determined prior to treatment is termed the *clinical stage* (cTNM or TNM). When stage is changed after surgery, the term *pathologic stage* (pTNM) is used.

Prior to 1992, gynecologic cancers were commonly classified using a separate system developed by the International Federation of Gynecology and Obstetrics (FIGO). Information from the FIGO system has been incorporated into the staging system published in the *Manual for Staging of Cancer*,[1] and a separate system is no longer necessary. Table 4-6 provides examples.

Staging of cancers of the central nervous system (CNS) varies from that for other disease sites. Important prognostic indicators in brain cancer are the biologic behavior, or rate of growth, and the location and size of the tumor (refer to Chapter 6). Staging for brain cancer, therefore, considers grade (G) and tumor size and location (T). A higher grade is a more malignant tumor; a grade 3 tumor (G3) will be classified stage III unless the tumor crosses the midline. Any tumor that crosses the midline (T4) or any CNS tumor with metastasis is classified stage IV. The brain is not supplied with lymphatic drainage, therefore "N" is not used.

Hematologic malignancies cannot be classified using the TNM system. Leukemias are classified according to cell type and differentiation but are not staged further. Leukemia research compares patients on the basis of remission or first, second, or third relapse and prognosis can be determined on that in-

Table 4–5   Selected TNM Staging Guidelines

STAGE	LUNG	BREAST	BONE
Occult	**TX-N0-M0** TX: primary proven only by cells (sputum)		
0	**Tis-N0-M0** Tis: carcinoma in situ	**Tis-N0-M0** Tis: carcinoma in situ	
I	**T1 or T2-N0-M0** T1: tumor $\leq$ 3 cm T2: >3 cm and/or involving main bronchus or pleura	**T1-N0-M0** T1: tumor $\leq$ 2 cm	**G1 or 2- T1 or 2** well or moderately differentiated T1, within cortex T2, outside cortex **N0-M0**
II	**T1 or T2-N1-M0** N1: peribronchial or hilar lymph node metastasis; same side as tumor	**T0 or T1-N1-M0** **T2-N0 or N1-M0** **T3-N0-M0** T2: tumor 2-5 cm T3: tumor > 5 cm N1: met. to movable axillary lymph node(s) same side	**G3 or 4- T1 or 2** **N0-M0** G3: poorly differentiated G4: undifferentiated
IIIA	**T1 or T2-N2-M0** **T3-any N-M0** N2: mediastinal or subclavian nodes. same side T3: tumor invades chest wall, diaphragm, mediastinal pleura, pericardium	**T0, T1, T2-N2-M0** **T3-N1 or N2-M0** N2: fixed axillary lymph nodes; same side	**Not defined**
IIIB	**Any T-N3-M0** **T4-any N-M0** N3: metastasis in lymph nodes opposite side T4: invades other organs (heart, mediastinum, etc.) or pleural effusion	**T4-any N-M0** **Any T-N3-M0** T4: tumor invades chest wall or skin N3: internal mammary node mets; same side	
IV	**Any T, any N, M1** M1: distant metastasis	**Any T-any N-M1** M1: distant metastasis	**Any G & T-N1-M0** **Any G & T-Any N-M1**
STAGE	**LARYNX**	**COLO-RECTAL/DUKE'S**	
0	**Tis-N0-M0** Tis: carcinoma in situ	**Tis-N0-M0** Tis: carcinoma in situ	
I	**T1-N0-M0** T1: tumor limited to vocal cord with normal mobility	**T1 or T2-N0-M0** T1: tumor invading submucosa T2: invading muscle layer	**Duke's A**
II	**T2-N0-M0** T2: extends to supraglottis and/or subglottis with impaired cord mobility	**T3 or T4-N0-M0** T3: invades through muscle layer, into subserosa T4: directly invades other organs or perforates visceral peritoneum	**Duke's B**
III	**T3-N0-M0** **T1, T2, or T3-N1-M0** T3: tumor limited to larynx with vocal cord fixation N1: single, same-side node < 3 cm	**Any T-N1, N2, or N3-M0** N1: 1-3 pericolic or perirectal lymph node metastases N2: $\geq$ 4 pericolic or perirectal lymph node metastases N3: any nodal metastasis along vascular trunk or apical node.	**Duke's C**

Continued.

Table 4–5 Selected TNM Staging Guidelines—cont'd

STAGE	LARYNX	COLO-RECTAL/DUKE'S	
IV	**T4-N0 or N1-M0** **Any T-N2 or N3-M0** **Any T, any N, M1** T4: tumor invades thyroid cartilage and/or tissues beyond larynx N2: single node, same side, 3-6 cm N3: any node > 6 cm M1: distant metastasis	**Any T- any N-M1** M1: distant metastasis	Duke's D

STAGE	GASTRIC	PROSTATE	
0	**Tis-N0-M0** Tis: carcinoma in situ	**T1a-N0-M0 (G1)** T1a: incidental finding < 5% of tissue G1: well differentiated	
IA	**T1-N0-M0** T1: tumor invades lamina propria or submucosa	**T1a, T1b, or T1c-N0-M0** T1b: incidental finding > 5% of tissue T1c: identified by needle biopsy	
1B	**T1-N1-M0** **T2-N0-M0** T2: invades muscle layer or subserosa N1: perigastric node within 3 cm of primary site		
II	**T1-N2-M0** N2: perigastric node > 3 cm form primary or any other nodes	**T2-N0-M0** T2: tumor confined within prostate	
IIIA	**T2-N2-M0** **T3-N1-M0** **T4-N0-M0** T3: penetrates visceral peritoneum without invasion of other structures T4: invades other adjacent structures	**T3-N0-M0** T3: extends through prostatic capsule	
IIIB	**T3-N2-M0; T4-N1-M0**		
IV	**T4-N2-M0** **Any T, any N, M1** M1: distant metastasis	**T4-N0-M0** **Any T-N1, N2, or N3-M0** **Any T-any N-M1** T4: tumor is fixed & invades adjacent structures N1: single node ≤ 2 cm N2: single node 2-5 cm N3: 1 or more nodes > 5 cm M1: distant metastasis	

STAGE	SOFT-TISSUE SARCOMA	PANCREAS	LIVER
0			
I	**T1 or 2-N0-M0** T1: tumor < 5 cm T2: tumor > 5 cm	**T1 or 2-N0-M0** T1: limited to pancreas T2: direct extension into duodenum, bile duct, or peripancreatic tissues	**T1-N0-M0** T1: single tumor 2 cm or less
II	**T1 or 2-N0-M0 (G2)** G2: moderately differentiated	**T3-N0-M0** T3: extends directly into stomach, spleen, colon, or large vessels	**T2-N0-M0** T2: single > 2 cm or multiple < 2 cm without vascular or single > 2 cm with vascular invasion

Table 4–5 Selected TNM Staging Guidelines—cont'd

STAGE	SOFT-TISSUE SARCOMA	PANCREAS	LIVER

III	**T1 or 2-N0-M0 (G3 or 4)**
	G3: poorly differentiated
	G4: undifferentiated
		Any T-N1-M0
		N1: regional lymph nodes
			T1 or 2-N1-M0
			T3-N0 or N1-M0
			T3: Single > 2 cm with
			    vascular, multiple
			    in one lobe
			N1: regional lymph
			    nodes involved

IV	**Any T-N1-M0**
	Any T- any N- M1
	N1: lymph nodes involved
	M1: distant metastasis
		Any T- any N- M1
		M1: distant metastasis
			T4-any N-M0
			Any T- any N-M1
			T4: multiple, more than
			    1 lobe or major
			    blood vessels
			M1: distant metastasis

STAGE	SMALL BOWEL	ESOPHAGUS	
0	**Tis-N0-M0** Tis: in situ	**Tis-N0-M0** Tis: in situ	
I	**T1 or 2-N0-M0** T1: tumor invades lamina propria T2: tumor invades muscularis	**T1-N0-M0** T1: tumor invades lamina propria or sub-mucosa	
II	**T3 or 4-N0-M0** T3: invades through muscularis T4: perforates peritoneum or invades other organs	**T2 or 3-N0-M0** T2: invades muscularis T3: invades adventitia into pancreas **T1 or 2- N1- M0** N1: regional lymph nodes	
III	**Any T-N1-M0** N1: regional lymph nodes involved	**T3 or 4-N1-M0** T4: invades adjacent structures	
IV	**Any T- any N- M1** M1: distant metastasis	**Any T- any N- M1** M1: distant metastasis	

Adapted from Beahrs O and others: Manual for staging of cancer, 4th edition, Philadelphia, 1992, JB Lippincott.

formation. Myeloma may be staged on the basis of clinical manifestations including hemoglobin, serum calcium, presence of lytic bone lesions, and serum protein levels. A patient with a hemoglobin less than 8.5, calcium level greater than 12 mg/dl, or several lytic bone lesions would be expected to have a large mass of myeloma cells and would be classified stage III.[14] Lymphomas, both Hodgkin's disease and non-Hodgkin's lymphoma, are staged according to the Ann Arbor system. Under the Ann Arbor system, lymphomas are staged I, II, III, or IV based on the area or region of lymph nodes involved. Stages are subdivided into A or B, A indicating absence of systemic symptoms, B indicating presence of systemic symptoms.[1] General principles of the Ann Arbor system are outlined in Table 4-7.

In addition to TNM staging, colorectal tumors may also be classified by the Duke's system,[1] outlined below:

Duke's Stage A Carcinoma limited to the mucosa

Stage B1 Carcinoma invades the muscle but is confined to the bowel wall

Stage B2 Carcinoma penetrates through the muscularis propria into the serosa and connective tissue

Stage B3 Same as B2 with adherence or invasion into adjacent organs, but with negative nodes

Stage C1 Lymph nodes positive for metastatic disease but main tumor confined to bowel wall

Stage C2 Lymph nodes positive for metastatic disease and tumor completely penetrates bowel wall

Stage C3 Same as B3, with positive nodes

Stage D Distant metastasis

Duke's stage in comparison to TNM is included in Table 4-5.

The prognosis for patients with malignant mela-

Nursing Management

The word *cancer* has frightening connotations for individuals who may associate a diagnosis of cancer with death or pain. Virually all diagnostic work-ups involve periods of waiting for information. Time may be perceived as endless and may be extremely anxiety provoking for the patient and family awaiting an unknown or feared diagnosis. The family shares this experience with the patient and frequently is the patient's major support system. Families must be an integral part of the care of oncology patients, especially during the stressful time of diagnosis and staging. The following section describes nursing assessments, diagnoses, and interventions for both patients and families during the difficult period of diagnosis and staging.

Initial nursing assessments during the diagnosis and staging phase include assessment of: the patient and family's feelings and beliefs about the diagnostic process and about cancer; knowledge of the diagnostic process; ability to understand information presented; support systems available and used in past crisis situations; and coping styles. The nurse must establish rapport before the patient and family can feel comfortable sharing this information. Sitting with them, maintaining eye contact, listening, and arranging uninterrupted time can be helpful in establishing rapport. The following responses may be experienced by the patient and family during this phase and may be identified as nursing diagnoses from a successful interview: fear, related to a possible diagnosis of cancer; anxiety, related to uncertainty about a diagnosis of cancer; ineffective individual coping; ineffective family coping; spiritual distress; knowledge deficit regarding procedure; knowledge deficit regarding cancer, disease and treatment; anticipatory grieving; and health seeking behaviors. Other nursing diagnoses may be identified depending on presenting symptoms, prior conditions, and individual and family responses.

Many patients undergoing diagnosis and staging are seen in the outpatient or clinic setting. These patients and their families also experience the responses described above. Time should be allotted for assessment of needs, answering questions, providing information, and providing support for those patients and families who will be going home following a procedure.

Nursing interventions depend on the identified nursing diagnoses. Basic information about the diagnostic process, what test is to be done (do not assume the patient understood the physician's expla-

nation), what may be learned, and how that information fits into the total picture is needed by most patients and families. Nurses can also correct misconceptions and provide reassurance. Most breast lumps biopsied, for example, are benign. This information may be helpful to the woman awaiting results of biopsy. Some cancers can be cured, others can be controlled for many years, with treatment based on appropriate staging information. The nurse can present information about the treatment plan once a diagnosis has been determined. Information about support groups and interaction with cancer survivors may also be helpful after a diagnosis has been confirmed.

NURSING DIAGNOSES

Fear related to possible cancer diagnosis

- Outcome Goals: Patient/significant others will acknowledge validity of feelings; identify effective means of dealing with diagnosis and treatment
- Assessments: Emotional response; knowledge base & misconceptions; support systems
- Interventions: Establish rapport; acknowledge validity of feelings; correct misconceptions, provide information; encourage use of support systems

Anxiety related to uncertainty/diagnosis of cancer

- Outcome Goals: Patient/significant other will identify source of anxiety and utilize effective skills for dealing with the perceived threat.
- Assessments: Uncertainty of diagnosis, situation, or prognosis; perceptions of the individual about the situation; psychosocial responses to the situation; physical responses (sweating, flushing, hyperactivity, sighing respirations or shortness of breath, rapid heart rate, elevated blood pressure); speech patterns (pressured speech, blaming, returning to a single topic, or refusing to talk about cancer)
- Interventions: Limit time waiting for information; provide information about disease and treatment; encourage exploration and verbalization of feelings; explore previous effective responses; encourage use of effective responses; teach behavioral interventions, including relaxation and distraction.[5]

Knowledge deficit related to procedure

- Outcome Goals: Verbalize knowledge of procedure, rationale, and information to be obtained.
- Assessments: Knowledge of procedure; cognitive level and reading ability; stress level

- Interventions: Explain procedure and rationale; explain what information may be gained; provide written information appropriate to the patient's cognitive and reading level; repeat and simplify information for those persons under stress

Ineffective family coping
- Outcome Goals: Family will utilize effective coping strategies
- Assessments: Coping styles; family communication patterns; support systems
- Interventions: Identify and encourage effective coping strategies; encourage effective family communication; encourage use of support systems; consult social worker, chaplain, other support services as appropriate.[6]

Health-seeking behaviors
- Outcome Goals: Patient/significant others will identify effective health seeking behaviors
- Assessment: Behaviors and questions aimed at seeking health; effectiveness of those behaviors
- Interventions: Encourage behaviors that are effective in the prevention of cancer or maintenance of a healthy lifestyle (stopping smoking, low-fat diet, increased exercise); answer questions openly and provide information

Table 4–6 Staging of Ovarian Cancer: Comparison of TNM and FIGO

TNM	Stage	FIGO
Stage 0	Tis-N0-M0 Tis: carcinoma in situ	
Stage I	T1-N0-M0 T1: tumor confined to corpus uteri	I
Stage II	T2-N0-M0 T2: tumor invades cervix but not extending beyond uterus	II
Stage III (A&B)	T3-N0-M0 T3: involves serosa or adnexa	IIIA &B
Stage IIIC	T1, T2, T3-N1-M0 N1: regional lymph node metastasis	IIIC
Stage IVA	T4-any N-M0 T4: invades bladder or rectal mucosa	IVA
Stage IVB	Any T-any N-M1 M1: distant metastasis	IVB

Adapted from Beahrs O and others: Manual for staging of cancer, 4th edition, Philadelphia, 1992, JB Lippincott.

Table 4–7 Ann Arbor Staging System for Lymphomas

Stage	
I	Single lymph node region or localized involvement of single organ
II	Two or more lymph node regions on same side of diaphragm or localized involvement of a single organ plus regional lymph nodes
III	Lymph nodes on both sides of diaphragm involved, may include localized involvement of single organ and/or spleen
IV	Disseminated involvement of extralymphatic organs, or isolated organ plus distant lymph nodes
A	**No systemic symptoms**
B	**Presence of systemic symptoms**

Adapted from Beahrs O and others: Manual for staging of cancer, 4th edition, Philadelphia, 1992, JB Lippincott.

Table 4–8   Melanoma Staging*

TNM	Clark's
Stage I pT1-N0-M0	
pT1: Tumor < 0.75 mm thickness and invading papillary dermis	Clark's level II
pT2: Tumor 0.75-1.5 mm and/or invades papillary-reticular dermal boundary	Clark's level III
Stage II pT3-N0-M0	
pT3: Tumor 1.5-4 mm thickness and/ or invades reticular dermis	Clark's level IV
Stage III pT4-N0-M0	
any pT-N1 or N2-M0	
pT4: Tumor > 4 mm thickness and/or invades subcutaneous tissue and/or satellite lesions	Clark's level V
Stage IV any pT-any N-M1	

Adapted from Beahrs, et al. Manual for staging of cancer, 4th edition, Philadelphia, 1992, Lippincott.
*Breslow's staging system incorporates measurements of tumor depth now incorporated into TNM system.

noma is largely dependent on the depth of penetration of the original lesion. Two classification systems, Clark's and Breslow's, have been used to classify melanomas on the basis of depth of penetration. Information from these systems has been incorporated into the TNM system, using a pathologic (after excision) T staging.[1] Table 4-8 compares the classifications for melanoma.

CONCLUSION

The diagnostic period can be confusing and frightening for both the patient and family. Overwhelmed patients and family ultimately look to the nurse to be their advocate and educator. Competent and confident delivery of nursing care can help reduce the anxiety experienced during this period.

BIBLIOGRAPHY

1. Beahrs O and others: Manual for staging of cancer, ed 4, American Joint Committee on Cancer, 1992, JB Lippincott Co.
2. Borg S and Rosenthal S: Handbook of cancer diagnosis and staging—a clinical atlas, New York, 1984, John Wiley & Sons.
3. Bragg D, Putnam C, and Hendee W: Oncologic imaging: state of the art and research priorities, Am J Clin Oncol 11:394, 1988.
4. Bristol-Meyers Oncology Division: The basics of cancer treatment, vol 2, Oncology: programmed modules for nurses, New York, LP Communications, 1986.
5. Clark J, McGee R, and Preston R: Nursing management of responses to the cancer experience. In Clark J and McGee R, editors: Core curriculum for oncology nursing, ed 2, Philadelphia, 1992, WB Saunders Co.
6. Dufault K and others: Ineffective family coping. In McNally J, Somerville E, Miaskowski C and Rostad M, editors: Guidelines for oncology nursing practice, ed 2, Philadelphia, 1991, WB Saunders Co.
7. Flam T and others: Diagnosis and markers in prostate cancer, Cancer 70:357, 1992.
8. Greco F and Hainsworth J: Tumors of unknown origin, CA 42:96, 1992.
9. Heberman RB: Tumor markers. American Association for Clinical Chemistry NCI, Triton Diagnostics, Inc., Alameda, CA, 1991.
10. Hellman S, Jaffe E, and DeVita V Jr: Hodgkin's disease. In DeVita V, Hellman S, and Rosenberg S, editors: Cancer: Principles and practice of oncology, ed 3, Philadelphia, 1989, JB Lippincott Co.
11. Markel D: Introduction to classics in oncology "Spectrophotometer: new instrument of ultra-rapid cell analysis by Kamentsky, Metamed, & Derman," CA 42:57, 1992.
12. Newman F, Ogburn-Russell L, and Rutledge J: Magnetic resonance imaging: the latest in diagnostic technology, Nursing 87:44, 1987.
13. Perkins A, Pimm M: Immunoscintography: practical aspects and clinical applications, 1987, New York, Wiley-Liss.
14. Salmon S and Cassady R: Plasma cell neoplasms. In DeVita V, Hellman S, and Rosenberg S, editors: Cancer: Principles and practice of oncology, ed 3, Philadelphia, 1989, Lippincott.
15. Schwartz M: Markers in diagnosis and screening. In Ting S, Chan J, and Schwartz M, editors: Human tumor markers, New York, 1989, Excerpta Medica.
16. Strohl R: Implications of diagnosis and staging on treatment goals and strategies. In Clark J and McGee R, editors: Core curriculum for oncology nursing, ed 2, Philadelphia, 1992, WB Saunders Co.

UNIT II

CLINICAL MANAGEMENT OF MAJOR CANCER DISEASES

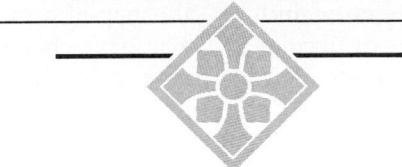

CHAPTER 5

Bone Cancers and Soft Tissue Sarcomas

Stephanie Chang

BONE CANCERS

Primary bone cancers are uncommon malignant lesions. They account for 0.2% of all malignant tumors in the United States today.[1] These tumors are diverse in their presentation and are comprised of many distinct histologic patterns. During the past two decades, major advances have been made in the management of these tumors. These advances can be attributed to new diagnostic imaging techniques, improved histologic evaluation, staging procedures, adjuvant therapies, and surgical reconstructive techniques. Management of these tumors involves a multidisciplinary team approach.

Epidemiology

It is estimated that 2000 new cases of bone cancer will be diagnosed in 1993. Men will account for approximately 1100 of these cases and women slightly less with an incidence of 900. The estimated number of deaths is 1050.[1] This disease exhibits a bimodal pattern with peak occurrences between the ages of 15 to 19 years and after the age of 65.[12]

Etiology

Very few risk factors have been associated with primary bone tumors. Most of these neoplasms arise for unknown reasons. It is therefore difficult to identify preventative or screening measures that could aid in detection of this malignancy.

Paget's disease, fibrous dysplasia, enchondromatosis, bone infarction, or prior exposure to radiation are all conditions known to be associated with bone tumors.[12] Identification of a sarcoma virus has been well documented in other species but not conclusively in humans. Circulating immune complexes have been described in patients with sarcoma and their relatives; however, there is no known causal association between viruses and human sarcomas.[10]

Classification

Primary bone malignancies are classified histologically by the cell or tissue type from which they originate. These include osseous, cartilaginous, fibrous, reticuloendothelial, and vascular (Table 5-1). Due to the low incidence of these neoplasms, only osteosarcoma, chondrosarcoma, fibrosarcoma, and Ewing's sarcoma will be discussed in this chapter.

Table 5-1 Common Malignant Bone Tumors

Tissue Type	Bone Malignancy
Osseous	Classic osteosarcoma (IIB) Parosteal osteosarcoma (IA) Periosteal osteosarcoma (IIA)
Cartilaginous	Primary chondrosarcoma (IIB) Secondary chondrosarcoma (IA)
Fibrous	Fibrosarcoma (IIB) Malignant fibrous histiocytoma (IIB)
Reticuloendothelial	Ewing's sarcoma (IIB) Multiple Myeloma (III)

Adapted from Enneking WF: Common bone tumors. Clinical Symposia 41:2, 1989.

Biological Behavior

Bone tumors have specific biological properties that can be categorized based on their ability to grow and extend beyond their natural barriers. Bone or fibrous tissue form a pseudocapsule around the tumor. This is seen most frequently at the periphery of the tumor where the cells are least mature. There is a reactive zone that forms between the pseudocapsule and the surrounding normal bone that is formed by reactive bone or fibrous tissue, neovascular, and inflammatory tissues. Tumors frequently break through the pseudocapsule and invade the reactive zone to form noncontiguous satellite lesions. These satellite lesions are called *skip metastases* and are usually associated with a poor prognosis.[12,27]

Staging

Enneking developed a surgical staging system for musculoskeletal tumors that reflects the biologic behavior of the lesion and its degree of aggressiveness (Table 5-2). It is based on the histologic grade (G), anatomic site (T), and the presence or absence of distant metastasis (M). Grade is divided into G1 (low grade malignant), and G2 (high grade malignant). Anatomic site is divided into T1 (intracompartmental), and T2 (extracompartmental). Regional or distant metastasis (M) are represented by either M0 or M1.[12,17,28]

Approximately 30% of patients with malignant lesions present as Stage I lesions, 60% as Stage II, and 10% as Stage III. Stage I lesions are more often intracompartmental (66%), while 90% of Stage II lesions are usually extracompartmental.[17]

OSTEOSARCOMA
Epidemiology

Osteosarcoma (osteogenic sarcoma) constitutes about 20% of all primary malignant bone tumors. It accounts for approximately 1.7 cases per million per year, representing 600 to 900 new cases annually. The disease most commonly affects adolescents in the second decade of life during the period of maximal growth. Males are affected more frequently than females by a ratio of 1.6 to 1.0.[21,27]

Biological Behavior

Osteosarcoma is composed of highly malignant spindle-shaped tumor cells that tend to be locally aggressive, have characteristic patterns of growth, and arise from primitive bone-forming mesenchyma in the medullary cavity. Metastatic disease develops by the hematogenous route, and usually appears first in the lungs. Because bones lack a lymphatic system, early spread to regional lymph nodes is rare. It is estimated that over 80% of patients have micrometastatic disease at diagnosis.[12,21,27]

Most osteosarcomas originate in the metaphysis of long bones, the area of highest growth. At the time of diagnosis, most of these tumors are Stage IIB lesions that have infiltrated the surrounding soft tissue. The most commonly affected sites are the distal femur, proximal tibia, and proximal humerus. Less common sites are the pelvis, vertebral column, mandible, clavicle, scapula, or bones in the hands and feet. More than 50% of cases occur in the knee region.[12,21]

Histologically, osteosarcoma is characterized by resorption of normal bone by reactive osteoclasts, causing tissue destruction. The bone involved may be sclerotic, lytic, or a combination of both. Usually there is an aggressive periosteal reaction that is accompanied by a soft tissue mass. Other periosteal reactions include a "sunburst" appearance due to a calcified mass of bone matrix.[21]

In about 50% of adolescent patients, the tumor penetrates the growth plate into the epiphysis. Skip metastases develop in approximately 20% of patients; pulmonary metastases are clinically detectable in about 10% of patients upon initial presentation.[12]

Clinical Features

Individuals most commonly present with complaints of pain and/or swelling in the affected extremity. Pain is usually worse at night and increases as the tumor expands in size. In some instances, an unrelated history of trauma or sport-related injury may call attention to the lesion. The most frequent abnormal laboratory finding is an elevated serum alkaline phos-

Table 5–2 Staging System for Malignant Bone Tumors

Stage		Grade	Site	Metastasis
IA	Low grade, intracompartmental	G1	T1	M0
IB	Low grade, extracompartmental	G1	T2	M0
IIA	High grade, intracompartmental	G2	T1	M0
IIB	High grade, extracompartmental	G2	T2	M0
IIIA	Low or high grade, intracompartmental with metastases	G1-2	T1	M1
IIIB	Low or high grade, extracompartmental with metastases	G1-2	T2	M1

Adapted from Enneking WF: Common bone tumors. Clinical Symposia 41:2, 1989.

phatase level, which is indicative of osteoblastic activity.[12,21]

A small number of osteosarcomas may occur in conjunction with Paget's disease of bone. Severe, unremitting pain and pathologic fracture are the primary clinical features upon presentation. It is not uncommon for individuals to wait several weeks to months before medical treatment is sought.

Treatment and Prognosis

The 5-year survival rate for individual's treated with surgery alone or a combination of surgery and radiation is approximately 10% to 20%. This high mortality rate has been attributed to microscopic metastatic disease, which is assumed to be present at time of diagnosis. Presently, 60% to 80% of patients presenting with osteosarcoma without metastases will be cured following appropriate surgery and chemotherapy.[12,21,27] Treatment options are discussed later in this chapter.

CHONDROSARCOMA
Epidemiology

Chondrosarcoma constitutes about 13% of all primary malignant bone tumors. It occurs most often in adults between 40 and 60 years of age and affects males twice as often as females.[12]

Biological Behavior

Chondrosarcoma is a malignant cartiliginous tumor that is characterized by the formation of cartilage by tumor cells. This tumor may arise in the medullary canal or peripherally on the external surface of the bone causing cortical destruction. Calcification occurs in portions of the intracellular matrix of the tumor cartilage.[12]

The most commonly affected sites are the pelvis, proximal femur, and shoulder girdle. Transformation of a preexisting enchondroma or osteocartilaginous exostosis to a chondrosarcoma occurs in approximately 25% of these cases.[12]

Histologically, chondrosarcomas are more cellular and pleomorphic and contain numerous plump cells with double nuclei. Cell nuclei are larger and have a more dispersed pattern of chromatin than their normal counterparts.[12,16]

Chondrosarcoma is often a slow-growing tumor but can metastasize to distant organs. Tumor growth rates range from slow growing to highly malignant metastasizing tumors. The histologic characteristics are based on the cellularity of the tumor tissue. Low-grade chondrosarcomas more closely resemble normal cartilage than high-grade tumors and tend to have a firmer consistency. High-grade chondrosarcomas often have a soft, viscous, jellylike appearance.[12,16]

Clinical Features

A persistent, dull, aching pain like that of arthritis is usually the initial symptom. Physical examination may reveal a firm, swollen area over the tumor site.[12]

Treatment and Prognosis

The treatment of chondrosarcoma is primarily surgical. Both chemotherapy and radiation therapy have proven to be relatively ineffective in the treatment of this tumor.[12,16,41]

Stage I tumors rarely metastasize or recur locally. The estimated 10-year survival rate for this stage is 87%. At 10 years, stage II tumors have an estimated survival rate of 41%, while the stage III rate is 27%.[12]

FIBROSARCOMA
Epidemiology

Fibrosarcoma accounts for less than 4% of all primary malignant bone tumors and is most often seen in adolescents or young adults.[12]

Biological Behavior

Fibrosarcoma is a malignant fibroblastic lesion usually arising within the medullary cavity. Radiographs reveal a poorly defined, destructive, radiolucent lesion of the metaphyseal area. The most commonly affected sites are the femur and the tibia.[12]

Histologically, the appearance varies with the degree of aggressiveness. Stage I (low-grade) tumors have a low cell-to-matrix ratio with less anaplasia and usually remain within the bone and have a distinct, well-defined margin. Stage II (high-grade) fibrosarcomas have less cellularity and more anaplasia, and they have poorly-defined margins with increased bone destruction, which resembles a "moth eaten" pattern.[12]

Clinical Features

The individual with fibrosarcoma usually presents with pain and swelling of the affected area. This presentation resembles that of the other primary bone malignancies. There are no abnormal laboratory findings that are associated with this type of tumor. Electron microscopy may be necessary to determine the histogenesis when the tumor is poorly differentiated.[12]

Treatment and Prognosis

Surgical resection is the optimal treatment for this neoplasm. Excision with a wide margin is indicated for stage IA tumors, whereas stage IIB fibrosarcomas require radical margins or wide margins with adjuvant chemotherapy or radiation therapy. The prognosis is guarded. The reported 5-year survival rate is 21.8%.[12]

EWING'S SARCOMA
Epidemiology
Ewing's sarcoma comprises approximately 6% of all primary malignant bone tumors. Children are affected more commonly than adults. The average age of patients with this neoplasm is lower than for any other primary malignant bone tumor. Ewing's sarcoma is seen most frequently in children between the ages of 10 and 15 years. This tumor is more common in males than in females and is rare in the black population.[12,29,32]

Biological Behavior
Ewing's sarcoma is a highly malignant bone tumor that originates from the nonmesenchymal elements of the bone marrow. The tumor arises most commonly in the shaft of the long bones. Lytic destruction is the most common finding due to reactive new bone formation, which produces dense areas. There may be multiple layers of subperiosteal reactive new bone, which radiographically gives this neoplasm an "onionskin" appearance. The formation of this new bone is the result of periosteal reaction to the tumor tissue that has invaded the cortex.[12,29]

The bones of the pelvis and lower extremity constitute the majority of sites involved, although any bone and/or portion of that bone may be affected. The femoral diaphysis is the most common site, followed by the ilium, tibia, humerus, fibula, and ribs.[32]

In most cases Ewing's sarcoma extends beyond the anatomic barriers of the bone into the adjacent soft tissues. The tumor consists of sheets of cells that are numerous, round, and have round nuclei. Cell borders are indistinct and nuclei may have a "ground-glass" appearance. The tumor may be solid or semiliquid and is not encapsulated. Areas of necrosis and hemorrhage are common.[12,32]

Metastases usually occur early and involve the lungs. Other sites of metastases include the bones and regional lymph nodes. While solitary metastases do occasionally occur, it is more common to have multiple metastatic lesions. The presence of metastatic disease has been reported in 14% to 35% of patients at time of diagnosis.[29,32]

Clinical Features
The presenting signs and symptoms of Ewing's sarcoma are often vague and may be indicative of other malignant or nonmalignant conditions. As with other bone tumors, pain and swelling of the affected area are the most common presenting symptoms. These symptoms tend to be progressive, with some patients experiencing them for months before they seek medical aid. Low grade fever is relatively common. The child may present with flu-like symptoms of malaise, tiredness, and/or weakness. Other symptoms include anemia, leukocytosis, and an elevated erythrocyte sedimentation rate.[12,29]

Treatment and Prognosis
The previous dismal outlook for patients with Ewing's sarcoma has improved considerably. Current studies indicate that prognosis is most affected by the presence of disseminated disease and the location or size of the primary lesion. Tumors in the pelvis are often detected late and are therefore larger, with a poorer prognosis. The estimated 5-year survival rates now range from 54% to 74%.[30]

Introduction of adjuvant systemic chemotherapy has markedly reduced the incidence of pulmonary metastases. Radiation therapy and surgery also play a role in the treatment of this tumor.[12,30,32]

Initial treatment begins with chemotherapy followed by wide surgical excisions versus radiation therapy for local control if (1) the involved bone is expendable (fibula, rib, clavicle) or can be reconstructed without disabling the patient; (2) radiation therapy would cause significant growth deformity; (3) successful rehabilitation is not feasible; and (4) previous local irradiation was unsuccessful.[12]

SOFT-TISSUE SARCOMAS
Malignant sarcomas of the soft tissue are an unusual primary malignant tumor representing only 1% of all neoplasms in adults in the United States today.[23] These tumors are characterized by their diverse histology, biologic behavior, and anatomic locations.[8,10] This uncommon and diverse presentation has contributed to the difficulty in treating these neoplasms. Significant progress has been made over the past 10 years in the diagnosis and treatment of soft tissue sarcomas. This can be attributed to new diagnostic imaging techniques, a standard system for grading these tumors, use of flow cytometry, and multimodality therapy with surgery, radiation, and chemotherapy, which has resulted in improved local tumor control.[10] Management of these tumors involves a multidisciplinary approach by the healthcare team.

Epidemiology
The American Cancer Society predicts 6000 new cases of soft tissue sarcomas will occur in 1993. Men will account for approximately 3300 of these cases and women slightly less with 2700. The estimated number of deaths is 3100.[1] Currently, twice as many individuals die of soft-tissue sarcomas each year as die of Hodgkin's disease, even though the incidence of the two neoplasms is similar.[8]

Etiology
Approximately 5% of sarcomas occur within ports of prior radiation therapy, which was delivered more

than 20 years prior to development of the sarcoma. This is seen most frequently in osteosarcoma, but it also has been reported in mixed mesodermal sarcomas of the uterus.[2]

Chemicals such as asbestos are associated with mesothelioma and polyvinyl chloride, arsenic, and hemochromatosis with angiosarcoma of the liver. Dioxin (Agent Orange) exposure has been associated with the development of soft tissue sarcomas.[2]

Individuals with neurofibromatosis have a 7% to 10% risk of developing malignant neurofibrosarcoma. Approximately 50% of all neurofibrosarcomas develop in patients with neurofibromatosis.[2]

Identification of a sarcoma virus has been well documented in other species but not conclusively in humans. Circulating immune complexes have been described in patients with sarcoma and their relatives.[19]

The majority of patients that present with soft tissue sarcomas have a history of trauma. Current studies have indicated that trauma is not associated with development of these tumors.[2]

Classification

Soft-tissue sarcomas are classified according to cell type or tissue of origin: for example, fat, smooth and striated muscle (Table 5-3). The majority of soft-tissue sarcomas are found in the lower extremity (40%), trunk (15%), retroperitoneum (15%), and the upper extremity including the head and neck region. Visceral sarcomas arise in the gastrointestinal and gynecologic tracts. Kaposi's and mesotheliomas are classified as miscellaneous sarcomas.[2]

Biological Behavior

Soft-tissue sarcomas are composed of connective tissue cells. Connective tissue arise from the mesoderm and include tendons, fat, muscles, and fibrous and synovial tissues. Therefore, these tumors can arise in any of these structures throughout the body.[2]

Soft-tissue sarcomas usually originate in deep-seated structures and present as an ill-defined, asymptomatic mass. These tumors tend to expand and infiltrate tissue spaces, producing a pseudocapsule of normal tissue as well as microscopic tumor infiltrates. These infiltrates are often considerable distances from the tumor. Soft-tissue sarcomas are characteristically known for their propensity for local recurrence following simple surgical resection. Recurrent tumors often grow deeper and larger, and may fungate or metastasize.[2]

Metastases are usually spread by hematogenous routes or local invasion into surrounding normal tissues by the tumor. This presentation generally indicates a poor prognosis. Presenting symptoms vary due to the anatomic location of the tumor. These may include peripheral neuralgias due to nerve impinge-

Table 5–3 Histologic Types of Soft Tissue Sarcomas

Tumors of fibrous tissue	Fibrosarcoma
Tumors of adipose tissue	Liposarcoma—well differentiated, myxoid, pleomorphic
Tumors of smooth muscle	Leiomyosarcoma
Tumors of striated muscle	Rhabdomyosarcoma—alveolar, pleomorphic, embryonal
Tumors of vascular origin	Angiosarcoma Lymphangiosarcoma Malignant hemangiopericytoma
Tumors of synovial tissue	Synovial sarcoma
Tumors of mesothelioma	Malignant mesothelioma
Tumors of neurogenic origin	Neurogenic sarcoma (malignant schwannoma)
Tumors of "histiocytic" origin	Malignant fibrous histiocytoma Giant cell tumor of soft tissue
Tumors of cartilaginous origin	Extraskeletal chondrosarcoma (choroid sarcoma)
Tumors of uncertain origin	Dermatofibrosarcoma protuberans Epithelioid sarcoma Clear cell sarcoma Kaposi's sarcoma Alveolar soft part sarcoma Ewing's sarcoma in soft tissue

ment, vascular ischemia, paralysis, bowel obstruction, and various other symptomatology.[2]

Staging

The staging of soft-tissue sarcomas is still a controversial issue among pathologists. There are difficulties with the reproducibility of tumor grade, which may be due to the lack of established uniform criteria for grading these tumors.[23]

The staging of soft-tissue sarcomas is largely dependent upon the number of mitoses per high-power field (Table 5-4). In 1969 the American Joint Committee on Staging and End Results applied a grading system that classified neoplasms as low (grade I), medium (grade II), and high (grade III). This grading system was based primarily on the number of mitosis per high-power field. Tumor grade (G) is recognized

Table 5–4   Clinicopathologic Staging for Soft-Tissue Sarcomas

Stage	Grade	Comments
1	Low	<1 mitoses/10 HPF
2	Intermediate	1-4 mitoses/10 HPF
3	High	>5 mitoses/10 HPF

HPF = high power field
Adapted from Eilber FR, and others: Progress in the recognition and treatment of soft-tissue sarcomas, Cancer 67:1169, 1990.

Table 5–5   Staging of Soft-Tissue Sarcomas

Stage Grouping:				
Stage I				
IA	G1	T1	N0	M0
IB	G1	T2	N0	M0
Stage II				
IIA	G2	T1	N0	M0
IIB	G2	T2	N0	M0
Stage III				
IIIA	G3	T1	N0	M0
IIIB	G3	T2	N0	M0
IIIC	Any G	T1-2	N1	M0
Stage IV				
IVA	Any G	T3	Any N	M0
IVB	Any G	Any T	Any N	M1-4

Adapted from Pories and others: Soft-tissue sarcomas. In Rubin P, editor, Clinical oncology: A multidisciplinary approach, New York, American Cancer Society, 1983.

as the most important prognostic indicator (Table 5-5). Several cooperative groups have utilized this staging system and compared their results (Table 5-5). For high grade lesions there is approximately an 80% to 90% agreement; however, for intermediate grade 2 lesions there is considerable variation in terms of agreement on the grade.[2]

New technologies are currently being utilized that look at histogenesis on a cellular basis rather than a histogenic pattern. These include electron microscopy, immunohistochemical staining for cellular products, and DNA analysis.[10]

LIPOSARCOMA

These tumors occur most frequently in adults and tend to involve the proximal lower extremities (i.e., thigh, buttocks, groin). The primary treatment is surgical resection. Liposarcomas rarely develop from previous lipomas.[13]

LEIOMYOSARCOMA

This malignant tumor arises from smooth muscle and occurs in visceral regions of the body. Common sites include the uterus, retroperitoneum, and gastroin-

testinal tract. Long-term survival is usually poor due to their early metastatic spread.[13]

RHABDOMYOSARCOMA

Rhabdomyosarcomas are malignant tumors of muscle origin and are divided into three types. The most common type is embryonal rhabdomyosarcoma and occurs most often in young children. Alveolar rhabdomyosarcoma is the second most common type and occurs in both children and young adults. The prognosis tends to be poor due to the aggressiveness of this tumor. The least common type is pleomorphic rhabdomyosarcoma, which occurs in late middle age. Treatment for this tumor group is surgical resection and chemotherapy. Embryonal rhabdomyosarcoma responds most favorably to these treatment modalities.

ANGIOSARCOMA

This tumor is of vascular origin and occurs most frequently in the liver, skin, and breast. These neoplasms are poorly defined and tend to have deep vascular extension. A common presenting sign is bruising over the affected area.[13]

SYNOVIAL SARCOMA

Synovial sarcoma arises from mesenchymal cells and occurs most frequently in tendons, bursae, or joints. This is a rare tumor that occurs most frequently in young adults and tends to involve the extremities.

MALIGNANT MESOTHELIOMA

Asbestos exposure has been implicated in this malignancy. The older male population is most commonly affected. This tumor occurs most frequently in the lung pleura and peritoneum and has a poor prognosis due to its unresponsiveness to standard forms of treatment.[25]

NEUROGENIC SARCOMA

Neurogenic sarcoma (NGS), also known as neurofibrosarcoma, malignant schwannoma, or malignant neurilemmoma, usually arises in the sheath tissue of a peripheral nerve. These tumors can occur at any age but are uncommon in the first 2 decades of life. Approximately 50% of all neurofibrosarcomas develop in patients with neurofibromatosis. The brachial plexus, sciatic, medial, and spinal nerves are most commonly affected. These tumors tend to recur locally and spread hematogenously to the lungs and bones. Surgical intervention is the only form of management known to be effective.[2,33]

DIAGNOSIS AND STAGING
Patient Evaluation

The evaluation of a patient with a suspected malignant primary bone tumor or soft tissue sarcoma in-

Nursing Management

Primary bone malignancies and soft tissue sarcomas involve all age groups. The diagnosis of cancer can be devastating to these individuals and their family members. The nurse plays an integral role as an information resource and support liaison.

NURSING DIAGNOSIS
- Knowledge deficit related to disease process

INTERVENTIONS
- Determine patient/family learning needs and knowledge levels pertaining to:
  - specific disease process
  - specific treatment modalities
  - specific diagnostic testing
- Assess patient/family views and beliefs about cancer.
- Observe patient/family coping mechanisms.
- Assess cultural background and belief systems.
- Determine what patient/family feels is important to know.
- Assess readiness of patient/family to learn.
- Provide and discuss information related to specific type of cancer (i.e., pamphlets and videos).
- Provide and discuss information related to specific diagnostic procedures (i.e., CT scan, bone scan, MRI).
- Teach about emotional reactions to cancer.
- Initiate referrals to other health team members if necessary.

PATIENT TEACHING PRIORITIES

Assess patient/family learning needs for:
   specific disease process (e.g., osteosarcoma, soft tissue sarcoma)
   specific diagnostic testing (e.g., arteriography, scan, MRI)
   specific treatment modalities (e.g., above/below knee amputation, and/or radiation therapy, chemotherapy)
Assess and monitor emotional reactions to cancer
Initiate referrals to multidisciplinary members: physical therapist, occupational therapist, prothesist, dietician, social services, rehabilitation services.

BONE CANCERS AND SOFT TISSUE SARCOMA CLINICAL FEATURES

Osteosarcoma	Pain, swelling in the affected extremity, elevated alkaline phosphatase level
Chondrosarcoma	Persistent, dull aching pain, firm, swollen area over tumor site
Fibrosarcoma	Pain, swelling of the affected area
Ewing's sarcoma	Vague symptoms, progressive pain and swelling of affected site, fever and anemia

---

BONE CANCERS AND SOFT TISSUE SARCOMA DISEASE AND TREATMENT RELATED COMPLICATIONS

Infection, skin necrosis, amputation, arthritic-type conditions, iatrogenic fractures, allograft and autograft nonunion, joint dislocation and/or dysfunction, post-operative: extensive blood loss and delayed wound healing

---

volves a multidisciplinary approach by the healthcare team. Nursing plays a pivotal role in the education and support of these individuals. The evaluation begins with a thorough history and physical examination. The individual's age, site and size of the lesion, occupation, and the presence of risk factors that are associated with these malignancies such as Paget's disease of the bone (osteosarcoma) or neurofibromatosis (neurofibrosarcoma) are identified. Selected laboratory studies and radiographs are obtained. Based on the results of these tests, further staging studies may be initiated to determine histologic diagnosis, local extent, and regional or distant spread.[12] See the boxes on this page.

Imaging Techniques
Significant progress has been made in the past decade with the advent of computed tomography (CT) and magnetic resonance imaging (MRI). These techniques have significantly enhanced diagnosis. Clear definition of primary bone tumors and delineation of soft tissue sarcomas has become possible.[10]

The purpose of radiographic staging of these tumors is twofold. The first is to obtain information regarding the probable diagnosis and the second is to define the anatomic extent of the tumor.[17]

RADIOGRAPHY. Screening or plain radiographs are the most important initial staging technique for primary bone malignancies. They give the most general diagnostic information about the tumor by demonstrating the bone involved, extent and type of destruction, and the amount of reactive bone formed. They are often helpful in defining a reliable area for biopsy. If malignancy is suspected a plain chest radiograph is usually indicated due to the high occurrence of pulmonary metastases.[12,17,27]

BONE SCANS. Radionuclide scanning (bone scan) assesses multiple sites of involvement, extent of local intraosseous involvement and activity of the tumor, and often skeletal metastases. The amount of radioisotope uptake in and around the tumor indicates its activity: the greater the uptake, the more aggressive and malignant the tumor.[12,27]

COMPUTED TOMOGRAPHY. Tomograms are used to determine intra- and extraosseous extension of the tumor. CT more accurately estimates local extent of the tumor, which is important when identifying surgical options. CT scanning is the most sensitive technique for detecting pulmonary metastases. When scanning focal bone lesions CT scanning is usually performed with and without contrast. Contrast aids in the identification of the major neurovascular structures and well-vascularized lesions. CT currently is the best technique for evaluating cortical penetration and osseous detail. It is more sensitive than plain radiographs in detecting small changes in mineralization of bone.[17,21,27]

MAGNETIC RESONANCE IMAGING. MRI is the most recent technologic development in the staging of musculoskeletal tumors. It is the most accurate method of evaluating the intramedullary extent of a bone tumor as well as detection of skip metastases. MRI is now accepted as the primary imaging method for estimation of tumor extent within the marrow space and with respect to muscle groups, subcutaneous fat, joints, and major neurovascular structures around the tumor. This technique is also extremely valuable in planning limb-sparing procedures.[17,27,28]

ARTERIOGRAPHY. Prior to the development of MRI and CT, arteriography was a major diagnostic technique in the staging of bone tumors. Arteriography is now used primarily in difficult anatomic locations such as the shoulder girdle or the pelvis where, after CT and MRI, the surgical margins between the tumor and the vessels remain unclear. This technique is also useful in limb salvage surgery when the neurovascular bundle must be resected and reconstructed due to tumor involvement.[17,21]

Biopsy

The biopsy should be performed only after a complete work-up is done. This includes a thorough history, physical examination, laboratory studies, and radiographic evaluation.[17,21]

The purpose of the biopsy is to obtain adequate tissue for an accurate histologic diagnosis and grad-

ing. The biopsy of a suspected bone tumor must be performed with great care. One of the most common causes for amputation is a poorly placed biopsy in which local tumor contamination occurs. It is recommended that the biopsy be done by the same surgeon or surgical team who will perform the definitive surgery.[17,21,27]

Biopsies can be performed in a number of ways. The biopsy site should be carefully planned and placed in a location where it can be excised when the definitive surgery is performed. This prevents contaminated tissue from being left behind.[17,21,27]

Historically, open incisional biopsy has been considered the procedure that afforded the greatest accuracy and reliability. Today, however, many other techniques may be employed such as closed percutaneous biopsy, either with fine needle aspiration cytology or tissue cores from a special cutting needle.

Needle biopsy can be performed on an outpatient basis. It is well tolerated by patients and carries a low risk of tissue contamination. As with open biopsy, potential contamination of the biopsy tract should be anticipated and the biopsy should be placed in an area that is surgically resectable when the definitive surgery is performed.[17,21]

There are certain complications associated with biopsies and in some cases treatment has to be altered. Complications associated with biopsies include inadequate tissue for definitive diagnosis, excessive contamination of uninvolved soft tissues by hematoma, infection of the biopsy site, and positioning of the biopsy in such a way that definitive surgical resection is compromised, therefore necessitating an amputation in a patient who would have previously been a candidate for limb salvage surgery. It is reported that these complications are three to five times more common when the biopsy is performed in the referring institution rather than when done in a center that specializes in musculoskeletal tumors and limb salvage surgery.[17]

TREATMENT
Surgical Management

Surgical management in conjunction with other treatment therapies is indicated for a majority of primary bone and soft tissue sarcomas. Surgery was the first treatment modality applied to these tumors and remains an essential element in the care of these patients.

Table 5–6 Patient Criteria for Limb-Salvage Protocol

- Specific location of tumor
- Proper placement of the biopsy incision
- Postoperative function of spared limb must be equal to or greater than function of a prosthetic device
- An individual's age

Local resection was utilized during the first half of this century but was largely abandoned due to a very high local recurrence rate. Therefore, amputation was adopted as the only procedure that offered a chance for local disease control. In the early to mid 1980s multiple research studies supported the validity of the limb-salvage protocol for high-grade sarcomas. This limb-sparing procedure resulted in excellent local control of tumor and a high salvage rate of functional limbs. This form of surgery in conjunction with chemotherapy and/or radiation therapy has proven to be as successful for long-term survival as that of amputation, utilizing the same adjuvant therapies. Approximately 90% of all sarcomas are salvageable. This approach provides a limb that is functional as well as cosmetically acceptable.[2,39]

The ultimate goal for all patients is to preserve their life. There are specific criteria that are utilized to identify those individuals who are candidates for limb-sparing procedure (Table 5-6). The first criterion is the location of the tumor. Soft tissue sarcomas are not encapsulated and are in direct contact with surrounding normal tissue. Therefore, it is important that the location of these tumors allow total surgical resection that will result in tumor-free surgical margins. Secondly, great care must be exercised when performing surgery on these patients. Proper placement of the biopsy incision is essential since the entire biopsy tract must be removed with the tumor in order to prevent implant of sarcoma cells along the tract. Third, the postoperative function of the spared limb must be equal to or greater than the function provided by a prosthetic device following amputation. The fourth criterion is age. Elderly individuals may not adapt to a prosthesis due to poor wound healing or lack of desire to partake in the vigorous physical therapy regimen that is required postsurgically.[14,39]

Previously, children less than 10 years of age were not considered candidates for limb-salvage surgery. The majority of these tumors involved the lower extremities. In order to excise the tumor it was also necessary to remove one or more major growth plates. Due to continuing growth of the unaffected leg this technique causes significant discrepancy in leg length.

Nursing Management

Preoperatively, the patient and family need information related to the surgical procedure. This information can be complex and highly technical. The patients receive copious amounts of information regarding their diagnosis and possible treatment options. The nurse plays a major role in educating the patient and family.

NURSING DIAGNOSIS
- Knowledge deficit related to surgery

INTERVENTIONS
- Assess prior experience with surgery.
- Determine knowledge base and major concerns regarding surgery.
- Gauge readiness to learn and assess barriers to learning.
- Review purpose of surgery (i.e., curative, palliative, evaluative).
- Describe the surgical procedure:
    incisional biopsy
    local excision
    excision with wide margin
    use of implants and special grafts
    en bloc resection
    amputation
    resection of metastases
    cytoreductive surgery
- Explain common terms and procedures related to pathology specimen.
- Discuss potential surgical outcomes:
    change in bodily appearance
    changes in bodily functions
    limitations in mobility
    loss of extremity
- Describe preoperative preparation:
    surgical prep (area to be shaved)
    bowel prep regimen
    removal of prosthetics and valuables
    dietary restrictions (i.e., clear liquid diet and nothing by mouth after midnight)
    preoperative medications
    scheduled time of surgery
    holding area in the OR (i.e., preoperative room)
    family waiting area
- Provide teaching materials/educational videos
- Explain postoperative routine
    pulmonary toilet
    mobility
    pain management
    potential devices such as drains, surgical wound dressings, chest tubes, nasogastric tubes, foley catheter, etc.
For nursing management associated with postoperative surgical pain refer to Chapter 28, Pain Management.

Today, however, surgeons are successfully treating these young people by the use of implantable, expandable lower extremity prostheses. If the tumor is located in the upper extremity or in the diaphysis of a bone in the lower extremity (not requiring excision of the growth plates), limb-salvage surgery has the same indication as for skeletally mature individuals.[11,14]

Cure is the long-term goal of surgical therapy, regardless of the type of surgical technique utilized. What has become clear, whether or not surgery is the primary method, or whether chemotherapy and radiation therapy are added as adjuvants, is that the total excision of the tumor with clear pathologic margins is the best method to achieve local tumor control.

Surgical Techniques

WIDE EXCISION.   The goal is to obtain tumor-free histologic margins but spare major neurovascular structures. During surgery great care is taken to maintain a margin of normal tissue between the plane of dissection and the tumor. In this operative procedure there is no origin to insertion resections of the entire muscle groups surrounding the tumor.[4,11]

AMPUTATION.   Amputation may be indicated when this method is the only technique able to obtain local tumor control. Indications for primary amputation are late presenting lesions with neurovascular involvement, pathologic fractures (especially in the proximal femur), infected or inappropriately placed biopsy incisions, or extensive muscle involvement.[9,27]

EN BLOC RESECTION.   This procedure is utilized most frequently for local tumor control. The choice for this surgical procedure is based on the ability to remove involved tissues while preserving vital structures. This technique involves wide excision of surrounding normal tissue, removal of entire muscle bundles at points of origin and insertion, and resection of involved bone as well as vascular structures. A whole block or "compartment" is surgically removed. A margin of at least 5 to 7 centimeters above and below the limit of tumor activity is necessary to ensure complete tumor removal.[4,18]

TIKHOFF-LINBERG   PROCEDURE.   This   surgical technique is utilized with lesions of the proximal humerus and encompasses en bloc resection of the scapula, part of the humerus, and clavicle. Following this procedure, the functions of the hand and elbow are preserved. This method of resection is performed as an alternative to forequarter amputation.[18,21]

Reconstruction Options

After extensive resection, reconstruction may be necessary to provide stability. This can be accomplished by the use of a variety of metal as well as synthetic

Table 5–7   Terminology for Limb-Salvage Surgery

Allograft—a graft from another individual (usually a cadaver)
Autograft—a graft taken from the patient
Vascularized graft—graft implanted with vessels supplying it intact
Arthroplasty—surgical formation or reformation of a joint
Arthodesis—surgical fusion of a joint
Endoprosthesis—artificial replacement of a joint or bone by a metallic implant

Adapted from Hockenberry MJ and Lane B. Limb salvage procedures in children with osteosarcoma. Cancer Nurs 11:2, 1988.

Table 5–8   Limb-Salvage Techniques

Distal femur
   Autologous arthrodesis (with tibia or femur intermedullary rod graft)
   Segmental prosthesis to restore skeletal continuity
   Prosthetic knee replacement for lesions involving the diaphysis
   Tibial rotation plasty
Proximal femur
   Endoprosthesis—long-stem Moore prosthesis with acrylic cement
   Total joint prosthesis—hip replacement or arthroplasty
Proximal tibia
   Resection arthrodesis
Proximal humerus
   Tikhoff-Linberg procedure
   Total shoulder replacement
   Endoprosthesis
   Proximal humerus allograft

Adapted from Hockenberry MJ and Lane B. Limb salvage procedures in children with osteosarcoma. Cancer Nurs 11:2, 1988.

materials. Tables 5-7 and 5-8 review common terms and techniques used in limb salvage surgery.

Allograft—This is a graft from another individual and is usually obtained from a cadaver. This graft may be used following excision of a primary skeletal tumor.[18,31]

Autograft—Bone is taken from one area and transplanted to another area in the same individual.

Vascularized Graft—Bone graft is implanted with the vessels supplying it intact. These grafts are able to bridge large gaps to allow for rapid bone ingrowth. The fibula is the most commonly used graft.[12]

Prosthesis

Metallic Endoprosthesis—Artificial replacement of a joint or bone by a metallic implant. There are a number of prosthesis that are currently being used and are custom-made for the individual.

Intermedullary Rod—Similar to an endoprosthesis and is utilized for stability to form a union between two sections of bone following en bloc resection.

Joint Reconstruction

Two of the most common methods of joint reconstruction following sarcoma resection are arthrodesis and arthroplasty, with use of metallic and/or allograft implants.

Arthrodesis—Fusion of the joint using part of the femur, tibia, or vascularized fibular grafts. This procedure is most useful in the knee, shoulder, hip, and wrist. The disadvantage is that this technique results in a stiff joint, but it is sturdy and permits activities such as running, jumping, and heavy lifting.[12,31]

Arthroplasty—Surgical formation of a joint using a custom metallic implant, bone allograft implant, or a combination of both to maintain joint function. The implant, however, is an artificial joint, and therefore jogging, racquet sports, or heavy lifting is prohibited.[18,31]

Soft-Tissue Reconstruction

Occasionally, after resection of a soft-tissue or bone sarcoma, a cavity can occur. It may be necessary for a plastic surgeon to perform a muscle flap to close this cavity.[31]

COMPLICATIONS

There are several factors that tend to increase the complications associated with limb-salvage surgery. These include a long operating time, lengthy anesthesia, extensive blood loss, and technically difficult procedures. These complications are what tend to prohibit elderly patients from being selected as candidates for this type of surgical procedure.

Many of the elderly have co-morbid illnesses, such as cardiovascular disease, pulmonary disorders, diabetes mellitus, and hypertension, which may impair healing. Rehabilitative therapy is very strenuous and

Nursing Management

Individuals (all age groups) often imagine that they will return to their normal physical activities after limb salvage. It is difficult for them to understand that they will be partially disabled regardless of the type of reconstruction they have. Individuals who have undergone amputation have a better understanding of their limitations but may have difficulty in adjusting to the physical loss of a limb. The nurse plays a major role in educating as well as offering emotional support to both the patient and family.

NURSING DIAGNOSIS

- Impaired physical mobility related to limb salvage or amputation

INTERVENTIONS

- Assess emotional status
- Determine and evaluate:
  growth and development (age related)
  range of motion (ROM) of joints
  muscle strength
  gait, balance, and coordination
  vascular status (circulation and sensation)
  posture
- Postoperative assessment includes:
  general physical status
  vital signs
  proper body positioning
  signs and symptoms of postop complications related to surgery (hemorrhage, infection, compartmental syndrome, pulmonary embolus, skin breakdown)
  signs and symptoms of complications related to impaired mobility (constipation, skin breakdown, pneumonia, urinary retention, anorexia)
  pain management (phantom pain for amputees)
  ability to perform ROM exercises and/or use of assistive devices (overhead traction bar, crutches, prosthesis, and others)
  ability to care for stump and prosthesis
- Coordinate rehabilitative measures with other multidisciplinary members (physical therapist, occupational therapist, prosthetist, dietition)
- Arrange for contact with rehabilitated patient if appropriate
- Patient education:
  Discuss importance of physical therapy (ROM exercises, mobility)
  Reinforce importance of proper nutrition and hydration
  Discuss with patient/family possible complications associated with amputation/limb salvage (irritation of skin, altered fit of cast, increased swelling or pain, fever, mechanical problems with prosthesis)
  Emphasize importance of open communication
  Provide information for support groups for patient/family

For nursing management associated with body image disturbance refer to Chapter 31, Sexuality.

many of these elderly individuals opt for less aggressive surgical intervention.[14,39]

Postoperatively, infection is the most immediate concern. There may be extensive wound incisions following large surgical resections. Many individuals have had chemotherapy and/or radiation therapy prior to surgery and this may compromise or delay wound healing. Other early complications may include iatrogenic fracture or penetration of the cortex by a metallic fixation device, skin necrosis, arterial and venous occlusion, neuropraxia, and joint dislocation.[14]

Delayed complications resulting from metallic endoprostheses include joint dysfunction, loosening of the prosthesis, infection, resorption of the bone, nerve palsies, penetration of the shaft, and stress fractures. Delayed complications associated with allografts and autografts include nonunion, fracture, and bony resorption. Arthritic-type conditions can occur as a late-effect following limb-salvage surgery, as well as local tumor recurrence.[14,18]

POSTOPERATIVE REHABILITATION

Rehabilitative treatment is necessary for individuals who have undergone either limb salvage or amputation as part of their surgical treatment. With the improved survival rate, the focus of rehabilitation is to improve the quality of these individuals' lives.

The immediate postoperative treatment for both above-knee (AK) and below-knee (BK) amputation is similar. A rigid dressing is applied at the time of surgery to reduce pain and swelling. Three to 4 days post-amputation, the rigid dressing is removed. A cast is then taken of the amputated limb for the temporary prosthesis.[22]

For the AK amputee, the original rigid dressing is reapplied. Extra prosthetic socks may be added to facilitate compression of the stump. In order to prevent hipflexion contractures, range of motion (ROM) and exercises in the prone position are instituted in the immediate postoperative period. The patient receives the temporary prosthesis 6 to 7 days after surgery. Gait training with partial weight bearing is then started. Upon discharge, 7 to 9 days after surgery, the patient is able to ambulate with assistance of crutches.[22]

Once the rigid dressing is removed, the BK amputee receives an immediate postoperative prosthesis (IPOP). Gait training with partial weight bearing is then started. Approximately 3 weeks after surgery, the IPOP is replaced with the temporary prosthesis and full weight-bearing training is begun.[22]

Both the AK and the BK amputees remain in temporary prostheses for the period that they are receiving chemotherapy treatments. During this time these individuals may experience weight fluctuations. Also during this period the residual limb matures and shrinks. One month after completion of chemotherapy, the permanent prosthesis is made.[22]

Rehabilitation of the amputee involves a multidisciplinary approach. This includes proper fitting of the prosthesis, gait training, and evaluation of functional status. The rehabilitative process is complete when the individual has achieved an optimal level of independence and is able to incorporate the prosthesis into his or her body image.

The initial postoperative rehabilitation process for limb salvage begins slowly. Institutions differ as to the type of program they utilize to assist these individuals in obtaining maximal function of the extremity. The healing process differs from one individual to another. Stabilization of the salvaged limb may occur as early as 2 months postoperatively or take as long as 10 months for proper healing to occur.[18] Rehabilitation programs are tailored to meet the individual patient's needs.

Individuals who have undergone limb-salvage surgery differ greatly in the methods of gait compensation that they use. Therefore, it has been difficult to measure and interpret gait performance based on motion analysis (Simon). Gait patterns differ from patient to patient. A recent study concluded that, in terms of energy expenditure during gait, reconstructions with mobile components were superior to arthrodesis, which, in turn, was superior to above-the-knee amputation. Yet, none of the reconstructions compare with normal knee function.[39] Patients often imagine that they will be able to resume their normal activities after limb salvage. The patients and their families must be made to realize that none of the surgical reconstruction approaches will enable them to have a normal limb, and that they will be partially disabled.[39]

CHEMOTHERAPY

The introduction of chemotherapy in the past two decades has made a dramatic impact on survival of individuals with sarcomas of the bone and soft tissue. Adjuvant chemotherapeutic agents are targeted at subclinical metastases. Improved survival has resulted from the eradication of overt as well as micrometastatic disease. This has resulted in less radical surgery for resection of the primary malignant lesion.[41]

Chemotherapy may be administered systemically as adjuvant (postoperative) therapy, or it may be given as neoadjuvant (preoperative) therapy, either intravenously or intra-arterially.

Neoadjuvant chemotherapy has become the standard approach to treatment and is designed to produce necrosis and shrinkage of the tumor. Theoretically, the chemotherapeutic agents are delivered to an undisturbed tumor bed with an excellent blood supply and adequate oxygenation, both of which are essential conditions for drug delivery effectiveness. The effectiveness of the chemotherapy regimen is evaluated at the time of surgical resection by the amount of necrosis the tumor displays. This necrosis is graded in the following manner: grade I, <50%; grade II, 50% to 90%: grade III, >90%; grade IV, 100%. The higher the percentage, the better the response. Recent trials indicate that 5-year disease-free survival rates ranging from 80% to greater than 90% have been achieved in patients who had a good tumor response, while rates of 60% or less have been achieved in those who had a poor tumor response.[10,12,41]

Adjuvant chemotherapy is frequently administered postoperatively. This may be given as an initial treatment or as follow-up treatment for patients who received neoadjuvant therapy. The chemotherapeutic agents chosen depend on the type of sarcoma and/or the response of the tumor to previous agents.

Doxorubicin (Adriamycin) is the most active single agent for soft tissue sarcomas. The addition of dacarbazine (DTIC) to the regimen has resulted in the highest response rate. Ifosfamide is currently the most active salvage agent for patients who have failed on doxorubicin-containing regimens. Current trials are now underway utilizing preoperative doxorubicin and cisplatinum.[2,8]

Osteosarcoma, Ewing's sarcoma, malignant fibrous histiocytoma of bone, and childhood rhabdomyosarcoma have all demonstrated sensitivity to chemotherapeutic agents. Chondrosarcoma remains resistant. The response of these various sarcomas to chemotherapy depends, to a great extent, on the biology of the specific tumor.[41]

Currently, doxorubicin, cisplatin, high-dose methotrexate, and ifosfamide are used as the primary agents for both osteogenic sarcoma and malignant fibrous histiocytoma. Other drugs, such as dactinomycin, bleomycin, and cyclophosphamide, are also used.[8,27,41]

A specific chemotherapy regimen has not been clearly identified in the treatment of Ewing's sarcoma. Successful regimens have used combinations of agents that include vincristine, actinomycin D, doxorubicin, and cyclophosphamide. Recent results support the use of ifosfamide and etoposide in the treatment of patients who have recurrent disease or those with metastatic disease at time of initial diagnosis. An Intergroup Ewing Sarcoma Study (IESS-III) is currently underway to determine the effect of the addition of ifosfamide and etoposide to standard therapy on disease-free and over-all survival.[41]

Multiagent chemotherapy has improved the 5-year disease-free survival of children with rhabdomyosarcoma from 20% to 60%. The most commonly used regimens include combinations of vincristine, actinomycin D, and cyclophosphamide.[41]

The primary treatment for chondrosarcoma is surgical resection of the tumor. This tumor is relatively resistant to chemotherapy. Patients with locally advanced or metastatic disease are treated with chemotherapy regimens, which include combinations of doxorubicin, cisplatin, and high-dose methotrexate.

Somatostatin, a growth-hormone inhibitor, has specific inhibitory effects on cell proliferation and appears to exhibit this effect on the growth of chondrosarcomas in rats. Recently, clinical trials have been initiated that are evaluating the efficacy of this drug on patients with high-grade chondrosarcoma or refractory mesenchymal chondrosarcoma.[41]

RADIATION THERAPY

Frequently, a combination of both chemotherapy and radiation therapy is utilized in the treatment of both soft tissue sarcomas and primary bone malignancies. This combination has been reported by several investigators to improve the local control rate.[8] The main advantage of these combination preoperative protocols is the reduced dose required for radiation therapy. Current trials for soft tissue sarcomas are now underway utilizing preoperative doxorubicin/cisplatin chemotherapy followed by 2800 cGy of radiation with subsequent surgical resection. Radiation therapy, like chemotherapy, causes tumor necrosis, which thereby facilitates limb salvage surgery. This form of treatment is most effective in tumors that originate from bone marrow. Connective tissue tumors are relatively radioresistant.[12] Other soft tissue sites, such as retroperitoneal and head and neck sarcomas, have not fared well with this multimodality approach. These tumors make complete surgical excision difficult due to their anatomic locations.[2,10]

Radiation therapy has limited effect on osteosarcoma, chondrosarcoma, and fibrosarcoma and is reserved for palliation of tumors that are inoperable. Ewing's sarcoma tends to be relatively radiosensitive.[27,32]

For nursing management associated with chemotherapy and radiation therapy refer to Chapters 21 and 22.

CONCLUSION

Nurses play a major role in caring for the individual with a primary bone malignancy or soft tissue sarcoma. Multimodality therapy may be utilized and this creates a tremendous need for teaching. These patients may require outpatient as well as inpatient therapy, so it is imperative that open communication exists between the nursing staff in these various health-care settings. Treatment involves extensive use of resources such as the medical oncologist, surgical oncologist, orthopedic surgeon, radiation oncologist, physical therapist, and nursing team.

Great strides have been made in the past decade with the addition of combination chemotherapy, radiation therapy, new surgical interventions, and the addition of new imaging techniques. Survival has improved and hopefully will continue to improve as more research is done and newer chemotherapeutic agents are developed.

BIBLIOGRAPHY

1. American Cancer Society: Cancer statistics, 1993, CA 43:1, 1993.
2. Antman KH, Eilber FR, and Shiu MH. Soft tissue sarcomas: current trends in diagnosis and management. In Haskell CM, editor: Current problems in cancer, Chicago, 1989, Year Book Medical Publishers, Inc.
3. Bell RS and others: Complications and functional results after limb-salvage surgery and radiotherapy for difficult mesenchymal neoplasms: a prospective analysis, Cancer 32:69, 1981.
4. Bowden L and Booher RJ: The principles and technique of resection of soft parts for sarcoma, Surgery 44:963, 1958.
5. Bramwell VH: Chemotherapy for metastatic soft tissue sarcomas—another full circle? Br J Cancer 64:7, 1991.
6. Carter SR and others: A review of 13-years experience of osteosarcoma, Clin Orthop Research 270:45, 1991.
7. Dalinka MK and others: The use of magnetic resonance imaging in the evaluation of bone and soft-tissue tumors, Radiol Clin North Am 28:461, 1990.
8. Dirix LY and Van Oosterom AT: The role of ifosfamide in the treatment of adult soft tissue sarcomas, Ewing's sarcoma, and osteosarcoma: a review, Semin Oncol 17:50, 1990.
9. Eckardt JJ and others: Endoprosthetic replacement for stage IIb osteosarcoma, Clin Orthop 270:202, 1991.
10. Eilber FR and others: Progress in the recognition and treatment of soft tissue sarcomas, Cancer 67:1169, 1990.
11. Eilber FR and others: Limb salvage for skeletal and soft tissue sarcomas, Cancer 53:2579, 1984.
12. Enneking WF and Conrad EU: Common bone tumors, Clin Symp 41:2, 1989.
13. Enterline H: Histopathology of sarcomas, Semin Oncol 8:133, 1981.
14. Finn HA and Simon MA: Limb-salvage surgery in the treatment of osteosarcoma in skeletally immature individuals, Clin Orthop 262:108, 1991.
15. Goodnight JE and others: Limb-sparing surgery for extremity sarcomas after preoperative intra-arterial doxorubicin and radiation therapy, Am J Surg 150:109, 1985.
16. Greenspan A: Malignant chondroblastic lesions, Orthop Clin North Am 20:358, 1989.
17. Heare TC, Enneking WF, and Heare MM: Staging techniques and biopsy of bone tumors, Orthop Clin North Am 20:273, 1989.
18. Hockenberry MJ and Lane B: Limb salvage procedures in children with osteosarcoma, Cancer Nurs 11:2, 1988.
19. Jaffe N: Chemotherapy for malignant bone tumors, Orthop Clin North Am 20:487, 1989.
20. Karakousis CP, Emrich LJ, and Vesper DS: Soft-tissue sarcomas of the proximal lower extremity, Arch Surg 124:1297, 1989.
21. Klein MJ, Kenan S, and Lewis MM: Osteosarcoma clinical and pathological considerations, Orthop Clin North Am 20:327, 1989.
22. Lane MJ and others: New advances and concepts in amputee management after treatment for bone and soft-tissue sarcomas, Clin Orthop 256:22, 1990.
23. Lawrence W and others: Adult soft tissue sarcomas, Ann Surg 205:349, 1987.
24. Lienard D, Roemans P, and Lejeune FJ: Resection of lung metastases from sarcomas, Eur J Surg Oncol 15:530, 1989.
25. Lind J: Lung cancer. In Clark JC, editor: Core curriculum for oncology nursing, Philadelphia, 1992, WB Saunders Co.
26. Link MP and others: Adjuvant chemotherapy of high-grade osteosarcoma of the extremity, Clin Orthop 270:8, 1991.
27. Meyer WH and Malawer MM: Osteosarcoma: Clinical features and evolving surgical and chemotherapeutic strategies, Pediatr Clin North Am 38:317, 1991.
28. Murphy WA: Imaging bone tumors in the 1990s, Cancer 67:1169, 1991.
29. Nirenberg A and Bridgewater C: Malignancies in adolescents, Semin Oncol Nursing 2:75, 1986.
30. O'Connor MI and Pritchard DJ: Ewing's sarcoma, prognostic factors, disease control, and the re-emerging role of surgical treatment, Clin Orthop 262:78, 1991.
31. Piasecki PA: The nursing role in limb salvage surgery, Orthop Nursing 26:33, 1991.
32. Pritchard DJ: Small round cell tumors, Orthop Clin North Am 20:367, 1989.
33. Raney B and others: Treatment of children with neurogenic sarcoma, Cancer 59:1, 1987.
34. Rosen G and others: Primary osteogenic sarcoma, the rationale for preoperative chemotherapy and delayed surgery, Cancer 43:2163, 1979.
35. Russell WO and others: A clinical and pathologic

staging system for soft tissue sarcomas, Cancer 40:1562, 1977.

36. Rydholm A and Rooser B: Surgical margins for soft-tissue sarcoma, J Bone Joint Surg 69-A:1074, 1987.

37. Saleh RA and others: Response of osteogenic sarcoma to the combination of etoposide and cyclophosphamide as neoadjuvant chemotherapy, Cancer 65:861, 1990.

38. Santoro A and Bonadonna G: Soft tissue and bone sarcomas, Cancer Chemother Biolog Response Modifiers, 10:344, 1988.

39. Simon M: Limb salvage for osteosarcoma in the 1980s, Clin Orthop 270:264, 1991.

40. Stotter AT and others: The influence of local recurrence of extremity soft tissue sarcoma on metastasis and survival, Cancer 65:1119, 1990.

41. Yasko AW and Lane JM: Chemotherapy for bone and soft-tissue sarcomas of the extremities, J Bone Joint Surg 73-A:1263, 1991.

CHAPTER 6

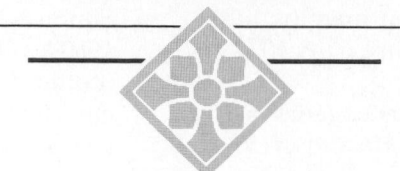

Cancer of the Brain and Central Nervous System

Mary E. Murphy

Cancer of the central nervous system (CNS) includes primary and metastatic tumors of the brain and spinal cord. Despite a relatively high ratio of primary tumors in the pediatric population, adult CNS tumors represent only 2.2% of all cancer deaths. Metastatic lesions continue to present symptom and treatment management concerns. This chapter deals with adult CNS tumors. Additional readings are recommended for the pediatric population.[6,7,25,29,31]

EPIDEMIOLOGY

Cancer of the CNS accounts for 1.5% of all malignancies with 17,500 diagnosed cases in 1993. Peak incidence occurs from birth to 6 years and after the age of 45. CNS tumors account for the fourth leading cause of cancer death in persons ages 15 to 34. Incidence is slightly higher in males.[31,32,38] Race differences have not been documented. Metastatic lesions represent 20% to 40% of all CNS neoplasms, with most arising from lung and breast cancers. Sarcomas, melanomas, and tumors may arise from the kidney and the colon.[4,6,10]

ETIOLOGY AND RISK FACTORS

Specific causes and risk factors have not been identified. Chemical carcinogens and some oncologic viruses have induced CNS tumors in laboratory animals. Genetic factors have been linked with neurofibromatosis, tuberous sclerosis, familial polyposis, Von Hippel-Lindau disease,[25] Turcot syndrome, and family cancer syndromes of breast, soft-tissue sarcoma, and leukemia.

Chemical exposures that have been implicated include vinyl chloride, radiation, petrochemical, inks,

solvents, acrylonitrile, lubricating oils, and solvents.[7] Viruses have also been implicated including the Epstein-Barr virus genome. Traumatic causes and environmental carcinogens have not been indicated at this time. Ongoing investigation is in progress.

PREVENTION AND SCREENING DETECTION

At this time no screening or prevention methods exist. Symptoms appear gradually and do not lend themselves to diagnostic prescreening methods.

CLASSIFICATION

In order to provide a simplistic understanding of the complexity of CNS tumors a variety of systems have been developed. Tumors of the CNS include both brain and spinal cord tumors. Tumors of the CNS are classified as primary and metastatic in nature. Primary tumors may exist as intracerebral or extracerebral. Major intracerebral tumors include those within the brain, neuroglia (Fig. 6-1), neurons, and cells of the blood vessels of the connective tissue. Extracerebral tumors originate outside of the brain and include meningeomas, acoustic nerve, pituitary, and pineal gland tumors. Metastatic tumors may exist either inside or outside of the body. The classification of benign versus malignant is not differentiated, since surgical accessibility determines the ultimate prognosis.

Within each specific location the classification of CNS tumors is based on all types of differentiation and location.[6,25] Detailed classifications were developed by the World Health Organization in 1979 and are available for use.[47] Table 6-1 represents a workover and modified system of common CNS tumors, cell type, occurrence, and malignant state.[2,12]

74

Ependymal cell   Astrocyte

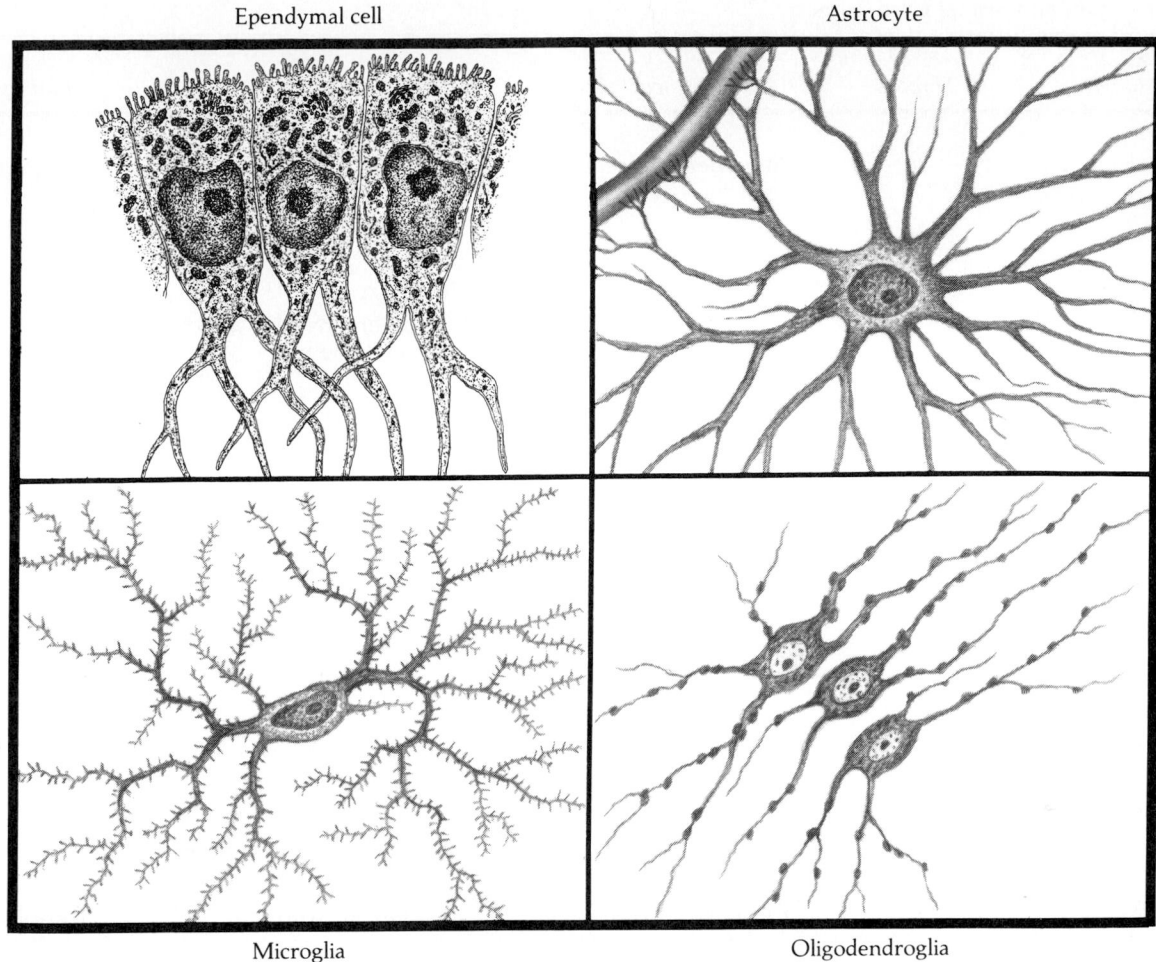

Microglia   Oligodendroglia

Figure 6–1   Types of neuroglia cells. (From McCance KL and Huether SE: Pathophysiology, The biologic basis for disease in adults and children, St. Louis, 1990, Mosby.)

Glial tumors represent two thirds of all types of CNS tumors with glioblastomas representing the largest subclass. Schwannomas and meningomas represent the largest classification of spinal cord tumors. CNS lymphoma are seen among immunosuppressed patients, particularly patients diagnosed with acquired immune deficiency syndrome (AIDS). Metastatic brain tumors may be as common as 35% in all cancer patients with the largest representation among patients with lung tumors.*

CLINICAL FEATURES

The clinical features manifested by CNS tumors vary according to their size and specific location. The most common symptom is headache and seizure activity. Headaches are commonly bifrontal and bioccipital and occur upon awakening. Episodes of nausea and vomiting may also present with the complaints of headache. Seizure activity is seen in 20% to 50% of

all patients with brain tumors and are most common in parietal and temporal tumors.[4,6,11,21,34] As tumor bulk increases in size cerebral edema accumulates and increased intracranial pressure and brain tissue hemorrhages may be seen. Displacement of cerebral structures may result in brain herniation, an emergency and often lethal complication of increased tumor size and local invasion.[22,35,41,44,45]

Structural changes, memory defects, speech, motor, and visual changes are also displayed and vary depending on tumor location and size. Figure 6-2 demonstrates the principal functional subdivisions of the cerebral hemisphere and the functions of specific cortical areas. Common sites of intracranial tumors are seen in Figure 6-3. Tumor related side effects can be expected and understood with knowledge of tumor type, location of tumor, and approximate size of the tumor at the time of diagnosis.

Spinal cord tumors are also related to the site and size of the lesion. Pain is the most common presenting symptom. Weakness, sensory loss, muscle spasms,

---

*References 6, 7, 25, 29, 31, 36, 45.

Table 6–1   Brain and Spinal Cord Tumors

Neoplasm	% of Tumors	Location	Characteristics	Cell of Origin
Gliomas Astrocytoma	20	Anywhere in brain or spinal cord	Grade I and II Slow-growing, invasive	Supportive tissue Astrocytes Glial
Glioblastoma multiforme	30	Common in cerebral hemispheres	Grade III, IV Highly invasive and malignant	Thought to arise from mature astrocytes
Oligodendrocytoma	4	Common in frontal lobes deep in white matter; may arise in brain stem, cerebellum, and spinal cord	Avascular, tends to be encapsulated; more malignant form called *oligodendroblastoma*	Oligodendrites and glial cells
Ependymoma	5	Intramedullary; wall of the ventricles; may arise in caudal tail of the spinal cord	Common in children, variable growth rates; more malignant, invasive form called *ependymoblastoma;* may extend into the ventricle or invade brain tissue	Ependymal cells
Neurilemmoma	4	Cranial nerves (most commonly vestibular division of cranial nerve VIII)	Slow-growing	Schwann cells
Neurofibroma		Extramedullary—spinal cord	Slow-growing	Neurilemma, Schwann cells
Pituitary Tumors	8	Pituitary gland; may extend to or invade floor of the third ventricle	Age-linked, several types slow-growing, macro- and micro-adenomas may be secreting or nonsecreting	Pituitary cells, pituitary chromophobes, basophils, eosinophils
Pineal Region	1	Pineal region; pineal parenchyma posterior or third ventricle	Several types (germinoma, pineocytoma, teratoma)	Several types with different cell origin
Blood Vessel Tumors Angioma	3	Predominantly in posterior cerebral hemispheres	Slow-growing	Arising from congenitally malformed arteriovenous connections
Neuronal Cell Medulloblastoma	1	Posterior cerebellar vermis, roof of fourth ventricle	Well-demarcated, rapid-growing, fills fourth ventricle	Embryonic cells

Table 6–1 Brain and Spinal Cord Tumors—cont'd

Neoplasm	% of Tumors	Location	Characteristics	Cell of Origin
Mesodermal Tissue Meningioma	20	Intradural, extramedullary; sylvian fissure region, superior parasagittal surface of frontal and parietal lobes, olfactory groove, wing of sphenoid bone, superior surface of cerebellum, cerebellopontine angle, spinal cord	Slow-growing, circumscribed, encapsulated, sharply demarcated from normal tissues, compressive in nature	
Choroid Plexus Papillomas	1	Choroid plexus of the ventricular system, lateral ventricle in children, fourth ventricle in adults	Usually benign, slow in expansion inducing hemorrhage and hydrocephalus; malignant tumor is rare	Epithelial cells
Cranial Nerves and Spinal Nerve Roots Hemangioblastomas	2	Arises from blood vessels Predominant in cerebellum	Benign Slow-growing	Embryonic vascular tissue
Lymphoma	1	Cerebral hemispheres	Metastasis common	B cells
Metastatic tumors	35 of all cancer patients	Cerebral cortex diencephalon	Malignant spread	From lung, breast, colon, kidney, thyroid, prostate

and loss of bowel and bladder control occur as the tumor invades local tissue causing nerve destruction.[44,45] Table 6-2 summarizes common clinical features of CNS tumors.

DIAGNOSTIC AND PATHOLOGIC STAGING

An initial assessment of a suspected CNS tumor would include a physical and neurological assessment. Pertinent data on emotional and physical changes may need to be obtained from family members. Computed tomography (CT) and magnetic resonance imaging (MRI) are the two most common and valuable diagnostic tests used to diagnose CNS tumors. CT is the most useful in low grade astrocytomas and small diameter tumors because of their increased visibility for tumor location and size. CT is also useful for spinal cord tumors and evaluation of tumor recurrence and treatment response.[44,45]

MRI provides exquisite detail to tumor location and reconstruction of images at three views at right angles (axial, sagittal, and coronal).[7,25,44,45] MRI also has the ability to detect edema but does not differentiate between edema and tumor (Figure 6-4).

Position emission tomography (PET) uses CT to detect the emission of positive electrons and some radioactive substances. Chemical substances such as glucose are distributed in tissues to evaluate the tumor response and activity. These metabolic activities are produced in a series of color pictures. PET has until now only been utilized as part of research protocols.

Cerebral angiograms and radionuclide (RN) angiograms are x-rays used to evaluate cerebral blood vessel flow near the tumor. These x-rays should only be used after CT and MRI. RN angiograms show various concentrations of injected material in the brain. Additional examinations that may be ordered include skull and spinal films and evoked-potentials. Evoked-potentials measure the electrode activity of nerves and may be important at the time of surgical removal of tumors that surround nerves.[6,11]

Electroencephalogram (EEG) is a rare test with little diagnostic ability. Tumor markers have only demonstrated usefulness in embryonal tumors in the pineal area. Alpha-fetoprotein and beta-HCG are found in cerebrospinal fluid.[6,25] Lumbar puncture examina-

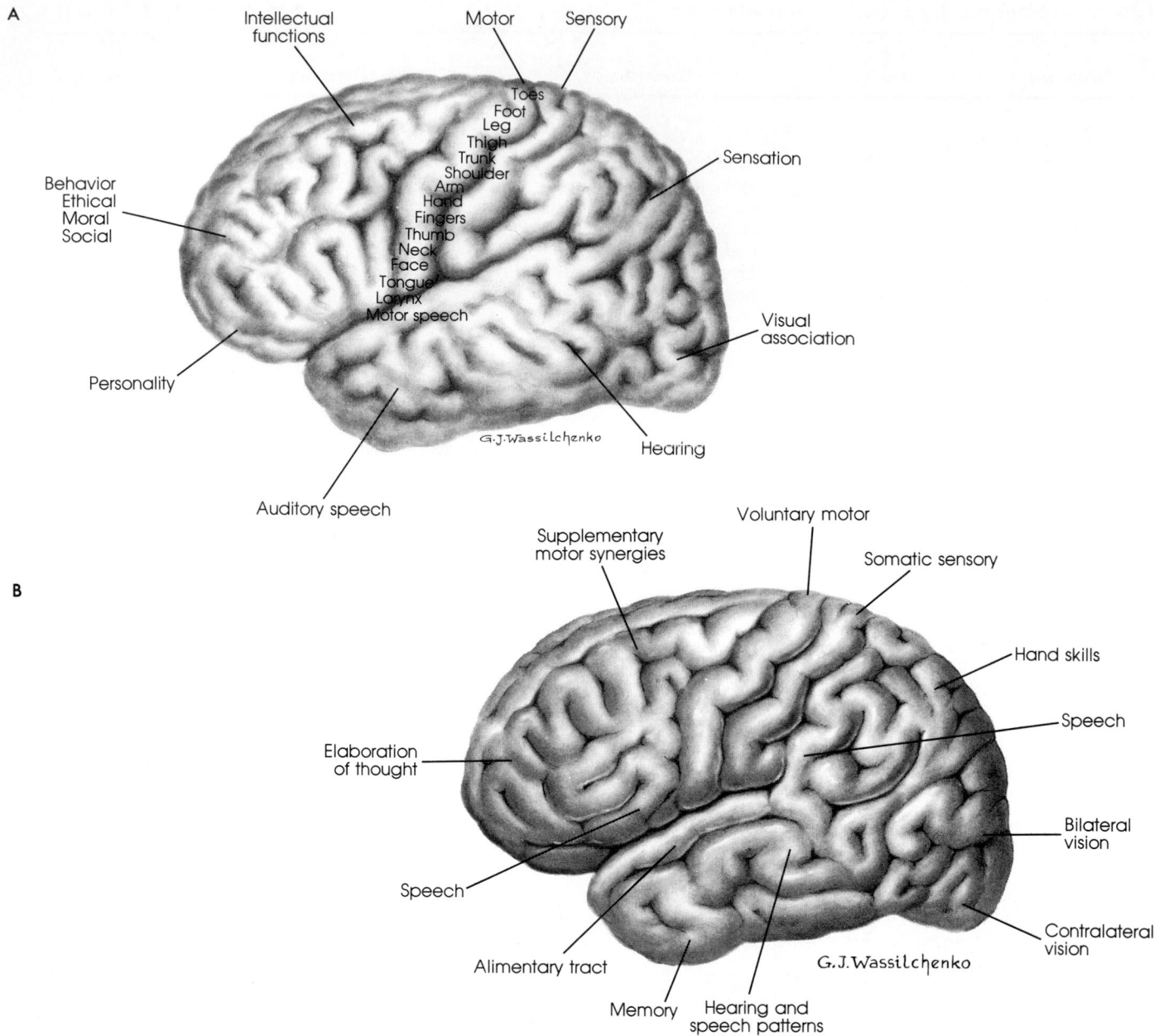

Figure 6–2 **A**, Principal functional subdivisions of the cerebral hemisphere. **B**, Functional areas of specific cortical areas. (From McCance KL and Huether SE: Pathophysiology, The biologic basis for disease in adults and children, St. Louis, 1990, Mosby.)

tions should only be performed when risk of increased intracranial pressure has been ruled out, and following MRI and CT. A lumbar puncture is useful in the diagnosis of meningeal involvement, periventricular tumors, and CNS lymphomas. Results from spinal fluid analysis that may indicate tumor involvement include increased spinal pressure readings, elevated white blood cell and protein count, and glucose level.

Diagnostic examinations are only tentative, a definitive diagnosis can only be made when the specific tumor type is identified. The identification of tumor cell type can only be done by a biopsy of tumor tissue. This can be accomplished by either open biopsy, such as a craniotomy, or through stereotactic needle biopsy, which is a closed system into a Burr hole opening. A biopsy probe in a three-dimensional space is utilized to visualize the tumor. Simple needle biopsies yield inadequate specimens and may result in bleeding complications. When biopsy specimens are not available due to tumor location interpretation must be done with only diagnostic examinations. Meta-

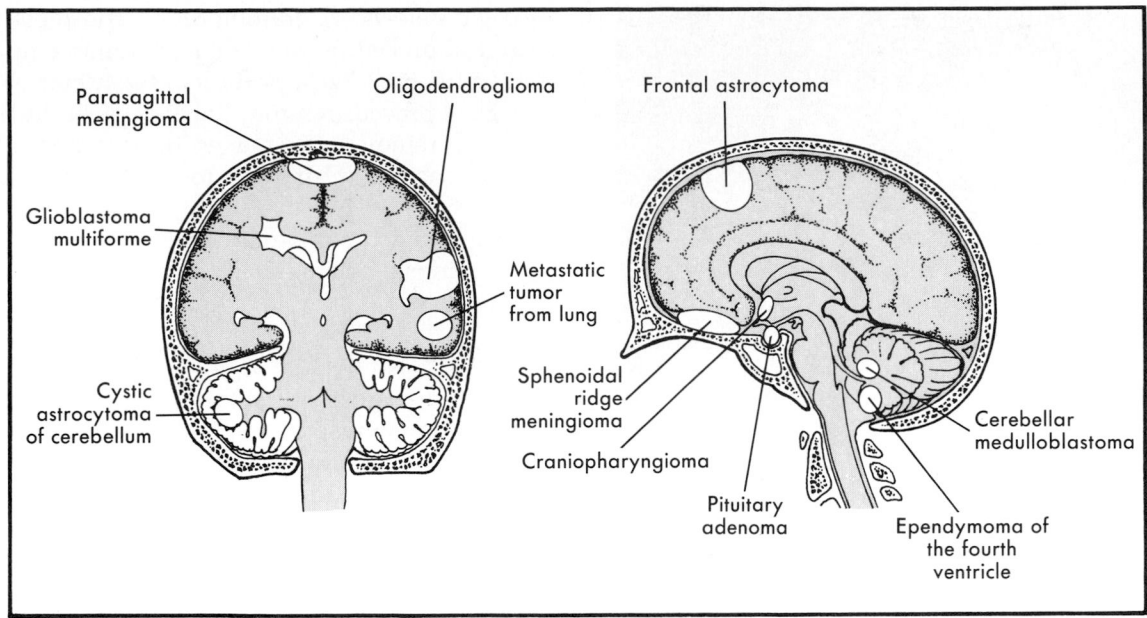

Figure 6–3   Common sites of intracranial tumors. (From McCance KL and Huether SE: Pathophysiology, The biologic basis for disease in adults and children, St. Louis, 1990, Mosby.)

Table 6–2   Common Clinical Features of CNS Tumors

Very Early	*Late*
Headache	Impaired cognitive skills
Seizures	Personality changes
Nausea	Short-term memory loss
Vomiting	Aphasia
	Sensory/motor defects
	Visual changes
	Loss of sphincter control

static CNS tumors are evaluated in a similar manner with the primary focus on the discovery of the tumor's primary site.

Pathologic staging is based on histology, grade, and the completeness of tumor removal. The TNM (tumor, nodes, metastatic disease) staging system is utilized to stage CNS tumors. Tumor locations are divided into supratentorial (above the tentorium cerebelli), intratentorial (below the tentorium cerebelli), and infratentorial. Category N (Node) is not applicable since lymph nodes do not exist in CNS tumors. Tumor grading is based on cell differentiation. Stages I through IV exist with subcategories A and B (see box on p. 81).[12,28]

METASTASIS

The spread of primary CNS tumors beyond the brain and spinal cord is rare. Seeding is the most common method of spread within the CNS and spinal cord.

Medulloblastoma tumors have the greatest potential to develop metastatic lesions within the CNS.[6,12,38,45]

TREATMENT MODALITIES

Surgery remains the treatment of choice for all CNS tumors. Nonresectable or partially resectable tumors may require additional treatment modalities such as radiation, chemotherapy, biotherapy oncogenes, and use of steroids and anticonvulsant therapy to treat tumor or treatment side effects.

Pretreatment techniques involve use of steroids such as Dexamethasone (Decadron) that are administered to assist with the reduction of cerebral edema, which may cause personality changes, altered level of consciousness, and sensory-motor defects. Anticonvulsant therapy may also be administered for those patients with focal changes that result in seizure activity. Steroidal and anticonvulsant therapy may be continued after surgery or radiation to minimize potential side effects.[6,12,22,25,38]

Surgery

Surgery serves as a diagnostic and treatment modality. Surgical intervention provides tissue sampling for histology, decreases the tumor burden for further treatment, and can provide a cure for low-grade tumors. The ability for complete resection varies with size and tumor location. Various types of surgical procedures may be performed depending on the ability to access the tumor and the patient's overall ability to tolerate the surgical procedure without gross neu-

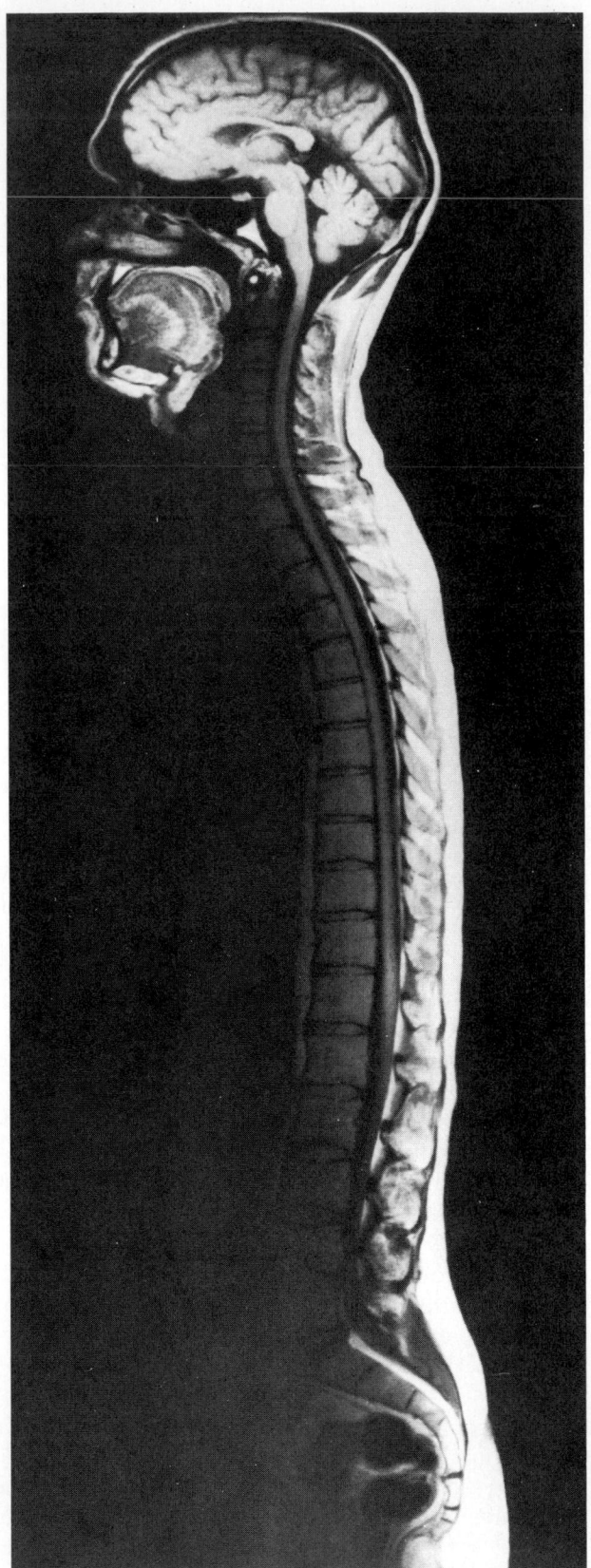

Figure 6—4 Midsagittal MRI image, demonstrating the extraordinary anatomic detail possible with this technique. (From McCance KL and Huether SE: Pathophysiology, The biologic basis for disease in adults and children, St. Louis, 1990, Mosby.)

rologic defects. A craniotomy is the most common surgical procedure performed to remove tumor mass or debulk the largest portion of the tumor. Additional surgical procedures may include stereotactic biopsy for the removal of smaller tumors and placement of radioactive substances to treat nonresectable tumors.[6,31,37]

Metastatic tumors may also lend themselves to surgical removal if benign lesions exist or favorable prognosis from the original primary tumor exists.

Radiation Therapy

Tumors that are inoperable or have only partial tumor resection may respond to radiation therapy if the tumor histology is radiosensitive. Tumors that are radiosensitive include medulla-blastomas, high-grade astrocytoma, and metastatic brain tumors of the breast, lung, metamona, and sarcoma.[40]

Radiation treatments may be administered in a variety of doses and methods. Conventional dose therapy is usually given over a series of weeks, allowing normal tissue to heal and hypoxic tumor cells to become more susceptible to treatment. Doses may also be given to the entire brain and spinal cord when there is risk of metastasis to surrounding tissue.

Additional methods of radiation may be given at the time of surgery and include interstitial implants of radioactive seeds directly to the tumor. Radiation may also be administered via the stereotactic route during surgery. This method allows a single dose of radiation to be administered to one area of the brain.[6,25,34,38]

Other methods of radiation administration include hyperthermia, a local treatment done during surgery, which utilizes catheters implanted into the tumor. These catheters administer heat throughout the tumor. Tumor cells are more sensitive to heat and therefore hyperthermia may enhance radiation therapy to the tumor site. Experimental treatment modalities include radioactive sensitizers, hyperfractionation, heavy particle radiation therapy, photodynamic therapy, and neutron capture therapy. These treatments are now under clinical investigation. A summary of these treatments can be found in Table 6-3.*

Chemotherapy

Chemotherapy may be utilized in combination with surgery and radiation for the treatment of gliomas and medulloblastomas. Response rate remains as low as 20% to 40% due to the blood-brain barrier mechanism.[33] The most commonly used drugs are the nitrosoureas (BCNU and CCNU). Additional agents are the alkylating (cisplatin, cyclophosphamide, and nitrogen mustard), antitumor antibiotics (bleomycin),

---

*References 8, 18, 19, 24, 27, 30.

TNM CLASSIFICATION OF BRAIN TUMORS

Primary tumor (T)

TX Primary tumor cannot be assessed
T0 No evidence of primary tumor

Supratentorial tumor

T1 Tumor 5 cm or less in greatest dimension; limited to one side
T2 Tumor more than 5 cm in greatest dimension; limited to one side
T3 Tumor invades or encroaches on the ventricular system
T4 Tumor crosses the midline, invades the opposite hemisphere, or invades infratentorially

Infratentorial tumor

T1 Tumor 3 cm or less in greatest dimension; limited to one side
T2 Tumor more than 3 cm in greatest dimension; limited to one side
T3 Tumor invades or encroaches on the ventricular system
T4 Tumor crosses the midline, invades the opposite hemisphere, or invades supratentorially

Regional lymph nodes (N)

This category does not apply to this site.

Distant metastasis (M)

MX Presence of distant metastasis cannot be assessed
M0 No distant metastasis
M1 Distant metastasis

Histopathologic grade (G)

GX Grade cannot be assessed
G1 Well differentiated
G2 Moderately well differentiated
G3 Poorly differentiated
G4 Undifferentiated

Stage grouping

Stage IA	G1	T1	M0
Stage IIB	G1	T2	M0
	G1	T3	M0
Stage IIA	G2	T1	M0
Stage IIB	G2	T2	M0
	G2	T3	M0
Stage IIIA	G3	T1	M0
Stage IIIB	G3	T2	M0
	G3	T3	M0
Stage IV	G1, G2, G3	T4	M0
	G4	Any T	M0
	Any G	Any T	M1

From Beahrs OH and others: Manual for staging of cancer, ed 3, Philadelphia, 1992, JB Lippincott Co.

Table 6–3 Investigational Treatments with Radiation Therapy

Type	*Definition*
Radiosensitizer	Uses radiosensitized drugs to substitute ingredient to repair cells
Fractional radiation therapy	Doses of radiation are given in fractional increments closer apart to allow for cell cycle vulnerability
Heavy particle therapy	Changed particles are superior to external rays by decreasing damage and increasing tumor cell kill
Photodynamic therapy	Drugs that concentrate in tumor cells; light activates the drug during a surgical procedure
Neutron capture therapy	Nonionizing radiation with a drug concentrates in tumor cells; radiation activates tumor cells and kills them

plant alkaloids (vincristine, etoposide), antimetabolites (methotrexate), and procarbazine.*

Common routes of administration include oral and intravenous. Additional methods include intra-arte-

*References 5, 6, 9, 20, 25, 26, 29, 39.

EXPERIMENTAL BIOTHERAPY

Interferon
Growth factors
Tumor necroses factors
Interleukens
Colony stimulating factors
Monoclonal antibodies
Lymphokine-activated killer cells
Tumor infiltrating lymphocytes
Immunotoxins
Bacterial derivatives
Retinoids
Cellular transfer

rial into the carotid or vertebrae artery, via timed-release biodegradable wafers impregnated with chemotherapy, into the spinal column. The use of the Ommaya reservoir, a surgically implanted pump placed in the ventricles, has eliminated numerous lumbar punctures.[42] (See Figure 20-1.)[6,25]

Experimental uses of biotherapy are listed in the box directly above.[6,25]

Metastatic tumors are treated based on the primary tumor location and the spread of the metastasis and may include all modalities. Management of CNS lymphomas and AIDS-related lymphomas follow normal protocols for that disease.[14]

SPINAL CORD TUMORS

The treatment of spinal cord tumors is similar to brain tumors. Surgical resection is used for diagnosis and tumor removal. Decompression laminectomy is used when tumor compression is present. Postoperative radiation may include the entire spinal column or cord segments. Chemotherapy may be given in the intrathecal route or systemically.[25]

DISEASE-RELATED COMPLICATIONS

Major disease related complications include increased intracranial pressure from cerebral edema and displaced brain structures resulting in brain herniation. A major complication of spinal cord tumors is spinal cord compression (see Chapter 19, Oncologic Complications).

Increased intracranial pressure is caused by an increase in intracellular volume from the expanding tumor mass and edema. Signs and symptoms can be seen in the box on this page. Cerebral edema results in tissue hypoxia and acidosis (Figure 6-5). If left to progress, brain stem compression occurs and herniation of the brain results. Ultimate respiratory arrest will follow. Management includes surgical removal and supportive therapy with diuretics and corticosteroids. Close nursing observation is required to monitor potentially fatal outcome (Figure 6-6).[6,11,12,25]

> **SIGNS AND SYMPTOMS OF INCREASED INTRACRANIAL PRESSURE AND BRAIN STEM HERNIATION**
>
> *Intracranial pressure*
> Headache
> Vomiting
> Mental acuity changes
> Seizures
> Alteration in motor or sensory response
> Changes in vital signs
> Ocular changes

TREATMENT-RELATED COMPLICATIONS
Radiation Therapy

Radiation treatment-related side effects are based on the dose and location of treatment. Local and long-term side effects can be experienced (see box on p. 83). Most side effects are temporary and related to local irritation or disruption of myelin formation. Radiation doses are cumulative and retreatment in the same manner is not recommended.[6,11]

Chemotherapy

Major side effects related to chemotherapy are based on the combination of drugs and their specific dose.

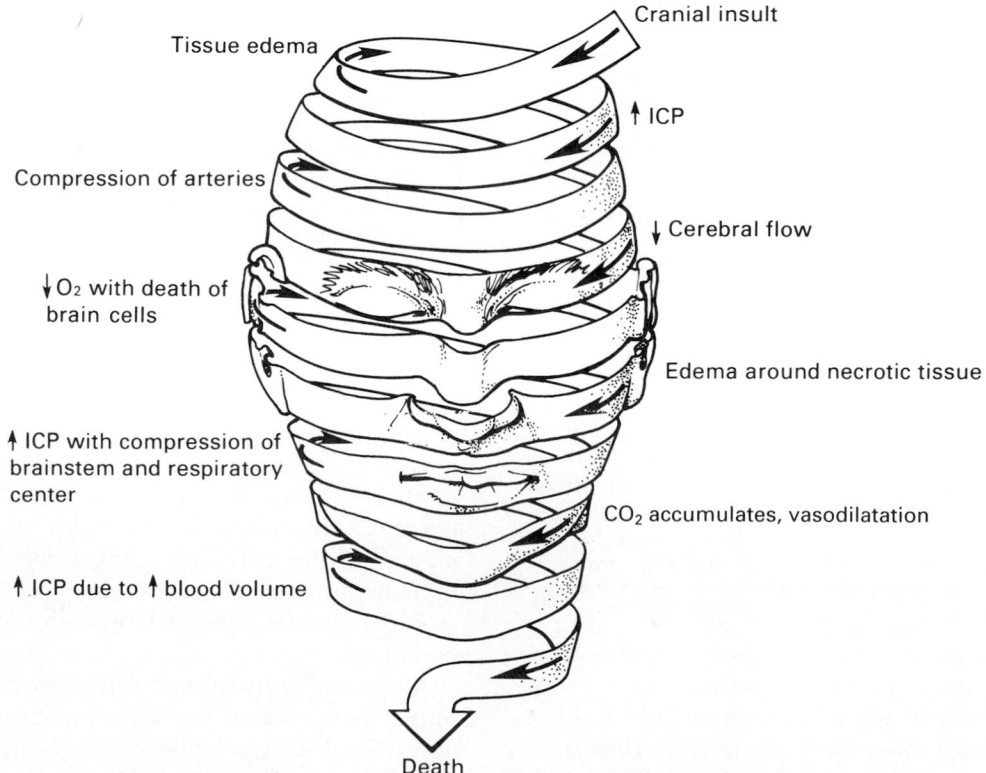

Tissue edema
Cranial insult
↑ ICP
Compression of arteries
↓ Cerebral flow
↓ O₂ with death of brain cells
Edema around necrotic tissue
↑ ICP with compression of brainstem and respiratory center
CO₂ accumulates, vasodilatation
↑ ICP due to ↑ blood volume
Death

Figure 6-5   Progression of increased ICP. (From Lewis SM and Collier IC: Medical-surgical nursing, ed 3, St. Louis, 1992, Mosby.)

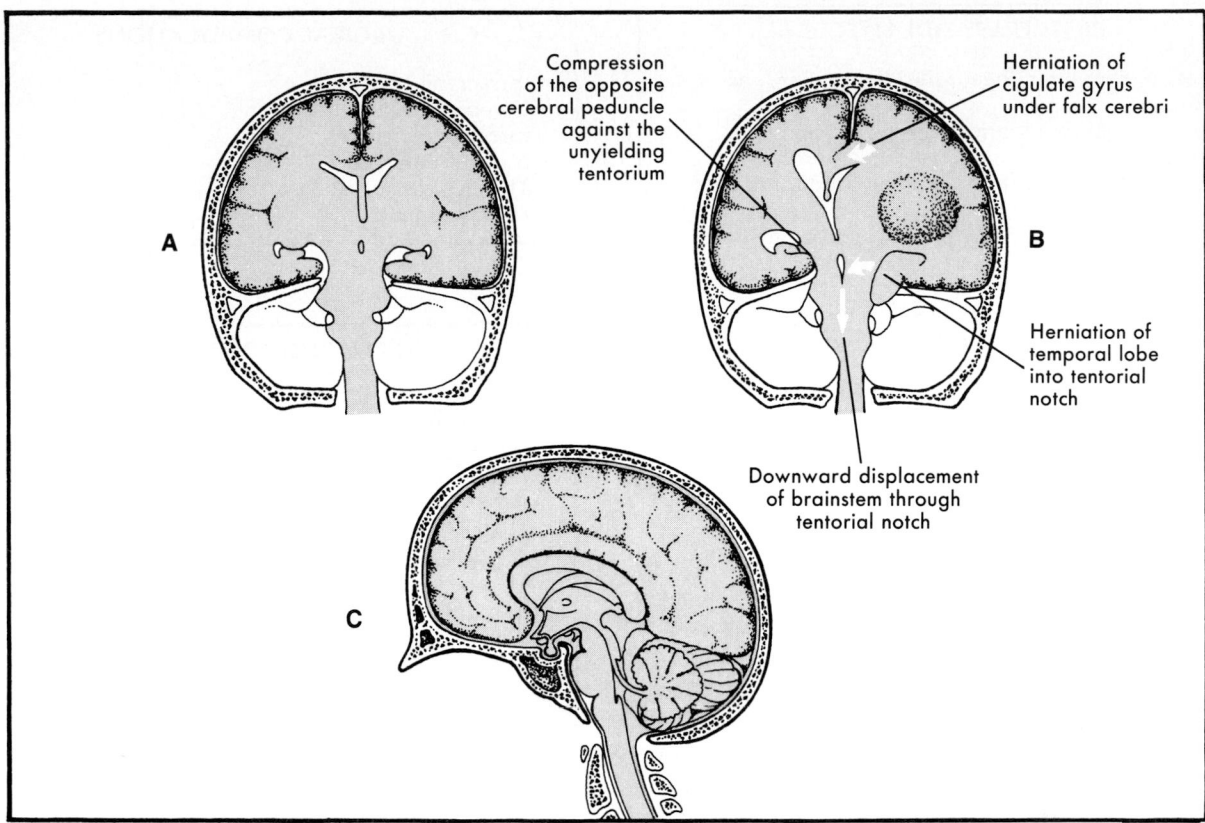

Figure 6-6 Herniation. **A**, The normal relationship of intracranial structures. **B**, Shift of intracranial structures. **C**, Downward herniation of the cerbellar tonsils into the foramen magnum. (From Lewis SM and Collier IC: Medical-surgical nursing, ed 3, St. Louis, 1992, Mosby.)

RADIATION THERAPY SIDE EFFECTS

Early
Hair loss
Skin changes (redness, darkness, itching)
Nausea
Inflammation around the ear
Edema (increased intracranial pressure)
Anorexia
Lethargy

Long term
Decreased intellect
Altered motor/sensory function
Pituitary dysfunction

Spinal cord
Radiation myelopathy

Major areas that are affected include the bone marrow, hair follicles, and gastrointestinal tract. Major side effects of common drugs used in CNS tumors are found in Table 6-4.[39,43]

Biotherapy

Side effects of biotherapy are related to dose and combined modality. Common side effects are listed in the upper left-hand box on p. 84.[6,12,25]

Table 6-4 Chemotherapy Drugs and Related Side Effects

BCNU	Bone marrow suppression
CCNU	Nausea, alopecia, pulmonary fibrosis
Cisplatin	Ototoxicity, renal dysfunction, bone marrow depression, anorexia, nausea, vomiting
Cytoxan	Nausea/vomiting, diarrhea, alopecia, bone marrow suppression
Nitrogen mustard	Nausea, vomiting, anorexia, alopecia, diarrhea, bone marrow suppression, hepatic/neurologic dysfunction
Bleomycin	Nausea, vomiting, stomatitis, hepatic/neurologic dysfunction, pulmonary fibrosis
Vincristine	Nausea/vomiting, anorexia, alopecia, neurologic dysfunction
Etoposide	Nausea, vomiting, anorexia, hypotension, bone marrow suppression
Methotrexate	Bone marrow suppression, renal tubular necrosis, stomatitis, diarrhea, hepatic dysfunction
Procarbazine	Nausea, vomiting, diarrhea, alopecia, myelosuppression, hepatic and neurologic dysfunction

---

BIOTHERAPY SIDE EFFECTS

Flu-like symptoms (headache, fever, chills, ar-
thralgia, myalgia)
Nausea/vomiting (varies with individual and
amount of dose)
Weight loss (amount depends on amount of side
effects)
Altered neurologic functioning (decreased short-
term memory concentration/attention)
Alopecia (partial)
Skin changes (erythema, rash, pruritus)
Fluid and electrolyte imbalances (hypocalcemia,
hypomagnesemia)
Bone marrow suppression (pancytopenia)

SURGICAL COMPLICATIONS

Intracranial bleeding
Cerebral edema
Infection
Neuromotor deficits
Thrombosis
Hydrocephalus

STEROID THERAPY SIDE EFFECTS

Hyperglycemia
Irritability
Insomnia
Psychotic reactions/mood swings
Hypokalemia
Hypernatremia
Depressed immune response
Elevated lipid and cholesterol levels
Fluid retention
Cataract formation
Osteoporosis
Thrombophlebitis
Steroid-induced gastric ulcers
Relocation of fat deposits (round face and thick
trunk)
Cutaneous striae
Withdrawal symptoms (doses must be reduced
from IV to oral and then in amount and fre-
quency)

Surgery

Postoperative surgical complications are included in
a box on this page. Size and location of tumor as well
as the overall preoperative state of the patient enhances the potential for complications.[44,45]

Steroidal Therapy

Use of steroids pre- and post-operatively can also produce a variety of treatment side effects that can produce local as well as systemic effects. Included in a
box on this page are major effects of steroidal therapy.[16,39] Steroids are administered to produce an antiinflammatory response and reduce cerebral swelling. Steroidal therapy may begin after an initial dose
of mannitol, which may be used before, during, or
after surgery to reduce immediate cerebral edema.
Postoperative management with titration will be done
with steroids such as dexamethasone.

Nursing Management

The diagnosis of cancer produces high levels of anxiety and fear in most patients and families; of particular concern are those patients diagnosed with CNS
tumors. Emotional distress is brought on by the rapid
onset of debilitation, physical and emotional changes,
and the ultimate poor prognostic factors. Preparation
time from the onset of symptoms to diagnosis and
surgery is limited and often allows little time for emotional support and education. Most information on
the treatment course will be provided after surgery
and is based on tumor size, type, location, and ability
to remove tumor mass.

Lack of past experience with hospitalization and
surgery will further increase the anxiety and fear patterns. Paralysis, coma, and neurologic defects may all
be a postoperative reality. For patients with metastatic
disease who have already undergone treatment, the
knowledge of cancer recurrences can be devastating.

NURSING DIAGNOSIS
• Fear and anxiety related to diagnosis and postoperative outcomes.
• Knowledge deficit related to limited experience with
diagnostic pre- and post-operative routines.

Interventions are based on providing emotional
support through information and teaching on expected outcomes. Assessment of past coping mechanisms and support systems within the family struc-

ture are needed. Education should be based on teaching learning principles and include visual information. A basic review of the anatomy and physiology of the CNS system will assist in the understanding of tumor locations and causes of present symptoms. Discussion should include an explanation of tests and procedures, their diagnostic indications, postoperative routines, monitoring devices, potential postoperative complications, and expected body image alterations. Patients with altered cognition from extensive CNS involvement may not be able to participate. These families will need additional support systems of family, clergy, or other hospital supports that may be available. The inclusion of a clinical nurse specialist in neurology is helpful and can provide ad-

ditional information on postoperative concerns. A summary of patient/family education needs are found in the box below.

PATIENT/SURGERY TEACHING PRIORITIES

Explanation of surgical diagnostic procedures
Basic review of anatomy and physiology of CNS
   system
   Tumor location
   Expected signs/symptoms
Postoperative monitoring
   Equipment
Postoperative nursing care routines
Postoperative complications
Body image concerns

POSTOPERATIVE CARE

Surgery for CNS tumors may be done by standard craniotomy or use of laser surgery. Use of laser surgery is limited but has several advantages: (1) it decreases the amount of dissection to surrounding tissue and (2) it has the ability to reach tumors that were formerly inaccessible. Spinal tumors can also be re-

moved by laser surgery or standard decompression laminectomy. Surgery is always indicated to assist with histologic typing and debulking of tumor mass. Inoperable tumors may respond by the relief of general symptoms of compression and intracranial pressure.

Nursing Management

The postoperative course will require extensive monitoring for complications. Further treatment will be based on operative results, tumor histology, and patient complications. Families will continue to need intense emotional support during the postoperative course. For those patients with inoperable tumors a referral for home care or hospice is appropriate.

NURSING DIAGNOSIS

- Self care deficit related to postoperative procedure
- Body image changes related to altered physical status
- Potential sensory/perceptual alterations related to neurologic deficits
- Potential for physical and cellular injury related to altered cognition and side effect of medications
- Pain related to surgical procedure
- Ineffective coping of family and patient related to prognostic factors

Postoperative care of the patient with a craniotomy will include frequent neurologic examinations, measurement of vital signs, supportive nursing care of positioning, administration of medications including pain, steroids, and anticonvulsant therapy. Observation of increased intracranial pressure and brain herniation is a critical factor in the postoperative course.[20,21] Common postoperative complications are included in a box on p. 84.

Neurologic examinations should include measurement of the level of consciousness, orientation, emotional response to surgery, and motor and sensory perception. Pupils are observed for inequality. Vital signs should be observed for decreased respirations and pulse and widened pulse pressure. The patient should be placed in a quiet nonstimulating environment and positioned according to physician protocol. The most common position will be with the head of the bed at a 30 degree angle to reduce cerebral edema

Continued.

and stress on the suture line. Dressings and drains are monitored for the type and amount of drainage. Coughing, deep breathing techniques, and suctioning are done in a nonaggressive manner so as to reduce increased intracranial pressure.

The patient will experience a self-care deficit for several days and require skin and mouth care as well as maintenance of bowel and urinary function. Assessment of the patient's comfort level is done during administration of care. Restlessness and moaning or increased head movement may indicate pain. Positioning, maintenance of a quiet environment, and low doses of mild pain medication are given. Safety measures for those patients with potential seizure activity may include seizure pads and the administration of anticonvulsant therapy.

Management of increased intracranial pressure is through administration of mannitol and corticosteroids such as dexamethasone.[16] Long-term use of steroids to reduce edema can cause serious side effects (box on p. 84) and therefore requires a titration schedule to reduce the amount and frequency of the drug.

Following the immediate postoperative care the patient and family will need further evaluation and continued support. Postoperative changes such as hair loss, edema, and generalized weight loss can cause extreme depression due to altered body image. Patients left with residual neurologic deficits may require nutritional supplements, tube feedings, or hyperalimentation depending on the ultimate prognosis. Rehabilitation and supportive equipment may also assist in caring for the patient at home.

Patients with primary spinal cord tumors experience a similar but a less aggressive postoperative course. Nursing observations include observation of neurologic function and level of motor and sensory function. Bowel and bladder control may be altered depending on the location of the tumor. Paralysis or motor deficits will require additional rehabilitative consults. Prognostic factors and the amount of deficit will determine the amount of aggressive rehabilitative therapy. Support and follow up are needed to assist patients and families during this critical period.

Metastatic spinal cord tumors represent an oncology emergency that requires immediate medical intervention. Early signs include neck and back pain, motor weakness, and loss of sensation. Treatment includes radiation therapy followed by surgery if the tumor does not respond to radiation and use of steroids.

RADIATION THERAPY

If the tumor excision has been incomplete and the histologic report reveals a radiosensitive tumor, a patient may be scheduled for radiation therapy treatments after postoperative healing has taken place. Patient and family will need information on the length of treatment and expected side effects (see box below).

Spinal cord tumors are also treated with radiation, although the dose and treatment time may vary. The most serious consequence of spinal cord radiation is radiation myelopathy, which results in paraplegia and loss of bowel and bladder control. This is usually a late occurrence (6 to 15 months posttherapy). Family and patients need to be instructed to notify their physician if any symptoms occur. Symptoms of therapy complication may also manifest tumor recurrence. Constant anxiety exists even for those patients with better prognostic factors. Assessment of the emotional stability of the family and patient is ongoing and a critical nursing factor.

CHEMOTHERAPY AND BIOTHERAPY

Nursing management of those patients receiving chemotherapy and biotherapy treatments will include providing knowledge about drugs and their expected side effects (see box below). Monitoring side effects and appropriate treatment can ensure patient comfort and safety.[1]

PATIENT TEACHING PRIORITIES
RADIATION THERAPY

Knowledge of treatment schedule
Knowledge of skin care routine and care
  Marks are not to be washed off
  No creams or lotions to treatment site
Knowledge of radiation complications

PATIENT TEACHING PRIORITIES
CHEMOTHERAPY AND BIOTHERAPY

Knowledge of drug administration route and
  schedule
Knowledge of side effects and supportive measures
  Weight changes/loss of appetite
  Nausea
  Bruising and bleeding episodes
  Temperature changes
  Oral hygiene routine

Nursing Management

NURSING DIAGNOSIS

- Knowledge deficit related to lack of experience with chemotherapy routine and side effects.
- Nutrition alteration less than body requirements related to chemotherapy induced nausea.
- Altered oral mucus membrane related to chemotherapy administration.
- Potential for infection related to altered immune status.

Knowledge of the limited use and experimental nature of chemotherapy and biotherapy is important for patients and family. Because of the blood-brain barrier a limited number of drugs are considered effective therapy for CNS tumors. Patients will need to understand drug treatment schedules, follow-up blood work, and expected side effects.[13]

Potential side effects of biotherapy are listed in a box on p. 84. Nursing interventions include assessment of the patient's nutritional status, administration of antiemetics, small frequent bland feedings, monitoring intake and output, weight checks, and providing nutritional consultations.

Blood counts will assist with monitoring the hematologic and immune status alterations produced by chemotherapy treatments. Limiting visitors with colds, vigilant handwashing, monitoring changes in temperature, and observation of signs and symptoms of infection all are critical for those patients with lowered white blood cell counts. Reduction of hemoglobin and platelets may produce cellular damage. Patients should be observed for shortness of breath, weakness, fatigue, bruises, petechiae, and signs of active bleeding. Applying pressure to injection sites and limited use of rectal medications are also methods of controlling increased trauma and induction of bleeding.

Oral hygiene is essential to reduce risk of infection and to promote cleanliness and comfort. Oral assessment for evidence of yeast infections or lesions should be done daily. Specific mouth care protocols should follow physician's routine.

The administration of steroids is a common occurrence for many chemotherapy protocols, particularly CNS tumors. Common side effects from steroidal therapy can be found in a box on p. 84.[16] The nurse monitors the patient's response to steroid therapy by continued observation of vital signs, blood sugars, changes in emotional state, and potential gastrointestinal bleeding. Administration of antacids or gastric antagonists will assist with potential gastric complications. Body image changes from steroidal therapy, hair loss, or residual neurologic deficits may cause increased depression and withdrawal. Supportive care is required for both patients and family.

Biotherapy treatment requires constant observation for side effects. Treatment with biotherapy may be part of an experimental or researcher protocol. A box on p. 84 includes common side effects of biotherapy. Patients who experience increased symptoms may require removal from treatment because of an effort to keep data collection complete. Patients and families may experience anger and frustration over removal from the last hope of treatment.

Nursing Management

NURSING DIAGNOSIS

- Knowledge deficit related to lack of experience with radiation routine and side effects
- Skin integrity impaired related to radiation treatment modality
- Self-concept disturbance related to change in physical appearance/Tx markings, skin changes, and hair loss
- Sensory/perceptual changes related to postradiation damage.

Patients and family should be informed of the number of treatments that will be required. Normal treatments are daily for a period of 4 to 8 weeks. Transportation arrangements may be indicated if mobility limitations are present. A brief introduction to the Radiation Department and an explanation of the use of radiation therapy helps to eliminate additional anxieties.

Included in teaching of side effects will be knowledge of skin markings, hair loss, and skin changes near the radiation site. Instructions on skin care include not washing marks off and no application of creams near treatment. If treatments are given near the ear or in a visual field, hearing and vision may become impaired. Radiation treatments may also cause an increase in intracranial pressure and may require additional steroidal therapy. Reporting signs and symptoms of headache or changes in personality are important considerations. Emotional support is needed to deal with additional self-concept concerns.

- Potential for cellular injury related to chemotherapy side effects/steroid administration
- Altered self esteem related to chemotherapy-induced side effects

GERIATRIC CONSIDERATIONS

Diagnostic difficulties
Increased assessment (preoperatively and post-operatively)
Treatment modality complications
Rehabilitation
Home care referral

GERIATRIC CONSIDERATIONS

The normal age related changes in the geriatric population may lead to a delay or misdiagnosis of CNS tumors. Altered ambulation patterns, sensory impairment, decreased visual and hearing acuity, and changes in cognition are similar to CNS tumor changes. Once diagnosed these normal physiologic changes will also interfere with adequate postoperative assessment and the speed of recovery. Response to extensive surgery and treatment modalities may also produce increased side effects in the elderly. Rehabilitation needs and expanded home care referrals will be required to assist the expansion needs of the geriatric population. The box above summarizes these specific concerns.

PROGNOSIS

The ultimate prognosis of CNS tumors is determined by the following factors, histologic type, tumor grade, size and extent of tumor, patient's age, performance status, and residual tumor.[5,25] Survival rates range from complete cure to rapid deterioration and death. Glioblastoma multiforme (grade IV) has the poorest prognosis and a life expectancy of 9 to 12 months. Younger individuals who are neurologically intact survive longer than the geriatric (elderly) patient.

Metastatic lesions present a different prognosis and vary depending on whether the tumor is a single lesion or disseminated, size and cell type of primary tumor, other metastatic lesions, patient age, performance status, and the time from the treatment of the primary lesions until the start of the metastasis.[5,25]

CONCLUSION

Despite the low incidence of CNS tumors they continue to produce rapid deterioration, debilitation, and higher mortality than most primary cancers. Metastatic CNS tumors represent a continued challenge to the medical community. New clinical trails and surgical modalities are under investigation in the hopes of providing relief of symptoms and increased survival rates.

BIBLIOGRAPHY

1. Abner B and Collins J: Cancer chemotherapy and practice, Philadelphia, 1990, JB Lippincott.
2. Alvarez F and others: Malignant and atypical meningiomas: a reappraisal of clinical, histological, and computer tomographic features, Neurosurgery 20:688, 1987.
3. Amato CA: Malignant glioma: coping with devastating illness, J Neuroscience Nursing 23:20, 1991.
4. American Cancer Society: Cancer facts and figures—1993, Atlanta, 1993, American Cancer Society.
5. American Joint Committee on Cancer: Manual of staging of cancer, ed 3, Philadelphia, 1992, JB Lippincott.
6. Association for Brain Tumor Research: A primer of brain tumors, The Association, ed 5, 1991.
7. Baird SB and others: A cancer source book for nurses, Atlanta, 1991, American Cancer Society.
8. Bernstein M and others: Interstitial brachytherapy for malignant brain tumors: preliminary results. Neurosurgery 26:371,1990.
9. Blaney SM, Balis FM, and Poplack DC: Pharmacologic approaches to the treatment of meningeal malignancy, Oncology 5:107, 1991.
10. Boring CC, Squires TS, and Tong T: Cancer Statistics, CA 41:19, 1991.
11. Boss BJ, Heath J, and Sunderland PM: Alteration of neurologic function. In McConce KL and Heuther SE, editors: Pathophysiology the biologic basis for disease in adults and children, St. Louis, 1990, Mosby.
12. Cammermeyer M and Appledome C, editors: Core curriculum for oncology nursing, ed 3, Park Ridge, Ill, 1990, American Association of Neuroscience Nurses.
13. Chemotherapy and you: a guide to self help during treatment: National Cancer Institute No. 91-1136, 1990.
14. DeAngelis LM and others: Primary CNS lymphoma: managing patients with spontaneous and AIDS-related disease, Oncology 1:52, 1987.
15. Doenges ME, Moorhowe MF, and Geissler AC, editors: Nursing care plans, ed 2, Philadelphia, FA Davis Co.
16. Dropcho EJ and Seng-jaw S: Steroid-induced weakness in patients with primary brain tumors, Neurology 41:1235, 1991.
17. Drummond BC: Preventing increased intracranial pressure: nursing can make a difference. Focus Crit Care 17:116, 1990.
18. Edwards DK, Stupperick TK, and Welsh DM: Hyperthermia treatment for malignant tumors: nursing management during therapy. J Neurosci Nursing 23:34, 1991.
19. Edwards MS and others: Hyperfractioned radiation therapy for brain-stem glioma: a phase I-II trial, J Neurosurg 70:691, 1989.

20. Gullatte MM and Graves T: Advances in antineoplastic therapy, One Nur Forum 17:867, 1990.
21. Hart S: Neurological care. In Shaw M and others, editors: Illustrated manual of nursing practice, Springhouse, PA, 1991, Springhouse Corp.
22. Hickey JV: The clinical practice neurological and neurosurgical nursing, ed 2, Philadelphia, 1986, JB Lippincott.
23. Kornblith P, Walker M, and Cassady JR: Neurologic oncology, Philadelphia, 1987, JB Lippincott.
24. Leibel SA and others: Survival and quality of life after interstitial implantation of removable high-activity iodine-125 sources for treatment of patients with recurrent malignant gliomas: Int J Rad Oncol Biol Phys 17:1129, 1989.
25. Levin VA, Sheline GE, and Gutin PH: Neoplasms of the central nervous system. In DeVita VT, Hellman S, and Rosenberg SP, editors: Cancer: principles and practice of oncology, ed 3, Philadelphia, 1989, JB Lippincott.
26. Levin VA and others: Superiority of post-radiotherapy adjuvant chemotherapy with CCNU, procardazine, vincristine (PCV) over BCNU for anaplastic gliomas: (NCOG final report), Int J Rad Oncol Biol Phys 18:321, 1990.
27. Loeffler JA and others: Radiosurgery for brain metastases, PPU Updates 5:1, 1991.
28. Manual of Staging of Cancer: American Joint Committee on Cancer, ed 3, Philadelphia, 1988, JB Lippincott.
29. Owens B: Neurological cancer. In Clark J and McGee R, editors: Core curriculum for oncology nursing, ed 2, Philadelphia, 1992, WB Saunders Co.
30. Radiation therapy and you: a guide to self help during treatment: National Cancer Institute, No. 91-2227, Oct, 1990.
31. Ransohoff R, Koslow M, and Cooper P: Cancer of the central nervous system and pituitary. In Holled AI, Fink DJ, and Murphy GP, editors: American Cancer Society textbook of clinical oncology, Atlanta, 1991, American Cancer Society Inc.
32. Robinson C, Roy C, and Seager M: Central nervous system cancers. In Baird S, McCorkle R, and Grant M, editors: Cancer nursing: a comprehensive textbook, Philadelphia, 1991, WB Saunders Co.
33. Rodriquez L and Levin V: Does chemotherapy benefit the patient with a central nervous system glioma? Oncology (USA) 1:29, 1987.
34. Rowland LP: Merritt's textbook of neurology, ed 8, Philadelphia, 1989, Lea and Febiger.
35. Saba MT and Magolan JM: Understanding cerebral edema: implications for oncology nurses, One Nursing Forum 18:499, 1991.
36. Saleman M and Kaplan RS: Intracranial tumors in adults. In Haskell CM, editor: Cancer treatment, ed 3, Philadelphia, 1990, WB Saunders Co.
37. Schein PS: Decision making in oncology, Philadelphia, 1989, BC Decker.
38. Schenk E: Management of persons with neurologic problems. In Phipps WS and others, editors: Medical surgical nursing, ed 4, St. Louis, 1991, Mosby.
39. Shalter M and Mariebe EN: The nurse, pharmacology and drug therapy, Redwood City, CA, 1989, Allison-Wesley Pub. Co.
40. Shaw EG and others: Radiation therapy in the management of low grade supratentorial astrocytomas, J Neurosurg 70:853, 1989.
41. Speea WG and McArthur JC: Headache. In Harvey AM and others, editors: The principles and practice of medicine, Norwalk, CT, 1988, Appleton and Lange.
42. Sunderson N and Suite ND: Optimal use of the Ommaya reservoir in clinical oncology, Oncology 3:15, 1989.
43. Tennebaum L: Cancer chemotherapy: a reference guide, Philadelphia, 1989, WB Saunders Co.
44. Walleck C: Intracranial problems. In Lewis SM and Collier IC, editors: Medical surgical nursing, ed 3, St. Louis, 1992, Mosby.
45. Wegmann JA and Hakius P: Central nervous system cancers. In Groenwald SL and others, editors: Cancer nursing: principles and practice, ed 2, Boston, 1990, Jones & Bartlett.
46. Yasko S: Care of the client receiving external radiation therapy, Reston, VA, 1982, Reston-Hall Co.
47. Zulch KJ: Histological typing of tumors of the central nervous system. International Histologic Classification of Tumors 21:19, 1979.

CHAPTER 7

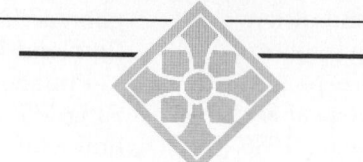

Breast Cancer

Rebecca Crane

Breast cancer is a major public health concern throughout the world. In almost all parts of Europe, and in North America, Australia, and New Zealand, breast cancer is the most frequent cancer in women as well as the leading cause of death for 35 to 54 year old women.[143] The incidence of breast cancer is increasing throughout the world for reasons not fully understood. It is predicted that by the year 2000 female breast cancer will be seen as often in developing countries as in developed countries.[113]

In the United States public awareness of breast cancer has grown considerably in recent years. Women in the public eye have spoken out about their experiences with breast cancer; media coverage has expanded to include breast health as well as breast cancer care information; legislative efforts have made screening mammography more available under insurance coverage; and grass roots movements have placed women's health care issues into the forefront in the competition for research dollars.[182]

It has only been in the last 15 years that the Halsted radical mastectomy has been replaced with more conservative surgery.[151,166,195] The "one-step" procedure (biopsy with frozen section diagnosis and immediate surgery) has been replaced with the two-step procedure. Women are expected to be involved in their treatment planning. The knowledge that breast cancer needed to be considered a systemic disease at the time of diagnosis led to increasing justification for the use of chemotherapy and hormonal manipulation as adjuncts to surgery to improve survival. Several questions regarding such adjuvant therapy continue to be addressed in ongoing national clinical trials:

(1) Which women with negative nodes should receive systemic treatment?

(2) What is the optimal timing for initiation of treatment?

(3) What is the best drug or combination of drugs to be used?

(4) What is the optimal duration of treatment?

(5) How does dose intensity impact survival?

Randomized clinical trials continue to assess the value of autologous bone marrow transplant in the treatment of women with breast cancer at high risk for recurrence and with advanced disease. New technologies in molecular genetics have enabled researchers to study the world of tumor suppressor genes and oncogenes, to begin to understand their effects on breast cancer initiation and development, and their role as prognostic variables.[103] Each of these endeavors lends hope that new and better methods for the treatment of breast cancer will lead to reductions in mortality. In addition, a "precedent-setting" randomized clinical trial launched in 1992 will assess the effects of tamoxifen for breast cancer prevention in 16,000 women at high risk for breast cancer.[103] The future in breast cancer prevention and treatment, as in all health care, is challenging clinically, economically, and emotionally.[62]

Focus will continue on early detection as the key to breast cancer control. Breast cancer screening guidelines continue to come under discussion, with efforts by major organizations to achieve widespread acceptance.[4,43] Mammography remains the mainstay for finding breast cancer before it has become clinically detectable. Coupled with regular and thorough breast self-examination (BSE) and regular periodic examination of the breasts by a professional, breast cancer can be found early, when it is more likely to be cured, often with conservative surgical management.

Studies of socioeconomic and ethnic differences in the practice of breast cancer control activities as well as stage at diagnosis and survival have pointed out the need for more attention to these factors in all phases of the breast care continuum.[61,69,98] As the population of women in the United States ages more consideration must also be given to the needs of an elderly population of women at risk for, diagnosed with, or followed after treatment for breast cancer.

The psychosocial impact of breast cancer screening, diagnosis, and treatment on the individual or family remains a major clinical and research responsibility for nursing, particularly in such challenging arenas as socioeconomic and ethnic diversity, the aging female population, and pregnancy after breast cancer. Because research results are at times confusing, conflicting, and controversial, women need help in integrating the information they are given whether regarding risk of developing breast cancer or treatment options after the diagnosis. Nurses have a key role in advocating for women whether in the political arena or at the bedside. Nurses need to be knowledgeable about current trends in breast cancer management so they can assist women throughout their treatment process. Nurses are also vital to public education efforts directed at breast cancer screening, teaching breast self-examination and guidelines for mammography and professional breast examinations, and portraying the hope of breast cancer cure with early detection.

EPIDEMIOLOGY

In 1991 the American Cancer Society revised the estimate of the average American woman's risk for developing breast cancer from one in ten to one in nine.[4,20] This translates into 182,000 newly diagnosed female cases in the United States during 1993. Men rarely develop breast cancer by comparison, accounting for only 1000 new cases during the same year. It is predicted that 46,000 women and 300 men will die from the disease in 1993.[4,20] These numbers reflect cases of invasive breast cancer. Carcinoma in situ (CIS) (discussed later in this chapter) will account for 25,000 additional new cases of breast cancer in women in 1993, increased from 5000 cases in 1988, 10,000 in 1989, 15,000 in 1990, and 20,000 in 1992.[4]

Overall, breast cancer incidence rates in women have continued to increase by about 3% per year since 1980.[4] This may be due, in part, to increased use of screening programs and therefore earlier detection, as well as to an aging population. However, other reasons for the increase remain unknown. Mortality rates have remained essentially unchanged over the past 50 years, despite improvements in treatment and earlier detection.[4] In contrast, lung cancer death rates

in women increased by 423% between 1955 and 1987 and surpassed breast cancer as the leading cause of cancer-related deaths in American women.[20] Breast cancer remains the most common site of cancer in American women.

The highest rates of breast cancer in the world are in the United States (by country), and specifically by population group, Hawaiians in Hawaii, white women in Hawaii, and white women in Alameda County in Northern California.[143] While black women generally have a lower incidence rate of breast cancer than white women in the United States, incidence rates have been increasing at a greater rate for black women.[121,143] While mortality rates for white women in the United States remain relatively stable, rates for black women have increased by 29% over the same period of time.[19] Black women in the United States are more likely to be diagnosed with breast cancer at a later stage, and subsequently have a 5-year relative survival rate that is nearly 13% lower than that for white women.[5] A disproportionate number of blacks in the United States are at lower socioeconomic levels; associated with an inadequate social and physical environment, inadequate information and education, a risk-promoting lifestyle, and impaired access to health care, this most likely accounts for more of the differences in cancer survival than race.[7,13,61]

ETIOLOGY AND RISK FACTORS

Research has shown that there is no known single cause of breast cancer. It is a heterogeneous disease, most likely developing as a result of many different factors that are not the same from woman to woman, and most of which are yet unknown. There are several characteristics that appear to increase the probability of a woman developing breast cancer.[44,173] These characteristics, or *risk factors*, when present have been shown to be associated with a greater incidence of breast cancer than when such factors are absent.[147] Women diagnosed with breast cancer may or may not have any of the risk factors. In fact, in one large prospective study by the American Cancer Society, 75% of the breast cancers detected occurred in women who had none of the most widely recognized higher risk factors.[181]

It is therefore understandable that the concept of risk in breast cancer is often confusing and frequently fear-inducing. Many women overestimate their risk of developing breast cancer.[105] This can lead to extremes of reaction from that of avoidance of health care to the opposite of worry and seeking of unnecessary repeated evaluations. Health care providers who do not understand risk may reinforce such fears. It is important for women and their nurses to understand the concept of risk and current knowledge of risk factors in order to develop individualized breast health plans of care.

Understanding Breast Cancer Risk

Breast cancer risk can be expressed as risk of development or risk of death from the disease. This chapter emphasizes risk as it relates to the development of breast cancer. *Absolute risk* is the number of breast cancer cases in a given population divided by the number of women in the population, expressed as an *average* risk for every woman in that population.[66] For white women in the United States today, this comes out to be about an 11% chance of developing breast cancer, most commonly expressed as the often quoted "1 in 9" statistic. This can be deceiving. This percentage is a cumulative lifetime risk, based on the sum of risks at different ages (age-specific risks) for all women from birth to 110 years of age![66,105] This does not take into account an individual woman's situation (her estimated lifespan, her current age, or the presence of other potentially high risk factors).

Absolute risk is sometimes expressed as age-specific risk for women in different age brackets. For example, white women ages 35 to 45 have a risk of developing breast cancer of 1%, whereas at ages 65 to 75 they have a 3% (age-specific) risk of developing breast cancer.[105] The risk is higher for older women because breast cancer occurs more frequently as age increases. The cumulative lifetime risk for white women 35 years of age (to the age of 110) is 10%, whereas at age 65 there is a 6.3% risk of developing breast cancer by the age of 110.[105] The cumulative lifetime risk is lower for the 65-year-old woman because she has fewer years left to be at risk (even if she did live to be 110, because it is still a comparison based on years of life remaining). This risk for developing breast cancer is also lower for black women in both groups because their overall incidence is lower.[105] Because absolute risk can be presented in different ways and does not take into account individual situations, it may be difficult to derive personal meaning from such numbers. Absolute risk may underestimate the risk to some women (e.g., those with a family history of breast cancer) and overestimate the risk for others (e.g., non-white women).[66] However, absolute risk is a very meaningful statistic when addressing the magnitude of the breast cancer problem in the United States, or for a very specific population.[66,105]

Relative risk is the incidence rate of breast cancer in a population of women with a known or suspected risk factor divided by the incidence rate of breast cancer in a population of women without that risk factor.[66,105] It is most often stated in studies addressing the epidemiology of breast cancer.[66] A woman with no risk factors would have a relative risk of 1.0; a relative risk greater than 1.0 indicates a greater likelihood of developing breast cancer than individuals without the risk factors.[124,187] For example, if the relative risk for a woman is 2.0, she is two times more likely than the population to develop breast cancer.[106] Relative risk expresses the excess risk of cancer that can be attributed to the risk factor.[66] The relative risk will increase as the number of risk factors increases.[181] To determine individual risk one cannot multiply the cumulative lifetime risk (absolute risk) by the relative risk and get a meaningful number. However, multiplying the *age-specific* risk by the *relative risk* will give a percent risk; for example, for the next 10 years of life (i.e., the woman age 35 with an age-specific risk of 1% between the ages of 35 and 45, and a relative risk of 2.0 would have about a 2% chance of developing breast cancer over the next 10 years).[66,105,124]

Attributable risk is the number of cancer cases in a population that are associated with given risk factors and that could potentially be prevented by alteration or removal of those factors.[124,181] It is most useful in public health policy and planning for cancer prevention and control. Unlike lung cancer, where there is a clear causal link with smoking, there are no such factors in breast cancer. Attributable risk does not account for the majority of breast cancer cases.[181] Where there is a known associated risk for some women, the factors involved (e.g., family history, nulliparity or late age at first birth) are ones over which they generally have little or no control.[106,142,181]

Risk Factors

The following information covers those risk factors most widely acknowledged or suspected to increase the probability of a woman developing breast cancer. GENDER.   Women are more likely than men to develop breast cancer. Breast cancer accounts for 32% of all cancers in women and less than 1% of the cancers in men.[20,44,173]

AGE.   The incidence of breast cancer increases with age. Most breast cancer cases are diagnosed in women 40 years of age and older.[8,31,105] Most women who develop breast cancer will have no known risk factor other than being female and over 40 years of age.

PERSONAL HISTORY OF CANCER.   A previous diagnosis of breast cancer increases a woman's lifetime risk for developing a second breast cancer in the opposite (contralateral) breast. Estimates are that this lifetime risk is approximately 15%,[66] or a relative risk in the range of 3.0 to 4.0.[106] The risk has been shown to be even higher in women who also have a family history of breast cancer.[66,106] In addition, a previous history of primary ovarian or endometrial cancer has been associated with an increased risk of breast cancer (relative risk under 1.5).[66,106,142]

FAMILY HISTORY OF CANCER.   Women with a family history of breast cancer in a first-degree relative (mother, sister, or daughter) have a relative risk of 2.0 to 3.0.[66,106] This is a risk two to three times that of the general population. Risk increases further if both the mother and sister have had breast cancer (relative risk greater than 4.0).[65,106] Risk is greatest in women with a familial history of premenopausal bilateral breast cancer or a familial cancer syndrome.[65] A paternal history of breast cancer also has been shown to increase an individual's risk of developing breast cancer.[105]

GENETICS.   There are very few families in which the incidence of breast cancer can be attributed to genetics alone; yet when that is the case, lifetime risk can reach 50%.[65] In some families the frequency of breast cancer can only be accounted for by chance, or by interactions between shared environmental and genetic factors that are less well understood.[65] It is important to study such families, because there is growing evidence that there may be genetic transmission of tumor suppressor genes in both hereditary and nonhereditary breast cancer.[106] Lynch has described the following clinical features of possible hereditary breast cancer:[128]

- Earlier age at diagnosis
- Bilateral breast cancer
- Predisposition to cancers in other sites (e.g., colon, ovary, uterus)
- Genetic transfer occurring through the mother's or father's genes (an autosomal dominant disease susceptibility gene[129])

No single test is currently available to determine who carries the specific gene(s) that increase the susceptibility to breast cancer.[105] Recent advances in molecular technology have enabled scientists to study in great detail the genetic structure of individual chromosomes and thus some of the mechanisms by which tumor suppressor genes work in cancer cell growth.[103,105] In 1990 the discovery was made of the tumor suppressor gene (oncogene) p53 on the short arm of chromosome 17, which is associated with an increased risk of breast and other cancers.[65,103,105] On the long arm of chromosome 17 several genes have been discovered that may influence breast cancer growth and invasion—one of these, the oncogene HER-2/*neu* (or c-*erb*B-2), is often overexpressed in breast and ovarian cancers and is associated with more aggressive disease.[103] It is possible that there will be new discoveries in the near future of other genes that may be responsible for the initiation or promotion of breast cancer growth.[65] This is perhaps the most exciting area of research, with the hope of improved understanding of breast cancer inheritance and development, associated risk factors and, potentially, prevention.[65,106]

EARLY MENARCHE AND LATE MENOPAUSE.   The exact role of hormones in the etiology of breast cancer has not been precisely determined. *Early onset of menarche* (before age 12) and *late menopause* (after age 50) are each associated with increased risk of breast cancer.[84,106] Studies have shown that risk also increases as the time interval lengthens between menarche and menopause.[84] Regular ovulatory cycles with cumulative exposure to estrogen therefore appears to be the major determinant of this risk.[84] The greater the number of years of menstrual activity (e.g., 40) the greater the risk of developing breast cancer.[66,84] The lifetime exposure of the breast to estrogen appears to be the most convincing factor,[84] though of great significance is the role of other circulating hormones and/or metabolites, such as estradiol, progesterone, and prolactin.[106] Factors that have contributed to trends toward a lowering of the age at menarche in countries such as the United States include better nutrition and infectious disease control.[84] Surgically or radiation-induced menopause (i.e., bilateral oophorectomy or pelvic irradiation) reduces breast cancer risk, perhaps slightly greater than with natural menopause.[84]

REPRODUCTIVE HISTORY.   Having no children (*nulliparity*) or the *first full-term pregnancy after age 30* places a woman at an increased risk.[106,173] The relative risk is higher for the woman who delays childbirth than for the nulliparous woman.[105,106] Childbirth at an early age (before age 20) has been shown to have a protective effect.[84,105,106] The mechanism behind this reduction in risk remains unknown, but most likely results from changes in the actual breast tissue or the hormones that make the breast tissue less susceptible to cancer formation.[106] The trend for more American women to delay pregnancy until a later age, thus increasing the exposure of breast tissue to estrogen, has potentially contributed to the increasing incidence of breast cancer.[142] Some authors[105,106] suggest that more studies of such women are needed, as most present day studies reflect benefits to women who became pregnant many years ago, or who were diagnosed with breast cancer after the age of 50.

Some studies have shown that as the number of months of breastfeeding increases there is an associated reduction in the risk of developing breast cancer, particularly for premenopausal women.[106,142] Such findings are not without question, though it would appear that if the number of ovulatory cycles and exposure to estrogens is related to breast cancer risk, this risk would also be reduced if lactation led to a reduction in the exposure to estrogen.[84]

BENIGN BREAST DISEASE.   The term *benign breast disease* is frequently misunderstood in discussions of risk.[105] The term encompasses a broad array of histopathologic diagnoses that are commonly experienced by women clinically at some time in their lives but that are never biopsied. Some question why such a common condition should be termed a "disease". Many of these so-called "diseases" are not associated with any increased risk of breast cancer. Fibrocystic disease is a catchall term to describe clinical symptoms and findings of local or generalized lumpiness, pain, or cystic changes. *Fibrocystic changes* may be a more appropriate term to describe these often normal breast changes.

Benign breast lesions, when pathologic diagnosis is made, are classified into three groups. *Nonproliferative lesions*, when found alone, are not associated with any increased risk of breast cancer. These include histologically diagnosed cysts, apocrine metaplasia, papillary apocrine change, epithelial-related calcifications, fibroadenomas, and mild hyperplasia.[177] The presence of gross cysts in women with a family history of breast cancer has been shown to be associated with increased risk.[177]

Proliferative lesions without atypia include moderate or florid hyperplasias of the usual type, sclerosing adenosis, and intraductal papillomas. There is some evidence that multiple as opposed to single papillomas, occurring peripherally rather than centrally, are susceptible to breast cancer development.[177] Occurring in the ductal or glandular tissue of the breast, proliferative lesions without atypia have been associated with only a slightly increased risk (1.5 to 2.0) of breast cancer during the 10 to 20 years after biopsy.[48,157,158,177]

Proliferative lesions with atypia, or *atypical hyperplasia*, constitute the third category of benign breast disease and are most associated with increased breast cancer risk.[157,158] Only 3% to 5% of benign breast disease biopsies are found to have atypical cells.[105,157] Atypical hyperplasia can be found in either ductal or lobular tissue. It is a proliferation of abnormal looking cells within the duct or lobule.[105,142,157,158,163] The diagnosis by biopsy of atypical ductal or lobular hyperplasia is associated with a relative risk of 4.0 to 5.0 during the 10 to 20 years after biopsy.[106,157,158]

If these cells continue to proliferate and take on the appearance of cancer cells the lesion then becomes "carcinoma in situ," or cancer confined to the site of origin, and further increases the risk of developing invasive breast cancer.[105,124,157,158] Treatment of women with this diagnosis will be discussed later in this chapter.

OBESITY AND DIETARY FAT. Obesity has been shown to be associated with increased risk of developing breast cancer in postmenopausal women.[106,142] Excess adipose tissue is rich in the necessary enzyme to convert estrone and estradiol from their precursors.[95] Consequently, obese women may have increased levels of circulating estrogens, which can af-

fect hormone-dependent breast cancer cells.[95] Another observation has been that obesity is associated with decreased levels of sex-hormone-binding globulin (SHBG), which normally binds estradiol and would prevent stimulation of breast cancer cells.[95,106] Seidman and others[181] used the measure of "relative weight index 110 or more" in their study of high risk categories, defined as 10 percent or more above the average weight for a given woman's height and age. Kelsey and Gammon[106] described being "heavy" as associated with a relative risk of 1.1 to 1.9. Others have described being 40 percent above ideal body weight as increasing one's risk of developing breast cancer.[8]

There is an increased incidence of breast cancer in industrialized countries with a high socioeconomic status and an increased consumption of dietary fat, suggesting a relationship. Migrant studies evaluating the daughters of immigrants from Japan (where incidence of breast cancer is low and dietary fat consumption is low) to California have shown rates of breast cancer similar to those for American white women.[143,186] Dietary factors said to be associated with these variations in breast cancer incidence also are different for pre- and post-menopausal women.[105,186] Yet the studies to date are difficult to interpret.[67,186] Dietary fat consumption in these studies has ranged from 25% to 49% or more of total calories from fat; the U.S. per capita fat intake was about 36.5% of total calories in 1985.[186] A reduction in fat intake to 20% to 30% of total calories and the addition of high fiber foods have been suggested as healthy dietary habits because of the potential for cancer risk reduction as well as risk reduction in other illnesses such as heart disease.[8,124,173] Further studies addressing the relationship between dietary factors and estrogen or other hormones and breast cancer risk are necessary to clarify the association with breast cancer.

RADIATION EXPOSURE. There has been a greater incidence of breast cancer than expected in women exposed to ionizing radiation for the treatment of tuberculosis or postpartum mastitis, or in survivors of the atomic bombs at Hiroshima and Nagasaki.[18,136,143] Sensitivity to the effects of radiation is greatest in childhood (ages 10 to 14) and decreased to almost negligible by age 40.[143] This susceptibility to radiation is important when considering potential risk from radiation with such procedures as mammography.[143] The current availability of low-dose mammography coupled with regular use in women *over 40* years of age makes the risk from radiation exposure almost negligible.[144]

EXOGENOUS HORMONES. Because breast cancers are thought to be hormone related, numerous studies have been done to evaluate the risk associated with the use of oral contraceptives (OC) and estrogen replacement therapy (ERT). Research results have been contradictory and inconclusive. The majority of these studies have shown no increased risk for the majority of women.[84,105,106,142]

Oral contraceptive use became widespread in the early 1960s. Adequate follow-up data are only recently becoming available to identify possible latent effects associated with OC use and to estimate the resulting breast cancer risk. Some studies have suggested an increased risk associated with early onset of use and long-term use (more than 6 years).[84] Important considerations in future studies include the differences in OC composition over time (earlier OC had higher estrogen content than many available today); age at onset of use; duration of use; and use by women with existing known other high risk factors.[66,84] Others suggest, after reviewing the data, that cautious use of OC might be prudent in the very young or perimenopausal.[66]

In January 1989, the Fertility and Maternal Health Drugs Advisory Committee of the Food and Drug Administration concluded no relationship exists between OC use and breast cancer, and recommended further studies. In the fall of 1989 the Committee on the Relationship Between Oral Contraceptives and Breast Cancer within the Institute of Medicine[96] was assembled to examine the etiology of breast cancer as related to OC. Its report recommended that no fundamental change in clinical practice with respect to the use of OC is supported by the knowledge to date about OC and risk of breast cancer.[96] It also recommended that women seeking contraception be given adequate information and counseling as to the current ambiguities in the knowledge to date of the relationship between OC and breast cancer.[96]

Estrogen replacement therapy (ERT) in postmenopausal women has been available in the U.S. since 1942, with widespread use by the 1960s.[105] With new concern about endometrial cancer risk in the late 1970s progesterone was added for a cyclic regimen.[84] In postmenopausal women such ERT has been used to manage the menopausal symptoms of hot flashes and dyspareunia secondary to atrophic vaginitis. In recent years ERT has also been employed for the prevention of osteoporosis and to reduce the risk of cardiovascular disease. Studies to date of the relationship between ERT and breast cancer remain controversial, with some suggestion of increased risk when use is prolonged (more than 9 years), with higher doses, and with the addition of progesterone.[47,66,84,106] Women who take unopposed estrogens have an increased risk for endometrial cancer.[173] Until further studies address these issues, women should be advised of current knowledge and should weigh the potential benefits and risks before undertaking ERT.[66,84,105,124]

ALCOHOL CONSUMPTION.   Several studies have shown a slight increased risk associated with alcohol consumption.[106] Unfortunately, the studies have been inconsistent with respect to the amount and type of alcohol use correlated with an increased risk. The age at which drinking begins (under 30 years of age), volume, and duration of use appear to be important variables in understanding risk with alcohol consumption.[105,106] The association with younger age at onset of alcohol consumption may be related to the developing and potentially susceptible breast tissue.[186] Heavy alcohol consumption may also be associated with poor nutrition.[105] Further study is needed of each of these variables.

OTHER.   Associations between mammographic parenchymal (tissue) patterns and breast cancer risk remain unclear.[66,106] Higher socioeconomic status is associated with a higher risk of developing breast cancer, but lower socioeconomic status is associated with a greater risk of dying from the disease.[19,61] Ethnicity also is associated with risk, with nonwhite women being less at risk of developing breast cancer, but at greater risk of dying from the disease.[19,61] No clear associations with increased risk of breast cancer have been found for cigarette smoking, stress, personality type, cerumen (ear wax), exposure to electromagnetic fields, caffeine, or hair dyes.[66,105,106]

For the woman who appears to have an increased risk based on family history or other factors, a detailed assessment should be conducted to determine actual individual risk. "Risk Analysis" services are available in many breast centers throughout the United States.[105,187] This risk assessment should thoroughly explore a woman's perceptions of risk, her attitudes toward and beliefs about early detection methods (BSE, CBE, mammography) as well as her participation in each, and her needs for information. An important message at this time is that risk relates to developing breast cancer and not dying from it.[187] Screening guidelines should be vigorously followed; some suggest an earlier age for beginning mammography, and more frequent CBE.[67,187] There is no clear preventive intervention. Reduction in alcohol and dietary fat intake, and weight loss if postmenopausal and obese, are some measures that the individual can take, but none have a clear association with breast cancer prevention. Prophylactic mastectomy is quite controversial.[67,187] It should probably only be considered in women with a clearly hereditary cancer and a history of biopsy-proven atypical hyperplasia or lobular carcinoma in situ (LCIS).[67]

There remains much to learn about risk factors for breast cancer and the effects of combinations of risk factors now known or suspected. New risk factors need to be identified, risk quantified, and control measures studied. Most women who will be diagnosed with breast cancer have no known risk factors. Current knowledge about risk factors in breast cancer will help the nurse guide the patient in obtaining personally meaningful information. In most cases interventions will need to be focused less on risk factor reduction and more on developing a plan of care for the early detection of breast cancer when it occurs.

PREVENTION, SCREENING, AND DETECTION

It is not known what causes breast cancer or how to prevent the disease. Breast cancer is a heterogeneous disease; in other words, it is a disease of many characteristics, varying from woman to woman in its potential for development, growth, and metastasis. The epidemiology of the disease indicates that it is hormonally influenced, with the duration of exposure to elevated levels of circulating estrogens being a primary factor in the promotion of cancer cell development over several years of time. This period of time of cell promotion is characterized by reversibility. If this exposure could be reduced or if the adverse effects of the exposure could be prevented, breast cancer might be prevented.[123] The breast cancer prevention trial described at the beginning of this chapter is one study to evaluate the role of tamoxifen for breast cancer prevention in a group of women at higher risk for breast cancer development. This is a placebo-controlled trial, meaning that women who consent to participate in the study are randomized to either the tamoxifen or a placebo. Because there is no known means to prevent breast cancer, the placebo is necessary to control for any bias that might result. To participate in the study women must be 60 years of age or older, or 35 years of age or older with a risk profile that meets pre-established criteria. Women who participate will be on the medication (tamoxifen or placebo) for 5 years and followed regularly thereafter as well. Because estrogens are known to have an important role in reducing rates of coronary heart disease and osteoporosis in postmenopausal women, these will be closely monitored as part of the study. The purpose of the trial is to test the effectiveness of long-term tamoxifen in preventing the occurrence of invasive breast cancer as well as in reducing mortality from the disease. It will be some time before the results of this or other studies evaluating prevention will translate into interventions that clearly have a major impact on the female population.

Early detection is therefore the most important means of control of breast cancer. Research has shown that survival is directly related to the stage of the disease at diagnosis. The American Cancer Society (ACS) has developed *screening guidelines* for asymptomatic women that incorporate three methods of early detection[4,43]:

1. *Breast self-examination (BSE)* should be performed monthly by all women beginning at age 20.
2. *Clinical breast examination (CBE)* by a health professional should be done every 3 years for women ages 20 to 40 and annually after age 40.
3. *Mammography* should begin by age 40. Routine screening mammography should be performed every 1 to 2 years for women ages 40 to 49, and then every year beginning at age 50.

A woman with known risk factors (e.g., family history) or chronic symptomatology should be advised to consult with her physician regarding the frequency and specificity of clinical examinations and mammography for her situation. Nurses have a major role in teaching these potentially lifesaving guidelines to all women. For greatest effectiveness, frequency (regular and periodic) and proficiency (skill and thoroughness) are key concepts to consider in each screening method.

Mammography

Mammography is the only proven means of detecting breast cancer before it can be detected by physical examination or BSE. Screening mammography is used to detect cancer in *asymptomatic* women. By the time a lesion is 1 cm in diameter and detectable by palpation, it has been estimated that it may have been present for 8 or more years.[81] Figure 7-1 depicts the average-size lump detected with BSE and mammography. Since the HIP (Health Insurance Plan of New York) study in the early 1960s and the Breast Cancer Detection Demonstration Project (BCDDP) in the 1970s, screening mammography has repeatedly been shown to be effective in reducing the number of deaths associated with breast cancer through the detection of clinically occult lesions less than 1 mm in size.[15,54,91,180]

Mammography is also useful in evaluating high-risk women and women with breasts difficult to palpate (e.g., breasts that are large and pendulous or with severe fibrocystic changes). Ultrasound is helpful in conjunction with mammography for diagnostic purposes to help differentiate a fluid-filled cyst from a solid mass. Other methods for imaging the breasts, such as thermography, diaphonography (transillumination), and magnetic resonance imaging (MRI) have been evaluated but have not been shown to be effective in screening for breast cancer.[173] When properly performed mammography can effectively detect 85% to 90% of breast cancers. It is possible for 10% to 15% of malignant lesions to be undetected.[15] Therefore, in women with clinical symptoms, a negative mammogram does not rule out the need for a biopsy. Dense breast tissue is the major reason for false-neg-

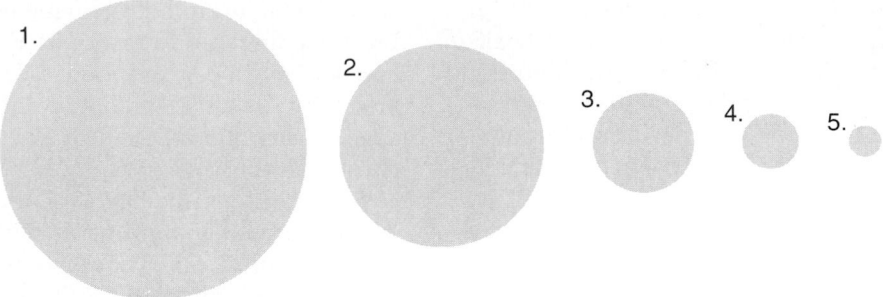

Figure 7–1 **1;** Average-size lump found by women untrained in BSE. **2;** Average-size lump found by women practicing occasional BSE. **3;** Average-size lump found by women practicing regular BSE. **4;** Average-size lump found by first mammogram. **5;** Average-size lump found by regular mammograms. (From Spence W: Breast care: the good news, Waco, TX, 1986, Health Edco, Inc.)

ative readings, but faulty equipment or skill of the technologist, or errors in interpretation can also be the cause.[15]

Screening mammography generally consists of two views of each breast: one from side to side (lateral or oblique) and one from top to bottom (craniocaudal).[15] For each view the breast is compressed in order to decrease the thickness of the breast and enable better visualization of the structures of the tissue, also reducing the amount of radiation.[15] It may be momentarily uncomfortable for women but explaining the rationale for the pressure may help them understand the importance of that discomfort. It is also helpful if premenstrual women do not have the screening mammogram immediately before their menses, for the similar concern about comfort. Xeromammography was popular for several years beginning in the early 1970s but has largely been replaced with film-screen mammography. Refinements in technology have made film-screen mammography the preferred breast imaging method because of its higher image contrast, lower radiation dose, and less equipment downtime.[15]

Concern has been expressed regarding the risks related to the radiation exposure from mammograms. The radiation dose delivered has been significantly lowered since the 1960s and, with equipment dedicated solely to mammography, the risk is negligible. The benefits must always be weighed against the potential risk. Because of this and other concerns about mammography, the American College of Radiology and other organizations joined together to issue a policy statement on mammography in breast cancer screening centers.[8] Their guidelines include recommendations for the presence of:

- Dedicated mammographic equipment with regular monitoring to ensure that the minimum necessary radiation dose is administered
- Radiologic technologists who are specially trained and experienced in mammography

- Radiologists with demonstrated experience and competence in mammography

Along with these guidelines the American College of Radiology now offers a voluntary accreditation program for mammography facilities.

Cost can prohibit some women from obtaining screening mammograms. The cost for a screening mammogram can range from $50 to over $200. Through efforts of the ACS, NCI, and other organizations, costs for screening mammography have been declining in many parts of the United States, and insurance coverage has increased.

Despite its value, mammography is still underutilized. One reason has been physician disagreement with following the ACS guidelines for mammography. A 1989 survey of over 1000 U.S. physicians revealed that while physicians reported a greater inclination (since 5 years previously) to order screening mammography in asymptomatic women, reasons given for not ordering a mammogram included concerns about affordability and cost; reliability of the test; availability of a qualified radiologist or equipment; doubt of need if no symptoms or family history; and radiation risk.[3] In studies of womens' attitudes about mammography, most have heard of the test but fewer (who are eligible) have had a mammogram.[8,15] One of the major reasons has been the lack of a referral or recommendation from their physician.[8,15,60,144] Fear of radiation, discomfort, or of cancer, the cost, belief one is not at risk, and sometimes the belief that other tests (such as the physical examination) are adequate have also been reported as barriers.[3,15,60,132] Physician and public education efforts are important to overcome such barriers.

Breast Self-Examination

BSE is a free, private, and relatively simple examination. Nearly 90% of all palpable breast lumps are discovered by the woman herself.[173] Most physicians advocate BSE as a useful health care practice, and the technique essentially has no adverse effects.[8,112,173] In areas of the world where mammography or health care is not readily available, BSE may have important applicability.[144] There is increasing evidence in the research literature that women who perform BSE sometimes or regularly are more likely to discover smaller tumors and to have a smaller number of positive lymph nodes at diagnosis compared to women whose cancer is discovered accidentally.[12,32,59,93,183] Estimates are that regular practice of BSE could reduce the overall breast cancer mortality by approximately 19%.[73] The first prospective randomized controlled trial to evaluate the effectiveness of BSE was begun in 1985 in Leningrad and Moscow with the World Health Organization (WHO) and has encouraging preliminary results.[113]

Most women in the United States know about BSE, yet only 19% to 40% of them report practicing BSE on a regular basis.[32] Many women who practice BSE do not do it thoroughly (proficiently). Compliance may be poor for a variety of reasons[11,26,27,33,46,57,171] such as: inadequate knowledge of how to do BSE; lack of confidence in ability to perform BSE and to detect abnormalities; fear of finding something; discomfort with touching breasts; lack of confidence in BSE as a means of detecting changes; forgetfulness; and lack of motivation. How effective will a woman be if she performs BSE monthly but poorly, or thoroughly but less often?

Through one-on-one education that is repeated at intervals, monthly reminders, and encouragement by health professionals, compliance rates may improve. Studies have shown that education needs to include factual information about normal breast changes, breast cancer, and early detection, and should promote positive attitudes or values.[32] Pamphlets and video instruction are passive teaching methods that have not been shown to be effective when used alone.[11] They also may not be ethnically sensitive, in the language of the woman being taught, or at a reading level that is appropriate.[140] BSE is a motor skill that entails coordination of palpation, movement, and sensation.[103] Opportunities for women to practice on silicone breast models and on themselves with feedback during the practice are crucial, and may also enhance self confidence in BSE performance.[11,32,33,46,130,172]

Women should be advised to perform BSE monthly. Premenopausal women should examine their breasts 5 to 7 days after their menstrual period begins. At this time their breasts may be less engorged and tender, thus allowing a more thorough and less distorted examination. Nonmenstruating or postmenopausal women should select the same day each month to do BSE. Selecting an anniversary or birth date is one suggestion to encourage women to remember. Women who are pregnant or breastfeeding should still examine themselves monthly, but the breastfeeding mother should do so soon after her breasts have been emptied. Women who have had breast cancer surgery should still perform BSE, with special attention to the surgical scar area and to the chest wall (postmastectomy).

BSE includes inspection and palpation of the breasts in both a standing and lying position. Attention is focused on evaluating for change. It is best done in an atmosphere that is unhurried and most comfortable for the individual woman. A thorough BSE will usually take 20 to 30 minutes. The ACS and NCI are two sources of patient and professional educational materials on BSE. The MammaCare® Learning System is perhaps the most comprehensive and researched program, emphasizing proficiency through individualized instruction, the use of specially designed breast palpation models, an instruction manual, and a video program for self-learning.[133] Use of this system as well as other reviews of BSE proficiency are in the literature.[8,33,57,160,172] The components of BSE for proficiency in practice include: *inspection* of the breasts in front of a mirror, *palpation* of the entire area of the breast using the flat *pads of the fingers* at different levels of *pressure*, in a specific *pattern* and *motion* within that pattern (i.e., small dime-sized circles in a vertical strip, wedge, or circular pattern), most easily done when in a flat or partial side-lying (upper body turned at 45-degree angle) *position* (Figure 7-2).[8,33,172]

Inspection of the breasts is best conducted standing in front of a mirror, with the arms at the sides, both breasts exposed for complete visualization of the skin surface, nipple/areola complex, and breast contour. Turning slightly side to side, the breasts are inspected for any evidence of skin retraction, puckering, dimpling, erythema, vein prominence, and presence of other characteristics such as nevi. The nipples should be noted as everted or inverted. Women with pendulous breasts should lift the breast on either side to inspect the skin on the lower side of the breasts and the chest area. It is normal that one breast may be slightly larger than the other. With hands on the hips pressing in and down, the same observation is repeated. This is further repeated with the arms over the head, and with the arms in front while leaning forward.

Palpation is then performed lying down as previously described. Lotion can be applied to the flat pads of the fingers in order to smooth the skin. With respect to areas of the breast that may warrant additional attention, the upper outer quadrant of the breast is the most common location of most types of breast cancer, followed by the central area of the breast around the nipple.[164] Common errors in technique include *not palpating deeply enough at different levels of pressure, not palpating the entire breast tissue area*

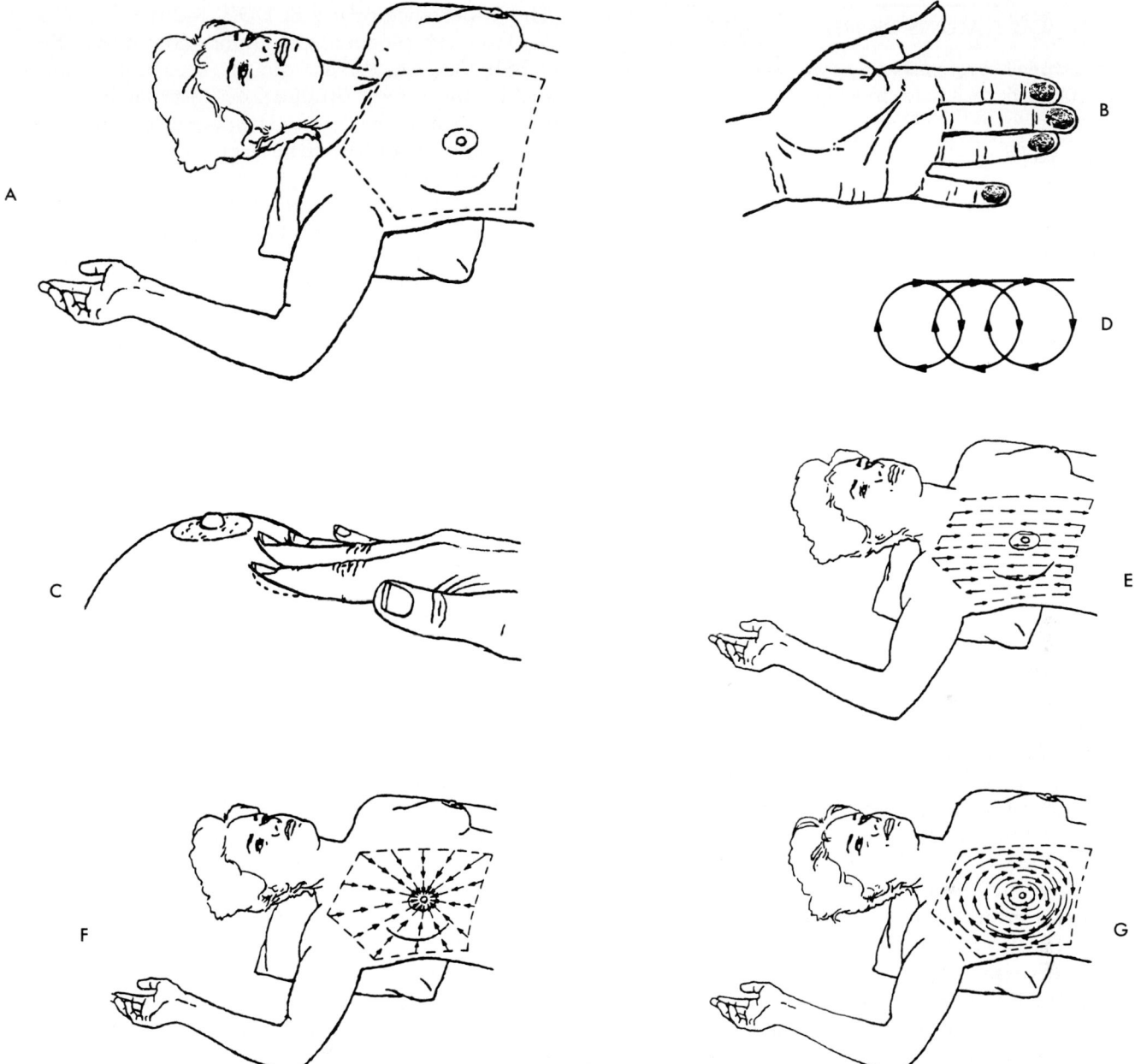

Figure 7–2 Breast self-examination. **A,** The perimeter of the area to be examined should include all breast tissue. This area is bounded by a line that extends vertically from the middle of the axilla (armpit) to the rib just beneath the breast and continues horizontally along the underside of the breast to the mid sternum (middle of the breast bone). It continues up the mid sternum to the clavicle (collarbone), and along the lower border of the clavicle to the shoulder and back to the mid-axilla. **B,** Palpation is performed with the pads of the fingers. **C** and **D,** Move your fingers (3 or 4) in small circles about the size of a dime. Varying levels of pressure (light, medium, and firm) should be applied to each spot palpated. Moderate pressure is illustrated. The following patterns can be used for the examination: **E,** Vertical strip. **F,** Wedge. **G,** Circle. (Courtesy American Cancer Society.)

including behind the nipple, & using the fingertips for palpation rather than the flat pads of the three middle fingers. Palpation needs to be done at three levels of pressure: light, medium, and deep. The light pressure will detect any changes in the skin that too firm pressure might push away. Medium pressure will enable a woman to feel the glandular and fatty tissue of the breast. Deep pressure allows examination of the breast to the underlying ribs and muscle. The fingertips should be avoided because they tend to push any lumps or changes away. Women should be reminded not to do the examination too hurriedly. Beginning at the axilla or in the upper outer quadrant, the entire breast, axilla, and supraclavicular areas need to be examined. This area extends from the axilla to the bra-line, over to the sternum, up to the supraclavic-

---

CLINICAL FEATURES OF BREAST CANCER

Most common symptoms at presentation

Mass (particularly if hard, irregular, nontender) or thickening in the breast or axilla

Spontaneous, persistent, unilateral nipple discharge that is serosanguineous, bloody, or watery in character

Nipple retraction or inversion

Change in size, shape or texture of breast (asymmetry)

Dimpling or puckering of the skin

Scaly skin around the nipple

Symptoms of local or regional spread

Redness, ulceration, edema, or dilated veins

Peau d'orange skin changes

Enlargement of lymph nodes in the axilla

Evidence of metastatic disease

Enlargement of lymph nodes in the supraclavicular (collar bone) cervical area

Abnormal chest x-ray with or without pleural effusion

Elevated alkaline phosphatase, elevated calcium, positive bone scan, and/or bone pain related to bone involvement

Abnormal liver function tests

---

ular notch, along the clavicle to the shoulder, and back to the axilla.[172] This completed pattern is followed by a gentle pressure, or milking action, on the breast and nipple to check for nipple discharge, and additional palpation in the axilla. Some women may additionally wish to repeat the entire BSE in the shower.

It is crucial to emphasize that when first performing BSE a woman is learning her normal breast characteristics so that any future variations or changes can be recognized and evaluated. If she notices a change on one breast, she may wish to check the other breast for symmetry. She should be encouraged to have a plan of action should she detect a change that needs evaluation. This might be to call her physician for an appointment. Prompt medical attention should be sought if any of the clinical features or common symptoms of breast cancer are noted in the box above. Although fear is a common feeling experienced when a new change or symptom is discovered, women can be encouraged that most breast lumps discovered are benign.[4,8,146]

Clinical Breast Examination

CBE is the most commonly employed screening technique for breast cancer today.[3,56] In the HIP study previously described, CBE contributed significantly to reductions in mortality for women in the 40 to 49 year old group who were diagnosed with breast cancer.[144]

The importance of the BCDDP findings was that each of the screening measures (mammography, CBE, and BSE) detected breast cancer cases not initially found by the other.[8] Studies have estimated that a lump of 0.3 cm can be detected by palpation in silicone breast models.[56] For CBE to be as effective as possible, the professional performing the examination needs to be proficient. Research suggests, however, that health professionals vary considerably in their confidence in and ability to perform CBE.[56,144,146] One study of registered nurses found an association between high confidence in their own BSE and utilization of CBE in elderly women.[127] Unfortunately many women relegate the examination of their breasts solely to their health care providers. A physician or other health professional does not have the advantage of being familiar with a woman's normal monthly breast irregularities when examinations are only performed yearly. The California Division of the American Cancer Society has piloted a program to help health professionals become more proficient in their performance of CBE, outlined in a publication describing seven areas of proficiency, modeled after those for BSE (Figure 7-2).[6]

During CBE the health professional can demonstrate BSE technique, explain the rationale for each step, and encourage women to be partners in their care by continuing monthly BSE at home. In addition, a woman's particular normal anatomic variations can be pointed out. Signs and symptoms of breast abnormalities can be discussed, and risk factors for breast cancer discussed, with particular attention to what that means to the individual woman. The establishment of a relationship of trust between the health professional and the patient may lead to improved participation in breast cancer screening activities.

In the United States the goal for breast cancer screening by the year 2000 is that 80% of women aged 50 to 70 will be receiving annual CBE and mammography. This is increased from 45% for CBE alone and 15% for mammography.[74] Particular attention needs to be paid to special populations for all aspects of breast cancer screening. Problems in access, knowledge, and priorities are evident in the socioeconomically disadvantaged, with resultant higher mortality.[7,61,203] Reports of cancer screening availability for women in public health clinics,[200] or rural settings,[72] studies of mammography utilization[23,100] and BSE practice by nonwhite women,[69,98,152,201] the elderly,[34,37,130] or high-risk women[90,102] graphically demonstrate the need to find improved ways of reaching these populations with breast cancer screening.

Regular mammograms for eligible women, regular physical examinations, and monthly BSE can detect

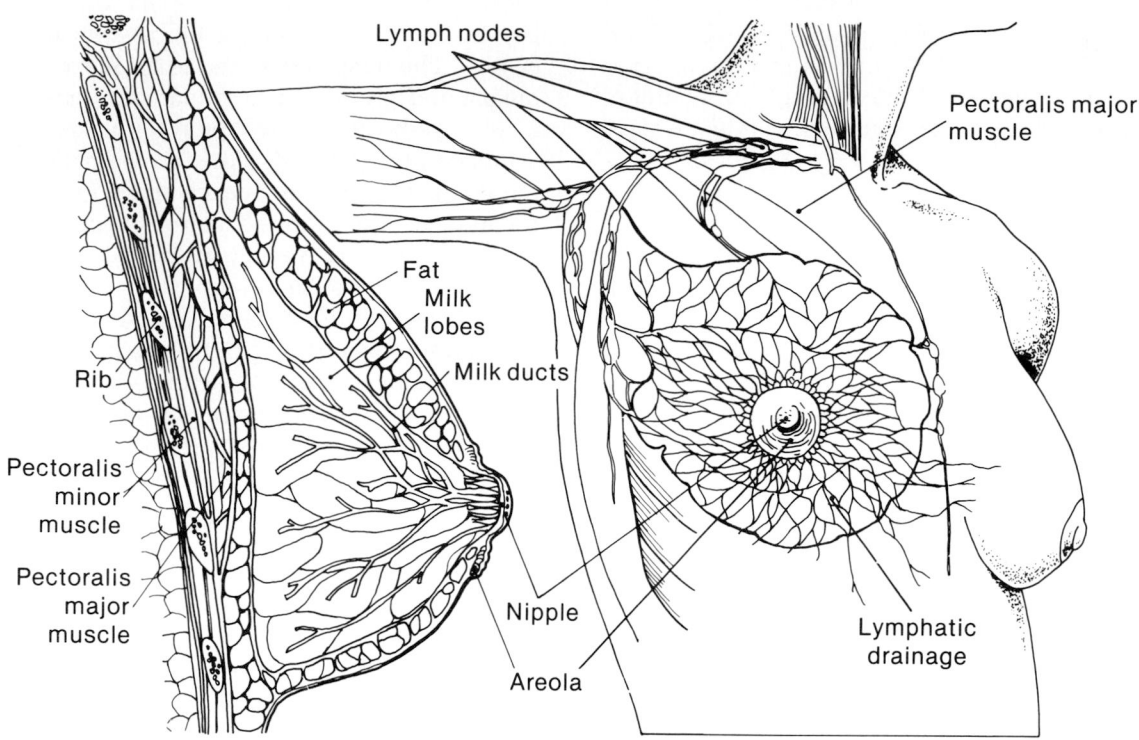

Figure 7–3   Anatomy of the female breast. (From DiSaia PJ: Clinical gynecological oncology, ed 3, St Louis, 1989, Mosby.)

early breast cancers. All three components must be included in breast cancer screening. None of them is as effective individually as when combined. Early detection provides the opportunity for women and their physicians to select treatment options for managing small breast cancers, and results in improved survival. These breast cancer detection recommendations are to be taught to all women, and women should be encouraged to incorporate these behaviors into their individual lifestyles.

CLASSIFICATION

Knowledge of the anatomy of the breast helps in understanding the classification of breast cancer. The breast is a gland located on the chest wall (Figure 7-3). The overlying skin contains hair follicles, sweat, and sebaceous glands. The pigmented area surrounding the nipple is known as the *areola*, and this has sebaceous glands that secrete a lubricant during breastfeeding. Fibrous strands called *Cooper's ligaments* pass through the glandular and fatty tissues from the skin to the underlying muscle, giving the breast support. The glandular tissue is made up of 15 to 20 lobes arranged in a radial pattern, capable of producing milk, connecting with ducts that drain into the nipple. An extensive lymphatic and vascular supply is present. Breast tissue extends to the clavicle, sternum, latissimus dorsi muscles, and up into the

axilla. The axillary lymph nodes drain approximately 60% of the lymph from the breast. They are distributed from low in the armpit, at the lateral border of the pectoralis minor muscle (level I), to midway behind the pectoralis minor muscle (level II), and above at the medial border of the pectoralis minor (level III). Lymph nodes located between the pectoralis major and minor muscles are known as *Rotter's nodes*. The remainder of the lymph is drained from the internal mammary nodes.[111,155,167]

Primary breast cancers are grouped as invasive or noninvasive. A malignancy confined to the ducts or lobules is classified as noninvasive, or *carcinoma in situ*. If it arose in the ductal system, it is referred to as *ductal carcinoma in situ* (DCIS); in the lobule system it would be called *lobular carcinoma in situ* (LCIS). Once the malignant cells penetrate the tissue outside the ducts or lobules, the cancer is described as infiltrating or invasive. Most breast malignancies are carcinomas and classified as ductal or lobular, with a small number of sarcomas and metastatic tumors reported. *Infiltrating ductal carcinoma* accounts for the majority (65% to 80%) of all breast carcinomas and *infiltrating lobular carcinomas* 10% to 14%.[168] *Paget's disease* of the nipple is uncommon (2% of all cases) and is most often associated with invasive carcinoma.[164] Also uncommon is *inflammatory carcinoma*, which is characterized by swelling, erythema, and invasion of the dermal lymphatics (giving the classic peau d'orange, or orange peel appearance). When noninvasive cancer is found with invasive cancer the staging and treatment planning is based on the characteristics of the invasive carcinoma.

CLINICAL FEATURES

In asymptomatic women, mammography serves to detect microscopic changes indicative of cancer such as a small irregular mass, microcalcifications, skin thickening, distortion of the ductal or ligament structures, or asymmetric density.[14] Palpable breast masses may also have these characteristics, often with peripheral spiculations, and nipple or skin retraction when underlying structures are involved.[14] Additional clinical signs and symptoms of breast cancer at presentation are noted in the box on p. 100.

DIAGNOSIS AND STAGING
Tissue Diagnosis

Breast cancer can be diagnosed following cytologic (cells) or histologic (tissue) evaluation. Examination of tissue will give a definitive diagnosis. *Fine needle aspiration (FNA) biopsy* for cytology is easily performed when dominant masses are palpable. It is a simple procedure involving the aspiration of material from the mass using a syringe and 22 gauge needle. The content of the aspiration is mounted on slides and processed for review. In skilled hands it is highly accurate; false negatives and false positives are rare. A negative result in the presence of a suspicious mass warrants further evaluation.[173] *Stereotactic FNA* is available in some centers. This involves the same procedure under radiographic direction, for nonpalpable lesions. Some advantages of the FNA are the ease with which it can be done in the office setting, using minimal local anesthesia, and the low incidence of damage to surrounding tissue.[109] When the results are cancer, it also prevents the necessity of surgical biopsy prior to treatment planning for definitive surgery.[109]

Core needle biopsy provides a core of tissue from a dominant mass. This procedure requires more local anesthesia and has been associated with bleeding and pain during the procedure, especially where deeper lesions are involved. False positives may be a greater problem than with FNA, though still low in incidence. For women who have already had an FNA or core needle biopsy diagnosis of carcinoma, a biopsy is usually performed intraoperatively to reconfirm the diagnosis just prior to the definitive surgical procedure.

In all other situations a two-step procedure is planned. *Incisional biopsy* is performed when the mass is large, and involves removal of only a portion of the mass. *Excisional biopsy* involves removal of the entire mass and a margin of normal tissue around it. Nonpalpable masses detected mammographically can also

be removed by excisional biopsy *(needle localization biopsy)*. The suspicious area is localized by the radiologist and, under x-ray guidance, a small wire with a hook on the end is directed into the lesion. The wire is taped to the patient's skin and the patient then sent to the operating room for excisional biopsy. The tissue removed is radiographed to verify removal of the suspicious area (or to direct further excision). The tissue is then examined microscopically in permanent sections. These techniques enable definitive diagnosis of cancer and opportunity for the woman to be involved in her treatment plan. Women need to be assured that the interval between diagnosis and definitive treatment, in order to obtain recommendations regarding management options, does not adversely affect survival.

Staging

Breast cancer is most frequently staged according to the TNM classification system, which evaluates the tumor size (T); involvement of regional lymph nodes (N); and distant spread of the disease or metastases (M) (discussed in detail in Chapter 4). The stages may be simply classified as follows[9]:

Stage 0:   Carcinoma in situ (TisN0M0)

Stage I: Tumor under 2 cm with negative nodes (T1N0M0)

Stage II: Tumor 0 to 2 cm with positive nodes, or 2 to 5 cm with negative or positive nodes, or greater than 5 cm with negative nodes (T0N1; T1N1; T2N0 or N1; T3N0; all M0)

Stage III: Lymph node involvement (nonmovable axillary nodes), or tumor of any size with direct extension to skin or chest wall

Stage IV: Any distant metastasis (includes ipsilateral supraclavicular nodes)

The historical classification of stage, still seen in national statistical reports, classifies stage as local (no lymph nodes involved), regional, and distant. Of breast cancer cases diagnosed between 1981 and 1987, 52% had local disease, 38% regional disease, and 7% had distant (metastatic) disease at diagnosis.[20] Black women (43%) were less likely than white women (52%) to have their breast cancer diagnosed at a local stage during that same period of time.[19]

Evaluating the extent of disease allows appropriate therapy to be planned, determines the overall prognosis, and permits comparison of research results related to treatment.[80] The clinical staging process routinely begins preoperatively with a thorough history and physical examination, bilateral mammography, renal function tests, alkaline phosphatase, and calcium. Pathologic staging is based on the histological review of the primary tumor from surgical specimens (type, size, and margins) and, when invasive carcinoma is present, the lymph nodes. Evaluation of a patient's bony structure, liver, and head is individualized according to the patient's specific symptoms, laboratory test results, and clinical evidence of enlarged axillary nodes. For example, elevated liver enzymes with or without hepatomegaly would warrant a CT of the abdomen or liver scan to rule out liver metastases. Specific complaints of bone pain or an elevated alkaline phosphatase or calcium level would be evaluated with a bone scan or bone survey. Extensive local surgery may not be performed if distant metastases are discovered at the time of the initial diagnosis.

A variety of substances known to be secreted by some tumors are being evaluated for their applicability in breast cancer. Presently they are not considered part of the staging process. The potential value is in monitoring response to therapy and/or detecting early recurrence. Serial levels that show a pattern of continued increase over time are evidence of metastasis.[83] Two of these *tumor markers* with some value in breast cancer are carcinoembryonic antigen (CEA) and CA15-3. CEA has been the most widely studied marker.[83] A normal value preoperatively provides a baseline by which to follow the patient with serial levels. This marker, however, is limited in its value because it can be elevated with other conditions, such as benign breast disease or smoking. Additionally, less than half of all patients with known breast cancer metastases show an elevation in the CEA (greater than 10 ng/ml).[83]

CA15-3 may also be elevated in benign breast conditions, but is not elevated in smokers. It appears, from studies to date, to be a more sensitive marker for breast cancer metastases than CEA, with elevated levels (greater than 22 U/ml) in 70% to 85% of such patients.[83] In patients with *primary* breast cancer, CA15-3 levels will be elevated in 20% to 50% of patients as compared with only 10% to 30% of patients who will have an elevated CEA.[83] Neither test is specific enough to be routinely used for staging and follow-up.

PROGNOSTIC FACTORS

Tumor size and lymph node status, incorporated into the staging system, have long been recognized as pathologic characteristics that alone have value in predicting survival. Yet the staging system, while it has provided direction for treatment, has not provided the means by which to predict which of the women in a particular stage group will have disease recurrence and which will not. It is now recognized that 20% to 30% of women with negative lymph nodes at the time of breast cancer diagnosis will develop dis-

---

PROGNOSTIC FACTORS IN BREAST CANCER

Tumor size
Lymph node status
Histologic and nuclear grade
Estrogen and progesterone receptors
DNA content analysis
  Ploidy
  S phase fraction (SPF)
Vascular and lymphatic invasion
Oncogenes (e.g., HER-2/*neu*)
Tumor suppressor genes
Epidermal growth factor (EGF)
Cathepsin D
Heat shock stress response proteins
Necrosis
Margins of resection
Inflammatory response
Multicentricity
Extensive intraductal component (EIC)
Demographic characteristics

Under investigation for many of these factors is their interaction with each other, and the influence of each on tumor growth, local recurrence, metastasis, or response to therapy.

---

tant metastases within 10 years. Adjuvant therapy would be most appropriately directed to those women if one could somehow identify them by additional pathologic studies of the tumor.[81] Several pathologic characteristics have been studied for their ability to determine risk of local recurrence, metastasis, response to therapy, and overall prognosis. These are known as *prognostic factors*, shown in the box above.

Tumor Size

Small tumor size at diagnosis is associated with (1) a decreased incidence of axillary nodal metastasis at diagnosis, (2) potential eligibility for breast-preserving surgery, and (3) less chance of tumor recurrence within the breast or axilla.[204] The 5-year survival rate is 99% when tumor size is less than 0.5 cm; 80% for tumors less than 2 to 5 cm, and 50% to 60% for tumors greater than 5 cm.[81,204]

Axillary Lymph Node Status

The larger the tumor the greater the likelihood that lymph nodes will be involved. The single most important predictor of disease recurrence and survival is the presence of axillary lymph node metastasis. When the lymph nodes are involved, there is a greater probability that distant micrometastases are present. Survival is influenced by the number of lymph nodes involved (Table 7-1). Women with negative lymph nodes have a higher rate of survival than women with involved lymph nodes. Similarly, women with one to three involved lymph nodes do better than women with four or more involved lymph nodes.[81,204] Involve-

Table 7–1 Ten-Year Survival According to the Number of Nodes Involved*

Number of Nodes	10-Year Survival (%)
0	68-80
1-3	38-63
4 or more	13-27

*For women not treated with radical mastectomy.
Adapted from Harris JR and Hellman S: Natural history of breast cancer. In Harris JR and others, editors: Breast diseases, ed 2, Philadelphia, 1991, JB Lippincott Co.

ment of the level I nodes has a better prognosis than involvement of the level III nodes.[81,204] Surgical evaluation of the nodes is important because clinically negative nodes will be pathologically involved in 30% of the cases.[81,111]

Estrogen and Progesterone Receptors (ER/PR)

Since 1971, a biochemical assay has been available to analyze breast cancer cells, removed at the time of diagnosis, for the presence of *estrogen and progesterone receptors (ER/PR)*. These receptors are located in the nucleus or on the surface of the cell and bind to circulating steroid hormones. The receptor-hormone complex then works within the cell nucleus to promote cellular growth and division.[154] Patients are said to be positive or negative for ER and PR based on the level of binding receptors present. If the primary lesion is too small, there may be an inadequate amount of tissue available to submit for this analysis. Newer assays that estimate ER and PR levels on smaller tissue specimens have been developed and are being evaluated.[154] Care should be taken at the time of biopsy and/or definitive surgery to ensure that tissue that is malignant is sent for ER and PR measurement. Approximately 60% to 70% of breast cancers are ER positive and 40% to 50% are PR positive.[154]

The presence of ER and/or PR receptors in breast cancer tissue has been utilized widely in planning treatment based on predicted responsiveness to hormonal therapy. The greatest likelihood of response to hormonal therapy is related to high levels of both ER and PR receptors. Tumors that are ER negative and PR positive have shown more responsiveness than ER and PR negative tumors.[154] In addition, receptor status correlates with a variety of clinical and biologic parameters, some of which are also noted as prognostic factors (Table 7-2). Only recently have ER and PR been considered for their role in predicting prognosis.[154,199] Receptor-positive tumors are seen more commonly in postmenopausal women, are associated with a lower recurrence rate, and generally have a better overall prognosis.[154]

Histologic and Nuclear Grade

Pathologists will also report the histologic grade (cellular arrangement) of the tumor, which includes mitotic index, defined as whether the cellular structure is well differentiated (grade I), moderately well differentiated (grade II), or poorly differentiated (grade III).[204] Poorly differentiated tumors (with high mitotic rate) are generally considered to be associated with a poorer prognosis. Nuclear grade refers to the differentiation of the tumor cell nuclei. In this grading system grade 1 shows the best differentiation, grade 2 shows moderate differentiation, and grade 3 shows the worst differentiation. Nuclear grade is considered to be more important than histologic grade as a prognostic factor. Both have been criticized because of the subjective means by which they are determined.[204] Computer technology that allows objective measurement has been evaluated and may enable more consistent reporting. Additionally, developing a standardized means for measuring the amount, for example, of ductoglandular differentiation or mitotic rate, would enhance objectivity.[204]

Lymphatic and Blood Vessel Invasion

The presence of lymphatic and blood vessel invasion by tumor cells is generally associated with a greater incidence of disease recurrence and a worse prognosis.[94] There is no specific completely objective laboratory method to identify lymphatic or blood vessel invasion.[94,204]

DNA Content

Recent advances have been made in understanding the proliferative potential of breast cancer cells. Flow cytometry evaluates the aggressiveness of a neoplasm by analyzing the cellular DNA content (ploidy) and the percentage of cells in the S phase of cellular division (S-phase fraction, or SPF). Tumors are classified as diploid (normal DNA content) or aneuploid (abnormal DNA content), and with high or low SPF.[35,88,199] Cutoff values for high versus low SPF have varied in studies to date; studies in patients with negative lymph nodes and values above 6.7% may lead to further understanding of cutoff determination.[35,88] A greater risk of recurrence and worse prognosis are associated with aneuploid tumors and cells with a high percentage of cells in the S phase. The combination of ploidy and SPF has greater prognostic value than ploidy alone.[94] Type I DNA histograms refer to diploid and low SPF tumors, type II are diploid and high SPF, and type III are aneuploid and high SPF, the latter being associated with poor differentiation and poorer prognosis.[35,70,94] Studies are currently in progress to evaluate the clinical applicability of these tests in determining prognosis. This information may

Table 7–2 Clinical and Biologic Differences between ER Positive and Negative Tumors

Biologic Parameter	ER Positive	ER Negative
Tumor differentiation	Well-differentiated (low grade)	Poorly differentiated (high grade)
DNA content	Normal (diploid)	Abnormal (aneuploid)
Nuclear grade	Cell nuclei well-differentiated	Poorly differentiated cell nuclei
S phase fraction	Low percentage of cells in S phase (DNA synthesis)	High percentage of cells in S phase
Age/menopausal status	≥50, postmenopausal	<50, premenopausal
Clinical course of disease	Prolonged disease-free survival and overall survival	Shorter time to recurrence and shorter overall survival
Type of metastases	Bone and soft tissue	Visceral involvement (lung, liver, brain)
Response to endocrine therapy	Responsive	Unresponsive

Adapted from Osborne CK: Receptors. In Harris JR and others, editors: Breast diseases, ed 2 Philadelphia, 1991, JB Lippincott Co.

be most useful in defining subsets of node-negative breast cancer patients who are not cured by surgery alone and, therefore, need systemic adjuvant therapy. The *Thymidine Labelling Index (TLI)* is another method of measuring cell proliferation, expressed as a percentage of cells taking up labelled thymidine. This method of evaluating proliferation has largely been replaced by flow cytometry.[88]

Oncogenes

Proto-oncogenes are normally involved in regulating cell growth and differentiation. When altered they become known as oncogenes, the genes responsible for cancer.[149] Abnormalities of amplification (multiple copies) or overexpression (multiple quantities) of the proto-oncogene HER-2/*neu* (or c-*erb*B-2) in the DNA of some breast cancers has been associated with tumor growth, more aggressive cancers, local or distant recurrence, and poorer overall survival.[149,199] Other proto-oncogenes under investigation are c-*myc* and Ha-*ras*. *Tumor suppressor genes*, or antioncogenes, may be absent or not functional. Normally inhibiting cancer growth, their absence has significance in cancer cell growth. Currently under study are p53, Rb-1, and nm23.[24] The study of oncogenes has promise for adding prognostic factors that will differentiate higher risk women with negative lymph nodes who will benefit from adjuvant therapy. In addition, therapies may be developed that are able to target the genetic aberrations.[24,88,199]

Epidermal Growth Factor

Epidermal growth factor (EGF) influences breast cancer growth by binding with receptors. The presence of increased numbers of receptors for EGF (EGF-R) has been associated with more aggressive tumors, metastases occurrence and location, and poorer prognosis.[88,199]

Cathepsin D

Cathepsin D is a glycoprotein that can be induced by estrogen and/or growth factors in breast cancer cells, resulting in effects on the extracellular matrix and basement membrane that may in turn mediate tumor proliferation, invasion, and metastasis.[88,199] Although the assay for measuring Cathepsin D is commercially available in the United States, further study is needed to determine cutoff values for determining good or poor prognosis in node-negative versus node-positive women.[88]

Other

Heat shock or stress response proteins are currently under study for their significance in measuring the biologic stress between the patient and cancer.[199] The associations of microscopic tumor necrosis, inflammatory response, and margins of resection have been inconclusively associated with prognosis.[204]

Tumor type and size, lymph node status, estrogen and progesterone receptor status, histologic and nuclear grade, and DNA content (ploidy and SPF) are the most commonly considered evaluations in use today for determining prognosis and treatment plans.[137] The heterogeneity of breast cancer complicates precise determination of prognosis and treatment given our present understanding of the prognostic factors described and the technology available.[88,149] Further study will refine laboratory methods of measurement, consistency in reporting, and measures of interactions among prognostic factors.

Mortality rates have not changed significantly during the past 50 years.[4] However, the number of women diagnosed at an earlier stage has increased. Fewer women are being diagnosed with large tumors (greater than 5 cm in diameter).[190] Most of the increase has been in women diagnosed with tumors less than 2 cm in diameter with negative lymph nodes.[190] Approximately two thirds of all cases of invasive breast cancer diagnosed today will not involve axillary nodes,[137,190] and approximately 70% of those patients will be cured without adjuvant therapy.[137] The use of prognostic factors will be most helpful in identifying high-risk groups of women in need of adjuvant therapy.[88,137]

METASTASIS

Adjuvant systemic therapy has been shown to improve overall survival and prevent or delay the development of metastatic disease. Once metastatic disease develops, the goal of treatment is palliation. Breast cancer spreads by direct invasion of surrounding tissues, along mammary ducts, or by way of lymphatic vessels. The major site of regional spread is the axillary lymph nodes. These nodes are positive in approximately 50% of patients who have palpable tumors at diagnosis.[81] Systemic or distant spread of the disease can occur in a variety of organs and tissues. The most frequent sites are bone, lung, pleura, liver, and adrenals. Other less common sites are the brain, thyroid, leptomeninges, eye, pericardium, and ovary.[81,89] Symptoms described by patients that should be considered potentially associated with the existence of metastasis include bone pain, shortness of breath, nausea and/or vomiting not associated with chemotherapy, loss of appetite, loss of weight, or neurologic changes.[89] Elevations of the serum alkaline phosphatase, calcium, and liver function tests may be indicative of site-specific metastases, when seen in combination with clinical and/or radiographic findings (see box on p. 100).

Two serious complications of metastatic disease, considered oncologic emergencies, are spinal cord compression and hypercalcemia. Metastatic tumor compressing the spinal cord results in motor weakness and progresses to autonomic or sensory deficits and paralysis. Preservation of neurologic function depends on early diagnosis and prompt treatment. Therapeutic options include radiotherapy alone or in combination with surgical decompression. Further palliative systemic treatment may be added. Hypercalcemia is generally a reversible metabolic problem. The symptoms are nonspecific: nausea, constipation, weakness, confusion, and lethargy. This problem may be the result of progressive bone metastases, compromised renal function, or as part of a "flare reaction." Another complication associated with breast cancer metastasis is malignant pleural effusion. Gradual to acute onset of increasing respiratory distress, particularly dyspnea on exertion, is the most common sign. (See Chapter 19 for further information on oncologic complications.)

The median survival from the appearance of metastases is approximately 2 to 3.5 years, though some patients (25% to 35%) may live for 5 years, and others (10%) may live for more than 10 years.[89] Patients who were diagnosed with metastases a longer time after their initial breast cancer diagnosis and who have metastases to the bone or soft tissue areas have a better prognosis.[89] Metastatic breast cancer is not curable, but therapies are usually available that will control or perhaps alleviate the symptoms altogether and prolong life.

TREATMENT MODALITIES
Surgery

Surgical management of breast cancer is centuries old, preanesthesia and preantisepsis, yet it has only been within the last century that surgical intervention has shown survival benefits.[111] The primary goal of surgery has always been to achieve local and regional control of the disease. The Halstedian view that breast cancer spread in an orderly fashion from the breast to the lymph nodes prompted the extensive resection characteristic of the radical mastectomy. Newer views of the nature of breast cancer as a systemic disease at diagnosis and the lack of support for the view that lymph nodes serve as a barrier to metastasis prompted further investigation into less extensive surgery and the role of adjuvant systemic therapy.[81] Early diagnosis and local/regional treatment may also be adequate for some patients. Modified radical mastectomy has replaced the radical mastectomy in the past 15 years, and currently breast conserving surgical procedures with axillary node dissection are the preferred treatment for many small invasive breast cancers. Removal of regional lymph nodes at levels I and II is suggested as the best method for determining nodal status in patients with clinically negative nodes, with full dissection to level III in patients with clinically positive nodes.[111,145,167] Axillary node sampling is not recommended.[111,145] Surgical procedures in the treatment of breast cancer are described in a box on the opposite page.[111]

PRIMARY THERAPY.   The type of surgery selected is based on clinical stage of the disease (tumor size, fixation, histology, nodes, metastases), mammographic findings (including evidence of cancer cells in other areas of the breast separate from the primary), the tumor location, patient history, available surgical and radiotherapeutic expertise, breast size and shape, and patient preference.

Some research has suggested the timing of breast cancer surgery during the menstrual cycle may influence outcomes. Hrushesky[92] reviews the results of some of these studies and emphasizes the need for further research that monitors this issue as well as other variables. While the timing of breast cancer surgery during the menstrual cycle may have some clinical application in the future, patients who desire

---

SURGICAL PROCEDURES IN THE TREATMENT OF BREAST CANCER[111]

Modified radical mastectomy (also referred to as total mastectomy with axillary node dissection)—The entire breast is removed along with axillary lymph nodes and the lining over the pectoralis major muscle. The pectoralis major muscle is not removed. The pectoralis minor muscle may or may not be removed.

Total mastectomy (also referred to as *simple mastectomy*)—All the breast tissue, including the nipple-areolar complex and the lining over the pectoralis major muscle is removed. There is no axillary node dissection. Chest wall muscles are not removed.

Lumpectomy (or excision; *tumorectomy*)—The tumor is removed and the major portion of the breast is left. A *tylectomy* refers to a wide excision with at least 3 cm of normal breast tissue around the tumor.

Wide excision (limited resection, partial mastectomy)—Excision of the tumor with grossly clean margins of normal breast tissue.[190]

Quadrantectomy (also referred to as *partial mastectomy*)—The entire quadrant of the breast containing the tumor is removed along with the overlying skin and the lining over the pectoralis major muscle.

Note: In each of the breast conserving surgical procedures (lumpectomy, wide excision, and quadrantectomy) axillary node dissection is usually performed through a separate incision, and surgical intervention is followed by radiation therapy to the remaining breast tissue to treat any undetected cancer and achieve local control.[190]

scheduling of surgery in accord with their menstrual cycle should be encouraged to discuss this option with their physician.

Nearly all patients with operable breast cancer are candidates for the modified radical mastectomy. In large tumors this procedure allows for local control and pathologic staging. For most women with smaller tumors (stages I and II disease), breast conserving treatment is now recognized as appropriate therapy with proven equivalence to modified radical mastectomy in terms of overall and relapse-free survival rates.[190,202] Adequate time should be allowed, in all cases, for full discussion with the patient as to her options, advantages, and disadvantages.[174] Critical to the success of breast conserving surgery is appropriate patient selection and a multidisciplinary approach. Patients are selected for breast conserving treatment based on the factors noted in the box on right.[111,202]

Studies of utilization patterns of breast conserving surgery in women with stage I or II disease have been undertaken to assess implementation of the National Institutes of Health Consensus Development Conference recommendations released in 1990.[118,156,190] Some studies indicate that in certain areas of the country breast conserving treatment is not being applied ap-

---

CONSIDERATIONS IN PATIENT SELECTION FOR BREAST CONSERVING TREATMENT[111,202]

1. *Tumor size*—Local control is best with relatively small tumors. Most published experience in treating patients has been with tumors a maximum of 4 to 5 cm in diameter. *Contraindications* are the existence of stage III or IV disease.
2. *Tumor location*—Peripheral tumors are best, with clinically negative axillary lymph nodes. *Contraindications* include two or more gross malignancies in other quadrants of the breast, or mammographic indications of suspicious diffuse calcifications (*multifocal*, or *multicentric* disease). Lesions located centrally in the breast, such as beneath the nipple area, usually necessitate removal of the entire nipple-areolar complex; cosmesis then is a consideration.
3. *Breast size*—The tumor-to-breast size ratio influences the cosmetic results. If lumpectomy will result in a large surgical defect, then a mastectomy followed by breast reconstruction may be more appropriate. A *contraindication* may be large pendulous breasts due to difficulties encountered with radiation therapy—reproducing the positioning of the patient, and availability of equipment to provide dose homogeneity.
4. *Patient preference and attitude*—A woman's desire to save her breast and a willingness to undergo 5 to 6 weeks of daily outpatient radiation therapy are important factors. A short hospital stay may also be required if radiation implants are used. Some women might consider this extended treatment an unacceptable cost and inconvenience, or they may achieve greater peace of mind with the physical certainty of surgical removal. Nurses can be supportive of patients in this decision-making process by facilitating communications, providing information, and helping them explore their personal values and relationships.[25,191,196,197] Many studies to date have shown no significant differences for general measures of emotional distress in women undergoing mastectomy or breast conserving surgery.[116,117,202] However, studies have shown that women undergoing breast conserving surgery may have a more positive sexual and body image and fewer problems with clothing, but may need additional psychosocial support during radiation therapy.[64,107,116,117,179]
5. Other *contraindications* are prior irradiation to the breast region that would limit therapeutic dosing for breast cancer treatment; a history of collagen vascular disorder, which has been associated with poor tolerance of radiation; and pregnancy. Women in first or second trimester pregnancies would be unable to undergo radiation therapy; women in their third trimester could feasibly receive breast irradiation after delivery.

propriately.[76,118,156] Availability of radiation facilities and of surgeons and radiation oncologists who specialize and are experienced in the management of breast cancer is important for optimal results. Lack of such expertise may be one factor of underutilization of breast-conserving surgery. Public and professional education and costs may be other reasons. The finding in one study that young and elderly women were more likely to receive breast conserving surgery but that the elderly were less likely to receive radiation therapy when indicated raises further questions for investigation.[118]

To prevent breast cancer in certain high-risk women, prophylactic total mastectomies (unilateral or bilateral) with reconstruction may be considered after careful discussion of potential risks and benefits. Women for whom this procedure may be appropriate include those with[114,115,138]:

1. Strong family history of breast cancer.
2. Biopsy proven ductal or lobular carcinoma in situ, or proliferative benign breast disease.
3. Personal history of contralateral multicentric carcinoma in situ or invasive breast cancer.
4. History of multiple breast nodules and biopsies.

Cancerophobia alone is not an indication for prophylactic mastectomy, though anxiety associated with any of the foregoing indications may be the factor prompting a woman to seek such a procedure appropriately.

Subcutaneous mastectomy, consisting of removal of breast tissue through an inframammary incision, removes 90% to 95% of the tissue, retaining the skin and nipple-areolar complex. Owing to the difficulty removing all of the breast tissue and problems with cosmesis most authors do not recommend its application in the aforementioned situations.[114,115,134]

Ductal and lobular carcinoma in situ (DCIS and LCIS), referred to earlier in this chapter, are noninvasive. In the past these were rarely seen. Because of mammography screenings DCIS is being seen much more frequently; LCIS is being seen more frequently but *incidentally* in biopsies of suspicious lesions or masses. DCIS is associated with a high risk of development of invasive ductal carcinoma at or near the biopsy site, whereas LCIS appears to be an indicator of the possible future development of invasive cancer anywhere in either breast. The management of each is different and controversial.[63,78,108,110,178]

DCIS is primarily discovered on mammography, read out by the radiologist as suspicious clustered microcalcifications.[78] As described previously, these lesions could be biopsied via the needle localization technique. It is not known whether all DCIS will progress to an invasive cancer, or when. DCIS and occult invasive cancer may also be found incidentally near an invasive cancer. When found outside the area of the primary tumor DCIS is referred to as *multicentric*

foci (sites outside the quadrant of the breast where the primary tumor was found) or *multifocal* (sites within the same quadrant as the primary tumor).[63] It is not known whether these are actually separate sites of disease or continuous disease spreading along the ducts. It is much more common as the size of the primary invasive tumor increases.[78]

Mastectomy has been the primary treatment for DCIS with a cure rate of nearly 100%.[78] Axillary node dissection is controversial; whether nodes at levels I and II or none should be removed.[63] Studies of breast conserving surgery and radiation therapy for these women have a short duration of follow-up. Studies are in progress by the National Surgical Adjuvant Breast and Bowel Project (NSABP) to evaluate breast conserving surgery with or without radiation therapy and/or tamoxifen, which hopefully will lead to a better understanding of DCIS and its treatment.

LCIS, when found incidentally on a biopsy specimen, presents different management problems. It is not truly a precancerous lesion but an indicator of the risk of future invasive cancer, most commonly invasive ductal carcinoma.[110] Treatment decisions for LCIS include no further surgery and close lifetime observation, or bilateral total mastectomies, or total mastectomy on the side where LCIS was found with a biopsy of the opposite breast in the same location, and subsequent mastectomy if LCIS is found there also.[110] Neither axillary node dissection nor radiation therapy would be necessary if only LCIS was present.[110]

METASTATIC DISEASE.   Surgery also have a role in the management of metastatic disease. Examples include procedures to excise local recurrences, drain pleural effusions, debulk and decompress spinal cord metastasis, and remove ovaries to eliminate that source of endogenous estrogen.

BREAST RECONSTRUCTION.   The disfigurement and loss associated with a mastectomy can be devastating for many women and their sexual partners. A woman's breasts are equated with femininity, sexual attractiveness, and nurturing behavior.[170] There is now increased recognition, by physicians and patients, of the psychosexual consequences related to breast cancer surgery.* Consequently, reconstruction has become an important element in a woman's rehabilitation following breast cancer surgery. Improved reconstructive techniques offer women hope for a more unaltered body image. A coordinated treatment approach by the surgeon, radiologist, and medical oncologist with the plastic surgeon will increase the likelihood of achieving the desired results.[114]

The debate about immediate versus delayed reconstruction continues. There are pros and cons with

---

*References 52, 53, 64, 107, 114, 116, 117, 148.

either approach. In the past there has been concern about reconstruction interfering with detection of local recurrence of breast cancer or with wound healing. If cancer does recur locally, it usually involves only the chest wall or the overlying skin, and recurrences in the pectoralis major muscle are rare.[165] Wound complications were found to be less in the immediate reconstruction group in one study.[192] Breast reconstruction has not been shown to hide or delay diagnosis of such local recurrence.[114,115,165] Other reasons for delaying reconstruction have been beliefs that women needed to first adjust to the mastectomy and diagnosis prior to making a decision about reconstruction, as if this might somehow enable them to make a better decision and thus better appreciate the reconstructed breast.[77,114] It appears that such beliefs have been unfounded.[114] Patients undergoing immediate reconstruction have been found to experience less overall trauma with their mastectomy and recalled less intensely the pain of their initial operation.[175,176] Another advantage of immediate reconstruction is the elimination of one other hospitalization and anesthesia for the first stage of reconstruction.[114]

Initially, many women express a desire to have reconstructive surgery, but the enthusiasm may diminish with the passage of time. Some reasons for not pursuing reconstruction include: fear of additional surgery, fear of recurrence of cancer, adjustment to their physical change, guilt feelings related to the desire to restore their breast, and reluctance to separate from their prosthesis.[175] Cost may be another variable. Costs for reconstruction vary based on the type of procedure and geographic area. Many insurance companies will cover reconstruction following mastectomy for breast cancer, though many will not cover reconstructive or cosmetic surgery on the opposite side to adjust for symmetry.[114] Women need to inquire whether their individual insurance policies will cover these procedures. Some cost savings may occur when hospitalization for mastectomy and reconstruction are combined.

Treatment of the breast cancer must remain the priority; thus treatment planning within the team will help clarify timing of reconstruction and/or adjuvant therapies. Scheduling of surgery should not be delayed unnecessarily because of coordination between the oncologic and plastic surgeons.[138] Unexpected complications can occur after mastectomy when combined with immediate reconstruction and thus can delay the onset of adjuvant chemotherapy or radiation therapy.[21,115] Such concern in itself may warrant a medical recommendation to delay reconstruction. Where chemotherapy is given postoperatively, reconstruction is usually delayed for 3 to 6 months following completion of this therapy so that the white blood cell count, tissue response, and metabolism can stabilize.[115]

A thoughtful discussion of the options for reconstruction should be incorporated into the initial treatment planning period. The amount of information about the diagnosis and treatment options, potential for adjuvant therapy, clinical trial participation, and the discussion of reconstruction can be overwhelming for the patient as she sifts through the details while experiencing distress over the diagnosis and potential losses. Whether or not she chooses to undergo reconstruction, having that information can inspire hope as well as show support that she does have options.

Most mastectomy patients, particularly those with a good prognosis, are candidates for reconstruction. The patient's motivation and desire for a restored breast is one of the most important indicators for reconstruction.[21] The reasons women seek breast reconstruction are varied and may include a desire to feel whole again, to maintain a sense of femininity and positive body image, to eliminate an external prosthesis, or to reestablish physical symmetry.[114] Some women will choose mastectomy with reconstruction over breast conserving surgery because of a desire not to worry about remaining breast tissue or having to undergo radiation therapy.

Advanced age is not a contraindication for reconstruction as long as the woman is in good enough health to tolerate the effects of surgery. Patients with unrealistic expectations that reconstruction will eliminate the physical and psychologic effects of mastectomy for a breast cancer diagnosis or will result in a perfect replication of the lost breast are more likely to be dissatisfied with the results. Women who are obese, smokers, or have a history of diabetes or debilitating disease have the highest rates of complications.[138]

The goals of reconstructive surgery are to (1) construct a breast mound, (2) achieve symmetry with the opposite side, and (3) build a nipple-areolar complex.[114,115] Considerations for type of surgery include the quality and amount of skin, the size and shape of the opposite breast, the initial surgical operation for cancer, the patient's goals, and general health.[115] Plastic surgery techniques are listed in Table 7-3.

The first implants developed were silicone gel-filled. Next came saline-filled silicone shells, and later *tissue expanders* consisting of an inner silicone gel in liner surrounded by a silicone liner that could be inflated with saline. Polyurethane foam-covered silicone gel prostheses were introduced in the early 1970s. Problems with deterioration of the polyurethane and concerns about safety resulted in those prostheses being withdrawn from the market. The most recent development has been silicone gel im-

Table 7–3 Plastic Surgery Techniques in Breast Cancer[77,114,115]

Reconstruction	Method
Implant (with or without tissue expander) Silicone gel-filled Saline-filled silicone shells Polyurethane foam-covered silicone gel Textured surface/silicone gel	Surgically placed under skin and muscle of chest.
Myocutaneous flaps Latissimus dorsi Transverse rectus abdominis (TRAM)	Transfer of skin underlying muscle and blood supply to chest.
Free flap transfer	Microsurgical resection of section of tissue connected to its main vascular supply, transferred to chest with reconnection of blood supply to existing artery and vein. Simple closure of donor site.
Nipple-areolar complex reconstruction	Areola: transfer of skin from inner thigh or opposite areola. Nipple: transfer of skin from labia minora, fat pad of toe, or behind the ear; raising skin flap from skin (e.g., breast mound). Tattooing (color)
Symmetry	Augmentation Mastoplasty (breast lift) Reduction

plants with a mechanically textured surface. Tissue expanders are gradually inflated over weeks or months. The shell-type expanders must be removed and replaced with a permanent prosthesis, whereas the gel-inflatable has a filling port that can usually be removed and thus leaves the implant as a permanent prosthesis.[115]

The most common complication of implants is capsular contracture, or hardening of the scar tissue, resulting in firmness of the breast tissue and sometimes distortion of shape. Mechanical problems with inflation or deflation can occur with the tissue expanders but are uncommon. Of greatest concern are reports of autoimmune diseases linked to rupture or leakage of silicone gel into the body tissues. The majority of women with implants have undergone breast augmentation and not reconstruction related to breast cancer. More studies are needed assessing the safety of implants for all women. In 1991 the Federal Drug Administration (FDA) asked manufacturers to stop selling any implants for which safety and effectiveness data had not been submitted. Until further information is available, reconstruction with implants for women with breast cancer should continue to be preceded by a full discussion of the available options, risks, and benefits.

The *latissimus dorsi myocutaneous flap* from the upper back often is supplemented with an implant for full symmetry. It effectively fills the defect beneath the clavicle present due to removal of the pectoralis major muscle in women who have had a radical mastectomy.[114] The *transverse rectus abdominis myocutaneous flap (TRAM)* from the lower abdomen accomplishes a simultaneous abdominoplasty (similar to a "tummy tuck") and does not require the use of an implant. Complications with either of these procedures include loss due to damage of the blood supply, skin necrosis, infection, hematoma, delayed wound healing, and fat necrosis or fibrosis, all being greater with the TRAM procedure.[114,115] Hernias at the donor site have occurred with the TRAM flap as well. In either procedure an additional scar is left, but the scar from the TRAM procedure is usually hidden within an acceptable "bikini" line. The TRAM flap can also be performed bilaterally. The TRAM procedure carries greater risk for the woman who has a history of smoking or obesity or is in otherwise compromised health.[115] *Free flap transfers* are rarely used because of the complexity of the surgical dissection and prolonged operating time, and a higher rate of failure than the myocutaneous flaps.[114,115]

Augmentation, mastopexy (breast lift), or reduction of the remaining breast is sometimes necessary to achieve symmetry. This and any further refinements in the reconstructed breast should be completed before the nipple-areolar complex reconstruction.[115] Saving the nipple-areolar complex at the time of mastectomy for later reconstruction is no longer recommended. Skin transfers as noted in Table 7-3 have been the primary means of nipple and areola reconstruction. However, newer and more satisfactory techniques involve the raising of a flap of skin from the reconstructed breast mound and folding back sections of the flap to create the projecting nipple.[77,114,115] In all cases tattooing of the nipple-areolar complex may be indicated to attain a satisfactory pigmentation effect.[77,114,115] A picture of optimal reconstructive results is shown in Figure 7-4.

Radiation Therapy

Radiation therapy has localized effects on breast cancer and as such has a role in local-regional control of disease as adjuvant therapy, and in combination ther-

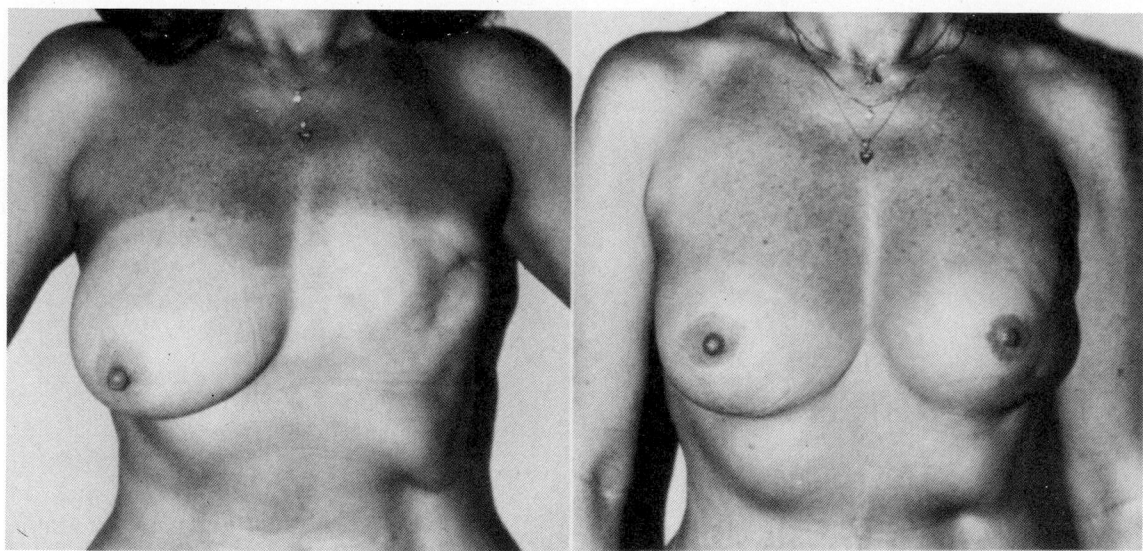

Figure 7–4 Breast reconstruction results. (From Bostwick J: Aesthetic and reconstructive breast surgery, St Louis, 1983, Mosby.)

apy for local-regional advanced or metastatic disease. In the past radiotherapy was routinely used after a modified radical mastectomy to decrease the risk of local/regional disease recurrence. The area irradiated included the chest wall, supraclavicular fossa, and the axilla. This practice is now less common, reserved for situations where there is a high risk for local recurrence of the disease (most commonly when the deep surgical margins of resection are involved). Other cases where benefit has been shown include those with tumors greater than 5 cm in size with four or more positive nodes.[79]

Radiation therapy in conjunction with breast-conserving surgery is administered to achieve local control of disease in women with early stage breast cancer. External beam radiotherapy begins 2 to 4 weeks after adequate healing after wide excision and axillary node dissection. Treatment planning is done to ensure homogeneity of dose through consistent reproducible positioning of the patient and the use of supervoltage equipment.[202] Each field should be treated daily, Monday through Friday, to a total whole breast dose of 4500 to 5000 cGy at 180 to 200 cGy per fraction. This therefore generally takes 4 to 5 weeks. A radiation boost to the original tumor site should always be given when surgical margins are involved or close, and it is usually delivered to all patients in spite of some controversy about the necessity. It can be delivered by two methods: electron beam (external boost) or iridium-192 implanted temporarily in the tumor site. The latter requires a short hospital stay. The external boost is generally preferred because of cost, convenience, and cosmesis. The boost increases the total dose to the primary tumor site to 6000 to 6600 cGy.[202] Systemic adjuvant therapy may addition-

ally be recommended. Future questions to be addressed include the optimal timing of adjuvant chemotherapy and radiation therapy postoperatively, with some consideration to early initiation of chemotherapy and delayed implementation of radiation therapy.

Radiation therapy in combination with chemotherapy can be used to shrink inoperable breast lesions enough to allow surgical removal. For patients unable to undergo a surgical procedure, radiotherapy may be used as the primary therapy. In metastatic cancer, radiation therapy is palliative for painful bony metastases, shrinks metastatic brain lesions or tumors compressing the spinal cord, and relieves the symptoms of superior vena cava syndrome.

The toxicities associated with radiation therapy are generally mild and reversible. They include local skin changes, generalized fatigue, pain related to temporary inflammation of the nerves or the pectoral muscles in the radiation field, and occasionally sore throat. Extended axillary irradiation can aggravate lymphedema and range of motion difficulties. (For a more detailed discussion of the radiation-associated toxicities and specific nursing interventions, see Chapter 21 and box on p. 118).

Systemic Therapy

Systemic treatment of breast cancer involves the use of chemotherapy or endocrine manipulation to treat patients with (1) axillary node involvement, (2) poor prognosis node-negative disease, (3) advanced local-regional disease, or (4) distant metastases. The specific therapy recommended is influenced by the prognostic factors discussed earlier as well as the patient's general medical condition. Dosages used and the du-

Table 7–4   Chemotherapy Regimens for Breast Cancer[85,87,89]

Acronym	Drugs
CMF	Cyclosphosphamide (Cytoxan)
	Methotrexate
	5-Fluorouracil (5-FU)
FAC/CAF	5-FU
	Doxorubicin (Adriamycin)
	Cytoxan
AC	Adriamycin
	Cytoxan
M-F followed by	Methotrexate
leucovorin	5-FU
CMF (P)	Cytoxan
	Methotrexate
	5-FU
	Prednisone
CMFVP	Cytoxan
	Methotrexate
	5-FU
	Vincristine
	Prednisone
CAFVP	Cytoxan
	Adriamycin
	5-FU
	Vinblastine
	Prednisone
VATH	Vinblastine
	Adriamycin
	Thiotepa
	Fluoxymestrone (Halotestin)

NOTE—Concurrent or sequential tamoxifen may also be recommended.

ration of therapy vary. Table 7-4 lists some common regimens used for breast cancer management.

ADJUVANT CHEMOTHERAPY.   Breast cancer can spread not only to axillary nodes but also to distant sites through the bloodstream. A percentage of women will therefore have micrometastases at diagnosis. Since 1972, adjuvant chemotherapy or hormone therapy has been given to prevent or delay the development of metastatic disease. It is given following the definitive surgical treatment while the tumor burden is small (micrometastases) and the cells are least likely to become drug resistant. Clinical trials have clearly demonstrated that adjuvant chemotherapy delays recurrence and improves overall survival, particularly in premenopausal, node-positive patients.[85,151] The medical decision to recommend adjuvant therapy and the patient's decision to receive it can be complex and difficult. As with decisions about the type of surgical procedure to have, patients need help understanding the concept of adjuvant therapy as well as information about the benefits and risks.[119,162,169]

The regimens most commonly used in adjuvant therapy contain a combination of cyclophosphamide (C), methotrexate (M), and 5-fluorouracil (F). Because doxorubicin is one of the most active single agents for the treatment of metastatic breast cancer, it is often used in the adjuvant setting in combination regimens.[85] The optimal drug combination, treatment schedule, and duration of therapy have not been established. Clinical trials to date have resulted in a gradual decrease in the total length of time recommended for adjuvant chemotherapy, to the current duration of 4 to 6 months as suitable for most patients.[85] Dose intensity and scheduling also remain under investigation. Clinical trials are in progress to determine the benefits of perioperative chemotherapy (begun within hours after surgery), neoadjuvant therapy (administered for a period of time before surgery), and short-course intensive chemotherapy.[55,85]

Standard practice recommendations, at this time, are to treat all premenopausal women with involved nodes with combination chemotherapy.[85,151] In the past, node-negative patients were considered to have a good prognosis, and no additional therapy after surgery was recommended. Evidence that 20% to 30% of these patients will develop recurrent disease led to further studies that might identify these patients and effective treatment.[81] Adjuvant chemotherapy clinical trials indicate that this therapy delays the time to recurrence for some patients.[85,190] The ideal regimen and duration, as well as characteristics of those women who benefit, are not yet known.[45,85,190] Reports of long-term toxicities of adjuvant chemotherapy indicate that much is still unknown.[39,85] The report of the 1990 National Institutes of Health (NIH) Consensus Conference, in summarizing the knowledge to date, recommended that outside of participation in a clinical trial, women with negative lymph nodes should be made aware of the risks and benefits of adjuvant chemotherapy so as to be able to make an informed decision about such treatment.[190] It was also recommended that, whenever possible, prognostic factors (tumor size, ER and PR status, nuclear grade, histologic type, and DNA content) should be considered in estimating an individual woman's risk of recurrence.[190] However, much remains to be learned about prognostic factors as well. Women with tumors less than 1 cm in diameter and negative lymph nodes do not warrant adjuvant chemotherapy outside of a clinical trial. Further studies in progress will identify the specific subsets of patients who need adjuvant therapy and the most appropriate regimen.[190]

ADJUVANT ENDOCRINE THERAPY.   Tamoxifen delays recurrence in postmenopausal breast cancer patients.[85] In studies of node negative patients it also reduces the incidence of cancers in the opposite breast.[190] In premenopausal patients, however, the long-term risks of tamoxifen therapy secondary to endocrine abnormalities are not fully known.[190] The optimal duration of therapy has yet to be established.

Table 7–5   Summary of 1985 and 1990 NIH Consensus Development Conferences[45,151,190]: Recommendations Regarding Adjuvant Breast Cancer Therapy For Patients Not Enrolled in Clinical Trials

Menopausal Status	Axillary Nodes	Hormone Receptor Status	Treatment
Premenopausal	Positive	Positive or negative	Combination chemotherapy
	Negative, high risk*		Combination chemotherapy
	Negative, low risk†		Tamoxifen?
Postmenopausal	Positive	Positive	Tamoxifen with or without chemotherapy
	Positive	Negative	Chemotherapy with or without tamoxifen
	Negative, high risk*	Positive or negative	Chemotherapy with or without tamoxifen
	Negative, low risk†		Tamoxifen

*Higher risk = tumor ≥2 cm, receptor negative, aneuploid or diploid with a high S phase.
†Low risk = tumor < 1 cm, generally regarded as lower risk are tumors that are smaller; receptor positive; tubular, colloid or papillary in histology; low S phase fraction, diploid.
Adapted from Glick JH: Meeting highlights: adjuvant therapy for breast cancer, J Natl Cancer Inst 80:471, 1988, and Refs 45, 151, 190.

Current studies indicate long-term treatment, closer to 5 years, is probably better than therapy of 2 years' duration.[85] Therapy in excess of 5 years is not recommended outside of a clinical trial.[85] Benefit from the addition of tamoxifen to multidrug chemotherapy in premenopausal women needs further study. While such a combination may be advantageous in the management of postmenopausal women, further research is needed to establish the fact. All patients on tamoxifen need to be monitored for infrequently reported toxicities but frequently experienced symptomatic side effects that may be disruptive enough to cause a woman to discontinue therapy. Primarily these are hot flashes and gynecologic problems such as vaginal discharge, irritation, or dryness.[123,184] For postmenopausal women a secondary benefit may be an increase in bone density; risks reported include endometrial cancer and changes in lipid values (cholesterol, triglycerides, and high density lipoproteins or HDL).[87,123,184]

In 1985, the NIH gathered a panel of experts to evaluate the results of adjuvant clinical trials and to make treatment recommendations.[151] The panel determined that optimal breast cancer therapy has not been established for any subset of women. However, some recommendations could be made for treatment of patients outside of the context of a clinical trial. A subsequent review in 1988 and a consensus panel for early stage breast cancer in 1990 further addressed adjuvant therapy for subsets of women.[68,190] While increased numbers of women have been given the opportunity to participate in clinical trials through the Community Clinical Oncology Programs (CCOP), emphasis should still be placed on participation by women and their physicians in clinical trials. For women not registered in a clinical trial, general treatment recommendations are summarized in Table 7-5. TREATMENT OF ADVANCED DISEASE.   Certain patients with features of *locally advanced disease* may be considered inoperable at diagnosis. This includes tu-

mors with direct extension to the chest wall or skin, fixed axillary nodes or metastases greater than 2.5 cm, skin ulceration, and inflammatory changes. While potentially resectable with radical mastectomy, the local recurrence rate is greater than 50% and, in the majority of cases, overall survival is zero at 5 years.[150] Some, but not all, of these patients will have distant metastases at the time of diagnosis. Patients with locally advanced disease benefit from combination chemotherapy with or without endocrine therapy, followed by radiation therapy and/or surgical intervention for local control. The presence of supraclavicular or infraclavicular nodes or large, nonmovable axillary nodes at the initial diagnosis, and response to chemotherapy will determine whether the subsequent treatment is high-dose radiation therapy, mastectomy, or both. Systemic therapy is then resumed following local therapy. The optimum therapy for locally advanced disease still has not been determined in spite of improved responses with this sequential therapy.[150]

The goal of therapy in metastatic disease is control of the disease and palliation of symptoms. Metastatic breast cancer is incurable with either chemotherapy or hormone manipulation. These modalities are able to achieve temporary regression of the disease in a majority of patients, but these responses rarely last a long time. Overall, the median survival after the development of metastatic disease is less than 3 years.[51,86,193,194] As noted previously, a small percentage of these patients will be alive at 5 years, and a very few will live 10 or more years.[89,193]

Women with receptor-positive cancers have more potentially beneficial treatment options available to them than those with receptor-negative cancers. Local/regional, soft tissue, and bony recurrences that are not life threatening are generally treated with endocrine therapy first. Radiation therapy may be used for local or symptomatic control. For more aggressive disease (liver, lymphangitic lung disease, and widespread, painful bony metastases), frontline treatment is chemotherapy. The regimen selected may be one of those listed in Table 7-4; selection is based on prior adjuvant treatment, prior response, and current physical condition.[193]

CHEMOTHERAPY.   Responses to combination drug therapy occur in approximately 50% to 80% of patients. These disease regressions generally last from 5 to 13 months.[86] Doxorubicin (Adriamycin) is the most effective single agent in the treatment of metastatic breast cancer. Other active single agents commonly employed in combination regimens include cyclophosphamide, methotrexate, and 5-fluorouracil.[86] Mitoxantrone, similar to doxorubicin but with less cardiotoxicity, is an effective drug more recently available. Once initial therapy for distant metastases fails, subsequent treatment regimens often use vinblastine, mitomycin C, thiotepa, etoposide (VP-16), and cisplatin. Taxol is the newest drug approved for use in breast cancer treatment (mid-1990). Because there is no "standard" therapy for metastatic disease, new approaches are regularly being tested in phase II and III research. Examples include noncross-resistant therapy, new phase II agents, standard versus intensified dose therapy, intensive chemotherapy and autologous bone marrow transplantation, chemoendocrine combinations, weekly low-dose chemotherapy, and continuous infusion regimens.

HORMONAL MANIPULATION.   The ability to quantify ER and PR receptors in breast cancer cells has allowed oncologists to predict with greater accuracy which women might respond to hormone manipulation. Receptor-positive patients respond 50% to 60% of the time while only 10% of receptor-negative patients will respond. A variety of endocrine approaches can be classified as *additive* or *ablative therapies*. Metastatic tumors responding to one form of hormone therapy are more likely to respond to subsequent hormone maneuvers.[87] This type of therapy requires several weeks to be effective. Therefore it is not recommended in women with life-threatening liver, lung, or brain metastases. The dosage and duration of these therapies vary. An interesting phenomenon seen with endocrine therapy is "withdrawal responses" (i.e., tumor regressions that occur just because the hormone therapy is stopped).[87]

Ovarian ablation via bilateral oophorectomy has been a treatment of choice for premenopausal women.[193] This procedure reduces the level of circulating estrogens available to stimulate breast cancer cells. Ovarian ablation has also been achieved with radiation therapy but the responses take longer than surgical removal of the ovaries. Studies are underway to evaluate the role of luteinizing hormone-releasing hormone (LHRH) agonists or antagonists (buserelin, leuprolide, goserelin).[87,193] Their mechanism of action resembles a medical oophorectomy.[87]

Tamoxifen is the primary *antiestrogen* used either as adjuvant therapy or to treat metastatic disease. It is primarily used in the management of postmenopausal women who are ER positive. Recent studies have shown that tamoxifen and oophorectomy are equally effective in treating premenopausal women with distant metastases. It is reasonable that tamoxifen may be selected as first-line therapy for metastatic disease in such patients.[87]

Tamoxifen binds to estrogen receptor sites in breast cancer cells, thereby blocking the uptake of estrogen necessary for cell proliferation. The drug is taken orally and has few toxicities. As with other types of endocrine therapy, "flare reaction" may occur during the first few weeks of treatment. The most frequent symptom of a flare reaction is abrupt onset of diffuse musculoskeletal pain hours to weeks after starting therapy. Hypercalcemia is the most serious manifestation of a flare reaction.[87] This reaction should not be confused with progressive disease, nor should the drug be discontinued. Women are to be monitored for this reaction and provided treatment for these symptoms. While this flare reaction has been thought to be associated with a subsequent therapeutic response, patients without a flare reaction may also have a therapeutic response.[87]

Adrenalectomy and *hypophysectomy* (surgical removal of the adrenals and pituitary glands, respectively) used to be therapies of choice for postmenopausal women. Surgical morbidity and mortality and long-term side effects have led to removal of these as primary treatment options. Medical adrenalectomy can be achieved with the use of the drug aminoglutethimide. Effect on the tumor is a result of inhibition of the enzyme that converts androgens produced by the adrenal glands from converting to estrogens.[193] Patients must receive hydrocortisone (HCT) to prevent adrenal insufficiency while on aminoglutethimide. They are encouraged not to discontinue the HCT abruptly while receiving aminoglutethimide or after it is discontinued. A gradual tapering of the dose is done until the patient's adrenal function returns. The most frequently experienced side effect on aminoglutethimide is lethargy, with less frequently occurrences of dizziness, skin rash, nausea/vomiting, and Cushingoid symptoms.[87] Aminoglutethimide is not effective in premenopausal women. The effect of removal of the pituitary glands has been demonstrated medically through the use of levodopa or bromocriptine, which suppresses levels of prolactin, normally secreted via the pituitary.[87] Further study is needed as to the role of such antiprolactin drugs.

Additive therapies include the use of estrogens, androgens, and progestins. *Estrogens* such as Premarin or diethylstilbestrol (DES) can also result in tumor regressions in postmenopausal women. High doses of estrogen act at the level of the hypothalamus to inhibit the release of luteinizing hormone, which normally stimulates the ovaries to produce estrogen. These drugs are as effective as tamoxifen but are associated with significant side effects (nausea, vomiting, anorexia, vaginal bleeding, breast engorgement, and edema).[87] Consequently, tamoxifen is the treatment of choice in the initial management of the patient.

Androgens, or male hormones, are effectively used in the treatment of breast cancer. They are not as effective as estrogens or tamoxifen.[87] Testosterone and fluoxymesterone (Halotestin) have been evaluated, but fluoxymesterone is preferred. The exact mechanism of action of androgens is unknown. While side effects are minimal, the usefulness of these compounds is limited because of the unacceptability of masculinizing effects (facial and body hair, deepening of the voice, alopecia).[87] The flare response and hypercalcemia have been associated more frequently with androgen therapy than with any other endocrine therapy.[87]

The *progestins* most commonly used are megestrol acetate (Megace) and medroxyprogesterone acetate (Depo-Provera). Recent studies have shown these drugs to be as effective as other forms of hormone manipulation. However, tamoxifen remains the first choice in postmenopausal women. The mechanism of action of progestins has not been established. There are relatively few side effects associated with their use; weight gain is the most commonly experienced side effect.[87]

AUTOLOGOUS BONE MARROW TRANSPLANTATION (ABMT). Chemotherapy for metastatic breast cancer in escalating dosages is limited presently by the myelosuppressive toxicity associated with higher doses. This could be circumvented if the patient's own bone marrow was removed prior to high dose treatment and reinfused after treatment. Several hundred women with high risk stage II and III disease (generally 10 or more positive nodes) or stage IV disease have been enrolled in such studies; most were treated with conventional agents with failure prior to ABMT. More recent studies have begun to address the role of ABMT for women in remission. Difficulties with this research in breast cancer include the selection of candidates (young, excellent performance status), complexity of the treatment, the cost, the expertise required, and the fact that breast cancer frequently metastasizes to the bone marrow.[86] Morbidity and mortality are high. The availability of colony stimulating factors (see Chapter 23) will undoubtedly contribute to a reduction in toxicities associated with marrow suppression. Until further research results are available, dose escalations and ABMT are not generally recommended outside of a clinical trial.[86]

Nursing Management

Selected nursing diagnoses and interventions are discussed below. Further nursing diagnoses and interventions are based on patient age, clinical history, specific problems and concerns, concomitant physical and psychosocial problems, visual or auditory deficits, educational level, ethnic and cultural influences, language, coping strategies, prior experience with illness, social support, medical diagnoses, and specific treatment goals and options planned. The role of nursing along a continuum of health care experiences for the woman at risk for or diagnosed with breast cancer was described by Thomas and is reflected in part here in the discussion of phases of care.[189]

PREDIAGNOSTIC PHASE

Nurses who work in public health clinics or outpatient facilities will have many opportunities to interact with women who are entering the health care system for routine screening procedures. A valuable role for nurses is to offer public education programs on breast health and to reinforce the positive health care maintenance behaviors of individual women. When a woman notices a change in her breast, or her health care provider finds a palpable mass, or she receives a report of an abnormal mammogram, anxiety and fear are likely to follow. Taking further action to learn the nature of the abnormality requires participation by the woman with her health care provider. Thomas describes many factors that might influence a woman's actions during this time, such as usual coping style, experience with the health care system, beliefs about cancer, and cultural and ethnic background.[189] Access to the health care system and the services necessary, a problem for the elderly and socioeconomically disadvantaged, may be a factor that could result in a delay in diagnosis.[61,76,169] Denial of the symptom or finding might result in a delay as well.[169,189] Her prior experience with breast problems, or knowledge of other women who have had breast problems requiring evaluation, may positively or negatively impact her response. Nurses can be advocates to support women in seeking this follow up.

DIAGNOSTIC PHASE

When a procedure is indicated to evaluate an abnormality, a woman may experience anxiety, fear, and even anticipatory grieving over the threat of the diagnosis of cancer and loss of the breast. Diagnostic procedures and tests can be overwhelming and frightening. Simply waiting for test results may seem unbearable. The main components of nursing care during this phase include (1) preparation of the patient for the procedures/tests, both physically and emotionally; (2) creation of a positive and supportive environment; and (3) provision of adequate information and resources to address patient concerns.

NURSING DIAGNOSIS

Anxiety related to fear of diagnosis of breast cancer

INTERVENTIONS

- Explain purpose, preparation, and steps of procedures required for diagnosis (mammography, ultrasound, fine needle aspiration, needle localization biopsy, excisional biopsy).
- Provide literature as appropriate.
- Allow patient to ventilate fears and concerns regarding malignant diagnosis.
- Explain postprocedure care.
- Encourage patient to bring spouse/significant other/friend when returning for test results.
- Be present, if possible, when patient is given test and biopsy results. Continuity of care and a relationship of trust established early in the treatment phase do much to allay anxieties about the health care system.
- Patients who do not have a diagnosis of cancer will need information about follow up specific to their diagnosis. Women with benign proliferative breast disease and/or a strong family history of breast cancer, who have concerns about personal breast cancer risk, should be referred to appropriate resources for counselling regarding risk.[105,187] Instruction in BSE and guidelines for follow up with mammography and CBE should also be given.

GOAL/OUTCOME

Anxiety will be manageable so that the patient will complete the diagnostic workup. Patients without a cancer diagnosis will have a plan of care that prepares them for early detection of cancer and reduces anxiety as much as possible. Patients with a diagnosis of cancer will be supported in adjusting to the next phase of care.

PREOPERATIVE PERIOD

Patients who have been diagnosed with breast cancer are faced with an onslaught of information that ranges from the basic fact of the diagnosis of cancer to the complexity of choosing a type of surgical procedure with or without a second treatment (radiation therapy), with or without chemotherapy or hormonal therapy and possibly within the context of a clinical research study. The decision about what to recommend to a patient and how that is subsequently explained to the patient can be equally complex for health care providers.[169] It is important that patients are given adequate information from which they can make informed decisions. Many states now mandate that patients be given information on surgical treatment options. Some states also require second surgical opinions before any elective surgery.[169] Repeated discussions are often necessary in order to clarify information previously given but forgotten or not heard due to the stress experienced during the discussions.

Rowland and Holland describe four potential responses of patients during this period[169]: (1) deferral to the physician to make the decision; (2) permitting physicians to only do a certain procedure; (3) temporarily indecisive or potentially unable to make any decision; and (4) decisive based on a thoughtful review of the options. Most women benefit from some time to think over the information provided, discuss that information with significant others in their support network, and review again with the physician and treatment team.[25,169,191,196,197] Continuity of care providers is important for the continuity of information provided. Potential nursing diagnoses during this time can include (1) anticipatory grieving related to threatened changes in body image, work, or personal role relationships; (2) powerlessness related to inability to control diagnosis and perceived inability to make decisions; and (3) ineffective individual coping. Most women find their coping mechanisms challenged during this time and respond appropriately.

NURSING DIAGNOSIS

Powerlessness related to decisional conflict and informational overload regarding breast cancer treatment options and plan of care

INTERVENTIONS

- Be present with medical team, if possible, when treatment plan is initially discussed and at subsequent discussions.
- Provide appropriate literature to supplement verbal discussion.
- Clarify information as appropriate.
- Act as liaison between the patient and medical team.
- Anticipate patient and family concerns and questions and involve significant others as indicated by patient and situation. Identification of the social support network of the patient will be helpful throughout treatment.[22,52,53]
- Allow the patient and family to verbalize concerns openly, and reinforce normalcy of responses.[162]
- Rabinowitz suggests this is a time to "demythologize," or to clarify misinformation that women may

have or receive through other sources about breast cancer and its treatment.[162]

- Decision-making may be aided by helping the patient review the pros and cons of her options, and thinking through how she has made decisions in the past.[162]
- Referral to recovered patients who have undergone a specific treatment, such as breast-conserving surgery with radiation, may be helpful for some women. The Reach to Recovery program of the ACS is one resource.
- Patients who have unusual difficulty processing the information and/or who do not follow through with making a treatment decision may need referral to professional resources for additional support in coping and adjustment.

GOAL/OUTCOME

The patient will have adequate information and support to make an informed decision about treatment, involving her significant other(s) as appropriate.

OPERATIVE PHASE

When Thomas described the periods of care in breast cancer in 1978 many women were still undergoing a one-step procedure, waking up after a biopsy only to discover that they had indeed undergone a mastectomy.[189] Fortunately today that is not the case, and women admitted to the hospital for surgical treatment are better prepared. Hospitalization and surgery alone are associated with stressors, such as separation from family, disruption in sense of control, and general anesthesia.[189] Feelings of sadness at the anticipated loss (whether part or all of the breast), a sense of readiness for the surgery, and relief (that the cancer will be removed) are often interspersed postoperatively with concern about the final pathology report and the involvement of lymph nodes.

Wound care and remobilization of the arm are physical tasks of this period.[22,139] There is some controversy as to the best time to begin mobilization of the arm and shoulder postoperatively and differences between patients undergoing mastectomy or breast conserving surgery.[41,75,99,122,161] Concerns about early mobilization (days 1 to 2 postoperatively) have been related to the potential for increased drain tube output, delay in drain removal, post-drain seroma formation, and potential for impaired wound healing and infection. Concerns about late mobilization are related to arm and shoulder motion difficulties that may occur when exercise is not begun sooner. Restricted mobility carries the potential risk of later development of a "frozen shoulder." Some postoperative exercise to include flexion and extension of the hand and wrist, and elbow and limited movement for simple activities (eating, brushing teeth) seem reasonable immediately

after surgery, with gradually increasing exercises beginning within 3 to 5 days after surgery designed to regain full range of motion of the shoulder joint. Often such exercise programs are designed by a treatment team of nursing, surgery, occupational, and/or physical therapy. Because surgical admissions are of much shorter duration, much preoperative preparation takes place in the clinic or office setting as does postoperative education. Nurses have an important role not only in education but in promoting the expression and exploration of feelings by the patient and her spouse or significant other. It is important to include both individuals in the treatment planning and follow up (see box on p. 118).

Possible nursing diagnoses during this phase include the following: (1) grieving related to changes in body and body image; (2) potential for infection related to surgical wound and axillary lymph node dissection; (3) impaired physical mobility related to imposed restriction, pain, or fatigue; (4) body image disturbance; and (5) anxiety regarding final pathology report.

NURSING DIAGNOSIS

Potential for injury (infection, delayed wound healing, immobility) related to surgical wound and impaired lymph drainage secondary to breast cancer surgery, complicated by failure to view and care for wound/drains.

INTERVENTIONS

- Inform patient and family about hospital and operative routines.
- Describe postoperative activity (positioning and care of the arm on the operative side, drains, intravenous line, and ambulation) before surgery so that patient will be prepared to participate appropriately.
- Position arm on operative side slightly elevated with flat pillow or folded towel behind upper arm, until patient fully awake and ambulatory. Maintain position when reclining.
- Reinforce importance of early ambulation, coughing and deep breathing.
- All intravenous access or venipunctures should be managed on the nonoperative side.
- Monitor wound for inflammation, tenderness, swelling, or purulent drainage. Change dressing when ordered using aseptic technique.
- Monitor drains: intact, secured to the skin or clothing so as not to dangle, color and amount of fluid output.
- Assess patient and medicate for pain or discomfort as ordered.
- Provide information on normal sensory sensations patient will experience postoperatively such as paresthesias of the inner aspect of the upper arm, and

---

DISEASE AND TREATMENT-RELATED COMPLICATIONS OF BREAST CANCER

Disease related

Local/regional recurrence
Ulceration
Lymphedema
Brachial plexopathy
Distant recurrence
Spinal cord compression
Brain/leptomeningeal metastases
Hypercalcemia
Pathologic fractures
Pleural effusion
Lymphangitic spread
Pericardial effusion/tamponade
Superior vena cava syndrome

Treatment related

Surgery
Impaired wound healing/seroma
Nerve injury
Lymphedema
Shoulder dysfunction
Radiation therapy
Skin reactions
Lymphedema
Shoulder dysfunction
Marrow suppression
Fatigue
Chemotherapy
Marrow suppression (bleeding/sepsis)
Stomatitis
Anorexia/nausea/vomiting
Extravasation/skin necrosis
Hemorrhagic cystitis

---

increased skin sensitivity.[36] "Phantom breast" experiences have also been reported.[120]

- Assess readiness to look at incision, and offer support when patient decides to view the incision. Description of the wound appearance may be helpful to some patients prior to actual viewing. Discuss possible response of patient's spouse/significant other toward viewing the incision and patient's readiness for this.
- Instruct patient in arm care and postsurgical arm exercises.[36,67,112,139] This will usually require further follow-up instruction in the outpatient setting, because the exercises should continue for a minimum of 6 weeks after surgery but may need to be continued for up to 6 months for full recovery and flexibility.[22] Examples of recommended exercises include squeezing a ball, brushing the hair, shoulder shrugs and circles, and finger climbing up a wall facing the wall (standing about 6 inches away from the wall) and turned perpendicular to the wall. All exercises should begin gently without the sensation of pain. Gentle stretching of muscles but not strain is encouraged. Reach to Recovery volunteers also provide exercise instruction. Referral to Occupational or Physical Therapy may be helpful if not initially involved in the exercise instruction.
- Instruct in avoidance of strenuous household tasks such as vacuuming, sweeping, moving or rearranging furniture, and lifting objects more than 10 pounds until full surgical wound healing has occurred and range of motion is improved.
- Instruct in use of temporary prosthesis and wearing of bra, and possible options for the woman postmastectomy for sense of symmetry and balance pending fitting for a weighted prosthesis or reconstruction.

GOAL/OUTCOME

The patient will be free of infection in the postoperative period, without delayed drain removal or excess fluid reaccumulation, without delayed wound healing, and able to successfully care for her wound at home. In addition, she will be able to view her operative site and begin to integrate this into her body image and sense of self, involving her spouse and significant others as appropriate. She will be able to describe arm care and demonstrate beginning range of motion exercises.

Breast Reconstruction

Preoperative nursing care of the patient who is to undergo immediate or delayed reconstruction focuses on the woman's perceptions and expectations of the specific reconstructive approach chosen. Problems and dissatisfaction can be minimized if the woman has realistic expectations of the procedure. Important aspects to reinforce from the physician's discussions with the patient include the appearance of the reconstructed breast, the type of scar(s), the surgical dressing and wound suction, and the use of a brassiere. A preoperative or postoperative visit by a woman who has had a successful breast reconstruction can be beneficial. Postoperative care will be dictated by the type of reconstructive procedure performed. Patients receiving breast implants will need to be taught wound care and bandaging, often inclusive of some type of external pressure support, eventual massage of the implants, and a restricted exercise routine (no heavy lifting or stretching for 4 to 6 weeks). Patients undergoing myocutaneous flap reconstruction will have more wound and drain care needs (as for major abdominal surgery with the TRAM flap) in the hospital.[139] Attention to skin care is vital because these patients may be restricted in mobility in the immediate postoperative period. Further discharge teaching should include the specifics of exercise appropriate to the surgical procedure.

Lymphedema

Lymphedema after breast cancer surgery is the accumulation of lymph fluid in the tissues of the upper extremity, extending from the upper arm potentially to the hand and fingers. It occurs in less than 6% to 7% of all patients undergoing modified radical mastectomy.[71] Risk of developing lymphedema is increased by complete lymph node dissection (levels I, II, and III), radiation therapy to the axilla, obesity, poor nutritional status, increased age, and wound infection.[22,71] It may occur at any time after surgery. It is caused by the interruption or removal of lymph channels and nodes after axillary node dissection or radiation therapy. These procedures result in less efficient filtration of lymph fluid and an impaired ability to fight infection. Prevention of cosmetic deformity, functional impairment, and discomfort are the goals. Nurses can teach the importance of reporting any swelling or red appearance of the affected arm. Intervention should be instituted as soon as lymphedema is noted, so as to prevent or reduce the extent of further progression. This includes elevation of the arm, range of motion exercises, not carrying heavy objects with the affected arm, and avoidance of skin breaks to the arm (venipunctures, harsh detergents,

etc.).[22] Mechanical decompression with a pneumatic pump and arm sleeve may be indicated to reduce swelling. Once a reduction in the swelling has been achieved the patient can be fitted for an elastic sleeve and gauntlet that provides gradient pressure to the upper extremity from the hand to the shoulder. With new onset of lymphedema the medical assessment includes evaluation for infection and other obstructive problems (vein thrombosis or tumor recurrence).[71] Specific arm care precautions to prevent trauma and infection in the arm on the operative side are listed in the box below.

ARM CARE PRECAUTIONS AFTER AXILLARY LYMPH NODE DISSECTION

Avoid sunburns or heavy sun exposure (and wear sunscreen)

Avoid burns while cooking, baking, or smoking

Wear protective gloves when gardening

Use the *unaffected* arm for injections, blood samples, intravenous access, or blood pressures

Use thimble when sewing

Watches, jewelry, and clothing should fit loosely on the arm and hand

Use creams and lotions to keep cuticles soft; do not pull cuticles

Treat cuts promptly and monitor for signs of infection

No chemotherapy is to be given in the affected arm

Nursing Management

ADJUVANT TREATMENT PHASE

During this period patients will need continued reinforcement of exercise routines so as to regain full shoulder function. Wound healing will be completed and final pathology reports discussed. Patients face new decisions about adjuvant chemotherapy and/or hormonal therapy and additional information needs to be clarified. Making a decision about treatment that potentially has side effects when one feels well is not easy. The discussion earlier in this chapter regarding facilitating a patient in decision-making is applicable here.[119,162,169] Patients undergoing breast conserving surgery will generally be receiving radiation therapy. Others will be receiving chemotherapy or hormonal therapy with tamoxifen.

The transition to this therapy phase and its completion is another important intervention period for

nurses.[28,139] Sociocultural and psychosocial factors continue to be important throughout a physical treatment phase.[2,169] The impact of the diagnosis and treatment may be felt more fully during this time by not only the patient but her spouse/significant other and family members. The patient and her family may face new challenges to work and role relationships and functioning. Loveys and Klaich described "demands of illness" in a study of women after the diagnosis of cancer.[124] Treatment issues, social interaction or support, change in life context or perspective, and acceptance of the illness were the most frequently identified concerns, although reconstructing the self, physical changes, uncertainty, financial or occupational concerns, loss, making comparisons, acquiring new knowledge, making choices, mortality issues, and making a contribution were also expressed as concerns. Interventions during this time are directed toward reducing the psychologic and physiologic distress these women experience.

Possible nursing diagnoses during this period include (1) potential for injury, infection, stomatitis, or bleeding secondary to chemotherapy, or skin impairment related to radiation therapy[49,112,139,169]; (2) fatigue related to radiation and/or chemotherapy treatments limiting energy and usual exercise routine[17]; (3) alteration in comfort, hot flashes, decreased/absent vaginal secretions related to chemotherapy or hormone therapy-induced ovarian suppression; (4) body image disturbance related to altered body image secondary to surgery, alopecia, weight gain or loss; (5) altered role performance related to disruption in life and work pattern secondary to treatments; (6) knowledge deficit related to chemotherapy side effects; and (7) anxiety related to completion of adjuvant therapy and transition to regular follow-up period.

NURSING DIAGNOSIS

Anxiety related to fear of side effects of additional treatment with chemotherapy and/or radiation therapy, and impact on resumption of usual activities in social and family life

INTERVENTIONS

- Explain the rationale for adjuvant systemic therapy.
- Promote participation in breast cancer treatment clinical trials as appropriate.
- Describe the specific treatment regimen schedule, route(s) of administration, anticipated side effects, and prevention or management of side effects.
- For premenopausal women, discuss effects of chemotherapy on menstrual function: irregularities, amenorrhea, and potential for pregnancy, with options for birth control while undergoing treatment.
- Postmenopausal women, or premenopausal women undergoing tamoxifen therapy, need information about potential side effects such as hot flashes and vaginal discharge and dryness. Patients should be informed to report such symptoms and subsequently be given guidance on the management of these problems.
- Emphasize and monitor compliance with the proposed treatment regimen.
- Monitor for potential side effects of treatment and intervene appropriately.
- Monitor for potential shoulder dysfunction secondary to decrease in exercises. Additionally assess involvement in other exercise activities.[205]
- Assist the patient and her significant other in identifying real or imagined barriers that may influence resumption of normal sexual relations.
- Assist patient in locating resources for support, such as specifically targeted breast cancer patient support

groups,[29,171,185] resources for fitting for a breast prosthesis, or other programs in the community. The "Women in Nature" program described by Johnson and Kelly incorporated outdoor activities in the wilderness, exercise, and keeping a journal for women diagnosed with cancer.[101] The benefits of exercise alone have also been described.[205]

- Encourage discussion of other psychosocial concerns such as role functions in the home, return to work, vocational retraining, and family and social relationships. Patients may need assistance in identifying their emotional strengths, sources of support, and positive qualities separate from their appearance at a time when they are feeling vulnerable, threatened, and undesirable. Facilitating open communication between the patient and her significant other can be enormously helpful in the couple's adjustment to the cancer diagnosis and treatment. Referral to appropriate resources may be indicated.[30,67]
- Further specific interventions for patients undergoing chemotherapy and radiation therapy are in Chapters 21 and 22, respectively.

GOAL/OUTCOME

The patient will be able to complete adjuvant therapy as close to schedule as possible with successful management of side effects and changes in role or daily activities.

RECOVERY/REHABILITATION/LONG-TERM FOLLOW-UP PHASE

During this period the patient will be adjusting to the completion of chemotherapy and/or radiation therapy and may remain on tamoxifen therapy. There are often feelings of loss and anxiety associated with stopping adjuvant therapy, or the fear that stopping such therapy may somehow allow the cancer to return. The patient, now free from regular frequent medical visits and beginning, perhaps, to feel more physically well again, faces a potential return to more usual patterns of living. The majority of breast cancer survivors who were employed before the diagnosis of cancer return to work.[30] It is usually not without some difficulty, however, including concerns about how co-workers will respond to her and about her own ability to withstand work pressures or physically being able to work the same schedule or type of work.[30] Loss of a job and loss of insurance benefits are of even greater concern in the 1990s. Job discrimination is also a very real fear for those seeking employment.[30,36] While discrimination against disabled persons is prohibited by The Rehabilitation Act of 1973 and the Americans with Disabilities Act of 1990, some courts have decided that recovered cancer patients are not disabled (Chapter 30). The California state law regarding handicapped and disabled persons specifically includes cancer patients.[67] But discrimination is not always so obvious. "Reintegration" describes the process of assisting women with a history of breast cancer to return to work via a program with their employers and organizations that is directed to understanding the needs of each and how to work together.[30] Women who find new employment is necessary may find help in vocational rehabilitation, often available via state or private industry programs.

After therapy is completed, premenopausal women often will resume menstrual function. The question of pregnancy after breast cancer has been well noted in recent literature.[40,82] Most studies of women who became pregnant after successful treatment of breast cancer have found that pregnancy did not negatively influence survival.[40,82] The greatest risk for recurrence of breast cancer is in the first 2 years, so one suggestion has been to delay pregnancy until after that time.[40] Hassey describes the genuine quality of life issues for a woman and her spouse facing this decision: the importance of reproductive counseling, discussion of the risk of recurrence, and discussion of the potential, if there is recurrence and disease progression, of single parenthood for the spouse.[82] The issue of pregnancy after breast cancer, with more women delaying childbirth, is likely to remain an integral aspect of the nursing care of premenopausal women with breast cancer.

NURSING DIAGNOSIS
Possible impaired social interaction

INTERVENTIONS
- Assist patient to verbalize fears and concerns.
- Provide supportive information regarding those concerns and to ease fears, as appropriate, such as plans for continued medical follow up, positive appraisal of her strengths, and services for vocational rehabilitation.
- Encourage and facilitate discussion with appropriate medical resources for pregnancy planning.
- Encourage participation in survivorship activities or group support, if desired.
- Encourage the patient and/or her family to resume participation in activities previously enjoyed.

GOAL/OUTCOME
The patient will effectively resume, re-establish, or begin anew personal and social relationships that are meaningful and rewarding, and integrate the concept of survivorship.

RECURRENCE/METASTASIS/TERMINAL PHASE[38,189]

Fortunately many women diagnosed with breast cancer today will not die from their disease. For those who face a recurrence, however, the experience may be much more traumatic than the initial diagnosis.[131,135] Local recurrences are often managed with local treatments, such as surgical resection or radiation therapy. For the woman experiencing a local recurrence after breast conserving surgery, mastectomy may be recommended. Nursing care in such circumstances has been addressed previously.

The patient with metastatic recurrence (or disease at diagnosis) may exhibit physical signs or symptoms such as bone pain, hypercalcemia, dyspnea, or fatigue, or the recurrence may be suspected before symptoms present (as in elevated liver function tests or an abnormal bone scan). This is a time when there is recognition that the previous treatment failed to control the disease completely. Coping strategies that worked well in the past may be stressed during this time. There is much uncertainty and there is anticipation of loss. The sense of hope may be challenged. It is a time when information about the next plan of action can give hope and direction. Many agents have demonstrated effectiveness in breast cancer and, while cure is no longer possible, palliation of symptoms and prolonged control of the disease are reasonable and worthwhile goals.

NURSING DIAGNOSIS
Anticipatory grieving related to possible losses including death

INTERVENTION
- Provide support when the patient is informed of diagnosis and treatment plan.
- Explain the rationale for treatments and the side effects to anticipate and their management.
- Encourage the patient and her significant other(s) to openly discuss their concerns. Many times when conventional treatment fails or is difficult, unproven therapies are sought; being able to discuss this with the health care team can help prevent complications (see also Chapter 25).
- Assist the patient and family to manage symptoms or complications of the disease and/or treatment, such as pain and hypercalcemia.[10,141]
- Assess coping and support needs of the patient and family. Assist the patient and family in the terminal phase to verbalize feelings about the meaning of illness and death.
- Referrals to supportive resources may be indicated, such as home nursing care and hospice programs, support groups, pastoral care, and/or professional counselors for therapeutic intervention.

GOAL/OUTCOME
The patient will effectively grieve the loss of the concept of cure, and will feel supported in resuming ther-

apy, if indicated. The patient will experience satisfactory control of side effects and/or complications or treatment. In the terminal phase the patient will come to some degree of acceptance of death (see also Chapter 30).

FOLLOW-UP

All patients with breast cancer require periodic follow-up evaluations for the remainder of their life. These evaluations are performed to monitor for recurrent disease and complications of treatment (see box on p. 118). They also allow opportunity to assess the patient's level of coping and that of her husband/significant other and family.

Because the risk for recurrence is highest during the first 2 years after diagnosis, physical assessments are recommended every 3 months for the first 2 to 3 years, biannually for the next 2 to 3 years, and then annually.[83] Serum chemistry tests are usually obtained at each evaluation, mammograms are done yearly, and chest x-rays and bone scans may be done annually or as indicated.[83] Any signs or symptoms the patient has at the time of each evaluation will influence what additional tests or imaging studies are ordered, or their frequency.

Northouse reported that difficulties in psychosocial adjustment to breast cancer are not confined to the early phase of the illness but persist over time for both patients and husbands.[153] Fear of disease recurrence, role adjustment problems, resource depletion, toxicities of therapy, as well as changes in body image, self-esteem, and patterns of sexuality are problems the patient and, to some extent, the husband/significant other may encounter. Cancer affects families, and children may need support also.[97] Emotional problems may require referrals to trained counselors or support groups available through the ACS, local hospitals, or community.

Husbands/significant others are to be encouraged to come to the follow-up evaluations with the patients. This allows them to be included in the discussion regarding concerns and problems they are experiencing individually and as a couple. Special consideration needs to be given to the elderly woman who may have a limited social support network (see box at right).

In addition to regular evaluations by a health professional, women are to be encouraged to begin or continue monthly BSE and regular mammograms. It is also important to identify high-risk family members to whom appropriate screening recommendations can be provided.

A summary of patient teaching priorities for breast cancer is given in the box on p. 123.

GERIATRIC CONSIDERATIONS

Prevention and detection*

- Health assessments need to incorporate cognitive function, physical limitations/sensory deficits, and support network
- Education efforts should address knowledge, skill, and confidence in BSE, mammography and CBE, and benefits of early detection
- Continuity and participation may be enhanced when health care is coordinated by one or few providers (e.g., advocate, case manager)
- Community-based breast cancer screening is beneficial
- The effectiveness of rescreening after age 70 is controversial
- Education of health care providers should emphasize continuing need for scheduled screening of elderly women in light of current data

Diagnosis and treatment[16,58,188]

- The importance of patient involvement in decision-making needs to be considered irrespective of age
- Age in and of itself ought not to determine type or extent of surgery or subsequent therapy
- Care throughout the operative phase includes careful preoperative assessment and intra- and post-operative physiologic monitoring
- Early *comprehensive discharge planning* should involve the patient and significant other
- Side effects with radiation and chemotherapy may be enhanced or prolonged
- Most trials of systemic therapy have excluded women over 70 years of age

Rehabilitation[50]

- Return to or maintenance of pre-cancer level of functioning is a reasonable goal
- Care should be taken to incorporate psychosexual assessment and intervention as appropriate for all ages
- Physical illness can impair developmental task completion
- Depression in the elderly may be masked by physical symptoms

Metastatic disease[50]

- Differential diagnosis of symptoms must differentiate normal or pathologic changes from signs of metastatic disease
- Chronic pain may be indirectly expressed via other physical changes (e.g., anorexia, irritability, aching, insomnia)
- Recurrent disease may exacerbate other felt losses of the elderly

*References 34, 37, 42, 60, 126, 127, 130, 144, 159, 188, 198.

CONCLUSION

Breast cancer presents nurses with many challenges along a continuum of prevention, early detection, and treatment. The nurse must be knowledgeable about breast cancer and its ever-changing management; honest, realistic, and creative when providing support and care; skilled at symptom management; and observant of the patient's unspoken needs and willing to involve herself/himself in the challenging opportunity of caring for the patient with breast cancer. Health care for the elderly will be a major concern for the next decade and breast cancer is of utmost interest in an aging female population. Likewise early detection outreach to socioeconomically disadvantaged women will prove to be beneficial in reducing the number of deaths from breast cancer. Nurses have a key role on all of these fronts.

BIBLIOGRAPHY

1. Alagna SW and Reddy DM: Predictors of proficient technique in successful lesion detection in self breast examination, Health Psychol 3:113, 1984.
2. Ali NS and Khalil HZ: Identification of stressors, level of stress, coping strategies, and coping effectiveness among Egyptian mastectomy patients, Cancer Nurs 14:232, 1991.
3. American Cancer Society: 1989 survey of physicians' attitudes and practices in early cancer detection, CA 40:77, 1990.
4. American Cancer Society: Cancer facts and figures—1993, Atlanta, 1993, American Cancer Society, Inc.
5. American Cancer Society: Cancer facts and figures for minority Americans—1991, Atlanta, 1991, American Cancer Society, Inc.
6. American Cancer Society: Clinical breast examination: proficiency criteria and guidelines, Oakland, CA, 1988, American Cancer Society, California Division, Inc.
7. American Cancer Society: Special report on cancer in the economically disadvantaged, New York, 1986, American Cancer Society, Inc.
8. American Cancer Society: Special touch breast health trainer's guide, ed 2, Oakland, CA, 1990, American Cancer Society, California Division, Inc.
9. American Joint Committee on Cancer: Manual for staging of cancer, ed 3, Philadelphia, 1988, JB Lippincott Co.
10. Arathuzik D: Pain experience for metastatic breast cancer patients. Unraveling the mystery, Cancer Nurs 14:41, 1991.
11. Assaf AR and others: Comparison of three methods of teaching women how to perform breast self-examination, Health Educ Q 12:259, 1985.
12. Baines CJ: Breast self-examination, Cancer 69:1942, 1992.
13. Baquet CR, Horm JW, Gibbs T, and Greenwald P: Socioeconomic factors and cancer incidence among blacks and whites, JNCI 83:551, 1991.
14. Bassett LW: Mammographic features of malignancy. In Mitchell GW and Bassett LW, editors: The female breast and its disorders, Baltimore, 1990, Williams & Wilkins.
15. Bassett LW and Gold RH: Introduction to mammography. In Mitchell GW and Bassett LW, editors: The female breast and its disorders, Baltimore, 1990, Williams & Wilkins.
16. Blesch KS: The normal physiological changes of aging and their impact on the response to cancer treatment, Semin Oncol Nurs 4:178, 1988.
17. Blesch KS and others: Correlates of fatigue in people with breast or lung cancer, Oncol Nurs Forum 18:81, 1991.
18. Boice JD Jr and Monson RR: Breast cancer in women after repeated fluoroscopic examinations of the chest, J Natl Cancer Inst 59:823, 1977.
19. Boring CC: Cancer statistics for African Americans, CA 42:7, 1992.

20. Boring CC, Squires TS, and Tong T: Cancer statistics, CA 42:19, 1992.

21. Bostwick J III: Breast reconstruction following mastectomy, CA 39:40, 1989.

22. Brown M, Eyles H, and Bland KI: Nursing care for the patient with breast cancer. In Bland KI and Copeland EM III, editors: The breast: comprehensive management of benign and malignant diseases, Philadelphia, 1991, WB Saunders Co.

23. Burack RC and Liang J: The acceptance and completion of mammography by older black women, AJPH 79:721, 1989.

24. Callahan R and others: Somatic mutations and human breast cancer, Cancer 69:1582, 1992.

25. Cawley M, Kostic J, and Cappello C: Informational and psychosocial needs of women choosing conservative surgery/primary radiation for early stage breast cancer, Cancer Nurs 13:90, 1990.

26. Champion VL: Attitudinal variables related to intention, frequency and proficiency of breast self-examination in women 35 and older, Res Nurs Health 11:283, 1988.

27. Champion VL: The relationship of selected variables to breast cancer detection behaviors in women 35 and older, Oncol Nurs Forum 18:733, 1991.

28. Chou A: Breast health nursing. In Gross A and Itto D, editors: Women talk about breast surgery, New York, 1990, Clarkson Potter/Publishers.

29. Christ GH and others: Educational and support programs for breast cancer patients and their families. In Harris JR and others, editors: Breast diseases, ed 2, Philadelphia, 1991, JB Lippincott Co.

30. Clark JC and Landis LL: Reintegration and maintenance of employees with breast cancer in the workplace, Am Assoc Occup Health Nurses 37:186, 1989.

31. Coleman CM and Crane R: Knowledge deficit related to prevention and early detection of breast cancer. In McNally JC, Somerville ET, Miaskowski C, and Rostad M, editors: Guidelines for oncology nursing practice, ed 2, Philadelphia, 1991, WB Saunders Co.

32. Coleman EA: Practice and effectiveness of breast self examination: a selective review of the literature (1977-1989), J Cancer Ed 6:83, 1991.

33. Coleman EA and Pennypacker H: Measuring breast self-examination proficiency, Cancer Nurs 14:211, 1991.

34. Coleman EA and others: Efficacy of breast self-examination teaching methods among older women, Oncol Nurs Forum 18:561, 1991.

35. Collins-Hattery AM and Blumberg BD: S phase index and ploidy prognostic markers in node negative breast cancer: information for nurses, Oncol Nurs Forum 18:59, 1991.

36. Cooley ME and Erikson B: Rehabilitation. In Fowble B and others, editors: Breast cancer treatment: a comprehensive guide to management, St Louis, 1991, Mosby.

37. Costanza ME: Breast cancer screening in older women: synopsis of a forum, Cancer 69:1925, 1992.

38. Coward DD: Self-transcendence and emotional well-being in women with advanced breast cancer, Oncol Nurs Forum 18:857, 1991.

39. Curtis RE and others: Risk of leukemia after chemotherapy and radiation treatment for breast cancer, N Engl J Med 326:1745, 1992.

40. Danforth DN: How subsequent pregnancy affects outcome in women with a prior breast cancer, Oncology 5:23, 1991.

41. Dawson I and others: Effect of shoulder immobilization on wound seroma and shoulder dysfunction following modified radical mastectomy: a randomized prospective clinical trial, Br J Surg 76:311, 1989.

42. Dellefield ME: Informational needs and approaches for early cancer detection in the elderly, Sem Oncol Nurs 4:156, 1988.

43. Dodd GD: American Cancer Society Guidelines on screening for breast cancer, Cancer (Supplement) 69:1885, 1992.

44. Donegan WL: Cancer of the breast in men, CA 41:339, 1991.

45. Dorr FA and Friedman MA: The role of chemotherapy in the management of primary breast cancer, CA 41:231, 1991.

46. Dorsay RH and others: Breast self-examination: improving competence and frequency in a classroom setting, AJPH 78:520, 1988.

47. Dupont WD and Page DL: Menopausal estrogen replacement therapy and breast cancer, Arch Intern Med 151:67, 1991.

48. Dupont WD and Page DL: Risk factors for breast cancer in women with proliferative breast disease, N Engl J Med 312:146, 1985.

49. Ehlke G: Symptom distress in breast cancer patients receiving chemotherapy in the outpatient setting, Oncol Nurs Forum 15:343, 1988.

50. Engelking C: Comfort issues in geriatric oncology, Semin Oncol Nurs 4:198, 1988.

51. Falkson G and others: Survival of premenopausal women with metastatic breast cancer. Long-term follow-up of Eastern Cooperative Group and Cancer and Leukemia Group B studies, Cancer 66:1621, 1990.

52. Feather BL and Wainstock JM: Perceptions of postmastectomy patients. Part I, Cancer Nurs 12:293, 1989.

53. Feather BL and Wainstock JM: Perceptions of postmastectomy patients. Part II, Cancer Nurs 12:301, 1989.

54. Feig SA: Decreased breast cancer mortality through mammography screening: results of clinical trials, Radiology 167:659, 1988.

55. Fisher B: A biological perspective of breast cancer: contributions of the National Surgical Adjuvant Breast and Bowel Project clinical trials, CA 41:97, 1991.

56. Fletcher SW, O'Malley MS, and Bunce LA: Physician's abilities to detect lumps in silicone breast models, JAMA 253:2224, 1985.

57. Fletcher SW and others: How best to teach women breast self-examination: a randomized controlled trial, Ann Intern Med 112:772, 1990.

58. Forrest APM: Primary breast cancer in older women. In Balducci L, Lyman GH, and Ershler WB, editors: Geriatric oncology, Philadelphia, 1992, JB Lippincott Co.

59. Foster RS and others: Breast self examination practices and breast cancer stage, N Engl J Med 299:265, 1978.

60. Fox SA, Murata PJ, and Stein JA: The impact of physician compliance on screening mammography for older women, Arch Intern Med 151:50, 1991.

61. Freeman HP: Cancer in the socioeconomically disadvantaged, CA 39:266, 1989.

62. Friedell GH: The 'squeaky wheel' and health care policy (Commentary), JAMA 265:3300, 1991.

63. Frykberg ER, Ames FC, and Bland KI: Current concepts for management of early (*in situ* and occult invasive) breast carcinoma. In Bland KI and Copeland EM III, editors: The breast: comprehensive management of benign and malignant diseases, Philadelphia, 1991, WB Saunders Co.

64. Ganz PA and others: Breast conservation *versus* mastectomy, Cancer 69:1729, 1992.

65. Garber JE: Familial aspects of breast cancer. In Harris JR and others, editors: Breast diseases, ed 2, Philadelphia, 1991, JB Lippincott Co.

66. Garber JE, Henderson IC, Love SM, and Gelman RS: Management of high-risk groups. In Harris JR and others, editors: Breast diseases, ed 2, Philadelphia, 1991, JB Lippincott Co.

67. Gaskin TA and others: Rehabilitation. In Bland KI and Copeland EM III, editors: The breast: comprehensive management of benign and malignant diseases, Philadelphia, 1991, WB Saunders Co.

68. Glick JH: Meeting highlights: adjuvant therapy for breast cancer, J Natl Cancer Inst 80:471, 1988.

69. Gonzalez JT: Factors relating to frequency of breast self-examination among low-income Mexican American women. Implications for nursing practice, Cancer Nurs 13:134, 1990.

70. Goodman M: Adjuvant systemic therapy of stage I and II breast cancer, Sem Oncol Nurs 7:175, 1991.

71. Gottlieb LJ and Patel P-KK: Lymphedema following axillary surgery: elephantiasis chirurgica. In Harris JR and others, editors: Breast diseases, ed 2, Philadelphia, 1991, JB Lippincott Co.

72. Gray ME: Factors related to practice of breast self-examination in rural women, Cancer Nurs 13:100, 1990.

73. Greenwald P and others: Estimated effect of breast self-examination and routine physician examination on breast cancer mortality, N Engl J Med 299:271, 1978.

74. Greenwald P and Sondik EJ: Cancer control objectives for the nation 1985-2000, NCI Monographs, No 2, 1986.

75. Gutman H and others: Achievements of physical therapy in patients after modified radical mastectomy compared with quadrantectomy, axillary dissection, and radiation for carcinoma of the breast, Arch Surg 125:389, 1990.

76. Hand R and others: Hospital variables associated with quality of care for breast cancer patients, JAMA 266:3429, 1991.

77. Handel N: Current status of breast reconstruction after mastectomy, Oncology 5:73, 1991.

78. Harris JR: Clinical management of ductal carcinoma in situ. In Harris JR and others, editors: Breast diseases, ed 2, Philadelphia, 1991, JB Lippincott Co.

79. Harris JR: Postmastectomy radiotherapy. In Harris JR and others, editors: Breast diseases, ed 2, Philadelphia, 1991, JB Lippincott Co.

80. Harris JR: Staging of breast carcinoma. In Harris JR and others, editors: Breast diseases, ed 2, Philadelphia, 1991, JB Lippincott Co.

81. Harris JR and Hellman S: Natural history of breast cancer. In Harris JR and others, editors: Breast diseases, ed 2, Philadelphia, 1991, JB Lippincott Co.

82. Hassey KM: Pregnancy and parenthood after treatment for breast cancer, Oncol Nurs Forum 15:439, 1988.

83. Hayes DF and Kaplan WD: Evaluation of patients following primary therapy. In Harris JR and others, editors: Breast diseases, ed 2, Philadelphia, 1991, JB Lippincott Co.

84. Henderson BE and Bernstein L: The role of endogenous and exogenous hormones in the etiology of breast cancer. In Harris JR and others, editors: Breast diseases, ed 2, Philadelphia, 1991, JB Lippincott Co.

85. Henderson IC: Adjuvant systemic therapy of early breast cancer. In Harris JR and others, editors: Breast diseases, ed 2, Philadelphia, 1991, JB Lippincott Co.

86. Henderson IC: Chemotherapy for metastatic disease. In Harris JR and others, editors: Breast diseases, ed 2, Philadelphia, 1991, JB Lippincott Co.

87. Henderson IC: Endocrine therapy of metastatic breast cancer. In Harris JR and others, editors: Breast diseases, ed 2, Philadelphia, 1991, JB Lippincott Co.

88. Henderson IC: Prognostic factors. In Harris JR and others, editors: Breast diseases, ed 2, Philadelphia, 1991, JB Lippincott Co.

89. Henderson IC and Harris JR: Integration of local and systemic therapies. In Harris JR and others, editors: Breast diseases, ed 2, Philadelphia, 1991, JB Lippincott Co.

90. Houts PS and others: Using a state cancer registry to increase screening behaviors of sisters and daughters of breast cancer patients, AJPH 81:386, 1991.

91. Howard J: Using mammography for cancer control: an unrealized potential, CA 37:33, 1987.

92. Hrushesky WJM: Timing of surgery in breast cancer (editorial), Lancet, 337:1604, 1991.

93. Huguley CM Jr and others: Breast self-examination and survival from breast cancer, Cancer 62:1389, 1988.

94. Hutter RVP: The role of the pathologist in the management of breast cancer, CA 41:283, 1991.

95. Ingram D and others: Obesity and breast disease. The role of the female sex hormones, Cancer 64:1049, 1989.

96. Institute of Medicine, Committee on the Relationship Between Oral Contraceptives and Breast Cancer, Division of Health Promotion and Disease Prevention: Oral contraceptives and breast cancer, Washington, D.C., 1991, National Academy Press.

97. Issel LM, Ersek M, and Lewis FM: How children cope with mother's breast cancer, Oncol Nurs Forum 17(S):5, 1990.

98. Jacob TC, Penn NE, and Brown M: Breast self-examination: knowledge, attitudes, and performance among black women, J Natl Med Assoc 81:769, 1989.

99. Jansen RFM and others: Immediate versus delayed shoulder exercises after axillary lymph node dissection, Am J Surg 160:481, 1990.

100. Jepson C and others: Black-white differences in cancer prevention knowledge and behavior, AJPH 81:501, 1991.

101. Johnson JB and Kelly AW: A multifaceted rehabilitation program for women with cancer, Oncol Nurs Forum 17:691, 1990.

102. Kaplan KM and others: Breast cancer screening among relatives of women with breast cancer, AJPH 81:1174, 1991.

103. Karp JE and Broder S: Oncology, JAMA 268:391, 1992.

104. Kegeles SS: Education for breast self-examination: why, who, what, and how? Prev Med 14:702, 1985.

105. Kelly PT: Understanding breast cancer risk. Philadelphia, 1991, Temple University Press.

106. Kelsey JL and Gammon MD: The epidemiology of breast cancer, CA 41:146, 1991.

107. Kemeny MM, Wellisch DK, and Schain WS: Psychosocial outcome in a randomized surgical trial for treatment of primary breast cancer, Cancer 62:1231, 1988.

108. Ketcham AS and Moffat FL: Vexed surgeons, perplexed patients, and breast cancers which may not be cancer, Cancer 65:387, 1990.

109. Kinne DW: Biopsy of a palpable lesion. In Harris JR and others, editors: Breast diseases, ed 2, Philadelphia, 1991, JB Lippincott Co.

110. Kinne DW: Clinical management of lobular carcinoma in situ. In Harris JR and others, editors: Breast diseases, ed 2, Philadelphia, 1991, JB Lippincott Co.

111. Kinne DW: Surgery. In Harris JR and others, editors: Breast diseases, ed 2, Philadelphia, 1991, JB Lippincott Co.

112. Knobf MT: Symptoms and rehabilitation needs of patients with early stage breast cancer during primary therapy, Cancer 66:1392, 1990.

113. Koroltchouk V, Stanley K, and Stjernsward J: The control of breast cancer. A World Health Organization perspective, Cancer 65:2803, 1990.

114. Krizek TJ: Breast reconstruction after mastectomy. In Harris JR and others, editors: Breast diseases, ed 2, Philadelphia, 1991, JB Lippincott Co.

115. LaRossa D: Reconstructive surgery. In Fowble B and others, editors: Breast cancer treatment: a comprehensive guide to management, St Louis, 1991, Mosby.

116. Lasry J-CM: Women's sexuality following breast cancer. In Osoba D, editor: Effect of cancer on quality of life, Boca Raton, 1991, CRC Press, Inc.

117. Lasry J-CM and Margolese RG: Fear of recurrence, breast-conserving surgery, and the trade-off hypothesis, Cancer 69:2111, 1992.

118. Lazovich D and others: Underutilization of breast-conserving surgery and radiation therapy among women with stage I or II breast cancer, JAMA 266:3433, 1991.

119. Levine MN and others: A bedside decision instrument to elicit a patient's preference concerning adjuvant chemotherapy for breast cancer, Ann Intern Med 1117:53, 1992.

120. Lierman LM: Phantom breast experiences after mastectomy, Oncol Nurs Forum 15:41, 1988.

121. Liff JM and others: Does increased detection account for the rising incidence of breast cancer? AJPH 81:462, 1991.

122. Lotze MT and others: Early versus delayed shoulder motion following axillary dissection, Ann Surg 193:288, 1981.

123. Love RR and others: Symptoms associated with tamoxifen treatment in postmenopausal women, Arch Intern Med 151:1842, 1991.

124. Love SM: Dr. Susan Love's breast book. Reading, Massachusetts, 1990, Addison-Wesley Publishing Co., Inc.

125. Loveys BJ and Klaich K: Breast cancer: demands of illness, Oncol Nurs Forum 18:75, 1991.

126. Ludwick R: Breast examination in the older adult, Cancer Nurs 11:99, 1988.

127. Ludwick R: Registered nurses' knowledge and practices of teaching and performing breast exams among elderly women, Cancer Nurs 15:61, 1992.

128. Lynch HT, Pennisi VR, and Lynch JF: Heredity in breast cancer. In Ariel IM and Cleary JB, editors: Breast cancer diagnosis and treatment, New York, 1987, McGraw-Hill Book Co.

129. Lynch HT and others: Natural history and age at onset of hereditary breast cancer, Cancer 69:1404, 1992.

130. Maddox MA: The practice of breast self-examination among older women, Oncol Nurs Forum 18:1367, 1991.

131. Mahon SM: Managing the psychosocial consequences of cancer recurrence: implications for nurses, Oncol Nurs Forum 18:577, 1991.

132. Mahon SM and Casperson D: Teaching women about mammography through use of a brochure, Oncol Nurs Forum 18:1375, 1991.

133. MammaTech Corporation: MammaCare learning system for breast self-examination. Gainesville, FL, 1990, MammaTech Corporation. MammaCare, P.O. Box 15748, Gainesville, FL 32604.

134. Marchant D: Surgery for breast cancer. In Mitchell GW Jr and Bassett LW, editors: The female breast and its disorders, Baltimore, 1990, Williams & Wilkins.

135. McEvoy MD and McCorkle R: Quality of life issues in patients with disseminated breast cancer, Cancer 66(S):1416, 1990.

136. McGregor D and others: Breast cancer incidence among atomic bomb survivors, Hiroshima and Nagasaki, 1950-1969, J Natl Cancer Inst 59:799, 1977.

137. McGuire WL and Clark GM: Prognostic factors and treatment decisions in axillary-node–negative breast cancer, N Engl J Med 326:1756, 1992.

138. McInnis WD: Plastic surgery of the breast. In Mitchell GW Jr and Bassett LW, editors: The female breast and its disorders, Baltimore, 1990, Williams & Wilkins.

139. McKenney S and Dow KMH: Patient rehabilitation and support: nursing. In Harris JR and others, editors: Breast diseases, ed 2, Philadelphia, 1991, JB Lippincott Co.

140. Meade CD, Diekmann J, and Thornhill DG: Readability of American Cancer Society patient education literature, Oncol Nurs Forum 19:51, 1992.

141. Meriney DK: Application of Orem's conceptual framework to patients with hypercalcemia related to breast cancer, Cancer Nurs 13:316, 1990.

142. Mettlin C: Breast cancer risk factors, Cancer (Supplement) 69:1904, 1992.

143. Miller AB: Causes of breast cancer and high-risk groups. In Harris JR and others, editors: Breast diseases, ed 2, Philadelphia, 1991, JB Lippincott Co.

144. Miller AB: Early detection of breast cancer. In Harris JR and others, editors: Breast diseases, ed 2, Philadelphia, 1991, JB Lippincott Co.

145. Mitchell GW Jr: Ambulatory surgery for diagnosis and treatment. In Mitchell GW Jr and Bassett LW, editors: The female breast and its disorders, Baltimore, 1990, Williams & Wilkins.

146. Mitchell GW Jr: History and physical examination. In Mitchell GW Jr and Bassett LW, editors: The female breast and its disorders, Baltimore, 1990, Williams & Wilkins.

147. Morra ME and Blumberg BD: Women's perceptions of early detection in breast cancer: How are we doing?, Seminars in Oncology Nursing 7:151, 1991.

148. Morris T: Psychosocial aspects of breast cancer; a review, Eur J Cancer Clin Oncol 19:1725, 1983.

149. Morrison BW: Oncogenes and breast cancer. In Harris JR and others, editors: Breast diseases, ed 2, Philadelphia, 1991, JB Lippincott Co.

150. Morrow M, Hoffman PC, and Weichselbaum RR: Locally advanced breast cancer. In Harris JR and others, editors: Breast diseases, ed 2, Philadelphia, 1991, JB Lippincott Co.

151. National Institutes of Health consensus development conference statement: adjuvant chemotherapy for breast cancer, September 9-11, 1985, CA 36:42, 1986.

152. Nemcek MA: Factors influencing black women's breast self-examination practice, Cancer Nurs 12:339, 1989.

153. Northouse L: A longitudinal study of the adjustment of patients and husbands to breast cancer, Oncol Nurs Forum 17(S):39, 1990.

154. Osborne CK: Receptors. In Harris JR and others,

editors: Breast diseases, ed 2, Philadelphia, 1991, JB Lippincott Co.

155. Osborne MP: Breast development and anatomy. In Harris JR and others, editors: Breast diseases, ed 2, Philadelphia, 1991, JB Lippincott Co.

156. Osteen RT and others: Regional differences in surgical management of breast cancer, CA 42:39, 1992.

157. Page DL and Dupont WD: Anatomic markers of human premalignancy and risk of breast cancer, Cancer 66:1326, 1990.

158. Page DL and Simpson JF: Benign, high-risk, and premalignant lesions of the mamma. In Bland KI and Copeland EM, editors: The breast. Comprehensive management of benign and malignant diseases, Philadelphia, 1991, WB Saunders Co.

159. Paul PB: The older woman: implications for care. In Proceedings of the Sixth National Conference on Cancer Nursing: Cancer prevention, early detection and screening, Atlanta, 1992, American Cancer Society, Inc.

160. Pennypacker HS and others: Toward an effective technology of instruction in breast self-examination, Int J Ment Health 11:98, 1982.

161. Petrek JA and others: Axillary lymphadenectomy. A prospective, randomized trial of 13 factors influencing drainage, including early or delayed arm mobilization, Arch Surg 125:378, 1990.

162. Rabinowitz B: Guidelines for facilitating patient decision making, Innovations in Oncology Nursing 5:4, 14, 1989.

163. Ramzy I: Pathology of benign breast disease. In Mitchell GW and Bassett LW, editors: The female breast and its disorders, Baltimore, 1990, Williams & Wilkins.

164. Ramzy I: Pathology of malignant neoplasms. In Mitchell GW and Bassett LW, editors: The female breast and its disorders, Baltimore, 1990, Williams & Wilkins.

165. Recht A and Hayes DF: Local recurrence following mastectomy. In Harris JR and others, editors: Breast diseases, ed 2, Philadelphia, 1991, JB Lippincott Co.

166. Robinson JO: Treatment of breast cancer through the ages, Am J Surg 151:317, 1986.

167. Rosato EF and Curcillo PG II: Surgical considerations in the management of breast cancer. In Fowble B and others: editors: Breast cancer treatment: a comprehensive guide to management, St Louis, 1991, Mosby.

168. Rosen PP: The pathology of invasive breast carcinoma. In Harris JR and others, editors: Breast diseases, ed 2, Philadelphia, 1991, JB Lippincott Co.

169. Rowland JH and Holland JC: Psychological reactions to breast cancer and its treatment. In Harris JR and others, editors: Breast diseases, ed 2, Philadelphia, 1991, JB Lippincott Co.

170. Sachs BC: Breasts: sex symbols and releasers, Diseases of the Breast 4:26, 1978.

171. Samarel N and Fawcett J: Enhancing adaptation to breast cancer: the addition of coaching to support groups, Oncol Nurs Forum 19:591, 1992.

172. Saunders KJ, Pilgrim CA, and Pennypacker HS: Increased proficiency of search in breast self-examination, Cancer 58:2531, 1986.

173. Scanlon EF: Breast cancer. In Holleb AI, Fink DJ, and Murphy GP, editors: American Cancer Society textbook of clinical oncology, Atlanta, 1991, American Cancer Society, Inc.

174. Schain WS: Physician-patient communication about breast cancer. A challenge for the 1990s, Surg Clin North Am 70:917, 1990.

175. Schain WS, Jacobs E, and Wellisch DK: Psychosocial issues in breast reconstruction: intrapsychic, interpersonal and practical concerns. In Scheflan MB, editor: Clinics in plastic surgery, Philadelphia, 1984, WB Saunders Co.

176. Schain WS and others: The sooner the better: a study of psychological factors in women undergoing immediate versus delayed breast reconstruction, Am J Psychiatry 142:40, 1985.

177. Schnitt SJ and Connolly JL: Benign breast disorders. In Harris JR and others, editors: Breast diseases, ed 2, Philadelphia, 1991, JB Lippincott Co.

178. Schnitt SJ and Harris JR: Ductal carcinoma in situ (intraductal carcinoma) of the breast, PPO Updates 2:1, 1988.

179. Schover LR: The impact of breast cancer on sexuality, body image, and intimate relationships, CA 41:112, 1991.

180. Seidman H and others: Survival experience in the Breast Cancer Detection Demonstration Project, CA 37:258, 1987.

181. Seidman H, Stellman SD, and Mushinski MH: A different perspective on breast cancer risk factors: some implications of the nonattributable risk, CA 32:301, 1982.

182. Sharp N: The politics of breast cancer, Nurs Management 22:24, 1991.

183. Shugg D and others: Practice of breast self-examination and the treatment of primary breast cancer, Aust N Z J Surg 60:455, 1990.

184. Speroff L: Tamoxifen: special considerations for gynecologists, Contemp OB/GYN 37:50, 1992.

185. Spiegel D: Facilitating emotional coping during treatment, Cancer 66:1422, 1990.

186. Stampfer MJ, Bechtel SD, and Hunter DJ: Fat, alcohol, selenium, and breast cancer risk, Contemporary OB/GYN 37:42, 1992.

187. Stefanek ME: Counseling women at high risk for breast cancer, Oncology 4:27, 1990.

188. Stewart JA and Foster RS Jr: Breast cancer and aging, Sem Oncol 16:41, 1989.

189. Thomas SG: Breast cancer: the psychosocial issues, Cancer Nurs 1:53, 1978.

190. Treatment of early-stage breast cancer. National Institutes of Health consensus development conference statement, 1990, June 18-21:8(6).

191. Valanis BG and Rumpler CH: Helping women to choose breast cancer treatment alternatives, Cancer Nurs 8:167, 1985.

192. Vinton AL, Traverso LW, and Zehring RD: Immediate breast reconstruction following mastectomy is as safe as mastectomy alone, Arch Surg 125:1303, 1990.

193. Vogel CL: Treatment of metastatic breast cancer, Sem Oncol Nurs 7:194, 1991.

194. Vogel CL and others: Survival after first recurrence of breast cancer. The Miami experience, Cancer 70:129, 1992.

195. Wagner FB: History of breast disease and its treatment. In Bland KI and Copeland EM, editors: The breast: comprehensive management of benign and malignant diseases, Philadelphia, 1991, WB Saunders Co.

196. Ward S and Griffin J: Developing a test of knowledge of surgical options for breast cancer, Cancer Nurs 13:191, 1990.

197. Ward S, Heidrich S, and Wolberg W: Factors women take into account when deciding upon type of surgery for breast cancer, Cancer Nurs 12:344, 1989.

198. Weisman CS and others: Cancer screening services for the elderly, Public Health Reports 104:209-214, 1989.

199. Weiss MC and Kelsten ML: Biologic markers of breast cancer prognosis. In Fowble B and others, editors: Breast cancer treatment: a comprehensive guide to management, St Louis, 1991, Mosby.

200. Whitman S and others: Patterns of breast and cervical cancer screening at three public health centers in an inner-city urban area, AJPH 81:1651, 1991.

201. Willis MA and others: Inter-agency collaboration: teaching breast self-examination to black women, Oncol Nurs Forum 16:171, 1989.

202. Winchester DP and Cox JD: Standards for breast-conserving treatment, CA 42:134, 1992.

203. Woolhandler S and Himmelstein DU: Reverse targeting of preventive care due to lack of health insurance, JAMA 259:2872, 1988.

204. Yeh I'T and others: Pathologic assessment and pathologic prognostic factors in operable breast cancer. In Fowble B and others, editors: Breast cancer treatment: a comprehensive guide to management, St Louis, 1991, Mosby.

205. Young-McCaughan S and Sexton DL: A retrospective investigation of the relationship between aerobic exercise and quality of life in women with breast cancer, Oncol Nurs Forum 18:751, 1991.

CHAPTER 8

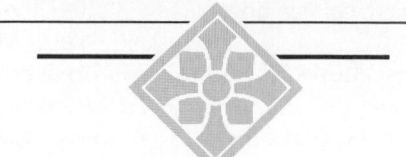

Colorectal Cancer

Mary E. Murphy

Colorectal cancer is the second most common malignant tumor in the United States, second only to lung cancer in its incidence and mortality. An estimated 6000 new cases develop each year with an annual death rate of 60,000. Cure rates remain at only 50% despite recent advancements in treatment technology.[1,3,6] Continued research to investigate the cause and treatment of this disease are under investigation and remain a medical priority.

EPIDEMIOLOGY

Colorectal cancer affects both sexes equally, with the incidence increasing significantly in persons over the age of 50. The mean age at the time of diagnosis is 62.[51] The disease occurs most frequently in Western industrialized countries of Northern America, Northern Europe, and New Zealand. Individuals from low incidence countries who move to Western countries develop colorectal cancer at the same rate as in Western countries.[4,10,15] There has been a continued increase in disease incidence among the black population.

ETIOLOGY AND RISK FACTORS

The cause of colorectal cancer is unknown, but recent research indicates that diet, genetics, and other predisposing factors such as bowel disorders may play an important role in the development of colorectal cancer.

Diet

The relationship between diet and colorectal cancer remains under investigation, but evidence shows that individuals with diets low in animal fats and high in fiber demonstrate a significantly lower incidence of disease.[17] Research indicates that fats and meat products may alter the concentration of normal body products such as cholesterol, fecal bile salts, and also change the normal intestinal flora of the bowel. This process may serve as a cancer promoter by damaging the colonic mucosa and increasing the proliferational activity of the epithelium of the colon.

Reduced dietary fiber may also serve as a promoter of the carcinogenic process by increasing the amount of contact time that the carcinogenic substance has with colonic mucosa, therefore increasing the potential for mutagenic changes in the bowel wall.

Other dietary factors that serve as promoters of the carcinogenic process include genotoxic carcinogens such as charbroiled meats, fish, and fried foods. Dietary deficiences of Vitamin A, C, E, selenium, and calcium have also been investigated and may demonstrate future dietary recommendations.[23,24,33,41,44]

Genetic Factors

Genetics play a role in the predisposition to colorectal cancer. Persons with first-degree relatives who have colorectal cancer have a threefold risk of having the disease themselves.[28] Polyposis syndromes such as Gardner's, Turcot's, and Plutz-Jegher's are linked with increased risks for the development of colorectal cancers. These autosomal dominant diseases are manifested by thousands of colonic adenomas that have a high malignant potential. As these adenomas grow and increase in size, cellular changes occur that result in a malignant transformation.

Other Predisposing Factors

Other predisposing factors include ulcerative colitis and Crohn's disease. These inflammatory bowel disorders are associated with dysplasia and associated malignant lesions. Potential for the malignant process is correlated to the duration of the disease. In addition to inflammatory bowel disease, adenomas polyposis represent most common types of bowel polyps and account for 80% of all of types of bowel polyps.[18,19] These polyps increase their malignant potential as they grow larger and demonstrate cellular changes. This process takes 10 to 15 years from the time of diagnosis. Villainous adenomas are another type of polyp that has been associated with increased malignancy and high fatality. These polyps produce excessive mucus and result in severe fluid and electrolyte disorders.

PREVENTION, SCREENING, AND DETECTION

The American Cancer Society recommends specific protocols for the screening and prevention of colorectal cancers, which include diet and diagnostic examinations.

Dietary considerations include a low-fat, high-fiber diet, including whole grain cereals, fruits, and vegetables. Cruciferous vegetables, such as brussels sprout, cauliflower, cabbage, kohlrabi, and broccoli, have been recommended to reduce colon cancer risk.[3,21,33,49] Although the relationship between diet and colon cancer continues to be investigated, additional research is needed to provide more definitive information. Current dietary recommendations are listed in the box below.

The American Cancer Society's recommendations for colon cancer screening for an asymptomatic person include an annual digital rectal examination for persons over age 40 and an annual stool guaiac test for persons over age 50. Proctosigmoidoscopy should be done every 3 to 5 years after age 50 after two negative annual examinations.[3,33] Persons at high risk

may need screening at an earlier age and more frequently than the general population (Table 8-1).[3,51,52]

Because many tumors are found in the lower rectum, abdominal and rectal exams should be performed at the time of a routine physical.

Guaiac screening is also an effective and inexpensive screening tool but is not without its limitations. False-negative and false-positive results may occur for a variety of reasons. The primary reason may be inadequate instruction on sample collection or poor compliance with specific directions. Instructions should include various dietary, medication, and collection procedures.

All individuals should be on a meat-free, high-residue diet for 2 days before specimen collection. Red meats may contain nonhuman hemoglobin, which yields false-positive tests. Foods with peroxidase activity, such as tomatoes, turnips, beets, radishes, and cherries, should be eliminated because their consumption will yield a false-positive test. High-residue diets are recommended to encourage bleeding from small colonic lesions.[3,44,51]

Medication ingestion may also yield false-negative or false-positive tests. Vitamin C and antacids produce false-negative test results even in the presence of active bleeding. Iron, aspirin, cimetidine, cytochromes, and halogens are known for false-positive results and should be avoided during the testing period. Diseases such as diverticulosis, hemorrhoids, and other gastrointestinal pathology have yielded false-positive tests resulting from an alternate bleeding source.

Sample collection also has a direct impact on test results. Diluted specimens obtained from toilet water may result in fecal blood loss from the sample or may be affected by the halogens, such as chlorine, that may be present in the water. Stool samples either too dry or wet may also alter results. Two separate samples from each stool should be collected in designated containers for 3 consecutive days for a total of six samples. Testing should be done within 5 days of sample collection.

DIETARY RECOMMENDATIONS FOR CANCER PREVENTION

1. Reduce the amount of saturated and unsaturated fats in the diet from 40% to 30% of total daily caloric intake.
2. Increase the amount of fiber in the diet by eating fresh fruits, vegetables (including cruciferous vegetables—cabbage, broccoli, brussel sprouts, kohlrabi, cauliflower), and whole grain breads/cereals.
3. Foods rich in vitamin C—citrus fruits, strawberries, currants, cabbage, tomatoes, walnuts, and rosehips.
4. Foods rich in vitamin A—peaches, cantaloupe, apricots, and the dark green and yellow vegetables (carrots, spinach, squash, asparagus, sweet potatoes).
5. Foods rich in vitamin E—vegetable oils (soybean, corn, cottonseed, sunflower seed), alfalfa, and lettuce leaves.

Table 8-1 Summary of American Cancer Society Recommendations for the Early Detection of Cancer in Asymptomatic People

Test or Procedure	Sex	Age	Frequency
Sigmoidoscopy	M & F	50 and over	Every 3 to 5 years based on advice of physician
Stool guaiac slide test	M & F	Over 50	Every year
Digital rectal examination	M & F	Over 40	Every year

Further methods of screening include a fecal blood test, the Hemo-Quant (Smith-Kline Bio-Science Laboratories). The advantages of Hemo-Quant are that it can detect hemoglobin in smaller amounts of stool and that it is unaffected by other factors that interfere with a guaiac test. Immunochemical stool screening is also being evaluated as a suitable method for colorectal screening and may show future benefits.[20]

Proctosigmoidoscopy is also an appropriate method of screening for cancerous lesions of the colon and rectum. Approximately 50% to 65% of all colorectal cancers can be found within the range of this particular instrument (25 cm). A flexible fiberoptic sigmoidoscope is available that can reach to the splenic flexure (60 cm). This instrument provides for increased visibility and patient comfort but requires additional time and cost for the procedure.[41,51,52,56]

CLASSIFICATION

The site of presentation is primarily the sigmoidorectal area. The vast majority (40% to 50%) of lesions occur in the rectum, and 20% to 35% occur in the descending and sigmoid colon. Only 8% occur in the transverse colon and 16% in the cecum and ascending colon. A small percentage (4% to 8%) may occur as a second primary site.[10,15,17,22,23]

The majority of bowel cancers are adenocarcinomas and are moderately to well differentiated cancers. Other forms of colorectal cancers consist of epithelioma, squamous cell carcinomas, sarcoma, lymphoma, leiomyosarcoma, and melanomas. Cancer of the anus is a rare phenomena, but recent research has shown an increase in males with a history of homosexual and bisexual activity or a history of anal condylomata acuminata. Other anal cancers include squamous, basal, and melanomas.

CLINICAL FEATURES

General signs and symptoms exist for all colorectal cancers and may include a change in bowel habits, blood in the stool, abdominal pain, anorexia, flatulence, and indigestion. Later symptoms include loss of energy, weight loss, and a decline in general health. Symptoms may vary greatly according to size, location, tumor type, and the individual patient (Figure 8-1). Specific variances are seen between the right and left colon and the rectum. Right-sided lesions do not display changes in bowel habits because of the liquid nature of the stool. Specific symptoms include a dull, vague abdominal pain radiating from abdomen to back. These tumors present as palpable masses in the right lower quadrant. Dark or mahogany red blood may be present in the stool. Anemia leading to weakness and malaise occurs and indigestion and weight loss are often present.

In contrast, left-sided lesions usually display a change in bowel habits because the area affected is

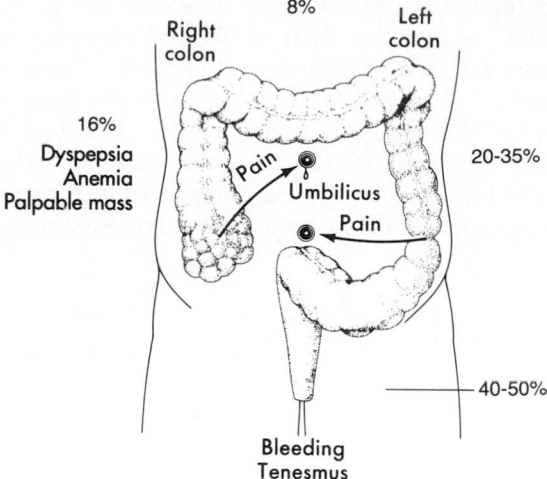

Figure 8–1 Signs and symptoms related to colon cancer. (From Beare P and Myers J: Principles and practice of adult health nursing, ed 1, St Louis, 1990, Mosby.)

COLORECTAL CANCER CLINICAL FEATURES

- General: Change in bowel habits, blood in the stool, abdominal pain, anorexia, flatulence, and indigestion
- Late symptoms: Weight loss, fatigue, decline in general health
- Right-sided lesions: Dull, vague abdominal pain radiating to the back, dark/mahogany red blood in stool, weakness, anemia, malaise, indigestion, weight loss, and liquid stool
- Left-sided lesions: Change in bowel habits—cramps, gas pains, decrease in the caliber of the stool, bright red bleeding, constipation, rectal pressure, and incomplete evacuation of stool
- Transverse colon: Palpable masses, obstruction, changes in bowel habits, and bloody stools
- Rectal: Changes in bowel habits, bright red bleeding, tenesmus, severe pain in groin, labia, scrotum, legs, or penis

---

the sigmoid colon and the rectum. Symptoms include cramps, gas pains, a decrease in the caliber of stool, bright red bleeding, constipation, and a feeling of rectal pressure or incomplete evacuation of stool. Obstruction may occur and result in emergency surgery. Transverse colon tumors present with palpable masses, obstruction, change in bowel habit, and bloody stools. Rectal cancers may display similar symptoms, such as change in bowel habits, bright red bleeding, tenesmus, and a late symptom of severe pain in the groin, labia, scrotum, legs, or penis (see box above). Unfortunately, colorectal cancer may be advanced before symptoms occur. Pain may only be

---

DIAGNOSTIC WORKUP

Barium enema
Colonoscopy
Chest x-ray
Liver scan
Bone scan
CBC, SGOT, LDH, alkaline phosphate, BUN
Carcinoembrogenic antigen (CEA)

---

the last symptom and metastasis may be present before treatment is sought.

DIAGNOSIS AND STAGING

Persons at high risk for disease or who have symptoms and are guaiac-positive require additional diagnostic testing. A barium enema provides a clear picture of the large intestine and has the ability to find smaller tumors. Colonoscopy may be performed at this time, especially if surgery is indicated. This exam provides increased visualization as well as the ability to biopsy lesions. Potential metastatic lesions are evaluated using chest x-ray, liver, bone, and other scans. Laboratory work includes CBC, SGOT, LDH, alkaline phosphate, and BUN. A carcinoembryonic antigen (CEA) test may be used. This biologic marker is elevated in later stages of colorectal cancer and may have a prognostic value at the time of diagnosis or disease recurrence. Additional tests currently being evaluated are antigens, such as colon-specific antigens (CSAs) and colon-specific antigen protein (CSAP), are currently being evaluated for their usefulness as a diagnostic tool.[18,47] Diagnosis is confirmed by tissue biopsy from the suspected site. Additional diagnostic evaluation includes a variety of procedures (see box above).

STAGING

The most widely used method for colorectal surgery is the Duke's classification or some modification of the original form, which was developed in 1932. The Duke's system classifies tumor into four major categories based on the degree and depth of tumor involvement and presence of lymph nodes. Subcategories were developed by Astler and Collier in 1954 in an attempt to delineate the importance of tumor wall penetration.

Duke's Classification:

Stage A—Carcinoma limited to the mucosa
Stage B1—Carcinoma invades the muscle but is confined to the bowel wall
Stage B2—Carcinoma penetrates through the muscularis propria into the serosa and connective tissue
Stage B3—Same as B2 with adherence or invasion into adjacent organs, but with negative nodes

Table 8–2 Comparison of Staging Systems

Tis-N0-M0 Tis: carcinoma in situ	

T1 or T2-N0-M0
   T1: tumor invading submucosa
   T2: invading muscle layer
	DUKES A

T3 or T4-N0-M0
   T3: invades through muscle layer, into subserosa
   T4: directly invades other organs or perforates visceral peritoneum
	DUKES B

Any T-N1, N2, or N3-M0
   N1: 1-3 pericolic or perirectal lymph node metastases
   N2: 4 pericolic or perirectal lymph node metastases
   N3: any nodal metastasis along vascular trunk or apical node
	DUKES C

Any T-any N-M1 M1: distant metastasis	DUKES D

Stage C1—Lymph nodes positive for metastatic disease but main tumor confined to bowel wall
Stage C2—Lymph nodes positive for metastatic disease and tumor completely penetrates bowel wall
Stage C3—Same as B3, with positive nodes
Stage D—Distant metastasis

The variances and minor modifications of various systems of colorectal staging resulted in the promotion of the TNM system by the International Union Against Cancer (UICC). In this system "T" refers to tumor, "N" node involvement, and "M" distant metastasis. Additional numbers are added to each letter to specify the extent of tumor growth. No uniform or widely accepted staging is used for anal cancers. A comparison of the Duke's system and TNM system is given in Table 8-2.[26]

METASTASIS

Most colorectal cancers spread by direct extension and penetration into layers of the bowel. Local invasion occurs to surrounding organs. Lymph node involvement and invasion into the vascular bed allow for disseminated disease. Lymphatic disease is present in 50% of all diagnosed cases. Nodal chains follow the pathway of the superior and mesenteric arteries. The colon and upper one half of the rectum spread by direct extension to the liver. The lower half of the rectum spreads to portal veins and the inferior vena cava. Venous invasion permits distant metastasis, with the liver and lung as the most common site.

Additional sites include brain, bone, and adrenal glands. Anal cancers spread directly in local muscles and to genitourinary organs. Metastasis spread at the time of diagnosis significantly alters prognosis and treatment modalities. Disease related complications are summarized in the box above.

TREATMENT MODALITIES
Surgery

Colon resection with disease-free margins remains the surgical goal. Tumor and associated blood vessels are resected en bloc with the vascular and lymphatic structures to prevent seeding of malignant cells. A biopsy of the liver and regional lymph nodes is taken at the time of surgery to evaluate the extent of disease.

Extensive procedures may be needed to attain the goal of reanastomosis and return to normal bowel function. Tumor size, location, and additional metastasis determine the type and the extent of surgery. Three major surgeries performed for colorectal cancer include resection of the tumor with reanastomosis, a colostomy (temporary or permanent), and an abdominal perineal resection[9,13,20,35] (Figure 8-2). Site-specific surgeries that may be done for various portions of the colon and rectum are outlined in Table 8-3.

The most questionable procedure is surgery of the middle rectal tumors, which requires judgment, surgical skill, and intense evaluation of the potential for cure over sphincter-sparing procedure (Figure 8-3). The use of the end-to-end stapler has permitted increased success with these lesions. This instrument facilitates an anastomosis from the low rectal area to the colon. Procedures such as this spare patients from the bladder and sexual dysfunction that result from radical abdominal perineal resection. Research continues to evaluate the success of these procedures versus the likelihood of disease return.

In addition to general tumor site surgical guidelines, each case must be evaluated individually to meet specific patient needs. Age, nutritional status,

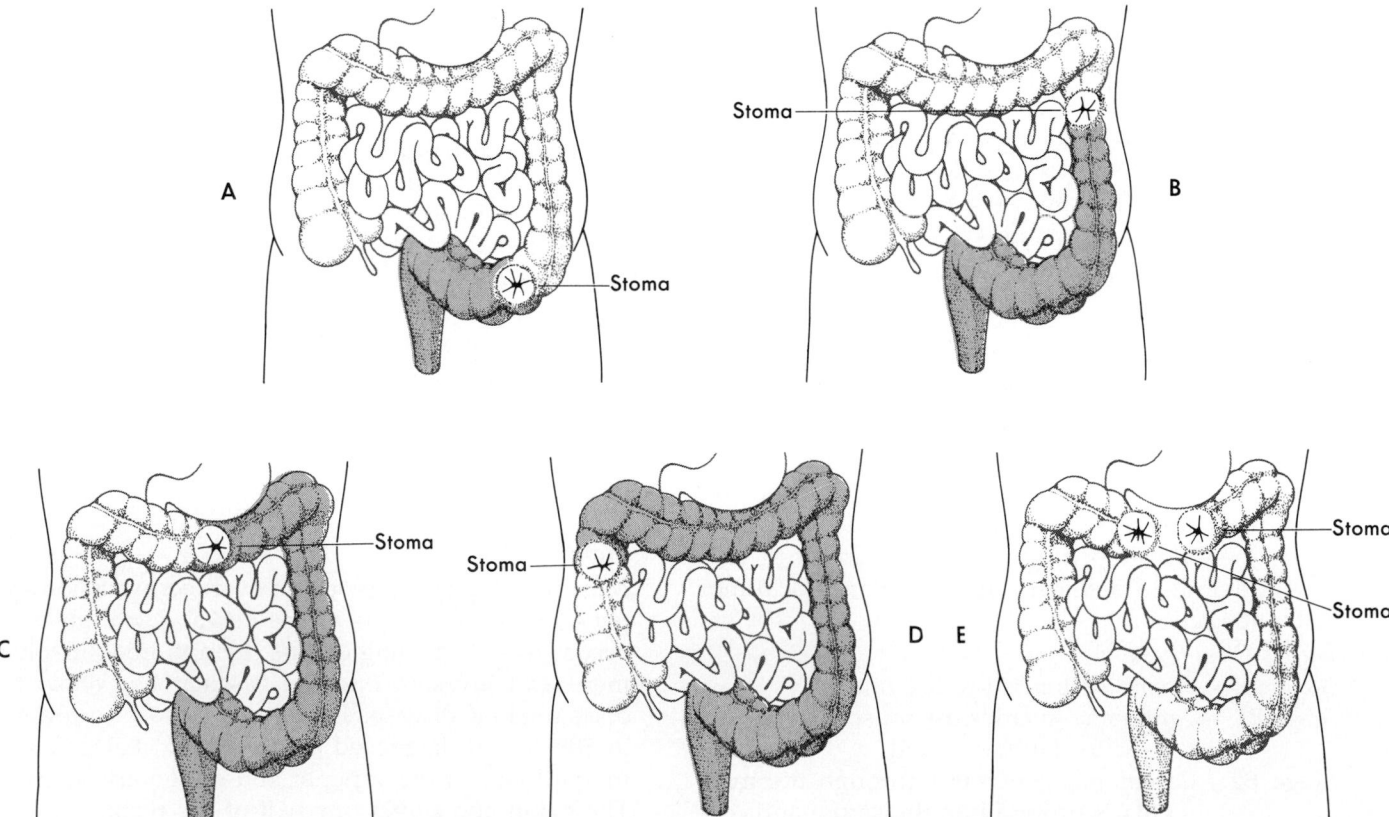

Figure 8–2 **A,** Sigmoid colostomy. **B,** Descending colostomy. **C,** Transverse colostomy. **D,** Ascending colostomy. **E,** Double-barrel colostomy. (From Beare P and Myers J: Principles and practice of adult health nursing, ed 1, St. Louis, 1990, Mosby.)

Table 8–3 Major Surgeries for Colorectal Cancer

Location	Tumor Site	Procedure
Right colon	Cecum, ascending colon, proximal and midtransverse colon	Right colectomy or colostomy
Left colon	Splenic flexure and descending colon	Colectomy or colostomy
Sigmoid colon	Sigmoid portion of the bowel	Sigmoid resection
Upper rectum	12 cm from the anal verge	Anterior colon
Middle rectum	7-11 cm from the anal verge	Pull-through procedure
Lower rectum	7 cm from the anal verge	Abdominal perineal resection and colostomy

tine (CCNU), mitomycin C, vincristine, cisplatin, methotrexate, and biotherapy such as bacille Calmette-Guérin (BCG), methanol-extractable residue (MER), and interferon. Leucovorin has been combined with 5-FU to enhance the effectiveness of 5-FU. Levamisole plus 5-FU given after surgery to reduce disease recurrence has shown a significant benefit to improve survival in patients with stage C disease. 5-FU continues to remain the drug of choice for treatment of colorectal cancer.[2,28–31,48]

metastases, and complications including perforation and obstruction may alter the surgical course. Additional surgical modalities may be required for palliation even when cure is not possible. Relief of pain, odor, or bleeding may be the ultimate goal. Extensive metastases may also require more radical surgeries such as pelvic exenteration where the entire bladder and rectum and other structures are removed and an ileal conduit and sigmoid colostomy are created. The best sites for ostomies are shown in Figure 8-4.

Chemotherapy

Chemotherapy alone has not been proven to be effective against colorectal cancer. Chemotherapy continues to be considered an adjunct to the initial surgical intervention. Various forms of combination drug therapy have been evaluated, including 5-fluorouracil (5-FU) alone and in combination with methyl lomus-

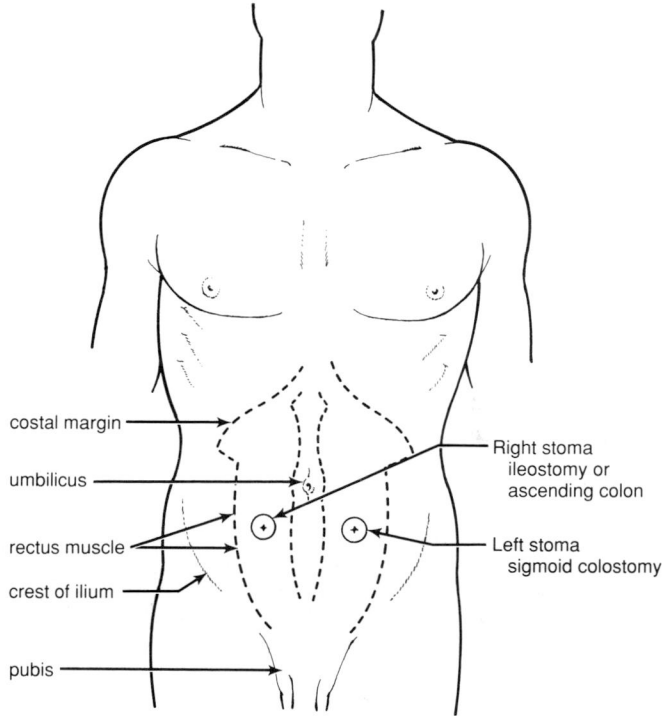

Figure 8–4 Best sites for ostomies.

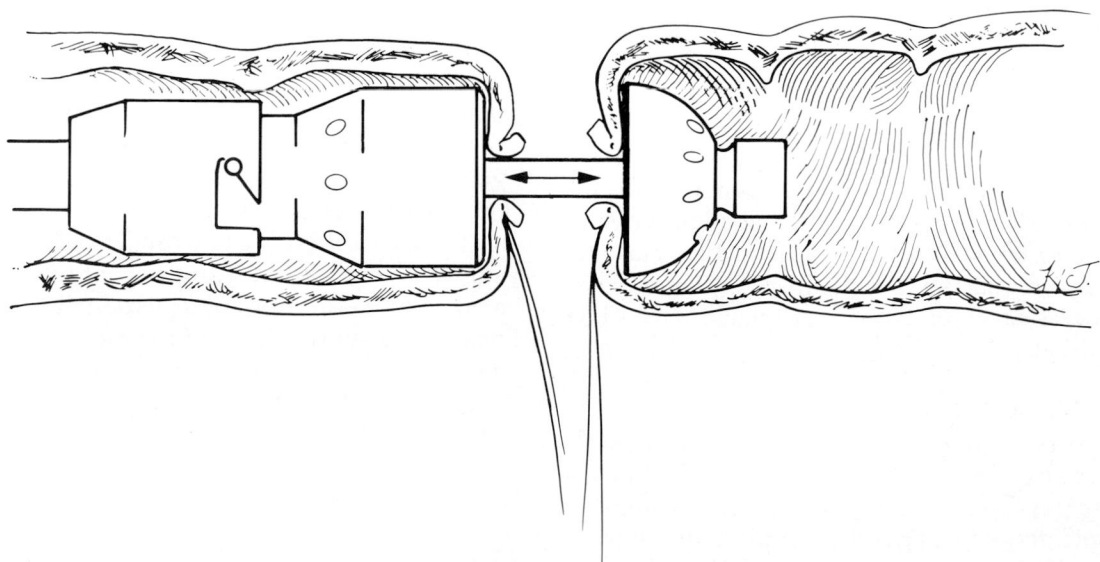

Figure 8–3 Sphincter-sparing procedure. (From Broadwell D and Jackson B: Principles of ostomy care, ed 1, St Louis, Mosby.)

<table>
<tr><td colspan="2">

**COMMON CHEMOTHERAPY DRUGS USED IN
THE TREATMENT OF COLORECTAL CANCER**

5-FU
Methyl lomustine (CCNU)
Mitomycin C
Vincristine
Cisplatin
Methotrexate
5-FU/levamisole
Advanced cancer:
  FUDR (via pump)
  5-FU and leucovorin
  Methotrexate 5-FU and leucovorin
</td></tr>
</table>

PROGNOSIS RATES FOR COLORECTAL CANCER

Duke's classification	Survival rate
A	80%-90%
B	60%
C	25%-45%
D	5%
Anal cancer	48%-66%

Table 8–4 Chemotherapy Drugs and Related Side Effects

Drug	Side Effects
5-FU	Anorexia, nausea, vomiting, stomatitis, diarrhea, bone marrow suppression, alopecia, dermatitis, skin hyperpigmentation
CCNU	Bone marrow suppression, nausea, alopecia, pulmonary fibrosis
Cisplatin	Anorexia, nausea, vomiting, stomatitis, bone marrow suppression, renal insufficiency, ototoxicity
Mitomycin C	Nausea, vomiting, anorexia, stomatitis, bone marrow suppression, alopecia, necrosis
Methotrexate	Bone marrow suppression, renal tubular necrosis, stomatitis, diarrhea, hepatic dysfunction
Vincristine	Extravasation, peripheral neuropathy, intestinal obstruction

Chemotherapy has also been used in attempts to prevent unresectable tumors confined to the liver from metastasizing. 5-FU has been administered by intra-arterial catheter into the hepatic artery, and floxuridine (FUDR), an analogue of 5-FU, has been administered by an implanted pump known as an Infusaid pump. The role of regional hepatic perfusion remains controversial in the treatment of metastatic disease. Additional studies with 5-FU, leucovorin, and methotrexate are under investigation (see box above and Table 8-4).

Radiation Therapy

The role of radiation therapy in the management of colon tumors remain under investigation, but radiation therapy is often used for patients with extensive microscopic tumor penetration, lymph node involvement, and direct tumor extension into the viscera or perineum. Various combination approaches have been attempted including preoperative radiation, postoperative radiation, and a combination of both known as the "sandwich technique." Preoperative radiation therapy may damage malignant cells that could disseminate during surgery and may help shrink unresectable lesions. Postoperatively, radiation has proven effective in prevention of disease recurrence in high-risk persons. Palliation may result from radiation treatment through reduction of tumor size, thereby relieving pain, bleeding, and pressure.*

PROGNOSIS

Persons diagnosed with colorectal cancer must receive follow-up treatment after initial surgery, including periodic physical examinations, colonoscopy, CEA levels, and traditional x-rays as needed. Symptoms of weight loss and pain should be evaluated immediately. Disease recurrence may be observed locally or regionally in distant organs. Local recurrence at the original tumor site is a possibility and may cause obstruction and hemorrhage. Penetration beyond the bowel wall may result in fistula formation. Further surgery or combined adjunctive therapy may be indicated.

Spread to distant organs has a direct impact on the prognosis and ultimate survival of the person. Survival time for persons with metastasis usually is less than 1 year. Age is an additional factor that affects the survival rate; persons under age 30 have a poorer prognosis and patients over age 70 have a higher surgical morbidity rate. High CEA titers before surgery, the presence of obstruction at the time of diagnosis, and poorly differentiated cancers also decrease the survival rate.[10] Rectal tumors continue to be associated with poor prognosis, especially those located near the lower one third of the rectum.[4,10,23] The overall survival rate of all stages is 40%. Survival rates continue to change as new treatment modalities and early detection methods are developed.[19] Specific prognosis rates are shown in the box above.

---

* References 11,12,36,38,43,53.

Text continued on p. 142.

Nursing Management

SURGERY
Preoperative Teaching

Patient teaching and preoperative counseling are essential elements of nursing care for the patient preparing for colorectal surgery. Many patients will have already had several diagnostic and laboratory tests in an outpatient setting before they reach the hospital. Often they are aware of their diagnosis but may be in the stage of denial or disbelief that this could be happening to them. Patients and their families may be anxious or even angry at the diagnosis and will require additional attention and reinforcement of teaching preoperatively and postoperatively.

Teaching may begin with the preparation of colon for surgery. Most protocols involve a regimen of 2 or 3 days of liquid diets, a combination of laxatives or enemas, and the use of oral antibiotics to sterilize the bowel before surgery.[22,44,45] Antibiotics suppress both anaerobic and aerobic colonic organisms and reduce septic complications after surgery. Patients with bowel obstructions do not receive the usual bowel preparation.

NURSING DIAGNOSES

- Knowledge deficit related to lack of experience in surgical routine and procedure
- Fear related to the diagnosis of cancer and operative procedure outcomes
- Knowledge deficit related to ostomy

INTERVENTIONS

The nurse must provide support to an already anxious patient by explaining the rationale of the bowel-prep regimen. Close observation of the patient's tolerance of laxatives and enemas must be reported, including the side effects of nausea, vomiting, abdominal discomfort, excessive diarrhea, and the symptoms of electrolyte imbalance. Elderly and debilitated patients are at the greatest risk for discomfort and complications.

Preoperative Care

Preoperative teaching may begin at this time and should include a review of the patient's past experience with surgery. Basic preoperative teaching should include a review of the preoperative routine; preoperative medications, IVs, recovery room procedures, placement of a Foley catheter, nasogastric tube, and abdominal dressings. Postoperative exercises, such as coughing and deep breathing, wound splinting, and leg exercises, should be reviewed and practiced. Con-

cerns about pain medication and diet restrictions may be discussed preoperatively. Basic review of anatomy is necessary for the person to understand the surgical procedure and colostomy placement.

It is essential that psychosocial issues and concerns are addressed as well as support systems identified. A review of past coping mechanisms provide the individual with the opportunity to evaluate strengths and weaknesses. Ample time to discuss fears and concerns must be permitted to evaluate the dynamics of interpersonal relationships between patients and their support systems. Proper preoperative assessment allows for more effective intervention postoperatively.

If a colostomy is performed, a referral to an enterostomal therapist or appropriate resource should be made as soon as possible. Preoperative teaching should review the type of surgery, understanding of what an ostomy is, various pouching methods available, and marking of the stoma site. The marking of the stoma site is important to eliminate the possibility of future skin problems and difficult pouch applications. One of the basic rules for stoma marking is that the stoma should be away from the waistline, folds, scars, or where the abdominal incision will be placed (Figure 8-4). The stoma should be placed so that the patient will be able to see and reach the pouch easily. The stoma site will be placed through the rectus abdominal muscle, which runs vertically through the abdomen. Approximately 3 inches of skin will be necessary to provide adequate pouch placement. Various positions should be attempted before marking the stoma. The stoma should be visualized in sitting, standing, and lying positions. The site is usually below the umbilicus and at the infraumbilical bulge. The stoma site is then marked with a dye such as methylene blue or gentian violet.[42] The marking of the stoma validates the reality of the ostomy. Documentation of the patient and family reaction is important to meet future emotional needs.

Postoperative Care

NURSING DIAGNOSES

- Alteration in comfort related to incisional discomfort
- Potential for infection related to improper wound healing
- Alteration in bowel elimination related to loss of normal bowel function
- Alteration in skin integrity related to abdominal incision and stoma drainage

INTERVENTIONS

The postoperative period includes meeting the physical and metabolic needs of the patient. Observation of the patient for initial complications includes the assessment of vital signs and lung and bowel sounds. The incision is inspected for drainage or bleeding and approximation. The nasogastric tube and Foley catheter, if present, are monitored for the amount of drainage, color, and patency. Accurate recording of intake and output is necessary to provide proper electrolyte balance. The stoma site is observed at each shift initially for color and size. A postoperative pouch usually covers the stoma, allowing for easy visibility. The stoma should appear pink and moist. Signs of necrosis and ischemia are present if the stoma appears blue, black, or has a dusky appearance. This observation should be reported at once because this indicates stoma death. Drainage from the stoma should be scant and bloodtinged. A strict postoperative routine of coughing, deep breathing exercises, early ambulation, and adequate pain control will assist the patient toward early recovery and limit potential complications.

Despite good nursing care, postoperative complications do occur, including infection, paralytic ileus, pulmonary complications, anastomotic leak, urinary problems, stoma retraction, and prolapse.[9,20,22,42] Fevers may result from infection, respiratory difficulty, urinary infections, or thrombophlebitis. Elderly patients with preexisting medical illness such as diabetes and lung disease are at greatest risk.

Anastomotic leaks are more common in lower resections and often result in fistula formation. Skin care and adequate nutrition are essential components of proper wound healing. Paralytic ileus, a common complication after bowel surgery, results from the surgical manipulation of the bowels in surgery and can last up to 14 days or more. Increased abdominal girth, distention, nausea, and vomiting are classic signs of an ileus. Decompression of the bowel with the use of a nasogastric tube and maintenance of the NPO status and increased activity usually return normal bowel function (see box below).

Postoperative wound infection is not usually a major concern because of prophylactic antibiotics and reduction of wound contamination with use of postoperative stoma pouching. Those patients with abdominal-perineal resections are at greater risk for wound complications and infections. Sitz baths, dressing changes, and topical ointments assist in the healing process. Healing may be very slow, and meticulous skin care remains necessary.

Postoperative Teaching

NURSING DIAGNOSES

- Sexual dysfunction potential related to body function alteration and body changes
- Self-concept disturbance related to altered body image
- Alteration in family process related to diagnosis of cancer and ostomy formation
- Alteration in health maintenance related to knowledge deficit of diet modifications and ostomy care

INTERVENTIONS

Postoperative teaching includes both the emotional and physical changes from the ostomy and appropriate referral to resources as needed. Postoperative pouch application and stoma care should be a step-by-step process moving from the simple to the complex components. Ostomy care includes pouch applications, emptying of the pouch, and use of skin products.

Pouch selection is based on the site of the stoma, manual dexterity, cost, and patient preference; all pouches should be well-fitted and odor-proof and should provide skin protection.[27,42] Special skin barriers may also be necessary, depending on the type of effluent discharged. Ileostomy drainage is particularly wet and contains enzymes that can cause skin irritation. Sigmoid colostomy effluent is solid but may also cause skin problems. Odor is managed with use of pouching, and ostomy deodorant sprays must be discussed. The enterostomal therapist is invaluable in selecting the appropriate product for the patient.

Colostomy irrigations may be an option for patients with a sigmoid colostomy. Patients should be told the advantages of both systems, that irrigation control takes patience, and that a daily schedule can be established over a period of time. Other types of ostomies cannot be regulated by irrigation because the effluent is constant and liquid.

The special dietary needs and restrictions of the ostomy patient are discussed, including adequate fluid intake and the avoidance of certain foods that may cause blockage, odor, or gas. A list of medications that are not absorbed in the intestine and may be expelled through the colostomy are also given to the patient. Foods that contain seeds, nuts, or excessive bulk should be avoided because there is a likelihood of blockage. Gas- and odor-producing foods are frequently the same foods that caused problems before surgery and usually are related to the cabbage

---

SURGICAL TREATMENT RELATED COMPLICATIONS

Infection (wound, urinary, lung)
Thrombophlebitis
Paralytic ileus
Pulmonary embolus
Hemorrhage
Anastomotic leaks

Trial-and-error and the use of commercial deodorant products assist with this problem. Discharge teaching includes specific problems that may be encountered, such as diarrhea or blockage. A Dietary Consult will also assist the patient in appropriate diet selection. A physician or enterostomal therapist should be notified if these problems arise. Stoma prolapse and stoma retraction may also occur if there is undue pressure on the stoma from an appliance or from edema or scar formation. Specific skin problems and use of products are discussed at this time. Discharge teaching may be an overwhelming task for a patient who is emotionally and physically drained from the events of surgery. Scheduling short visits with repetition is the most reliable method of teaching. Readiness to learn has the greatest impact on ostomy teaching.

Body image and sexuality concerrns are both discussed preoperatively and postoperatively. Signs of difficulty dealing with the new ostomy may include failure to look at the stoma, making remarks about the stoma, or not permitting the significant other to assist with care of the appliance. Common concerns are fear of rejection, shame, a sense of disfigurement, and concerns of others' reactions. Continued feelings of low self-esteem lead to depression, withdrawal, and sexual dysfunction.[34,39,40] An ostomy visitor with a similar background may provide the additional support and encouragement needed at this time. Meeting a person who is able to work and continue with outside activities provides the patient with a positive outlook and encouragement.

Sexual counseling begins while the patient is in the hospital. Communication about sexuality concerns includes a discussion with the patient, ultimately including the spouse or significant other.[33] Suggestions to assist couples to deal with sexuality issues should begin with open communication and gradual introduction of sexual activity. Body image concerns may be dealt with by the use of pouch covers, nightgowns and shirts, or other methods to conceal the ostomy until the patient is comfortable with the issue. Altered sexual positions that are more comfortable and less traumatic on the stoma should also be discussed.[39,40] Patients with abdominal-perineal resections require referrals for further counseling, because 30% to 100% of all men with this surgery experience erectile impotence. Damage to the parasympathetic nerve and loss of sensation have a severe impact on sexual performance. Referral to a urologist for a semirigid or inflatable penile implant is necessary if the patient finds he is unable to perform sexually and desires further medical intervention. Research on females with abdominal-perineal resections is not conclusive, but reports include changes in sensation that alter the orgasmic process.[39,40]

Rehabilitation

Rehabilitation of the patient with colorectal cancer requires the combined effort of a number of professionals. Physical, emotional, and spiritual concerns must be met to return the patient to the preoperative state of functioning. Rehabilitation concepts stress reaching the maximum capabilities within the limits of the disease. The ultimate goal is to provide the patient with the knowledge and support to live within the capabilities of the disability and to maximum potential.[42] The United Ostomy Association and the American Cancer Society can provide additional support and knowledge for the patient and the family. Additional referrals for counseling to deal with emotional and sexual concerns may also be necessary for long-term support. The availability of an enterostomal therapist and adequate access to ostomy supplies are additional supports for those patients who have had ostomy surgery.

RADIATION THERAPY

NURSING DIAGNOSES

- Impairment of skin integrity: potential related to radiation treatment effects
- Alteration in bowel elimination: diarrhea related to treatment side effects
- Fluid volume deficit: potential related to nausea and vomiting
- Health maintenance alteration related to knowledge deficit of radiation side effects

INTERVENTIONS

Patients receiving radiation therapy to the abdominal cavity require emotional and physical support throughout the course of their treatment. Preradiation instruction reviews the frequency and length of treatments, skin markings and their care, and potential side effects and their management. Patients who have an ostomy may need additional information about skin care to their stomas. Side effects experienced by patients receiving abdominal radiation include nausea, vomiting, diarrhea, cystitis, sexual dysfunction, bone marrow suppression, local skin reaction, and fatigue (see box below).[32,43,54,55]

RADIATION THERAPY TREATMENT RELATED COMPLICATIONS

Skin irritation
Proctitis
Nausea/vomiting
Cystitis
Sexual dysfunction
Bone marrow suppression
Fatigue

Nausea and vomiting are of particular concern to those patients receiving radiation therapy over the abdominal area. This is primarily related to the destruction of the epithelial lining of the bowel wall. The toxic waste production from cellular destruction produces increased stimulus to the nausea receptors in the medulla. Prolonged nausea and vomiting may produce weight loss and dehydration. Appropriate nursing measures include use of antiemetics, 1 to 2 hours before radiation therapy and up to 12 hours after each treatment. Small frequent meals are encouraged with high protein and liquid supplements if needed. Weights as well as dietary intake and hydration status should be monitored weekly. For those patients with an ostomy, significant weight loss causes stoma shrinkage. Measurement of the stoma size and pouch sizes may be needed.[42]

Diarrhea is another symptom frequently experienced by a majority of individuals. Diarrhea begins about 1 or 2 weeks after the start of radiation treatment and is caused by the rapid cellular proliferation of the epithelial cells in the intestinal wall. Patients experiencing diarrhea should be instructed to eat low-residue, high-protein, carbohydrate diets. Fluids high in potassium are encouraged; milk products are discouraged. Antidiarrheal products are effective in controlling diarrhea. Patients are instructed to record the number and consistency of bowel movements. Rectal irritation from bowel movements or from radiation therapy to the rectum require sitz baths, topical creams, and assessment by the radiologist and enterostomal therapist. Ostomy patients require increased pouch changes, assessment of peristomal skin, and use of a skin barrier to protect their skin. Severe excoriation of the peristomal skin requires a referral to the enterostomal therapist or the discontinuation of treatments until symptoms subside.[42]

Abdominal radiation causes inflammation of the bladder, resulting in symptoms of cystitis, burning, back pain, hematuria, and foul-smelling urine. Instructions should be given on increasing fluid intake to 2 to 3 quarts of liquids and limiting caffeine products. Urine cultures, sensitivity specimens, and monitoring intake and output may be necessary.

Sexual dysfunction occurs for a variety of emotional and physical reasons. Changes in self-concept, decreased libido, impotence, fertility concerns, and vaginal lining changes may all occur as a result of radiation therapy. Instructions include alternative forms of sexual contact, use of a water-based lubricant, and appropriate referrals for severe sexual concerns and fertility issues.

Bone marrow suppression may also occur because of the close proximity to the treatment site and the pelvic bones. The significance of suppression depends on the treatment size, number of treatments, and dose delivered. Patients are monitored for fatigue, infection, bleeding, and fever. Weekly laboratory work should be obtained. Patients instructions include prudent handwashing to minimize the potential for infection.

Local skin reactions may occur at any time, resulting from the destruction of epithelial tissue. Reactions include itchy, dry skin, darkened areas near the radiation site, and mild excoriation. Patients are instructed to avoid excessive heat or cold and to avoid using creams or lotions near the treatment site. Only skin products applied by the radiologist are to be used because an increased skin reaction occurs with nonprescribed creams.

Patients with ostomies experience increased radiation dermatitis near the peristomal skin site, because of the direct exposure of mucous membrane to treatment field. Pouches are often removed before treatments and cause the patient increased concern about skin exposure. Assessment of the peristomal skin is done at this time. Careful cleansing of the skin and protective skin barriers assist with adequate protection. Severely excoriated areas require the use of additional creams or powders near the stoma site. A referral to the enterostomal therapist should always be made if the skin condition worsens. Treatments are often delayed if symptoms progress.

CHEMOTHERAPY
NURSING DIAGNOSES
- Knowledge deficit related to potential chemotherapeutic side effect
- Oral mucous membrane alteration related to side effects of chemotherapy drugs
- Nutrition alteration to less than body requirements related to nausea and vomiting
- Infection potential related to altered immune status
- Injury potential related to alteration in clotting factor
- Alteration in bowel function: diarrhea related to chemotherapy side effects
- Self-concept disturbance in body image related to hair loss and body changes

INTERVENTIONS
Patients receiving chemotherapy for colorectal cancer may be treated with a single or multidrug protocol as well as a combination of chemotherapy, radiation, and biotherapy. Side effects are usually dose, drug, and patient specific. General side effects include nausea, vomiting, diarrhea, and myelosuppression. Specific drugs and their side effects in the treatment of colorectal cancer are listed in Table 8-4.

Nursing measures include adequate instructions on potential drug side effects. Diarrhea is of particular concern to the ostomy patient because skin breakdown may easily occur. Use of a protective barrier and additional paste or powder may be necessary. Recording the number and consistency of stools is of vital importance to assess hydration status. Small, frequent, high-protein meals rich in potassium are encouraged. Antidiarrheal agents may become necessary if bowel movements are too frequent.[1,7]

Constipation is treated with the use of fluids, stool softeners, laxatives, and irrigations of the stoma if necessary. Stomatitis is also found around the peristomal skin and the stoma itself. Irrigation from chemotherapy agents requires the use of protective skin barriers, careful pouch changes, and proper skin cleansing. Fungal infections near the stoma site may also result from prolonged myelosuppression. Antifungal powders near the peristomal skin assist in wound healing. Local trauma from low platelet counts may also be experienced near the stoma. Careful pouch removal is necessary to avoid trauma.[42]

Nausea and vomiting cause excessive weight loss that changes stoma size. This often requires a pouch change or size variance. Consultation for the appropriate pouch should be done before any significant changes.

Alteration in self-concept requires emotional support to deal with the additional body alteration changes of hair loss and ostomy formation. Support groups and counseling should be provided for these individuals.

Metastatic disease to the liver is common in advanced colorectal cancer. Treatment of these unresectable tumors requires perfusion of chemotherapy agents to the liver by the hepatic artery. Nursing management of external intraarterial lines requires observation for thrombosis, embolism, catheter breakage, clotting, and infection. Placement of standard hepatic arterial lines requires monthly hospitalizations and x-ray fluoroscopy.

The Medtronics Infusion Pump allows patients increased freedom from hospitalization but requires extensive patient teaching concerning the pump's placement and management. The placement of the Medtronics Infusion Pump is a surgical procedure; a disk-shaped pump is placed into a subcutaneous pocket allowing access to the hepatic artery. The pump contains an access port, a chamber for the fluid to be infused, and a chamber filled with fluorocarbon. The vapor pressure of fluorocarbon at normal body temperature allows for expansion of the pump and release of the drug (see Figure 20-8).[14,37,46]

Postoperative complications include development of a seroma, an accumulation of sterile fluid in the pump pocket. Seromas may require draining. Infections may also occur within the pocket site and may require surgical removal of the pump.

Percutaneous access is employed to fill the pump on a 2- to 4-week schedule. Each patient's schedule will vary. FUDR and a heparin solution are infused every 2 weeks. Between the doses of FUDR, a solution of normal saline and heparin is used to keep the pump open. Access to the pump for filling is done by a perfusion scan and injection of radioactive material to assist with proper placement.

NURSING DIAGNOSIS

- Knowledge deficit related to care and side-effect management of infusion pump

Specific teaching concerning the pump includes understanding of its use and particular filling schedule. Side effects of FUDR must also be discussed and managed. Common side effects include nausea, vomiting, abdominal pain, diarrhea, fatigue, and chemical hepatitis. Symptoms are treated systemically except hepatitis, which requires the removal of the drug from the pump. Patients must also be instructed to avoid blunt trauma to the pump site and to limit exposure to extremes of temperature and altitude, which may

---

PATIENT TEACHING PRIORITIES

Surgery (preoperative care)
Turn, cough, deep breathing
Wound splinting
Ambulation
Pain management
Pouch application
Bowel preparation
Postoperative complications

Chemotherapy
Drug name/routine
Side effects
Complications
Follow-up schedule

Surgery (postoperative care)
Ostomy care
Skin care
Pouch application
Diet modifications
Complications
Sexuality
Rehabilitation
Community support

Radiation
Schedule
Side effects and treatments

interfere with drug administration. The effect of intra-arterial chemotherapy and its effectiveness in hepatic metastasis are still under evaluation. Continued patient teaching is needed to support the patient with colorectal cancer through the postoperative course and through various treatment modalities. A summary of teaching implications for this population is included in the box on p.141.

Geriatric Considerations

Special consideratons should also be given to the geriatric population, who may demonstrate a lack of awareness of increased risk factors, signs and symptoms, and recommended screening. Awareness of the American Cancer Society guidelines and the availability of community screening programs is imperative to early diagnosis. Once a diagnosis is made and treatment is indicated the geriatric patient may experience increased side effects due to pre-existing medical conditions and lack of physical stamina to tolerate aggressive therapy.

Postoperatively there is an increased potential for pulmonary, circulatory, and bowel complications in the geriatric population. Added treatment modalities of radiation and chemotherapy impose greater complications of fluid and electrolyte imbalance, infection, and skin concerns. Monitoring the immune and nutritional status of this population is of great importance.

Postoperative teaching of geriatric patients may also require added time to allow for any vision and hearing impairment as well as dexterity with pouch applications. Community resources and referrals should be made to assist with physical and financial support. A summary of geriatric considerations can be found in the box below.

GERIATRIC CONSIDERATIONS

Education needs
Awareness of screening recommendations
Knowledge of signs and symptoms
Understanding of risk factors

Treatment complications
Surgery
  Pulmonary
  Circulatory
  Bowel

Chemotherapy and radiation
  Fluid and electrolyte imbalance
  Infection
  Skin impairment

Teaching concerns
  Vision/hearing impairment
  Dexterity for pouch applications

Community resources
  Financial/home care referral

CONCLUSION

Colorectal cancer provides an exciting challenge to the medical profession. Knowledge of the impact of dietary and environmental factors on colorectal statistics is a critical goal of research. Promotion of the American Cancer Society guidelines and large-scale, cost-effective screening may improve statistics and survival rates. Clinical trial research also provides hope for new treatment modalities with drug protocols and combined radiation therapy. Nursing will play an important role in health-care teaching and promotion of future health-care practices.

BIBLIOGRAPHY

1. Abner B and Collin J: Cancer chemotherapy and practice, Philadelphia, 1990, JB Lippincott Co.
2. Adjuvant therapy for patients with colon rectum cancer, Natl Inst Health Consensus Dev Conf Consensus Statement 8:1, 1990.
3. American Cancer Society: Cancer facts and figures—1993, Atlanta, 1993, American Cancer Society.
4. Beart R: Colorectal cancer. In Holleb AI, Link DJ, and Murphy GP, editors: American cancer society textbook of clinical oncology, Atlanta, 1991, American Cancer Society.
5. Boarini J: Gastrointestinal cancer: Colon, rectum, and anus. In Groenwald SL, Frogge MH, Goodman M, and Yanbro HC, editors: Cancer nursing principles and practice, Boston, 1990, Jones and Bartlett Publishers, Inc.
6. Boring CC, Squires TS, and Tong T: Cancer statistics, CA 41:19, 1991.
7. Cancer of the Colon and Rectum, Nat'l Cancer Institute Research Report, US Dept of Health and Human Services NH #88-95, 1988.
8. Chemotherapy and you: a guide to self help during treatment, National Cancer Institute No. 91-1136, 1990.
9. Clark JC and Gwin RR: An overview of cancers in bowel and bladder diversions, Progressions 4:15, 1992.
10. Cohen AM, Shank B, and Friedman MA: Colorectal cancer. In DeVita VT, Hellman S, and Ro-

senburg SA, editors, ed 3, Cancer: Principles and practice of oncology, Philadelphia, 1989, JB Lippincott Co.

11. Douglass HO: Adjuvant therapy of colorectal cancer. In Moossa AR, Schimpff SC, and Robson MC, editors, ed 2, Comprehensive textbook of oncology, Baltimore, 1991, Williams & Wilkins.

12. Ernstoff MS: Advances in adjuvant therapy for colorectal cancer: Clinical oncology quiz, Oncology and Virology 3:1, 1990.

13. Fazio VW: Surgery of colonic carcinoma: Techniques and tactics, Sem in Colon Rectal Surg 2:36, 1991.

14. Gullatte MM and Graves T: Advances in antineoplastic therapy: Oncol Nurs Forum 17:867, 1990.

15. Haskell CM, Selch MT, and Ramming KP: Colon and rectum. In Haskell CM, editor, ed 3, Cancer treatment, Philadelphia, 1990, WB Saunders Co.

16. Hernsby-Lewis L and Windawer SJ: Natural History and current management, colorectal polyps, Oncology 4:139, 1990.

17. Heuther SE, McCance KL, and Tarmina MS: The digestive system. In McCance KI and Heuther SE, editors: Pathophysiology the biologic basis for disease in adults and children, St Louis, 1990, Mosby.

18. Hodyoke ED: The role of the carcinoembryonic antigen in management of colorectal cancer. In DeVita VT, Hellman S, and Rosenberg SA, editors, Cancer: Principles and practice of oncology, 2-1, 1988.

19. Jagelman DG: Extra-colonic manifestations of familial adenomatous polyposis, Oncology 2:23, 1991.

20. Kodner IJ: Colostomy: Indications, techniques for construction and management of complications, Sem in Colon Rectal Surg 2:73, 1991.

21. Kritechvsky D: Diet and Nutrition, CA 41:328, 1991.

22. Long BC and Roberts RA: Management of persons with problems of intestinal nature. In Phipps WS and others, editors, ed 4, Medical surgical nursing, St Louis, 1991, Mosby.

23. Luk GD: Colorectal cancer, Gastroenterol Clin North Am 17:654, 1988.

24. Luk GD: Colorectal cancer, in Harvey AM and others, The principles and practices of medicine, Norwalk, CT, 1988, Appleton-Lange.

25. MacDonald JS and Schnall SF: The role of 5-FU plus levamisole in therapy of colon cancer, PPO Updates 5:1, 1991.

26. Manual of Staging of cancer: American Joint Committee on Cancer, ed 4, Philadelphia, 1992, JB Lippincott Co.

27. Masson M: Gastrointestinal care. In Shaw M and others, editors, Illustrated manual of nursing practice, Springhouse, PA, 1991, Springhouse Corp.

28. Mellsteat H, Frodin JE, and Masucci G: Clinical status of monoclonal antibodies in the treatment of colorectal cancinoma, Oncology 12:25, 1989.

29. Moertel CG and others: Levamisole and fluorourasil for adjuvant therapy of resection colon carcinoma, New Engl J Med 2:352, 1990.

30. Pazdur R and others: 5-Fluorourasil and recombinant interferon Alfa-2a: Review of activity and toxicity in advanced colorectal carcinomas, Oncol Nurs Forum 18:11, 1991.

31. Poon MA and others: Biochemical modulation of flurouracil with leucovorin in confirmatory evidence of improved therapeutic efficacy in advanced colorectal cancer, J Clin Oncol 9:1967, 1991.

32. Radiation therapy and you: a guide to self help during treatment, National Cancer Institute No. 91-2227, Oct, 1990.

33. Redfield C and Reilly N: Colorectal cancer. In Baird SB and others, editors, A cancer source book for nurses, ed 6, Atlanta, 1991, American Cancer Society.

34. Rhedume A and Gooding BA: Social support, coping strategies, and long-term adaptation to ostomy among self-help members, J Enterstom Ther 18:11, 1991.

35. Schein DS: Decision making in oncology, Philadelphia, 1989, BC Decker.

36. Schilsky RL and Brachman DG: Adjuant chemotherapy and radiation therapy in colorectal cancer, PPO Updates 6:1, 1992.

37. Shalfer M and Marieb EN: The nurse pharmacology and drug therapy, Redwood City, CA, 1989, Addison-Wesley Publishing Co.

38. Shank B, Cohen AM, and Kelsen D: Cancer of the anal region: In DeVita VT, Hellman S, and Rosenberg SA, editors, ed 3, Cancer: Principles and practice of oncology, Philadelphia, 1989, JB Lippincott.

39. Shell JA: The psychosexual impact of ostomy surgery, Progressions 4:3, 1992.

40. Shipes E: Sexual function following ostomy surgery, Nurs Clin North Am 22:303, 1987.

41. Sleisenger MH and Fortan JS: Gastrointestinal disease, pathology, diagnosis and management, ed 4, Philadelphia, 1989, WB Saunders Co.

42. Smith DB and Johnson DE: Ostomy care and the cancer patient, Orlando, Fl, 1986, Grune & Stratton.

43. Stevens KR: The colon and rectum: In Moss WT and Cox JD, editors, ed 6, Radiation oncology: Rationale, technique, results, St Louis, 1989, Mosby.

44. Strohl RA: Colorectal cancers: In Clark JC and

McGee RF, editors, Core curriculum for oncology nursing, ed 2, Philadelphia, 1992, WB Saunders Co.

45. Swatske ME, Whittaker K, and Young M: Care of the intestinal stoma: preoperative, postoperative, long-term, Semin Colon Rectal Surg 2:148, 1991.
46. Tennebaum L: Cancer chemotherapy: a reference guide, Philadelphia, 1989, WB Saunders Co.
47. Torosian MH and Daly JM: An evaluation of the clinical usefulness of CEA in colorectal cancer, Oncology 5:41, 1991.
48. Wadler S: The treatment of advanced colorectal carcinoma, Oncoline 6:1, 1991.
49. Weinhouse S and others: American Cancer Society guidelines on diet, nutrition, and cancer, CA 41:324, 1991.
50. Weinlich SP and others: Timely detection of colorectal cancer in the elderly, Cancer Nursing 12:170, 1989.
51. Weinrich SP: Predictors of older adults' participation in fecal occult blood screening, One Nurs Forum 5:715, 1990.
52. Winawer SJ, Schottfeld D, and Flehinger BJ: Colorectal cancer screening, J Natl Cancer Inst 83:1, 1991.
53. Willett CG and others: Adjuvant postoperative radiation therapy for colonic carcinoma, Ann Surg 206:694, 1987.
54. Witt ME: Questions on colon and rectum radiation therapy, One Nurs Forum 3:79, 1987.
55. Yasko J: Care of the client receiving external radiation therapy, Reston, VA, 1982, Reston-Hall Co.
56. Zanca JA: If people understood what to do, they'll do it, Cancer Nursing (American Cancer Society) 10:1, 1992.

CHAPTER 9

Gastrointestinal Cancers

Betty Thomas Daniel

Gastrointestinal (GI) cancers will account for 21% of the new cases of cancer diagnosed in the United States in 1993, and 23% of the cancer deaths in the same period. This represents a total of 236,900 new cases and 120,325 cancer deaths.[11] Progress has been made in treating some of the GI cancers, but others remain difficult to control. Symptoms of many of these cancers are vague and nonspecific until advanced disease develops, which makes treatment difficult and long-term survival rates low. Prevention and early detection can reduce the impact of the disease and prolong survival, however.

Nurses have an important role to play in the prevention, early detection, diagnosis, and treatment of GI cancers. In some instances, prevention and early detection are not possible, but knowledge of the course of disease may improve the patient's quality of life.

CANCER OF THE ESOPHAGUS

EPIDEMIOLOGY

Cancer of the esophagus is a fairly uncommon cancer in the United States, but its incidence varies greatly throughout the world. It is considered endemic in the Lin Xian region of central China and along the east coast of southern Africa, where its incidence is reported to be as high as 50 cases per 100,000 men.[19] In the United States the estimated number of new cases in 1993 is 11,300, and 10,200 of these patients will die of their disease.[11] Esophageal cancer is most common in elderly males, and the male-to-female ratio is approximately 3:1.[22] The incidence and mortality rates are over three times higher among blacks than whites.[6]

ETIOLOGY AND RISK FACTORS

Although the etiology of esophageal cancer is not well defined, some identified risk factors are associated with chronic irritation of the esophagus. In the United States and Western Europe, smoking and alcohol ingestion are the most prominent factors.[25] In some Asian countries and South America, the consumption of hot tea and a hot beverage called *mate* have been identified as risk factors. Other factors that are implicated include a previous history of squamous cell carcinoma of the head and neck, the presence of Barrett's esophagus, a history of lye ingestion, esophageal achalasia, Plummer-Vinson syndrome, tylosis, and a variety of nutritional deficiencies.[19,22,25,35]

PREVENTION, SCREENING, AND DETECTION

Prevention of the disease focuses on counseling regarding alcohol and tobacco usage and instructing patients with risk factors to report any problems with dysphagia (difficulty in swallowing) or odynophagia (pain on swallowing). These patients must be evaluated immediately so that any cancer present may be diagnosed as early as possible.[35] In areas where esophageal cancer is endemic, mass screening by brushing techniques is feasible, but in the United States the incidence of the disease does not justify this approach.

CLASSIFICATION

The most common types of esophageal carcinomas are squamous cell carcinoma (60%) and adenocarcinoma (35%).[33] Squamous cell carcinomas arise from the surface epithelium and are found most often in the middle and lower esophagus. Adenocarcinoma most often occurs in the lower third of the esophagus and probably arises from the gastric fundus. It is rarely found in the upper and middle esophagus. Fewer than 1% of all esophageal tumors are sarcomas.[22]

CLINICAL FEATURES

Dysphagia and weight loss are the most common presenting symptoms of this disease, occurring in 90% of patients.[43] Many of the patients do not seek medical attention at first, but instead adjust their diets to soft and then to liquid foods. Odynophagia is present in about 50% of cases.[43] A 40- to 50-pound weight loss over a period of 2 to 3 months is not uncommon before the patient is seen by a physician. Because of this delay, most patients present with advanced disease. The symptoms of advanced disease are usually due to the invasion or involvement of surrounding organs and structures (see box above).

DIAGNOSIS AND STAGING

All patients complaining of dysphagia should be tested by a barium swallow and an upper GI endoscopy.[35] Esophageal tumors have a characteristic irregular, ragged mucosal pattern with narrowing of the lumen.[22] Endoscopy is required to confirm the presence of a malignant tumor. Biopsies and brushings can be obtained through the endoscope to confirm the diagnosis. Endoscopic ultrasonography may be used to identify invasion of the tumor into the tissue layers and involvement of lymph nodes to aid in staging of disease. Computed tomography (CT) provides information about the enlargement of lymph nodes and involvement of neighboring organs.[35]

The American Joint Committee on Cancer's Tumor, Node, Metastasis (TNM) staging system is used for staging both cervical and thoracic esophageal carcinomas (see box, top right).

TNM SYSTEM FOR CLASSIFICATION AND STAGING OF CANCER OF THE ESOPHAGUS

Primary tumor (T)

T1	Tumor invades lamina propria or submucosa
T2	Tumor invades muscularis propria
T3	Tumor invades adventitia
T4	Tumor invades adjacent structures

Regional lymph nodes (N)

N0	No regional lymph nodes metastasis
N1	Regional lymph node metastasis

Distant metastasis (M)

M0	No distant metastasis
M1	Distant metastasis

Stage grouping

Stage I	T1	N0	M0
Stage IIA	T2	N0	M0
	T3	N0	M0
Stage IIB	T1	N1	M0
	T2	N1	M0
Stage III	T3	N1	M0
	T4	Any N	M0
Stage IV	Any T	Any N	M1

METASTASIS

Esophageal cancer can spread to almost any part of the body, but distant metastases do not usually present on initial diagnosis. They are almost always found during autopsy, however. Primary sites of metastasis include the lung, stomach, peritoneum, kidney, adrenal gland, brain, and bone.[43] Cancer of the esophagus is characterized by extensive invasion of local or adjacent tissue and organs. The aorta and trachea are threatened by this invasion, exacerbating the poor prognosis of these patients.

TREATMENT MODALITIES

The most effective approach to the treatment of esophageal cancer is a combined modality therapy. Chemotherapy with surgery or radiation therapy appears to be the most promising approach. Frequently, the patient's weakened cardiopulmonary status makes him or her a poor surgical risk.[43] Metastasis to the liver, peritoneum, or neck glands is often considered a contraindication to radical surgery.[29]

Surgery

The choice of surgical approach to an esophagectomy and esophagogastrostomy depends on the extent and location of the tumor. Lesions involving the esophagogastric junction or lower thoracic esophagus are approached by a left thoracotomy (Figure 9-1). For lesions of the upper esophagus, a total esophagectomy using an upper midline incision and right tho-

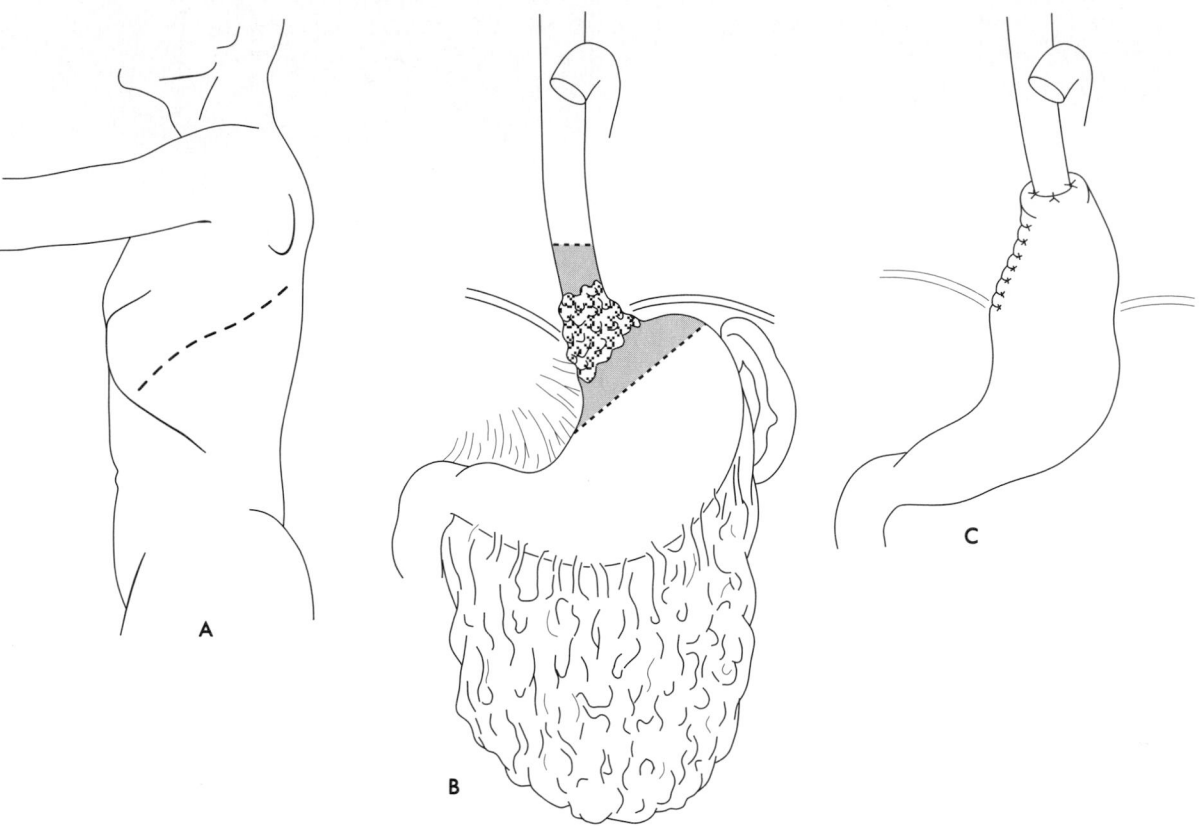

Figure 9–1   Technique of esophagogastrectomy and esophagogastrostomy for carcinoma of the cardia. **A,** site of incision; **B,** extent of resection (shaded area); **C,** completed esophagogastrostomy. (From Ellis HF Jr and Shahlan DM: Tumors of the esophagus. In Glenn WWL, Baue AE, Geha AS, Hammon GL, and Laks H, editors, Thoracic and cardiovascular surgery, ed 4, Norwalk, Conn, 1983, Appleton & Lange.)

racotomy (Ivor Lewis) or a transhiatal approach may be used (Figures 9-2 and 9-3). The transhiatal approach has been used for lesions at every level of the esophagus. If the patient has had an operation involving the stomach, or the tumor extends so far as to require a total esophagectomy, the esophagus must be reconstructed using a portion of the small or large intestine. The left colon is most commonly used (Figure 9-4).[11]

Radiation Therapy

Both squamous cell carcinoma and adenocarcinoma of the esophagus are sensitive to radiation therapy, which is used most often as palliation for obstruction and for pain control for patients who are not candidates for surgical procedures.[35] Unfortunately, this relief is short term for more than 50% of the patients.[43] Radiation therapy is seldom used as a primary therapy, because a course of treatment usually lasts 6 to 8 weeks and median survival for these patients is only a few months. Patients offered radiation therapy alone are those with widespread metastasis, advanced and obstructing tumors, or a poor functional status that does not permit combined modality therapy.[35]

Both preoperative and postoperative radiation therapy are commonly used. Preoperative radiation therapy is used to reduce large tumors to a resectable size and to decrease the risk of dissemination of viable cancer cells during surgical manipulation.[40] Postoperative radiation therapy is used to eliminate microscopic disease and reduce local tumor. Results of clinical trials show that relapse occurs in at least 80% of patients treated with combined therapy, again making palliation an important application of radiation therapy.[27]

Chemotherapy

Single agent chemotherapy has shown some effectiveness in treating squamous cell carcinoma but not in adenocarcinoma of the esophagus and cardia.[35] Both patients with local and patients with advanced disease respond to single-agent or combination chemotherapy, but the response duration is measured only in months.[32] Cisplatin appears to be the most effective agent, and many of the combination proto-

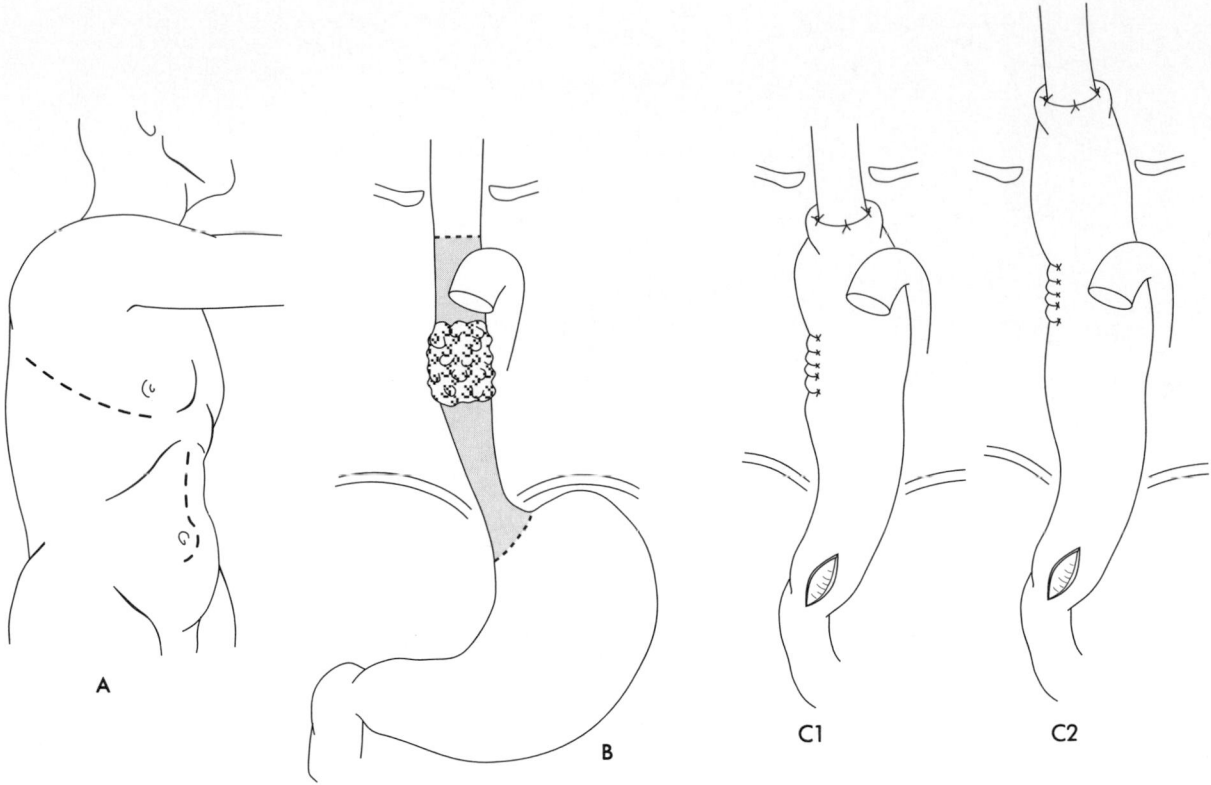

Figure 9–2 Esophagogastrectomy with thoracoabdominal approach. **A,** combined abdominal incision and right thoracotomy for lesions of the upper thoracic esophagus; **B,** extent of resection (shaded area); **C1,** esophagogastrostomy in the chest; **C2,** if submucosal spread is great, cervical anastomosis can be performed through a third incision. (From Ellis FH Jr: Esophagogastrectomy for carcinoma: technical considerations based on anatomic location of lesion, Surg Clin North Am 60:273, 1980.)

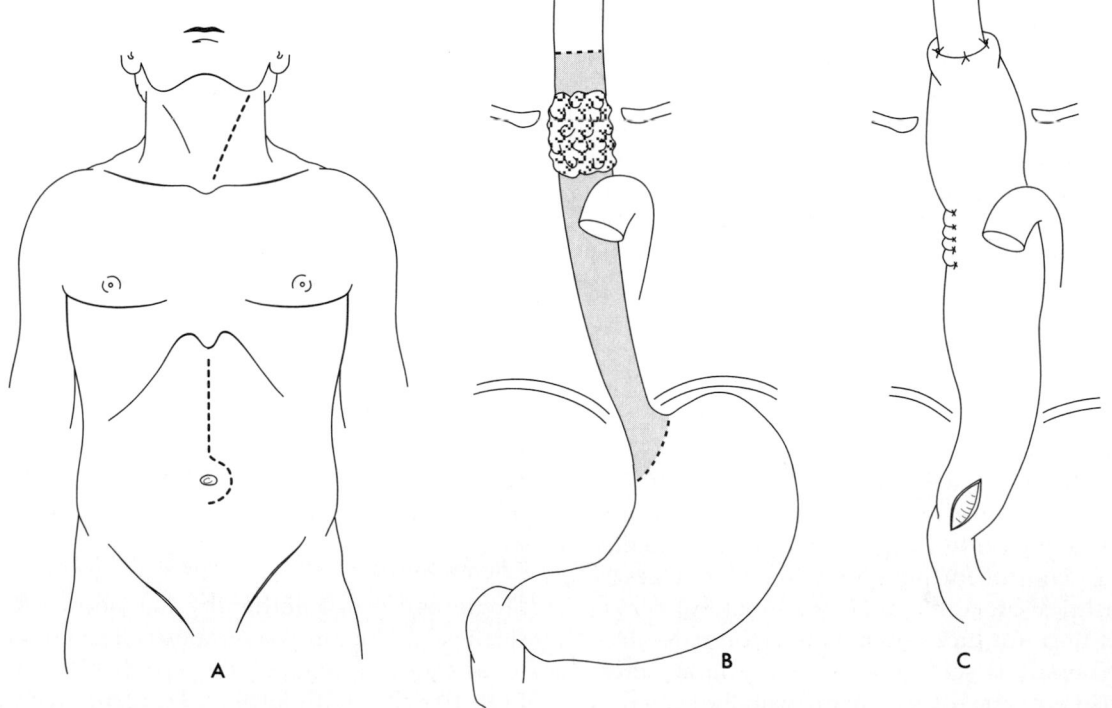

Figure 9–3 Transhiatal approach (esophagectomy without thoracotomy). **A,** upper midline and left cervical incision; **B,** extent of resection; **C,** Completed anastomosis. (From Ellis FH Jr: Esophagogastrectomy for carcinoma: technical considerations based on anatomic location of lesion, Surg Clin North Am 60:276, 1980.)

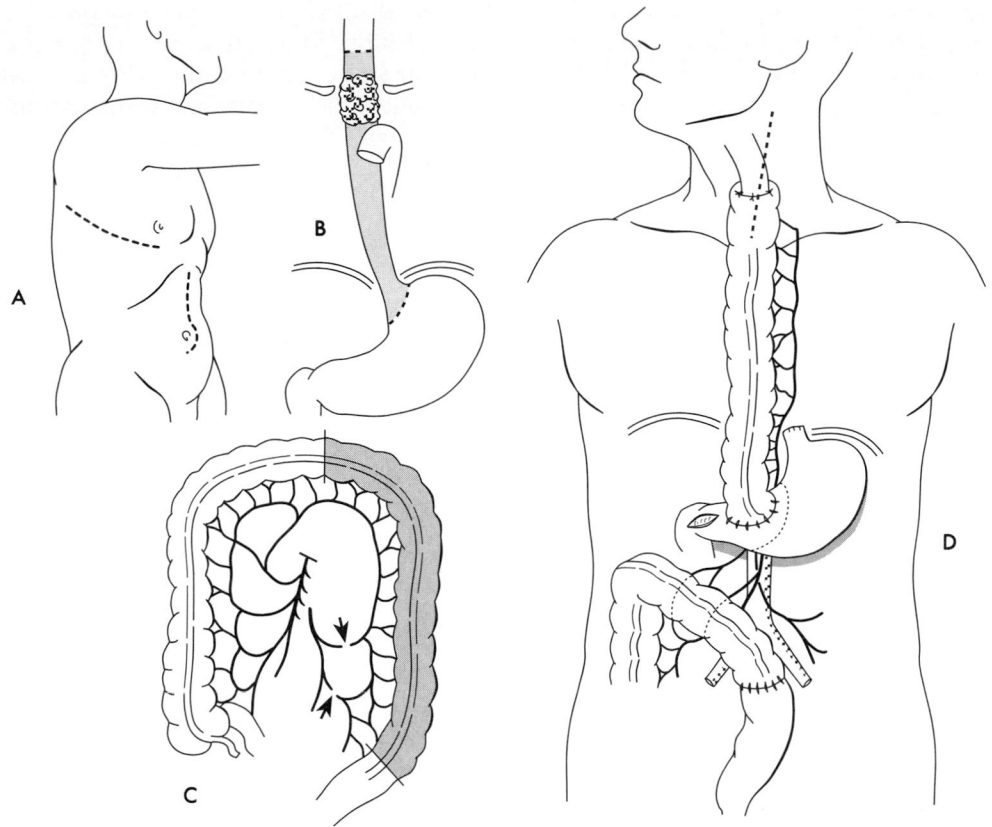

Figure 9–4 Esophagectomy with colon interposition. **A,** right thoracotomy and midline incision; **B,** extent of resection; **C,** segment of left colon used; **D,** completed resection. (From Ellis FH Jr: Esophagogastrectomy for carcinoma: technical considerations based upon anatomic location of lesion, Surg Clin North Am 60:277, 1980.)

cols are based upon this drug. Other agents commonly in use, both as single agents and in combination, include bleomycin, mitomycin, doxorubicin, methotrexate, and 5-fluorouracil (5-FU).[43]

The chemotherapy may be given prior to surgery or radiation therapy. Preoperative (neoadjuvant) chemotherapy may provide the advantages of enhancing surgical outcome by reducing the tumor burden, minimizing the probability of developing drug resistance, and allowing in vivo evaluation of the effectiveness of the agents given.[44] Toxic effects depend on the agents used, and may include nausea, vomiting, myelosuppression, nephrotoxicity, and peripheral neuropathy.

A number of studies have used concurrent neoadjuvant chemotherapy and radiation therapy. The purpose of preoperative radiation therapy is to control local recurrence while improving the resectability of the primary tumor. The purpose of chemotherapy is to eliminate metastatic disease. A large percentage of esophageal cancer patients die of metastatic disease, but most have locoregional recurrence as well, which explains the increase in the number of clinical trials

---

ESOPHAGEAL TREATMENT RELATED COMPLICATIONS

Following esophageal resection[43]
   Anastomotic leak or stricture
   Respiratory insufficiency
   Congestive heart failure
   Pulmonary embolism
   Wound infection or dehiscence
   Obstruction at esophageal hiatus
   Ruptured spleen
   Phlebitis
   Subphrenic abscess
   Torsion, gangrene, or rupture of GI replacement
   Hemorrhage

Related to radiation therapy[43]
   Radiation pneumonitis
   Pericarditis
   Myocarditis
   Spinal cord damage
   Stricture
   Fistula formation
   Hemorrhage

of preoperative chemoradiotherapy.[2] Researchers have learned that not only does thoracic radiation therapy control local recurrence but a number of the chemotherapeutic agents used to treat esophageal cancer, such as 5-FU and cisplatin, act to potentiate the effect of radiation. However, patterns of failure in the reported trials show that the majority of patients had only distant disease. This leads researchers to believe that a more intensive chemotherapy component in multimodality therapies is needed.[2] The box on p. 149 summarizes potential treatment-related complications.

PROGNOSIS

The prognosis for persons with esophageal cancer is very poor. For the period from 1981 to 1987 the 5-year survival rate reported was 9% for whites and 6% for blacks.[11] Therefore, 90% to 95% of patients are in need of palliative care at diagnosis or shortly thereafter. The major problems experienced by patients with ad-

vanced disease include dysphagia, chest pain, and malnutrition.[12] Palliative surgery is not always an option; alternatives include peroral dilation, peroral esophageal prosthesis, and laser ablation of obstructing lesions. These procedures usually allow the patient to continue oral feedings of liquids and possibly soft foods. If the patient develops anorexia or is unable to continue oral feedings, enteral feedings may be used. Percutaneous endoscopic gastrostomy is a low-risk method of placing a feeding tube. It avoids the need for a laparotomy and general anesthesia in severely ill patients.[12] Total parenteral nutrition is not commonly used in these patients if another route is possible. Chronic severe mediastinal and posterior chest pain is indicative of regional spread of cancer and is very incapacitating. If the patient is unable to take oral sustained-release analgesics, he or she may require a patient-controlled analgesia pump for maximum comfort.

Nursing Management

The nurse can assume a significant role in identifying persons at risk of esophageal cancer and providing counseling on the signs and symptoms of esophageal cancer, lifestyle modifications to eliminate or reduce risk factors, and importance of annual health examinations by a health care professional. Because there are few or no early signs of esophageal cancer, other than vague GI symptoms of pressure, indigestion, or heartburn, nurses should be aware of persons who are chronic users of home remedies or over-the-counter medications for GI distress. Nurses should urge these persons to seek medical attention immediately.

NURSING DIAGNOSIS

• Knowledge deficit. Prevention and early detection of esophageal cancer related to unfamiliar information.

Patient outcome

• Identify risk factors associated with development of esophageal cancer.
• Identify measures to minimize risks.
• Identify signs and symptoms to be reported to health care professionals related to early detection of esophageal cancer.

INTERVENTIONS

1. Assess for high-risk factors such as heavy alcohol and cigarette use or history of reflux esophagitis, hiatus hernia, or Barrett's esophagus.

2. Provide instructions on healthy lifestyle behaviors:
   • Annual health examination by a health care professional
   • Stop use of cigarettes through a smoking cessation program
   • Eliminate or reduce consumption of alcoholic beverages
   • Eat balanced diet with adequate portions of recommended food groups
3. Provide instructions to report these signs and symptoms: persistent GI distress (regurgitation, reflux, heartburn, epigastric pain) requiring use of antacids, difficulty swallowing requiring changes in diet, or weight loss.

Many persons with esophageal cancer have had a significant weight loss just before they are diagnosed. They usually are experiencing dysphagia and have had to make some dietary adjustments. Depending on the severity of the dysphagia, they will need to change their oral intake, take enteral feeding, or even take total parenteral nutrition.

NURSING DIAGNOSIS

• Altered Nutrition: Less than body requirements related to dysphagia

Patient outcomes

1. Identify signs and symptoms to report to the health care professionals.
2. Identify measures to obtain adequate nutrition.
3. Demonstrate a stable nutritional status.[26]

INTERVENTIONS: MILD DYSPHAGIA

1. Assess the patient for choking or regurgitation during and after meals.
2. Obtain dietary consult for calorie count and dietary modification as needed.
3. Weigh patient every other day.
4. Instruct patient to sit upright for meals and 30 minutes after meals. If in bed, raise head to at least 45 degree angle.
5. Offer six to eight small feedings per day of high protein and high-calorie liquified foods and nutritional supplements.
6. Avoid feedings within 2 hours of bedtime.
7. Teach patient to use oral suction if he or she is afraid of aspiration.
8. Provide oral and written instructions of measures to maintain stable nutritional status and prevent aspiration.

INTERVENTIONS: SEVERE DYSPHAGIA (IN ADDITION TO MILD DYSPHAGIA)

1. Monitor food and fluid intake daily.
2. Weigh patient daily.
3. Assess for fatigue, altered mental status, weight loss of 2 pounds or more, and decreased serum albumin.
4. Dietary consult for alternate routes of nutrition (enteral feedings via nasogastric or gastrostomy tubes, or total parenteral nutrition).
5. Administer feedings per physician's orders.
6. Instruct patient/caregiver to administer feedings.
7. Instruct patient/caregiver to provide oral hygiene frequently
8. Instruct patient/caregiver in signs and symptoms to report to the health care professionals.

CANCER OF THE STOMACH

Although cancer of the stomach has shown a significant decline in incidence, about 60% from the 1930s to the 1970s, it remains the eighth most common cause of cancer deaths in the United States.[36,37] The reason for the decline in incidence in some parts of the world but not in others remains an enigma. It is postulated that the increased consumption of refrigerated foods rather than spiced, smoked, and pickled foods may be a factor.[18] Although the United States reports an incidence of 10 per 100,000 population, Japan's incidence is 90 per 100,000. Iceland and certain parts of Central and South America report incidences similar to that in Japan.[36]

EPIDEMIOLOGY

In the United States, it has been estimated that in 1993, 24,000 new cases of stomach cancer will be diagnosed, and a total of 13,600 deaths will be attributed to the disease.[11] Gastric cancer is more common in men than women; the ratios range from 3:2 to 2:1.[18] It is found more commonly in people between 50 and 70 years of age,[33] and is three times more common in semiskilled and unskilled labor groups than in executive and professional groups.[18]

ETIOLOGY AND RISK FACTORS

Several dietary factors have been associated with the development of cancer of the stomach. Immigrant studies show that the second generation of families emigrating from countries of high incidence to low incidence have fewer cases of gastric cancer. This decrease may be attributed to changes in dietary habits. High consumption of smoked or salted foods or foods contaminated with aflatoxin has been associated with increased incidence of stomach cancer.[37]

Occupational risk factors have also been associated with higher incidence of stomach cancer. Workers in coal mining, farming (in Japan), nickel refining (in Russia), rubber processing, timber processing, and asbestos processing have all been shown to have higher than normal incidence.[37] This may be associated with social class rather than the actual occupational hazard, however.

Familial occurrence of gastric cancer is rare, but a small increase in incidence has been noted in direct relatives of some people who have had gastric cancer. The most notable family with this disease is that of Napolean Bonaparte.[33] It has been reported that diffuse gastric cancer is significantly more common in patients with blood group A, in relatives of patients with diffuse gastric cancer, and in cases of familial hypogammaglobulinemia.[18]

Pathologies or past medical history associated with the development of gastric cancer include gastric polyps, especially the villous adenoma; pernicious anemia; chronic reflux esophagitis; and gastric resection for benign peptic ulcer disease.[37] It is suggested that the presence of atrophic gastritis and achlorhydria in persons with pernicious anemia may contribute to the development of gastric cancer.[36]

PREVENTION, SCREENING, AND EARLY DETECTION

The key to prevention of cancer of the stomach lies in dietary intake. As previously indicated, people of geographic areas and socioeconomic groups associated with the lowest incidence consume a diet different from those of highest incidence. Nutrition counseling to prevent gastric cancer should stress the importance of consuming a balanced diet high in fresh fruits and vegetables and moderate in amount of animal protein and fats. Salted, smoked, and pickled foods should be consumed in low quantities.

Screening and early detection programs have been very successful in Japan. Upper GI endoscopic examinations and upper GI series are the techniques used most. The diagnosis of early gastric cancer in Japan increased from 1.3% in 1941 through 1945 to 36% in 1965.[23]

In Western countries, where the incidence of gastric cancer is low, widespread screening programs are not considered useful because of the low yield. It is important, however, to identify persons at high risk and follow them with annual endoscopic examinations. The high-risk group includes those with atrophic gastritis, pernicious anemia, intestinal metaplasia, gastric polyps, familial hypogammaglobulinemia, previous gastric surgery, or dysplasia.[18]

CLASSIFICATION

Adenocarcinomas represent almost 90% of the malignant tumors of the stomach.[37] Lymphoma accounts for up to 8%, leiomyosarcoma makes up from 1% to 3%. Other, rarer types of malignant gastric tumors include carcinoids, plasmacytomas, and metastatic cancers.[33]

Several classification systems are used for stomach cancer. One developed by Borrmann identifies five different types of stomach cancer: type 1 includes polypoid or fungating cancers; type 2 includes ulcerating lesions with elevated borders; type 3 includes ulcerating lesions infiltrating the gastric wall; type 4 includes diffusely infiltrating carcinomas; and type 5 includes unclassifiable cancers.[33,36,37] Lauren developed the DIO system, which identifies two main groups of gastric cancers: diffuse gastric cancer (D) and intestinal gastric cancer (I). These two groups account for 90% of all stomach cancers; the remainder are referred to as "other" (O). Intestinal gastric cancers are characterized by polypoid or fungating lesions that may ulcerate centrally. Diffuse gastric cancers infiltrate the gastric wall without forming large discrete masses and are associated with a very poor prognosis. They are frequently seen in patients with pernicious anemia and familial hypogammaglobulinemia. A classical example is linitis plastica.[18] Broder's classification system is based on degree of histologic differentiation. Tumor cells are graded from 1 (well differentiated) to 4 (anaplastic). An example of grade 4 is linitis plastica, typically a poorly differentiated cell type. Polypoid tumors are most likely to have well-differentiated grade 1 tumor cells.[37]

CLINICAL FEATURES

One of gastric cancer's most frustrating aspects is that it has no early symptoms. Most patients present with locally advanced or metastatic disease.[36] The symptoms are vague and may have been present for several months. They include indigestion and epigastric discomfort (which the patient may have been treating with antacids), malaise, early satiety, postprandial fullness, and loss of appetite.[18] Back pain may indicate that the cancer has spread to the pancreas. Dysphagia is associated with lesions in the cardia. Vomiting after meals is seen in obstructing tumors of the middle third and pyloric regions of the stomach.[18] Hematemesis is not common with gastric carcinoma, but may indicate leiomyosarcoma of the stomach.[36]

DIAGNOSIS AND STAGING

Physical examination of the patient suspected of having gastric cancer should include palpation of the abdomen for masses and nodules around the umbilicus. Attention should also be paid to whether the supraclavicular and axillary nodes are enlarged. A digital rectal examination should be performed to assess for the presence of a shelf of metastatic deposits.

The two most useful diagnostic procedures for gastric cancer are the upper GI endoscopy and the double-contrast upper GI series.[18,36,37] The latter is able to identify the site of the lesion and, with special compression techniques, detect depressions and elevations of the gastric mucosa. The fiberoptic gastroscope permits the skilled endoscopist to obtain multiple biopsies of all suspicious lesions and brush cytologic specimens. In patients with a stiffened stomach that insufflates poorly, an exploratory laparotomy is usually indicated to make a diagnosis.[36] CT scans and ultrasonography are helpful in defining sites of metastatic spread, but not the primary tumor. Endoscopic ultrasonography is used to stage gastric cancer and the presence of adenopathy.[36]

The American Joint Commission on Cancer's Staging TNM criteria for classification and staging of cancer of the stomach are shown in a box on p. 153.[8]

METASTASIS

In addition to local extension to nearby organs and tissue, cancer of the stomach metastasizes most frequently to the liver, lungs, bone, and brain. Stomach cancer also spreads to local lymph nodes, Virchow's node in the left supraclavicular area, and the left axillary node (Irish's node). Peritoneal metastasis is also known to occur, and Krukenburg tumor (metastasis to the ovary) is one indication of metastasis to the peritoneum. Another is the identification of periumbilical nodules (Sister Joseph nodes). Blumer's rectal shelf is another form of peritoneal metastasis that may

TNM CLASSIFICATION AND STAGING FOR CANCER OF THE STOMACH

Primary tumor (T)

T1	Tumor invades lamina propria or submucosa
T2	Tumor invades the muscularis propria or the subserosa
T3	Tumor penetrates the serosa (visceral peritoneum) without invasion of adjacent structures
T4	Tumor invades adjacent structures

Regional lymph nodes (N)

N0	No regional lymph node metastasis
N1	Metastasis in perigastric lymph node(s) within 3 cm of the edge of the primary tumor
N2	Metastasis in perigastric lymph node(s) more than 3 cm from the edge of the primary tumor, or in lymph nodes along the left gastric, common hepatic, splenic, or celiac arteries

Distant metastasis (M)

M0	No distant metastasis
M1	Distant metastasis

Stage grouping for cancer of the stomach

Stage IA	T1	N0	M0
Stage IB	T1	N1	M0
	T2	N0	M0
Stage II	T1	N2	M0
	T2	N1	M0
	T3	N0	M0
Stage IIIA	T2	N2	M0
	T3	N1	M0
	T4	N0	M0
Stage IIIB	T3	N2	M0
	T4	N1	M0
Stage IV	T4	N2	M0
	Any T	Any N	M1

be identified by rectal examination. It is described as a stony-hard indurated area of prerectal tumor that feels like a shelf.[36]

TREATMENT MODALITIES

Surgery, chemotherapy, and radiation therapy are all used to treat cancer of the stomach. They all have potential complications, however (see box at right).

Surgery

Surgery is the major treatment modality and is used for both cure and palliation. It is recommended that any patient with biopsy-proven gastric cancer and no evidence of distant metastasis should undergo an exploratory laparotomy or celiotomy to determine whether the patient should undergo a curative procedure or a palliative one. Fewer than 40% of patients who have a laparotomy are determined to be curable.

The operative procedure chosen depends upon the anatomic location of the tumor and knowledge of the pattern of spread from that particular location.[47] For selection of procedure, the stomach may be divided into thirds. The proximal third includes the gastroesophageal junction and the fundus; the middle third includes the fundus to mid-section of the lesser curvature; and the distal third includes the remaining portion to the pylorus.[47] For tumors in the proximal third, choice of surgical procedure remains controversial, but usually either a radical subtotal gastrectomy[47] or a total gastrectomy is used.[52] Tumors in the middle section usually require a total gastrectomy to obtain tumor-free margins.[47] Tumors located in the distal third are usually treated with a radical subtotal gastrectomy.[47,52] Figure 9-5 illustrates the sur-

GASTRIC CANCER DISEASE AND TREATMENT RELATED COMPLICATIONS

Disease-related complications
  Pain
  Obstruction
  Bleeding
  Dysphagia

Treatment-related complications
Postoperative complications[52]

Early	**Late**
Anastomotic leak	Dumping syndrome
Infection	Reflux esophagitis
Hemorrhage	Chronic weight loss
Acute pancreatitis	Anemia
Ileus, jaundice	Hypoproteinemia

Radiation therapy complications

During treatment[14]	**Late**[37]
Anorexia	Radiation nephritis
Nausea	Hypertension
Vomiting	GI bleeding
Weight loss	Duodenal ulcers

Chemotherapy complications
  Myelosuppression
  Stomatitis
  Nausea/vomiting
  Diarrhea

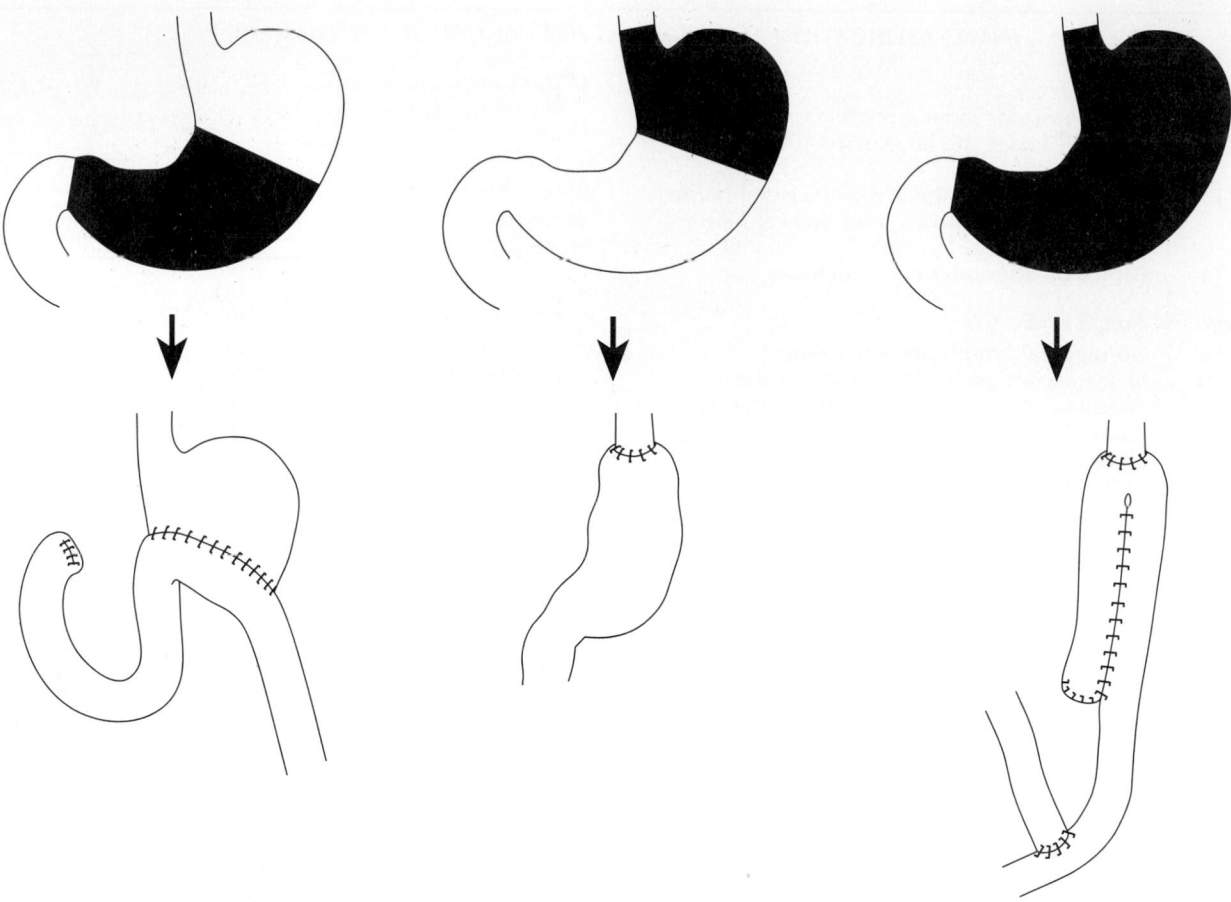

Figure 9–5 Surgical resections and reconstruction for the three locations of gastric cancer. (From Lawrence W Jr: Gastric neoplasms. In Holleb AI, Fink DJ, and Murphy GP, editors: Textbook of clinical oncology, Atlanta, 1991, American Cancer Society, Inc.)

gical resections and reconstruction for each procedure.[33]

Chemotherapy

Gastric cancer does seem more responsive to chemotherapy than some of the other malignancies.[28,54] Chemotherapy is now being studied as adjuvant therapy for fully resected tumors, for advanced gastric cancer, and in combination with radiation therapy. One of the older regimens that has been widely studied is FAM (5-FU, doxorubicin, and mitomycin-C). It shows a consistent response rate of approximately 35%, but has a minimal impact on survival.[28] A newer regimen in use is EAP (etoposide, doxorubicin, and cisplatin), but this regimen is associated with significant dose-limiting myelosuppression.[28] A third regimen that is currently showing good responses is ELF (etoposide, leucovorin, and 5-FU).[28] EAP and ELF are newer protocols that show encouraging response rates, but need further testing on the impact on long-term survival.

Radiation Therapy

Radiation therapy is important in the treatment of locally advanced or recurrent gastric cancer. Although radiation therapy has been used alone with some response, it has greatest benefit when combined with chemotherapy.[37] Controversy exists regarding the preferred method of combining radiation with surgery; preoperative, intraoperative, and postoperative schedules have all been proposed. A tolerable dose is 45 to 50 Gy delivered in 1.8 Gy fractions per day.[14] Intraoperative radiation therapy (IORT) has been useful in the control of microscopic disease with a maximum tolerated dose of 15 to 20 Gy.[14] The advantage of IORT is that radiosensitive normal tissue can be removed from the field. Combining IORT and postoperative radiation has been studied and may increase the long-term survival of patients with stage II, III, or IV disease.[1] Another method that increases the effectiveness of radiation therapy is administering 5-FU as a radiosensitizer over the first 3 days of the radiation schedule.[38]

PROGNOSIS

The prognosis for patients with gastric cancer depends on the extent of the disease and on the treatment. The 5-year survival rate reported for the period of 1981 to 1987 is 16%.[11] Therefore the prognosis for these patients remains poor. It has been reported that two thirds of patients are not candidates for curative surgery at the time of diagnosis.[33] The only option for these patients is palliative resection of the tumor, which may alleviate the symptoms of obstruction, bleeding, and pain.[47] Patients experiencing dysphagia with tumors of the proximal stomach unable to undergo a resection may benefit temporarily from dilations, laser ablation of tumor, or placement of an endoprosthesis.[52]

Nursing Management

Like patients with cancer of the esophagus, these patients experience profound weight loss caused by the disease process and the treatment modalities, particularly radical subtotal or total gastrectomy. The preoperative patient assessment should include a nutritional evaluation encompassing a diet and weight loss history (especially the type and consistency of diet consumed), laboratory values (serum albumin, leukocyte count, total iron binding capacity, ferritin, and electrolytes), and calorie intake.[45]

NURSING DIAGNOSIS

- Altered nutrition (less than body requirements) related to gastrectomy

Patient outcomes

- Explain rationale for altered nutrition and factors that contribute to malnourishment.
- Demonstrate measures to manage nutritional status.
- List signs and symptoms to report to the health care team.
- Demonstrate a stable nutritional status consistent with stage of disease.

INTERVENTIONS[15]

1. Weigh daily.
2. Accurate intake and output every 24 hours.
3. Monitor laboratory values including electrolytes and leukocyte count.
4. Provide patient/caregiver dietary instructions:
   a. Six small feedings per day
   b. Limit fluids at meal time, drink fluids between meals
   c. Progress slowly from liquid to soft diet
   d. Choose high protein and moderate carbohydrate foods
   e. Avoid greasy foods
   f. Eat slowly
5. Provide instructions on signs and symptoms to report to health care team:
   a. Diarrhea
   b. Clay colored stools
   c. Fatty stools
   d. Abdominal cramps
   e. Weakness
   f. Faintness
   g. Rapid heartbeat
6. Provide instructions for diet if diarrhea occurs:
   a. Choose low-residue, bulk-forming foods (refined breads and cereals, pasta, rice, cheese, fish, chicken, bananas, applesauce, cooked vegetables)
   b. Avoid foods such as whole-grain breads or cereals, fresh fruits and vegetables, gas-forming foods, citrus fruits, and juices
   c. Eat slowly
   d. Notify health care team of need for antidiarrheal and/or antispasmodic agents
7. Provide instructions for diet if dumping syndrome occurs:
   a. Choose foods high in protein and fat, low in carbohydrates
   b. Avoid concentrated sweets
   c. Drink liquids between meals
   d. Rest after meals for at least 30 minutes
   e. Notify health care team if symptoms continue
8. Obtain dietary consult for assistance, evaluation, and diet planning.
9. Administer enteral/parenteral feedings if ordered and provide instructions to patient/caregiver if necessary prior to discharge.

CANCER OF THE LIVER

Hepatocellular carcinoma (HCC) is relatively uncommon in the United States but is one of the most common malignancies in some parts of the world, especially parts of Africa and Asia. There are no effective controls against this disease, and it continues to be rapidly fatal in areas of high incidence.

EPIDEMIOLOGY

For reporting purposes in the United States, HCC is combined with biliary tract cancers (gallbladder carcinoma, cholangiocarcinoma, and periampullary carcinoma). Therefore, the incidence data are not completely reliable for primary liver cancer (HCC) alone. The estimated number of new cases of liver and biliary tract cancers in 1993 is 15,800, which will result in 12,600 deaths.[11] It has been estimated that the number of deaths from HCC is around 4000 annually in the United States; black men have a three times higher risk of getting the disease than women or white men.[4]

This situation is quite different in Asia and Africa. In Mozambique, the incidence is 500 times that in the United States. In Japan, HCC is the third leading cause of cancer deaths among men and fifth among women.[4]

ETIOLOGY AND RISK FACTORS

Because of the widespread geographic variations in incidence, researchers have been particularly interested in studying the environmental factors implicated in the development of HCC. The box on this page summarizes the etiologic and risk factors known to be associated with primary liver cancers. Hepatitis B and C infections are probably the most important cause worldwide. There exists a positive correlation between the presence of hepatitis B surface antigen (HBsAG) in the serum of patients and HCC. Hepatitis C is also associated with an increased risk of developing HCC. Hepatitis A, however, does not appear to be related to the development of HCC.[4]

Cirrhosis and alcohol consumption have been associated with the development of HCC. Cirrhosis associated with chronic hepatitis B infection and hemachromatosis a major risk factor in Asia and Africa. In the Western world, however, alcoholic cirrhosis is more common and therefore may be a more important risk factor. Once cirrhosis has developed, the risk of developing cancer does not diminish, even if alcohol consumption is stopped.[4]

Aflatoxin is a carcinogen produced by fungus growing in contaminated grain and other foods improperly stored in warm, moist places. This is a widespread problem in humid regions of Africa and Asia where HCC is most common.[4]

A number of chemical agents have been implicated in the development of primary liver cancer. These include 16 different pesticides and herbicides, along with industrial chemicals such as cycasin and nitrosamines that are known to produce liver cancer in laboratory animals.[4] Thorotrast, a contrast medium used until the 1950s, is associated with the development of angiosarcoma of the liver.[53] The use of oral contraceptives has also been reported to lead to HCC, but this is very rare; benign liver adenomas and focal nodular hyperplasia are more common in users of oral contraceptives, however.[4]

SUMMARY OF CONDITIONS ASSOCIATED WITH HCC	
Hepatitis B virus	Aflatoxins
Hepatitis C virus	Alcoholism
Hemochromatosis	Occupational exposure
Cirrhosis	to pesticides and herbicides

PREVENTION, SCREENING, AND DETECTION

Technological advances in the agricultural field and in storage of grains have reduced contamination of food by aflatoxin in developed countries, but these advances have not yet been made in the developing countries. The advent of the vaccine against hepatitis B may significantly reduce morbidity and mortality from HCC in high-risk areas.[9] High-risk patients with chronic hepatitis B or cirrhosis may be screened for the tumor marker alpha-fetoprotein (AFP) and by abdominal ultrasonography.[53]

CLASSIFICATION

The histopathologic types of primary cancers of the liver include hepatomas or hepatocellular carcinomas, intrahepatic bile duct carcinomas or cholangiocarcinomas, and mixed types.[8] Almost 95% of all primary liver tumors are malignant. The benign liver tumors include adenomas, focal nodular hyperplasia, hamartomas, and hemangiomas.[7] In the United States, almost 90% of the primary liver cancers are HCC, and intrahepatic cholangiocarcinomas represent about 7%; the remainder are angiosarcomas, hepatoblastomas, and primary lymphomas.[4]

CLINICAL FEATURES

The most common presenting symptoms of HCC are a right upper quadrant abdominal mass, pain, and epigastric fullness.[20] The pain is usually located in the right upper quadrant of the abdomen, and may be described as dull or aching and may radiate to the right shoulder.[4,53] Other signs and symptoms are listed in a box on p. 157.[4] HCC is also associated with several paraneoplastic syndromes, including hyperglycemia, hypoglycemia, Cushing's syndrome, precocious puberty, hyperlipidemia, polycythemia, microangiopathic hemolytic anemia, leukocytosis, and disseminated intravascular coagulation.[9]

PRESENTING SIGNS AND SYMPTOMS OF HCC

Symptoms
   Abdominal pain
   Weight loss
   Anorexia
   Nausea/vomiting
   Abdominal mass
   Weakness, fatigue, malaise
   Gastrointestinal bleeding
   Diarrhea
Signs
   Abdominal mass/hepatomegaly
   Jaundice
   Ascites
   Fever

DIAGNOSIS AND STAGING

Diagnosis of liver cancer can be challenging. Patients presenting with a right upper quadrant abdominal mass should begin a diagnostic work up at once. The initial studies should include blood tests, x-rays, and ultrasound.

Blood tests should include AFP and hepatitis surface antigens. AFP is the principal tumor marker associated with HCC and is elevated in over 70% of patients with the disease.[53] The normal value for AFP is 40 ng/ml, and elevations to greater than 400 ng/ml are almost diagnostic for HCC. It is important to note, however, that a significant number of patients with HCC will have normal AFP.[4]

Radiologic studies should specifically include an ultrasound and CT. The ultrasound is inexpensive, noninvasive, and nontoxic[53]; it will detect lesions less than 3 cm in size. CT is able to detect and demonstrate the extent of the liver tumors and is helpful in identifying any metastatic disease.[4,53] For any tumor that appears to be resectable, an arteriogram is necessary to provide information regarding arterial and venous involvement. This information is also invaluable if the patient requires hepatic artery infusions.

A biopsy is ultimately necessary to make a definitive diagnosis. If the tumor appears resectable, a surgical approach is best for obtaining a tissue specimen. Resection should be attempted only for local lesions limited to one lobe or segment that is without extrahepatic spread.[53] For unresectable tumors, the percutaneous route is preferred and may be done with either sonographic or CT guidance. Hemorrhage is a risk for vascular lesions but is usually self limiting. Peritoneoscopy is another approach for obtaining a specimen that allows direct visualization of the liver and decreases the risk of hemorrhage.[53]

In 1988, the American Joint Commission on Cancer adopted a staging system based on degree of liver involvement, extent of vascular invasion, nodal involvement, and the presence or absence of distant metastasis (TNM).[8] A box on this page summarizes this system.

TNM CLASSIFICATION AND STAGING FOR LIVER CANCER

Primary tumor (T)

T1 Solitary tumor 2 cm or less in greatest dimension without vascular invasion

T2 Solitary tumor 2 cm or less in greatest dimension with vascular invasion, or
Multiple tumors limited to one lobe none more than 2 cm in greatest dimension without vascular invasion, or
A solitary tumor more than 2 cm in greatest dimension without vascular invasion

T3 Solitary tumor more than 2 cm in greatest dimension with vascular invasion, or
Multiple tumors limited to one lobe, none more than 2 cm in greatest dimension, with vascular invasion, or
Multiple tumors limited to one lobe, any more than 2 cm in greatest dimension, with or without vascular invasion

T4 Multiple tumors in more than one lobe or Tumor(s) involve(s) a major branch of portal or hepatic vein(s)

Lymph node (N)

N0 No regional lymph node metastasis
N1 Regional lymph node metastasis

Distant metastasis (M)

M0 No distant metastasis
M1 Distant metastasis

Stage grouping

Stage I	T1	N0	M0
Stage II	T2	N0	M0
Stage III	T1	N1	M0
	T2	N1	M0
	T3	N0	M0
	T3	N1	M0
Stage IVA	T4	Any N	M0
IVB	Any T	Any N	M1

METASTASIS

The usual sites for HCC metastasis are the regional nodes, lung, bone, adrenal gland, and brain. Approximately 40% of the HCC patients have tumor cells in the regional nodes, but other metastatic sites are rare. At the time of surgery few patients have metastasis, but more than 50% have metastasis at the time of autopsy.[53] Spread also occurs by direct invasion of adjacent structures such as the stomach and diaphragm.[45]

TREATMENT MODALITIES
Surgery

Surgery is the only potentially curative treatment modality for patients with HCC. Unfortunately, only 25% of the patients meet the criteria for liver resection. Patients with extrahepatic involvement of major vessels or structure are ineligible, as are those with poor hepatic reserve or severe coagulopathy.[4,34] Patients with cirrhosis are not usually candidates for resection

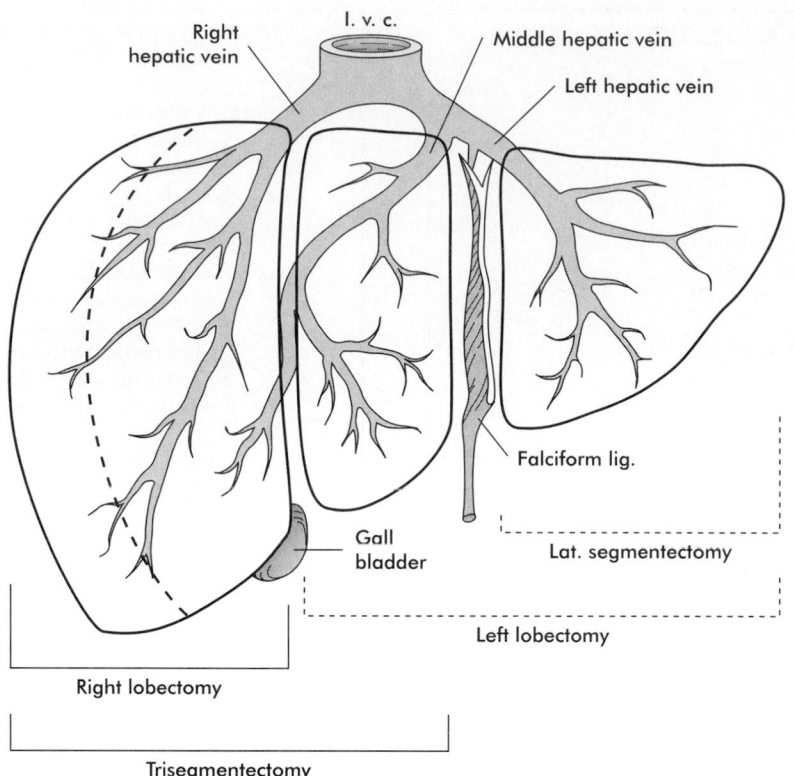

Figure 9–6 Four approaches to liver resection. (From Starzl TE, Bell RH, Beart RW, and Putnam CW: Hepatic trisegmentectomy and other liver resections, Surg Gynecol Obstet 141:729, 1975.)

because of the risk of intraoperative hemorrhage and postoperative hepatic failure.[50]

Hepatic resection involves either a bilateral subcostal or a thoracoabdominal incision. Following the incision, there are four recognized resection techniques: the right and left lobectomy, the trisegmentectomy, and the lateral segmentectomy. The lateral segmentectomy involves the removal of the outer portion of the left lobe. The trisegmentectomy is the removal of the right lobe and the inner portion of the left lobe.[4] Figure 9-6 illustrates the four approaches to liver resection.

Chemotherapy

No single-system chemotherapeutic agent has shown high activity against HCC. Doxorubicin has been the most active, but the true response rate is substantially below 20%.[4] A number of combinations of agents have been studied, but none has been recognized as a standard therapy, and none has demonstrated a survival advantage over any other.[4]

Because a large number of HCC patients have significant unresectable liver tumors without extrahepatic spread, regional chemotherapy has been investigated. Regional chemotherapy involves infusion of agents that are highly metabolized by the liver via the hepatic artery. This greatly increases the dose of drug delivered to the tumor but minimizes the systemic side effects.[4] Intraarterial chemotherapy can be administered through temporary catheters placed into the axillary or femoral arteries. This method requires that the patient remain in bed for the duration of the infusion, which may be up to 5 days. Complications of this method include thrombosis of the hepatic and other intra-abdominal arteries, catheter displacement, sepsis, and hemorrhage. Drugs may also be administered via an implantable pump, which offers the advantages of allowing the patient to remain ambulatory and reducing catheter-related complications. The most common problems associated with the implantable pump have been gastroduodenal ulceration and inflammation.[34] The agents used most commonly for intra-arterial chemotherapy are floxuridine (FUdR) and 5-FU. Other drugs used include cisplatin, doxorubicin, mitomycin-C, and dichloromethotrextate.[4] Combination therapy via the hepatic artery is currently being investigated.

Embolization and Chemoembolization

Embolization is the selective occlusion of hepatic vessels by injecting nondegradable particles, typically Gelfoam and Ivalon. Embolizations usually need to be repeated because of the fomation of collateral circulation. Chemoembolization involves occlusion by particles into which chemotherapeutic agents have been adsorbed. Drugs used in this application include doxorubicin, cisplatin, mitomycin-C, aclarubicin, and carmustine (BCNU).[4,53]

Radiation Therapy

Even though HCC is considered a radiosensitive tumor, the use of radiation therapy is restricted by the relative intolerance of the normal liver parenchyma. The whole liver will tolerate 3000 cGy. At this dose the incidence of radiation hepatitis is 5% to 10%. A cure or long-term remission of HCC requires significantly higher doses. In order to improve results, radiolabeled antibodies have been used with some success. The high concentration of ferritin in HCC has led to the use of antiferritin antibodies labeled with iodine 131; this technique allows tolerance of high doses. The dose-limiting toxicity is thrombocytopenia, because the bone marrow has a significant uptake of the antiferritin antibodies.[4] A summary of typical treatment-related complications is provided in the box at right.

PROGNOSIS

Overall prognosis for the patient with primary liver cancer is poor. The relative 5-year survival rate for cancer of the liver is 5%.[11] For those with resectable disease this rate increases to 10%.[42]

HEPATIC TREATMENT RELATED COMPLICATIONS

Surgery-related[24]
  Hemorrhage
  Coagulapathy
  Liver failure
  Hypothermia
  Acute respiratory distress
  Renal failure
Hepatic artery infusion-related[5]
  Acid peptic disease
  Catheter occlusion, migration
  Arterial thrombosis
  Pseudoaneurysm of hepatic artery
  Pump pocket seroma
  Drug toxicities
  Chemical hepatitis
  Hemorrhage
  Stenosis of hepatitic artery
  Localized infection
  Hepatic abscess
Hepatic artery or chemoembolization-related (1-3 days)[4]
  Fever
  Right upper quadrant pain
  Nausea, vomiting
Radiation therapy-related
  Nausea
  Anorexia
  Occasional vomiting
  Fatigue

Nursing Management

The nursing care of the patient with primary liver cancer is very challenging. Because most patients with HCC are not candidates for liver resection, many will be treated by hepatic artery infusion therapy via an implanted infusion pump. The nurse's primary responsibility is educating the patient and family to manage this form of therapy.[17]

NURSING DIAGNOSIS

• Knowledge deficit: management of hepatic artery infusion therapy related to lack of exposure

Patient outcomes

• State rationale for use of hepatic artery infusion.
• Demonstrate measures for care of implanted pump and management of side effects of chemotherapy.
• Identify signs and symptoms to report to the health care team.

INTERVENTIONS

1. Assess the patient's understanding of treatment goals, and the patient's ability to manage care post-

operatively, the availability of support from family and friends.
2. Provide both verbal and written instructions regarding the implanted pump and chemotherapy:
   • Purpose of the pump and where the catheter is placed anatomically in the liver.
   • Management of the pocket site: keep incision clean and dry until healed; resume usual activities when healed; avoid activities that may lead to blunt trauma to the pump pocket or those which may cause increased temperature, pressure, or altitude.
   • What to report to health care team: temperature greater than 101 degrees fahrenheit for more than 24 hours; air travel; or change in residence requiring a change in altitude.
   • Side effects of the chemotherapy drug(s) being infused and other medications.
3. Provide written list of phone numbers of health care team members and schedule of treatment cycles.

CANCER OF THE PANCREAS

Pancreatic cancer is the second most common GI cancer and the fourth leading cause of cancer death in the United States.[10] Cancers of the pancreas fall into three different categories: those in the exocrine pancreas, those around the ampulla of Vater, and those in the islets of Langerhans. The pathologic and etiologic characteristics of the three types differ. The term *pancreatic cancer* usually refers to cancer of the exocrine pancreas.

EPIDEMIOLOGY

The estimated number of new cases of cancer of the pancreas reported in 1993 is 27,700, which will result in 25,000 deaths. This represents 3% of the cancers diagnosed and 5% of the cancer deaths in women, and 2% of the cancers diagnosed and 4% of deaths in men. Over the past 60 years, the incidence of cancer of the pancreas has been slowly but steadily increasing.[11] The median age of patients with pancreatic cancer is about 70. The incidence is about 35% higher in the black population than in the white population; the American black male is the person at highest risk worldwide.[3]

ETIOLOGY AND RISK FACTORS

Cigarette smoke is the most clearly identified carcinogen in pancreatic cancer. Several dietary carcinogens have been implicated, but no conclusive data have appeared. High-risk dietary components include excessive consumption of meat, coffee, and alcohol. Occupational exposure to solvents and petroleum compounds is associated with increased risk of pancreatic cancer, as is history of chronic pancreatitis and diabetes mellitus.[13]

PREVENTION, SCREENING, AND DETECTION

Since no specific risk factors have been conclusively identified for pancreatic cancer, it is impossible to determine how to prevent the disease. Avoiding cigarette smoke and eating a healthy balanced diet would probably reduce risk. The occupational exposure is decreased if safety precautions are employed when working with known carcinogens. No cost-effective test has been found that could be used to screen the asymptomatic population and identify patients for more invasive procedures.[39]

CLASSIFICATION

Ninety-five percent of cancers involving the pancreas arise from the exocrine gland.[3,13] Ductal adenocarcinoma accounts for 80% of all pancreatic cancers. Other less common types include squamous cell carcinomas, giant cell carcinomas, and carcinosarcomas.[13] Primary lymphomas and plasmacytomas occur rarely.[3] The majority of the carcinomas occur in the proximal gland, which includes the head, neck, and uncinate process of the pancreas. Twenty percent occur in the body of the pancreas, and 5% to 10% occur in the tail.[13]

CLINICAL FEATURES

Pain is the most common symptom in patients with pancreatic cancer and is often the reason the patient seeks medical attention. The pain is generally described as gnawing and is located in the epigastrium. Occasionally the pain may be relieved with meals, mimicking the pain associated with peptic ulcer disease. Severe pain is usually indicative of invasion of the splanchic plexus and is a sign of unresectability.[13]

Two other common symptoms are anorexia and weight loss. A typical patient has lost more than 10% of his body weight at diagnosis. The exact cause of the weight loss is unknown, but it may be related to malabsorption. Table 9-1 summarizes signs and symptoms according to the location of the tumor.[3]

DIAGNOSIS AND STAGING

Ultrasonography is an effective and relatively inexpensive means of demonstrating a mass in the pancreas, but CT may be necessary for the diagnosis of pancreatic cancer. The CT can show a mass in the pancreas, involvement of the liver or bile ducts, ascites, and the presence of metastases.[13] It is also used for staging.[3] Endoscopic retrograde cholangiopancreatography (ERCP) is used to identify tumors of the ampulla or obstructed stenotic or sclerosed ducts. Angiography is helpful in determining any abnormal vasculature and whether the tumor is resectable. To confirm the diagnosis of pancreatic cancer, a biopsy

Table 9-1 Signs and Symptoms of Pancreatic Cancer According to Site of Lesion

Sign or Symptom	Percent of Patients	
	Head	*Body & Tail*
Symptom		
Weight loss	92	100
Pain	72	87
Anorexia	64	33
Nausea	45	43
Vomiting	37	37
Diarrhea	18	
Sign		
Jaundice	87	23
Palpable liver	83	33
Palpable gallbladder	29	
Abdominal tenderness		27
Abdominal mass	13	23
Ascites	14	20

Adapted from Ahlgren JD, Hill MC, and Roberts IM: Pancreatic cancer: patterns, diagnosis, and approaches to treatment. In Ahlgren J and MacDonald J, editors, Gastrointestinal oncology, Philadelphia, 1992, JB Lippincott Co.

is needed. If the patient is not a candidate for a laparotomy, a percutaneous biopsy may be obtained using ultrasound or CT guidance.[3]

The American Joint Commission for Cancer has accepted a staging system for pancreatic cancer based upon local, regional nodal, and distant metastatic involvement using the TNM system. The box below lists the established staging criteria.[8]

METASTASIS

Because of the location of the pancreas, early invasion of adjacent organs by pancreatic tumors is common. These adjacent organs include the major vessels, duodenum, stomach, bile duct, retroperitoneum, spleen, kidney, and colon. Widespread carcinomatosis and ascites are common because of intraperitoneal seeding.[3] Distant metastasis occurs most commonly to the liver, but other sites are the lung, bone, and brain.[13]

TNM CLASSIFICATION AND STAGING FOR CANCER OF THE PANCREAS

Primary tumor (T)

T1	Tumor invades mucosa or muscle layer
T1a	Tumor invades mucosa
T1b	Tumor invades muscle layer
T2	Tumor invades perimuscular connective tissue; no extension beyond serosa or into liver
T3	Tumor invades beyond serosa or into one adjacent organ, or both (extension 2 cm or less into liver)
T4	Tumor extends more than 2 cm into liver, and/or into two or more adjacent organs (stomach, duodenum, colon, pancreas, omentum, extrahepatic bile ducts, any involvement of liver)

Regional lymph nodes (N)

N0	No regional lymph node metastasis
N1	Regional lymph node metastasis
N1a	Metastasis in cystic duct, pericholedochal, and/or hilar lymph nodes (i.e., in the hepatoduodenal ligament)
N1b	Metastasis in peripancreatic (head only), periduodenal, periportal, celiac, and/or superior mesenteric lymph nodes

Distant metastasis (M)

M0	No distant metastasis
M1	Distant metastasis

Stage grouping

Stage I	T1	N0	M0
Stage II	T2	N0	M0
Stage III	T1	N1	M0
	T2	N1	M0
	T3	Any N	M0
Stage IV	T4	Any N	M0
	Any T	Any N	M1

TREATMENT MODALITIES

Even with the advances in treatment in recent years, pancreatic cancer continues to be the most difficult to treat of all GI cancers. Surgery is probably the only effective treatment. Unfortunately, the cancer is unsymptomatic until it invades adjacent organs or metastasizes. Only 15% of patients meet the criteria for curative surgery. Radiation therapy offers a chance for extended survival to patients with locally advanced disease, but the majority of patients are not candidates for curative surgery or radiation therapy. These will be in need of palliative therapy to relieve pain and maintain quality of life.[3]

Surgery

The majority of pancreatic cancers occur in the head of the pancreas. Patients who are amenable to curative resection will undergo either a pancreatoduodenectomy (or Whipple operation) or a total pancreatectomy. The pancreatoduodenectomy involves the removal of the distal stomach, the gallbladder, the common bile duct, the head of the pancreas, the duodenum, and the upper jejunum.[39] Figure 9-7 illustrates the pancreatoduodenectomy or Whipple resection of the pancreas.[51] Reconstruction following the pancreatoduodenectomy involves three steps. As part of the choledochojejunostomy, the jejunum is anastomosed to the common hepatic duct. A pancreatojejunostomy attaches the remaining pancreas to the small bowel. The standard gastrojejunostomy is then performed.[30]

A total pancreatectomy is an extension of the pancreatoduodenectomy and involves, in addition, removal of the body and tail of the pancreas and the spleen and a more extensive regional lymphadenectomy. Controversy continues over the advantages and disadvantages of the two procedures.[39]

Palliation for cancer of the head of the pancreas is the objective of surgery more often than is cure. Jaundice, gastric outlet obstruction, and pain are the problems most often relieved through surgical intervention. If the patient is a candidate for an operative procedure, but not a curative resection, palliative surgery is warranted to relieve symptoms and improve quality of life.[39] A laparotomy may be performed to establish tissue diagnosis. At this time the biliary tract is internally decompressed to relieve jaundice and pruritus and prevent ascending cholangitis, progressive liver failure, and coagulopathy.[39] A choledochojejunostomy or cholecystojejunostomy may be indicated to bypass distal obstruction of the biliary tree.[3] Duodenal obstruction is a late symptom of pancreatic cancer, but a gastrojejunostomy may be performed prophylactically or if compression or invasion of the duodenum is present.[39] A chemical splanchnicectomy may also be indicated for relief of pain.[39]

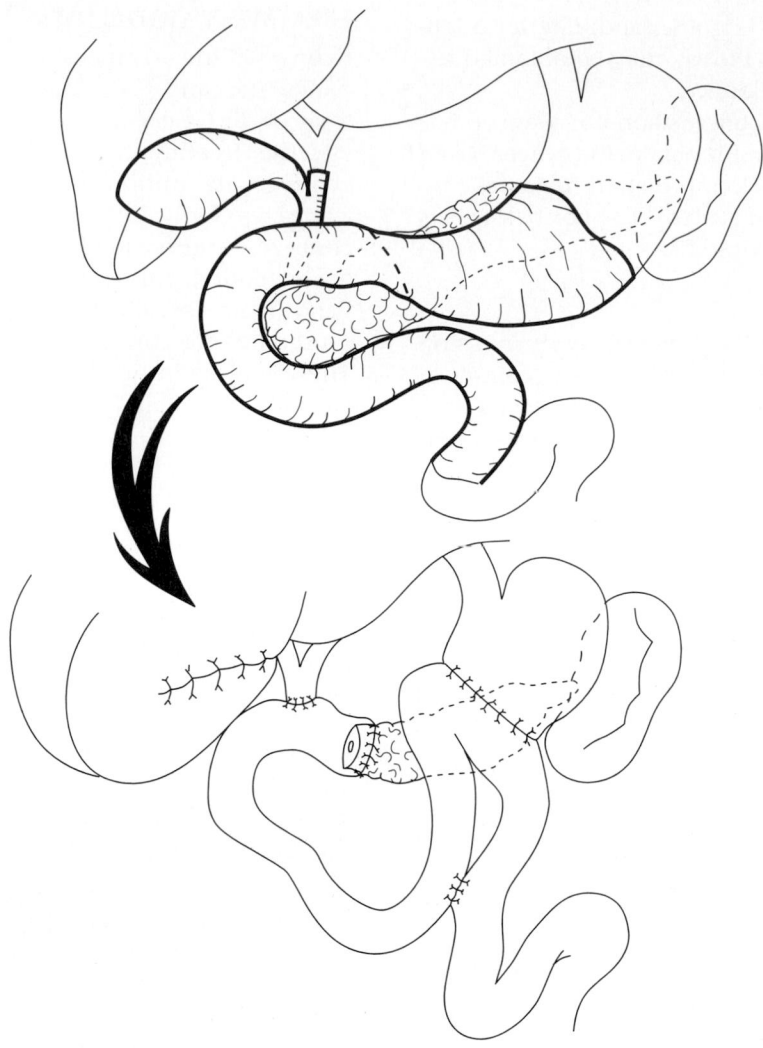

Figure 9–7   Extent of pancreatoduodenectomy or Whipple resection (above) and technique of resection (below). (From Trede M, Schwall G, and Saeger H: Survival after pancreatoduodenectomy, Ann Surg 211:454, 1990.)

If surgery is not an option for the patient, obstructive jaundice may be relieved by either the endoscopic placement of a stent, which will provide internal drainage of bile, or the placement of percutaneous transhepatic catheter, which will provide either external or internal-external drainage. The percutaneous transhepatic catheter may be used to internalize the drainage via a stent. Complications of these procedures include cholangitis, hemorrhage, bile leak, and catheter obstruction.[3]

Chemotherapy

For unknown reasons, pancreatic cancer cells are relatively chemoresistant.[13] Both single and multiple chemotherapeutic agents have been tried with generally poor results. 5-FU and mitomycin-C are the most responsive single agents,[39] but combinations now in use that show improved responses include streptozotocin, mitomycin-C, and 5-FU (SMF); 5-FU, doxorubicin (Adriamycin), and mitomycin-C (FAM);

and FAM with the addition of streptozotocin.[39] Studies are also in progress investigating the usefulness of biological therapies in treating pancreatic cancer.[13]

Radiation Therapy

The use of radiation therapy in treating cancer of the pancreas is limited by the close proximity of the pancreas to dose-limiting structures such as the kidneys, bowel, liver, and spinal cord. With the development of new techniques, however, radiation is now being used to improve local disease control and long-term survival.

Adjuvant radiation therapy is being studied for resectable tumors. Researchers are using postoperative external beam radiation with or without 5-FU as a radiosensitizer. Intraoperative radiation therapy (IORT) is also being studied. IORT has the advantage of being able to deliver tumor-specific high-dose radiation therapy while avoiding adjacent normal tissue.[3] Radiation therapy is the primary treatment for

---

PANCREATIC TREATMENT RELATED COMPLICATIONS

Surgery-related complications[30]
 Hemorrhage, intraoperative and postoperative in first 24-48 hours
 Fistula (pancreatic or biliary)
 Cardiovascular problems (myocardial infarction, congestive heart failure, rhythm disturbances)
 Vascular thrombosis, most commonly in the portal vein
 Infection (lung, urinary tract, incisional wound, peritoneal cavity)
 Renal or hepatic failure
 Pancreatitis
 Gastric retention
 Late complications (jaundice, gastrointestinal ulceration, diabetes mellitus, dumping syndrome)

---

patients with unresectable disease. External beam therapy, IORT, and combinations of these continue to have a 50% probability of local failure. The standard treatment remains 5-FU and external beam radiation therapy, because it consistently has extended median survival from the range of 6 months to 1 year.[3] The box at left summarizes treatment-related complications.

PROGNOSIS

The prognosis for persons with cancer of the pancreas is relatively poor. The reported 5-year survival rate for pancreatic cancer is 3%.[16] This figure has increased only slightly from that reported in the early 1960s.[11] Improved surgical techniques and supportive care have not led to improved survival. Median survivals in patients who have had a pancreatoduodenectomy range from 16 to 30 months.

Nursing Management

Patients who have had surgical intervention for pancreatic cancer have complex and challenging nursing needs. Preoperative assessment includes both psychological and physical parameters, including nutritional history, elimination problems, pain, jaundice, pruritis, fatigue or weakness, depression, or anxiety; laboratory values must be monitored for anemia and coagulation abnormalities. Postoperatively, nurses should be aware of the extent of the surgical resection and the reconstruction the patient has undergone in order to anticipate potential problems and plan for the care of the patient.

NURSING DIAGNOSIS

• Fluid volume deficit related to extensive abdominal surgery

Patient outcomes

1. State rationale for potential and actual fluid loss.
2. Demonstrate measures to correct or maintain adequate fluid volume.
3. Maintain fluid volume evidenced by normal laboratory parameters.

INTERVENTIONS FOR POTENTIAL FLUID LOSS

1. Assessment parameters:
   a. Monitor fluid intake and output, and note fluid preferences.
   b. Examine mucous membranes for moistness and integrity.
   c. Monitor weight and vital signs.
   d. Monitor laboratory values: BUN, creatinine, electrolytes, serum osmolality, and hematocrit.

2. Patient instructions:
   a. Signs and symptoms to report to health care team: thirst, dry skin and mucous membranes, fatigue, constipation, nausea/vomiting, diarrhea, or fever
   b. Appropriate fluid intake per day, as well as type and timing of fluid intake, to avoid possible problems such as dumping syndrome
   c. Administration of medications to minimize fluid loss

INTERVENTIONS FOR ACTUAL FLUID LOSS

1. In addition to above assessment parameters, monitor type and amount of output (diarrhea, wound drainage, emesis) and weigh patient daily.
2. Administer intravenous fluids per physician's orders.
3. Offer small amount of fluids by mouth as appropriate.
4. Administer replacement electrolytes per physicians' orders.
5. If tube feedings or total parenteral nutrition is ordered, administer and provide instructions to patient/caregiver as appropriate.
6. When oral feedings are resumed, administer pancreatic enzymes per physician's orders, and provide instructions on same to the patient.

NURSING DIAGNOSIS

• Potential for injury related to unstable blood glucose levels

Patient outcomes

1. State rationale for potential changes in blood sugar.
2. Demonstrate self blood glucose monitoring, urine testing, and insulin injection.
3. Identify signs and symptoms of hypoglycemia and hyperglycemia and measures to prevent/treat.

INTERVENTIONS

1. Assess patient for signs and symptoms of hypoglycemia and hyperglycemia, report to physician if occurs.
2. Test urine for acetone every 4 to 6 hours or as ordered by physician.
3. Monitor blood glucose levels every 6 hours and administer sliding scale insulin per physician's order.
4. If patient is not on total parenteral nutrition, blood glucose may be monitored before breakfast and evening meal with a daily dose of neutral protamine Hagedorn (NPH) insulin in the morning and sliding scale regular insulin in the evening.
5. Provide patient with written and verbal instructions regarding diabetic management.
6. Evaluate for the need for home health referral.

CANCER OF THE SMALL INTESTINES

Neoplasms of the small intestines are rare. They comprise only 1% of GI malignancies. The estimated number of new cases for 1993 is 3,600, which will result in 925 deaths.[11] Small bowel cancers have been reported in patients from 1 year to 84 years of age, but the average age is 57 years.[46] The types of neoplasms found in the small intestines include adenocarcinoma, lymphoma, leiomyosarcoma, liposarcoma, neurofibrosarcoma, malignant schwannoma, carcinoid, fibrosarcoma, hemangiosarcoma, and lymphangiosarcoma.[48] Risk factors that have been associated with small bowel cancers include inflammatory bowel disease, Crohn's disease, Peutz-Jeghers syndrome, familial polyposis, Gardner's syndrome, celiac disease, and neurofibromatosis.[46]

Symptoms of cancer of the small intestine are vague and not localizing,[48] occurring late in the disease course. There is usually a delay of months before a diagnosis is made. Symptoms may include pain, symptoms of small bowel obstruction, bleeding, and weight loss. Because the signs and symptoms are not specific, diagnosis may not be confirmed until surgery is performed. Treatment depends on the histologic type of tumor, but surgery is indicated in all symptomatic tumors. Radiation therapy and chemotherapy have little impact on primary small intestinal cancer, although adjuvant therapy is currently being investigated. Nursing care guidelines follow the practices recommended for the patient's particular therapy (see boxes below and on p. 165).

GERIATRIC CONSIDERATIONS

Factors related to cancer prevention and early detection
  Encourage low fat high fiber diet within ethnic, social, and economic limitations
  Encourage smoking cessation and avoidance of exposure to other health hazards (e.g., sun, chemicals, petroleum products)
  Be suspicious of symptoms such as malaise, fatigue, anorexia, weight loss, and altered bowel habits as possible indicators of cancer and not automatically attributed to nonmalignant illnesses associated with aging
Factors related to modalities of therapy
  Alterations in hepatic and renal function may necessitate adjustment of dosage and schedule of chemotherapy protocols
  Decreased bone marrow cellularity may place the patient at risk for prolonged myelosuppression following chemotherapy with toxic effects on the bone marrow

Decreased nutritional intake may be exacerbated due to the nausea and taste changes associated with many of the chemotherapeutic agents commonly used for GI malignancies
Fatigue may be increasing problem following courses of therapy requiring additional assistance with ADLs
Co-morbid disease (e.g., obesity, poor nutritional status, lung and cardiovascular disease, altered immune function) places the older adult at greater risk regarding surgical morbidity and mortality
Teaching should be tailored to take into account the older adult's life experiences and cognitive and physical impairments (e.g., reading comprehension, decreased vision and hearing, altered tactile sense, misconceptions regarding cancer and cancer treatment, past experience with cancer and family members)

From Boyle DM and others: Oncology nursing society position paper on cancer and aging: the mandate for oncology nursing, Oncol Nurs Forum 19:913, 1992.

PATIENT TEACHING PRIORITIES

Prevention and early detection
  Risk factors
  Dietary habits
  Avoidance of cigarette smoking
  Moderate or no alcohol consumption
  Signs and symptoms to report to health care
    professional (e.g., dysphagia, odynophagia,
    chronic indigestion, jaundice, weight loss not as-
    sociated with dieting, and change in bowel hab-
    its)
  Annual physical examination, and cancer checkup
Diagnostic procedures
  Purpose of procedure
  Preparation needed by patient
  Procedure description
  Post procedure care by patient

Treatment modalities
  Surgery—preoperative instructions include opera-
    tive experience and immediate postoperative pe-
    riod; discharge instructions include self care
    needs and any further treatment plans
  Chemotherapy—name of agent, possible side ef-
    fects and measures to control, route of adminis-
    tration, dose, schedule, and any directions
    needed for self administration
  Radiation therapy—description of the procedure
    and schedule and duration of treatment, skin care
    measures, and management of any side effects
Supportive care
  Community resources (e.g., home health care
    agencies, inpatient and outpatient hospice care)
  Use of any medical equipment in the home
  Referrals necessary for psychosocial support for
    patient and caregiver
  Referrals for financial assistance if needed

CONCLUSION

Gastrointestinal cancers remain a nursing practice challenge. The overall prognosis ranges from 5% to 15%. Progress has been made in treatment modalities. However, prevention, early detection, and the seeking of health care early when initial symptoms occur can reduce the impact and prolong the survival of the disease.

BIBLIOGRAPHY

1. Abe M and others: Japan trials in intraoperative radiotherapy. Intl J Radiat Oncol Biol Phys 5:1431, 1979.
2. Ahlgren JD: Esophageal cancer: chemotherapy and combined modalities. In Ahlgren JD and McDonald JS, editors: Gastrointestinal oncology, Philadelphia, 1992, JB Lippincott Co.
3. Ahlgren JD, Hill MD, and Roberts IM: Pancreatic cancer: patterns, diagnosis and approaches to treatment. In Ahlgren JD and McDonald JS, editors: Gastrointestinal oncology, Philadelphia, 1992, JB Lippincott Co.
4. Ahlgren JD, Wanebo HF, and Hill MC: Hepatocellular carcinoma. In Ahlgren JD and McDonald JS, editors: Gastrointestinal oncology, Philadelphia, 1992, JB Lippincott Co.
5. Ahmed T and Friedland ML: Chemotherapy of primary and metastatic hepatic neoplasms. In Hodgson WJB, editor: Liver tumors: Multidisciplinary management, St. Louis, 1988, Warren H. Green, Inc.
6. American Cancer Society: Cancer facts and figures, Atlanta, 1993, The American Cancer Society.
7. Anderson BB and others: Primary tumors of the liver, J Natl Med Assoc 84:129, 1992.
8. Beahrs OH, Henson DE, Hutter RV, and Myers MH: Manual for staging of cancer, ed 4, Philadelphia, 1989, JB Lippincott Co.
9. Beazley RM and Cohn I Jr: Tumors of the liver. In Holleb AI, Fink DJ, and Murphy DP, editors: Textbook of clinical oncology, Atlanta, 1992, American Cancer Society, Inc.
10. Beazley RM and Cohn I Jr: Tumors of the pancreas, gallbladder, and extrahepatic ducts. In Holleb AI, Fink DJ, and Murphy DP, editors: Textbook of clinical oncology, Atlanta, 1991, American Cancer Society, Inc.
11. Boring CC, Squires TS, and Tong T: Cancer statistics, CA Cancer J Clin 42:19, 1992.
12. Boyce HW: Palliation of advanced esophageal cancer, Semin Oncol 11:186, 1984.
13. Brennan MF, Kinsella T, and Friedman M: Cancer of the pancreas. In DeVita VT Jr, Hellman S, and Rosenberg SA, editors: Cancer: Principles and practice of oncology, ed 3, Philadelphia, 1989, JB Lippincott Co.
14. Caudry M: Gastric cancer: radiotherapy and approaches to locally unresectable or recurrent disease. In Ahlgren JD and McDonald JS, editors: Gastrointestinal oncology, Philadelphia, 1992, JB Lippincott Co.
15. Cimprich B: Esophagogastrectomy. In Brown MH, Kiss ME, Outlaw EM, and Viamontes CM, editors: Standards of oncology nursing practice, New York, 1986, John Wiley & Sons, Inc.
16. Connolly MM and others: Survival in 1001 patients with carcinoma of the pancreas, Ann Surg 206:366, 1987.
17. Cozzi E, Hagle M, McGregor ML, and Wood-

house D: Nursing management of patients receiving hepatic artery chemotherapy through an implanted infusion pump, Cancer Nurs 7:229, 1984.

18. Cuschieri A: Tumors of the stomach. In Moossa AR, Schimpff SC, and Robson MC, editors: Comprehensive textbook of oncology, ed 2, Baltimore, 1991, Williams & Wilkins.

19. Douglas HO Jr: Overview of gastrointestinal cancer: two decades of progress. In Moossa AR, Schimpff SC, and Robson MC, editors: Comprehensive textbook of oncology, ed 2, Baltimore, 1991, Williams & Wilkins.

20. Edmondson HA and Craig JR: Neoplasms of the liver. In Schiff L and Schiff ER, editors: Diseases of the liver, ed 6, Philadelphia, 1987, JB Lippincott Co.

21. Ellis FH Jr: Esophagogastrectomy for carcinoma: technical considerations based upon anatomic location of lesion, Surg Clin North Am 60:265, 1980.

22. Ellis FH, Levitan N, and Lo TCM: Cancer of the esophagus. In Holleb AI, Fink DJ, and Murphy GP, editors: Textbook of clinical oncology, Atlanta, 1991, American Cancer Society, Inc.

23. Farley DR and Donohue JH: Early gastric cancer, Surg Clin North Am 72:401, 1992.

24. Foster JH Jr: Liver resection techniques, Surg Clin North Am 69:235, 1989.

25. Frank-Stromberg M: The epidemiology and primary prevention of gastric and esophageal cancer: a worldwide perspective, Cancer Nurs 12:53, 1989.

26. Grady R, Farnen J, and Ascheman P: Nutrition, alteration in: less than body requirements related to dysphagia. In McNally JC, Somerville ET, Miaskowski C, and Rostad M, editors: Guidelines for oncology nursing practice, ed 2, Philadelphia, 1991, WB Saunders Co.

27. Hancock SL and Glatstein E: Radiation therapy of esophageal cancer, Semin Oncol 11:144, 1984.

28. Havlin KA and McDonald JS: Gastric cancer: chemotherapy of advanced disease. In Ahlgren JD and McDonald JS, editors: Gastrointestinal oncology, Philadelphia, 1992, JB Lippincott Co.

29. Jackson JW: Operations for carcinomas of the thoracic and oesophagus and cardia. In Jackson JW and Cooper DKC, editors: Rob & Smith's operative surgery, thoracic surgery, ed 4, London, 1986, Butterworths.

30. Jordan GL Jr: Pancreatic resection for pancreatic cancer, Surg Clin North Am 69:569, 1989.

31. Kellum JM, Clark J, and Miller HH: Pancreaticoduodenectomy for resectable malignant periampullary tumors, Surg Gynecol Obstet 157:362, 1983.

32. Kelsen DP: Chemotherapy of esophageal cancer.

In Roth JA, Ruckdeschel JC, and Weisenburger TH, editors: Thoracic Surgery, Philadelphia, 1989, WB Saunders Co.

33. Lawrence W Jr: Gastric neoplasms. In Holleb AI, Fink DJ, and Murphy GP, editors: Textbook of clinical oncology, Atlanta, 1991, American Cancer Society, Inc.

34. Lightdale CJ and Daly J: Management of primary and metastatic cancer of the liver. In Schiff L and Schiff ER, editors: Diseases of the liver, ed 6, Philadelphia, 1987, JB Lippincott Co.

35. Little AG and McGregor BD: Tumors of the esophagus. In Moossa AR, Schimpff SC, and Robson MC, editors: Comprehensive Textbook of Oncology, ed 2, Baltimore, 1991, Williams & Wilkins.

36. McDonald JS, Hill MC, and Roberts JM: Gastric cancer: epidemiology, pathology, detection, and staging. In Ahlgren JD and McDonald JS, editors: Gastrointestinal oncology, Philadelphia, 1992, JB Lippincott Co.

37. McDonald JS, Steele G, and Gunderson LL: Cancer of the stomach. In DeVita VT Jr, Hellman S, and Rosenberg SA, editors: Cancer: Principles and practice of oncology, ed 3, Philadelphia, 1989, JB Lippincott Co.

38. Moertel CG and others: Combined 5-FU and radiation therapy as a surgical adjuvant for poor prognosis gastric carcinoma, J Clin Oncol 2:1249, 1984.

39. Moossa AR: Tumors of the pancreas. In Moossa AR, Schimpff SC, and Robson MC, editors: Comprehensive textbook of oncology, ed 2, Baltimore, 1991, Williams & Wilkins.

40. Naden G and Phillips TL: Radiation therapy for cancer of the esophagus. In Roth JA, Ruckdeschel JC, and Weisenburger TH, editors: Thoracic oncology, Philadelphia, 1989, WB Saunders Co.

41. Nerenstone SR, Friedman MA, and Ihde DC: Primary liver cancer. In Moossa AR, Schimpff SC, and Robson MC, editors: Comprehensive textbook of oncology, ed 2, Baltimore, 1991, Williams & Wilkins.

42. Niederhuber JE and Ensminger WD: Surgical considerations in the management of hepatic neoplasia, Semin Oncol 10:135, 1983.

43. Rosenberg JC, Lichter AS, and Leichman LP: Cancer of the esophagus. In DeVita VT Jr, Hellman S, and Rosenberg SA, editors: Cancer: Principles and practice of oncology, ed 3, Philadelphia, 1989, JB Lippincott Co.

44. Roth JA and Kelsen DP: Surgery and adjuvant chemotherapy for carcinoma of the esophagus. In Roth JA, Ruckdeschel JC, and Weisenburger TA, editors: Thoracic oncology, Philadelphia, 1989, WB Saunders Co.

45. Sandor C: Nutrition, alteration in: less than body

requirements related to disease process and treatment. In McNally JC, Somerville ET, Miaskowski C, and Rostad M, editors: Guidelines for oncology nursing practice, ed 2, Philadelphia, 1991, WB Saunders Co.

46. Sindelar WF: Cancer of the small intestines. In DeVita VT Jr, Hellman S, and Rosenberg SA, editors: Cancer: Principles and practice of oncology, ed 3, Philadelphia, 1989, JB Lippincott Co.

47. Smith JW and Brennan MF: Surgical treatment of gastric cancer, Surg Clin North Am 72:381, 1992.

48. Smith LE and Hill MC: Cancer and other tumors of the small bowel. In Ahlgren JD and McDonald JS, editors: Gastrointestinal oncology, Philadelphia, 1992, JB Lippincott Co.

49. Starzl TE, Bell RH, Beart RW, and Putnam CW: Hepatic trisegmentectomy and other liver resections, Surg Gynecol Obstet 141:429, 1975.

50. Stone MD and Benotti PN: Liver resection: pre-operative and postoperative care, Surg Clin North Am 69:383, 1989.

51. Trede M, Schwall G, and Saeger H: Survival after pancreatoduodenectomy, Ann Surg 211:447, 1990.

52. Vezeridis MP and Wanebo HJ: Gastric cancer: surgical approach. In Ahlgren JD and McDonald JS, editors: Gastrointestinal oncology, Philadelphia, 1992, JB Lippincott Co.

53. Wanebo HJ, Falkson G, and Order SE: Cancer of the hepatobiliary system. In DeVita VT Jr, Hellman S, and Rosenberg SA, editors: Cancer: Principles and practice of oncology, ed 3, Philadelphia, 1989, JB Lippincott Co.

54. Wooley PV and Treat J: Nonsurgical treatment of gastric cancer. In Moossa AR, Schimpff SC, and Robson MC, editors: Comprehensive textbook of oncology, ed 2, Baltimore, 1991, Williams & Wilkins.

CHAPTER 10

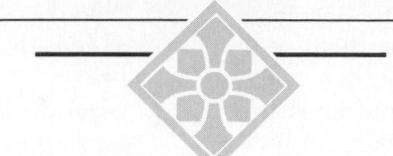

Genitourinary Cancers

Marilyn Davis

Genitourinary malignancies include cancer of the urinary and genital organs in males and urinary organs in females. As a group, genitourinary tumors in the United States represent 33% of all cancers in males and 17% of male deaths, 4% of cancers in females and 3% of cancer-related deaths in females.[5] Advancements in diagnosis include new applications of ultrasonography and magnetic resonance imaging (MRI), pathology refinements exemplified by whole mount techniques for prostate gland visualizations, and elucidation of a range of biologic markers including α-fetoprotein, human chorionic gonadotropin, and prostatic specific antigen. With refinements in the traditional therapeutic modalities, and sophistication in newer treatment maneuvers including laser therapy and biologic response modifiers, enormous progress has been achieved in the management of genitourinary tumors. This chapter reviews principles and practices in the diagnosis and management of genitourinary malignancies, including prostate, testis, bladder, and kidney cancer, with special emphasis on issues related to prevention, early detection, and continuing care.

PROSTATE CANCER

EPIDEMIOLOGY

Prostate cancer is the most common tumor in men in the United States. Approximately 165,000 new cases are diagnosed each year.[5] The third leading cause of cancer deaths in men, with an estimated annual mortality of 35,000, it has a devastatingly morbid as well as mortal impact on the aging American male population. The global distribution of prostate cancer reveals a predominance in the United States and northern European countries, most notably Sweden, followed by a moderate incidence in South America, southern Europe, and Israel, and a lower incidence

in eastern Europe and Asia.[6] However, Asians living in the United States are beginning to experience a rate of prostate cancer approaching that of U.S. white males. Of particular concern is the higher rate of prostate cancer in black males with a correspondingly higher mortality also documented.[32] It is projected that one in nine black North American males will develop prostate cancer, while one in 11 white North American males will develop the disease. North American males of Native American or Hispanic origin have lower rates of prostate cancer.

ETIOLOGY AND RISK FACTORS

The influence of endogenous hormones is the only clear factor implicated in the promotion and subsequent development of prostate cancer. Specifically, prostate cancer cells depend to some extent on dihydrotestosterone (DHT), the intracellularly active metabolite of testosterone. In 1922, Deaver observed that prepubertal removal of endogenous testosterone sources by bilateral orchiectomy eradicated the risk of prostate cancer.[11] The absence of prostate cancer in androgen deficient males as well as the induction of prostate cancer in experimental animals by prolonged administration of male sex hormones implicate the hormonal mileau.

Various promoting and initiating factors, including genetic influences, sexual history, exposure to viruses, pathogens, cadmium, industrial chemicals, and urbanization, have been postulated. Dietary habits, specifically the high-fat Western diet, which alters hormone metabolism, are suggested as associative factors. Documented familial patterns may reflect genetic or lifestyle influences.

Prostate cancer is associated with the aging process because fewer than 1% of cases occur under age 50. However, a man's risk of developing prostate cancer

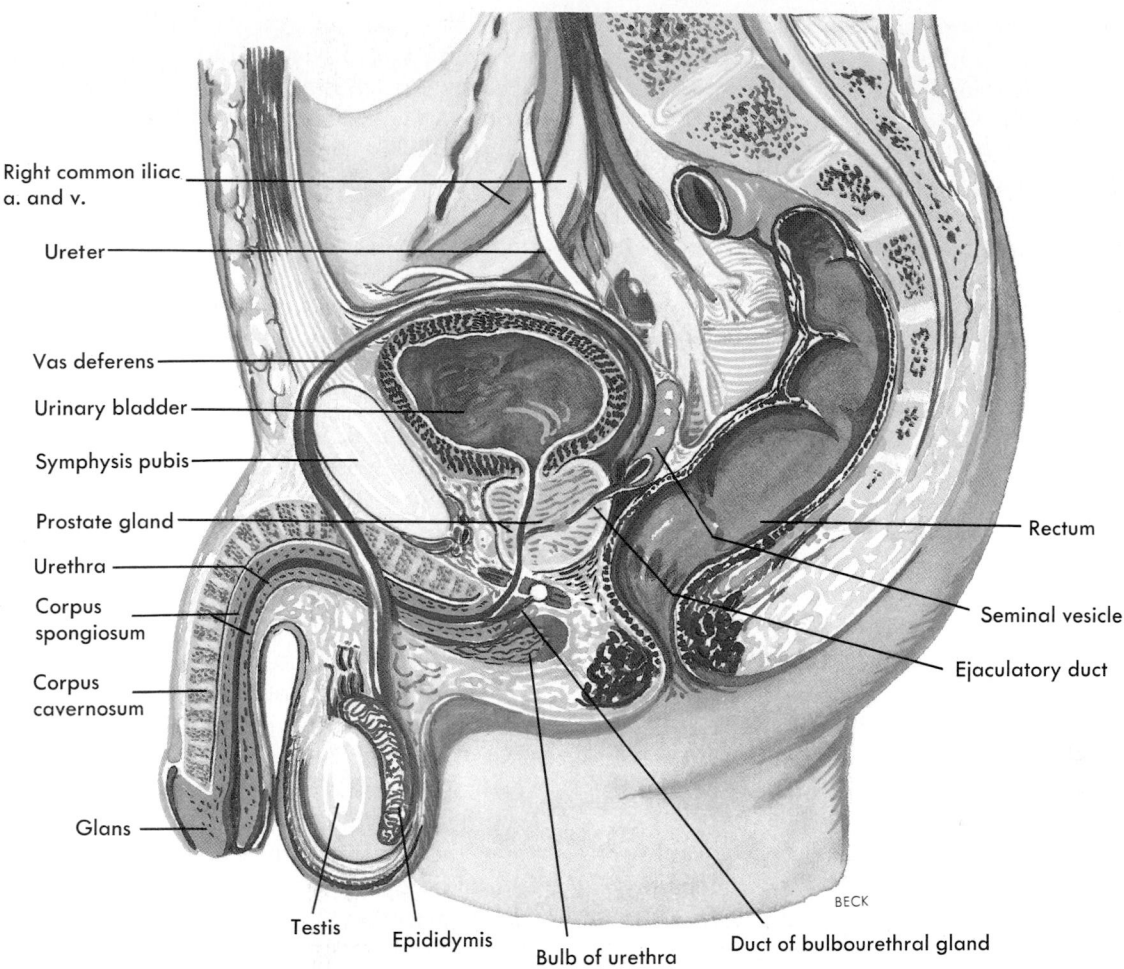

Right common iliac a. and v.

Ureter

Vas deferens

Urinary bladder

Symphysis pubis

Prostate gland

Urethra

Corpus spongiosum

Corpus cavernosum

Glans

Testis   Epididymis

Bulb of urethra

Duct of bulbourethral gland

Rectum

Seminal vesicle

Ejaculatory duct

BECK

Figure 10–1   Male pelvic organs. (From Anthony C and Thibodeau G: Textbook of anatomy and physiology, ed 12, 1987, St Louis, Mosby.)

increases exponentially after the age of 50 years. Autopsy series report that the true incidence of occult prostatic tumors microscopically identified may be as high as 30% in men over 50 years of age while approaching 80% in men over 80 years of age.[33]

ANATOMY

The prostate gland is a small, walnut-sized, firm organ weighing about 20 g and shaped like an inverted pyramid. The superior surface referred to as the base lies at the neck of the urinary bladder; the inferior apex rests on the urogenital diaphragm (Figure 10-1). The portion of the urethra passing centrally from the superior base to the inferior apex is referred to as the prostatic urethra. Dense, fibrous tissue surrounds the gland. The ejaculatory ducts penetrate the gland posteriorly and superiorly. There are no true lobar divisions in the prostate gland. Visualizing the prostate gland as having a central area or zone, a submucosal or transitional zone, and a horseshoe-shaped peripheral area may help with understanding disease distribution, and the area accessible to digital rectal ex-

amination (DRE).[10] Palpable areas include posterior or posterolateral region of the peripheral zone with a median furrow, which is felt as a shallow midline depression, and the two superiorly positioned seminal vesicles are identifiable landmarks on rectal palpation.[40] The prostate serves as a sex accessory gland with the seminal vesicles contributing viscous secretions to semen.

PREVENTION, SCREENING, AND DETECTION

Because there are no known etiologic factors, prevention is not a reasonable expectation. Therefore, the major challenge in prostate cancer is the promotion of early detection when the cancer is confined to the prostate gland and is curable. This can be accomplished most easily by a simple, cost-effective, and high-yield examination (DRE). The American Cancer Society (ACS) suggests annual DRE of the prostate gland for men beginning at age 40. Recent guidelines issued by ACS recommend prostate specific antigen (PSA) level quantification annually for men 50 years of age and older.

To perform a DRE, wearing a lubricated glove, the examiner inserts the index finger approximately 2 to 3 cm into the anal orifice and gently presses against the lower wall of the rectum systematically palpating the accessible surface of the prostate gland. This examination is facilitated when the subject is leaning forward with arms resting on the examination table, toes pointed inward, and knees slightly flexed.

Any change in size, consistency, or contour detected in the gland may represent an inflammatory process, infarction, or calculus, in addition to tumor. When a suspicious area is identified in the prostate, a biopsy is indicated. Prostatic needle biopsy for a core of tissue is accomplished easily with good yield and low morbidity by either the transperineal or transrectal approach. Fine needle aspiration of sheets of cells for cytologic review has been extensively used in European medical centers. Previous enthusiasm generated by this technique, however, has been tempered by the introduction of a spring-loaded bioptic device that permits relatively painless collection of multiple prostate tissue specimens while providing excellent material for pathology review and such ancillary studies as flow cytometry to assess DNA content and morphometry to assess nuclear configuration.

High-frequency transducers in transrectal ultrasonography have enabled the visualization of internal prostatic anatomy—an opportunity previously available only to pathologists studying radical prostatectomy or autopsy specimens. Transrectal ultrasonography shows most prostatic lesions, both malignant and benign, as hypoechoic. The role of transrectal ultrasonography in early detection of prostate cancer remains controversial because with no data clearly demonstrating its impact on prostate cancer mortality, it is used primarily in assessment of prostate diseases and guidance for biopsy of suspicious areas. Magnetic resonance imaging (MRI), with its ability to illustrate glandular subtleties and determine capsular penetration and seminal vesicle involvement, may be helpful in the staging of prostate cancer. Computed tomography (CT) continues to be the primary modality for evaluation of nodes, tissue, and organs; radionuclide scanning continues to be a primary modality for detecting or confirming metastatic bone involvement.

In response to recent developments in the diagnosis of prostate cancer as well as disease prevalence, the Southwest Oncology Group has initiated an intergroup prostate cancer prevention trial, anticipated to register over 12,000 men over a 2-year period. Eligible participants will include males 55 and older with normal prostates and PSA levels within normal range. At registration, participants will be randomized to receive finasteride (Proscar), a 5-alpha reductase inhibitor that prevents conversion of testosterone to DHT, or a placebo. Annual DRE and PSA level measurement will be done. Biopsy will be performed if PSA level reaches 4.0 ng/nl or greater in the placebo group; an equal percentage of men in the finasteride group will also be biopsied.

CLASSIFICATION

Ninety-five percent of prostate cancers are adenocarcinomas. Ductal carcinomas including transitional and squamous cell carcinomas, endometrioid carcinomas, and sarcomas account for the remainder. The classically employed Gleason system ascertains degree of glandular differentiation and tumor growth pattern in relation to prostate stroma. A score is assigned both to the predominant pattern of differentiation, ranging from well-formed to undifferentiated tumor, and to any secondary pattern of differentiation observed microscopically. The histologic grading systems assign grade based on the most undifferentiated portion or on the predominant pattern observed. The Gaeta grading system assigns numbers ranging from I to IV for both glandular structure (I representing normal and IV representing predominant or complete loss of organization) and nuclear configuration (I indistinguishable from normal nuclei and IV representing unusual, increased mitotic activity, or bizarre or giant nuclei). Recently, ductal-acinar dysplasia, identified by nuclear and cytoplasmic abnormalities, has been characterized as prostatic intraepithelial neoplasia (PIN). Early studies suggest that PIN meets the criteria for premalignant lesions, defined as those with the ability to progress to invasive cancer.[4]

DIAGNOSIS, STAGING, AND CLINICAL FEATURES

Clinically, prostate cancer is staged A through D by the Whitmore-Jewett System, first introduced by Whitmore in 1956 and modified by Jewett in 1975. The Tumor, Node, Metastasis (TNM) system was adopted by the American Joint Committee for Cancer Staging (AJCC) and End Results Reporting in 1975. Both systems are described in the box on p. 171.

Stage A, T1, disease is asymptomatic unsuspected at a digital rectal examination and found incidentally on pathologic examination of resected prostate tissue for management of prostatic hypertrophy. Stage A is further subdivided into A_1, T1a, which is pathologically graded well-differentiated tumor or tumor foci representing 5% or less of resected tissue; and A_2, T1b, which is moderately or poorly differentiated tumor involving greater than 5% of the resection. Stage B, T2, disease is palpable tumor confined to the prostate. B_1, T2a, disease is a focal lesion 1.5 cm less in diameter; B_2, T2b, is diffuse disease over 1.5 cm in diameter or 2 or more foci of tumor foci at a time. Stage B_1, T2, prostate cancer may also be asymptomatic. Clinically determined involvement of seminal

PROSTATE CANCER STAGING SYSTEMS

Whitmore-Jewett	Description	AJCC
A	*Incidental finding of carcinoma upon examination of prostate tissue after prostatectomy or transurethral resection*	T1
A_1	Histologically well- or moderately well-differentiated tumor or tumor consisting of <5% of resected specimen	T1a
A_2	Histologically poorly differentiated or anaplastic tumor or tumor consisting of >5% of resected specimen	T1b
B	*Clinically palpable tumor confined to prostate*	T2
B_1	Focal ≤1.5 cm	T2a
B_2	Diffuse >1.5 cm > 2 foci	T2b
C	*Extension beyond the prostate capsule to seminal vesicles or contiguous tissue*	T3
D	*Metastatic tumor*	N, M
D_1	Regional nodal involvement	M1-3
D_2	Metastasis to any of the following: Bone Lymph nodes above the aortic bifurcation Other organ(s)	M

vesicles or adjacent structures is staged as C, T3, disease. At this stage, local irritative symptoms including painful urination, frequency, and hematuria. Stage D, N,M, represents metastatic disease with D_1, N 1-3, limited to regional involvement and D_2, M, indicative of tumor metastatic to bone, other organs, or nodes above the aortic bifurcation.

Symptoms associated with advanced disease may include painful urination, frequency, hematuria, bone, back, or joint pain, weight loss, and fatigue. Prostate cancer spreads by direct extension to the seminal vesicles and contiguous structures, the bladder, membranous urethra, and pelvic sidewalls. The rectum is essentially spared because it is offered a degree of protection by Denonvilliers' fascia. Lymphatic spread to pelvic nodes or hematogenous deposition to bone is frequently encountered.

BIOLOGIC MARKERS

Laboratory quantification of acid phosphatase levels provides a marker for monitoring response to therapy. However, acid phosphatase is not specific to the prostate gland because, in addition to being produced by prostatic acinar cells, it is also present in liver, erythrocytes, and disintegrating platelets. This enzyme is rarely elevated in early disease and may also be within normal limits in up to 40% of patients with metastatic disease. Acid phosphatase values are subject to diurnal (daily, cyclic) variations and prostatic manipulations, and may be elevated in a wide variety of hematologic, bone, liver, kidney, and thromboembolic conditions. PSA, a glycoprotein produced by normal and neoplastic ductal epithelium, serves to lyse the seminal coagulum. First purified from normal prostate tissue in 1979, PSA has since been found in seminal fluids, in benign hypertrophied prostate tissue, and in cancerous tissue.[24] Monoclonal and polyclonal antibodies that react with PSA have been developed to provide laboratory determination of the level of PSA present.[1] The ability of PSA to predict localized disease reliably is being evaluated. Because PSA is specific for prostatic cellular activity, it offers the clinician an additional marker to assess the likelihood of disease recurrence after definitive therapy. For example, a rising PSA after radical prostatectomy suggests clinical recurrence. In men without prostatic disease, the normal range in the Tandem-R assay is 0 to 40 ng/ml.[4]

TREATMENT MODALITIES

Therapeutic maneuvers viewed with optimism in all stages of prostate cancer are also surrounded by controversy. In disease confined to the prostate gland, complete response to therapy and attainment of a normal life span are reasonable goals. More extensive disease involvement can be managed effectively with results varying from a complete response to partial remission. In contrast to many other tumors, the therapy of advanced disease can be accompanied by partial remission or stable disease for a gratifying period of time.

Surgery

Surgery has historically been the primary therapy for prostate cancer in the form of radical prostatectomy for localized cancer, transurethral resection for tumor causing bladder outlet obstruction, or bilateral orchiectomy for management of metastatic disease. Stage A, B_1, B_2, T1, and T2 lesions may be treated surgically by radical prostatectomy. The technique of radical prostatectomy by perineal approach, introduced in this country by Hugh Hampton Young in

---

PROSTATE CANCER DISEASE AND TREATMENT RELATED COMPLICATIONS

Disease related complications: Infection, painful urination, frequency, hematuria, impotence

Treatment modalities	*Treatment complications*
Surgery (Prostatectomy)	Impotence, difficulty with urination
Radiation	
External	Impotence, diarrhea, cramps, rectal irritation, difficulty with urination
Internal	Impotence, diarrhea, cramps, rectal irritation, difficulty with urination

---

1903, demonstrated the feasibility of removal of the prostate and seminal vesicles in the management of prostatic malignancy. This is still used, particularly in patients with early stage clinical disease. It offers advantageous exposure and a shorter operating time, a consideration in many elderly men.

The retropubic approach is employed most often because it provides access to regional lymph nodes in the pelvis. Regional node sampling permits assessment of presence or absence of tumor in adjacent nodes. If tumor is present in nodes, radical prostatectomy may be deferred. For patients with prostate cancer confined to the gland, radical prostatectomy is one of the most effective methods for definitively eradicating the tumor. Postoperative complications of incontinence and urethral stricture are seen in less than 5% of patients. Previously, impotence was a major complication of radical prostatectomy; postoperatively 85% to 90% of men were incapable of sustaining an erection adequate for vaginal penetration. However, new surgical techniques popularized by Walsh spare the cavernous nerves and retain the physiologic responses required to maintain potency.[40] Pharmacologic erection or surgical implantation of a penile prosthesis may manage disease- or treatment-related impotence. After radical prostatectomy, whole mount techniques add a new dimension to pathologic assessment of the prostate capsule and seminal vesicles because the pathologist can reconstruct the gland, allowing for accurate measurement of tumor volume, visualization of foci of tumor, and analysis of surgical margins. Potential disease and treatment related complications are summarized in the box above.

Radiation Therapy

For males who are not candidates for radical prostatectomy based on performance status, concomitant medical conditions, or preference, external beam radiotherapy with or without interstitial radiation implantation may result in long-term complete remissions with disease-free survival rates paralleling those achieved with radical prostatectomy for clinical stage A, B_1, B_2, T1, and T2 disease. Complications of curative radiotherapy include urethral stricture, incontinence, and proctitis. Degrees of erectile dysfunction after external beam radiotherapy ranging from 22% to 84% have been reported.[8,11] Many patients have experienced complete responses to external beam megavoltage radiotherapy or interstitial implants.

The treatment of stage C (T3, T4) prostate cancer presents a clinical dilemma. As a number of prostate cancers initially thought to be stage C are ultimately determined to be stage D_1, the curative potential of either surgery or radiotherapy decreases dramatically.

Hormonal Therapy

Even patients with metastatic disease appear to offer equivalent outcomes as measured by survival with potentially different outcomes as gauged by quality of life.

Established therapeutic interventions including orchiectomy and oral estrogens have effectively managed the disease process for long periods of time without compromising quality of life for the majority of patients. Because prostatic epithelial cells depend on dihydrotestosterone for growth and differentiation, an understanding of the hypothalamic-pituitary-gonadal axis that regulates the physiologic balance of circulating testosterone is essential (Figure 10-2). Removal of the testes as a source of 95% of the major circulating androgen, testosterone, through bilateral orchiectomy as introduced by Huggins and Hodges in 1941, is a cost-effective, well-tolerated intervention that interrupts the gonadal portion of the axis.[20]

In 1971, a decapeptide, luteinizing hormone-releasing hormone (LHRH) was described by Schally.[30] Luteinizing hormone, released from the anterior pituitary in response to pulsatile release of LHRH, which is synthesized in the supraoptic nucleus of the hypothalamus, results in the testicular secretion of a physiologic level of testosterone with corresponding spermatogenesis (production of spermatozoa). Administration of exogenous estrogens such as diethylstilbestrol (DES) profoundly inhibit pituitary LH secretion, thereby reducing circulating testosterone to castrate level while increasing sex steroid–binding globulin and promoting prolactin secretion. This mechanism led to widespread application of DES in varying daily doses in the treatment of metastatic prostate cancer.

Subsequently, a synthetic LHRH analogue was produced with a potency of up to 100 times that of naturally occurring LHRH. Initially, it was felt that the synthetic LHRH would stimulate pituitary release

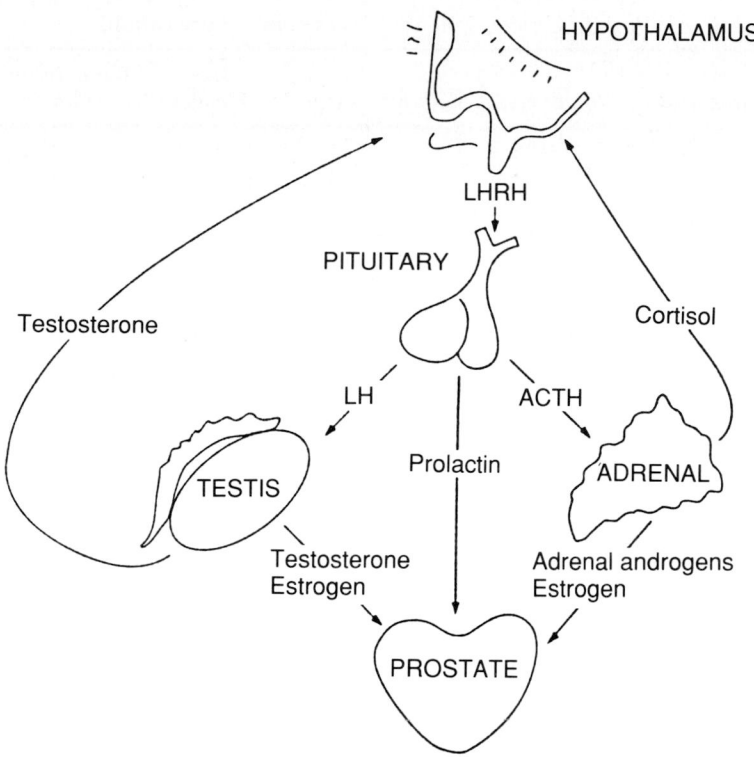

Figure 10–2 The hypothalamic-pituitary-testicular-adrenal axis. (Adapted from Crawford ED: Combined androgen blockade, Urology 34 [suppl]:24, 1989.)

of follicle-stimulating hormone and luteinizing hormone. However, it was discovered that in hypophysiologic concentration, the LHRH analogues actually demonstrated a paradoxic effect. After an initial stimulation of gonadotropin release, long-term administration of LHRH analogues results in an enduring inhibition with corresponding gonadal down-regulation, including inhibition of prostatic growth. This may be the result of pituitary desensitization to the overabundance of LHRH. After an initial rise, serum testosterone falls to castrate levels with chronic LHRH therapy. LHRH agonists (e.g., Leuprolide, Zoladex) have been established as effective options in the treatment of advanced prostate cancer.

Peripheral tissue sources and adrenal androgens account for the remaining 5% of circulating testosterone. Pharmacologic therapy directed at ablating the adrenals as a source of androgens results in a reversible medical adrenalectomy. High-dose ketoconazole (1200 mg daily), an antifungal agent, affects both gonadal and adrenal androgens, rapidly lowering unbound testosterone to castrate levels within 1 to 2 days. However, its cost as well as the gastrointestinal intolerance and potential for hepatotoxicity associated with it limits its clinical use. Aminoglutethimide effectively blocks adrenal steroidogenesis, synthesis of mineralocorticoids, glucocorticoids, and sex steroids, but must be coupled with hydrocortisone to circum-

vent moderate to fatal adrenal insufficiency. Surgical adrenalectomy and surgical hypophysectomy are not cost-effective or therapeutically advantageous options.

Antiandrogens, both steroidal and nonsteroidal agents, such as flutamide (Eulexin), compete with dihydrotestosterone for binding sites on prostatic cells. Through this action, antiandrogens do not alter the level of circulating male hormone but rather block the hormone from reaching the target tissue, the prostate gland. The antiandrogens do not interfere with sexual potency because they do not alter testosterone levels.

Chemotherapy

Chemotherapeutic agents and biologic response modifiers (BRM) have been extensively investigated in clinical trials either as single agents, in combination regimens, or in conjunction with hormonal agents. Single agents, including cyclophosphamide, 5-fluorouracil, doxorubicin, methotrexate, and cisplatin, have been associated with subjective responses and disease stabilization in 25% to 50% of patients.[38] Combination chemotherapy does not appear to offer any significant clinical advantages and is associated with significant morbidity. Potential treatment complications associated with hormonal therapy for prostate cancer are summarized in Table 10-1.

Table 10–1   Hormone Therapy for Prostate Cancer: Potential Treatment Complications

	Cardiovascular	Impotence	Gastrointestinal	Hot Flashes	Testosterone Flare	Permanent	Cost
Bilateral orchiectomy	—	↑↑↑	—	↑↑	—	↑↑↑	$
Estrogens	↑	↑↑↑	↑	↑	—	—	$ to $$$*
LHRH analogues	—	↑↑↑	—	↑↑	↑↑	—	$$$
Antiandrogens	—	↑	↑↑↑	↑	—	—	$$$
Progestational agents	—	↑↑↑	↑	↑	↑	—	$$
Ketoconazole	—	↑↑↑	↑↑↑	↑	—	—	$$$
Aminoglutethimide	—	↑↑↑	↑↑	—	—	—	$$

*Thromboembolic management.
From Davis MA, Crawford ED: Unpublished data. 1991.

PROGNOSIS

New imaging and diagnostic techniques, laboratory quantification of tumor markers, and pathology refinements have greatly advanced knowledge of prostate cancer and its biologic behavior. Refinements in surgical technique for complete tumor removal and advances in the delivery of radiation therapy for maximum tumorcidal activity have greatly decreased treatment-associated morbidity, thus offering the possibility of long-term remission with overall survival rates paralleling that of the general male population. The introduction of new hormonal agents and the continuing quest for effective chemotherapeutic and immunotherapeutic strategies offer considerable optimism in the management of advanced stage disease.

Nursing Management

Nurses and physicians must promote compliance with screening recommendations, especially in men with a family history of prostate cancer. Black men, in particular, need to be aware of their increased risk for disease and disease-associated mortality.

Because prostate cancer has become a major tumor afflicting the American male, a corresponding awareness of the disease and its potential for morbidity needs to be emphasized. Clinical support services of a multidisciplinary professional team with expertise in diagnosis and management of prostate cancer must address the issues of pain control, nutritional support, financial impact, sexuality, and emotional support. See boxes below and on p. 175 for geriatric considerations and clinical features.

GERIATRIC CONSIDERATIONS

As approximately 87% of prostate cancer patients are 65 years of age or older, awareness of the concerns of this population is appropriate. With the transition to older adulthood and accommodation to the gradual shift in family responsibilities, retirement, and declining economic opportunities as described by Havighurst, the aging adult is challenged to achieve ego integrity as defined by Erikson.[15,18] Along with the acceptance of age-related limitations, the senior adult is adjusting to physiologic aging, retirement, reduced income, deaths of relatives, friends and conceivably spouse, while maintaining a safe and solvent environment often in a relocation setting.[18] The older person is customarily concerned about finances, loss of independence, and placing a burden on family or society. Frequently the senior adult approaches the health care system and care providers from a docile perspective and may not aggressively pursue or report symptoms, thus resulting in delay of diagnosis or lack of symptom resolution. The older adult with Medicare has acute-care coverage but may not have comprehensive coverage for preventive or supportive care, including oral and subcutaneous medications. Intellectual function is usually maintained in older adulthood although short-term memory may gradually decline, underscoring the need for application of recall and repetitive techniques. Special attention to establishing a framework for open communication and identifying components of the individual's dilemma such as reimbursement are suggested for facilitating compliance and rehabilitation for the older adult.

TESTICULAR CANCER

EPIDEMIOLOGY

Although testicular tumors are rare, accounting for 1% of all cancer in U.S. males, they are the most common cancers in young men between the ages of 15 and 35.[5] Testis tumors occur more commonly in white males than black males in the United States. With the advent of biologic serum markers with the dual capacity of indicating presence of disease and response to therapy, as well as chemotherapeutic refinements, overall cure has exceeded a remarkable 90%.

ETIOLOGY AND RISK FACTORS

The etiology of testis cancer is unknown, but certain conditions are associated with an increased incidence of this malignancy. Specifically, testicular tumors are more likely to occur in an atrophic testis or a cryptorchid (undescended) testis. With 12% of all testis tumors originating in cryptorchid testis, the likelihood of subsequent development of a testis cancer in an undescended testis is 40 times greater than in a normal testis. Orchiopexy, surgical descent of the cryptorchid testis, before a boy is 2 years old may reduce the probability of subsequent development of testis tumor. Tesk's tumors occur more commonly in white males than black males in the United States.[16]

PREVENTION, SCREENING, AND DETECTION

Prevention of testicular cancer is not a reasonable expectation because etiologic factors are unknown. However, early detection is an achievable goal in testis tumors. As recommended by the ACS, young men from puberty through age 40 need to be taught and encouraged to perform monthly testicular self-examination (TSE; see Figure 10-3). The examination is facilitated by the heat of a warm bath or shower. Each testicle is examined with both hands. The index and middle fingers are placed on one side of the testicle; the thumbs are placed on the other side. A gentle rolling motion allows for complete palpation of each testicle. The epididymis, which collects and carries sperm, is felt as a cordlike structure at the back of each testicle. One testicle may be larger than the other. Any lump, new finding, or worrisome area needs to be reported.

The classic presentation of a testis tumor is a nontender, enlarged testis. However, a scrotal mass may represent a variety of conditions including varicocele, hydrocele, spermatocele, torsion, chronic or acute epididymitis or testicular trauma, and testicular malignancies. In many instances, there is a delay in diagnosis of a testis tumor either because of the man's reluctance to seek medical attention for a troublesome testis condition or the clinician's assumption that a scrotal mass represents an infectious or inflammatory process. A history of trauma, mumps orchitis, episodic testicular pain, low back, groin, or abdominal aching, or breast enlargement or tenderness is often reported. More than half of testicular tumors are initially considered to represent epididymitis. If symptoms persist after completion of antibiotic prescribed for suspected epididymitis, testicular cancer must be considered. Ultrasonic examination of both testes may confirm the clinical impression.

Proper examination of a scrotal mass, including digital separation of the anterior testis within the tunica albuginea from the posterior adnexal elements including the epididymis and the cord, must be performed so that the intrascrotal contents may be palpated (Figure 10-3). A hard mass deep within the testicular substance is highly suspicious for malignancy. Properly performed testicular ultrasonography may be diagnostic even for small intratesticular tumors. The pathologic confirmation of a testicular tumor is made after the involved testis is surgically removed. An inguinal incision rather than a transscrotal incision is made to approach the mass. Violation of the scrotal lymphatic vessels is to be avoided because testicular tumors metastasize primarily by the lymphatic route, with the exception of choriocarcinoma, which is disseminated venously and lymphatically. This exploratory process is based on the lymphatic drainage of the testis. Because the right testicular lymphatics drain along the right testicular vein into the vena cava, this will be the initial area of tumor involvement. The lymphatic drainage from the left testis follows the left spermatic vein into its drainage into the left renal vein, which will be the site of the first nodal involvement. Of note is the presentation of some testis tumors in extragonadal tissues, primarily the mediastinum. This process reflects the embryologic route of migration from the yolk sac endoderm at the primordial location of the kidneys along the urogenital ridge to the gonads. Careful monitoring of the testes is recommended in this type of patient because occult disease may be harbored.

CLASSIFICATION

Ninety-seven percent of all testicular tumors are germ cell tumors originating in the primordial germ cells essential for spermatogenesis. The remaining 3% are nongerminal in origin or metastatic foci of other tumors, primarily lymphomas and leukemias. Pure

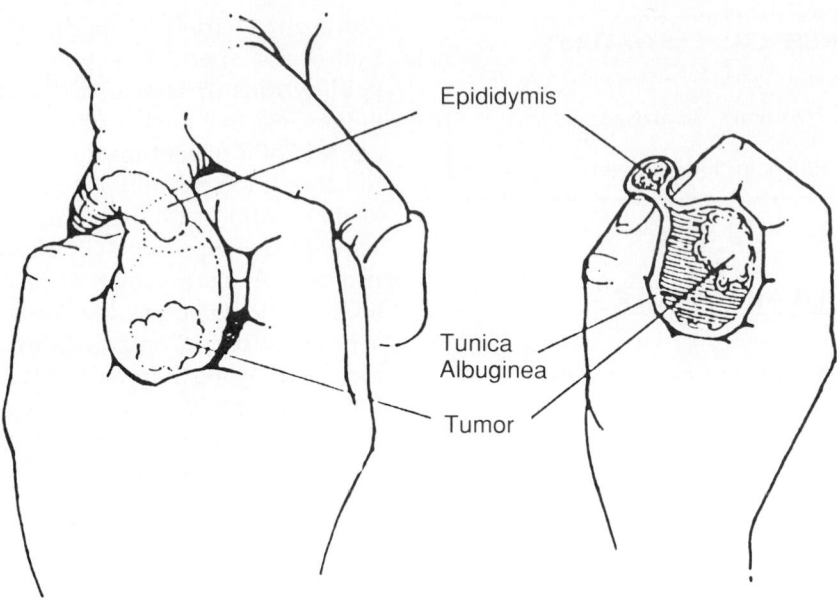

Figure 10–3 Male scrotal examination. Care is taken in the digital separation of the testis from posterior elements including the epididymis and cord for thorough palpation of intrascrotal contents. (Adapted from Donohue JP: The testis. In Paulson, editor: Genitourinary surgery, 1984, Churchill Livingstone, Inc.)

seminomas account for 40% of testis tumors; 15% to 20% are pure embryonal carcinoma. The rest of the tumors are usually mixed types. Pure choriocarcinoma is a rare finding. Most clinicians distinguish primarily between pure seminoma and nonseminoma. This distinction is critical because it influences treatment selection. Seminomas exhibit dramatic radiosensitivity. Approximately 70% of patients with seminoma have disease confined to the testis.[16]

DIAGNOSIS, STAGING, AND CLINICAL FEATURES

The evaluation of the metastatic disease status of the patient is a pivotal element in treatment planning. Approximately 60% of males have evidence of lymphatic or other sites of metastatic involvement at diagnosis. CT has largely replaced lymphangiography in many centers for assessment of nodal status and definition of areas of abnormality. Whole lung tomography and lung CT scans are sensitive diagnostic methods for evaluation of the lungs. A standard chest x-ray is also necessary. Intravenous pyelography (IVP) may be used to assess the kidneys, ureters, and bladder.

The staging system most commonly used in the United States for testicular cancer labels tumors confined to the testis as stage A. Stage B disease, metastases to the retroperitoneum, is further categorized as B_1, microscopic metastases to five or fewer lymph nodes; B_2, metastases to more than five lymph nodes, any node larger than 5 cm, or extracapsular spread; and B_3, bulky or palpable retroperitoneal disease. Stage C encompasses metastatic activity beyond the retroperitoneum.

TESTIS CANCER CLINICAL FEATURES

Classic presentation
　Non-tender, enlarged testis
History
　Trauma
　Mumps orchitis
　Episodic testicular pain or heaviness
Symptoms
　Abdominal aching
　Low back pain
　Gynecomastia
　Breast tenderness

Clinical features associated with testis cancer are in the box above.

BIOLOGIC MARKERS

Serum marker proteins for testicular tumors have added greatly to the clinical assessment of the patient's disease status. These can also be used to gauge the response to therapy. Both the α-fetoprotein (AFP) and the β subunit of human chorionic gonadotropin (HCG) as serum markers provide valuable information for the assessment of testicular malignancies. Any elevation in AFP or HCG in a patient with a testicular mass raises the clinical index of suspicion. Therefore, serum marker proteins need to be obtained before an orchiectomy so that the efficacy of the removal of the primary testicular malignancy may be assessed. The half-life of AFP is approximately 5 days; the half-life of HCG is approximately 16 hours. Elevation in serum marker proteins after appropriate attention is given to the half-life curve indicates the persistence of metastatic disease.

Not all patients will have elevated serum marker proteins. Therefore, these serum marker proteins are useful only when they are initially abnormal or when one or both illustrate a rising pattern after normalization, indicating disease recurrence. Elevated HCG is possible with pure seminoma. An elevated AFP is never observed in pure seminoma. If the AFP is elevated, the tumor is not pure seminoma but rather a mixed cell type. High levels of HCG are suspicious in the patient considered to have pure seminoma. The debate continues as to whether HCG levels of greater than 100 or 200 in a patient with seminoma indicate presence of nonseminomatous elements type.

TREATMENT MODALITIES
Seminoma Therapy

Seminomas exhibit dramatic radiosensitivity. Stage A seminoma confined to the testis is treated with regional radiation designed to eliminate micrometastatic tumor. After orchiectomy, radiotherapy is delivered to the periaortic area and the ipsilateral pelvic lymph nodes. An approximate dose of 165 cGy daily is given for a total dose of 2500 cGy over 3 weeks. The small percentage of patients relapsing after radiotherapy (3% to 5% in clinical stage A disease) may often be effectively "salvaged" with combination platinum-based chemotherapy. Approximately 5% of stage A seminomas will metachronously develop a contralateral testis tumor. Stage B seminoma, or evidence of regional nodal adenopathy, may be treated with radiotherapy to the infradiaphragmatic periaortic chain and the ipsilateral pelvic nodes. Generally, stage B seminoma is cured with radiotherapy. However, stage B_3 patients with a palpable tumor demonstrate a less successful response to radiotherapy. Chemotherapy is the treatment of choice for stage C disease, advanced supradiaphragmatic adenopathy or metastases to brain, bone, lung, or liver. Seminoma is sensitive to platinum-based chemotherapy regimens.[12]

Nonseminoma Therapy

Controversy regarding the initial management of stage A nonseminoma, confined to the testis, continues. In the United States, radical retroperitoneal lymph node dissection (RPLND) has been the classic therapy for pathologic staging of nonseminomatous disease and removal of all nodes involved in lymphatic drainage of the testis. However, with the dramatic results achieved with platinum-based chemotherapy, surveillance programs are commonly employed with initiation of salvage chemotherapy in event of recurrence. Surveillance programs consist of programmed follow-up usually monthly for 12 months including physical examination, tumor markers including AFP, HCG, and LDH, and chest x-ray.

If all parameters are negative after 12 months, follow-up is every 2 months for the second year, then every 6 months for life. Surveillance in stage A disease patients is predicated on the premise that unnecessary node dissections are avoided in the majority of patients who would be both clinically and pathologically negative. Also, for patients who have experienced a relapse, salvage combination chemotherapy can be successfully employed. Critical to surveillance programs is patient compliance. Surveillance outside of a protocol setting can be fraught with patients lost to follow-up. Proponents for RPLND feel that patients in need of chemotherapy will be identified, whereas potential loss of patients to follow-up on surveillance programs will be avoided. Those who argue against RPLND cite morbidity and unnecessary surgery.

The Indiana University approach in the management of clinical stage A tumor confined to testis and clinical stage B regional nodal involvement nonseminomas employs serum markers after orchiectomy, whole lung tomography with or without chest CT, and CT of the abdomen and pelvis.[12] If there is no evidence of disease, the patient is advised of his options, including surveillance or RPLND, and relative risks. If RPLND is selected, surgical planes and margins are determined based on the presentation of the primary tumor, right-sided versus left-sided. Subsequent management is based on nodal status. If no evidence of tumor is found in nodes (negative), the patient is followed with monthly chest x-rays and serum markers for 1 year postoperatively and once every 2 months in the second year postoperatively, then at 6-month intervals, similar to the surveillance pattern. If tumor is present (positive) but all tumor is felt to be eradicated, either postoperative surveillance or adjuvant chemotherapy is advocated. The cure rate in this group of patients has been truly impressive— it approaches 100%. Retroperitoneal lymph node dissection in patients (including those with Stage B_3 disease) results in complete removal of tumor from the retroperitoneum. Therefore, retroperitoneal relapses are not anticipated. Relapses generally occur in the chest. The cure rate with this group, defined as patients with minimal pulmonary disease, approaches 100% when chemotherapy is a part of the treatment regimen. In the Indiana series, excellent results have been achieved in terms of survival with either primary retroperitoneal lymph node surgery with or without adjuvant chemotherapy or primary chemotherapy with or without postchemotherapy surgery.[12] Questions of toxicity, morbidity, and clinician and patient acceptance are still being addressed. The efficacy of surgery, radiation therapy, and chemotherapy has been convincingly demonstrated.

A number of centers now employ preoperative aggressive chemotherapy in the management of stage C advanced unresectable, retroperitoneal disease. Although chemotherapy makes the subsequent dissection more difficult because of the fibrous reaction, it also frequently converts a nonresectable tumor into a tumor that can be resected safely. Therefore, preoperative chemotherapy may be advocated as the first line of treatment in this group of patients. The surgical management of bulky disease following chemotherapy depends on the clinical, radiologic, and serum marker protein testing status. If retroperitoneal disease or pulmonary masses persist after chemotherapy, RPLND is often performed to manage the disease surgically. If serum marker proteins were elevated preoperatively and remain elevated, the prognosis is unfavorable and salvage chemotherapy is initiated. In the patient who experiences a complete remission after chemotherapy, dissection of the retroperitoneum may not be necessary. Persistent elevation of serum marker proteins may indicate the need for chemotherapy. Rising serum marker proteins after chemotherapy indicate the need for salvage chemotherapy before any surgical intervention may be attempted.

Chemotherapy

Considerable excitement has been generated with the success of chemotherapy in testis tumors. Cisplatin was discovered to have a profound inhibitory effect on bacteria replication by Rosenberg in 1965.[28] Before that, a number of single agents had demonstrated activity in disseminated testicular cancer, most notably actinomycin D, methotrexate, chlorambucil, vinblastine, mithramycin, and bleomycin. However, enduring complete remissions were enjoyed by less than 20% of patients. With the introduction of cisplatin-based chemotherapy, this percentage dramatically increased to 80% to 90%. The coupling of cisplatin with vinblastine and bleomycin rendered a substantial number of patients disease free.[14] Etoposide and ifosfamide have demonstrated exciting activity in germ cell tumors. No other tumor type appears to have so many viable chemotherapeutic agents for induction and, if necessary, for salvage therapy. Meticulous attention needs to be paid to the selection of appropriate combinations of drugs with proven efficacy, employing dosages and schedules as determined in clinical trials. Patients need to comply with their therapeutic regimens, and clinicians need to encourage these patients in their compliance efforts.

The box at right summarizes testicular cancer treatment modalities and potential complications.

Fertility after Treatment

Many of the patients successfully treated for testis tumors are interested in parenthood, and the effects of therapy including surgery, radiation, and chemotherapy on fertility have been questioned. In one prospective study of 41 patients before therapy, 77% were oligospermatic (sperm deficient), 17% were azoosper-

---

TESTICULAR CANCER DISEASE AND TREATMENT RELATED COMPLICATIONS

Potential organ system, body image, and reproductive capacity complications associated with testis cancer and treatment are serious and significant. Compliance is paramount to achievement of optimal success in the management of testis tumors. With cure a likely expectation, the individual with a testis tumor, his support network, and his clinicians are encouraged to maintain an outcome-focused approach while mandating compliance with proven therapeutic regimens with their acceptable and generally reversible profile of complications. Key elements in potential complications are highlighted.

Treatment modality	*Treatment complications*
Orchiectomy	Body image concern
RPLND	Body image concern
	Spermatogenesis deficiency
Chemotherapy	Body image concern
	Bone marrow suppression
	Organ function impairment
	Renal
	Neurologic
	Otologic
	Pulmonary
	Alopecia
	Fatigue
	Spermatogenesis impairment
Radiation therapy	Body image concern
	Spermatogenesis impairment
	Skin integrity compromise

---

mic (completely lacked sperm), and only 6.6% could meet requirements for sperm banking.[13] In this same group of patients, 96% were azoospermic after 2 months of therapy. Retrospective review of a group of 28 patients indicated normal sperm counts in 46% of patients after chemotherapy.[23] Reviews also indicate that combination chemotherapy does affect spermatic function, rendering most patients azoospermic. However, a high degree of recovery of spermatogenesis is experienced 2 to 3 years after initiation of chemotherapy. Subsequent to successful pregnancies, no increased incidences of fetal abnormalities or tumors in offspring have been reported.

PROGNOSIS

With the cure rates seen in both seminomatous and nonseminomatous disease, testicular tumors are truly a model of success for combination agent chemotherapy and multimodality therapy. At this time, we have the luxury of striving for achieving a higher percentage of early stage diagnoses through promoting testicular self-exam and motivating males to seek clinical evaluation upon discovery of a mass in the scrotum. Proper management of the primary tumor, evaluation for metastatic disease status, and the proper coordination of the appropriate therapeutic interventions of surgery, chemotherapy, and radiotherapy will guarantee dramatic successes. With current economic constraints and quality of life issues, persons with cancer are being treated in their local communities outside of the referral and university-based centers. We are starting to see a slight, but troubling decline in the percentage of complete and enduring cures for testis tumors. The tendency to consider a milder dose of chemotherapy adhering to the patient's work and social schedules needs to be tempered with the realization that any reduction in dosages or disruption in timing may compromise the patient's chance for a complete remission and a cure.

Nursing Management

There is no doubt that diagnostic and therapeutic maneuvers for the management of testicular tumors are indeed harrowing. However, the results are so dramatic and exciting that encouraging persons to comply is not just suggested but rather mandated. Compliance with treatment regimens of appropriate drugs, dosages, and sequencing of timing will result in enduring disease-free remissions in an extraordinarily high percentage of patients. Although the group at risk for developing testis tumors is at an age when body image concerns are paramount, temporary body image distortions, although deeply troubling, are a small price to pay for what appears to be the promise of a normal life span once appropriate therapy, with subsequent resolution of tumor, has been completed. See pp. 186-188 for detailed nursing interventions.

RENAL CELL CANCER

EPIDEMIOLOGY

Approximately 18,000 tumors of the kidney are diagnosed in the United States each year, representing 2% of all malignancy in adults[5] and 20% of childhood malignancy. Wilms' tumors, usually diagnosed in children under age 5, account for approximately 4% of all kidney cancers. In adults, kidney cancer occurs more commonly in men than women (2:1 radio). Cancer of the kidney is most commonly encountered in adults over age 40, with a median age at diagnosis of 64.3 years for whites and 58.2 years for blacks.[10]

ETIOLOGY AND RISK FACTORS

Etiologic factors include cigarette, cigar, or pipe smoking; chewing tobacco; urbanization; obesity; and exposure to petrochemical products. Studies report an increased risk of 1.5 to 2.2 for tobacco users. A high-fat diet may be responsible for the obesity and renal cell cancer relationship.

CLASSIFICATION

Renal cell or clear cell adenocarcinoma (hypernephroma) is the most common kidney cancer. Transitional cell cancers, the most commonly occurring cancer of the renal pelvis, also occur in the kidney. Squamous cell carcinoma and nephroblastoma are also identified. The growth of the kidney carcinoma may be well defined, surrounded by perinephric fat rather than infiltrating. Very often the renal vein is invaded, which may extend into the main renal vein and the inferior vena cava in the form of tumor thrombus. Although contiguous organs may be displaced, invasion and obstruction of surrounding organs are very unusual. Occasionally, the primary lesion may reach an enormous size in the absence of dissemination. Predicting the pattern of dissemination is difficult because it may spread by the lymphatics or by the venous route. The most common sites of a nonlymphatic metastases are lung, bone, liver, and brain.

CLINICAL FEATURES

Approximately 40% of all people with advanced renal cell carcinoma will experience pain directly related to their primary tumor. Analgesics generally will relieve the pain. Pain unresponsive to traditional maneuvers may indicate invasion of adjacent muscle and nerve routes. Hematuria is experienced by most patients during their disease process. Anemia is frequently encountered and is probably an anemia of chronic disease rather than persistent hematuria. Uncontrollable hematuria may be an indication for infarction with or without nephrectomy. Nonspecific disorders including fever and fatigue occur in a large percentage of patients. A box on p. 180 lists the clinical features of renal cell carcinoma.

Paraneoplastic processes associated with renal malignancies are listed in a box on p. 180. Erythrocytosis not associated with a leukocytosis or thrombocytosis may result from the secretion of erythropoietic stim-

---

**RENAL CELL CARCINOMA
CLINICAL FEATURES**

Pain
Hematuria
  intermittent
  uncontrolled
Anemia
Fever
Fatigue

**SYNDROMES ASSOCIATED WITH
RENAL CARCINOMAS**

Syndromes
Hypercalcemia
Nonmetastatic hepatopathy
Hypertension
Erythrocytosis
Pyrexia
Galactorrhea
Cushing's syndrome
Gynecomastia
Serum glucose abnormalities

Serologic factors and other syndromes
Prostaglandins
Alkaline phosphatase
Neuromyopathy
Amyloidosis
Coagulation factors
Iron metabolism
Gamma enolase
AFP
Vasculitis
Fibroblast growth factor

From Sufrin G and others: Paraneoplastic and serologic syndromes of renal adenocarcinoma, Semin Urol 7(3):159, 1989.

ulating substance in approximately 3% of the patients.[34] Approximately 5% of the patients may have hypercalcemia without osseous metastasis resulting from the secretion of a variety of hormonal agents.[25] Hypertension is commonly encountered and may be mediated by tumor secretion of renin.[19] Hepatic dysfunction is also encountered. Abnormal liver functions are frequently seen. An elevated alkaline phosphatase level is commonly observed and may be accompanied by symptoms.

DIAGNOSIS

Initially, a renal mass may be detected on IVP, although many tumors are now coincidentally detected by CT, cardiac angiography, or gallbladder ultrasonography being done for other purposes. When a renal mass has been demonstrated, its nature can be determined by ultrasonography as cystic or solid. If it is solid, further diagnostic tests are warranted. If the results of the standard diagnostic tests are equivocal, the effort to determine the diagnosis preoperatively is continued. However, surgical exploration of a questionable mass may be considered appropriate.

TREATMENT MODALITIES

Although in the majority of patients with metastatic involvement tumors experience rapid progression, some patients do survive for long periods of time. The often poor prognosis for a patient with metastatic renal cell carcinoma is a result of the tumor's lack of sensitivity to existing chemotherapy and radiation therapy. This is demonstrated by a short survival if the tumor is not completely eradicated surgically.

Surgery

In the 19th century and the early part of the 20th century, simple nephrectomy, the removal of the kidney leaving perirenal fat, adrenal gland, and regional lymph nodes, was the standard operation for renal cell carcinoma. For tumors suspected to be confined to the kidney, nephrectomy is the therapy of choice. Radical nephrectomy with ligation of the renal vessels before kidney manipulation, removal of Gerota's fascia and its contents, including the kidney, adrenal gland and perinephric fat, is the universal standard for achievement of the widest surgical margin. Renal tissue sparing may be considered when there are bilateral synchronous presentations or a small, incidentally discovered tumor. Simple nephrectomy removes the kidney while sparing the perineal fat, adrenal gland, and regional lymph nodes. The operative mortality associated with partial nephrectomy, simple nephrectomy, or radical nephrectomy is small, ranging from 0 to 6%, and the incidence of morbidity is approximately 10%. Nephrectomy in patients with disseminated renal cell carcinoma is rarely employed in consideration of prolonging survival or improving the quality of survival. Preoperative, percutaneous angioinfarction of the kidney may be done particularly in event of large, vascular tumors. Steel coils, absorbable gelatin sponges, or a 95% solution of ethanol may be introduced into the renal artery with subsequent tissue necrosis. A clinical picture of fever, pain, and, in some cases, leukocytosis predictably follows within several days, with resolution 3 to 7 days after infarction. The potential benefits derived from preoperative infarction include decreased blood loss allowing for an easier and shorter technical procedure. However, the value of infarction has not been clearly established.

The potential for surgical cure depends on a number of factors including stage, size, grade, and histologic type of the tumor, and the procedure performed. Involvement of regional lymph nodes portends a significantly decreased survival rate. In the absence of postoperative adjuvant therapeutic options, a radical nephrectomy is generally carried out even in the presence of enlarged lymph nodes. In selected patients with a solitary metastatic site or several metastatic depositions confined to one organ system, radical nephrectomy with surgical resection of metastatic foci may result in an enduring disease-free survival. Palliative nephrectomy may offer symptom alleviation for select patients. Kidney infarction alone may offer equivalent palliative results while avoiding surgical morbidity.

Systemic Therapy

A number of chemotherapeutic agents have been employed in the management of metastatic renal cell carcinoma. However, vinblastine continues to be the most active single agent with objective responses, defined as shrinkage of measurable tumor dimensions by at least 50%, observed in about 15% of patients.[10] The expectation of a complete response, which is total eradication of tumor, is unrealistic in the setting of metastatic disease. Prolongation of survival with chemotherapy has not been clearly demonstrated. Combinations of chemotherapeutic agents do not appear to offer any advantage.

In clinical trials, biologic response modifiers (BRM), including the interferons, interleukins, and the lymphokine activated killer (LAK) cells, have been aggressively evaluated.

To date, objective response rates to BRM therapy greater than 20% have not been achieved. Interleukin-2, a glycoprotein primarily produced by activated T-helper cells, has recently been approved for the treatment of metastatic renal cell cancer. The durability of responses to IL-2, most notable in the complete responders, has led to continuing research investigation with this cytokine alone or in combination with autologous tumor vaccine or alpha interferon.[29] Activated, cytotoxic, tumor-infiltrating T-lymphocytes (TILS), demonstrated to be more active than LAK cells in inducing tumor regression in animal models, are being studied.[2] The rationale for continuing investigations in the BRM field is that the individual's immune system may regulate the growth and dissemination of renal cell carcinoma.

PROGNOSIS

Renal cell cancer limited to the kidney and completely surgically resected offers a hopeful prognosis of long-term remission or cure. In the event of documented metastasis, the likelihood of dramatic improvement following nephrectomy is small. Quality of life issues are of major concern in patients with metastatic renal cancer. Pain and symptom control may enhance the person's emotional well-being. Because most patients are aware of the gradual nature of their declining process, unrealistic hope for a long-term survival is not commonly encountered. However, the rapid advancements in the field of biologic response modifiers is creating optimism for the therapy of selected tumors including renal cell carcinoma. Unique features of renal cell cancer including its suggestion of host-immune factors, responsiveness to BRM, and divergence of local, regional, and metastatic behaviors along with its resistance to chemotherapy and radiotherapy have made this tumor the model for systemic investigation of new therapies. Therefore, hope may be comfortably and honestly encouraged in all persons faced with the challenge of living with metastatic renal cell carcinoma.

Nursing Management

With the identification of certain etiologic factors, lifestyle or environmental modification to decrease the risk of kidney cancer development is a reasonable goal. Specifically, encouraging cessation or moderation of tobacco use, promoting avoidance of the development of a tobacco habit in youth, along with dietary modification to decrease or limit high fat content are positive steps in decreasing cancer risk. Minimizing occupation or lifestyle exposure to petrochemicals is also suggested. See pp. 186-188 for detailed nursing interventions.

BLADDER CANCER

EPIDEMIOLOGY

With approximately 51,600 new cases anticipated each year, primary bladder cancer is responsible for approximately 4% of cancer deaths reported in the United States annually.[5] Of historic interest, there has been a 50% increase in bladder cancer in the past 4 decades. Previously bladder cancer was predominantly a disease of aging men; it is now being seen increasingly in women and in younger patients, both males and females.

ETIOLOGY AND RISK FACTORS

Tobacco habits are clearly implicated in the initiation and promotion of 30% to 40% of bladder cancers.[7] As many as one third of all bladder cancers are felt to be related to industrial chemical exposure. Benzidine, B-naphtylamine, 4-aminobiphenol, and 4-nitrobiphenyl are implicated. These carcinogens may be present in chemical and dye manufacturing, petrochemical plants, and rubber, cable, printing, and paint occupations. Genetic factors may be involved. Detoxification of aromatic amines in cigarette smoke may be mediated by the hepatic enzyme M-acetyltransferase. Individuals found to be "slow-acetylators," roughly half the population, may be at increased risk for development of bladder cancer as they are unable to rapidly excrete toxic by-products.

CLASSIFICATION

In the United States, 90% of all cancers of the bladder are transitional cell carcinomas. The remainder of the cancers are squamous cell. In Egypt, there is a much higher incidence of squamous cell carcinomas of the bladder secondary to bladder irritants such as schistosomiasis, a parasitic infection.

CLINICAL FEATURES

Hematuria is usually the presenting sign. Approximately 75% of patients will report one or more episodes of hematuria experienced over 6 months to a year before seeking medical attention. The intermittency of the hematuria does not seem to have any relationship to the extent of the carcinoma of the bladder. Because urinary tract infection is often seen, many patients with cancer of the bladder have a history of being treated with antibiotics, with episodes of hematuria being considered hemorrhagic cystitis. This is particularly common in females. Another large group of patients will describe vesical irritability including frequency, spasms, and pain. The box below lists the clinical features of bladder cancer.

BLADDER CANCER CLINICAL FEATURES

Classic presentation
  Hematuria
    solitary
    recurrent
  Infection
    absent
    present
History
  Exogenous exposure
    present
    absent
  Tobacco habit(s)
    present
    absent
Symptoms
  Vesical irritability possible
    frequency
    spasms
    pain

DIAGNOSIS AND STAGING

Superficial papillary tumors account for approximately 70% of all primary tumors of the bladder with carcinoma in situ (CIS) accounting for 5% to 10%. CIS is felt to represent the reaction of the uroepithelium to a diffuse neoplastic stimulus. Its ability to persist, recur, or progress into invasive disease is well recognized.

These superficial tumors confined to the bladder mucosa may recur in up to 75% of patients, with progression in stage being more likely in CIS presentations. The primary goals in the management of superficial papillary tumors are to prevent tumor invasion into the bladder wall muscle and to reduce or prevent recurrences. Because there are very few blood lymphatic vessels in the more superficial layers of the bladder wall, tumors pathologically determined to be confined to the mucosal and lamina propria rarely have associated metastatic disease foci. In a patient with unexplained hematuria or suspected tumor of the bladder, IVP is performed. This is done before cystoscopy so that the upper urinary tracts, the kidneys and the ureters, can be visualized. IVP can indicate a persistent bladder filling defect or the presence of abnormality of the upper urinary tract. CT is reserved as an additional staging examination in patients with invasive tumors. Cystoscopy remains the main diagnostic method in patients suspected of having a bladder tumor. All areas of the bladder may be visualized during cystoscopy, with biopsies taken of suspicious areas. This can be performed readily under local anesthesia, usually an intraurethral topical anesthetic, with or without intravenous sedation. Facilitation of associated procedures such as transurethral resection, bimanual examination, or retrograde studies of the upper urinary tract are more readily accomplished in the sedated patient.

In addition, random bladder biopsies are routinely performed. The term, selected bladder biopsies, more accurately reflects the process of taking biopsies from predetermined areas of the bladder where tumors are most likely to occur. In addition to tissue biopsies, cells may be captured from bladder mucosa by bladder wash or voided urine for cytologic evaluation. Urinary cytology, a diagnostic technique similar to Pap smear for cervical tissue evaluation, was introduced in 1864 when unstained tumor cells were recognized in voided urine. Because malignant cells from the urinary epithelial surface will exhibit characteristic morphologic changes, urinary cytology is relatively reliable, inexpensive, safe, and adds to the management of tumors of the bladder. It complements but does not replace endoscopic and radiographic studies.

Paramount to treatment planning is the degree to which bladder carcinoma has penetrated. Tumor limited to the mucosa is designated as stage O by the

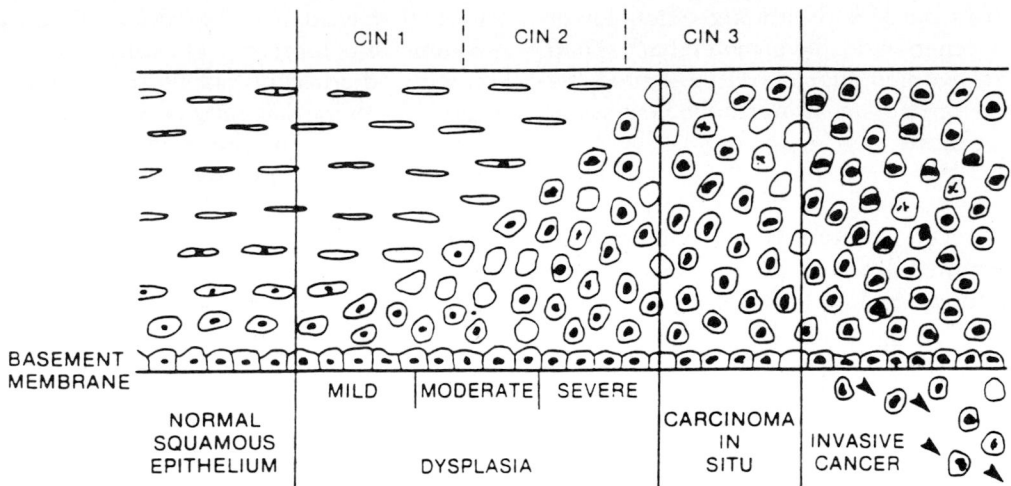

Figure 11—1 Progression of cervical intraepithelial neoplasia. (From Jones HW, Wentz AC, and Burnett LS: Novak's textbook of gynecology, ed 11, Baltimore, 1988, Williams & Wilkins Co.)

in the diet, tobacco use, and alcohol abuse. The role of genital hygiene also is being explored as a possible cofactor in the development of cervical cancer.[13]

In the late 1960s, an increase in the incidence of clear cell adenocarcinoma of the cervix was noted in women under 30 years of age. On review of medical histories for these women, a commonality was noted. Most of the women had been exposed in utero to diethylstilbestrol (DES), a synthetic estrogen given to women with high-risk pregnancies. Although the use of DES during pregnancy was discontinued in the early 1960s, a study of the incidence of cervical and vaginal carcinomas among DES-exposed women continues.[8]

PREVENTION, SCREENING, AND DETECTION
Prevention
Prevention is the key strategy for eradication of cervical cancer. Based on available knowledge about factors that place women at high risk for cervical cancer, the nurse can develop cervical cancer prevention programs for the public. Programs for teenagers may include strategies such as avoidance of penile-vaginal intercourse and use of contraceptives to prevent pregnancy and sexually-transmitted diseases. For women of all ages, the limitation of the number of sexual partners, and the use of barrier-type contraceptives, such as condoms and diaphragms, are recommended to reduce the risk of cervical cancer. Dietary modifications that may reduce the risk of cervical cancer include increased ingestion of foods high in vitamins A and C and folic acid. In addition, strategies to prevent initiation or to encourage discontinuation of tobacco and/or alcohol use could be included.[4,7,10] Since invasive cervical cancer is preceded by a preinvasive stage in most cases, the ACS guidelines for screening

should be taught as a cancer prevention strategy.

The target population for teaching prevention of cervical cancer is teenagers. Points to be stressed include an overview of normal physiologic changes that occur on the cervix during puberty and adolescence, the importance of using barrier contraception, and initiation of routine Pap smears and pelvic examinations whenever the teenager becomes sexually active. Emphasis on the ability to diagnose preinvasive lesions of the cervix and on the effectiveness of conservative treatment in eradicating preinvasive disease may lessen the fear of cancer and enhance compliance.

Screening
The primary screening test for cervical cancer is the Papanicolaou smear. The specimen is obtained by collecting a sample of cells from the squamocolumnar junction with a cotton swab, wooden spatula, or a cytobrush. The lowest false-negative rate and the highest predictability are achieved by sampling cells from the exocervix and the endocervical canal.[13] A pelvic examination is also recommended to evaluate the shape and consistency of the cervix and adjacent tissues.

The ACS recommendations for screening of asymptomatic women for cervical cancer include an annual Pap smear and pelvic examination for all women who are or have been sexually active or who are 18 years of age. After three or more normal, consecutive, annual Pap smears, the Pap smear and pelvic examination can be performed less frequently at the discretion of the physician.[1] Although debate continues about the cost-effectiveness of the Pap smear for women over 65 years of age, data indicate that the incidence of invasive cervical cancer increases with age in general and particularly among older, lower socioeconomic women who have never had a Pap smear. Therefore, women should not be denied the opportunity to get a Pap smear and pelvic examination based on age alone.

Detection

The detection of cervical cancer in symptomatic women is determined by a thorough history and physical examination. A clinical examination is per-formed to visualize the cervix, obtain a Pap smear, conduct a colposcopic examination, and palpate the cervix and adjacent tissues. The majority of invasive cervical carcinomas may be visualized on inspection. Cervical carcinoma presents in two primary patterns. The most common presentation is an exophytic lesion. These lesions occur primarily on the portio of the cervix, are polyp-like, spread superficially across the cervix, and bleed easily. Endophytic lesions invade toward the endocervical canal. These tumors

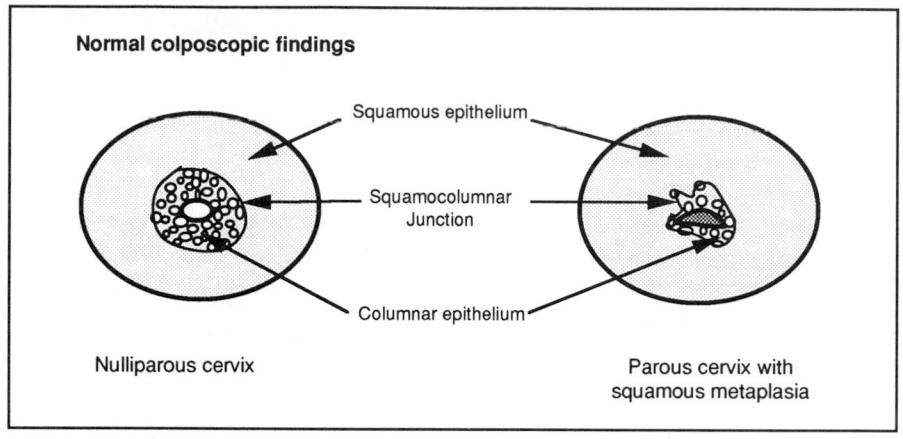

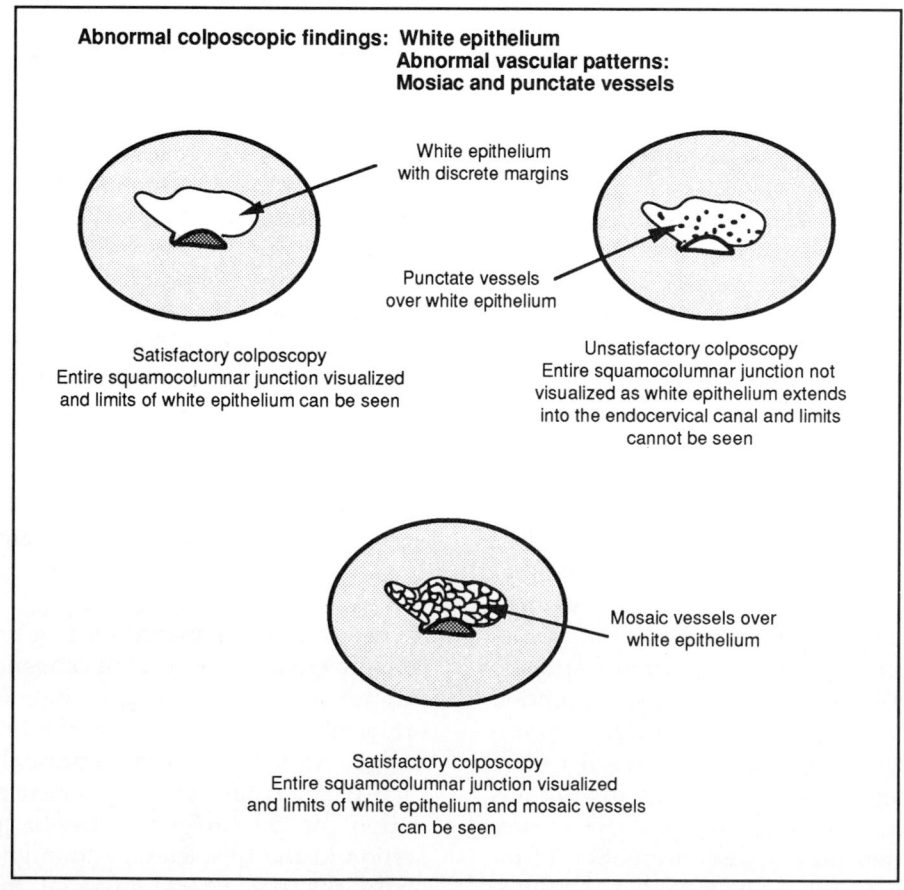

Figure 11–2 Graphic representation of cervical findings using the colposcope.

often go undetected as they expand within the endocervical canal and form a barrel-shaped lesion.[3,8,13]

A colposcopic examination may be performed in women with significant symptoms or grossly suspicious lesions on the cervix. The colposcope is a binocular optical device used to magnify and illuminate the cervical tissues. After application of a 3% to 5% acetic acid solution, the clinician evaluates the transformation zone and the squamocolumnar junction, if visible, for abnormalities in color and contour of tissues and vascular patterns (Figure 11-2). The clinician obtains a colposcopically-directed biopsy from the most abnormal areas for evaluation.

The rectovaginal, bimanual examination allows the clinician to evaluate the size, contour, and consistency of the cervix, corpus, ovaries, and vaginal and rectal tissues. Gross extension of the tumor to adjacent structures such as the rectum, vagina, and paracervical tissues also can be evaluated.

CLASSIFICATION

Cervical carcinomas are classified histologically by the tissue of origin. Historically, more than 90% of cervical carcinomas are squamous cell type. Squamous cell carcinomas have been divided further into keratinizing, nonkeratinizing, and small cell types based on histological descriptors. Adenocarcinomas and adenosquamous carcinomas account for an increasingly greater proportion of cervical cancers (11% to 16%), particularly in women under 35 years of age. The increase in cervical cancers with adenomatous features is important because of the poorer prognosis associated with the disease.[4,8,13]

CLINICAL FEATURES

The most common presenting symptom of women with cervical cancer is abnormal vaginal bleeding that may present as a decrease in the interval between the menstrual periods, an increase in the length or amount of menstrual flow, or intermenstrual bleeding. The woman also may describe episodes of "contact" bleeding after intercourse or douching. Less commonly, the woman may complain of a persistent, thin, watery, blood-tinged, odoriferous vaginal discharge.*

Symptoms of more advanced disease include urinary complaints such as difficulty starting the stream of urine, urinary urgency, hematuria, or pain with urination. Advanced disease resulting in pressure or invasion of the rectum may result in constipation, rectal tenesmus, or rectal bleeding. Involvement of regional lymph nodes may result in edema of the lower extremities. Pain of the lower back, groins, and

lower extremities also may be present with advanced disease.* See box below.

DIAGNOSIS AND STAGING

Diagnosis and staging form the basis of treament for cervical carcinomas. A tissue biopsy is required for the diagnosis of cervical cancer. The exocervix and the endocervical canal are easily accessible to punch biopsy and curettage, respectively. As the treatment of preinvasive cervical disease is more conservative, the tissue biopsy is needed to rule out or confirm the presence of invasive cancer. If an adequate tissue sampling for making the determination is not obtained, a more extensive tissue sampling with conization of the cervix is required (Figure 11-3). Pathologic confirmation of preinvasive or invasive disease is mandatory prior to the initiation of treatment.[8,13]

Staging for cervical cancer is done clinically. Data obtained from the clinical examination (inspection,

---

**GYNECOLOGIC CANCERS
CLINICAL FEATURES**

Cervical: Abnormal vaginal bleeding—increase in the amount, frequency, and/or length; contact bleeding related to intercourse; urinary urgency, dysuria, and hematuria
Endometrial: Bleeding—may be prolonged, irregular, and/or excessive; pain in the hypogastric, pelvis, and/or lumbosacral area
Ovarian: Dyspepsia, indigestion, anorexia, and/or early satiety; urinary frequency, constipation, pelvic pressure, and pain
Vulvar: Pain, pruritis, bleeding, discharge, dysuria, presence of lump or mass in vulvar area
Vaginal: Vaginal bleeding—perimenopausal and postmenopausal; foul smelling vaginal discharge, pain, and dyspareunia
Fallopian: Vaginal bleeding; intermittent, colicky, dull, aching pain; profuse, watery vaginal discharge
Gestational trophoblastic disease: First trimester vaginal bleeding, hyperemesis, abnormal enlargement of uterus, absence of fetal heart sounds and movement

DISEASE-RELATED COMPLICATIONS

Sexual dysfunction, infertility, sterility, alteration in bowel and bladder function, and loss of pregnancy

TREATMENT-RELATED COMPLICATIONS

Infertility, sterility (temporary/permanent), fistula formation, infection, bleeding, wound dehiscence, vaginal fibrosis/stenosis, ureteral obstruction, myelosuppression, alopecia, alteration in bowel and bladder function, termination of pregnancy, and altered sexual function

---

*References 3, 8, 11, 13, 18, 19.

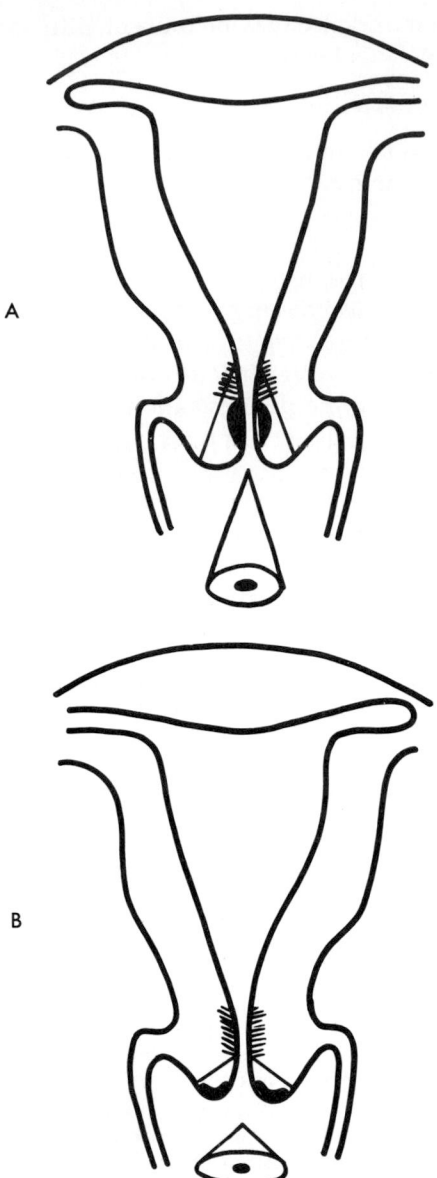

Figure 11–3 Cone biopsy for endocervical and exocervical disease. **A,** Endocervical disease—increased depth of cone biopsy to remove all abnormal areas. **B,** Exocervical disease—increased width of cone biopsy to remove all abnormal areas. (From DiSaia PJ and Creasman WT: Clinical gynecologic oncology, St Louis, 1993, Mosby.)

palpation, and colposcopy), radiographic examinations (chest, kidneys, sigmoid colon and rectum, and skeleton), and pathologic evaluation of biopsy and curettage materials are used to determine the extent of disease and ultimately plan treatment. Staging systems for cervical cancer have been developed by the American Joint Committee on Cancer and the International Federation of Gynecology and Obstetrics (FIGO) and are presented in Table 11-1.[8,11,13,18,19]

METASTASIS

Cervical carcinomas are slow-growing tumors that invade by direct extension to adjacent tissues of the uterus, vagina, rectum, bladder, and parametrial tissues. Lymphatic invasion also occurs in regional and distant lymphatic channels. Cervical cancer rarely spreads hematologically; however, metastatic disease can occur in the lungs or liver.[8,13,18,19]

TREATMENT MODALITIES

The treatment of preinvasive cervical disease is based on the extent of disease (Figure 11-4). Women with preinvasive disease may be treated conservatively with cryosurgery, electrocautery, or laser vaporization. Each of these techniques allows destruction of superficially abnormal cells with cold, heat, or light-energy, respectively. Of the three methods, the laser vaporization allows for more control of the pattern as well as the depth of tissue destruction.[8,13]

A cold-knife conization or Loop Electrosurgical Excision Procedure (LEEP) of the cervix may be used as treatment. With either procedure, the entire transformation zone and squamocolumnar junction are removed (Figure 11-3). Conization of the cervix often is recommended as treatment for women who desire to maintain fertility. However, many physicians recommend hysterectomy following completion of childbearing. For women with preinvasive disease who do not desire to maintain fertility or who are high-risk for noncompliance with follow-up examinations, hysterectomy may be considered as definitive treatment.[8,13]

Localized cervical carcinoma (stages I to IIA) may be treated with surgery alone, radiation therapy alone, or a combination of surgery and radiation therapy. Comparable survival rates have been demonstrated among the three treatment plans. The choice of treatment is based on extent of disease, the general health status, desire to maintain childbearing function, and indication of intent to comply with follow-up recommendations. Ideally, the treatment decision should be made jointly by the woman, the gynecologic oncologist, and the radiation therapist after review of the risks and benefits of treatment alternatives.*

Surgical treatment of women with invasive cervical cancer most commonly includes a radical hysterectomy with bilateral pelvic lymphadenectomy. Advantages of a radical approach to treatment include the gathering of additional pathologic information about the spread of the disease to local and regional lymph nodes and the need for adjuvant radiation therapy, and maintaining ovarian function. Disadvantages of radical surgical treatment include the high costs of hospitalization, risks of intraoperative and postoperative complications, and the loss of childbearing function. For a select number of women with stage

---

*References 3, 8, 13, 18, 19, 24.

Table 11–1 Staging Classification for Cervical Cancer

TNM	FIGO	Definition
Primary Tumor (T)		
TX		Primary tumor cannot be assessed
T0		No evidence of primary tumor
Tis	0	Carcinoma in situ
T1	I	Cervical carcinoma confined to uterus (extension to corpus should be disregarded)
T1a	Ia	Preclinical invasive carcinoma, diagnosed by microscopy only
T1a1	Iaa1	Minimal microscopic stromal invasion
T1a2	Ia2	Tumor with invasive component 5 mm or less in depth taken from the base of the epithelium and 7 mm or less in horizontal spread
T1b	Ib	Tumor larger than T1a2
T2	II	Cervical carcinoma invades beyond uterus but not to pelvic wall or to the lower third of vagina
T2a	IIa	Without parametrial invasion
T2b	IIb	With parametrial invasion
T3	III	Cervical carcinoma extends to the pelvic wall and/or involves lower third of vagina and/or causes hydronephrosis or nonfunctioning kidney
T3a	IIIa	Tumor involves lower third of the vagina, no extension to pelvic wall
T3b	IIIb	Tumor extends to pelvic wall and/or causes hydronephrosis or nonfunctioning kidney
T4	IVa	Tumor invades mucosa of bladder or rectum and/or extends beyond true pelvis
M1	IVb	Distant metastasis

Regional Lymph Nodes (N)

Regional lymph nodes include paracervical, parametrial, hypogastric (obturator), common, internal and external iliac, presacral and sacral.

NX	Regional lymph nodes cannot be assessed
N0	No regional lymph node metastasis
N1	Regional lymph node metastasis

Distant Metastasis (M)

MX	Presence of distant metastasis cannot be assessed
M0	No distant metastasis
M1 IVb	Distant metastasis

Stage Grouping

Stage	T	N	M
Stage 0	Tis	N0	M0
Stage IA	T1a	N0	M0
Stage IB	T1b	N0	M0
Stage IIA	T2a	N0	M0
Stage IIB	T2b	N0	M0
Stage IIIA	T3a	N0	M0
Stage IIIB	T1	N1	M0
	T2	N1	M0
	T3a	N1	M0
	T3b	Any N	M0
Stage IVA	T4	Any N	M0
Stage IVB	Any T	Any N	M1

From American Joint Committee on Cancer: Manual for staging cancer, ed 4, Chicago, 1992, The Committee.

IA disease who desire to maintain fertility, conization of the cervix may be used as definitive treatment. Follow-up with cervical cytology, colposcopy, and pelvic examination at 3-month intervals is recommended for early detection of recurrent invasive cervical cancer.[8,13]

Radiation with external beam (teletherapy) and internal or interstitial beam (brachytherapy) offers women with early stage disease equally effective treatment. Advantages of radiation are that the treatment can be given on an outpatient basis, intraoperative and postoperative complications are avoided, and treatment time is shorter.[19] Disadvantages include long-term effects of radiation on normal tissues such as radiation enteritis, bladder damage, fistula formation, vaginal stenosis, and ureteral obstruction.[8,19]

Advanced cervical carcinoma (stages IIB to IV) is treated primarily with radiation therapy alone although recent clinical trials include antineoplastic, radiosensitizing agents, hyperbaric oxygen, and hyperthermia administered in conjunction with radiation. Coordination between the medical oncologist and the radiation oncologist is mandatory to maximize therapeutic benefit while carefully monitoring immediate and long-term consequences of combined therapy.

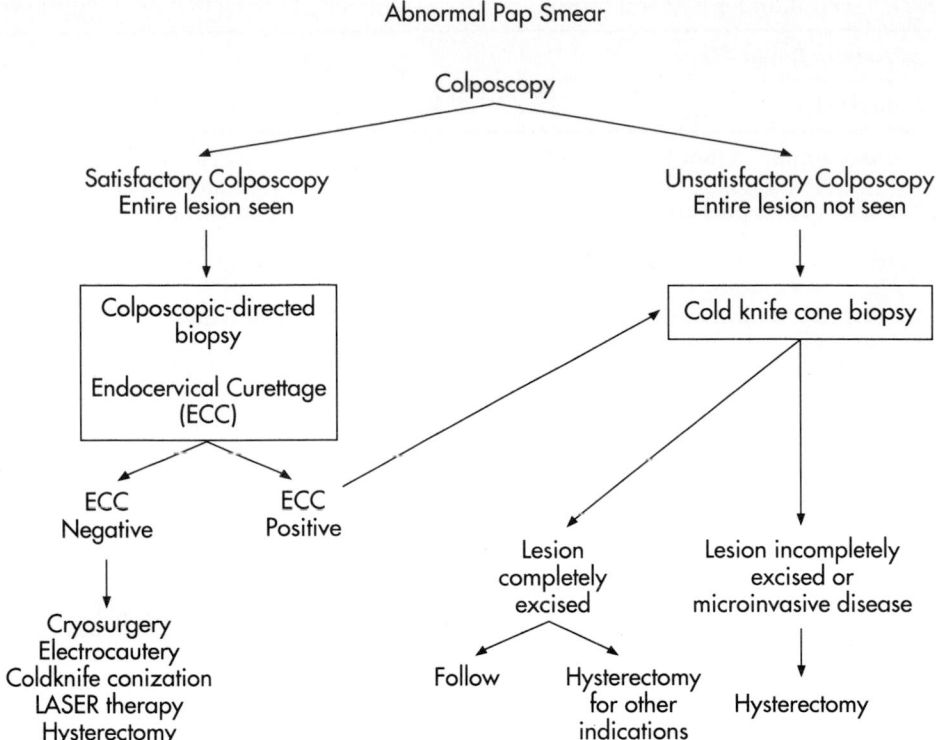

Figure 11–4 Decision tree for management of cervical intraepithelial neoplasia. (From Flannery M: Reproductive cancers. In Clark JC and McGee RF, editors: Core curriculum for oncology nursing, Philadelphia, 1992, WB Saunders Co.)

The rate of persistent or recurrent cervical cancer is approximately 35%. Women with advanced stage disease at diagnosis are in the highest risk group. For locally recurrent or persistent disease, treatment options include pelvic exenteration, radiation therapy to previously nonradiated areas, and antineoplastic therapy.

Pelvic exenteration is considered for curative treatment for women with recurrent disease if no evidence of extrapelvic disease, tumor fixed to the pelvic wall, or ureteral obstruction due to tumor is present preoperatively.[8,13] The procedure consists of removal of the uterus, cervix, vagina, rectum, bladder, urethra, and lateral supporting tissues and carries significant morbidity.[8,13] In women whose disease has not spread to the bladder or rectum, variations on the procedure may be performed, a posterior pelvic exenteration or anterior pelvic exenteration, respectively (Figure 11-5). Patients must be monitored carefully after the surgery for potential complications of the procedure such as infection, bleeding, wound dehiscence, and fistula formation.[8,13,18] In addition, the patient is faced with learning new self-care skills (ostomy care), evaluating components of self-image and body-image, and learning new sexual expression behaviors and attitudes.

Radiation therapy is used to treat some women with recurrent disease. Women with a central recur-

rence who have not received prior radiation therapy to the area are candidates for this form of treatment.

Antineoplastic agents, as single agents or in combination, have been used to treat women with recurrent cervical cancer; however, responses to treatment have been modest, ranging from 10% to 40%. Researchers and clinicians postulate that the low response rates are due to three primary factors: (1) Previous radiation therapy to the pelvis may result in fibrosis of the bone marrow and a decreased tolerance of the hematologic effects of the agents; (2) decreased vascularization of recurrent tumors may limit the ability of the agents to reach the target tissues; and (3) finally, fibrosis from previous radiation therapy can also damage and obstruct the ureters. The combination of ureteral obstruction and nephrotoxicity of many of the antineoplastic agents may result in the kidneys being unable to clear the drug metabolites from the body. The goal of current treatment with antineoplastic agents for recurrent cervical cancer is palliation.[3,8,13,19] See box on p. 193.

TREATMENT DURING PREGNANCY

As the incidence of preinvasive and invasive cancer is increasing in younger women of childbearing age, the issue of treatment for the woman who is pregnant has become more common. Careful discussion among

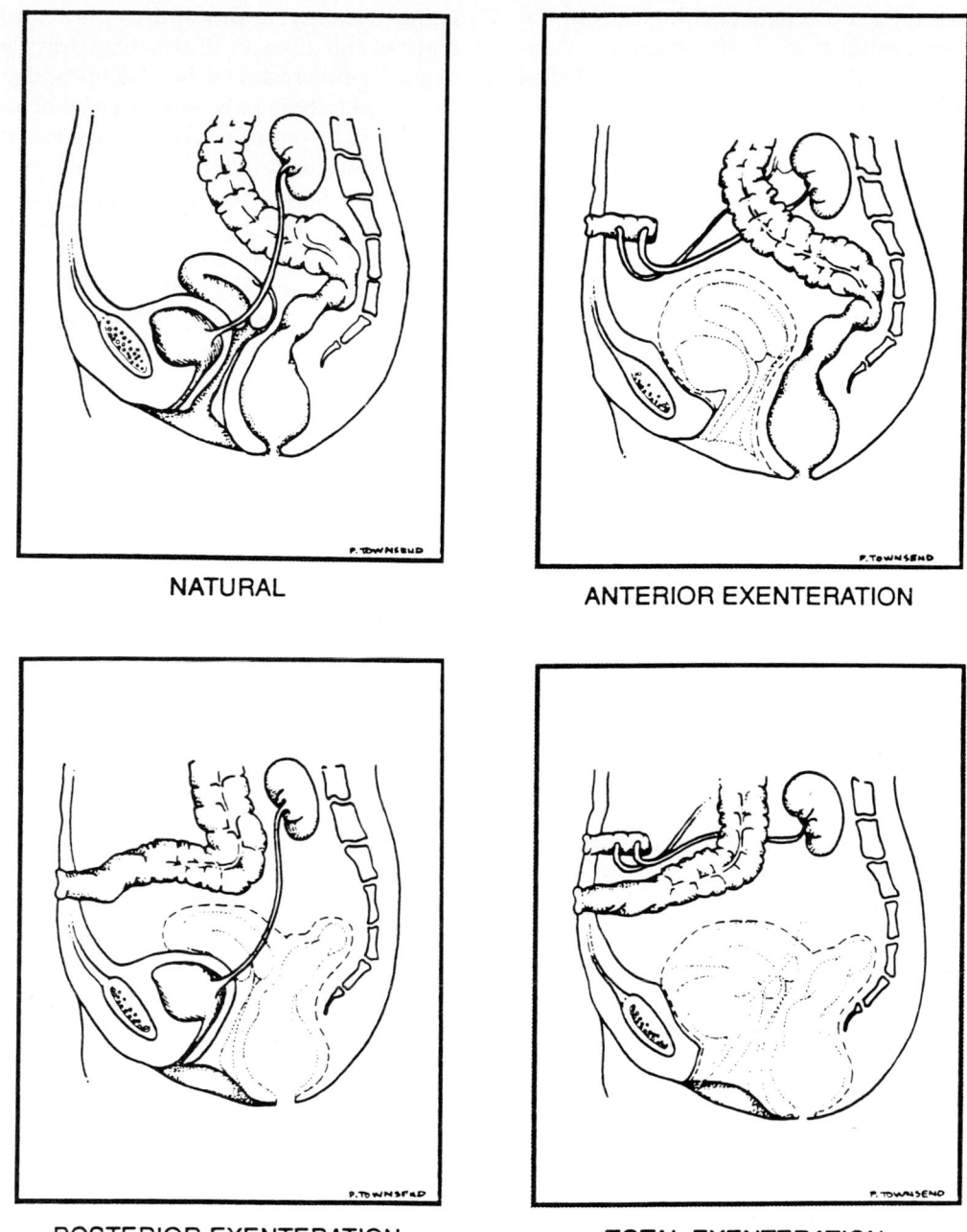

NATURAL

ANTERIOR EXENTERATION

POSTERIOR EXENTERATION

TOTAL EXENTERATION

Figure 11–5   Pelvic exenteration for treatment of cervical cancer. (From Martin LK and Braly PS: Gynecologic cancers. In Baird SB, McCorkle R, and Grant M (Eds.), Cancer nursing: A comprehensive textbook, Philadelphia, 1991, WB Saunders Co.)

the woman, partner, gynecologic oncologist, and obstetrician about potential risks of the disease, evaluation procedures, and treatment is recommended at each step of the evaluation and treatment process.[8,13]

Pregnant women with an abnormal Pap smear are evaluated with colposcopy and biopsies. If the squamocolumnar junction can be visualized entirely on colposcopy and directed biopsies are sufficient to rule out the presence of invasive cancer, the clinician can follow the woman to term with interval Pap smears and colposcopy examinations. Appropriate treatment is deferred until after delivery. If, however, the limits of the colposcopically abnormal area are not visualized or biopsies cannot rule out invasive cancer, a conization of the cervix is recommended. Profuse bleeding and spontaneous abortion of the fetus are potential complications of the procedure.[8,13]

Invasive cancer of the cervix occurs in 1 of 2205 pregnancies. Women with stage IA disease usually can be followed with Pap smears, colposcopy, and biopsies to term. In the presence of invasive cancer, immediate treatment is recommended. For women at less than 24 weeks gestation, the pregnancy is terminated. Radical hysterectomy or radiation therapy can be used as primary treatment. Treatment of women between 24 and 28 weeks gestation is more complicated. The risk of delaying treatment to allow for fetal development must be weighed carefully against the risk of progressive disease. After 28 weeks of gestation, the fetus is considered viable and is delivered by cesarean section to decrease the risk of maternal bleeding and spread of the disease. Radical hysterectomy is performed for definitive treatment after delivery.[13]

PROGNOSIS

Prognosis in cervical cancer is determined primarily by stage of disease. The 5-year survival rate for patients diagnosed with carcinoma in situ approaches 100%, with local disease 88%, regional disease 52%, and distant metastasis 14%. Overall survival trends have improved since the 1940s.[1]

ENDOMETRIAL CANCER

EPIDEMIOLOGY

Endometrial cancer is the most common gynecologic malignancy among women over 50 years of age. Of the estimated 31,000 women diagnosed with endometrial cancer in 1993, approximately 70% were over 50 years of age.[1,8,13] For reasons that are not clear, the incidence of the disease is increasing, particularly among women less than 50 years of age.

ETIOLOGY AND RISK FACTORS

Although the etiology of endometrial cancer is unknown, abnormal balance of endogenous and exogenous estrogen is thought to play a role in development of the disease. With advancing age, the amount of estrogen produced by the body decreases. However, researchers have suggested that as estrogen production is lowered, the body increases the production of estrogen precursors. These estrogen precursors are known to have carcinogenic potential and may play a role in the development of adenomatous hyperplasia, a premalignant condition.[13,18,19]

Additional evidence of the association of estrogen to the development of endometrial cancer is found clinically in situations where the endometrium is exposed to unopposed estrogen stimulation. Women who have Stein-Leventhal syndrome or who have an intact uterus and are receiving hormone replacement therapy with estrogen alone, as opposed to estrogen and progesterone combination therapy, are at higher risk of developing endometrial cancer.

Risk factors for cancer of the endometrium include advancing age, early onset of menstruation, late menopause, and concurrent conditions. Women who have a history of postmenopausal bleeding and have never been pregnant are at higher risk for cancer of the endometrium. Concurrent conditions, such as obesity, diabetes, hypertension, endometrial hyperplasia, or previous history of breast, colon, or ovarian cancer, also increase the risk for endometrial cancer.[3,8,13,18,19]

PREVENTION, SCREENING, AND DETECTION
Prevention

As knowledge of the etiology of endometrial cancer evolves, the primary focus of prevention is targeted toward high-risk women. Maintenance of ideal body weight is recommended to avoid obesity and to decrease the risk of hypertension and diabetes. Treatment of premalignant changes of the endometrium such as endometrial hyperplasia with progesterone is suggested as a prevention strategy. To control the symptoms of menopause in women with an intact uterus, the addition of cyclic progesterone to the estrogen replacement regimen is recommended to reduce the risk of development of endometrial cancer.[8,13]

Screening

No reliable, valid, and cost-effective tests are recommended for periodic screening of asymptomatic women for endometrial cancer. However, the ACS recommends that asymptomatic, high-risk women have an endometrial tissue sampling done at menopause.[1]

Detection

The detection of endometrial cancer in symptomatic women is guided by a complete history, physical examination, and diagnostic evaluation. The history includes a review of risk factors and the presence of clinical signs and symptoms for endometrial cancer. The physical examination includes evaluation of the size, consistency, and shape of the uterus. The uterine size, shape, and consistency is determined by palpation on the rectovaginal, bimanual examination. The depth of the uterine cavity is determined by inserting a uterine sound. An endometrial biopsy is obtained for histologic confirmation of the disease.

CLASSIFICATION

Five primary types of endometrial cancer are seen: adenocarcinoma, mixed mullerian tumors, sarcomas, clear cell carcinoma, and epidermoid carcinoma.[13] More than 90% of endometrial cancers are adenocarcinomas. These exophytic or polypoid lesions tend to invade the uterine muscle. Variants of adenocarcinoma include adenocanthoma (contains benign squamous elements) and adenosquamous carcinoma (contains malignant squamous elements). The aggressive nature of these lesions results in a higher incidence of invasion of the myometrium and lymph nodes, distant metastases, and a lower survival rate when compared to adenocarcinomas. Mixed mullerian tumors, sarcomas, clear cell carcinomas, and epidermoid carcinomas are rare and are associated with higher incidences of local and distant metastases and lower survival rates than adenocarcinomas.[3,8,13]

CLINICAL FEATURES

The most common presenting symptom in women with endometrial cancer is prolonged, excessive, or irregular premenopausal or postmenopausal bleeding. Additional symptoms may include a yellow, watery vaginal discharge, pyometria (accumulation of pus in the uterus), hematometria (accumulation of blood in the uterus), or pain in the hypogastric or lumbosacral areas or the pelvis. Women with advanced disease may present with intestinal obstruction, ascites, jaundice, respiratory distress, or hemorrhage.[8,10,13,18,19]

On physical examination, the uterus may be enlarged or have an irregular contour. In advanced stages, extension of tumor into the vagina, bladder, or bowel may be palpated on bimanual, rectovaginal examination. Enlarged inguinal lymph nodes also may be palpated. See box on p. 193.

DIAGNOSIS AND STAGING

The diagnostic evaluation includes physical examination, tissue sampling, and laboratory and radiographic studies to determine the histologic type, degree of differentiation, and extent of the disease. Ideally, the gynecologic and radiation oncologist collaborate on the physical examination and a thorough evaluation of potential sites of metastatic disease: cervix, vagina, tissues surrounding the urethral meatus, parametria, and regional lymph nodes.

Cervical biopsies, endocervical curettage, endometrial biopsy, and/or a fractional dilatation and curettage (D & C) are done to rule out the presence of a cervical malignancy and to obtain a tissue sample for diagnosis. Cervical biopsies and endocervical curettage are collected first to minimize the risk of contamination of the cervical specimen with endometrial tissue that may be dislodged by the uterine sound or dilator.[8,13] Although obtaining the necessary specimens can be uncomfortable for the patient, the diagnostic evaluation usually can be performed in the outpatient setting.

Laboratory studies routinely include a complete blood count (CBC), blood chemistry profile (SMA), and liver and renal chemistries. Additional radiographic studies to determine the presence of metastatic disease may include a chest x-ray, magnetic resonance imaging (MRI), and computed tomography (CT). If involvement of the bladder or rectum are suspected, intravenous pyelogram, barium enema, proctosigmoidoscopy, and cystoscopy may be done.

Endometrial cancer is staged surgically. Staging is based on the depth of myometrial invasion, degree of cellular differentiation, and the extent of metastatic disease. The schema for staging cancer of the endometrium is presented in Table 11-2.

METASTASIS

The majority of endometrial cancers originate in the fundus of the uterus and spread by direct extension to the entire endometrium, through the layers of the uterine wall (myometrium and serosa), or through the endocervical canal to the cervix. The disease may also spread outside the uterus to the structures of the parametria and abdominal cavity, such as the ovaries, fallopian tubes, vagina, bladder, rectum, omentum, or bowel. Lymphatic metastases occur primarily to the pelvic and para-aortic lymph nodes. The endometrium is highly vascular; therefore, hematogenous spread, particularly with sarcomas, is common. Lung, liver, bone, and brain metastases may occur.[3,8,13,18,19]

TREATMENT MODALITIES

Development of a plan for treatment of endometrial cancer is a collaborative effort between the gynecologic and radiation oncologist. Factors that influence the treatment plan selected include the type of tumor, degree of differentiation, stage of disease, and the general health status of the woman.

Surgery

Since abnormal bleeding brings the majority of women to the health care system with early stage

Table 11–2 Staging Classification for Endometrial Cancer

CARCINOMA OF THE UTERINE CORPUS

The Committee decided that corpus cancer should be surgically staged and as a result additional factors of prognostic importance are included in the staging. The Committee also decided to change the current definitions of tumor grading to coincide with the new recommendations of the International Society of Gynaecological Pathologists. The recommended staging is as follows:

STAGE

IA	G123	Tumor limited to endometrium
IB	G123	Invasion to <½ myometrium
IC	G123	Invasion to >½ myometrium
IIA	G123	Endocervical glandular involvement only
IIB	G123	Cervical stromal invasion
IIIA	G123	Tumor invades serosa and/or adnexa and/or positive peritoneal cytology
IIIB	G123	Metastases to pelvic and/or para-aortic lymph nodes
IVA	G123	Tumor invasion of bladder and/or bowel mucosa
IVB		Distant metastases including intra-abdominal and/or inguinal lymph nodes

HISTOPATHOLOGY: DEGREE OF DIFFERENTIATION

Cases of carcinoma of the corpus should be grouped with regard to the degree of differentiation of the adenocarcinoma as follows:

G1   5% or less of a nonsquamous or nonmorular solid growth pattern
G2   6%-50% of a nonsquamous or nonmorular solid growth pattern
G3   More than 50% of a nonsquamous or nonmorular solid growth pattern

NOTES ON PATHOLOGIC GRADING

1. Notable nuclear atypia, inappropriate for the architectural grade, raises the grade of a grade I or grade II tumor by one.
2. In serous adenocarcinomas, clear-cell adenocarcinomas, and squamous-cell carcinomas, nuclear grading takes precedence.
3. Adenocarcinomas with squamous differentiation are graded according to the nuclear grade of the glandular component.

RULES RELATED TO STAGING

1. Since corpus cancer is now surgically staged, procedures used previously for the differentiation of stages are no longer applicable, such as using dilatation and curettage findings to differentiate between stage I and stage II. (It is appreciated that there may be a small number of patients with corpus cancer who will be treated primarily with radiation therapy. If that is the case, the clinical staging adopted by FIGO in 1971 would still apply but designation of that staging system would be noted.)
2. Ideally, the thickness of the myometrium should be measured along with the depth of tumor invasion.

From American Joint Committee on Cancer: Manual for staging cancer, ed 4, Chicago, 1992, The Committee.

disease, the use of localized treatment is common. Surgery, usually a total abdominal hysterectomy and bilateral salpingo-oophorectomy (TAH-BSO), is the most common primary treatment for women with early stage disease. More extensive surgery, radical abdominal hysterectomy and bilateral pelvic lymphadenectomy, has been used for treatment, but surgical risks are higher and no significant improvement in survival rates has been reported.[3,8,13]

Radiation Therapy

Radiation therapy is used as primary treatment for women with other health problems that increase the risks of surgical complications. However, survival rates for women treated with radiation therapy alone, even with early stage disease, are not as high as those observed when surgery alone is used as the primary treatment. In women with bulky disease, poorly differentiated tumors, or greater depth of myometrial invasion, the addition of preoperative or postopera-tive radiation therapy may be recommended. Radiation may consist of brachytherapy, teletherapy, or a combination of the two. Advantages of preoperative and postoperative radiation therapy are detailed.[3,8,13]

Hormone Therapy

Endometrial cancer is a hormone-dependent tumor. Increased levels of progesterone and estrogen receptors have been identified in more well-differentiated tumors. Therefore, clinicians are using estrogen and progesterone receptor analyses as one factor to determine those women who may benefit from hormone manipulation either as an adjuvant therapy or as treatment for recurrent disease. Depo-provera, provera, dilalutin, and megace are the most common progestational agents currently used for women who are estrogen and progesterone receptor positive. Response rates with hormonal manipulation range from 30% to 70% with the highest response rate occurring in women with well-differentiated tumors.[3,8,13]

Chemotherapy

Antineoplastic agents are reserved for women who have estrogen/progesterone negative tumors, who have failed hormone therapy, or who have disseminated disease. However, antineoplastic agents, used either as single agents or in combination, have resulted in no significant improvement in survival rates from endometrial cancer. Agents commonly used include doxorubicin, 5-fluorouracil, vincristine, cisplatin, and cyclophosphamide. Evaluation of the effectiveness of combined hormone and antineoplastic agents in women with endometrial cancer is ongoing. See box on p. 193.

PROGNOSIS

Relative 5-year survival rates associated with a diagnosis of endometrial cancer have improved significantly between 1974-1975 and 1981-1987.[1] The 5-year survival rate for patients with all stages of endometrial cancer is 83%; with localized disease, 93%; with regional disease, 70%; and with distant metastasis, 27%.[1]

OVARIAN CANCER

EPIDEMIOLOGY

The 22,000 new cases of ovarian cancer account for only 25% of all gynecologic cancers diagnosed in the United States in 1993.[1] Yet, the disease is the leading cause of death (13,300 deaths in 1993) in women diagnosed with gynecologic cancers.[1] The highest incidence of ovarian cancer is reported in highly industrialized countries. The disease occurs less frequently in women from Asia and Latin America.[3,8,25]

The ACS estimates that 1 out of every 70 women will develop ovarian cancer during her lifetime.[1] This statistic is particularly alarming, since early disease is not symptomatic and no cost-effective, reliable, and valid screening tests are available.

ETIOLOGY AND RISK FACTORS

The etiology of ovarian cancer is unknown. However, age, genetics, history of other cancers, and menstrual history have been associated with an increased incidence of the disease. The majority of ovarian cancers are diagnosed in the 50- to 59-year age group. Families with a history of ovarian cancer across multiple generations have been identified but are uncommon. A familial or personal history of other cancers, including breast, colon, and uterine, increases the risk of ovarian cancer. The incidence of ovarian cancer is greater among women who are single, nulliparous, and infertile; the incidence is lower among women who use oral contraceptives. Researchers are currently evaluating the role of uninterrupted ovulation in the pathogenesis of ovarian cancer.[3,8,25]

PREVENTION, SCREENING, AND DETECTION
Prevention and Screening

As the etiology of ovarian cancer remains a mystery, no recommendations exist for prevention of the disease. Women in higher risk categories, as described previously, are encouraged to seek routine gynecologic care including an annual pelvic examination. Palpatation of a normal-sized ovary in postmenopausal women is cause for a further diagnostic evaluation. However, the overall yield of 1 case of ovarian cancer in 10,000 pelvic examinations is low. Furthermore, the occurrence of widely disseminated metastatic disease in women with palpable disease is high and survival rates in this group are low.[3,8,19,25]

Recently, the cost-effectiveness of the use of tumor markers and vaginal ultrasound to screen high-risk women for ovarian cancer has been studied. Researchers have noted variable specificity and sensitivity outcomes with tumor markers, such as the alpha-fetoprotein (α-FP) for rare endodermal sinus tumors, carcinoembryonic antigen (CEA), and CA-125 for epithelial ovarian tumors. Because of the variability in results, none of the tests are recommended for screening asymptomatic populations. However, serial CA-125 levels have been used to monitor selected high-risk women with a strong familial history of ovarian cancer. A third method of screening women at high risk for ovarian cancer has been with the use of serial vaginal ultrasounds. No long-term, large, prospective studies have been done to date that demonstrate cost-effectiveness of the procedure in detecting ovarian carcinoma in asymptomatic women.[3,8,18,25]

In summary, ovarian cancer is "silent" in the early stages. No effective methods of screening have been identified. Therefore, the majority of women continue to be diagnosed with ovarian cancer after the disease has spread throughout the abdominal cavity, lymphatic channels, and the vascular system.

Detection

Most women with early stage ovarian cancer are asymptomatic. Therefore, the clinician must maintain an index of suspicion for ovarian cancer. A careful personal and family history is important to identify women at high risk for the disease. Attention to generalized, vague complaints among women during their middle years often will alert the clinician to the possibility of ovarian cancer. Finally, a pelvic examination and palpation of an adnexal mass or a postmenopausal ovary raise suspicion for ovarian cancer.

CLASSIFICATION

Ovarian carcinomas are classified as epithelial, sex cord-stromal, or lipid cell tumors. Epithelial tumors, most frequently found in women 40 to 65 years of age, account for 85% of all ovarian malignancies diagnosed in the United States. Sex cord-stromal tumors occur much less frequently than the epithelial tumors. These tumors often are associated with femininizing or masculinizing effects. Women with sex cord-stromal tumors have a better prognosis than women with epithelial malignancies. Lipid cell tumors account for less than 5% of all ovarian malignancies. These tumors, particularly dysgerminoma, endodermal sinus tumors, and embryonal carcinoma, occur most frequently in younger women.[25] Since the majority of ovarian malignancies are epithelial tumors, the remainder of this section focuses on this specific ovarian neoplasm.

CLINICAL FEATURES

Vague gastrointestinal symptoms such as dyspepsia, indigestion, anorexia, and early satiety may be some of the first symptoms of ovarian cancer. Pressure of the tumor on the rectum and bladder may result in symptoms of urinary frequency, constipation, or pelvic pressure and discomfort. Progressive disease is marked by an increase in abdominal girth, pain, shortness of breath, intestinal or ureteral obstruction, and muscle wasting.* See box on p. 193.

DIAGNOSIS AND STAGING

Diagnosis and staging (Table 11-3) of women with ovarian cancer are achieved by tissue sampling and inspection of the abdominal cavity at the time of exploratory laparotomy. The initial approach and exploration of the abdomen are well-defined and methodical to allow careful evaluation of the extent of disease and to remove (debulk) as much of the tumor burden as possible. However, prior to surgical exploration, a series of laboratory and radiographic tests is recommended. A CBC, biochemical profile, and CA-125 are obtained. In addition, a chest x-ray, cystoscopy, proctoscopy, intravenous pyelogram, barium enema, CT, MRI, or ultrasound may be ordered.[3,8,13,25]

METASTASIS

Ovarian carcinoma spreads by direct extension to adjacent pelvic organs such as the opposite ovary, uterus, fallopian tubes, bladder, rectum, and peritoneum, seeding of the peritoneal cavity, and lymphatic and vascular channels (Figure 11-6). Spread occurs primarily by shedding of malignant cells that float within and form micrometastases throughout the peritoneal cavity. Common sites of metastatic disease include the omentum and surfaces of the bowel, uterus, bladder, and peritoneum. Free-floating malignant cells are washed beneath the diaphragm and

removed through lymphatic channels located in the diaphragm. This pattern of flow of peritoneal fluid accounts for the high incidence of metastatic ovarian disease found on the undersurfaces of the diaphragm.[25]

Lymphatic invasion can occur in the pelvic, para-aortic, and aortic nodes even in early stage disease. Partial or complete obstruction of lymphatic channels in the diaphragm result in the accumulation of malignant ascitic fluid.

Although rare, metastasis can occur through vascular invasion to distant sites. The most common sites of hematogenous spread include the liver, lung, and pleura.[3,8,11,19,25]

TREATMENT MODALITIES

Treatment of ovarian cancer is based on surgical staging of the disease, malignant potential of the tumor, and the bulk of remaining disease. Surgery, radiation therapy, and chemotherapy may be used as single or combined modalities.

Surgery

Surgery plays a role in the diagnosis, primary treatment, evaluation of response to therapy, and palliative care for women with ovarian cancer (see box on p. 205). In addition to the exploratory laparotomy required for staging, surgery is used as primary treatment for women with borderline and malignant tumors of the ovary. For younger women with tumors of borderline malignant potential, conservative treatment with unilateral oophorectomy may be considered definitive treatment. However, in women beyond childbearing years, every attempt is made to remove the uterus, cervix, fallopian tubes, and ovaries if the disease is considered surgically resectable. Beyond a total abdominal hysterectomy and bilateral salpingo-oophorectomy, surgical resection of the bulk of remaining tumor is attempted. Resection of the bladder, colon, or omentum may be indicated. The extent of the debulking procedure is based on evaluation of potential risks of more extensive resection and potential benefits in terms of survival and quality of life.[3,8,25]

The use of surgical exploration (second-look procedure) to evaluate the response to primary therapy for ovarian cancer is controversial. Advocates of second-look procedures indicate that the procedure allows for direct inspection of the abdominal cavity, sampling of ascitic fluid, and sampling of abdominal tissues at risk for persistent microscopic disease. Should persistent disease be found, the surgeon is able to debulk the tumor burden prior to retreatment. If no disease is documented, therapy is usually discontinued and the woman enters a clinical follow-up scheme. Opponents of the second-look procedure ar-

*References 1, 3, 8, 11, 18, 19, 24, 25.

Table 11–3 Staging Classification for Ovarian Cancer

TNM	FIGO	Definition (Primary Tumor (T))	Regional Lymph Nodes (N)
TX		Primary tumor cannot be assessed	Regional lymph nodes include hypogastric (obturator), common iliac, external iliac, internal iliac, lateral sacral, para-aortic, and inguinal.
T0		No evidence of primary tumor	
T1	I	Tumor limited to ovaries	NX — Regional lymph nodes cannot be assessed
T1a	Ia	Tumor limited to one ovary; capsule intact, no tumor on ovarian surface	N0 — No regional lymph node metastasis
T1b	Ib	Tumor limited to both ovaries; capsules intact, no tumor on ovarian surface	N1 — Regional lymph node metastasis
T1c	Ic	Tumor limited to one or both ovaries with any of the following: capsule ruptured, tumor on ovarian surface, malignant cells in ascites, or peritoneal washing	**Distant Metastasis (M)**

TNM	FIGO	Definition
MX		Presence of distant metastasis cannot be assessed
M0		No distant metastasis
M1	IV	Distant metastasis (excludes peritoneal metastasis)

TNM	FIGO	Definition (Primary Tumor (T) continued)
T2	II	Tumor involves one or both ovaries with pelvic extension
T2a	IIa	Extension and/or implants on uterus and/or tube(s)
T2b	IIb	Extension to other pelvic tissues
T2c	IIc	Pelvic extension (2a or 2b) with malignant cells in ascites or peritoneal washing
T3 and/or N1	III	Tumor involves one or both ovaries with microscopically confirmed peritoneal metastasis outside the pelvis and/or regional lymph node metastasis
T3a	IIIa	Microscopic peritoneal metastasis beyond pelvis
T3b	IIIb	Macroscopic peritoneal metastasis beyond pelvis 2 cm or less in greatest dimension
T3c and/or N1	IIIc	Peritoneal metastasis beyond pelvis more than 2 cm in greatest dimension and/or regional lymph node metastasis
M1	IV	Distant metastasis (excludes peritoneal metastasis)

Stage Grouping

Stage IA	T1a	N0	M0
Stage IB	T1b	N0	M0
Stage IC	T1c	N0	M0
Stage IIA	T2a	N0	M0
Stage IIB	T2b	N0	M0
Stage IIC	T2c	N0	M0
Stage IIIA	T3a	N0	M0
Stage IIIB	T3b	N0	M0
Stage IIIC	T3c	N0	M0
	Any T	N1	M0
Stage IV	Any T	Any N	M1

From American Joint Committee on Cancer: Manual for staging cancer, ed 4, Chicago, 1992, The Committee.

gue that the procedure requires hospitalization, a major abdominal surgery, and disruption of the normal activities of the patient. In addition, the ultimate benefit of the procedure is questioned given the high incidence of recurrent disease (15% to 20%) among women who have had negative findings at second-look procedure.[3,8,19,25]

Surgery has also been used in providing palliative care to women with advanced ovarian cancer. Bowel resection and bowel or urinary diversion may be done to relieve obstructive symptoms in selected patients.

The relative risks and benefits of such procedures are weighed carefully prior to surgical intervention.

Radiation Therapy

Teletherapy to the pelvis and abdomen and the instillation of radioactive isotopes in the peritoneal cavity have been used in the treatment of women with early stages (I and II) of ovarian cancer. Although adequate doses of radiation can be delivered to the pelvis and abdomen to eradicate the disease, the tolerance of normal tissues within the treatment field to

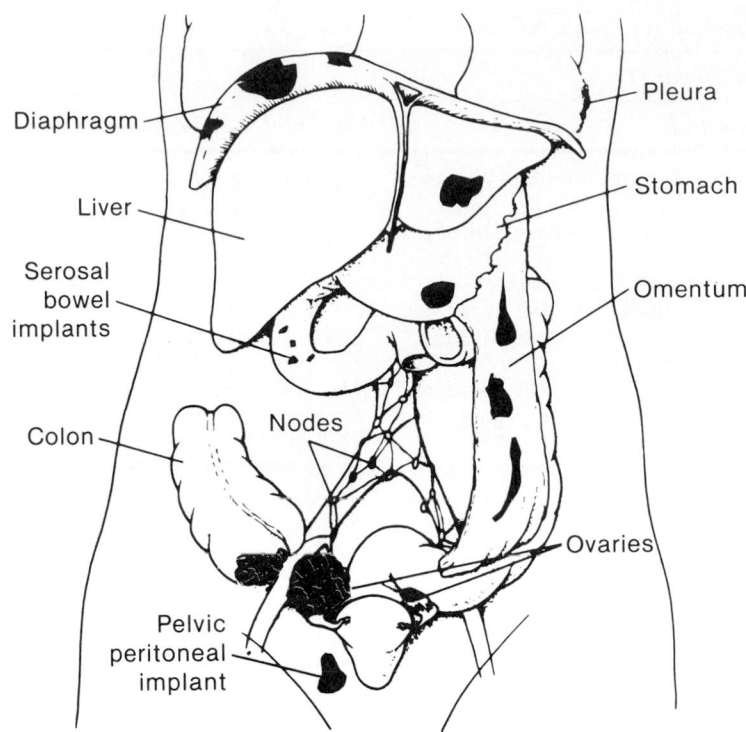

Figure 11–6   Patterns of metastasis for ovarian cancer. (From DiSaia PJ: Hosp Pract 22(4).)

the tumoricidal doses is limited. To overcome this barrier, shielding techniques for vital organs such as the kidneys and liver, multifield, and various fractionation techniques have been used to limit damage to normal tissues and organs.

The response to radiation therapy is determined by the extent of residual disease and the differentiation of the tumor. Women with well-differentiated tumors that are less than 2 cm in size have the best response rates.[8,19,25]

Radioactive isotopes (P^{32}) have been used to treat residual disease in the peritoneal cavity. Women who have limited residual disease, less than 2 cm, are the most likely candidates for P^{32} therapy. Disadvantages of the treatment include potential inability of the entire peritoneal cavity to be exposed to the isotope due to adhesions or loculation and the occurrence of small bowel obstruction or stenosis.[3,8,25]

Chemotherapy

For women with high-risk, early stage, epithelial ovarian tumors and for women with disseminated disease, antineoplastic therapy has resulted in improved length of survival. Historically, alkylating agents have been used most commonly as either single agents or in combination regimens for treatment of women with ovarian cancer. Systemic melphalan, 5-FU, thiotepa, and cyclophosphamide have shown activity. Altretamine, cisplatin, carboplatin, doxorubicin, ifosfam-

ide, and etoposide also have been used with response rates ranging from 27% to 78%.[8,19,25] In general, systemic combination therapy with cisplatin and cyclophosphamide has resulted in improved response rates, increased disease-free survival, and/or increased survival when compared to other multiagent regimens with significantly more severe toxicities.[25]

The fact that metastasis in ovarian cancer occurs primarily through exfoliation of malignant cells within the peritoneal cavity has lead researchers to explore the use of antineoplastic agents intraperitoneally to treat the disease. For individuals with no residual disease but who are at high risk for recurrence, intraperitoneal chemotherapy has been used as adjuvant therapy. In women with minimal residual disease, the intraperitoneal route of administration has been used to provide high concentrations of antineoplastic agent(s) to disease within the peritoneal cavity while limiting the concentrations of the agent(s) in the circulation and thus limiting systemic toxic effects. However, controversy still exists about the use and benefits of intraperitoneal chemotherapy in the treatment of ovarian cancer.[3,19,25] See box on p. 193.

Other Therapies

Since ovarian cancer is usually diagnosed in an advanced stage, many new therapies are being investigated for responsiveness. Studies with hormonal therapy, megace, tamoxifen, and leuprolide acetate

---

STEPS IN SURGICALLY STAGING OVARIAN CANCER

Step 1. If ascites is present, remove as much as possible for cytology. If no ascites is present, obtain cell washings from the pelvis, both abdominal gutters, and both subdiaphragmatic areas.

Step 2. Determine whether the mass is malignant; if malignant, perform appropriate pelvic procedure (total abdominal hysterectomy and bilateral salpingo-oophorectomy unless patient desires further childbearing and there is no evidence of spread beyond the ovary).

Step 3. Carefully examine pelvic peritoneum; if lesions are present, remove as much as possible and biopsy any lesion that cannot be removed. If no lesions are seen, sample at a minimum the peritoneum of the lateral pelvic sidewalls, the bladder, the rectosigmoid, and the cul-de-sac.

Step 4. Examine the paracolic gutters, and remove any lesions seen. If no lesions are seen, obtain a 1 × 3-cm strip of peritoneum on either side.

Step 5. Examine the omentum, and remove any that contains visible tumor (including the supracolic omentum if involved by tumor). If no lesions are seen, remove the infracolic omentum.

Step 6. Examine and palpate both diaphragms and the surface of the spleen and liver. If lesions are present, remove as much as possible; biopsy if they cannot be removed. If no lesions are seen, a strip of peritoneum 1 × 2 cm should be carefully excised from the right hemidiaphragm. (*Note:* Only peritoneum is needed, and care should be taken not to create a pneumothorax.)

Step 7. Beginning at either the rectum or cecum, carefully inspect the entire large colon and remove and/or biopsy any suspicious lesion of the intestine or mesentery.*

Step 8. Beginning at either the ileocecal valve or ligament of Treitz, carefully inspect the entire small bowel and mesentery, removing and/or biopsing any lesions.*

Step 9. If, after all of the above procedures, no gross disease larger than 1 or 2 cm is left, the pelvic and para-aortic lymph nodes should be sampled.

*If resection of intestine is necessary to cytoreduce the tumor optimally or to relieve obstruction, this should be performed.
From Young RC, Fuks Z, and Hoskins WJ: Cancer of the ovary. In DeVita VT Jr, Hellman S, and Rosenberg SA, editors: Cancer: Principles & practice of oncology, ed 3, Philadelphia, 1989, JB Lippincott Co.

---

are in progress. Taxol is in phase I and II clinical trials for ovarian cancer. Biologic response therapy with interferon, interleukin-2, monoclonal antibodies, and lymphokine-activated killer cells has been used in the treatment of ovarian cancer with varying results. Additional prospective, clinical trials are needed to determine the relative effectiveness of these therapies when compared to current treatment protocols.[3,8,25]

PROGNOSIS

Although the relative 5-year survival rates improved significantly from the mid-1970s to the mid-1980s, the rates remain dismally low (39%). Prognosis improves (87%) when the disease is diagnosed at an early stage and treated aggressively. Since early ovarian cancer is commonly asymptomatic, only 23% of patients are diagnosed with localized disease. Patients with distant metastasis at the time of diagnosis have a 19% 5-year survival rate.[1]

VULVAR CANCER

EPIDEMIOLOGY

Vulvar carcinoma accounts for approximately 5% of all gynecologic malignancies. Although the incidence of invasive vulvar cancer is small, the incidence rates of vulvar intraepithelial neoplasia (VIN) and carcinoma in situ are increasing. VIN occurs most commonly in women in their 40s, carcinoma in situ in women in their 50s, and invasive disease in women in their 60s. No ethnic or geographic variations have been noted in the incidence rates. The most frequent sites for vulvar carcinoma include the labia majora, labia minora, and the clitoris.*

ETIOLOGY AND RISK FACTORS

The etiology of vulvar carcinoma is unknown. However, several factors have been associated with an increased incidence of the disease. These include concurrent diseases such as hypertension, diabetes, cardiovascular disease, obesity, cervical cancer, early menopause, and chronic vulvar irritation.[3,13,16,18,24]

PREVENTION, SCREENING, DETECTION
Prevention and Screening

No specific measures are recommended for the prevention of vulvar cancer. In recent years, emphasis has been placed on teaching women vulvar self-examination as a strategy for screening in asymptomatic women.[13]

Detection

Many women with vulvar cancer are asymptomatic. Therefore, a thorough history and physical examination are required to identify women with existing

---

*References 3, 8, 13, 18, 19, 24.

GYNECOLOGIC-GERIATRIC CONSIDERATIONS

Vulvar and vaginal cancer disease onset occurs in the late fifth decade to the sixth decade of life.

Teaching the patient the need for annual ongoing health examinations that include bimanual pelvic exam with a thorough inspection and palpation of the perineal and vaginal areas

Other chronic diseases (hypertension, diabetes, arthritis) may exacerbate with the onset/progression of the disease and/or the side effects of the multiple therapies

Age-related modifications may require drug/therapy reduction

Elderly women may live alone and have limited financial/social/healthcare resources—assess needs and intervention strategies and consult with multiple referral systems (American Cancer Society, Social Services, Meals on Wheels, Home Health Care Agencies)

---

risk factors and to inspect and palpate vulvar tissue for abnormalities. Physical examination of the vulva, groins, and pelvis is mandatory.[8,13] See box above.

CLASSIFICATION

Invasive cancers of the vulva are classified as squamous cell, basal cell, adenocarcinoma, and malignant melanoma. Ninety percent of all malignancies of the vulva are squamous cell carcinomas.[13]

CLINICAL FEATURES

Symptomatic women with vulvar cancer most commonly present with a vulvar lump or mass, pain, or pruritus of several months duration. Vulvar tissues may be reddened, white, warty, or abnormally pigmented. Vulvar bleeding, discharge, and dysuria may be present. See box on p. 193.

DIAGNOSIS AND STAGING

Diagnosis of vulvar cancer is made by biopsy of abnormal areas noted on inspection, palpation, or colposcopic examination. Once a diagnosis of invasive disease is made, the woman undergoes a metastatic workup that may consist of cystoscopy, proctoscopy, barium enema, intravenous pyelogram, lymphangiogram, CT, and MRI.[3,8,13]

Staging for vulvar carcinoma is done clinically. The classification system for staging is presented in Table 11-4.

METASTASIS

Carcinomas of the vulva follow a predictable, slow pattern of spread by direct extension to local tissues and by lymphatic spread to inguinal and pelvic lymph nodes. With the exception of melanomas of the vulva,

hematogenous spread rarely occurs. Approximately one third of women with disease confined to the vulva will have nodal metastasis.[8,13,19]

TREATMENT MODALITIES

Treatment of women with vulvar cancer is based on the size and extent of the lesion as well as depth of invasion. The clinician also considers functional and cosmetic results when planning treatment. For women with preinvasive disease, VIN or carcinoma in situ, in a limited area, a conservative approach with topical 5-FU, cryotherapy, laser therapy, wide local excision, skinning vulvectomy, or simple vulvectomy can be used for primary treatment. With each treatment, the chance for control of disease with minimal disruption of function or cosmesis in carefully selected women is good. Women undergoing conservative treatment must be followed at 3- to 6-month intervals.

In women with invasive disease less than 2 cm in diameter, less than 5 mm of invasion, and negative inguinal lymph nodes on frozen section, wide local excision alone may be done. If the inguinal lymph nodes are positive, a radical vulvectomy with complete, bilateral groin dissection is done.[8,25] For women who are not candidates for surgical intervention, radiation therapy for early stage disease has been used successfully.

Historically, clinicians have used a surgical approach to the treatment of vulvar carcinoma although the risks of wound breakdown, lymphedema, and sexual dysfunction were high. Radiation therapy was not used because of the high incidence of short-term side effects (moist desquamation and maceration) of the skin over the vulvar, perineal, and groin areas. Given the advanced age of women commonly diagnosed with the disease, concurrent health problems that increase surgical risks, and improved techniques of delivering high doses of radiation therapy while sparing the skin, clinicians again are evaluating the role of radiation therapy in the treatment of women with vulvar cancer.

The treatment plan for women with locally advanced disease can consist of a combination of surgery, radical surgery (vulvectomy, anterior exenteration, posterior exenteration), and preoperative or postoperative radiation therapy. For women with distant metastasis, a combination of radiation therapy to control central disease and chemotherapy for systemic disease is commonly used as palliative treatment.

Chemotherapy has been used to treat limited numbers of women with vulvar cancer. Other than the use of topical agents to treat preinvasive disease, results have been disappointing. Clinical trials are currently in progress to evaluate the effectiveness of mi-

Table 11–4 Staging Classification for Vulvar Cancer

Primary Tumor (T)		Staging Grouping: Definitions of the Clinical Stages in Carcinoma of the Vulva			
TX	Primary tumor cannot be assessed	(Correlation of the FIGO, UICC, and AJCC nomenclatures)			
T0	No evidence of primary tumor	*Stage 0*			
Tis	Preinvasive carcinoma (carcinoma in situ)	Tis Carcinoma in situ, intraepithelial carcinoma			
T1	Tumor confined to the vulva, 2 cm or less in greatest dimension	*Stage I* T1	N0	M0	Tumor confined to the vulva; 2 cm or less in greatest di-
		T1	N1	M0	mension. Nodes are not palpable or are palpable in
T2	Tumor confined to the vulva, more than 2 cm in greatest dimension				either groin, not enlarged, mobile (not clinically suspi- cious of neoplasm)
T3	Tumor invades any of the following: urethra, va- gina, perineum, or anus				
T4	Tumor invades any of the following: bladder mu- cosa, upper part of the urethral mucosa, rectal mu- cosa, or tumor fixed to the bone	*Stage II* T2	N0	M0	Tumor confined to the vulva; more than 2 cm in greatest
		T2	N1	M0	dimension. Nodes are not palpable or are palpable in either groin, not enlarged, mobile (not clinically suspi- cious of neoplasm)
Regional Lymph Nodes (N)					
NX	Regional lymph nodes cannot be assessed				
N0	No nodes palpable	*Stage III*			
N1	Nodes palpable in either groin, not enlarged, mobile (not clinically suspicious of neoplasm)	T3	N0	M0	Tumor of any size with
		T3	N1	M0	(1) Adjacent spread to the
		T3	N2	M0	lower urethra and/or the
		T1	N2	M0	vagina, the perineum, or
N2	Nodes palpable in either groin, enlarged, firm and mobile (clinically suspicious of neoplasm)	T2	N2	M0	the anus, and/or (2) nodes palpable in either one or both groins (en-
N3	Fixed or ulcerated nodes				larged, firm, and mobile, not fixed but clinically suspicious of neoplasm)
Distant Metastasis (M)					
MX	Presence of distant metastasis cannot be assessed	*Stage IV*			
		T4	N0	M0	Tumor of any size
M0	No clinical metastasis	T4	N1	M0	(1) infiltrating the bladder
M1a	Palpable deep pelvic lymph nodes	T4	N2	M0	mucosa and/or the upper part of the urethral mu- cosa and/or the rectal
M1b	Other distant metastases				mucosa and/or
		Any T	Any N	M1a	(2) fixed to the bone or other
		Any T	Any N	M1b	distant metastases, and/or
		Any T	N3	M0	(3) fixed or ulcerated nodes either one or both groins

From American Joint Committee on Cancer: Manual for staging cancer, ed 4, Chicago, 1992, The Committee.

tomycin C, 5-FU, and cisplatin in combination with radiation therapy in the treatment of women with advanced disease.[3,13,19,24] See box on p. 193.

PROGNOSIS

Survival of patients with vulvar cancer is associated with the stage of disease at diagnosis and more spe- cifically the status of pelvic lymph nodes. Survival for patients with Stages I and II range from 90% to 98%.

If nodes were negative, regardless of stage, survival rates range from 69% to 100%. A marked decrease in survival (21% to 53%) is noted for patients with pos- itive nodes.[8]

VAGINAL CANCER

EPIDEMIOLOGY

Carcinoma of the vagina accounts for approximately 2% of all gynecologic cancers. The disease, preinvasive and invasive, occurs primarily in the fifth and sixth decades of life, respectively. Incidence rates have been declining with the use of screening cytology for cervical disease and development of more rigid diagnostic criteria for vagina carcinoma.[3,8,13] However, 300 deaths related to vaginal cancer were estimated for 1993.[1]

ETIOLOGY AND RISK FACTORS

The etiology of vaginal cancer is unknown. However, prior radiation to a field including the vagina, DES exposure in utero, and increasing age, place a woman at higher risk for the disease.[8,13,19]

PREVENTION, SCREENING, AND DETECTION
Prevention and Screening

No recommendations for the prevention and screening of women for vaginal cancers exist. However, a thorough physical examination including inspection and palpation of the vaginal tissues, cervical cytology, and bimanual examination should be done routinely as part of a gynecologic examination for women who are sexually active or 18 years of age or older.

Detection

Many women with vaginal carcinoma are asymptomatic. Detection of preinvasive and invasive lesions is accomplished by thorough inspection of the vaginal tissues, colposcopic examination, and palpation of the tissues along the length of the vaginal wall. Preinvasive lesions of the vagina may only be visualized by colposcopic examination that reveals areas of whitened tissues or atypical vascular patterns. Lesions occur most commonly on the posterior wall and the upper third of the vagina.[3,8,13,19,24]

CLASSIFICATION

The majority of carcinomas of the vagina are squamous cell cancers (93% to 97%). Other cell types include clear cell carcinomas associated with exposure to DES in utero, malignant melanomas, and sarcomas.[13]

CLINICAL FEATURES

Symptomatic women with vaginal cancer present with one or more of the following symptoms: abnormal perimenopausal, postmenopausal, or postcoital vaginal bleeding, dyspareunia, and foul-smelling vaginal discharge. With advanced disease, changes in patterns of urination and pelvic pain may occur. See box on p. 193.

DIAGNOSIS AND STAGING

Diagnosis of preinvasive and invasive carcinoma of the vagina is made by biopsy. Usually, the biopsy can be obtained in the outpatient setting.

Staging is done clinically based on inspection of the vagina, and palpation of pelvic structures on rectovaginal, bimanual examination. The clinician pays special attention to the location and size of the primary lesion. Metastatic disease is assessed by review of findings from laboratory and radiographic studies including biochemical profile, chest x-ray, intravenous pyelogram, barium enema, cystoscopy, and proctoscopy. MRI, CT, and lymphangiography may be used to rule out metastatic disease.[3,8,13] The FIGO staging system for carcinoma of the vagina is presented in Table 11-5.

METASTASIS

Squamous cell carcinoma of the vagina spreads primarily by direct extension to adjacent tissues including the urethra, bladder, rectum, parametria, and the pelvic side wall. In addition, spread can occur through extensive lymphatic channels surrounding the vagina and can extend to the rectal, pelvic, para-aortic, and femoral lymph nodes.

Other types of vaginal cancer have a greater tendency to spread through the lymphatic and hematogenous routes. Frequent sites of metastasis include the supraclavicular nodes and lungs.[3,8,13]

TREATMENT MODALITIES

Treatment of vaginal neoplasia is based on the stage of disease and general health status of the woman. For women with premalignant lesions of the vagina, local excision, CO_2 laser, or topical chemotherapy (5-FU) may be used for primary treatment. Partial or total vaginectomy may be done for treatment of women with multifocal disease involving more than a single portion or the full length of the vagina. Radiation therapy for treatment of preinvasive vaginal neoplasia is reserved for women who are poor surgical candidates.[3,8,13]

Surgery

Surgery is recommended as treatment for women with early stage disease (stage I). Based on the location, size, and extent of the lesion, a total hysterectomy, radical hysterectomy, partial vaginectomy and pelvic lymphadenectomy, or in very selected cases anterior or posterior exenteration (Figure 11-5) may be recommended. Surgery may also be recommended for women who have locally recurrent disease following primary treatment with radiation therapy.

Radiation Therapy

Because of the proximity of the bladder and rectum as well as the potential for local and regional lymph node metastasis, radiation therapy alone or in combination with surgery is recommended as treatment for women with stage II and higher carcinoma of the

Table 11–5　Staging Classification for Vaginal Cancer

Primary Tumor (T)		
TNM	*FIGO*	*Definition*
TX		Primary tumor cannot be assessed
T0		No evidence of primary tumor
Tis	0	Carcinoma in situ
T1	I	Tumor confined to vagina
T2	II	Tumor invades paravaginal tissues but not to pelvic wall
T3	III	Tumor extends to pelvic wall
T4	IVa	Tumor invades mucosa of bladder or rectum and/or extends beyond the true pelvis
M1	IVb	Distant metastasis

Regional Lymph Nodes (N)

NX　Regional lymph nodes cannot be assessed
N0　No regional lymph node metastasis

Upper two thirds of vagina:
N1　Pelvic lymph node metastasis

Lower one third of vagina:
N1　Unilateral inguinal lymph node metastasis
N2　Bilateral inguinal lymph node metastasis

Distant Metastasis (M)		
TNM	*FIGO*	*Definition*
MX		Presence of distant metastasis cannot be assessed
M0		No distant metastasis
M1	IVb	Distant metastasis

Stage Grouping

Stage	T	N	M
Stage 0	Tis	N0	M0
Stage I	T1	N0	M0
Stage II	T2	N0	M0
Stage III	T1	N1	M0
	T2	N1	M0
	T3	N0, N1	M0
Stage IVA	T1	N2	M0
	T2	N2	M0
	T3	N2	M0
	T4	Any N	M0
Stage IVB	Any T	Any N	M1

From American Joint Committee on Cancer: Manual for staging cancer, ed 4, Chicago, 1992, The Committee.

vagina. Teletherapy with or without brachytherapy may be used.[8,13]

Chemotherapy

The results of chemotherapy in treating women with advanced or recurrent vaginal carcinomas, including clear cell and melanoma, have been disappointing. Cisplatin, 5-FU, vincristine, cyclophosphamide, and doxorubicin have been used as single agents and in combined protocols with minimal response rates. More promising results have occurred with chemotherapy used to treat women with vaginal sarcomas and endodermal sinus tract tumors.[8]

PROGNOSIS

A marked improvement in the survival rates in patients with vaginal cancer has occurred in the past 3 decades. Survival at 5 years after diagnosis for all stages ranges from 42% to 56%. The most promising results occur in women who have been diagnosed with stage I (65% to 100%) and stage II (42% to 75%) disease.[8]

FALLOPIAN TUBE CANCER
EPIDEMIOLOGY

Cancer of the fallopian tubes accounts for only 0.1% of all cancers of the female reproductive system. The disease occurs in women 19 to 80 years of age, with the majority of women being diagnosed between 40 and 65 years of age. Fallopian tube carcinoma occurs in both tubes in 5% to 31% of women diagnosed with the disease.[8,13]

ETIOLOGY AND RISK FACTORS

The etiology of cancer of the fallopian tubes is unknown. Researchers have hypothesized that chronic inflammation of the tubes and tubal tuberculosis may contribute to the development of the disease. However, the number of cases of fallopian tube cancer is so small, meaningful data with respect to etiology and risk factors are limited.[8,13]

PREVENTION, SCREENING, AND DETECTION
Prevention and Screening

Currently, no recommendations are made specifically for the prevention and screening of women for cancer of the fallopian tubes. However, as the pelvic examination is done for screening for other gynecologic malignancies, the clinician must always be alert to the possibility of a pelvic mass being cancer of the fallopian tube. The presence of persistent positive cervical cytology in a woman without evidence of cervical, endometrial, or vaginal cancers should alert the clinician to the possibility of cancer of the fallopian tube.[3,8,13]

Detection

Clinical examination is done to detect the presence of ascites and a pelvic mass. A pelvic mass is palpable in over 50% of women with fallopian tube cancer.[3,8,13] Since fallopian tube carcinoma is rare and symptoms and clinical findings are similar to ovarian carcinoma, the diagnosis is rarely made prior to surgery.

CLASSIFICATION

Adenocarcinoma is the most common histologic type of cancer of the fallopian tube. Sarcomas, mixed mesodermal tumors, lymphomas, hydatidiform moles, and choriocarcinoma have also been reported. As the number of cases of carcinoma of the fallopian tube is so small, the clinical significance of both histology and grade of the tumor is unknown.[8,13]

CLINICAL FEATURES

The postmenopausal women may present with symptoms of vaginal bleeding; intermittent, colicky, dull, aching pain; and profuse, watery, vaginal discharge. If the tumor is large, pressure or a sense of heaviness on the bladder or rectum may be reported. In women with metastatic disease, ascites may be present and the woman may complain of abdominal fullness and pressure. See box on p. 193.

DIAGNOSIS AND STAGING

Diagnosis of fallopian tube carcinoma is made at the time of surgery for definitive treatment of a pelvic mass. Since the disease has a pattern of spread much like that of ovarian cancer, a similar surgical approach is recommended. Although many clinicians use the FIGO system for ovarian cancer, no official staging system for cancer of the fallopian tube exists.

METASTASIS

Carcinoma of the fallopian tube metastasizes primarily by direct extension to adjacent tissues and organs, seeding of the abdominal cavity, and lymphatic spread to local and regional nodes. The pattern of metastasis is thought to be related to the site of the primary lesion. For women with lesions in the proximal portion of the tube, metastasis is more likely to occur in the myometrium and endometrium. For women with lesions in the lateral position of the tube,

metastasis is more likely to occur to the ovaries and aortic nodes.

TREATMENT MODALITIES

Surgery, total abdominal hysterectomy, bilateral salpingo-oophorectomy, and omentectomy, is the treatment of choice for fallopian tube carcinoma. Debulking of the tumor burden is the primary goal. For women with residual disease, treatment with interperitoneal radioactive isotopes (P^{32} or Au^{198}), pelvic and/or abdominal teletherapy, or systemic single agent or combination chemotherapy with cyclophosphamide, doxorubicin, progestins, cisplatin, or chlorambucil, is recommended.[3,8,13]

PROGNOSIS

The prognosis for patients with cancer of the fallopian tube is similar to that of patients with ovarian cancer and is related to stage of disease in general and to depth of penetration of the tubal wall, specifically. The survival rate for all stages has been reported as 38%, with the rate as high as 88% in patients with stage I disease. Survival data are not as reliable for fallopian tube cancer as for other gynecologic malignancies because the number of cases is low and treatment varies considerably across published reports.[8]

GESTATIONAL TROPHOBLASTIC DISEASE

EPIDEMIOLOGY

Gestational trophoblastic disease (GTD) can occur with a molar pregnancy or after an abortion, ectopic pregnancy, or normal term delivery. Although the disease accounts for only 1% of all cancers of the female reproductive system in the United States, incidence rates in Asia and South America have been reported as high as 1:120 pregnancies.[8,13]

ETIOLOGY AND RISK FACTORS

GTD includes a variety of tumors that originate in the trophoblastic layer of the chorionic villae during pregnancy. The tumors may range from benign hydatidiform moles to locally invasive moles to choriocarcinomas. Although the etiology is unknown, empirical data indicate that low protein diets, poverty, and increasing age may contribute to development of the disease.[8,13]

PREVENTION, SCREENING, AND DETECTION
Prevention and Screening

No recommendations for prevention or screening of asymptomatic women for GTD are available.

Detection

The detection of GTD is based on careful review of findings on history, clinical examination, and laboratory studies. Disparities in gestational dates, uterine size, and hCG levels are keys to the early detection of GTD.

CLASSIFICATION

GTD is classified morphologically as either hydatidiform moles, invasive moles, or choriocarcinoma. Invasive moles and choriocarcinoma have a higher incidence of metastasis to surrounding tissues and thus carry a poor prognosis.[8,13]

CLINICAL FEATURES

The most common symptom of GTD is vaginal bleeding, particularly during the first trimester. A history of hyperemesis may be reported. Clinical examination reveals enlargement of the uterus in excess of the estimated length of gestation. Fetal heart sounds are absent and fetal parts cannot be palpated. Finally, elevations of the human chorionic gonadatropin (hCG) titers that exceed those found during the course of a normal pregnancy and postpartum period should alert the clinician to the possibility of the disease.[8,13] See box on p. 193.

DIAGNOSIS AND STAGING

Diagnosis of GTD is confirmed by tissue examination from expulsion of grape-like villi, vaginal bleeding, or evacuation of tissues from the uterus. Clinical examination of the uterus, pelvis, and vagina prior to and during surgery for evidence of metastasis is recommended. The lungs, brain, and liver are evaluated by laboratory and radiographic studies to rule out the presence of metastatic disease.

No uniform system of staging for GTD exists. However, clinicians commonly use a system developed by the New England Trophoblastic Disease Center (Table 11-6).

METASTASIS

Metastasis from GTD occurs primarily by local extension to surrounding tissues of the pelvis or through hematogenous spread. The most common sites of distant metastasis include the lungs, brain, and liver.[8,13]

Table 11–6 Staging Classification for Gestational Trophoblastic Disease

Stage 0	Molar pregnancy
	A. Low risk
	B. High risk
Stage I	Confined to uterine corpus
Stage II	Metastases to pelvis and vagina
Stage III	Metastasis to lung
Stage IV	Distant metastasis

From Goldstein DP and Berkowitz RS: The management of gestational trophoblastic neoplasms, Curr Prob Obstet Gynecol 4(1), 1980.

TREATMENT MODALITIES

Treatment of GTD is based on the staging. For women with local disease, surgery is the primary treatment. For women at high risk or with invasive disease and metastasis, a combination of surgery, chemotherapy, and radiation therapy may be used.

Surgery

Surgery, including evacuation of the uterus and dilatation and curettage, is the primary treatment for women with hydatidiform moles. Surgery, including hysterectomy, also plays a role in the treatment of women with other types of GTD. Radical surgery has not been shown to be beneficial in terms of increasing survival rates.

Chemotherapy

Treatment with antineoplastic agents is used for women with hydatidiform moles who have a plateau or elevation of weekly B-hCG titers postevacuation or the development of metastatic disease and for women with invasive moles or choriocarcinoma who present with metastatic disease. The most effective agents include methotrexate, with or without leucovorin rescue, actinomycin D, and chlorambucil. Salvage treatment with combination drug regimens including methotrexate, cisplatin, vincristine or vinblastine, bleomycin, and etoposide has been recommended.[3,8,13]

Radiation Therapy

Radiation therapy also plays a role in the treatment of women with metastatic disease. Women with metastasis to the brain or elevated levels of hCG in the spinal fluid receive whole brain radiation. Metastatic lesions to the liver may be treated with radiation therapy.[8,13]

Response to Therapy

Response to treatment is based on serial B-hCG levels. Postevacuation of hydatidiform moles, B-hCG levels are monitored weekly. For approximately 80% of women diagnosed, the levels return to normal and no additional treatment is needed.

For women with metastatic disease, B-hCG levels are evaluated prior to each course of treatment. Once the B-hCG levels have returned to normal and have remained within normal levels for 3 weeks, monitoring at monthly intervals is begun and is continued for 1 year. Current recommendations include measures to prevent pregnancy during the 1-year follow-up period.

PROGNOSIS

Prognosis for patients with GTD is reported based on the percentage of patients that achieve remission with treatment. For patients with nonmetastatic disease, remission (hCG levels within normal range for 3 consecutive weeks) rates with single agent chemotherapy range from 90% to 100%. Remission rates for patients with metastatic disease are related to the site(s) of metastasis. With combined chemotherapy and radiation therapy, patients with metastatic disease to the lungs or vagina had higher remission rates (74%) than those with metastatic disease at other sites.[8]

Text continued on p. 219.

Nursing Management

Women at risk or with a diagnosis of gynecologic malignancy present a range of challenges to the nurse. Prevention, screening, and early detection activities are nursing interventions that have the potential to improve both survival and quality of survival for these women.

Counseling on healthy life-style choices that can reduce cancer risks, teaching and valuing the importance of routine gynecologic surveillance and care including self-examination skills, Pap smear, and bimanual pelvic examination, and educating women about the early signs and symptoms of gynecologic cancers are critical elements of the role the nurse plays in prevention and early detection. Specific content for a teaching plan for women at risk for selected gynecologic malignancies is presented in the box below and on p. 213.

Throughout the diagnostic phase, the nurse becomes an advocate and resource for the woman and her significant others. The nurse is responsible for instruction on the rationale for, procedures involved in, and sensations experienced during diagnostics and pre-test and post-test care. The nurse also assumes a role in listening to concerns that the woman and her significant others may have about the requirements and results of the diagnostic evaluation.

During the treatment phase, the nurse assists the woman in meeting the physical and psychosocial demands imposed by the disease and treatment. In collaboration with the patient, significant others, physician, social worker, physical, respiratory, and occupational therapists, nutritionist, and chaplain, the nurse develops and coordinates implementation of a plan of care designed to provide a safe environment, minimize the incidence of complications from disease and/or treatment, monitor for signs and symptoms of complications of the disease and/or treatment, promote independence in self-care, include significant others in the plan of care, and promote coping strategies that foster self-worth and a positive self-concept.* Elements common to the nursing care of patients receiving surgery, radiation therapy, chemotherapy, biotherapy, and bone marrow transplantation are included in Chapters 20, 21, 22, 23, and 24, respectively.

Women facing gynecologic cancers have the potential to experience many common responses to the disease and treatment. Structural changes in anatomy resulting from surgery and/or radiation therapy for gynecologic cancers may result in altered sexuality patterns. Nursing care for patients experiencing this problem is detailed in the box on p. 214.

Aggressive treatment and progressive disease place the patient at risk for complications. Common complications associated with progressive disease include altered bowel elimination related to obstruction, fluid volume excess:ascites related to intraabdominal metastasis, and fluid volume excess: lymphedema related to blacked lymphatic channels. Nursing care for patients experiencing these problems is focused on maintaining safety, comfort, and mobility. Specific nursing assessments and interventions for each problem are presented in the boxes on p. 215.

Aggressive treatment for gynecologic cancers carries increased risks of complications. Since the bladder and bowel lie in proximity to the female reproductive system, altered bowel and urinary elimination related to treatment may result. Problems experienced include decreased sensation to defecate or void, enteritis, cystitis, and fistula formation. Nursing assessments and interventions to address these problems are described in the boxes on pp. 216 and 217. Radical surgery and radiation therapy, particularly involving the vulva, may result in impaired skin integrity. Nurs-

---

PRIORITIES OF PATIENT TEACHING

Prevention, screening, and detection practices for all the gynecologic cancers; disease symptomology (cervical, endometrial, ovarian, vaginal, vulvar, fallopian and gestational trophoblastic disease); treatment modalities with the pertinent side effects; discuss purpose, rationale, potential schedule, monitoring of blood counts, wound management, bowel and bladder elimination, self-care management, signs of infection (fever, chills, erythema, bleeding, drainage with odor), and sexual dysfunction issues (infertility, sterility, libido, intercourse)

---

*References 2, 5, 6, 9, 12, 14, 15, 20-23.

TEACHING PLAN FOR WOMEN AT-RISK FOR GYNECOLOGIC MALIGNANCIES

KNOWLEDGE DEFICIT related to prevention and early detection of gynecologic malignancies

Cervix

Assessments

Assess baseline knowledge of personal risk factors for cervical cancer.

Identify personal risk factors for cervical cancer: Age at onset of sexual activity, number of sexual partners, sexual history of partners, number of pregnancies, history of sexually transmitted diseases, history of cervical dysplasia, method of contraception, genital hygiene measures, history of alcohol or tobacco abuse.

Identify any concerns the woman may have related to personal risks for cervical cancer.

Interventions

Teach advantages of barrier contraception use.

Teach methods to discontinue smoking: "cold" turkey, nicotine patch or gum, I Quit, hypnosis.

Educate woman about the benefits and schedule of routine Pap smears and pelvic examinations.

Review signs and symptoms of cervical cancer: Abnormal menstrual, intramenstrual, or postcoital bleeding; vaginal discharge; pain.

Provide age- and culturally-sensitive written materials about cervical cancer.

Provide a list of community resources for information and services available to women at risk or with a diagnosis of cervical cancer.

Vulva

Assessments

Assess knowledge of personal risk factors for vulvar cancer.

Identify personal risk factors for vulvar cancer: Age, chronic vulvar irritation, concurrent diseases such as hypertension, diabetes, cardiovascular disease, and obesity, history of cervical cancer.

Identify any concerns the woman may have related to personal risks for vulvar cancer.

Interventions

Teach steps of vulvar self-examination: Inspection and palpation.

Encourage woman to report significant changes in the texture, color, or sensations of the vulva to a physician: a lump, pruritus, bleeding, or discharge.

Educate women about the benefits of an annual health examination, including evaluation of the vulva and groins.

Provide age- and culturally-sensitive written materials on vulvar cancer.

Provide a list of community resources for information and services available to women at risk or with a diagnosis of vulvar cancer.

Endometrium

Assessments

Assess baseline knowledge of personal risk factors for endometrial cancer.

Identify personal risk factors for endometrial cancer: Young age at onset of menstruation, menopause after 52 years of age, nulliparity, obesity, history of Stein-Leventhal syndrome, diabetes, or hypertension, family history of breast, colon, or endometrial cancer, and use of exogenous estrogens.

Identify concerns that the woman may have related to personal risks for endometrial cancer.

Interventions

Discuss life-style choices that can reduce endometrial cancer risks: Maintenance of ideal body weight, reduction of fat intake to 30% of total caloric intake.

Describe health promotion activities to screen for endometrial cancer: Annual Pap smear and bimanual pelvic exam, endometrial biopsy in women who are high-risk for endometrial cancer.

Review signs and symptoms of endometrial cancer: Prolonged, excessive, or intramenstrual bleeding in premenopausal women, postmenopausal spotting or bleeding, or a yellow, watery, vaginal discharge.

Provide age- and culturally-sensitive written materials about endometrial cancer.

Provide a list of community resources for information and services available to women at risk or with a diagnosis of endometrial cancer.

Ovary

Assessments

Assess baseline knowledge of personal risk factors for ovarian cancer.

Identify personal risk factors for ovarian cancer: History of infertility, nulliparity, personal or family history of breast, ovarian, colon, or uterine cancer.

Identify concerns that women may have related to personal risks for ovarian cancer.

Interventions

Discuss life-style choices that can reduce ovarian cancer risks: Use of oral contraceptives, serial CA-125s, or vaginal ultrasounds for high-risk women.

Describe health promotion activities to screen for ovarian cancer: Annual bimanual pelvic exam.

Review signs and symptoms of ovarian cancer: Dyspepsia, indigestion, loss of appetite, early satiety, pelvic pressure or discomfort, urinary frequency, increasing abdominal girth, weight loss.

Provide age- and culturally-sensitive written materials about ovarian cancer.

Provide a list of community resources for information and services available to women at risk or with a diagnosis of ovarian cancer.

ALTERED SEXUALITY PATTERNS RELATED TO THE IMPACT OF STRUCTURAL, FUNCTIONAL, AND PSYCHOLOGICAL CHANGES ASSOCIATED WITH TREATMENT FOR GYNECOLOGIC CANCERS

Assessments

Assess woman's and significant other's perception of patient as a sexual being.

Evaluate factors that contribute to woman's self-concept and expression of sexuality.

Identify perceived threats to sexuality imposed by disease and treatment.

Assess factors that may facilitate or hinder adaptation to the structural, functional, and psychological changes resulting from treatment.

Interventions

Review normal anatomy and physiology of the reproductive system with woman and significant other.

Describe strategies recommended for minimizing effects of treatment that can influence sexuality patterns.

Discuss the potential structural, functional, or psychological effects of treatment—surgery, radiation therapy, and/or chemotherapy.

Surgery

Only a small portion of the vagina is resected as a component of either a simple or radical hysterectomy. The edges of the vagina are sutured to form a closed tube. The vagina has the ability to stretch during penile/vaginal intercourse.

Removal of the ovaries results in lack of estrogen. The vaginal tissues may become dry and loose elasticity. Oral estrogen replacement therapy or vaginal estrogen creams may be ordered by the physician unless contraindicated by the presence of a hormone-dependent tumor, i.e., endometrial or breast cancer.

Radiation therapy

Radiation also can affect the vaginal tissues making them thinner, dryer, and less elastic over time. If the woman is not sexually active, vaginal stenosis may occur after radiation therapy.

Teach use of vaginal dilators to prevent vaginal stenosis.

Lubricate dilator with water-based lubricant or estrogen cream.
Insert dilator gradually to the full length of the vagina.
Leave dilator inserted in the vagina for 10 minutes each day.
Remove and wash the dilator thoroughly with soap and water.

Chemotherapy

Common side effects of chemotherapy including hair loss, stomatitis, nausea, vomiting, and fatigue can influence both perceptions of body-image and self-concept as well as the desire for sexual intimacy.

Encourage open discussions about perceptions of body-image and self-concept with health care team and significant others.

Encourage patient to assume an active role in decision-making about care.

Recognize incremental achievements in progress toward patient outcome goals.

Recommend participation in American Cancer Society's Look Good, Feel Better program.

Encourage open discussions with patient and partner about potential effects of treatment on sexuality patterns.

Teach patient and partner strategies to re-explore pleasurable experiences during intimacy.

Suggest increasing the length of time for foreplay to allow for adequate vaginal lubrication.

Suggest use of vaginal water-based lubricant or vaginal estrogen cream.

Describe sexual positions that provide the woman with more control over the depth of penetration.

Discuss benefits of engaging in sexual behaviors that require minimal energy (hugging, kissing, closeness) and that are initiated when well rested.

Recommend a schedule for resuming sexual activity.

Review signs and symptoms of altered sexuality patterns to be reported to the health care team: Feelings of decreased self-worth, negative feelings about body-image or self-concept, any changes in expression of sexuality that are not satisfying or pleasurable to self or partner.

Evaluate the impact of disease, treatment, and effectiveness of suggestions in maintaining a satisfactory sexuality pattern.

Refer for sexual counseling if problems persist.

FLUID VOLUME EXCESS: ASCITES RELATED TO INTRA-ABDOMINAL METASTASIS

Assessments

Assess weight and abdominal girth daily.

Assess condition of skin over the abdomen, buttocks, bony prominences, and back for changes in color, temperature, or texture.

Evaluate the effect of ascites on level of comfort, mobility, respiratory effort, and activities of daily living.

Interventions

Position patient with head elevated 30 to 90 degrees to allow for maximum respiratory expansion with minimal effort.

Monitor intake and output ratio each day.

Assist patient with activities of daily living as needed.

Encourage wearing loose clothing around the trunk and abdomen: Larger size bra, bikini-cut panties, pantyhose made for pregnant women.

Encourage compliance with low-salt diet.

Monitor for signs and symptoms of respiratory or gastrointestinal distress that requires medical intervention: Marked shortness of breath, protracted nausea or vomiting, acute changes in pattern of pain.

Provide supportive care as physician performs palliative paracentesis:

Instruct patient in terms of what will be involved in the procedure, what sensations may be experienced during and after the procedure, and elements of postprocedure care.

Position patient in comfortable position.

Administer any premedications ordered for anxiety.

Measure the amount of ascitic fluid removed and prepare specimen for laboratory as ordered.

Monitor subjective (pain, relief of shortness of breath) and objective responses (blood pressure, pulse, respirations) of the patient to the procedure.

Observe site post procedure for continued drainage, discharge, redness, pain, or warmth.

FLUID VOLUME EXCESS: LYMPHEDEMA RELATED TO BLOCKED LYMPHATIC CHANNELS

Assessments

Assess for predisposing factors that could contribute to the occurrence of lymphedema of the lower extremities: Concurrent cardiac, renal, or liver disease, previous lymphadenectomy or radiation therapy of pelvic nodes, diet

Assess pattern of lymphedema: Onset, location, aggravating and alleviating factors.

Evaluate impact of lymphedema on life style, comfort, skin integrity, and activities of daily living.

Evaluate serial measurements, presence on peripheral pulses, and range of motion of the affected extremities.

Interventions

Protect the affected extremity: Wear loose, protective clothing, avoid restrictive jewelry, irritants, and temperature extremes.

Avoid invasive procedures to the affected extremity.

Elevate the extremity as much as possible.

Monitor for and report changes in the color, temperature, intactness of skin over the affected extremity, and quality of peripheral pulses to the physician.

Consult physical therapy to evaluate the use of compression equipment and to develop a program of exercise to maintain range of motion in the extremity.

ALTERED BOWEL ELIMINATION RELATED TO DISEASE OR TREATMENT FOR GYNECOLOGICAL CANCERS

Assessments

Assess characteristics of the stool: Amount, consistency, odor, and color.

Assess bowel elimination patterns: Frequency, presence of constipation, diarrhea, pain with defecation, or incontinence.

Identify factors that contribute to bowel elimination patterns: Dietary intake, fluid intake, activity level, medication history

Interventions

Discuss changes that may occur in bowel elimination patterns after surgery or radiation therapy: Adhesions with bowel obstruction, decreased sensation of need to defecate, radiation enteritis, or rectovaginal fistula.

Surgery

Women treated with hysterectomy or radical hysterectomy will note decreased bowel function postoperatively due to manipulation of the bowel during surgery. The bowel is kept at rest postoperatively by avoiding oral fluid and food intake until bowel sounds return. Flatulence is common and may be uncomfortable. Attention to the pattern of bowel elimination is necessary in the first weeks postsurgery to minimize the risk of constipation associated with use of pain medication, changes in fluid and food intake, and inactivity.

Instituted bowel regimen as ordered by physician prior to surgery to cleanse the bowel of stool.

Encourage strategies to stimulate bowel function: Walking, heating pads, and bowel stimulants.

Monitor bowel sounds every 8 hours.

Instruct patient to notify team of presence of flatulence or passage of stool.

For women undergoing a total or posterior pelvic exenteration, a bowel diversion will be constructed.

Instruct the patient in skills to evaluate the condition of the stoma, application of collection devices, care of the peristomal skin, and irrigation techniques

Teach critical changes in the character of the stool, condition of stoma or peristomal skin, or functioning of the diversion to report to the health care team.

Radiation therapy

The most common immediate side effect of radiation therapy to the bowel is diarrhea.

Observe for signs and symptoms of dehydration.

Assess the condition of the perianal and perineal skin.

Teach women elements of good perineal hygiene after each bowel movement: Cleanse the area with water, pat area dry thoroughly, apply barrier cream as needed to maintain skin integrity.

Instruct in dietary changes to increase bulk of stool: Avoid fresh fruits and vegetables.

Administer antidiarrheals as ordered by the physician.

Long-term effects of radiation therapy on the bowel include radiation enteritis and rectovaginal fistula formation.

Place the bowel at rest.

Instruct in dietary changes to increase bulk of stool: Avoid fresh fruits and vegetables.

Administer antidiarrheals as ordered by the physician.

Administer anti-inflammatory agents to decrease inflammation in the bowel.

Teach significant changes to be reported to the health care team: Blood in stool, marked increase in the volume of diarrhea, symptoms of dehydration, or passage of stool from the vagina.

Progressive disease

Bowel obstruction is a common symptom of progressive disease.

Monitor of signs of bowel obstruction: Colicky, cramping, lower abdominal pain, alternating diarrhea and constipation, abdominal distention, vomiting, hyperactive, high-pitched bowel sounds above the obstruction and absent bowel sounds below the obstruction.

Prepare patient for nasogastric tube as ordered by the physician.

Report significant changes in character of symptoms that indicate need for immediate medical attention: increase in severity of pain, decrease in abdominal girth, rebound tenderness, and acute absence of bowel sounds.

ALTERED URINARY ELIMINATION RELATED TO DISEASE OR TREATMENT FOR GYNECOLOGIC CANCERS

Assessments

Assess urinary elimination patterns prior to initiation of treatment: Frequency, nocturia, incontinence

Identify factors that contribute to urinary elimination patterns: Volume and timing of fluid intake, concurrent diseases such as diabetes, medications

Interventions

Discuss changes that may occur as a result of surgery or radiation therapy: Decreased sensation to void, incomplete emptying of the bladder, cystitis, and vesicovaginal fistula formation

Surgery

After hysterectomy or radical hysterectomy innervation to the bladder may be damaged. Decreased sensation of need to void and incontinence are common effects. A suprapubic catheter is usually placed after surgery. Bladder retraining occurs with the catheter in place until residual urines of <50 cc are achieved after voiding.

Encourage to drink as much fluid as possible

Limit fluid intake after 7:00 PM

Establish a regular schedule for voiding.

For women undergoing a total or anterior pelvic exenteration, a urinary diversion will be constructed.

Teach skills to evaluate the condition of the stoma, application of collection devices, care of the peristomal skin.

Discuss critical changes in the character of the urine, condition of stoma or peristomal skin, or functioning of the diversion to report to the health care team.

Radiation therapy

The primary short-term effect of radiation on bladder tissues include radiation cystitis. Frequency, dysuria, and bleeding are common symptoms.

Encourage a daily fluid intake of 3000 cc.

Consult the physician to order medications to minimize discomfort.

Reassure patient that symptoms will improve with time.

The primary long-term effect of radiation therapy is weakening of the tissues between the vagina and bladder and formation of a fistula. Depending on the size of the fistula, urine may leak or flow through the vagina. Approaches to treatment range from catheter placement to surgical repair.

Institute care strategies to keep patient dry: Pouching, indwelling catheter, protective clothing.

Teach perineal care measures: Rinse perineum thoroughly with warm water after each voiding, pat area dry, apply skin barrier as ordered.

Monitor condition of perineal skin daily.

Review signs and symptoms of alteration in urinary elimination to report to the health care team: Frequency, pain, changes in the amount or character of the urine, inability to void, or passage of urine through the vagina.

---

ing care designed to address the needs of the patient receiving treatment for impaired skin integrity related to treatment of the vulva is presented in a box on p. 218.

Women with gynecologic cancers are often faced with adjusting to significant structural, functional, and cosmetic changes as a result of the disease and/or treatment. The nurse assumes a key role in addressing rehabilitation concerns that may range from care of ostomies resulting from pelvic exenteration, sexual counseling (Chapter 31), health maintenance issues (box on p. 218), and psychological concerns (Chapter 30). In collaboration with others on the

health care team, identification of rehabilitation needs for both the woman and her significant others and referral to appropriate rehabilitation services and agencies can occur. Potential agencies include the United Ostomy Association, National Coalition for Cancer Survivorship, American Cancer Society, and the National Lymphedema Network. Women can be encouraged to participate in support programs or groups such as CanSurmount. The nurse also plays an important continuous role in long-term evaluation of the success of rehabilitative efforts. See boxes on pp. 193 and 206.

IMPAIRED SKIN INTEGRITY RELATED TO SURGERY OR RADIATION THERAPY FOR TREATMENT OF VULVAR CANCER

Assessments

Assess the skin over the vulva, perineum, gluteal folds, and groin areas prior to initiation of treatment.

Evaluate for factors that predispose the woman to impaired skin integrity: Presence of diabetes, obesity, and age.

Assess steps in routine perineal hygiene measures.

Evaluate perceived and actual ability (skill and range of motion) of the patient to provide self-care during treatment.

Intervention

Discuss potential structural and functional effects of treatment of cancer of the vulva with surgery (wound breakdown) and radiation therapy (erythema, dry to moist desquamation).

Develop a plan of care to minimize risks of side effects of treatment.

Surgery

Wounds from a radical vulvectomy are difficult to heal particularly if preoperative radiation therapy has been given. Key elements of wound care for these patients are keeping the wound clean and dry.

Irrigate surgical wounds with one-half strength hydrogen peroxide.

Pack wounds with gauze.

Dry perineum with a hairdryer on the coolest setting.

Use bed cradles and positioning to increase circulation of air to the wound.

Radiation therapy

Tissues of the vulva, perineum, and groin areas are extremely radiosensitive. Erythema often occurs early in the course of therapy and is associated with edema, warmth, and tenderness of the tissues. Moist desquamation occurs later in the course of treatment and is accompanied by marked redness of tissues, serous drainage, and pain. Radiation is usually stopped until changes subside.

Suggest comfort measures such as wearing loose cotton panties or no panties, avoiding pantyhose, using cool compresses to the perineum, and taking pain medications as ordered by the physician.

Recommend measures to keep the tissues clean and dry.

Discourage use of any topical agents other than those recommended by the radiation oncologist.

Review signs and symptoms of infection and skin breakdown that should be reported to the health care team: Redness, increased pain, purulent drainage, foul-smelling discharge, fever, swelling, and ulceration.

ALTERATION IN HEALTH MAINTENANCE RELATED TO LACK OF ENDOGENOUS ESTROGEN IN THE PRESENCE OF AN ESTROGEN/PROGESTERONE DEPENDENT MALIGNANCY

Assessments

Assess lifestyle factors that contribute to health maintenance: Diet, activity, stress reduction techniques.

Assess woman's perception of physical and psychological changes experienced attributed to lack of estrogen.

Evaluate the extent to which changes have a negative impact on quality of life.

Evaluate personal and family history for presence of osteoporosis, cardiac disease, psychiatric problems.

Interventions

Discuss rationale for avoiding estrogen replacement therapy in the presence of an estrogen-progesterone dependent cancer.

Describe potential risks to health maintenance from lack of estrogen: Increased risks of osteoporosis, cardiovascular disease, psychiatric disease, and vasomotor changes.

Instruct in strategies to maintain bone integrity: Diet rich in calcium-containing foods, calcium supplements, regular exercise program, modifications in home environment to decrease risk of falls, periodic evaluation of bone density in high-risk women.

Teach strategies to minimize the risk of cardiovascular disease: Low-fat diet, regular exercise program, periodic evaluation of serum cholesterol and triglyceride levels.

Discuss alternate methods to minimize postmenopausal symptoms: Diet, exercise, and medications such as Bellergal®.

Suggest use of water-based lubricants for vaginal dryness.

Encourage expression of psychological responses to disease and treatment. If depressive symptoms persist or if woman has suicidal ideations, refer to psychologist or psychiatrist for medical management.

CONCLUSION

The specialty of gynecologic oncology has enjoyed some of the most impressive successes in the use of screening, early diagnosis, and treatment techniques to modify the natural history and incidence of selected gynecologic cancers. These successes have resulted in a significant decrease in mortality. Throughout the phases of care, prevention, screening, diagnosis, treatment, and rehabilitation, nurses play a critical role in improving the quantity and quality of survival. Challenges remain, but the rewards are seen in the daily lives of the many survivors of gynecologic cancers. Patients are often faced with adjusting to significant structural, functional, and cosmetic changes as a result of the disease and/or treatment. The nurse assumes a key role in addressing rehabilitation concerns. In collaboration with others on the health care team, identification of rehabilitation needs for both the woman and her significant others and referral to appropriate rehabilitation personnel and services can occur. The nurse also plays an important role in the long-term evaluation of the success of rehabilitative efforts.

Throughout the course of prevention, screening, diagnosis, treatment, and rehabilitation, the focus of nursing care is improving the quantity and quality of survival for women with gynecologic cancers. The challenges are great, but the rewards are seen in the daily lives of the many cancer survivors.

BIBLIOGRAPHY

1. American Cancer Society: Cancer facts & figures—1993. Atlanta, 1993, American Cancer Society.
2. Anderson BL: Psychosexual adjustment following pelvic exenteration, Obstet Gynecol 61(3), 331, 1983.
3. Barber HRK: Manual of gynecologic oncology, ed 2, Philadelphia, 1989, JB Lippincott Co.
4. Cashavelly BJ: Cervical dysplasia: An overview of current concepts in epidemiology, diagnosis, and treatment, Cancer Nurs 10(4):199, 1987.
5. Clark J: Mucous membrane integrity, impairment of: Related to vaginal changes. In McNally JC, Somerville ET, Miaskowski C, and Rostad M, editors: Guidelines for oncology nursing practice, ed 2, Philadelphia, 1991, WB Saunders Co.
6. Clark JC, McGee RF, and Preston R: Nursing management of responses to the cancer experience. In Clark JC and McGee RF, editors: Core curriculum for oncology nursing, Philadelphia, 1992, WB Saunders Co.
7. Davis M: Secondary prevention in oncology nursing practice. In Clark JC and McGee RF, editors: Core curriculum for oncology nursing, Philadelphia, 1992, WB Saunders Co.
8. DiSaia PJ and Creasman WT: Clinical gynecologic oncology, ed 4, St. Louis, 1993, Mosby.
9. Donovan MI and Girton SE: Cancer care nursing, ed 2, Norwalk, CT, 1984, Appleton-Century-Crofts.
10. Fanslow J: Knowledge deficit related to prevention and early detection of cervical and uterine (endometrial) cancer. In McNally JC, Somerville ET, Miaskowski C, and Rostad M, editors: Guidelines for oncology nursing practice, ed 2, Philadelphia, 1991, WB Saunders Co.
11. Flannery M: Reproductive cancers. In Clark JC and McGee RF, editors: Core curriculum for oncology nursing, Philadelphia, 1992, WB Saunders Co.
12. Fleming C, Scanlon C, and D'Agostino NS: A study of the comfort needs of patients with advanced cancer, Cancer Nurs 10(5):237, 1987.
13. Hoskins WJ, Perez C, and Young RC: Gynecologic tumors. In DeVita VT Jr, Hellman S, and Rosenberg SA, editors: Cancer: Principles and practice of oncology, ed 3, Philadelphia, 1989, JB Lippincott Co.
14. Jenkins B: Patients report of sexual changes after treatment for gynecological cancer, Oncol Nurs Forum 15(3):349, 1988.
15. Krouse HG: A psychological model of adjustment in gynecologic cancer patients, Oncol Nurs Forum 12(6):45, 1985.
16. Lamb M: Vulvar cancer: Patient information booklet, Oncol Nurs Forum 13(6):79, 1986.
17. Lovejoy NC: Precancerous lesions of the cervix, Cancer Nursing 10(1):2, 1987.
18. Martin LK and Braly PS: Gynecologic cancers. In Baird SB, McCorkle R, and Grant M, editors: Cancer nursing: A comprehensive textbook, Philadelphia, 1991, WB Saunders Co.
19. Otte DM: Gynecologic cancers. In Groenwald SL, Frogge MH, Goodman M, and Yarbro CH, editors: Cancer nursing: Principles and practice, ed 2, Boston, 1990, Jones and Bartlett Publishers.
20. Richards S and Hiratzka S: Vaginal dilatation post pelvic irradiation: A patient education tool, Oncol Nurs Forum 13(4):89, 1986.
21. Spencer MM: Bowel elimination, alteration in: Diversional methods. In McNally JC, Somerville ET, Miaskowski C, and Rostad M, editors: Guidelines for oncology nursing practice, ed 2, Philadelphia, 1991, WB Saunders Co.
22. Spencer MM: Urinary elimination, alteration in: Diversional methods. In McNally JC, Somerville ET, Miaskowski C, and Rostad M, editors: Guidelines for oncology nursing practice, ed 2, Philadelphia, 1991, WB Saunders Co.
23. Swihart J: Bowel elimination, alteration in: Bowel obstruction. In McNally JC, Somerville ET, Miaskowski C, and Rostad M, editors: Guidelines for oncology nursing practice, ed 2, Philadelphia, 1991, WB Saunders Co.
24. Tombes MB: Gynecologic malignancies. In Baird

SB, Donehower MG, Stalsbroten VL, and Ades TB, editors: A cancer source book for nurses, Atlanta, 1991, American Cancer Society.

25. Young RC, Fuks A, and Hoskins WJ: Cancer of the ovary. In DeVita VT Jr, Hellman S, and Rosenberg SA, editors: Cancer: Principles and practice of oncology, ed 3, Philadelphia, 1989, JB Lippincott Co.

CHAPTER 1 2

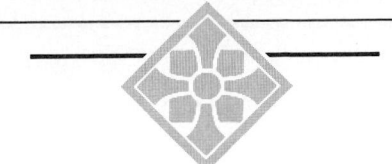

Head and Neck Cancers

Jeanne Parzuchowski

The old adage "a picture is worth a thousand words" is applicable in the treatment and care of patients diagnosed with head and neck cancer. It is the face, even more than the voice, the words we speak, the emotions we keep in or let out, or involuntary and unconscious mannerisms, that presents each one of us to the world. Although not among the five leading causes of death from cancer in the United States, cancers of the head and neck present the patient, family, and professional with a very visible and disabling threat. Left untreated, cancers in this area hold the potential to be disabling and fatal, and, even if treated, a patient may face potential loss of physiologic function, sensory loss, changes in body image, or death. Nurses are faced with significant challenges when providing education and care to these patients and their families and are placed in a unique position to support the patient and family in their adjustment to illness, treatment, and rehabilitation. Because the management of head and neck cancer is such a challenge, nursing care is presented in greater detail in this chapter. Nursing care guidelines are included throughout the chapter for cosmesis, surgery, and radiation therapy.

EPIDEMIOLOGY AND ETIOLOGY

Carcinoma of the upper aerodigestive tract accounts for 5% of all human tumors, with 95% of cases being of squamous cell histology.[11,12,33,34] These tumors typically occur in patients between the ages of 40 and 70 years. The most common sites are the oral cavity and

The author wishes to acknowledge Dr. M-Alsarraf, J.A. Kish, MD, J.E. Ensley, Dr. Richard Arden, Donna Howath, MD, and Jason V. Parzuchowski for support in the writing of this chapter.

the larynx. At the time of diagnosis, the majority of the patients have locally advanced (Stage III and IV) cancer.

The aerodigestive tract serves as a conduit for air, fluid, and food. Therefore, the body is constantly exposed to a broad range of potential carcinogenic agents. The etiologic factors that can produce cancer in the general population in the United States have not been well researched. Occupational exposures have been studied and do correlate positively to head and neck cancer. Various etiologic factors implicated in the incidence of head and neck cancer are summarized in Table 12-1.

PREVENTION, SCREENING, AND DETECTION

Major risk factors for the development of cancer in the oral cavity, pharynx, and larynx include the use of tobacco products (smoked and smokeless) and alcohol. Each factor alone accounts for a twofold or threefold increase in risk; jointly they can increase the risk more than 15 times that experienced by persons who neither smoke nor drink.[71] The primary constituent responsible for oral cancers is thought to be N^1-nitrosonor nicotine, which has tumor promoting properties in animals and is present in cigarette smoke condensate, chewing tobacco, and snuff. The risk factors of alcohol and tobacco have a maximum effect in the oral cavity and oropharynx in the horseshoe-shaped area extending from the anterior floor of the mouth to the tonsillar pillar-retromolar trigone where saliva pools. Precancerous lesions, leukoplakia or erythroplakia, are associated with cancers of the oral cavity, alveolar ridge, gums, and floor of the mouth in people who have dipped or chewed tobacco.[134] Evidence indicates that certain types of human viruses, such as the papilloma virus and herpes simplex virus

Table 12-1   Etiology of Head and Neck Cancer—Specific Sites

Site	Carcinogens	Other Factors
Skin	Inorganic arsenics in drugs, water, or occupational environment Ultraviolet rays of sun, ionizing radiation Polycyclic aromatic hydrocarbons, coke ovens, gas workers Chloroprene (neoprene) in synthetic rubber	Burns Riboflavin deficiency Syphilis—lip
Nose and sinuses	Wood dust (furniture industry) Shoe industry (leather manufacturing) Textile workers Radiochemical (Thorotrast) Radium dial painters and chemists (osteogenic sarcomas) Mustard gas Nickel refining Isoprophyl oil Bcme-bis (chloromethyl) ether-alkylating agent (produces esthesioneuroepithelioma in animals)	?Chronic sinusitis ?Cigarette smoke
Nasopharynx	Nitrosamines (N-nitrosodimethylamine)	Epstein-Barr virus Genetics: Chinese 25 times from Kwantung province Vitamin C deficiency Salted fish
Oral cavity	Cigarettes, reverse smoking Ethyl alcohol Snuff, chewing tobacco, betel nut Textile industries Coke ovens Leather manufacturing	Syphilis—tongue Nutrition: vitamin B, riboflavin deficiencies
Hypopharynx-larynx	Cigarettes Asbestos (ship builders) Mustard gas Polycyclic aromatic hydrocarbons (coke ovens) Ethyl alcohol Wood exposure	Nutrition: riboflavin deficiency
Esophagus	Ethyl alcohol Cigarettes	Nutrition: riboflavin, nitrosamines Race and nationality: Eskimos, Iranians, blacks
Thyroid	Radiation exposure	Iodine deficiencies Genetics
Salivary glands	Radiation	Genetics: Eskimos

Modified from Jesse TC: Etiology of head and neck cancer. In Suen JW and Myers EN, editors: Cancer of head and neck, New York, 1981, Churchill Livingstone.

(HSV), may be involved in the development of cancers in the aerodigestive tract.[76,91] Cancers of the thyroid have been found to occur more frequently in persons who received small doses of radiation therapy 20 years ago for acne, chronic tonsillitis, enlarged thymus, or middle ear disease. Ten percent of patients diagnosed with head and neck cancer develop a second malignancy.[63,115,147,165] Second or third primary cancers are common (e.g., esophagus, lung) and are explained by the concept of a diffuse mucosal atypia called "field cancerization." This concept poses that once mucosal surfaces of the upper aerodigestive tract have undergone changes (initiation, promotion, and proliferation), changes in surrounding tissues remains different. A small percentage of patients neither smoke nor drink: the risk factors in this group are unknown.

CLASSIFICATION

Carcinomas arising in the head and neck region are classified according to anatomic regions rather than cell type. These regions include: (1) nasal cavity, (2) nasopharynx, (3) oral cavity, (4) oropharynx, (5) larynx, and (6) hypopharynx. Each of these regions is subdivided into specific sites (Figure 12-1 and Table 12-2). The tumor characteristics of each area, therapeutic management, and results may differ depending on the natural history of the disease, the sites of metastases, and the biologic behavior of the disease.

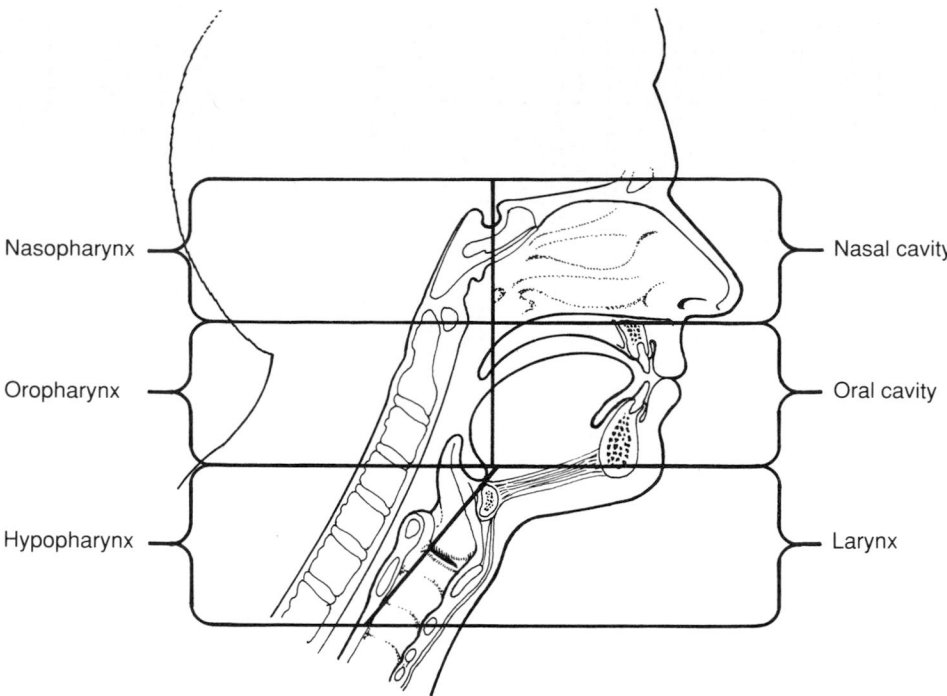

Figure 12–1   Regions of head and neck.

DIAGNOSIS

All patients should undergo a thorough oral and head and neck examination. Specified x-rays should be completed before obtaining a biopsy. A biopsy can alter the mucosa and bone detail and can cause the radiologist to misinterpret the film. The patient may undergo an incisional biopsy or triple endoscopy (laryngoscopy, flexible esophagoscopy, and bronchoscopy) with multiple biopsies.[154,165] The essential element in head and neck staging is the physician's documentation including a precise diagram and written description of the extent of the disease, to provide all consulting disciplines with accurate data.

STAGING

Head and neck tumors are classified by the American Joint Committee for Cancer Staging and End Results Reporting. Patient information that affects clinical staging of head and neck tumors is listed in the box at right. Head and neck T classifications are a general indication of the extent of the primary tumor. Additionally, these T classifications can be subclassified according to how the tumor affects other anatomic sites. Tumors of the oral cavity and lip are classified primarily by the T stage of the lesion. Cancer staging of tumors of the pharynx (nasopharynx, oropharynx, hypopharynx), larynx, and paranasal sinuses is determined by the extent of the primary tumor, depth of tumor invasion, and the number of sites involved. The depth of invasion can significantly affect normal

---

PATIENT INFORMATION NEEDED FOR STAGING HEAD AND NECK TUMORS

Facts about the tumor
- Exact location
- Histologic type
- Estimated degree of local invasion
- Local behavior (e.g., exophytic or invasive)
- Cytologic grade
- Involvement of other structures

Local lymph node involvement
- Location of all suspicious nodes (unilateral/bilateral)
- Size
- Firmness

Distant metastases
- Organ system involved
- Degree of tumor replacement

Presence or absence of second cancer

---

function and mobility of involved and neighboring structures such as in the hypopharyngeal, laryngeal region, where the tumor may invade bone or affect cranial nerves as in nasopharyngeal cancer. The N classifications indicate location (unilateral or bilateral), number, and size of cervical lymph node metastasis and is uniform for all sites. M classifications, which indicate distant spread of disease, are determined by clinical and radiographic findings.[12,77,135] In

Table 12-2 Major Subdivisions of Aerodigestive Tract

Site	Function	Anatomic Relationship	Clinical Features
Oral cavity	Maintain oral competency for swallowing, articulation	Sensory motor innervation of tongue is bilateral. Central chamber of the salivary system. Sensory innervation mediated by lingual nerve (V). Motor innervation to muscles by hypoglossal nerve (XII). Lymphatic drainage to the submaxillary and upper cervical lymph nodes and retropharyngeal lymph nodes	Early symptoms: painless "white spot," persistent ulcerations, difficulty with denture fit, difficulty swallowing, blood-tinged sputum
Oropharynx	Mouth and pharynx perform together in alimentary functions of swallowing, emesis, and respiratory functions of crying, speaking, coughing, and yawning	Boundaries include the soft palate, tonsils, tonsillar fossa, base of tongue. The glossopharyngeal nerve (IX) mediates the motor and sensory innervation to the pharynx and posterior one third of tongue. Soft palate and pharynx innervated by vagus nerve (X). Lymphatic drainage to the jugulodigastric (tonsillar) node, retropharyngeal lymph nodes	Irregular ulcerations of the mucosal surfaces, painless growth, dysphagia, pain on swallowing, otalgia, persistent sore throat Late symptoms: speech difficulties, palatal resultant incompetence with nasal regurgitation, dysphagia with or without aspiration, trismus
Nasal cavity	Conditions inspired air before entrance—olfaction humidification, temperature control, cleansing, antibacterial and antiviral protection	First cranial nerve (olfactory) innervates the mucous membranes to mediate a sense of smell Drain into submandibular nodes	Similar to chronic sinusitis
Nasopharynx	Anatomic boundary that lies behind nasal cavities and above the soft palate	Open space situated just below the base of the skull behind the nasal cavity. Inferior wall is bordered by soft palate, pharyngeal orifice of eustachian tube, abducen nerve (VI), oculomotor nerve (III), trochlear nerve (IV), optic nerve (II). Behind eustachian tube lies the internal carotid artery, internal jugular vein, and glossopharyngeal (IX), vagus (X), spinal accessory (X), and hypoglossal (XII) nerves Lymph node chain that drains these areas: posterior cervical triangles, supraclavicular nodes, jugular chain	Persistent poorly localized frontal headaches; temporal, parietal, orificial pain; decreased hearing, tinnitus; multiple nerve palsies, sensory losses Blood in a postnasal drip very significant Profuse epistaxis is an infrequent presenting symptom

	Function	Anatomy	Signs and symptoms
Paranasal sinuses	Air-filled cavities within the bones of the skull lined by mucous membranes that drain into the nasal cavities	Four pair/maxillary, ethmoid, frontal sphenoid tumors drain into submaxillary, retropharyngeal, jugular lymph nodes	Chronic sinusitis, bump on the hard palate, swelling, numbness and/or pain of the cheek, swelling gums, toothache, increased lacrimation, visual changes — diplopia exophthalmus. Persistent unilateral rhinorrhea — epistaxis
Hypopharynx	Anatomic boundary extending from the tip of the epiglottis to the lower border of the cricoid cartilage. Structures are important for swallowing, airway protection	Lower subdivision of oropharynx also called laryngopharynx divided into (1) pyriform sinuses, (2) posterior cricoid area; posterior and lateral pharyngeal walls. Pharyngeal constrictions innervated by glossopharyngeal (IX) and vagus (X) nerves. Lymphatic drainage — primary along internal jugular vein, retropharyngeal and paratracheal nodes.	Painless enlarged cervical lymph nodes. Odynophagia accompanied with progressive dysphagia and rapid weight loss. Otalgia on same side of tumor. Hoarseness, dysphagia
Larynx	Serves for speech production, maintaining airway, airway protection	Located directly below hypopharynx; sensory innervation supplied from the internal laryngeal branch of superior laryngeal nerve of vagus and recurrent laryngeal nerve. Divided into three anatomic sites: (1) supraglottic, (2) glottic, and (3) subglottic. Lymph drainage to anterior jugular nodes	Persistent hoarseness; change in quality, pitch, voice; pain; hemoptysis; dysphagia; cough; aspiration
Salivary glands	Production of saliva	Divided into major glands — paired parotid, submandibular, sublingual, and minor salivary glands. Lymphatic drainage usually to the deep jugular or intraglandular or paraglandular lymph nodes; innervation of this area includes mandibular branch of 7th cranial, lingual, and hypoglossal nerve (XII)	Painless, rapidly growing mass with or without associated nerve paralysis
Thyroid gland	Endocrine gland	Highly vascular gland located in the anterior and lower part of neck. Composed of a small central part, isthmus, and two lobes; isthmus covers second, third, and fourth tracheal rings; thyroid related medially to the esophagus and recurrent laryngeal nerve and laterally to the carotid sheath, containing the carotid artery; internal jugular vein and vagus nerve. Lymphatic drainage of the thyroid gland mainly by the lymphatic vessels that accompany the arterial blood supply	Neck pain tightness or fullness in the neck, hoarseness, dysphagia, dyspnea

the concept of the greater the T size the greater the stage, increased extension/invasion results in a greater stage; increased stage of disease is directly related to a poorer prognosis.

PRETREATMENT EVALUATION
Rationale for Treatment Options

The therapeutic measures available for the management of head and neck cancer include surgery, radiation therapy, and chemotherapy. Treatment modalities may be used alone or in combinations. Surgery or radiation therapy is used as standard treatments for patients with very early limited or advanced resectable head and neck cancers. The ultimate goal of all head and neck therapy is patient survival and quality of life. Treatments may be given in an attempt to achieve cure, control, or palliation. If the goal is cure, then treatment focuses on local control of the disease and prolonged relapse-free survival. When cure is no longer possible, palliation and control of symptoms become the focus of therapy. The advantages and disadvantages of each of the three therapeutic measures will be briefly discussed and are outlined in Table 12-3.

SURGERY.   Surgery is as effective as radiation in eliminating limited cancers of the head and neck region. Surgery may be done effectively without functional and cosmetic loss in small early cancers, which are easily accessible. Surgical failures are usually related to the inability of the surgeon to remove the tumor en bloc. A disadvantage of surgery is the potential for structural, functional, or cosmetic loss.

RADIATION THERAPY.   Radiation therapy has the ability to control the disease in situ, avoids surgical sacrifice of anatomic parts, and preserves functions of speech, swallowing, smell, and cosmesis. In spite of acute and long-term sequelae, radiation is classified as the best "tissue and organ sparing" treatment available. Radiation therapy has excellent cure rates for patients with limited disease (e.g., stages I and II).[40,57,75,77] Radiation failures in head and neck cancers are different from surgery or chemotherapy. Cancer cells that are hypoxic are insensitive to radiation and do not respond well to treatment. Local failure can also occur when occult malignant cells outside the irradiated field are present, when distant metastases through lymphatic and hematogenous spread are present at the time of treatment, or when tissue and organ tolerance to radiation is less than that of the tumor.

CHEMOTHERAPY.   Chemotherapy is being used in the treatment of patients with advanced or recurrent disease. The curative role of chemotherapy is still undergoing evaluation; however, its adjuvant or palliative roles in the treatment of this disease have been recognized. Normal epithelial tissues depend on certain substances to maintain their integrity and for cellular renewal. The role of chemotherapy is not being evaluated for its preventative potential in premalignant lesions (leukoplakia or erythroplasia of the oral cavity). Vitamin A and its natural analogues, retinoids, are necessary for the normal development and differentiation of epithelial tissues. Further discussion of drug side effects can be found within Chapter 23. The specific chemotherapy and biotherapy agents, treatment combinations, and side effects are discussed in Chapters 22 and 23.

COMBINED RESEARCH.   The ultimate goal of clinical head and neck research is to provide optimal therapies for each patient. Historically, treatment recommendations may have been based on limited experience and knowledge. The Southwest Oncology Group, Radiation Oncology Group, Veterans Administration Head and Neck Study Group, and other intergroup study groups have attempted to answer questions about the natural history, treatment, and

Table 12–3 Advantages/Disadvantages of Treatment

Treatment Modality	Advantage	Disadvantage
Surgery	Ability to remove central-resistant hypoxic tumor cells Immediate reconstruction	Potential for structural, functional, cosmetic loss
Radiation therapy	Ability to kill well-oxygenated cancer cells Used for T_1N_0 larynx cancers. Acute side effects generally disappear following treatment	Not effective as single treatment for large tumors Potential long-term sequelae radiation soft tissue damage, osteonecrosis
Chemotherapy/biologic therapy	Potential chemoprevention systemic treatment potential for killing lymphatic/hematogenous metastasis. May have potential to convert inoperable tumors to operable Less surgical resection	Normal tissue tolerance and tumor responsiveness are limiting factors

rehabilitation of head and neck cancer. These diversified groups are evaluating new therapies, including drugs, surgical techniques, radiation delivery systems, and biologic approaches to treating head and neck cancer. The strength of the cooperative group studies is the fact that larger populations are evaluable, which hold the potential to support statistically significant findings that will direct diagnosis and treatment of patients diagnosed with head and neck cancer.*

Factors Affecting Treatment Decisions

Treatment decisions are always affected by factors related to the tumor, patient, and the health-care provider. In choosing a treatment option, especially in head and neck cancer, the treatment team must place in perspective what is to be achieved. Clearly, survival is important and easily measured, but the quality of life during that survival is even more important.[1,20,26,54] The choice of treatment modalities depends on many factors: (1) site, (2) extent of lesion, (3) histology, (4) patient's physical and emotional condition, (5) availability of health-care providers and resources to provide comprehensive treatment and rehabilitation programs, and (6) quality of life. Quality of life is relevant to head and neck treatment studies, because the patient's adjustment to illness can be significantly affected by its symptoms and the side effects of the disease and treatment. Quality of life issues emphasize the impact of these symptoms on the patients' physical, physiological, emotional, and social functioning, in contrast to the standard performance status scales currently used (Karnofsky or Zubrod).[108,109] Since the potential for recurrence of the disease still remains high, quality of life could be of value when making treatment decisions.

TUMOR-RELATED FACTORS.   Appropriate therapy requires an accurate assessment of the tumor. The size and extent of the primary tumor are equally as important as type and site in determining the treatment to be employed. A guide to size and extent of primary head and neck tumors may be found in the American Joint Commission on Cancer Staging and End Results Reporting 1989.[12,77] In general, smaller cancers without metastases (T_1, or T_2, N_0) do not require multiple modality treatment. For larger primary tumors (T_3 or T_4), combined modalities offer a greater chance for quality survival. Patients with regional metastasis classified as N_1, or that have extension into soft tissue of the neck, have benefited by the addition of radiation, which has been shown to prevent recurrence within the neck. Primary lesions that present with regional metastases or distant disease may be best approached by combination therapy incorporating surgery, radiation, and systemic or regional chemotherapy.*

PATIENT-RELATED FACTORS.   Patient-related factors that affect treatment decisions include general health, previous therapy, dental health, social habits, motivation, economic resources, and individual needs. Many patients have other health conditions (e.g., chronic lung, cardiovascular, hepatic, or renal disease) that limit the clinician's ability to perform surgery or give maximum doses of chemotherapy. The patient brings a unique set of psychosocial experiences to the treatment milieu. An evaluation of the psychosocial status of the patient and significant others may be more important and more difficult to obtain than an evaluation of the physical status of the patient.† Many patients with head and neck cancer are chemical (alcohol/tobacco) abusers and may have associated personality disorders. An evaluation of the patient's smoking and drinking habits is essential in forming the treatment plan. The nurse must assess the patient for orientation to current medical status, appropriateness of responses to questions and health-care directions, and interactions with family or significant others.

Often the choice of therapy is influenced by myths and misconceptions the patient or family hold based on previous health-related experiences. Within the initial assessment, the nurse should attempt to determine how motivated the patient is to comply with the demands of illness and treatment and to survive. Insight into motivation may be gained by obtaining information related to the previous ability to work and work habits, lifestyle, economic status, social networks, perceived resources, and health seeking behaviors and history.‡ Finally, the nurse must remember that treatment cannot be administered if patients choose not to have therapy. The treatment team has the responsibility to educate patients who elect to take their "chances" about the natural course of their disease and the ultimate outcome. Regardless of the patient's decision, physical support and symptom control should be offered and continued. Offering educational materials and activating support systems early within the course of disease provides the patient with opportunities for control and self-care and facilitates the nurse-patient relationship.

HEALTH-CARE RESOURCES.   Treatment of head and neck cancers is influenced by availability of specialists, facilities, equipment and resources, health-

---

*References 5, 8, 9, 47, 60, 78, 85, 119.

*References 3, 5, 8, 9, 13, 14, 47, 52, 60, 75, 78, 79, 88, 102, 103, 119, 130, 152.
†References 26, 56, 61, 67, 87, 96, 136.
‡References 30, 42, 68, 74, 96, 132, 133.

care reimbursement, and the patient's ability to access care. The skills and experience of the head and neck surgeon, radiotherapist, and medical oncologist vary in each treatment center. Patients receiving treatment in centers that participate in clinical research trials are afforded opportunities to participate in treatment protocols otherwise unavailable. Patients should ideally receive treatment where a comprehensive rehabilitation team is readily available, including dentists, maxillofacial prosthodontists, speech pathologists, nurse specialists, social workers, physical and occupational therapists, and clinical dieticians. If these opportunities are limited, it may be efficacious for the physician to refer the patient to centers that provide such services.

Treatment/Rehabilitative Planning

Treatment and rehabilitative planning will always be dictated by the anatomic location and extent of the primary tumor. Before initiation of treatment, the patient should be evaluated by an interdisciplinary team.[42,68] Pretreatment assessment by the interdisciplinary groups can accomplish several goals: establish the diagnosis, stage the disease, plan treatment, and integrate prescriptive rehabilitative programs.* Nursing assessment in the pretreatment phase identifies any potential or actual nursing diagnoses that can minimize complications of therapy and promote adjustment of patient, family/significant other to the illness, treatment, and rehabilitation.†

PSYCHOSOCIAL ASSESSMENT. In general, patients with head and neck cancer and their families respond to the diagnosis of cancer with shock, anxiety, fear, denial, and grief.[28,54,56,81,93] The patient is faced with a potential threat to body image and self-esteem. The patient with head and neck cancer has the potential for severe and permanent facial disfigurement and functional loss that closely resembles that experienced by the burn patient.[15] The face and neck left uncovered by clothing are subject to full view of others. Physical disfigurement or functional loss may pose a threat to the patient's coping, sexuality, and socialization patterns.[15] Patients may feel stigmatized and may become socially isolated. Depression related to the prognosis, altered body image, or decreased self-esteem can become a major impediment to the rehabilitative process.[68] If surgery is planned, the patient may experience fear of undergoing anesthesia or dying during the surgical procedure. Potential altered body image or a patient's perception of distortion in body image often plays a significant role in the ability to cope with the illness and the treatment plan.[20,26,27,54,56]

A person's body image is a picture or concept of the physical and emotional self, which is incorporated into the person's psychologic construct. Many head and neck cancer patients initially refuse surgery in an attempt to preserve or maintain the concepts of self and function.[56] Body image, self-esteem, and sexuality can be threatened by the results of the surgical procedure. The patient who faces loss of cosmesis, structure, or function (e.g., laryngectomy, tongue, jaw/neck dissection) experiences a major adjustment in body image and may have problems coping. The degree of disfigurement and perceptions of the patient associated with the surgery may intensify the emotional response. The nurse must remember that patients diagnosed with early stage disease may not face the same issues as those with advanced or recurrent disease. A nursing diagnosis of potential altered patterns of sexuality can be related to changes in appearance, fear of the partner, or nonacceptance of surgery. Salient questions that should be incorporated into a psychosocial nursing assessment and suggested interventions are listed as follows. These nursing interventions support both patient and family and assist the patient to cope with and adjust to illness.*

PULMONARY ASSESSMENT AND HEALTH HISTORY. Patients with head and neck cancer may have other significant medical problems. The physician will evaluate the patient for a history of cardiopulmonary disease, diabetes, bleeding disorders, and renal disease. Careful review and documentation of preexisting medical disorders, along with routine paraclinical data, blood chemistries, cardiograph, and chest x-rays, should be evaluated. Disorders such as hypertension, end-stage cardiopulmonary disease, uncontrolled or labile diabetes, or bleeding disorders may preclude or significantly modify surgical interventions. Prognostic signs associated with cardiac disease that carry a high surgical risk for patient include (1) history of poor exercise tolerance, (2) increasing angina, (3) chronic diabetes, uncontrolled or acute congestive heart failure, (4) severe uncontrolled hypertension, (5) arrhythmias, (6) acute ECG changes indicating injury or ischemia, and (7) myocardial infarction within 6 months of surgery. Patients with respiratory insufficiency or with a significant smoking history should undergo a respiratory evaluation. Patients with respiratory insufficiency or chronic obstructive lung disease cannot adequately meet the body's oxygenation needs during stress. An aggressive pulmonary hygiene and rehabilitation program can be implemented by the nurse or respiratory therapist.[117] To circumvent complications of atelectasis or aspiration pneumonia, the patient should be in-

---

*References 30, 42, 66, 68, 74, 89, 99, 133, 162.
†References 15, 42, 56, 61, 66, 68, 93.

*References 15, 27, 61, 81, 93, 96, 97.

structed on proper posture, lung expansion techniques, and breathing exercises. Nicotine ingestion is clearly a source that contributes to poor wound healing and loss of reconstructive flaps. Some patients are more sensitive to the peripheral vasoconstrictive and ischemic effects of nicotine than others and in these patients the harmful microcirculatory effects of nicotine may persist weeks after cessation of smoking. When cessation of smoking is critical to the survival of the flap, as in the case of a free island flap, the physician may order preoperative urine nicotine levels. Treatment decisions may be significantly influenced by the patient's ability to successfully quit smoking.[55,64,73,80,161] A lengthy discussion of smoking cessation programs is not within the scope of this text, but programs such as "Fresh Start" (American Cancer Society) and "In Control" (American Lung Association) are among the available resources. A thorough nursing assessment should include documentation of use of drugs or chemicals.

Alcoholism is common in this patient population; thus a large percentage of these patients will also have associated medical and psychologic problems related to acute and chronic abuse (e.g., chronic liver disease, peripheral neuropathies, and damaged central nervous systems). Liver functions and standard coagulation screening tests, which include platelet count and partial thromboplastic and prothrombin time should be evaluated. If chronic alcohol abuse is suspected, the nurse should monitor the patient for clinical problems and signs and symptoms related to withdrawal. The alcohol withdrawal syndrome, which includes symptoms ranging from mild tremulousness to delirium tremens, represents the defense reaction of the body to withdrawal of the CNS depressant. Anxiety, tremulousness, increased visual imagery, and tachycardia are compensatory mechanisms that are no longer depressed by alcohol. Manifestations of symptoms may be quite variable from time of cessation of alcohol. Agitation, increased anxiety, and mild tremulousness usually occur within the first 24 to 36 hours. Seizures related to withdrawal most frequently occur within 24 to 48 hours, and delirium tremens is often preceded by tremulousness and agitation. In some patients, severe manifestations may be delayed for 3 to 5 days following the cessation of drinking. The medical management of alcohol withdrawal syndrome should include (1) maintenance of patient hydration, (2) providing adequate calories, (3) vitamin supplementation, (4) suppression of CNS hyperactivity with sedation, and (5) monitoring for electrolyte imbalance, metabolic imbalance, and acidosis.

NUTRITIONAL ASSESSMENT. Each of the three major treatment modalities used singly or in combination may affect the patient's nutritional status. Limited caloric intake for extended periods can deplete protein stores.[53,65,122,127] A pretreatment nutritional assessment should be completed because weight loss is common among these patients before, during, and following treatment.[19,24,29,127,138] A recent loss of 10% or more of actual body weight unrelated to dieting or other concurrent medical conditions (e.g., diabetes, infection, or alcoholism) is a critical indicator for continued nursing assessment and implementation of a nutritional plan.[37,44,65,74] The aim of nutritional support in head and neck cancer patients is twofold—to rebuild or maintain protein and to maintain fat stores. Reduced nutritional intake places the patient at risk for a physiologic state of negative nitrogen balance with a resultant loss of protein stores. A reduction in total plasma volume places the patient at risk for blood loss and hypotension, and poor wound healing. If the patient is unable to maintain adequate nutrition, the physician may prescribe oral high-calorie, high-protein supplemental feedings. Most physicians will choose the oral or enteral route if the patient has a functional gastrointestinal tract. Patients may require placement of a nasogastric, gastrostomy, or jejunostomy feeding tube.[131,138,160] Jejunostomy tubes are placed when the patient has or is at high risk for aspiration. The nurse may need to prepare the patient psychologically and educationally if placement of feeding tube is required. The psychologic and social impact of not being able to eat normally can be devastating to the patient and can result in ineffective coping or social isolation. Nursing education and interventions directed at assisting the patient to cope with these physical changes can help the patient circumvent feelings of not being "normal" or of being "socially unacceptable." Patients should be afforded the opportunity to continue experiencing all sensory input (e.g., smell and sight) and maintaining normal socialization patterns and lifestyle. The nurse and clinical dietitian may encourage the patient and family to puree normal high-calorie, high-protein meals in the blender before administration. Prepackaged supplements are also available if normal food preparation and blenderized meals are not a practical option. A complete review of nursing diagnoses, assessment, interventions and care plans related to nutrition are provided in Chapter 27.

COMMUNICATION/COGNITIVE MOTOR SKILLS. A thorough nursing assessment of the reading, comprehension, and communication skills of the patient should be accomplished before the initiation of the definitive therapy. Patient education should be tailored to the specific need and educational level of the patient. If patients have limited reading or writing skills, education may need to be accomplished by using simple explanations, pictures, or videos. Explanations without medical jargon facilitate effective communication. Alternative forms of communication will need to be established with the patient before undergoing definitive surgical procedures such as laryngectomy, glossectomy, or palatal resection. Additionally, a thorough hearing, speech, and visual examination should be accomplished in patients undergoing these procedures. Deficits in any of these functional areas need to be identified before surgery to facilitate appropriate rehabilitation. Functional losses related to the four types of laryngectomies are listed in Table 12-4. Pretreatment consultation with a speech pathologist facilitates communication among the patient, family, and nurse; establishes a trusting relationship among professional, patient, and family; and decreases anxiety. Meeting members of the re-

habilitation team before treatment serves as a nonverbal statement to the patient that wellness and rehabilitation are the primary treatment foci. If the patient is scheduled for a laryngectomy, a presurgical visit by a trained laryngologist prior to hospital admission may allay the patient's fears and/or anxieties.

Dental Assessment

Dental care is important before and during head and neck cancer treatment.[72,83,92,111] Assessing the dental history will give the nurse insight into the patient's knowledge, beliefs, and resources toward preventive care, as well as susceptibility to dental disease. Oral pathology may be present if the patient has not been evaluated or treated by a dentist. An accurate dental

Table 12–4 Functional Loss Associated with Laryngectomy

Procedure	Structures Removed	Structures Remaining	Functions
Total laryngectomy Loss of laryngeal sphincter mechanism may lead to aspiration. Swallowing mechanism must be intact so that when food lands on vocal cords, patient coughs to get it out and swallows instantly.	Hyoid bone Entire larynx Epiglottis, false, true cords Cricoid cartilage Two/three rings of trachea	Tongue Pharyngeal walls Lower trachea	Loss of voice (resulting from trachea-laryngectomy) Normal swallowing
Supraglottic/horizontal laryngectomy—partial During supraglottic laryngectomy, muscles that elevate the larynx are transected, thereby limiting the elevation of larynx. This, along with loss of supraglottic structures, further downgrades swallowing. Because cough is necessary to clear larynx, patient's pulmonary functions must be adequate.	Hyoid bone Epiglottis False cords	True cords Cricoid cartilage Trachea	Normal voice Increased risk for aspiration Normal airway
Hemivertical laryngectomy Interferes very little with swallowing. Removal of arytenoid cartilage may cause aspiration in a small percentage of patients. Free or pedicled muscle or submucosal cartilage grafts may prevent aspiration. *If surgical resection extends to base of tongue,* swallowing may be affected related to inability to move bolus. Aspiration may occur.	One true cord, one false cord Arytenoid cartilage One half thyroid cartilage	Epiglottis One true cord, one false cord Cricoid	Hoarse but serviceable voice Normal airway Normal swallowing
Partial laryngectomy laryngofissure Potential to affect predominantly deglutition and phonation	One vocal cord	All other structures	Hoarse, but serviceable voice Normal airway Normal swallowing

history is critical to prevention of oral complications during therapy. The following questions should be incorporated into a nursing dental history:

1. When was patient's last dental visit and what type of procedures were done?
2. How often does patient see a dentist?
3. Does the patient have a relevant history of:
   - Sore swollen gums, drainage, boils?
   - Toothaches or sensitive teeth to hot, cold or chewing?
   - Loose teeth?
4. Does the patient have loose, ill-fitting dentures or recurring problems of denture sores?
5. Does the patient have bad odor of breath?
   - What kind of toothpaste or dental floss does patient use?

Oral assessment by the dentist, hygienist, or nurse can facilitate identification of oral disease. The hard and soft oral tissue should be systematically and thoroughly examined. Equipment needed for an oral exam includes good light source, gloves, tongue blade, and unsterile 2 × 2 gauze square. Labial mucosa, vestibule, anterior dentition, and gingiva can be examined by retracting the lips. Buccal mucosa, vestibule, posterior dentition, and gingiva can be examined by retracting the cheeks. Dorsum and lateral surfaces of the tongue can be inspected by grasping the tip of the tongue, using a 2 × 2 gauze. Wrapping tongue to palate allows for examination of the floor of the mouth and lingual frenulum. By tilting the patient's head back, with chin up and mouth wide open, the hard palate, maxillary dentition, and gingiva can be inspected. All patients with dentures should have them evaluated for proper fit. Instability and excessive movement of the dentures potentially cause irritation and may become a source of infection. The nurse should pay particular attention to all denture-bearing surfaces: floor of mouth, hard and soft palate, lateral borders of the tongue. Demonstrated gingival recession, hypertrophy or decayed teeth, denture sores, or exposed roots should be documented and the dentist should be consulted. An individual dental treatment plan that reflects the patient's present and future dental needs should be developed. All corrective procedures should be completed before initiation of any treatment. The dentist or hygienist will take a full mouth x-ray (panorex), scale the teeth, and evaluate the roots. A pretreatment panorex x-ray identifies the presence of teeth in edentulate patients when radiation to this area is planned. Teeth should be extracted and restored, dental plaque and calculus should be removed, and periodontal disease should be corrected before initiation of treatment. If advanced periodontal disease exists on the teeth, it is best to extract the teeth in the involved area. Periodonatal disease and poor oral care

are major sources of infection during treatment. All of these procedures should be completed 1 to 10 days before the initiation of therapy. This waiting period allows for adequate healing of extraction sites. The nurse should enlist the patient's active participation in his or her dental care and oral hygiene. Patient education should include (1) oral hygiene instructions emphasizing the importance of cessation of use of tobacco and alcohol products; (2) fluoride application and oral hygiene instructions taught initially and on an individual basis or as outlined on radiation care plan; (3) nutritional counseling, limiting sucrose intake; and (4) avoiding commercially available mouthwashes that contain alcohol. The type of floss is not as important as compliance. The mechanical action of vertically moving the floss against the tooth disrupts bacterial colonization. Daily fluoride application should be encouraged as part of a preventive dental/oral care regimen. Fluoride is an anticaries agent with antibacterial properties that promote remineralization of the enamel. Three types of fluoride are available for use: acidulated phosphate fluoride, neutral sodium fluoride, and stannous fluoride.[72] The fluoride of choice, like oral rinses and toothpastes, should be nonirritating to the mucosa, readily available, and convenient. Patients undergoing radiation therapy with teeth included in the treatment field should have custom fluoride carrier trays, which will need to be prescribed by the dentist. These fluoride-filled trays are placed over dry teeth for at least 5 minutes to obtain a therapeutic effect (Figure 12-2). The patient should spit out the excess fluoride after removing the tray, but should not rinse, eat, or drink for 30 minutes following application. When patients are experiencing episodes of severe mucositis or xerostomia, the patient may need to convert to brush-on technique if placement of carrier trays is painful. Regardless of the fluoride delivery method employed, fluoride must be used daily and continuously when patients undergo radiation.

Most dentists will recommend a neutral sodium or stannous fluoride gel. It is important for the nurse to understand the differences in fluoride preparations and application techniques (Table 12-5). All patients with dentures should be instructed to keep the dentures and denture-soaking containers clean. Ideally, soaking containers should be disposable, and the cleaning solution (any commercial brand) should be discarded and replaced daily.[38,83] Common soaking solutions that have been found to inhibit microbial growth include chlorhexidine gluconate (Stuart Pharmaceuticals, Wilmington, DE), Chloroseptic (Norwich Eaton Pharmaceuticals, Norwich, NY), or Efferdent (Warner-Lambert Company, Morris Plains, NJ). Chlorhexidine oral rinse is used as an anticaries agent. S-mutans, a component of caries-producing dental

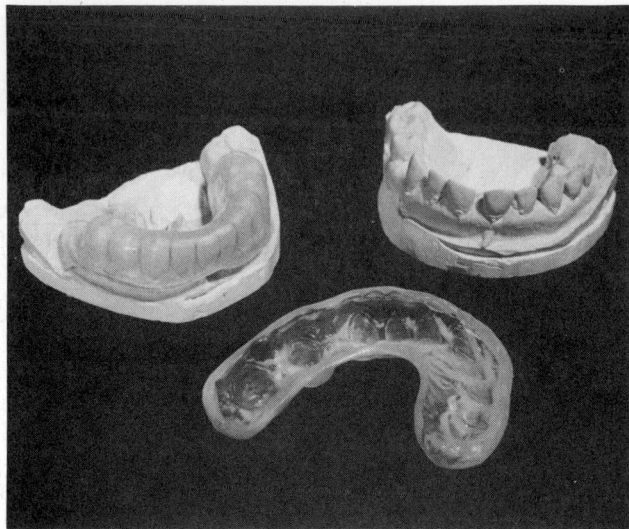

Figure 12–2 Oral cavity molds used to prepare individual carrier fluoride trays.

Table 12–5 Fluoride Sources

Type	Method of Application
Sodium fluoride	Carrier technique
Stannous fluoride	Mixed with water and brushed on
Acidulated phosphate fluoride	Brushed on

plaque, has been proven sensitive to chlorhexidine rinse solutions.[38,83,145] Mouth rinses with 0.1% or 0.2% aqueous solution of chlorhexidine used twice a day have proven effective in inhibiting plaque formation. In addition to a meticulous oral care program, the nurse should educate the patient about the importance of a balanced diet that emphasizes limiting sucrose intake. Sugarless gum and mints are acceptable and should be encouraged.[44]

TREATMENT MODALITIES

Marked improvements in the treatment of head and neck cancer have been made in the 1990s in comparison to therapies offered in the 1960s. New surgical techniques, radiotherapeutic approaches, and chemotherapy are now used earlier in patient management. However, only 30% of patients with resected cancers are alive after 5 years. Unfortunately the incidence of local regional failures is as high as 60%, with systemic metastases developing in more than 10% of this patient population. The sites of occurrence for second primary tumors vary from 10% in the larynx to 40% in the oropharynx, with the remainder in the esophagus, lung, and bladder. The second tumors usually prove to be the cause of death.

Surgery

The primary goal of surgery for head and neck cancer is removal of the primary disease and all metastatic lymph nodes in hope of controlling local disease and preventing recurrent disease. A secondary goal is to preserve structure and function as much as possible without compromising the treatment.[36] A final goal is to maximize the cosmetic and functional outcome.*

Surgery plays a major role in the diagnosis and staging of head and neck tumors. Surgical approaches to the treatment of these tumors depend to a great extent on the site and size of the primary lesion, the presence of cervical lymph nodes, and whether the patient has distant metastases.[77,165] While surgical management of benign lesions usually involves local excision, malignant lesions require wide resections with or without regional lymphadenectomy and reconstruction at the time of definitive procedure. When cure is no longer within the scope of treatment, the physician can offer palliative surgical options (e.g., tracheostomy, gastrostomy, jejunostomy placement, venous access, or implantable ports).

PRESURGICAL ASSESSMENT. Preoperative patient assessment, medical evaluation, and healthteam communication focused on rehabilitation can minimize postoperative complications and facilitate coping with illness. Additional time spent in preoperative education and planning may actually decrease postoperative complications, decrease the period of inpatient convalescence, and improve the overall quality of postoperative survival. Guidelines for preoperative and postoperative nursing care are presented later in this section.

A presurgical nutritional evaluation is essential because patients with head and neck cancer often experience interference with food and fluid intake, and weight loss. A reduction in nutritional intake, protein stores, and total plasma volume places the patient at risk for blood loss and hypotension. The nurse should monitor the patient for clinical signs and symptoms of hypovolemia, such as persistent tachycardia, dizziness, or syncope. The physician may order a volume replacement with red blood cells, albumin, or normal saline. The most efficient tissue oxygenation in microcirculation takes place in normal persons with a hemogloblin level above 10 g and a hematocrit level above 30%.† The nurse should be aware that, if volume depletion has occurred rapidly, a false increase in the hemoglobin and hematocrit level may be present for a short period of time. Preoperatively, the nurse should initiate a dietary consultation. It may be necessary to give the patient oral supplements, en-

---

*References 25, 31, 55, 69, 70, 73, 82, 87, 94, 95, 98, 110, 123, 125, 161, 163.
†References 19, 24, 44, 53, 64, 65, 80, 86, 122.

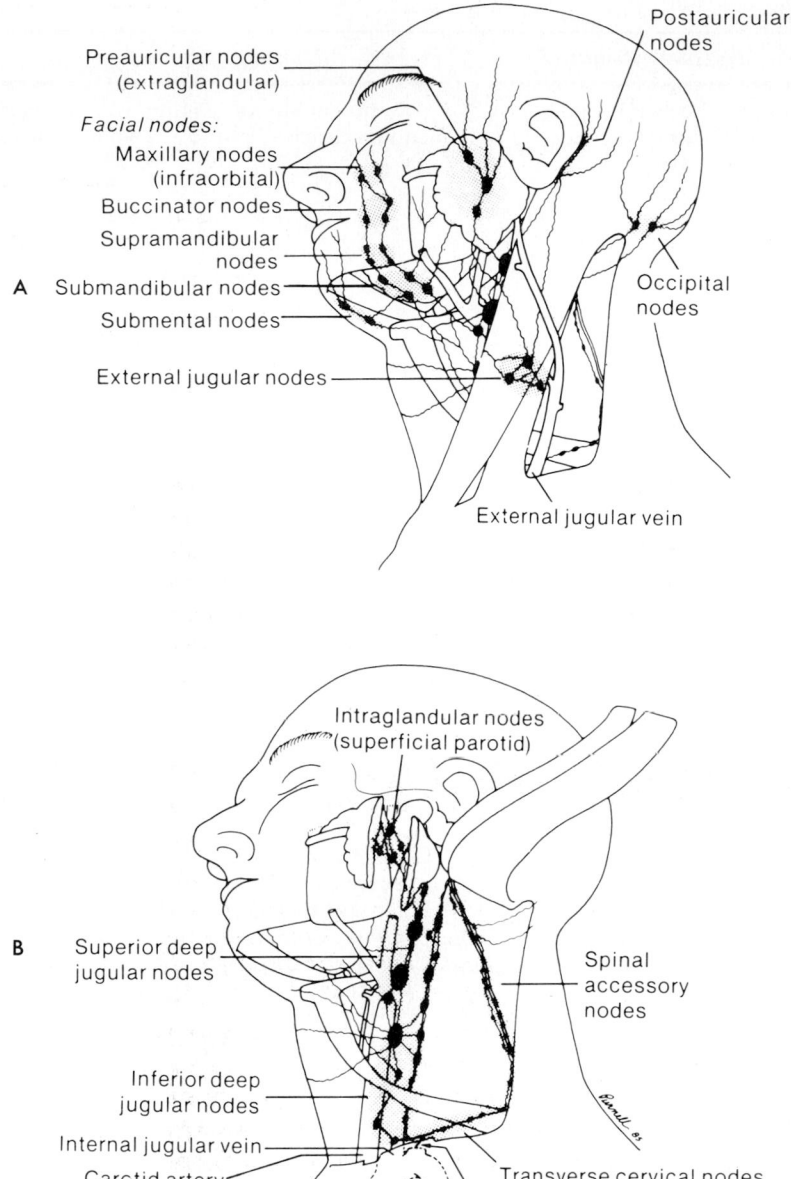

Figure 12-3   **A,** Superficial cervical and facial nodal drainage patterns. **B,** Deep cervical lymphatic drainage patterns. Note that sterno-cleidomastoid muscle is reflected. (From Cummings CW: Otolaryngology–head and neck surgery, Vol 3, Fredrickson JM, editor, St. Louis, 1986, Mosby.)

teral feedings by tube, or short-term parenteral therapies before surgery. Follow-up nutritional support should be evaluated on an ongoing basis by the nurse, dietitian, physician, and patient.

During the preoperative phase, the nurse will need to assess the patient's cognitive skills, motor skills, and ability to communicate. Any potential sensory deficits (e.g., vision, hearing, or fine motor writing skills) could affect the patient's ability to participate in the postoperative rehabilitative process.

SURGICAL PROCEDURES.   Cosmesis, body image, and function can be affected significantly by the type of primary and reconstructive procedures.* In addition to the primary surgery, the patient may require a lymph node dissection. The head and neck has about 300 lymph nodes, about 30% of the total lymph nodes in the body. Approximately 75 nodes are present on each side of the neck, most of which are in the deep jugular and spinal accessory chains (Figure 12-3). The nodes most frequently involved in metastatic

*References 2, 17, 18, 25, 31, 36, 70, 73, 94, 95, 105, 110, 113, 126, 128, 129, 141-144, 148, 161.

Table 12–6   Radical Neck Procedures

Procedure	Structures Removed	Advantage	Disadvantage
Classic, Complete, Radical Bilateral or unilateral (Crile, 1906)	Unilateral cervical nodes Sternomastoid, digastric muscle, styloid hyoid muscle Submaxillary salivary gland, tail of parotid gland Internal jugular vein Connective tissue of the carotid sheath, all lymph nodes, and lymph-bearing tissues of the anterior, posterior triangles, and deep jugular chain en bloc. Transverse cervical vessels/carotid Spinal accessory nerve and associated lymphatic chain with the deep layers of the cervical fascia Vagus, hypoglossal, phrenic lingual	Low probability of leaving nodal disease behind	Trapezius muscle dysfunction with shoulder drop; resulting in pain and limitation in motion Mild to moderate neck deformity If bilateral procedure is performed cerebral edema can persist Painful neuromas can occur Loss of carotid artery
Modified Neck Dissection Approximately six variations (Bocca, 1967)	Selective removal or preservation of the spinal accessory nerve (Roy: Bearns) Only lymphatic structures removed. Sternocleidomastoid muscle usually saved Carotid sheath opened; internal jugular vein saved	Low incidence of shoulder drop and shoulder disability Carotid artery not sacrificed Cosmetic deformity not as severe as CNN If cervical plexus is preserved, decreased incidence of sensory deficit and painful neuromas	Possible omission of occult positive nodes. Increased risk of hematoma under sternocleidomastoid muscle Increased risk of surgeon cutting into positive nodes and seeding neck Increased difficulty in performing a secondary and if disease occurs.

carcinoma are those in the deep jugular chain, which extends from the base of the skull to the clavicle. The decision to perform a neck dissection is based on the presence of lymph nodes or in a clinically negative neck, based on the probability of metastasis.[77,102,115,165] Table 12-6 lists the types of radical neck procedures, structures removed, and advantages and disadvantages of each procedure. Modified neck dissection is a term used to describe several different procedures that are modified from the classic, complete, or radical neck dissections.

Patients who have had a radical or modified procedure may benefit from a preoperative physical therapy evaluation. Functional parameters that are evaluated include head rotation and arm and shoulder mobility.

When the spinal accessory has been sacrificed, the head and shoulder range of mobility is significantly affected, and the patient faces the potential for permanent disability and chronic pain.[39,128]
RECONSTRUCTION.   The primary goal of most head and neck surgery prior to 1981 was to remove the cancer, replace the anatomic structure, and restore cosmesis. With the advent of muscle, musculocutaneous and free tissue transfer, more attention is being dedicated to restoration of functional losses and rehabilitation. Surgeon and communication scientists are coordinating efforts to identify and improve reconstructions of the oral cavity that focus on function of swallowing/speech. Videofluoroscopic studies are done to evaluate the patient's communicative ability, tongue strength, and range of motion. These studies when done pre- and post-operatively can help measure the patient's progress in rehabilitation. Patient education is the sine qua non to a patient's adjustment to illness, empowerment, and rehabilitation when considering reconstructive surgery.

The goals of reconstructive surgery are better accepted if the patient understands the reasons for considering various surgical options, such as flap versus graft or secondary wound healing. It is essential that the patient should understand that *no* restorative surgery can return them to complete normalcy and that function and imperfection in contour are an expected

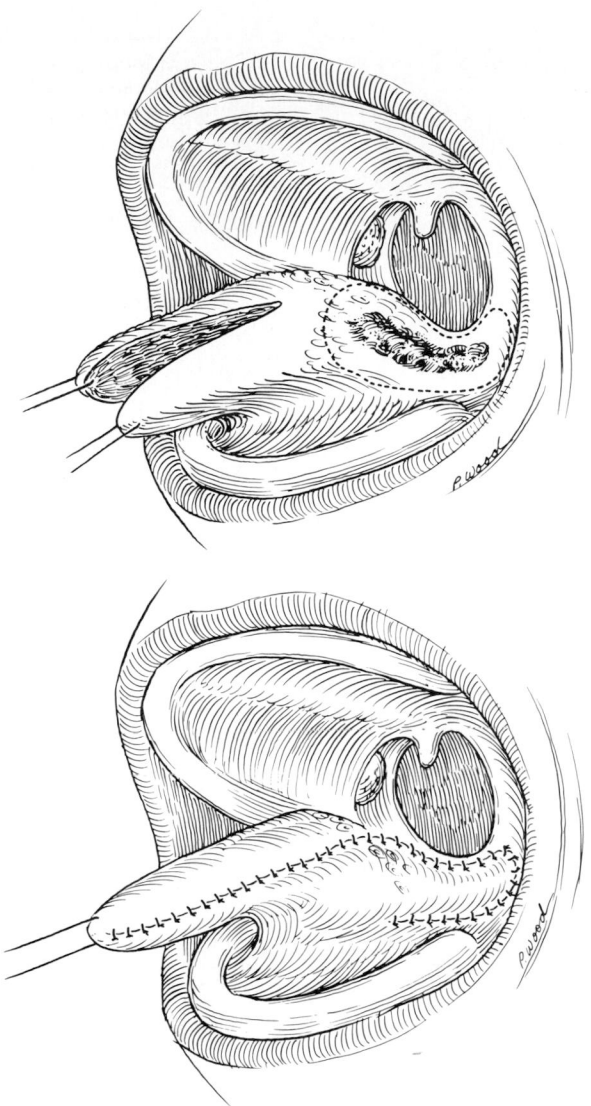

Figure 12–4 Tongue flap used for reconstruction of lateral oropharynx. (From Cummings CW: Otolaryngology-head and neck cancer, St. Louis, 1986, Mosby.)

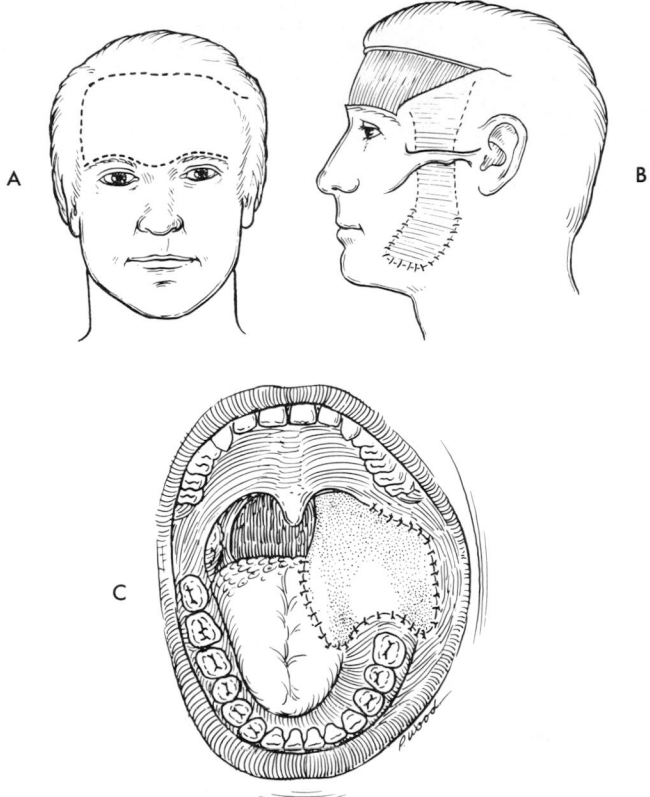

Figure 12–5 **A,** Forehead flap based on superficial temporal artery and portions of occipital artery. **B,** Rotation of forehead flap medial to zygomatic arch for reconstruction of oropharynx. Flap is pulled inferiorly to fill resected area. **C,** Completion of forehead flap reconstruction. (From Cummings CW: Otolaryngology-head and neck cancer, St. Louis, 1986, Mosby.)

Table 12–7 Factors that Affect Surgeon's Choice of Flaps

Tissue Considerations	*Physician Considerations*
Size of arc	Will the flap cover the defect?
Vascular supply	Will the flap survive?
Accessibility	How close to defect is the new tissue?
Donor site	Functional loss/contour of donor site.
Sensation	Maintain nerve supply

outcome. When immediate reconstruction is performed it is important and reasonable to anticipate possible need for revisions or future procedures. Surgical removal of head and neck tumors can result in functional, as well as socially unacceptable cosmetic deformities. Many patients will undergo immediate reconstruction. Patients may be faced with more than one surgical procedure for reconstruction. These include autogenous tissue and all aplastic material.* Normal physiology is best achieved when the surgeon uses autogenous tissue. Soft tissue defects can be closed by direct approximation (suturing), free skin grafts, pediculed tissue (using local, regional, or dis-

tant flaps), or by free flaps transferred by microvascular anastomoses. Skeletal tissue is best provided by living vascularized bone grafts or flaps.* Nonvascularized bone grafts or all aplastic material can be used for bone replacement.[128,129] Small defects can usually be covered by primary closure.

Moderate-sized defects may require skin grafting or local skin flaps (Figures 12-4 and 12-5). Factors that affect the surgeon's choice of flap are outlined in Table 12-7. There are several types of flaps available for

---

*References 16, 18, 31, 41, 69, 70, 73, 82, 94, 98, 110, 112, 113, 121, 123, 124, 128, 129, 139, 143, 148, 163.

---

*References 16, 18, 121, 139, 142, 161, 163.

Text continued on p. 241.

Nursing Management

NURSING CARE GUIDELINES
- Patients undergoing head and neck surgery.

NURSING DIAGNOSES
- Knowledge deficit related to surgery, preoperative/postoperative procedures
- Self-care deficit, related to postoperative treatments
- Anxiety related to the surgical experience and unpredictable outcome

PREOPERATIVE INTERVENTIONS
- Review purpose of surgery and rationale (temporary, permanent).

- Explain common terms and procedures, provide written literature (show videos), and show actual equipment. Patient will need to be familiar with terminology/equipment.
- Discuss potential sequelae of surgery:
    Change in bodily appearance
    Change in bodily function (e.g., breathing, speaking, swallowing, coughing, mobility)
- Explain roles of various medical and nursing personnel and purpose of visits.
    Medicine
    Respiratory therapy
    Nursing/Case manager
    Home care coordinator
- Instruct and have patient give verbal return demonstration on all self-care: coughing, deep breathing, ambulation.
- Document (in nursing notes):
    Patient's level of understanding
    Patient's ability to perform self-care behavior
    Patient education materials given

PREOPERATIVE OUTCOME CRITERIA
- Patient will demonstrate decreased anxiety and be knowledgeable about planned surgical procedure. The patient will effectively communicate feelings, demonstrate ability to do self-care, and seek assistance as necessary.
- Patient will name surgery and describe it.

- Patient will state reason for surgery, physical changes and expected outcome.

- Patient will state expectations of intraoperative care and professionals involved.

- Patient will state immediate postoperative care and will perform self-care behaviors.

- Patient will state he or she is less anxious when questioned.

POSTOPERATIVE INTERVENTIONS
- Instruct patient on self-care behaviors:
    Provide patient education materials.
    Teach patient to report symptoms of discomfort.
    Teach patient the importance of ambulation, coughing, deep breathing, and rehabilitation.
- Document:
    Patient's response to surgery, functional level, self-care level, and ability to perform procedures
    Patient's level of understanding
    Patient's ability to perform self-care
    Patient education materials given

POSTOPERATIVE OUTCOME CRITERIA
- Patient will demonstrate decreased anxiety and be knowledgeable about postoperative care and rehabilitation; effectively communicate feelings, and demonstrate ability to perform self-care. Patient's expectations for assistance that will be needed for postoperative care will be realistic.

POSTOPERATIVE INTERVENTIONS — cont'd

- Discharge patient with written instructions:
  Specific self-care behaviors (e.g., tracheostomy/ laryngectomy care exercise, wound management, oral/dental hygiene)
  Emergency procedures (list of appropriate nursing/medical personnel to contact in case of emergency)
  Home care referral

NURSING DIAGNOSES

- Breathing patterns, altered related to diversional methods (tracheostomy, laryngectomy)
- Airway clearance, ineffective, related to tracheal edema, secretions.
- Injury, potential for related to hematoma formation between flap and underlying tissue
- Tissue perfusion, alteration in: related to arterial erosion rupture around/at surgical site
- Skin integrity, impairment of: actual related to surgery flap reconstruction, flap failure
- Swallowing, impaired related to superior laryngeal nerve injury, loss or weakness of tongue.

POTENTIAL CLINICAL/COLLABORATIVE PROBLEMS

- Respiratory distress
- Hypoxia, airway obstruction, tracheal edema, aspiration
- Hemorrhage
- Hematoma
- Arterial rupture
- Failure of flap survival
- Nerve damage

POSTOPERATIVE INTERVENTIONS

- Monitor signs and symptoms of respiratory distress:
  Restlessness, agitation, confusion
  Individual complaint of air hunger, inability to breathe
  Diminished or absence of air exchange in breath sounds over tracheostomy, laryngectomy tube
  Use of accessory muscle retractions of soft tissues around airway
- Monitor signs and symptoms of hemorrhage:
  Continuous oozing of blood/or bleeding around surgical site, drains, tracheostomy, laryngectomy, unrelated to manipulation of suctioning, reconstruction

POSTOPERATIVE OUTCOME CRITERIA — cont'd

- Patient will state emergency procedures and names of personnel to contact.

- These instructions ensure a safe homebound environment even if patient demonstrates independence in hospital setting. It is not unusual for patient to become overwhelmed with information and experience difficulty processing it upon discharge.

- If tracheostomy is not placed during surgical procedure, tissue swelling (tracheal edema) may occur during the first 24 hours — patient should be observed for airway obstruction. Intrinsic laryngeal edema or hematoma, increased anxiety or apprehension can increase potential for obstruction. Elevate the head to facilitate lymphatic arterial flow — reduces edema.

- Continuous oozing of blood after first 24 hours postoperatively is not normal. May require surgical intervention for control.

POSTOPERATIVE INTERVENTIONS — cont'd

Presence of unusual edema around wound, stoma, reconstructive site, drainage tubes

- Monitor signs and symptoms of hematoma:
    Check drains for patency.
    Notify physician immediately if presence of air, serum, milky fluids.
    Normal, excessive absence.
  Air indicates dead space; milky drainage may indicate fistula formation with thoracic duct.
  Leakage can lead to severe fluid/electrolyte loss.

- Monitor signs and symptoms of infection:
    Vital signs
    Drainage/odor
    Intake/output
- Monitor wound and surrounding tissue for signs and symptoms of arterial erosion/rupture:
    Evidence of arterial erosion
    Color (red, pallor, black)
    Vascularity (evidence of bleeding and/or bruising, pulsations, arterial exposure)
    Temperature changes (warm, cool, unilateral)
    Edema (presence or absence)
    Turgor (taut, mobile)

- Monitor signs and symptoms of thoracic duct leakage:
    Milky white drainage often mixed with serous fluid in drainage tubes
- Monitor signs and symptoms of fluid and electrolyte imbalance.

- Monitor signs and symptoms of nerve injury:
    Superior laryngeal nerve dysphagia

    Recurrent laryngeal nerve

    Lingual nerve
    Hypoglossal nerve

POSTOPERATIVE OUTCOME CRITERIA — cont'd

- Surgical incision should be assessed carefully the first 24 hours for bleeding drainage and patency of drainage tubes. Serious complications can lead to skin flap wound breakdown. If suction apparatus and tubes are not functioning, skin flaps may not adhere, and necrosis may occur.

- If drains' suction becomes plugged, malfunctions, has excessive oozing, bleeding, vascular link-up occurs and fluid collects. Sets site for compromised circulation, infection.
- Drains prevent development of dead space. Continuous bloody drainage may indicate formation of hematoma or fistula formation.
- Hematoma formation is prevented by placement of suction catheter draining superiorly and anteriorly or of flap to recipient site eliminating dead space. Fluid or air collects between flap and underlying tissue. Gravity permits venous drainage through flap.
- Meticulous wound care as ordered by physician should be provided.
- Careful monitoring of intake and output avoids overhydration or underhydration.

- Exposure of the adventitial layer of artery to atmosphere facilitates drying and destroys blood supply of layers. Once artery is exposed to the air, destruction of wall occurs in approximately 6 to 10 days.
- Contributing factors to arterial erosion include poor wound healing, exposure of artery at the time of surgery, tumor growth invasion, previous radiation, fistula formation or infection.
- Raising head of patient's bed facilitates venous drainage; raising it 30 to 45 degrees promotes lymphatic venous drainage.

- Major lymphatic leak from thoracic duct represents loss of fluid and protein and may require surgical closure or protein replacement.

- Branch of vagus that innervates base of tongue may cause swallowing impairment.
- Responsible for adduction/abduction of vocal cords. Bilateral pareses requires immediate tracheostomy.
- Numbness on ipsilateral tongue can occur if severed.
- If severed, unilateral tongue paralysis results, which causes impairment of speech mastication. Innervates the genioglossus muscle and is responsible for movement of the tongue.

POSTOPERATIVE INTERVENTIONS — cont'd

Glossopharyngeal nerve

Facial nerve

Phrenic nerve
Spinal accessory nerve

- Monitor signs and symptoms of flap reconstructive failure:
    Monitor wound, flap, surrounding tissue every 2 hours × 72 hours, then every 4 hours
    Color (redness, pallor, cyanosis), tension, kinking, pressure, hematoma
    Vascularity (presence or absence of blanching)
    Temperature (warm, cool, unilateral)
    Edema (presence or absence)
    Turgor (taut, mobile, shiny, wrinkled)
    Odor (not malodorous)
    "Red Flap" — The flap will appear bright red and when tested for capillary filling will feel tense or thick on digital palpation. This occurs when blood flow is excessive. A red flap occurs when there is partial venous obstruction.
    "White Flap" — One that has limited or no blood supply. Related to tension, constriction, pressure, or occlusion can cause stop of blood flow. With dearterialization, the flap has no capillary refill, is cool to touch, and becomes white.
    "Blue Flap" — Occurs when the input of blood exceeds the output. This imbalance occurs when arterial pressure remains the same and venous pressure increases (e.g., hematoma) or constriction of the vascular pedicle related to the patient lying on flap, tight pressure dressing, or formation of a clot at the venous anastomotic site occurs.

- Monitor signs and symptoms of infection:
    Tenderness
    Thickness (inspect level of tissue repair, presence or absence of tumor)
    Moisture (dry, drainage — amount, color, odor — fistula formation)
- Monitor pressure — external pressure

Postoperative nursing care should focus on preventing and minimizing complications. Immediate postoperative care will be to maintain and monitor the airway. The head should be elevated to reduce

POSTOPERATIVE OUTCOME CRITERIA — cont'd

- Innervates posterior two thirds of the tongue. Damage can result in altered taste sensation on ipsilateral side and difficulty in swallowing.
- Result of trauma, especially in the area of parotid, may result in droop or asymmetry of musculature around the mouth (drooping periostosis).
- If severed, paralysis of diaphragm can result.
- Innervates trapezius muscle, which stabilizes and supports shoulder; allows lateral abduction of arm.
- Often affected in neck dissections. Injury results in painful shoulder, droopy atrophy of trapezius muscle, immobility of head and shoulder movement.
    - Major surgery can create deficits that may not be approximated and closed by direct suture. Skin flaps with or without muscle provide tissue, bulk protection to vital structures (e.g., carotid artery). Purpose is to maintain vascular integrity. Maximum redness should first occur 8 to 12 hours and decrease after 2 to 3 days. If arterial or venous supply is hindered, flap may necrose or slough. Flap and recipient sites should survive if no unusual kinking, pressure, hematoma, or infection occurs. Tension compromises blood supply; kinking causes decreased blood supply to distal portion of flap and compromises venous outflow resulting in increased capillary permeability and occlusion of lymphatic and arterioles. Pressure compromises blood supply. Position patient to permit gradual flow of lymph and blood. Elevate head of bed 30 to 45 degrees.
    - Normal tissue/flaps will be warm to touch. Recovers color slowly after tested for blanching. Flaps will have fine wrinkles — indication of minimal edema.
    - Abnormal findings indicate circulatory embarrassment, venous congestion. Shiny, taut, reddish. After testing for blanching, flap will recover color quickly.
    - Foul purulent drainage is seen.
    - Room temperatures that are extreme cold can be a contributing factor to flap loss (maintain room temperature).
- Flap necrosis can lead to formation of fistula, septicemia, arterial rupture, and prolonged hospitalization.
- External pressure on muscle flap compromises circulation, facilitates venous congestion, and leads to decreased permeability and occlusion of lymphatics.

edema. The nurse should make sure that drains are kept functional and clear to avoid accumulations of fluid under the surgical site or reconstructed flap. The intake and output must be monitored to avoid overhydration or underhydration. If the patient has a nasogastric tube, the first postoperative day the patient is kept NPO, and the tube is placed on suction to avoid gastric contents, air, vomiting, or aspiration from occurring. Feedings usually are initiated on the second or third postoperative day. Early ambulation is encouraged, and the upper aerodigestive system may require frequent gentle suction to prevent atelectasis, infection, and aspiration. If the patient has undergone a mandible/tongue or palatal or larynx resection, the nurse must provide the patient with paper or magic slate or a picture board to facilitate communication. Speech rehabilitation should be started as soon as the patient's surgical condition is stable. Whether or not the patient is to receive any additional therapy, he or she should be monitored for local or regional recurrence or new disease. The nurse should instruct the patient on the importance of maintaining all scheduled appointments; most physicians will follow the patient monthly for the first year. During this period, the patient should be prepared to undergo additional tests to evaluate the patient's response to treatment or identify any recurrences or new disease (e.g., chest x-ray and blood chemistries).

It is generally recommended that the patient be seen every 3 months for the first 3 years, and then every 6 months thereafter. Early detection of local or regional recurrences or a new primary lesion provide the patient with the best opportunity for cure or control of disease.

Nursing Management*

NURSING CARE GUIDELINES
- Cosmesis/body image/sexuality of head and neck cancer patient undergoing surgery

NURSING DIAGNOSIS

Body image disturbance, self-esteem disturbance, sexual dysfunction
- Potential sexual dysfunction related to altered self-esteem and change in appearance
- Disturbance in self-esteem related to: anatomic changes, role disturbance, disruption of lifestyle, uncertain future, sexuality patterns, altered related body image changes.[15]

PREOPERATIVE INTERVENTIONS
- Review purpose of interview, obtaining information, a sexual history early in a relationship with a patient validates to patient/partner that sexuality is an important part of health and rehabilitation and therefore it is appropriate for concerns to be discussed.
- Progress from less sensitive questions. Ask patient/partner if they have any questions at conclusion of history.
- Components of preoperative nursing assessment included in interview:
  Specific sexual needs of the patient/partner
  Sexual history (provide privacy, assure confidentiality)
  Coping style adjustment to previous illness or surgery
  Attitudes about sex
  Patient's attitudes about altered body image and perception of sexuality
  Effects of illness on partner/patient. Does patient's present or postoperative physical condition limit the ability for sexual expression by partner

PREOPERATIVE OUTCOME CRITERIA
- Patient and/or partner will identify aspects of sexuality/sexual function, that may be threatened by the surgical procedure (e.g., tracheostomy, laryngectomy, tongue, jaw/neck dissection/reconstruction).
  State factors that influence sexual identity
  Identify behaviors that facilitate acceptance of surgery
  Maintain satisfying social and sexual/role concept
  Verbalize importance of seeking professional assistance if normal lifestyle, socialization, or sexual function is impaired

---

*Modified from McPhetride LM: Nursing history: one means to personalize care, Am J Nurs 68:68-75, 1968.

PREOPERATIVE INTERVENTIONS — cont'd

Demonstration of nurse's acceptance. Facilitation of patient's comfort and adjustment to illness and surgery

Determination of involvement of partner in providing actual physical care and whether or not partner is fatigued

Assessment of whether partner feels guilty about initiating or making sexual demands

Evaluation of patient's physical condition (permit and its impact) on patient's usual form of sexual expression

Patient's/partner's reactions to impending physical change

Existence of pain, fatigue, depression, limited mobility that would affect normal expressions of sexuality

Interference by illness on patient's roles. Has being ill interfered with (mother, father, wife, husband, etc.)?

Impact of surgery on patient's self-perception

Effect of illness/disability on patient's sexual function

POSTOPERATIVE INTERVENTIONS

- Assess that patient/partner wants to know about surgical procedure, changes in function that may be related to surgical procedure
- Assess patient's attitude about altered body image and perception of sexuality
- Do pain, fatigue, limited mobility affect normal expressions of sexuality?
- What is patient's/partner's reaction to altered body image?

POSTOPERATIVE OUTCOME CRITERIA

- Provide patient/partner with factual information; give assurance that it is okay to share feelings and concerns; assist with coping/adjustments to illness

reconstruction: (1) tongue flaps are used to cover internal mucosal defects such as floor of mouth, pharyngeal wall, or cheek; (2) skin flaps consist of skin, the subcutaneous tissues, and the fascia of the underlying muscle; and (3) myocutaneous flaps incorporate an island of desired skin and underlying subcutaneous tissue, and fascia is severed from all surrounding tissues (Figure 12-6). A full thickness of underlying muscle is lifted with its blood supply. When reconstruction is not technically feasible, the patient may require fitting with a prosthesis (e.g., externally for a total ear or nose, or internally for a palate). Preoperative consultation with a maxillofacial prosthodontist is necessary. This preoperative consultation allows the patient and professional to evaluate all options for reconstruction. The surgeon and prosthodontist must work collaboratively. Appropriate planning for surgical resection and reconstruction allows for the anchoring and stabilization of a prosthesis. See pp. 236-240.

Radiation Therapy

Radiation therapy for head and neck tumors can be divided into three treatment categories: curative, palliative, or as an adjunct to surgery or chemotherapy.* Treatment planning is based on the nature, size, location, and growth of the tumor, volume of disease, the organs to be spared, and the purpose of treatment.[156] Radiation energies at or above 1 million V or radioactive isotopes are usually the primary source of treatment in head and neck cancers. These are termed megavoltage radiation sources, and they possess some very important physical advantages in the treatment of head and neck cancers, such as skin-sparing

*References 60, 75, 78, 79, 88, 102, 152, 164.

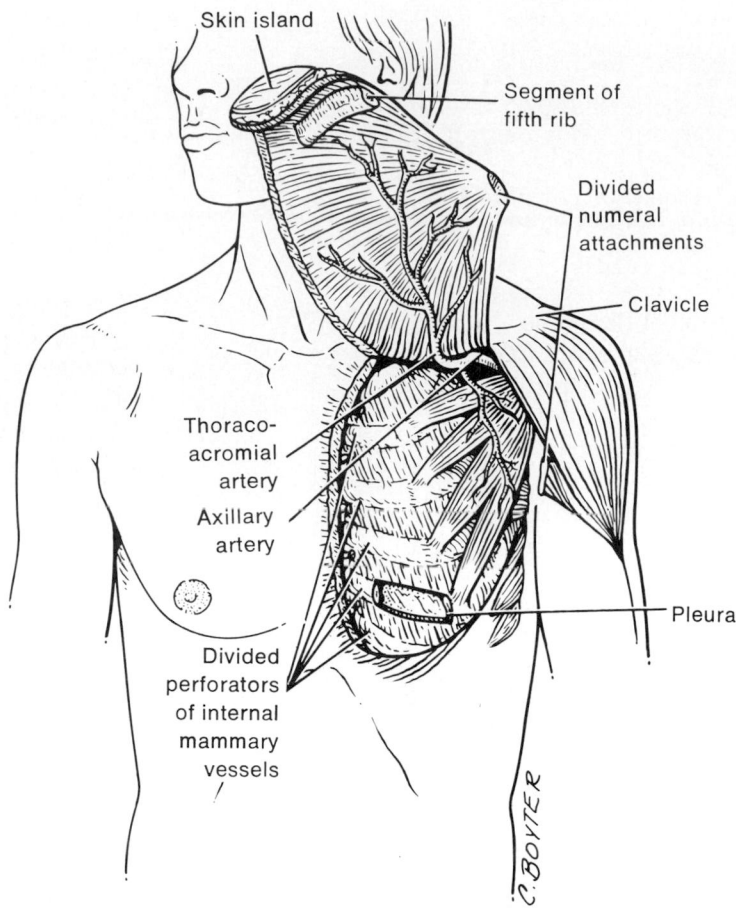

Skin island

Segment of fifth rib

Divided numeral attachments

Clavicle

Thoraco-acromial artery

Axillary artery

Pleura

Divided perforators of internal mammary vessels

C. BOYTER

Figure 12-6 Diagrammatic representation of myocutaneous flap procedure. (From Mathes S and Nahai F: Clinical applications for muscle and musculocutaneous flaps, St. Louis, 1982, Mosby.)

effects, increase in depth dose, formation of a sharp beam (which minimizes unnecessary damage to adjacent tissues and organs), and a bone-sparing effect related to decreased absorption by soft tissue and bone.[59,150,152,164]

In treatment of head and neck cancers radiotherapy may be given preoperatively to prevent marginal recurrences and to control subclinical disease at the primary site or in the nodes. It is also used to convert technically inoperable tumors to operable ones. The combination of preoperative irradiation and surgery is successful in decreasing both local and regional recurrence.* However, the major disadvantages of preoperative radiation are that the normal tissue reaction to radiation may obscure the surgeon's ability to determine the exact extent of the tumor margin and that the risk for postoperative complications are higher. Preoperative radiation is usually given for 1 month, followed by a 1-month rest period, which allows time for the acute tissue reaction to subside, yet stays within a timeframe when radioactive cell kill is still occurring.[156]

*References 5, 8, 9, 14, 59, 103, 118.

Postoperative radiation therapy may also be given to treat residual disease at the surgical margins and subclinical disease in the lymph nodes or may be implanted in the wound. Radiation treatments are usually given about 3 or 4 weeks after surgery to allow wound healing. Treatment usually lasts 6 to 8 weeks.

In addition to external beam radiation, radioactive isotopes and intracavitary implants are sources of radiation that may be applied closely to tumors by hollow containers loaded with radioactive sources. These techniques are beneficial when treating tumors of the antrum, sinuses, and nasal cavity. These interstitial or intracavitary implants can be used for the treatment of tongue, tonsil, nasopharynx, oral cavity, and metastatic neck nodes.[75,120] Interstitial irradiation is often used in the management of early localized T_1 lesions of the nasal vestibule with no detectable lymph nodes. Larger and more infiltrating (T_2) squamous cell carcinomas are treated by implants alone or with external beam radiation. This technique is termed *brachytherapy*. The advantage of brachytherapy is that it permits the delivery of irradiation at a high volume over a short period of time while delivering a relatively low dose to surrounding tissues.[100] Interest in protocols

INTERVENTIONS — cont'd

> Place bristles at an angle to where your gums and teeth meet.
>
> Use short back and forth strokes to clean front, back, and all chewing surfaces of teeth and tongue.
>
> Tongue can harbor bacterial plaque and should be gently brushed.
>
> Use toothpaste that contains fluoride.
>
> Use dental floss at least once a day to clean sides of teeth where toothbrush does not reach. Ease the floss between teeth so that it is close to the tooth as you guide it up and down. Do not snap floss between teeth because it may damage your gums.

- Provide instructions for edentulous patients:
> Oral hygiene — cleanse inside of mouth gently with moist clean gauze or toothette. Massage gums gently with finger.
>
> Clean dentures or partials every day with denture brush and denture cleaner (e.g., soap and water or baking soda and water).
>
> Change dental soaking cup and brush frequently — every 2 weeks.
>
> Store dentures in container of water to keep shape when not in mouth.
>
> Remove dentures several hours daily as prescribed by dentist.

- Instruct dentulous and edentulous patients to rinse mouth often:
> Rinse mouth several times daily. This helps relieve dryness, and promotes comfort, cleansing, healing.
>
> Mix solution (1 teaspoon table salt, 1 teaspoon baking soda, and 1 quart warm water), swish in mouth, and expectorate.
>
> Instruct dentulous patient on fluoride application — daily application of topical fluoride.
>
> Instruct on rationale/application of daily fluoride application after brushing, flossing, and rinsing.
>
> Instruct patient not to eat or drink anything for 30 minutes after application.

- Instruct patient to report to physician/nurse/dentist clinical problems early related to:
> Xerostomia
>
> Loss of taste
>
> Inability to maintain nutritional intake
>
> Inability to maintain hydration
>
> Infection

OUTCOME CRITERIA — cont'd

- The Bass Technique of brushing in which the toothbrush bristles are adapted to the teeth and gingiva at a 45-degree angle and vibrated in short back strokes. This method is effective in cleaning gingival sulcus.

- Toothpaste is not necessary to remove plaque from teeth. Fluorinated paste is recommended if used.
- Patient uses dental floss to cleanse the interproximal tooth surfaces inaccessible to toothbrush.

- Edentulous patients with or without prostheses cleanse soft tissues of oral cavity gently to stimulate circulation.

- Patient frequently changes denture storage container and brush to decrease potential for infection/ colonization of bacteria.

- Patient removes dentures from oral cavity to allow oral tissues to rest.

- Frequent oral irrigations with alkaline lavage will help buffer acidity of oral cavity/promote cleansing lubrication of oral mucosa. Variations or other rinses may be recommended by physician and/or dentist.

- Patient states self-care behaviors and performs application.
- Patient obtains a fluoride prescription and fluoride carrier tray from dentist.
- Five minute application daily decreases radiation caries and dental sensitivity.
- Fluoride is available in gel, rinses, and tablets. A 1.23% neutral sodium gel applied in custom carrier is most commonly used.
- Edentulous patients do not require fluoride application.
- Patient states expectations and rationale for regular dental visits and early reporting of symptoms.
- Patient states reason for maintaining nutritional intake and self-care behaviors.

INTERVENTIONS — cont'd

- Instruct patient on nutritional stomatitis/taste loss — maintenance and foods to be avoided.
  Consult dietitian.
  Encourage patient to substitute aroma of foods for taste to stimulate appetite. Eat frequent smaller meals. Avoid extreme temperatures.
  Apply soothing ointments to lips for dryness/cracking.
  Moisten foods with sauces, gravies, creams, and other liquids.
  Puree food.
  Chew sugarless gum.
  Take vitamin B complex if prescribed.

  Restrict all sucrose intake (i.e., candies, cakes, pastries).

POTENTIAL COLLABORATIVE/CLINICAL PROBLEMS

- Mucositis
- Xerostomia
- Radiation caries
- Soft tissue necrosis and osteoradionecrosis

During the course of radiation therapy and at follow-up visits:

INTERVENTIONS FOR MUCOSITIS

- Monitor signs and symptoms of mucositis:
  Oral pain
  Burning
  Discomfort
  Difficulty chewing/swallowing/speaking
  Sensitivity to temperature extremes/highly seasoned foods
  Unable to tolerate wearing dentures

Medical interventions

- Have patient take systemic analgesic as prescribed
  Apply viscous lidocaine to produce topical anesthesia.
  Note: viscous lidocaine application may adversely affect patients' taste sensation. Patients may be unable to detect temperature extremes and inadvertently bite themselves.

Nursing interventions

- Maintain patient comfort:
  Use moist gauze, toothette, or water rinse to cleanse teeth and mouth if toothbrush causes discomfort.
  Temporarily suspend fluoride application if discomfort occurs.

OUTCOME CRITERIA — cont'd

- Patient maintains weight/hydration. States reason for nutritional maintenance and expected outcome and rationale for avoiding:
  All forms of tobacco
  All forms of alcohol, including mouthwashes
  Having teeth pulled after radiation
- Damage to microvilli and outer surface taste cells of tongue and their innervating nerve fibers decreases ability to taste. Taste loss, xerostomia, soreness, dryness, difficulty chewing, swallowing, and sucrose restrictions can result in weight loss and nutrition.
- Taste acuity will return following therapy.
  Vitamin B complex therapy is effective for patients that experience angular cheilosis and lingual manifestation related to malnutrition. Angular cheilosis may also be caused by a loss of vertical dimension between the mandible and maxilla.
  Sucrose intake for dentulous patients has little nutritional value, promotes radiation caries.

- Mucosal erythema is usually expected within 1 to 2 weeks after initiation of treatment. Radiation destroys the basal cell layer thereby thinning the mucosa. Ulcerations can occur spontaneously or as a result of trauma from brushing, dentures, food, or teeth. Swallowing can become difficult if pharyngeal mucosa is involved.

INTERVENTIONS FOR MUCOSITIS — cont'd

Avoid alcohol or mouthwashes containing alcohol (alcohol drys, irritates mucous membranes).

Suggest methods to assist patient with cessation of alcohol and tobacco consumption.

Avoid coarse, spicy, acidic foods, extreme temperatures. Consult with dietitian.

Maintain soft bland or liquid diet.

Remove dentures or prosthesis that rests within the radiation field (exception: mealtime if tolerated).

INTERVENTIONS FOR XEROSTOMIA

- Monitor signs and symptoms of xerostomia:
  Dry mouth
  Burning sensation
  Difficulty swallowing
  Difficulty speaking
  Decreased ability to tolerate wearing a prosthetic appliance

Medical interventions

- Refer patient to physician/dentist.

Nursing interventions

- Encourage use of prescribed synthetic salivas to lubricate mouth and buffer oral microflora.
- Carry out frequent oral irrigations as prescribed.
- Have patient drink water and sugar-free beverages throughout the day as prescribed.
- Puree foods or use food processor.
- Moisten foods with gravies, sauces.
- Have patient use humidifier at home.
- Encourage use of sugarless gum and candy, ice chips.
- Have dentist instruct on wearing dentures.

INTERVENTIONS FOR RADIATION CARIES

- Monitor signs and symptoms of radiation caries:
  Tooth sensitivity
  Pain
  Destruction of teeth

OUTCOME CRITERIA — cont'd

- Radiation to the major and minor salivary glands results in a significant decrease in salivary secretions, changes in pH, viscosity, volume, and inorganic constituents of saliva. Alterations in quality and quantity of saliva inhibit the saliva to cleanse, lubricate, and buffer the oral cavity, predisposing the patient to caries and periodontal disease. Salivary flow decreases, and saliva is thick, viscous, and stringy. Saliva contains microbial compounds important in the mechanical removal of pathogens from mouth.

- Xerostomia and associated changes in salivary flow related to radiation can create environment for a highly acidic and cariogenic oral microflora. The total output of salivary production results in reduction of caries-protective electrolytes and immunoproteins. Reduced consumption of high detergent foods (coarse/roughage) that cleanse teeth also contributes to caries formation. Carious lesions can occur up to 3 months following completion, appear on the cervical margin of teeth, and progress to complete destruction of the crown. Patients are at risk for caries for their entire lives.

INTERVENTIONS FOR RADIATION CARIES — cont'd

Medical interventions

- Refer patient to physician/dentist.
    Maintenance of oral hygiene program
    Frequent alkaline lavage
    Restriction of sucrose intake

Nursing interventions

- Reinforce all prescriptions.

INTERVENTIONS FOR TISSUE NECROSIS

- Monitor signs and symptoms of tissue necrosis and osteoradionecrosis:
    Throbbing pain
    Bleeding
    Suppuration
    Fetid odor in breath
    Difficulty eating

INTERVENTIONS FOR INFECTION

- Monitor signs and symptoms of infection:
    Complaints of pain, burning, tenderness
    Bleeding (gingiva) tooth mobility
    Elevated temperature

Medical interventions

- Use topical nystatin mouth rinses daily.
- Ensure frequent physician/dental visits.
- Administer antibiotics if indicated.

Nursing interventions

- Maintain meticulous oral hygiene.
- Carry out oral irrigations.
- Provide for consistent monitoring of oral cavity.
- Monitor vital signs, specifically temperature.

INTERVENTIONS FOR TRISMUS

- Monitor signs and symptoms of trismus:
    Impaired ability to open mouth widely
    Impaired ability to chew
    Impaired ability to speak

Medical interventions

- Use prosthetic appliances and elastics prepared by dentist/prosthodontist.

OUTCOME CRITERIA — cont'd

- Soft tissue necrosis is the progressive enlarging of mucosal ulcers that become necrotic and may develop in radiated soft tissue as a result of radiation-induced fibrosis and impaired blood supply. Osteoradionecrosis is a progressive condition as a result of radiation on the osteocytes, regional blood supply, and bone marrow. Bony exposure, infection, and necrosis can occur, resulting in bone sequestration and fracture. Osteoradionecrosis is common in the mandible, usually results from trauma, and usually occurs within a year of treatment. This process can progress to pathologic fracture, infection of surrounding soft tissues, and oral-cutaneous fistula formation.

- Infection can occur during or following radiation. Oral infections are most common (such as candidiasis [thrush], periodontal disease [pyorrhea]). Periodontal disease is manifested by hyperemic and edematous gingiva.

- Muscles of mastication undergo fibrosis related to radiation. This may be indicative of disease recurrence — occurs 3 to 6 months after completion of therapy. Fibrosis of the muscles of mastication and the temporomandibular joint, while uncommon, may result in trismus.

INTERVENTIONS FOR TRISMUS — cont'd

Nursing interventions
- Refer patient to physician/dentist.
- Instruct patient to exercise masticatory muscles before, during, and after treatment—opening and closing mouth 20 times in row tid.
- Maintain meticulous oral hygiene.

fungal, or viral in origin. One of the most common acute infections seen in patients is moniliasis, resulting from radiation-induced changes of the normal oral flora. The nurse should monitor the patient for the classic white patches that scrape off, leaving burning tissue.

Fungal Infections

Topical and systemic antifungal agents may be prescribed by the physician. Antifungal agents are commonly mixed with sucrose to make the drug more palatable. A nonsucrose-containing antifungal agent should be used by head and neck cancer patients to prevent caries formation. A patient who wears a dental prosthesis or uses fluoride carrier trays must be instructed that these are to be removed from the oral cavity and immersed in an antifungal agent for 8 hours to avoid reintroduction of fungal organisms into the oral cavity. Toothbrushes and denture-soaking containers should be changed frequently.

The nurse should perform a weekly routine oral examination of patients to detect new lesions early in their development; the nurse must note carefully size, shape, location, and appearance. Cultures or smears of new lesions may be ordered by the physician to document and facilitate treatment of any superimposed infection.

Palliative treatment of mucositis related to radiation includes oral rinses and application of topical anesthetics. Sodium bicarbonate oral rinse (1 teaspoon of baking soda in 32 ounces of water or normal saline) should be used at least six times a day. Topical anesthetics can be used, progressing from the least potent and toxic to the more potent and toxic (see pp. 244-249).

Dermatitis

Dermatitis, an acute condition characterized by a "sunburned" appearance, results from radiation inhibiting mitosis of epithelial cells. The patient may experience significant pain or discomfort and become reluctant to perform any self-care. Treatment of this condition is discussed in detail in Chapter 29.

Xerostomia

Xerostomia (dry mouth) occurs when radiation therapy causes sclerosis of the acini of the salivary gland. Saliva regulates the pH in the oral cavity, which controls bacterial flora, and lubricates and cleanses the teeth. When the amount of saliva and consistency (thick) are changed, generalized oral disease can occur, and an environment conducive to caries formation is created. The oral pH becomes more acidic when salivary flow decreases and allows a major caries-forming organism, *Streptococcus*, to grow. Salivary flow can be accurately measured before and following radiation by having the patient undergo sialometric testing. With this measurement capability the clinician can measure the patient's ability to produce saliva when stimulated, either in total or by stimulation of paired major salivary glands.

Radiation therapy also affects taste bud function. Alteration in taste (dysgeusia) and decreased taste (hypogeusesthesia) can occur. The degree of taste alteration and impairment depends on the site and dose of radiation. Taste sensations are decreased because food must be in solution to be tasted. Taste buds, like other normal cells, will regenerate following the completion of radiation, if adequate nutrition is maintained. Most patients experience a degree of return of function within 4 to 12 months; however, in some patients taste alterations may be permanent. Most patients undergoing radiation therapy state that the taste sensation of sweetness lasts the longest. This is related to the fact that there are normally more taste buds devoted to detection of sweets than sour, or salt. The nurse must remember that with this alteration in taste sensation the patient may naturally increase sugar intake to obtain the same level of sweetness. Alternative sources for sugar should be identified to prevent radiation caries.

Palliation of xerostomia, hypogeusia, and impaired swallowing can be achieved by adequate hydration of the oral cavity with nonsucrose liquids. Most salivary substitutes consist of sodium carboxymethyl cellulose combined with fluoride and other agents. In 1992 a multi-institutional randomized double-blind study demonstrated that pilocarpine HCL may have a direct treatment benefit for hyposalivation in post-radiated patients. Pilocarpine is a cholinergal parasympathomimetic agent that acts as an agonist on the muscarinic receptors. When given orally it stimulates salivary flow (personal communication, Harper Hospital Department of Dentistry, F. Leveque DDS).

If the patient prefers not to carry a thermos of water or some other liquid to sip on frequently, then several artificial saliva products are commercially available, such as Moi-Stir (Kingswood Laboratory, Carmel, Indiana), Orex (Young Dental, Maryland Heights, Maryland), Salivart (Westport Pharmaceuticals, Westport, Connecticut), and Xerolube (Scherer Laboratories, Dallas, Texas). In addition, the patient should be instructed to moisten the lips with lanolin or cocoa butter. Rinses or creams containing synthetic steroids (e.g., Kenalog) should be avoided because they have the potential to facilitate fungal growth in preexisting conditions conducive to fungus. Patients may stimulate unaffected salivary glands by sucking or chewing on sucrose-free sour candies or gum. A dietary consult will aid the patient in learning additional food preparation techniques to facilitate chewing and swallowing (e.g., addition of sauces and gravies to dry foods, stimulation of taste sensations by the aroma of warm foods).*

Radiation Caries

Radiation caries can result from radiation-induced xerostomia, poor oral hygiene, and high sucrose intake. These lesions form within 2 to 3 months compared to several months in the normal patient. Classically, radiation caries occur in areas of the tooth that are normally self-cleaning, such as the incisional edges of the anterior teeth, near the gum line, and the cuspids. The preventive treatment regimen for radiation caries should include five key segments: pretreatment evaluation, periodontal care, oral hygiene instructions, daily fluoride application, and limited sucrose intake.[72] Once radiation caries form, teeth are at a high risk for fractures, and actual extractions are not recommended.[51,111]

Osteoradionecrosis

Osteoradionecrosis (infection into the bone) is by far the most devastating of all the chronic sequelae of radiation to the head and neck. In spite of improved technology of shielding and treatment delivery, patients remain at risk for this long-term side effect.[14,23,51,78]

Radiation causes hypoxic, hypocellular hypovascularization, resulting in tissue breakdown, cellular breakdown, cellular death, and collagen lysis that ex-

ceeds synthesis. Marx and co-workers describe this phenomena: "osteoradionecrosis is not a primary infection of irradiated bone, it is a complex metabolic and tissue hemostasis deficiency created by radiation-induced cellular injury and replication." This radiation-induced cellular injury weakens the bone and tissue, decreasing the ability to respond to injury, and produces favorable conditions for trauma and infection to occur. The mandible, with its single-source blood supply has a higher incidence of osteoradionecrosis than the maxilla, which has a broad-based blood supply.[23,51,111]

Monitoring the patient for osteoradionecrosis is extremely important. Nurses play a significant role in prevention of this phenomenon. Patient education, postradiation follow-up appointments, and the importance of regular examinations should be presented as *essential* and *nonoptional*. At these visits, the nurse should perform a thorough oral examination, documenting the presence or absence of chronic oral ulcerations, defective teeth, caries, defective restorations, or poorly fitting dentures. If any of these are identified, the patient should be immediately referred to the dentist for an examination. Follow-up visits should include concurrent medical and dental evaluations. Although prevention is the best approach to managing this potential clinical problem, local irrigations, high-dose extended antibiotics, and surgical procedures to remove dead bone tissue may be indicated.

Trismus

Patients that receive radiation that directly affects the muscles of mastication or the temporomandibular joint (TMJ) may develop trismus. Trismus may occur during therapy or may become problematic up until 6 months after completion of radiotherapy. Patient education about mouth-opening exercises is extremely important. A simple exercise of opening the mouth as widely as possible 20 times, three to four times a day, should minimize muscle fibrosis and loss of mobility. If trismus is noted, the degree of opening must be recorded and monitored at the patient's regular follow-up appointments. The dentist or maxillofacial prosthodontist may prescribe special appliances similar to those prescribed by an orthodontist, such as wedges, or appliances with screws, springs, or elastic for the patient to wear. Most physicians use all possible conservative measures to treat this side effect, leaving surgical interventions to the last. Any surgical procedure on devitalized tissue/bone holds the potential for poor healing and/or infection.

Chronic Side Effects

Chronic side effects of radiation include anorexia, alteration in taste (dysgeusia), and generalized leth-

---

*References 29, 44, 127, 133, 137, 138.

argy.[137] Ideally, every patient undergoing radiation for head and neck cancer should be seen by a nurse and registered dietitian before, during, and after radiation. Nutritional evaluation and support should be provided for at least 6 months after completion of radiation. Weight loss or potential for weight loss less than body requirements should be anticipated during radiation therapy. Weight loss will continue after radiation, being maximal at 3 months and remaining virtually unchanged for 6 months after treatment.[19,22,24,29,138]

Health-care education for patients undergoing radiation therapy should include the following:
- Importance of returning for all appointments
- Maintaining individualized oral hygiene program—brushing, flossing, fluoride, ongoing dental assessment
- Nutrition/weight maintenance/monitoring/gain
- Maintaining/return to normal lifestyles, work, recreation, family, social life

A comprehensive nursing care plan and guidelines for monitoring for potential collaborative/clinical problems are listed on pp. 244-249.

Chemotherapy

The role of chemotherapy in the treatment of head and neck cancer has changed since more single active agents and combinations have been discovered.[4,5,80] In the past, systemic chemotherapy was used as a palliative treatment or for patients who had persistent, recurrent disease, or disseminated metastases after standard therapy (surgery/radiation).[3,47,50,60] A brief discussion of agents under evaluation for the treatment of head and neck cancers is included in this chapter. Individual agents, classification, metabolism, toxicity, and indications are discussed in Chapter 22.

Medical oncologists are using chemotherapy in conjunction with standard therapy, surgery, and radiation. Clinical trials designed to answer questions related to efficacy timing, and sequencing of treatment are currently underway in national cooperative and intergroup studies.* Chemotherapy sequencing and timing may be given in three ways and are listed in the box on this page.

These sequences and combinations seek to answer questions related to treating head and neck cancer.
- What is the best combination to use?
- When should chemotherapy be included in the treatment plan?
- When and in what sequence should chemotherapy be used (e.g., preoperatively, before radiation, or in conjunction with radiation)?
- Is there a benefit of using chemotherapy as part of multimodality therapy?

*References 4, 5, 8, 9, 47, 50, 58, 78, 79, 84, 88, 119.

> **CHEMOTHERAPY SEQUENCING AND TIMING**
>
> Induction chemotherapy—used before standard treatment; also called neoadjuvant, prostandard, or prestandard therapy.
> Concurrent chemotherapy—used as total treatment or postoperatively in patients with resectable tumors.
> Sandwich chemotherapy—used after surgery or before radiotherapy.
> Maintenance chemotherapy—used after standard therapies.

- Does giving chemotherapy first delay or lessen the need for extensive radiation or surgery?
- Does chemotherapy have an effect on disease-free survival, overall survival, quality of life?
- What is the incidence of chronic or delayed side effects?
- Does chemotherapy cause a change in patterns of recurrence?

The physician monitors the patient's response to chemotherapy by clinical and physical examination, by x-rays, and by validating absence of tumor by having the surgeon obtain multiple biopsies. Nurses are responsible for educating and monitoring the patient for clinical problems related to the chemotherapy, such as adjustment to illness, knowledge deficits, potential for effective individual/family coping, comforts, and potential for infection.

Chemotherapeutic drugs that have demonstrated significant activity in head and neck cancer include methotrexate, bleomycin, Oncovin, cisplatin, carboplatin, and 5-fluorouracil (5-FU). These first-line agents are currently being used singly or in combinations for the treatment of head and neck cancer. If the patient fails to respond clinically, the physician may prescribe second-line therapies such as WR 2721 with high-dose cisplatin and 5-FU, or weekly IV methotrexate.[6,9,58,85] The nurse and patient will need to monitor for transient, acute, subacute, and chronic side effects related to these agents. One of the most important aspects of nursing care is educating and reinforcing to the patient the importance of maintaining scheduled appointments. Response to therapy and early detection of toxicities or new lesions can only be determined if the patient keeps the appointment. Patients may be tempted to delay or skip a treatment until they "get stronger," "feel better," "gain weight," or "conduct personal business." Early detection of side effects related to chemotherapy can facilitate patient comfort and safety. Documentation of toxicities and side effects is critical because subsequent therapies are determined and calculated by the patient's tolerance to treatment.[67]

PRETREATMENT ASSESSMENT. The general clinical status of the head and neck cancer patient is one of the best predictors of the patient's ability to tolerate chemotherapy, respond well to it, and survive. A pretreatment assessment of the patient's clinical status must be thoroughly evaluated, and should include age; nutritional status; disease staging (TNM); documentation of other disease processes (e.g., cardiac, pulmonary, TB); function and reserve of lung, liver, kidney, bone marrow; and prior therapies (e.g., chemotherapy, radiation, or surgery). The treatment of squamous cell carcinoma of the head and neck has reached the stage where chemotherapy may be potentially curative. Successful development of chemotherapeutic regimens that are curative in patients with advanced stages of disease hold the potential for effectively treating many nonadvanced patients.

Two techniques, MRI and solid flow cytometry, hold the potential to identify head and neck tumors or cellular characteristics that may direct the course of therapy. The use of flow cytometry to detect and measure tumor parameters has doubled over the last 4 decades. This technique involves passing a beam of light through a head and neck cancer cell. In theory, any part of the cell that can be caused to fluoresce by interruption of a beam of light when it passes through all of the DNA/RNA structures can be measured and studied. These techniques have proven efficacious in hematologic malignancies and may be able to identify tumor characteristics that could predict how head and neck tumors will respond to chemotherapy, radiotherapy, or surgery.[33,34,45,46,48-50]

The patient's overall performance status is consistently associated with prognostic outcome, including determining the response to systemic chemotherapy and survival. The better the patient's performance status, the greater the patient's ability to tolerate therapy, and the greater the likelihood that he or she will respond and survive longer.

Al-Sarraf and co-workers identified and reported two groups of prognostic factors that play an important role in determining the overall survival of the patient with recurrent or systemic disease (see the box on this page).

Up to 30% of patients who are unwilling to alter their lifestyles, particularly those who continue to smoke and drink, experience the occurrence of second cancers.

A complete nursing biopsychosocial evaluation should be included in the pretreatment evaluation. Emphasis should be placed on determining the patient's level of education, educational needs, literacy, and ability to learn/comprehend. Toxic effects related to chemotherapy can be life-threatening in patients who are unable to understand and monitor for these side effects.[35]

PROGNOSTIC FACTORS IN RECURRENT AND/OR SYSTEMIC HEAD AND NECK CANCER

Good prognosis factors
- Good performance status
- Minimal disease
- Local recurrence only
- No bony erosion
- Good response to induction (adjuvant) chemotherapy
- Good response to previous chemotherapy
- Long disease-free interval (DFT)
- First line chemotherapy
- Good organ(s) function
- CR (complete response) to chemotherapy

Poor prognosis factors
- Poor performance status
- Bulky disease
- Systemic/visceral disease
- Bone metastasis and/or hypercalcemia (and local bone invasion)
- Lymphangitis spread (skin)
- Failure of radiotherapy (persistent disease)
- Failure of induction (adjuvant) chemotherapy
- Patients receiving first line chemotherapy for recurrent and/or systemic cancer
- Organ(s) impairment
- Less than a complete response (CR) to chemotherapy

Modified from Al-Sarraf M: Head and neck cancer: chemotherapy concepts. Semin Oncol 15:70, 1988.

REHABILITATION

As treatment protocols improve, more patients are being diagnosed with secondary primary lesions or distant metastasis. The patient who has been treated for head and neck cancer is at significant risk for recurrent disease at the primary site or the neck.[110,115,134] The patient should also be monitored for a metachronous primary in the head and neck area, lung, or esophagus.[71] Ongoing assessment and evaluation of response to treatment are essential for early diagnosis of disease and validation of health. Routine follow-up of patients should include a thorough examination of the head and neck with indirect laryngoscopy once a month for the first year, every 2 months during the second year, and every 3 months the fifth year after treatment. Patients with new symptoms of significant weight loss, dysphagia, chronic soreness, or persistent hoarseness should have an endoscopic examination with biopsy when tumor is not visible by examination. Nurses share the responsibility to educate patients and reinforce the importance of maintaining scheduled appointments. Careful and meticulous follow-up is a significant link to long-term survival in this patient group. Nurses should emphasize the importance of maintaining a healthy lifestyle. The patient should be educated on the importance of ces-

Nursing Management

Individualized nursing care plans addressing lack of knowledge related to chemotherapy, and monitoring for potential side effects related to chemotherapy should be established. Family or significant others should always be incorporated into the teaching and care plan, because they can assist in monitoring the patient's response to treatment as well as adjustment to illness.

Routine home care nursing referral for patients receiving chemotherapy is recommended after the initial treatment and for those persons who continue to demonstrate knowledge deficits related to chemotherapy. The home care nurses can monitor for side effects of chemotherapy, reinforce patient teaching, validate the patient's ability to perform self-care, and monitor for adequate hydration and nutrition.

DENTAL EVALUATION

The goal of dental therapy for patients undergoing chemotherapy is the same as with radiation therapy and surgery,[1] to reduce potential infections and morbidity and avoid unnecessary delays of chemotherapeutic treatments. Chemotherapeutic agents such as 5-FU, methotrexate, or bleomycin, alone or in combination with radiation therapy, affect tissues with high turnover rates, such as the oral mucosa. Mucosal tissues, in general, are subject to chronic physical trauma and infection. As discussed previously, when the patient experiences decreased host resistance, changes in normal bacteria, viral and fungal flora, have the potential to become pathogens and infect the patient.

Once chemotherapy has been initiated, the focus of dental therapy should be directed at maintaining oral hygiene and decreasing the potential for infection. Guidelines for oral hygiene and dental care are similar to the patient undergoing radiotherapy.

NUTRITIONAL ASSESSMENT

Common nutritional problems experienced by these patients relate to not only the treatment modality, but also to altered physiologic function related to tumor involvement. A pretreatment nursing nutritional assessment is important to identify any anticipated problems related to the patient's ability to maintain weight and hydration. The nutritional assessment should include a careful dietary history (including previous alcohol exposure) and daily intake, weight loss, and patient completion of a 3-day dietary recall. These data enable the professional and patient to develop a reasonable pretreatment nutritional plan. The nutritional plan ideally should be implemented before initiation of chemotherapy and monitored closely throughout the entire course of treatment. Having the patient complete the 3-day recall provides the nurse and clinical dietitian with an excellent tool for patient education. Patient education booklets such as "Eating Hints" and other dietary materials are available free from the NIH and American Cancer Society.

Fluctuations of 2 to 3 lb between monthly visits is acceptable, but any rapid weight loss unrelated to infection or chemotherapy side effects may require the physician to place the patient on short-term or long-term enteral or parenteral nutrition. Head and neck patients undergoing combinations of chemotherapy that incorporate platinum or platinum derivatives should be monitored for signs and symptoms of dehydration and fluid and electrolyte imbalances.[67] These agents are extremely nephrotoxic, and a key nursing intervention to circumvent toxicity is to maintain hydration and have the patient maintain a strict intake and output record. Likewise, patients should be provided with written guidelines for the monitoring of their hydration and should know when to notify the nurse or physician if they are unable to maintain hydration. Patients should be provided information on alternative sources of fluid such as ice cream, jello, popsicles, and milkshakes. Symptom control (e.g., nausea and vomiting) and prescriptive therapies will depend on the chemotherapeutic agent given and the patient's response to treatment.[108,109]

sation of alcohol and tobacco, notifying physician of early symptoms, and keeping appointments.

RECURRENT DISEASE

Treatment options of recurrent disease are limited. The clinical management and treatment of recurrent disease depend on accurate specific site and staging of the disease. Recurrent head and neck cancer is, by definition, a failure to the standard definitive local therapy. Approximately 40% of these patients will recur overall, 20% locoregionally, 10% with distant metastasis, and another 10% with both local and distant disease. Many of these patients relapse within 6 to 24 months after treatment and have a median survival of 6 months from initial diagnosis to recurrence. In the past, reirradiation of recurrent tumors in the head and neck was performed with extreme caution. In select patient populations reirradiation has been combined with surgery and/or chemotherapy in attempts to control the disease.[118] Managing the psychosocial consequences of cancer recurrence provides nursing with a unique opportunity to implement interventions that can fulfill the emotional and spiritual needs of both the patient and families.[97,160]

In addition to recurrent disease, the physician is often challenged with other common clinical problems, which may significantly limit treatment options. The physician must identify the treatment regimen that holds the highest therapeutic value and lowest risk/benefit ratio.* Diseases related to lifestyles, chronic obstructive pulmonary disease, liver/renal disease substantially affect the physician's ability to deliver adequate therapeutic doses of chemotherapy such as cisplatin, bleomycin, or methotrexate. Age-related diseases, such as underlying cardiac problems, hypertension, and diabetes, can limit tolerance to chemotherapy.

Common tumor-related factors can impact the timing and choice of treatment such as fluorouracil and cisplatin. Malnutrition secondary to tumor or alcohol can have a major negative influence on treatment. Meningeal carcinomatoses and cranial nerve involvement may occur when the patient's tumor involves the base of the skull. These patients may require lumbar punctures and placement of Ommaya reservoir for intrathecal instillation of methotrexate. Hypercalcemia related to bone or tumor involvement will require aggressive hydration and furosemide treatment before chemotherapy can be administered. Infection related to local wound cellulitis or recurring aspiration pneumonia may result in sepsis, requiring antibiotic therapy and delaying the administration of chemotherapy. In addition, bleeding from the carotid or small vessels can produce a significant obstacle. Chemotherapies that cause nausea and vomiting can precipitate bleeding. Many patients may require surgical intervention for fulguration, or occasional embolization of the artery to control bleeding.

Choice of treatment for recurrent head and neck cancer will also be significantly influenced by the patient's previous exposure to radiotherapy or chemotherapy and ability to tolerate further bone marrow suppressive treatments.[85,88]

The boxes on this page and the next page list side effects, patient teaching priorities, and geriatric considerations.

CONCLUSION

Cancers of the head and neck are estimated to be the most prevalent cancers in the world. Whereas the

*References 3, 5, 8, 9, 60, 85.

HEAD AND NECK CANCER TREATMENT RELATED SIDE EFFECTS

Surgery
- Potential for structural, functional, or cosmetic loss: e.g., changes in bodily appearance and function (breathing, speaking, swallowing, coughing, and mobility)
- Respiratory distress; hypoxia, airway obstruction, tracheal edema, aspiration; hemorrhage; hematoma; arterial rupture; failure of flap survival; nerve damage.

Radiation therapy

Mucositis	Xerostomia
Pain	Radiation caries
Infection	Osteoradionecrosis
Dermatitis	Fungal infections
Trismus	Dysgeusia

Chemotherapy

Mucositis	Dehydration
Infection	Electrolyte imbalance
Immunosuppression	Nausea and vomiting
Weight loss	Diarrhea

General considerations
Patients with head and neck cancers receiving multimodality therapy may experience severe and permanent facial disfigurement and functional loss that resembles what is experienced by the burn patient.

PATIENT TEACHING PRIORITIES

- Rationale for pretreatment evaluation:
    Psychosocial assessment—potential changes in body image (structural, functional, and cosmetic changes)
    Cardiopulmonary assessment and health history
- Nutritional assessment; communication/cognitive motor skill dental assessment
- Rationale for treatment:
    Surgery—Review purpose, rationale, and potential sequelae; explain common terms and procedures; discuss preoperative and postoperative nursing interventions.
    Radiation therapy—Review purpose, rationale, and potential side effects of the therapy; explain the procedures, purpose of positioning the body, and scheduling of the radiation therapy treatments.
    Chemotherapy—Review purpose, rationale, and potential side effects of the therapy, discuss the chemotherapy treatment schedule and the need for weekly blood tests to monitor the side effects of the drugs.
    Rehabilitation—Initiate referrals to social worker, speech pathologist, physical therapist, occupational therapist, clinical dietician, and nurse specialist.

GERIATRIC CONSIDERATIONS

- *Age-related losses* such as vision, hearing, communication, fine motor skills (writing), and swallowing/eating functions will be further compromised by effects of surgery/radiation therapy and/or chemotherapy.
- *Nutritional and dental assessment* with appropriate interventions will need to be adapted to age-related changes (diet history-likes/dislikes; dentures and/or lack of due to age or finances)
- *Pretreatment evaluation:* psychosocial, cardiopulmonary, health history will require age-related adjustments and appropriate interventions
- *Treatment-related factors:* surgery, radiation therapy, chemotherapy, and rehabilitation will require age-related adjustments and appropriate interventions. Patients with chronic diseases such as hypertension, cardiopulmonary insufficiency, diabetes,

chronic obstructive pulmonary disease, arthritis, and chronic renal disease will require medical treatment adjustments.
   Surgery: potential for longer recovery and rehabilitation period.
   Radiation therapy: treatment schedule may require adjustment for recovery of side effects; fatigue/immunosuppression, weight loss, stomatitis, and infection.
   Chemotherapy: drug dosage, frequency of infusion, and monitoring of blood count will require adjustment (drug toxicities may increase related to the aforementioned chronic diseases).
- Transportation, financial, family resources, and home care responsibilities will require assessment and intervention based on the deficits and/or availability.

---

physician's goals are improving treatment and patient survival, the nurse is challenged with assisting the patient to adjustments related to the disease, treatment, and rehabilitative living. The most important nursing challenge, however, is in the areas of early detection, prevention, patient education, and quality of life.[26-28,42,81,99] The incidence of head and neck cancers will never significantly decrease until patient use of the most common cocarcinogen (tobacco) ceases. Herein lies a challenge to all medical professionals.

BIBLIOGRAPHY

1. Aaronson NK and Beckman J: The quality of life for cancer patients, New York, 1987, Raven Press.
2. Allison GR, Rappaport I, and Salibian AH: Adaptive mechanisms of speech and swallowing after combined jaw and tongue reconstruction in long-term survivors. Am Surg 154:419-422, 1987.
3. Al-Kourainy K and others: Excellent response to *cis*-platinum based chemotherapy in patients with recurrent or previously untreated advanced nasopharyngeal carcinoma. Am J Clin Oncol 11:427-430, 1988.
4. Al-Sarraf M: Head and neck cancer: Chemotherapy concepts, Semin Oncol 15(1):70, 1988.
5. Al-Sarraf M and others: Concurrent radiotherapy and chemotherapy with *cis*-platinum inoperable squamous cell carcinoma of the head and neck: An RTOG study, Cancer 59:259-265, 1987.
6. Al-Sarraf M and others: Current progress in head and neck cancer: The Wayne State Experience. In Jacobs JR and others, editors: Head and neck cancer: Scientific perspectives in management and strategies for care, New York, 1987, Elsevier.
7. Al-Sarraf M: Management strategies in head and neck cancer: The role of carboplatin. I carboplatin (JM-8). Current perspective and future directions. In Bunn PA, Canetta R, Ozols RF, and Rosenweig M, editors: Philadelphia, 1990, WB Saunders Co.
8. Al-Sarraf M and others: Combined modality therapy (CMT) in patients with head and neck cancer (HN-CA): Timing of chemotherapy, (CT). In Salton, sie JT editor: Radiation therapy oncology group (RTOG)6 study adjunct therapy of cancer, Philadelphia, 1990, WB Saunders Co.
9. Al-Sarraf M and others: Concurrent radiotherapy and chemotherapy with cistplatin inoperable squamous cell carcinoma of the head and neck. RTOG study. Cancer 54:259-265, 1987.
10. Al-Sarraf M: Head and neck cancer. Mediguide to oncology 8:1-6, 1988.
11. Ali S and others: Incidence of squamous cell carcinoma of the head and neck, J Laryngol Otol 100:315, 1986.
12. American Joint Committee on Cancer: Manual for staging of cancer, ed 4, Philadelphia, 1992, JB Lippincott Co.
13. Amerin PC, Fingert H, and Weitzman SA: Cis-platin-vincristine-bleomycin therapy in squamous cell carcinoma of the head and neck, J Clin Oncol 1:421, 1983.
14. Amour RJ and others: Postoperative irradiation for squamous cell carcinoma of the head and neck: An analysis of treatment results and complications. Int J Radiat Oncol Biol Phys 16:25-36, l989.
15. Anderson BL: Sexual functioning morbidity among cancer survivors, Cancer 55(7):1835, 1985.
16. Ariyan S: The pectoralis mycutaneous flap, Plast Reconstr Surg 63:73, 1979.

17. Baker SR, editor: Microsurgical reconstruction of the head and neck, New York, Edinburgh, London, Melbourne, 1989, Churchill Livingstone.
18. Barton FE, Spicer TE, and Byrd HS: Head and neck reconstruction with the latissimus dorsi myocutaneous flap: Anatomic observations and report of 60 cases, Plastic Reconstr Surg 71:1999, 1983.
19. Basset MR and Dobie RA: Patterns of nutritional deficiency in head and neck cancer, Otolaryngol Head Neck Surg 91:119, 1983.
20. Belcher AE: Nursing aspects of quality of life enhancement in cancer patients, Oncol 4(5):197-199, 1990.
21. Bertott JA: Trapezius musculocutaneous island flap in repair of major head and neck cancer. Plastic Reconstr Surg 65:16-21, 1980.
22. Beumer J, Curtis TA, and Morrish RB: Radiation complications in edentulous patients, J Prosthet Dent 36:193, 1976.
23. Beumer J and others: Osteonecrosis: predisposing factors and outcomes of therapy, Head Neck Surg 6:819, 1984.
24. Brookes GBH: Nutritional status: A prognostic indicator in head and neck cancer, Otolaryngol Head Neck Surg 93:69, 1985.
25. Buchbinder D and others: Functional mandibular reconstruction of patients with oral cancer, Oral Surg Oral Med Pathol 68(4):499-504, 1989.
26. Cassileth BR and others: The satisfaction and psychosocial status of patients during treatment of cancer, J Psychosoc Oncol 7(4):47-57, 1989.
27. Cella DF: Cancer and survival: psychosocial and public issues, Cancer Invest 5:59, 1987.
28. Cella DF and Lesko IM: Cancer survivors: Watch for signs of stress even years later, Oncol Rounds March 1, 1988.
29. Chencharick JD and Mossman KL: Nutritional consequences of radiotherapy of the head and neck cancer, Cancer 51:811, 1983.
30. Conti J: Cancer rehabilitation: Why can't we get out of first gear? J Rehabilitation 56(4):19-22, 1990.
31. Cook TA and others: Cervical rotation flaps for midface resurfacing, Arch Otolaryngol Head Neck Surg 117:77-82, 1991.
32. Crane L: Infections in patients with head and neck cancer. In Jacobs JR and others, editors: Head and neck cancer: Scientific perspectives in management and strategies for care, New York, 1987, Elsevier.
33. Crissman JD and others: Histopathologic diagnosis of early cancer, Head Neck Cancer 1:134, 1985.
34. Crissman JD: Prognostic value of histopathologic parameters in squamous cell carcinoma of the oropharynx, Cancer 54:2995, 1984.
35. D'Acquisto RW and others: The influence of chronic high alcohol intake on chemotherapy induced nausea and vomiting, Proc Am Soc Clin Oncol 5:257, 1986.
36. David DJ, Tan E, Katsaros J, and Sheen R: Mandibular reconstruction with vascularized crest: A 10 year experience, Plastic Reconstr Surg 82:792, 1988.
37. Deitel M and To TB: Major intestinal complications of radiotherapy, Arch Surg 122:1421, 1987.
38. Depalo LG and Minah GE: Isolation of Pathogenic Microorganisms from dentures and denture soaking containers of the myelosuppressed cancer patients, J Prosthet Dent 49:20, 1983.
39. DeSanto L and Beahrs OH: The modified and radical neck dissection for squamous cell carcinoma of the upper aerodigestive system. In Jacobs J and others, editors: Scientific and clinical perspective of head and neck cancer management strategies for cure, New York, 1987, Elsevier.
40. Douglas BG: Superfractionation: Its rationale and anticipated benefits, Int J Radiat Oncol Biol Phys 8:1143, 1982.
41. Duchateau J, Declty A, and Lejour M: Innervation of the rectus abdominous muscle implications for rectus flaps, Plast Reconstr Surg 223-227, 1988.
42. Dudas S and Carlson CE: Cancer rehabilitation, Oncol Nurs Forum 15:183, 1988.
43. Elias EG: Surgical management of head and neck neoplasia. In Peterson DE and others, editors: Head and neck management of the cancer patient, Boston, 1986, Martinus Nijhoff.
44. Elias EG and McCaslin DL: Nutrition in the patient with compromised oral function. In Peterson DE and others, editors: Head and neck management of the cancer patient, Boston, 1986, Martinus Nijhoff.
45. Ensley JF and others: The significance of pretreatment identification of prognostically important subgroups of squamous cell cancers of the head and neck. In Jacobs JR and others, editors: Scientific and clinical perspectives of head and neck cancer management strategies for cure, New York, 1987, Elsevier.
46. Ensley J and others: The impact of conventional morphological analysis on response rates and survival in patients with squamous cell cancers of the head and neck. Cancer 57:711-717, 1986.
47. Ensley J and others: Improved responses to radiation and concurrent cisplatin (CACP) in patients with advanced head and neck cancer (SCCHN) that fail induction chemotherapy. Proceedings of Sixth International Conference on Adjuvant Therapy of Cancer, March 7-10, 1990, Tucson, Arizona.

48. Ensley JF and others: Cellular DNA content parameters in untreated squamous cell cancers of the head and neck. Cytometry 10:334-338, 1980.

49. Ensley JF, Kish JA and Al-Sarraf M: The pretherapeutic identification of prognostically important parameters predictive of tumor response in squamous cell cancers of the head and neck. In Vog SE, editor: Contemporary issues in clinical oncology, head and neck cancer, Vol 7, New York, 1988, Churchill Livingstone.

50. Ensley JF and others: The correlation of specific variables of tumor differentiation with response rate of survival in patients with advanced head and neck cancer treated with induction chemotherapy. Cancer 63:1487-1492, 1989.

51. Epstein JB and others: Osteonecrosis: Study of relationship of dental extractions in patients receiving radiotherapy, Head Neck Surg 10:48, 1987.

52. Ervin TJ and others: An analysis of induction and adjuvant chemotherapy in the multidisciplinary treatment of squamous-cell carcinoma of the head and neck, J Clin Oncol 5:10, 1987.

53. Fearon KCH and others: Influence of whole body protein turnover rate on resting energy expenditure in patients with cancer, Cancer Res 48:2590, 1988.

54. Ferrans C: Quality of life: Conceptual issues. Semin Oncol Nurs 6:248-254, 1990.

55. Fisher J and Jackson T: Microvascular surgery as an adjunct to craniomaxillofacial reconstruction, Br J Plast Surg 42:146-154, 1989.

56. Fisher S: The psychosexual effects of cancer and cancer treatment, Oncol Nurs Forum 10(2):63-67, 1983.

57. Fletcher GH and Jesse RH: The place of irradiation in the management of the primary lesion in the head and neck cancer, Cancer 39:862, 1977.

58. Forastiere AA and others: Phase II trial of AZQ in head and neck cancer, Cancer Treat Rep 66:2097, 1982.

59. Fowler JF: Rationales for high linear energy transfer radiotherapy. In Steel GG, Adams GS, and Peckman MJ, editors: The biological basis of radiotherapy, New York, 1983, Elsevier.

60. Fu KK and others: Combined radiotherapy and chemotherapy with bleomycin and methotrexate in advanced inoperable head and neck cancer: update of a Northern California oncology group randomized trial, J Clin Oncol 5:1410, 1987.

61. Germino B: Cancer and the family. In Baird SB, McCorkle R, and Grant M, editors: Cancer nursing: A comprenhensive textbook, Philadelphia, 1991, WB Saunders.

62. Giunta JL: Pathology of malignancy. In Peterson DE and others, editors: Head and neck management of the cancer patient, Boston, 1986, Martinus Nijhoff.

63. Gluckman JL and Crissman JD: Survival rates in 548 patients with multiple neoplasms of the upper aerodigestive tract, Laryngoscope 93:71, 1983.

64. Goltrup F and others: The dynamic properties of tissue oxygenation in healing flaps, Surgery 95:527, 1984.

65. Goodwin WJ and Torres J: The value of the prognostic nutritional index in the management of patients with advanced carcinoma of the neck, Head Neck Surg 6:932, 1984.

66. Gotay C: Research in cancer rehabilitation. In McGarvey C, editor: Physical therapy for the cancer patient, New York, 1990, Churchill Livingstone.

67. Gralla RJ and others: The management of chemotherapy-induced nausea and vomiting, Med Clin North Am 71:289, 1987.

68. Grayden JE: Factors that predict patients' functioning following treatment for cancer, Int J Nurs Stud 25(2):117, 1988.

69. Gullane PJ and Arena S: Extended palatal island mucoperiosteal flap, Arch Otolaryngol 111:330, 1985.

70. Guillamondequi OM and Larson DL: The lateral trapezius musculocutaneous flap: Its use in head and neck reconstruction, Plastic Reconstr Surg 67:143-150, 1981.

71. Guinta JL: Pathology of malignancy. In Peterson DE and others, editors: Head and neck management of the cancer patient, Boston, 1986, Martinus Nijhoff.

72. Harriot JC and others: Dental preservation in patients irradiated for head and neck tumors: A 10 year experience with topical fluoride and a randomized trial between two fluoridation methods. Radiother Oncol 1:72, 1983.

73. Hidlago D: Aesthetic improvements in free flap mandible reconstruction, Plastic Reconstr Surg 88(4):574-584, 1991.

74. Hooper JA and Sigler BA: Nursing care of the head and neck cancer patient. In Myers EN and Suen JY, editors: Cancer of the head and neck, New York, 1988, Churchill Livingstone.

75. Housset M and others: A perspective study of three treatment techniques for T1-T2 base of tongue lesions: Surgery plus post op radiation, external radiation plus interstitial implantation and external radiation alone, Int J Rad Oncol Biol Phys 13:511-516, 1987.

76. Hou M, Chiou J, and McCabe BF: Anti-Epstein-Barr virus antibody in nasopharyngeal carcinoma, Ann Otol Rhinol Laryngol 83:19, 1974.

77. Jacobs J, Spitznagel E, and Sessions D: Staging parameters for cancer of the head and neck: A multifactorial analysis, Laryngoscope 95:1378, 1985.

78. Jacobs JR and others: Chemotherapy following definitive surgery for advanced squamous cell carcinoma of the head and neck: A Radiation Therapy Oncology Group study, Am J Clin Oncol 12:185-189, 1989.

79. Jacobs JR and others: Cisplatin and 5-fluorouracil infusion therapy before definitive treatments in advanced head and neck carcinoma: A RTOG Study, Arch Otolaryngol 113:193-197, 1987.

80. Jobsis FF, Boyd JB, and Barwick WJ: Metabolic consequences of ischemia and hypoxia. In Serafin D and Buncke HJ, editors: Microsurgical composite tissue transplantation, St. Louis, 1974, Mosby.

81. Johnson JL and Lane CA: Helping families respond to cancer. In Baird SB, McCorkle R, and Grant M, editors: Cancer nursing: A comprehensive text book, Philadelphia, 1991, WB Saunders Co.

82. Katsaros J and others: Further experience with lateral arm free flap, Plastic Reconstr Surg, pp 902-910, 1991.

83. Katz S: The use of fluoride and chlorhexidine for prevention of radiation caries, J Am Dent Assoc 104:164, 1982.

84. Kies MS and others: Analysis of complete responders after initial treatment with chemotherapy in head and neck cancer, Otolaryngol Head Neck Surg 93:199, 1985.

85. Kish J and others: Clinical results in recurrent head and neck carcinoma. In Jacobs J and others, editors: Scientific and clinical perspective of head and neck cancer management strategies for cure, New York, 1987, Elsevier.

86. Klein S and others: Total parenteral nutrition and cancer clinical trials, Cancer 58:1378, 1986.

87. Komisar A: The functional result of mandibular reconstruction. Laryngoscope 100:364, 1990.

88. Kramer S and others: Combined radiation therapy and surgery in the management of advanced head and neck cancer: Final report of Study 73-03 of the Radiation Therapy Oncology Group, Head Neck Surg:19, 1987.

89. Kudsk EG and Hoffman GS: Rehabilitation of the cancer patient, Primary Care 14:381, 1987.

90. Leen K, Goepfert H, and Wendt CD: Supraglottic laryngectomy for intermediate stage cancer. U.T.M.D. Anderson cancer center experience with combined therapy, Laryngoscope 100:831-836, 1990.

91. Levine PH and others, editors: EBV DNA content and expression in nasopharyngeal carcinoma, Amsterdam, 1985, Martinus Nijhoff.

92. Little W and Falace DA: Dental management of the medically compromised patient, St. Louis, 1980, Mosby.

93. Loescher LJ and others: Physiologic and psychological implications of surviving adult cancer (2 parts), Ann Intern Med 111:411, 1989.

94. Lukash FN and Sachs SA: Functional mandibular reconstruction: Prevention of the oral invalid, Plast Reconstr Surg 84:227, 1989.

95. McConnel FMS, Teichgraeber JF, and Adler RK: A comparison of three methods of oral reconstruction, Arch Otolaryngol Head Neck Surg 113:496-500, 1987.

96. McPhetride L: Nursing history: One means to personalize care, Am J Nurs 68:68, 1968.

97. Mahon SM: Managing the psychosocial consequences of cancer recurrence: Implications for nurses, Oncol Nurs Forum 16:39-43, 1989.

98. Matloub HS and others: Lateral arm free flap in oral cavity reconstruction: A functional evaluation, Head and Neck 11(3):205, 1989.

99. Mayer D and O'Connor L: Rehabilitation of persons with cancer: An ONS position statement, Oncol Nurs Forum 16:433, 1989.

100. Mendenhall W, Parsons J, Mendenhall N, and Million R: Brachy therapy in head and neck cancer: Selection criteria and results at the University of Florida, Oncology 5(1):87-93, 1991.

101. Mendenhall W, Parsons J, Stringer S, and Million R: The role of radiation therapy in laryngeal cancer, CA 40(3):150-165, 1990.

102. Mendenhall W and others: Is elective neck treatment indicated for T2 squamous cell carcinoma of the glottic larynx? Radiation Ther Oncol 14:199-202, 1989.

103. Mendenhall W and others: The role of radiation therapy in laryngeal cancer, CA 40(3):150-165, 1990.

104. Million RB, Cassiann J, Parsons JT, and Mendenhall WM: Radiation therapy in the management of carcinoma of the larynx. In Frei MD, editor: The Larynx: A multidisciplinary approach, Boston, 1988, Little Brown and Co.

105. Mitrani M and Krespi YP: Functional restoration after subtotal glossectomy and laryngectomy, Otolaryngol Head Neck Surg 98:5-9, 1988.

106. Moinpour CM and others: Quality of life end points in cancer clinical trials review and recommendations, J Natl Cancer Inst 81:485-495, 1989.

107. Morrish RB and others: Osteonecrosis in patients irradiated for head and neck carcinoma, Cancer 47:1980, 1981.

108. Morrow GR: Management of nausea in the cancer patient. In Rosenthal S, Carignam JR, and Smith BD, editors: Medical care of the cancer patient, Philadelphia, 1987, WB Saunders Co.

109. Morrow GR and Dobkin PL: Anticipatory nausea and vomiting in cancer patients undergoing chemotherapy treatment: Prevalence etiology and

behavioral interventions, Clin Psych Rev 8:517, 1988.

110. Muldooney JB, Cohen JJ, Porto DD, and Maisel RH: Oral cavity reconstruction using the free arm radial flap, Arch Otolaryngol Head Neck Surg 13:1219-1224, 1987.

111. Murray CG, Daly TE, and Zimmerman SO: The relationship between dental disease and radiation necrosis of the mandible, Oral Surg 49:99, 1980.

112. Netterville JL and Wood DE: The lower trapezius flap vascular anatomy and surgical technique, Arch Otolaryngol Head Neck Surg 117:73, 1991.

113. Netterville JL, Panje WR, and Maves ME: The trapezius myocutaneous flap: Dependability and limitations, Arch Otolaryngol Head Neck Surg 113:271-281, 1987.

114. Northhouse LL: Family issues in cancer care, Advance Psychosom Med 18:82-101, 1988.

115. Parker RG and Enstrom JE: Second primary cancers of the head and neck following treatment of initial primary head and neck cancer, Int J Radiat Oncol Biol Phys 14:561-564, 1988.

116. Pearlman NW, Johnson FB, and Kennaugh RC: Modified radical neck dissection and postoperative radiotherapy in squamous cell head and neck cancer, Am J Surg 150:448, 1985.

117. Pennington JE: Respiratory tract infections: Intrinsic risk factors, Am J Med 76(suppl SA):34, 1984.

118. Pomp J, Levendag PC, and Putten WLJ: Reirradiation of recurrent tumors in the head and neck, Am J Clin Oncol 11:543-549, 1988.

119. Poplin E and others: Combined therapies for squamous cell carcinoma of the esophagus: A Southwest Oncology Group study (SWOG-8037), J Clin Oncol 5:622, 1987.

120. Puthawala AA and others: Limited external beam and interstitial iridium-192 irradiation in the treatment of carcinoma of the base of tongue: A 10 year experience, Int J Rad Oncol Biol Phys 14:839-848, 1988.

121. Reuther JF, Steinau H, and Wagner R: Reconstruction of larger defects in the oropharynx with re-vascularized intestinal grafts: An experimental clinical report, Plastic Reconstr Surg 73:345, 1984.

122. Reynolds JV and others: Arginine, protein calorie malnutrition and cancer, J Surg Res 45:513, 1988.

123. Rirken M and others: Rectus abdominis free flap in head and neck reconstruction. Arch Otolaryngol Head Neck Surg 117:857-866, 1991.

124. Rivet D and others: The lateral arem flap: An anatomic study, Reconstr Microsurg 3(2):121-131, 1987.

125. Robson MC: The physiologic basis of reconstruction of the head and neck defect. In Jacobs J and others, editors: Scientific and clinical perspective of head and neck cancer management strategies for cure, New York, 1987, Elsevier.

126. Schuller DE and others: Analysis of disability resulting from treatment including radical neck dissection or modified neck dissection, Head Neck Surg 6:551, 1983.

127. Schulmeister L: Nutrition. In Otto S, editor: Oncology Nursing, St. Louis, 1991, Mosby.

128. Schusterman MA, Reece G, Kroll S, and Weldon M: Use of the AO plate for immediate mandibular reconstruction in cancer patients, Plastic Reconstr Surg 88(4):588-593, 1991.

129. Schwartz HC: Mandibular reconstruction using Dacron-Urethane prosthesis and autogenous cancellous bone: A review of 32 cases, Plast Reconstr Surg 73:387, 1984.

130. Seligman M and others: Combined therapy for recurrent or metachronous squamous cell carcinoma of the head and neck. Head and Neck Oncology Research Proceedings of the 2nd International Head and Neck Oncology Research Conference, Arlington, VA, 10-12 September, 1987, Kugler Publications Amsterdam-Berkeley/Ghendini Eds-Milano.

131. Shellito PC and Malt RA: Tube gastrotomy: Techniques and complications, Ann Surg 201:180, 1985.

132. Sigler BA: Nursing care of the head and neck cancer patient, Oncology Dec:49, 1988.

133. Sigler BA: Nursing care for head and neck tumor patients. In Thrawley SE and Panye WR, editors: Comprehensive management of head and neck tumors, Philadelphia, 1987, WB Saunders Co.

134. Silverman S, Gorsky M, and Lozuda F: Oral leukoplakia and malignant transformation, Cancer 53:563, 1984.

135. Sisson G and Pletzer H: Staging system by site: Problems in refinement, Otolaryngol Clin North Am 18(3):397, 1985.

136. Smith K and Lesko IM: Psychological problems in cancer survivors, Oncology 2:33, 1988.

137. Sonis ST: Oral complications of cancer therapy. In DeVita VT, Hellman S, Rosenberg SA, editors: Cancer: Principles and practice of Oncology, ed 2, Philadelphia, 1985, JB Lippincott Co.

138. Szeliga D, Groenwald S, and Sullivan D: Nutritional disturbances. In Groenwald S, and others, editors: Cancer nursing: Principles and practice, ed 2, Boston, 1990, Jones and Bartlett Publishers.

139. Taylor I, Graeme D, Miller M, and Ham F: Free vascularized bone graft: Plastic and reconstruction of patients with oral cancer, Oral Surg Oral Med Path 68(4):499-504, 1992.

140. Tchekmedyian NS, Cella DF, editors: Quality of life in current oncology practice and research, Oncology 4(5):21-232, 1990.

141. Teichgraeber J, Bowman J, and Goetert H: New test series for functional evaluation of oral cavity cancer, Head Neck Surg, 8:819, 1985.

142. Tiwari RM: Masseter crossover flap reconstruction of oral-oropharyngeal defects. In Wolf T and Carey TE, editors: Head and neck oncology research. Proceedings of the 2nd International Head and Neck Oncology Research Conference, Arlington, VA, September 10-12, 1987, Amsterdam-Berkeley/Gnedin Etoire-Milano, 1987, Kugler Publication.

143. Tiwari RM: Masseter muscle crossover flap in primary closure of oral oropharyngeal defects, J Laryngol Otol 101:172, 1987.

144. Tiwari RM and Snow GB: Role of myocutaneous flaps in reconstruction of the head and neck, J Laryngol Otol 97:441, 1983.

145. Tonelli PM, Hume WR, and Kenny EB: Chlorhexidine: A review of the literature, J West Soc Periodontal 31:5, 1983.

146. Urken MD and others: Rectus abdommis free flap in head and neck reconstruction, Arch Otolaryngol Head Neck Surg 117:501-511, 1991.

147. Vi Kram B and others: Failure at the primary site following multimodality treatment in advanced head and neck cancer, Head Neck Surg 6:720, 1984.

148. Wallis DP: Lateral face reconstruction with the medal-based cervicopectoral flap, Arch Otolaryngol Head Neck Surg 114:729-733, 1988.

149. Wang CC: Radiation therapy for head and neck neoplasms: Indications, techniques and results, Boston, 1983, John-Wright PSG.

150. Wang CC, Blitzer PH, and Siuit HD: Twice-day radiation therapy for cancer of the head and neck, Cancer 55:2100, 1985.

151. Wang CC, Busse J, and Gitterman MS: A simple after loading applicator for intracavitary radiation of carcinoma of the nasopharynx, Radiology 115:737, 1975.

152. Wang ZN and others: Treatment with preoperative irradiation and surgery of squamous cell carcinoma of the head and neck, Cancer 64:32-33, 1989.

153. Watson P: Cancer rehabilitation: The evolution of a concept, Cancer Nurs 13:2-12, 1990.

154. Weaver AW: Problems with multiple primary: role of endoscopy. In Jacobs JR and others, editors: Head and neck cancer: Scientific perspectives in management and strategies for cure, New York, 1987, Elsevier.

155. Weems DH, Mendenhall WM, Parsons JT, and others: Squamous cell carcinoma of the supraglottic larynx treated with surgery and/or radiation therapy, Int J Radiat Oncol Biol Phys 13:1483-1487, 1987.

156. Weichselbaum R and Beckett MA: The maximum recovery potential of human tumor cells may predict clinical outcome in radiotherapy, Int J Radiat Oncol Biol Phys 13:709, 1987.

157. Welch-McCaffery D: Cancer anxiety and quality of life, Cancer Nurs 8:151, 1985.

158. Welch-McCaffery D and others: Surviving adult cancers: Part 2—psychosocial implications, Ann Intern Med 111:517-524, 1989.

159. Wells R: Rehabilitation: Making the most of time, Oncol Nurs Forum 17:503-507, 1990.

160. Weing B and Keller AJ: Microvascular free flap reconstruction for head and neck defects, Arch Otolaryngol Head Neck Surg 115:118-120, 1989.

161. Weiland AJ: Vascularized bone grafts: Reconstructive surgery. In Green DP, editor: Operative hand surgery, New York, 1988, Churchill-Livingstone.

162. Wil TK, Pietrocola D, and Welch HF: A new method of percutaneous endoscopic gastrotomy using anchoring devices, Am J Surg 153:230-232, 1987.

163. Wong CS and Cummings BJ: The place of radiation therapy in the treatment of squamous cell carcinoma of the nasal vestibule, Acta Oncologila 27:203-208, 1988.

164. Zarbo RJ and Crissman JD: The pathologist's role in diagnosis and staging of upper aerodigestive tract carcinoma. In Jacobs JR and others, editors: Head and neck cancer: Scientific perspectives in management strategies for cure, New York, 1987, Elsevier.

CHAPTER 13

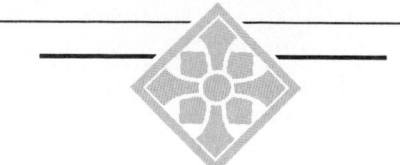

HIV and Related Cancers

Cynthia Brogden

On June 5, 1981, the first cases of an illness later defined as acquired immunodeficiency syndrome (AIDS) were reported by California health care providers to the Centers for Disease Control (CDC).[4] This first cluster of five Los Angeles men presented with unusual opportunistic infections and were thought to represent a geographically localized epidemic of an unknown infectious disease. Just 4 years later in 1985, 14,049 cases of AIDS were reported in the United States. Later that same year, the human immunodeficiency virus (HIV) was identified as the causative agent of AIDS—more than 7000 Americans had already died of the disease.[4]

We are now in the second decade of this epidemic, which has claimed the lives of 1.1 million people across the globe.[18] Although there has been scientific and clinical progress as well as development of new treatments and comprehensive models of care, HIV disease remains an incurable illness spreading rapidly throughout the United States and the world.

Nurses play a pivotal role in treatment and prevention of this disease. Patient education about risk behaviors and risk reduction techniques will help prevent new infections and will undoubtedly save countless lives. Appropriate, compassionate nursing care for those already infected may extend survival and will most certainly improve the quality of life for those afflicted with HIV disease.

HUMAN IMMUNODEFICIENCY VIRUS
EPIDEMIOLOGY

HIV infection has occurred in approximately 1.5 million Americans and progressed to AIDS in 284,840. This epidemic has killed 141,223 Americans, and the numbers increase daily.[5] Throughout the world, more than 12 million people are infected with HIV and

nearly 2 million have progressed to an AIDS diagnosis. It is estimated that greater than one million people have died of AIDS worldwide. While changes in risk behaviors have slowed the spread of HIV infection in some areas of the United States, HIV transmission has accelerated in others. More than 40,000 new infections are expected this year in the United States alone.[8] Early estimates of worldwide infection rates suggested approximately 40 million infections by the year 2000 (World Health Organization, 1991). That estimate has been revised and now many experts report there will be greater than 110 million persons infected with HIV by the end of this decade.

Throughout the epidemic, the numbers of those infected have steadily increased each year. Early in the U.S. epidemic, greater than 80% of those infected were homosexual men. Currently, less than 50% of infections occur in this population. Those persons now at greatest risk for acquiring HIV infection in the United States include heterosexual women and their children and intravenous drug users. African-Americans and Hispanic-Americans are at greater risk than Caucasian Americans.[5]

Worldwide, HIV continues to ravage heterosexual men, women, and their children. New infections in Asia have increased dramatically in the past 2 years and areas of Africa have infection rates as high as 35% to 50% among the general population.

Mortality rates in the United States currently approach 80% within 2 years of an AIDS diagnosis and may be even higher in undeveloped countries where treatment is virtually nonexistent.[18]

ETIOLOGY AND RISK FACTORS

Since the first description of AIDS in 1981, an extraordinary scientific adventure has ensued. In just over a decade, we have produced remarkable advancements in our understanding of the disease and its causative agent, HIV. The origin of HIV is still largely unknown, although evidence appears to support the hypothesis of an African origin. The first reports of an AIDS-like illness date back to the early 1960s in central Africa. HIV in humans likely has an animal origin, most likely nonhuman primates.

The causative agent of AIDS is infection with HIV. HIV is a human retrovirus and belongs to the lentivirus subfamily. Currently, five human retroviruses have been identified: HTLV-1, HTLV-2, HTLV-5, HIV-1, and HIV-2. HTLV-2 has not been conclusively associated with human disease. HTLV-1 and HTLV-5 have been associated with human T-cell leukemia and lymphoma, conditions characterized by proliferation of CD4+ (T4) helper cells. HIV-1 and HIV-2 both cause depletion of T4 helper cells, resulting in loss of cellular immunity, characterized by AIDS. HIV-1 is the predominant cause of AIDS in the United States, accounting for greater than 95% of AIDS cases. HIV-2 seems to be limited to geographic distribution and is most prevalent in West Africa.[11]

The life cycle of HIV is similar to that of the other retroviruses. Mature virions interact with specific host receptors and then use the host cell for viral replication. HIV interacts with the CD4 glycoprotein, which occurs on the membrane of specific cells, the CD4+ (T4) helper lymphocytes. These specific white blood cells contain the CD4 glycoprotein on their membranes, allowing the virus to fuse. The viral core is subsequently injected into the cell cytoplasm where the viral RNA genome is translated into DNA by a retroviral enzyme called reverse transcriptase. Infection and subsequent viral replication eventually depletes the host's T4 helper cells, resulting in a dramatic loss of the protective immune response against invading microorganisms.

The routes for transmission of HIV are well documented: (1) intimate sexual contact; (2) parenteral exposure to blood, blood-containing body fluids and blood products; and (3) from mother to child during the perinatal period. Although HIV has been identified in a variety of body fluids, those that have been consistently shown to be infectious are blood, semen, and vaginal secretions. Transmission has also been associated with breast milk, although this occurrence appears to be relatively uncommon. HIV is transmitted directly from person to person by sexual contact; direct innoculation with contaminated blood products, needles, or syringes; and from an infected mother to her newborn. HIV is not transmitted by casual contact including sneezing, coughing, or spitting; handshakes; toilet seats, bathtubs, showers, or swimming pools; or utensils, dishes, or linens used by an infected person. HIV disease is a blood borne,

sexually transmitted disease. Although certain sexual practices may be associated with higher risks for infection than others, any practice that exposes one to infected blood, semen, or vaginal secretions has the potential for viral transmission.

The natural history of HIV infection is associated with an unpredictable course of disease progression. Most patients undergo a prolonged period of clinically silent infection, often lasting for more than 10 years.[12] Although virus is consistently detectable throughout this time, patients typically have only subtle immunologic alterations. Once the patient becomes symptomatic, however, decreases in the number of T4 helper cells can be detected and viral replication increases.

It is postulated that there are several potential cofactors that may be associated with HIV disease progression. These cofactors, which may be of viral, host, or environmental nature, are thought to directly influence the replication of HIV or the severity of its pathogenic effects. Viral cofactors that may influence the progression of the disease include herpes simplex, cytomegalovirus, and Epstein-Barr virus. Host cofactors may include a variety of cytokines and intracellular mediators. Environmental cofactors may include repeated exposure to HIV, which may induce hyperactivation of the immune system, resulting in an expansion of the pool of HIV replicating cells.

As viral replication increases, depleting the body of T4 helper lymphocytes, the body's defense mechanisms are progressively weakened. Infections that were once disarmed by the healthy immune system are eventually able to cause serious and potentially life-threatening disease. These "opportunistic" infections include a wide variety of organisms such as viruses (herpes simplex, Epstein-Barr, cytomegalovirus), protozoans (*Pneumocystis carinii*, toxoplasma), mycobacteria (tuberculosis and avium complex), and fungi (histoplasma, cryptococci). In addition to the various opportunistic infections, the profound immune dysfunction also allows for the development of several neoplasms including non-Hodgkin's lymphoma, Kaposi's sarcoma, and cervical carcinomas.

PREVENTION, SCREENING, AND DETECTION

HIV disease is a blood borne, sexually transmitted disease. As such, prevention efforts must be focused on techniques to avoid exposure to contaminated blood and body fluids. With less than 3% of AIDS cases attributed to exposure with contaminated blood products, the greatest exposure risk is via sexual contact. AIDS prevention efforts must therefore be focused on ways to reduce sexual transmission.

Historically, it has been difficult to talk about sexuality in the American culture. It has been a subject laden with moral judgments and has been an area seldom addressed in our health care system. Nurses are in an excellent position to discuss sexuality with patients. Typically, it is the nurse who has an intimate rapport with the patient, talking about sensitive subjects and related health concerns. It is usually the nurse with whom the patient feels most at ease and it is the nurse who is most accessible to patients. The nurse plays a major role in the education of individuals and groups in the prevention of HIV disease.

Prevention efforts must include accurate, reliable, and clear information about risk factors for HIV disease and ways to decrease these risks. Prevention education programs must include the topics of safer sexual techniques and using clean drug paraphernalia as well as public health measures such as blood product screening and perinatal counseling. Prevention efforts must be focused on behaviors that put patients at risk for infection.

Safe Sex Counseling

Any exchange of blood, semen, or vaginal secretions can potentially put an individual at risk for HIV disease. Common sexual practices that are therefore risky behaviors include vaginal or anal penetration without a condom and possibly oral sexual practices. Use of barrier products such as latex condoms while engaging in these behaviors markedly reduces the likelihood of exposure to potentially infectious blood, semen, or vaginal secretions. In addition, education about condom use should include the use of prelubricated condoms. Non-oxynol-9, a commonly used spermicidal lubricant, may also have some antiviral properties. Use of condoms prelubricated with non-oxynol-9 may therefore further increase the protection afforded by condoms. Use of additional water-based lubricants should also be encouraged. Petroleum-based lubricant use should be discouraged, since these agents may cause latex breakdown.

Prevention education must also include risk reduction techniques such as minimizing the number of sexual partners and engaging in a mutually monogamous sexual relationship. In addition, sexual practices that do not put the individual at risk for potentially infectious fluids should be discussed. Mutual masturbation, massage, and body rubbing are safe sexual practices with no exchange of body fluids.

Intravenous Risk Reduction

The use of contaminated needles for subcutaneous, intramuscular, or intravenous injection represents a serious risk for HIV infection. Prevention education must include ways to clean needles and other paraphernalia used to inject drugs. While educational efforts may include information about substance abuse counseling and programs, use of a bleach solution to disinfect needles and paraphernalia must also be discussed.

Perinatal Transmission

Women who are HIV infected may pass the virus on to their newborns via three potential routes: during gestation, during delivery, and via breastfeeding. While the exact mechanism of perinatal transmission is unknown, the current estimate of risk to the newborn from an infected mother is approximately 30% in the United States.[19]

Public Health Measures

Prevention programs must also educate the public about the measures that are currently in place to screen and protect the blood supply from contamination. Currently, each unit of donated blood is tested for HIV infection as well as several other blood borne infections such as hepatitis. Because HIV screening of blood products has been conducted since 1985 in the United States, only recipients of transfusions prior to this time are at significant risk for infection via the blood supply.

Screening

HIV antibody testing plays an essential role in prevention and treatment of this disease process. The most common form of screening for HIV disease is the use of the antibody test with the enzyme-linked immunosorbent assay (ELISA) technique and the Western blot technique. The ELISA test uses spectrophotometry to detect serum antibody reactions to specific HIV viral proteins. The ELISA is highly sensitive and specific with a sensitivity of 98.4 to 99.6%. A positive ELISA test must be confirmed by the Western Blot technique.

Both the ELISA and the Western Blot techniques depend on antibody formation. Approximately 90% of the population will form antibodies in response to HIV exposure within 6 weeks to 3 months postexposure. A negative antibody test may occur in the "window phase" between the dates of actual exposure leading to infection and development of detectable serum antibodies. While approximately 90% of the population will form antibodies in response to HIV exposure within 6 weeks to 3 months postexposure, this period of time may be as long as 6 months.[9]

Since newborn infants maintain maternal antibodies for as long as 18 months, antibody testing is unreliable until the infant is 18 months of age. A newer test, the polymerase chain reaction (PCR), is now available. The PCR does not rely on antibody formation; instead, genetic subunits of the virus are identified, confirming infection. While this test is relatively new and sensitivity studies are still being con-

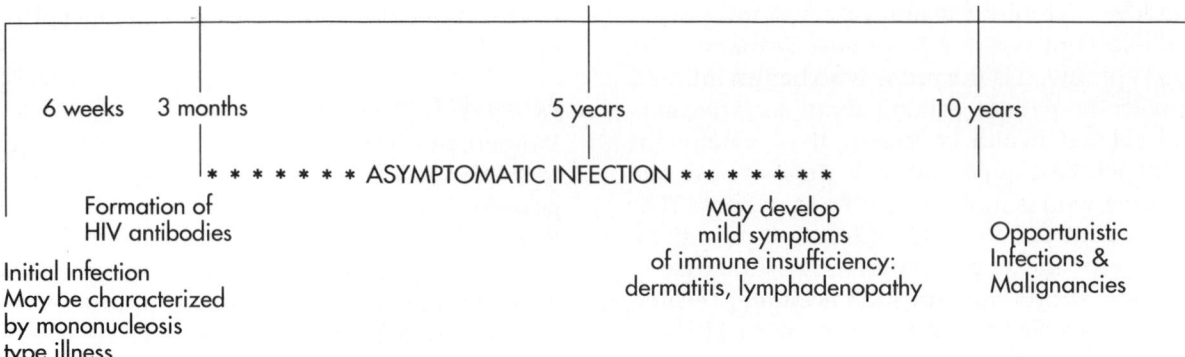

Figure 13-1   Usual progression of HIV disease in the United States.

ducted, it will undoubtedly prove valuable in a wide variety of patient populations such as newborns.

Maintaining patient confidentiality is essential in HIV testing. Every measure possible should be taken to insure that privacy is guaranteed. Unauthorized disclosure, stigmatization, and discrimination against HIV-positive individuals continue to occur with unfortunate regularity.

CLINICAL FEATURES

It has been estimated that there are 1.5 to 2 million Americans who are infected with HIV; approximately one half of those infected are unaware they carry the virus that causes AIDS. Although some (less than 50%) of those infected will develop a viral syndrome resembling mononucleosis or influenza within a few days or weeks of infection, most are unaware the symptoms are related to the initial infection with HIV. Acute infection is followed by a period of asymptomatic HIV infection. In these early stages of HIV disease, there are no symptoms of infection. Infected persons may remain asymptomatic for several years, with half of all persons remaining asymptomatic for 10 years or longer.[21]

As HIV depletes the body of sufficient numbers of T4 helper cells, subtle symptoms of immune deficiency may emerge. Patients may develop persistent generalized lymphadenopathy or minor dermatologic manifestations such as seborrhea. During this time, there is a slow, persistent destruction of the immune system with gradual decline in the number of T4 helper cells.

With continued destruction of the immune system, opportunistic infections and malignancies begin to develop and cause clinical symptoms. Clinical findings that appear to predict rapid progression to end-stage HIV disease (otherwise known as AIDS) include unexplained weight loss greater than 10% of usual body weight and persistent fever, diarrhea, or night sweats of greater than a 2-week duration.

Figure 13-1 provides an explanation of the usual progression of HIV disease in the United States.

Table 13-1   Opportunistic Infections

Opportunistic Infection	Clinical Features
Bacterial Infections	
Mycobacterium avium	General: persistent fever, night sweats, fatigue, weight loss, abdominal pain, weakness, lymphadenopathy, hepatosplenomegaly
Fungal Infections	
Candidiasis	Oral: white patches on tongue or buccal mucosa
	Vaginal: vulvar pruritis, vaginal discharge
Cryptococcosis	Meningitis: headache, fever, progressive malaise, altered mental status, seizures
	Pneumonia: fever, shortness of breath, cough
Histoplasmosis	Fever, weight loss, shortness of breath, lymphadenopathy
Protozoal Infections	
Cryptosporidiosis	Diarrhea, abdominal cramping, nausea, vomiting, fatigue, weight loss, dehydration
Pneumocystis	Pneumonia: Fever, nonproductive cough, shortness of breath, weight loss, nights sweats, fatigue
Toxoplasmosis	Encephalitis: altered mental status, seizures, fever, coma
Viral Infections	
Cytomegalovirus	Retinitis: unilateral visual deficit or change
	Gastrointestinal: dysphagia, wasting, nausea, fever, diarrhea
Herpes simplex	Painful blisters or ulcers

Specific clinical features of various opportunistic infections are listed in Table 13-1.

DIAGNOSIS AND STAGING

The spectrum of HIV infection ranges from asymptomatic infection to potentially life-threatening op-

Table 13–2   CDC Classification System for HIV Infections in Adults

Stage I	Acute Infection:	Occurs at the time of the initial HIV infection and may last from days to weeks. Characterized by a mononucleosis-like or influenza-like syndrome with approximately 50% of patients reporting or recalling symptoms.
Stage II	Asymptomatic Infection:	Occurs after stage I and may last for several years.
Stage III	Persistent Generalized Lymphadenopathy (PGL):	Characterized by palpable lymph node enlargement of 1 cm or greater at two or more extrainguinal sites, persisting for greater than 3 months.
Stage IV	Other Diseases:	PGL not prerequisite.

Subgroup A: Constitutional Disease—fever persisting for greater than 1 month, involuntary weight loss greater than 10% of usual body weight, diarrhea persisting for greater than 1 month.
Subgroup B: Neurologic Disease—dementia, myelopathy, peripheral neuropathy.
Subgroup C: Secondary Infectious Diseases—specific infectious diseases identified by CDC; commonly referred to as *opportunistic infections.*
Subgroup D: Secondary Cancers—includes Kaposi's sarcoma, non-Hodgkin's lymphoma, primary lymphoma of the brain.
Subgroup E: Other Conditions—includes other conditions specified by CDC (e.g., chronic lymphoid interstitial pneumonitis).

portunistic infection. In the past, many clinicians have used an informal staging system categorizing patients as falling into one of three categories: (1) HIV positive, (2) AIDS related complex (ARC), and (3) AIDS. In this staging system, HIV positive referred to those patients who were completely asymptomatic but HIV positive. Those patients classified as ARC exhibited constitutional symptoms including persistent generalized lymphadenopathy, persistent fevers, involuntary weight loss, and/or diarrhea. Any patient who had experienced an opportunistic infection (OI) was classified as AIDS.

Today, clinicians have become much more sophisticated about the stages of HIV disease and realize that it is a chronic, progressive illness characterized by four distinct categories. Although we commonly refer to end stage HIV disease as AIDS, most clinicians also use the staging system recommended by the CDC. The CDC Classification System for HIV infection in Adults is currently the most widely used staging system; Table 13-2 delineates this classification system.

METASTASIS

HIV disease is a chronic, systemic infection. The infection itself primarily infects a specific group of lymphocytes (the T4 helper cells) but also has the potential for direct infection of the monocytes and macrophages, and possibly muscle and nerve cells. In addition, many patients experience HIV infection directly affecting the central nervous system. As the disease progresses, nearly every organ system is affected by one or more of the opportunistic infections that occur secondarily to the profound immune deficiency that results from the original HIV infection. The majority of patients experience illness affecting the skin and mucous membranes, the respiratory tract, the gastrointestinal tract, and the central nervous system.

TREATMENT MODALITIES
Chemotherapy

While we have several treatment options now available to slow the progression of the illness, there is currently no cure for HIV disease. We are able, however, to treat and in some cases, to prevent, the associated opportunistic infections that occur as a result of HIV infection.

In general, patients with HIV infection may remain relatively free of clinical symptoms for several years. Because of the variability of the disease progression, immune system surveillance on a regular basis is an important component of HIV treatment. It is recommended that patients with stable T4 helper counts above 500/mm^3 obtain a physical examination and laboratory evaluation every 3 to 6 months. Currently, the T4 helper count is the single most important indicator in tracking progressive deterioration of immune system function in HIV infected individuals.

If the T4 helper cell count falls below 500 cells/mm^3, initiation of antiretroviral therapy is indicated. Zidovudine (also called Retrovir or AZT) was the first drug approved to treat HIV infection and remains the first choice of therapy for patients with less than 500 T4 helper cells. If patients fail to tolerate zidovudine or the disease progresses despite zidovudine therapy, two other similar drugs are now available: Videx (also called ddI) and Hivid (also called ddC). All three of these antiretrovirals belong to a class of drugs known as the nucleoside analogs and work to slow the rate of viral replication. These drugs are not cures for HIV infection.

There are several other drugs available to treat specific opportunistic infections that occur as the immune system is depleted. A varied degree of success has been achieved with these regimens in treating the opportunistic infection. In several cases, prophylaxis for recurrent or even primary opportunistic infections may be effective.

Pneumocystis carinii infection is the most common opportunistic infection occurring in HIV infected patients. This protozoan is a ubiquitous organism acquired by the majority of persons during childhood. Most commonly in HIV infection, *Pneumocystis carinii* causes pneumonia. Until recently, *Pneumocystis carinii* pneumonia (PCP) was an almost universally life-threatening OI in patients with HIV disease. Although it remains the most common OI, occurring in as many as 85% of HIV patients, the mortality rate has been markedly reduced since the use of intravenous trimethoprim-sulfamethoxazole or pentamidine therapy. Oral trimethoprin-sulfamethoxazole has now been shown to be highly effective in preventing recurrence of PCP as well. In addition, initiation of oral PCP prophylaxis in patients known to be at high risk for PCP infection has reduced the primary occurrence rate.

Biotherapy

Anemia, leukopenia, and thrombocytopenia are part of the natural history of HIV disease. These cytopenias can result from marrow failure or cell destructive processes. They can also be caused by drugs used to treat HIV disease and associated infections or malignancies. A number of HIV drug therapies have been shown to be myelotoxic. Many drugs used to treat opportunistic infections as well as Retrovir may have to be interrupted in certain patients secondary to myelotoxicity. Use of colony stimulating factors (CSFs) such as granulocyte and granulocyte-monocyte colony stimulating factors (G-CSF and GM-CSF) has proven useful in decreasing myelotoxicity and often allow successful completion of therapy.

Erythropoietin (EPO) can be used for treatment of Retrovir-induced marrow suppression. Although this therapy has not proven successful in all patients, a significant number of patients have required fewer transfusions and have been able to continue antiviral, anti-infective, or antineoplastic therapy while receiving EPO.[14]

Future Therapies

In the early years of the epidemic there was steadfast hope that a vaccination could be developed to stop the spread of this deadly virus. Multiple researchers across the country have conducted countless trials of various vaccines, but none has yet proven to be successful. The rapid rate of mutation of HIV has proven difficult for scientists to match with a vaccine that would stimulate appropriate antibody responses. Although vaccine research is continuing, most researchers feel that a vaccine for the general population will not likely be available before the end of the decade.[20]

Vaccine research historically has focused on the prevention of infection. A great deal of current vaccine research, however, is evaluating administration of a vaccine to patients who are already HIV infected. Through the use of an inactivated virus vaccine, researchers hope to spur the body's production of antibody specific for fighting HIV as well as the production of T4 helper cells. By stimulating the immune system's response to HIV, researchers hope that the vaccine might be able to halt or even reverse the spread of the virus in newly infected individuals.[7]

An increasing number of researchers now believe that gene therapy represents the only hope of cure for HIV disease. Gene therapy involves the insertion of a gene into a human cell. The new gene would direct the natural, antiviral human cell response. Theoretically, the new gene would program the human cell to destroy HIV. Although research is now only in the early stages in this new arena, the therapy appears promising.

HIV has potential disease and treatment related complications. See box below.

Prognosis

Although HIV disease appears to be a universally fatal illness, the time to progression of profound immune deficiency varies widely among patients. As more information and treatment options become available, HIV disease is likely to become a manageable, chronic illness. The nurse plays a primary role in educational efforts to prevent this disease as well as in the provision of compassionate and appropriate care to those already infected.

HIV DISEASE AND TREATMENT RELATED COMPLICATIONS

Disease Related Complications
  Profound immune suppression
  Development of various opportunistic infections/malignancies
  Constitutional symptoms: fever, night sweats, weight loss
  Persistent generalized lymphadenopathy
  Financial loss including employment, health insurance, housing
  Societal stigmatization and discrimination
Treatment Related Complications
  Anemia, neutropenia, thrombocytopenia
  Fatigue
  Nausea, vomiting, weight loss

Nursing Management

The nursing management of the patient with HIV disease is complex and demanding. Because the disease has such an unpredictable course, the nurse must be prepared to provide appropriate care to those with early, asymptomatic disease, to those who are suffering from acute opportunistic infections, to those battling AIDS related malignancies and to those in the terminal stages of their illness (see box on p. 266).

NURSING DIAGNOSIS: POTENTIAL FOR INFECTION

Risk of infection may be related to disease process with viral destruction of T4 helper cells; neutropenia related to medication, treatment, or infection; knowledge deficit regarding infection control precautions; or impaired skin integrity.

ASSESSMENT

People with HIV infection are at risk for developing infections due to a number of factors, at any stage of the disease. A variety of signs and symptoms may alert the nurse to an impending or current infection: neutropenia; decreased T4 helper count; fever, chills; impaired skin integrity with or without draining wounds; shortness of breath, cough; mental status change; nausea, vomiting, or diarrhea.

OUTCOME CRITERIA
- The patient will remain free of infection.
- Infections will be identified early and treatment initiated quickly.

INTERVENTIONS
- Carefully monitor vital signs and laboratory results for signs of possible infection.
- Institute a low microbial diet for patients with an absolute neutrophil count below 500 cell/cm^3. Patients should receive only pasteurized dairy products and no fresh fruits or vegetables.
- Perform appropriate physical assessment including careful examination of skin integrity and respiratory and gastrointestinal status.
- Perform appropriate mental status examinations.
- Maintain asepsis when caring for patient, including appropriate handwashing, limiting of infectious visitors.
- Educate patient in protective strategies such as handwashing, diet precautions such as thorough cooking of meat products, pet care precautions, avoiding rectal thermometers and suppositories.

NURSING DIAGNOSIS: INEFFECTIVE INDIVIDUAL COPING

Patients with HIV disease face a chronic, life-threatening illness. In addition, they face stigmitization and often overwhelming discrimination. Ineffective coping may be related to anxiety secondary to having a life-threatening illness, multiple losses secondary to the illness and resultant debilitation, changes in lifestyle secondary to HIV infection, or changes in self concept.

ASSESSMENT

Ineffective coping occurs when the individual is unable to successfully manage stressors secondary to lack of personal or external resources.[9] Ineffective coping can be evidenced by:
- Behavioral changes including sudden mood swings, social withdrawal, anger, depression, anxiety.
- Decreased self-esteem.
- Inability to solve problems.

OUTCOME CRITERIA
- The patient will devise new coping strategies and enhance current strategies.
- The patient will express feelings and maintain relationships.

INTERVENTIONS
- Establish a therapeutic nursing relationship using empathy, acceptance, and support.
- Facilitate expression of patient's feelings.
- Assist patient in identification of past and current coping strategies, effective and ineffective skills.
- Identify resources available to patient including family members, friends, clergy, support groups.
- Utilize multidisciplinary resources including social services, clergy, and psychiatry.

NURSING DIAGNOSIS: KNOWLEDGE DEFICIT RELATED TO DISEASE AND TREATMENT

Patients with HIV disease often have an overwhelming amount of information to assimilate regarding their illness and treatment. Knowledge deficits may be related to disease process, various treatment modalities, infection control, or protective mechanisms.

ASSESSMENT

Patients exhibit knowledge deficits in a variety of ways. Signs and symptoms that may alert the nurse to potential and actual deficits include new HIV diagnosis, institution of new treatment, inability to perform procedures correctly (such as failure to wash hands), failure to maintain infection control mechanisms (such as using condoms during sexual contact), repeated infections.

OUTCOME CRITERIA

- Patient will verbalize correct knowledge of illness and treatments.
- Patients will practice appropriate infection control precautions for protection of self and others.

INTERVENTIONS

- Assess patient knowledge and learning patterns.
- Provide a variety of educational resources including videos, printed materials, one-on-one instruction.
- Provide baseline education to patient regarding illness trajectory, infection control, protective mechanism, laboratory evaluation, and medication administration.
- Explain all procedures and treatments to patient.
- Encourage patient and family to ask questions.

HIV RELATED CANCERS

The HIV epidemic has been characterized not only by the occurrence of opportunistic infections but by the development of specific cancers. Kaposi's sarcoma and non-Hodgkin's lymphoma are the primary types of cancer associated with HIV infection. More recently, the occurrence of cervical and anal carcinomas has been noted in HIV infected patients. As patients with HIV disease experience increased survival, it is anticipated that an increased frequency of HIV related cancers will occur.[17]

KAPOSI'S SARCOMA

AIDS was first reported to the CDC in 1981 as a combined epidemic of *Pneumocystis carinii* pneumonia (PCP) and Kaposi's sarcoma (KS). KS remains the most common neoplasm in HIV infected patients. Although we have made some progress in understanding this malignant process, there is much that remains to be understood.

Epidemiology

In a San Francisco cohort of gay men diagnosed with AIDS from 1981 to 1982, KS accounted for over 75% of the AIDS defining illnesses. By 1988, however, only 19% of patients with AIDS were diagnosed with KS as their presenting illness.[1] This curious decline in the proportion of patients presenting with KS as their initial AIDS-defining illness is currently unexplained. Although all types of patients with AIDS have been found to have KS (heterosexual, homosexual, and IVDU), the incidence is greatest in homosexual HIV positive men.

Etiology and Risk Factors

KS is a tumor of vascular origin. Although little is known of the nature of the malignant cells, KS is a multifocal neoplasm, capable of arising simultaneously at multiple sites. The cause of KS in patients with HIV infection (AIDS-KS) is not yet known. It is suspected, however, that AIDS-KS may not be secondary to infection with HIV disease itself, but may

in fact be another sexually transmitted infection. Cytomegalovirus has long been suspected as a possible etiology.[1]

In addition to HIV disease, other immunodeficient states such as iatrogenically induced immunosuppression, as seen in renal transplant patients, have also been the setting for KS. It is possible, however, that immune deficiency is not a prerequisite for the development of KS. The genetic make-up of the host may be a factor contributing to the development of KS in AIDS patients. An increased frequency of major histocompatibility antigens DR-5 and DR-2 has been reported in some studies of HIV associated KS. The absence of the HIV genome in the KS tumor lends further support to an indirect role for HIV in AIDS-KS.[17]

Prevention, Screening, and Detection

Since AIDS-KS is either a result of HIV infection or is itself a sexually transmitted disease, prevention must include education about risky sexual behaviors. As with prevention of HIV disease, prevention of KS must involve barrier protection such as condoms and avoidance of potentially infectious body fluids including blood, semen, and vaginal secretions.

Since HIV infected patients are at significant risk for AIDS-KS, all HIV patients would be screened routinely for potential signs and symptoms of KS. Such screening requires visual inspection of all body surfaces including oral mucosa. Since there is no laboratory test for KS, patients must be educated to report any suspicious lesions immediately to their health care providers.

Classification

Prior to the advent of the HIV epidemic, KS was seen as an indolent cutaneous vascular tumor in elderly men, particularly of Jewish or Mediterranean descent. This classical or endemic form of KS is rarely life threatening.

AIDS-KS (also called *epidemic KS*) is usually characterized by multifocal, widespread lesions at the onset of the illness. AIDS-KS has a wide range of virulence in patients with HIV disease, ranging from limited stable involvement to fulminant disease with rapid, continuous development of new lesions. AIDS-KS is usually classified based on the site of the lesions. Nodular KS is characterized by subcutaneous nodular lesions that vary in size from several millimeters to several centimeters in diameter. Lymphadenopathic KS primarily affects the peripheral lymph nodes. Oral KS lesions can produce bleeding, tooth displacement, and pain. Visceral KS most commonly affects the lungs and gastrointestinal tract.[6]

Clinical Features

AIDS-KS is usually characterized by mutifocal, widespread lesions at the onset of illness. These lesions may involve the skin, oral mucosa, lymph nodes, or visceral organs including the lung, liver, spleen, and gastrointestinal tract. Most patients present with skin lesions appearing as flat or raised plaques ranging in size from a few millimeters to several centimeters. Colors range from blue-purple to red-brown. Although lymph node involvement occurs frequently, it is often difficult to distinguish from HIV associated lymphadenopathy. Visceral involvement may affect as many as half of reported cases.[6] Gastrointestinal involvement may be asymptomatic although advanced disease may result in blood loss, diarrhea, and weight loss. Pulmonary involvement, although uncommon, may result in radiographic abnormalities and symptoms of cough, dyspnea, and fever. Although lesions from KS have been observed at autopsy in all organs, including brain, pancreas, heart, and major vessels, these lesions remain generally asymptomatic.

Diagnosis and Staging

AIDS-KS is generally diagnosed by examining biopsies of skin or mucous membrane lesions. Although AIDS-KS has often been diagnosed without biopsy, it should be noted that the visual appearance may be similar to several other dermatologic presentations including fungal infection, lymphoma, dermatofibroma, and bacillary epithelioid angiomatosis (cat-scratch disease). AIDS-KS involving the lungs or gastrointestinal tract is usually diagnosed by endoscopic examination.[15]

Several staging systems have been proposed for AIDS-KS but none has achieved universal acceptance. The Oncology Committee of the National Institute of Allergy and Infectious Diseases (NIAID) has developed a proposal for staging criteria utilizing a description of the extent of the tumor, the status of the patient's immune system, and presence or absence of other HIV-related disease manifestations. Table 13-3 details the proposed staging system.

Table 13–3 Staging Classification for AIDS-KS

TUMOR (T)	
T-0	Confined to skin and/or lymph nodes
	Minimal oral KS
T-1	Tumor associated edema or ulceration
	Extensive oral KS
	Gastrointestinal KS
	Other visceral KS
IMMUNE SYSTEM (I)	
I-0	T_4 helper cells greater than or equal to 200
I-1	T_4 helper cells less than or equal to 200
SYSTEMIC ILLNESS (S)	
S-0	No history of opportunistic infection or thrush
	No constitutional symptoms
	Karnofsky performance score equal to or greater than 70
S-1	History of opportunistic infection and/or thrush
	Constitutional symptoms
	Karnofsky performance less than 70
	Other related HIV illness

Metastasis

Despite the overall progressive course of AIDS-KS, there may be a wide range of disease progression. A rapid course with short survival is seen in patients with opportunistic infections, systemic symptoms, and low T4 helper cell counts. This rapid course is typically associated with aggressive, disseminated disease involving the lungs and visceral organs. In patients with no history of opportunistic infections or systemic symptoms, and in those with T4 helper counts above 200, the disease may be limited to cutaneous lesions and relatively slow progression.

Treatment Modalities

Curative therapy for AIDS-KS does not exist. AIDS-KS, however, is rarely life threatening. Most patients with AIDS-KS ultimately die of opportunistic infections related to the profound immunodeficiency produced by HIV infection. Treatment of AIDS-KS is therefore usually instituted for the relief of symptoms and to eliminate or reduce cosmetically unacceptable lesions.

In those patients who have minimal cutaneous disease, a number of treatment options exist. Observation alone is a possibility, since the lesions themselves are not usually painful and typically cause no morbidity or mortality. Patients, however, may choose one of the local modalities to reduce unacceptable cosmetic appearance. Local modalities include surgical excision, electrodessication, and radiation therapy.

KS is generally very responsive to radiation therapy and good palliation can usually be obtained. Excellent responses can be obtained in treatment of cutaneous KS using whole-body electron beam therapy, fractionated focal x-ray therapy, or single dose treatments. Radiation therapy is particularly useful when a prompt local response is desired. It is important to note, however, that patients with AIDS-KS seem to be unusually sensitive to radiation in specific areas, including the oral cavity, pharynx, and feet.[15]

Patients with more rapidly progressive disease may benefit from chemotherapy. Chemotherapy is most appropriate for patients who have relatively limited disease and for those with relatively intact immune function. Single agent chemotherapy can produce cosmetic and symptomatic improvement with little toxicity or significant immune impairment. Overall, single agent chemotherapy may control disease in approximately 30% of patients. Single agent chemotherapy regimens may employ vinblastine, bleomycin, VP-16, or doxorubicin.

Combination chemotherapy has also been used successfully in the treatment of AIDS-KS. Since combination chemotherapy has not been shown to be consistently superior to single agent chemotherapy, combination therapy is usually reserved for patients with widespread KS, which results in functional impairment secondary to edema, pain, or disfigurement. Visceral KS may also be managed with combination chemotherapy. Combination regimens may include: vinblastine and vincristine; vinblastine and bleomycin; doxorubicin, bleomycin, and vinblastine; doxorubicin, bleomycin, and vincristine; or vinblastine, vincristine and methotrexate.

Chemotherapy has not been shown to increase survival in patients with AIDS-KS. Myelotoxicity and neurotoxicity have been the major adverse effects. The availability of hematopoietic growth factors (G-CSF and GM-CSF) may alleviate the myelotoxicity in a number of patients, however, and a survival advantage may be obtained in the future.

A number of clinical trials have confirmed the efficacy of alpha-2 recombinant interferon (IFN-2). Patients with relatively high numbers of T4 helper cells without prior opportunistic infections are more likely to respond to interferon therapy. Unfortunately, at doses required to produce responses in AIDS-KS, significant toxicities of interferon are common. Flu-like symptoms, weight loss, rash, and leukopenias occur in most patients. Combination therapy with IFN-2 and Retrovir may improve the chances for response to therapy, particularly in patients with T4 helper cell counts above 200 prior to treatment initiation.

Potential disease and treatment related complications are given in the box on this page.

AIDS-KS DISEASE AND TREATMENT RELATED COMPLICATIONS

Potential Disease Related Complications
  Disfigurement related to skin lesions
  Airway obstruction related to pulmonary lesions
  Nausea, vomiting, diarrhea related to GI lesions
Potential Treatment Related Complications
  Radiation
    Skin: erythema, dry/wet desquamation
    Abdomen: gastritis, nausea, vomiting
    General: fatigue
  Chemotherapy
    Neutropenia
    Increased risk of opportunistic infection
    Nausea, vomiting
    Alopecia
  Interferon therapy
    Flulike syndrome
    Weight loss
    Rash
    Neutropenia and resultant increased risk of opportunistic infection

---

Prognosis

Despite the fact that significant progress has been made in the treatment options available for patients with AIDS-KS, this has unfortunately not translated into an improvement in overall survival. Since optimal therapy of all stages is still in an early phase of development, patients are encouraged to enter into clinical trials whenever possible. Although curative therapy for AIDS-KS does not yet exist, KS is rarely life threatening. Most patients with AIDS-KS ultimately die of opportunistic infections that develop as a result of the profound immunodeficiency that develops secondary to HIV infection.

NON-HODGKIN'S LYMPHOMA

As we have improved the survival of patients with HIV disease, new clinical complications are developing. HIV related non-Hodgkin's lymphoma (NHL) appears to be increasing in frequency as we extend the lifespan of patients with HIV disease. These tumors appear most frequently at the end stages of AIDS, when the immune system is most profoundly impaired.

Epidemiology

It has been estimated that of the approximately 43,000 cases of NHL to be diagnosed in 1993, up to 27% will occur in individuals infected with HIV. The incidence of NHL among the population with advanced HIV infection has been estimated at 1.6%. It is clear that NHL cases will continue to increase as HIV infection

Nursing Management

NURSING DIAGNOSIS: SELF-CONCEPT DISTURBANCE RELATED TO CUTANEOUS LESIONS

ASSESSMENT

A person's self-concept results from thoughts and feelings related to his/her identity, self esteem, role performance, and body image.[9] Changes in physical appearance often accompany AIDS-KS and place the patient at risk for disturbance in self concept. Indications of this disturbance include: social withdrawal or isolation, statements of low self-worth, and depression.

OUTCOME CRITERIA

- The patient will have an improved self-concept.
- The patient will identify and implement strategies for coping with the physical disturbance of lesions.
- The patient will maintain social and intimate relationships.
- The patient will verbalize statements reflecting self-worth.

INTERVENTIONS

- Establish a therapeutic nursing relationship based on acceptance and encouraging open sharing of feelings.
- Identify sources of threats to self-concept.
- Educate the patient in the use of self-affirmation techniques.
- Facilitate incorporation of past adaptive coping behaviors.
- Involve family and significant others in support of the patient.
- Utilize multidisciplinary group such as dermatology, psychology, social work, and support groups.
- Educate patient in techniques to reduce visibility of lesions.

NURSING DIAGNOSIS: IMPAIRED SKIN INTEGRITY

Impairment of skin integrity may be related to KS lesions, poor nutritional status secondary to chemotherapy/radiation treatment, or radiation therapy.

ASSESSMENT

Signs and symptoms of actual or impaired skin integrity include erythema, scaling, or broken skin.
- Draining wounds
- Radiation therapy recipient
- Limited activity patterns

OUTCOME CRITERIA

- The patient will remain free of skin breakdown and associated infection.
- Breaks in skin integrity will heal.

INTERVENTION

- Assess skin surfaces at least every 8 hours for erythema, breakdown, excessive moisture, or other changes.
- Keep skin clean and dry; provide skin care at least every 4 hours.
- Provide appropriate beds, mattresses, or other appliances for pressure relief.
- Maintain adequate hydration and nutrition.
- Utilize multidisciplinary team including dermatology, skin care speciality nurse.

NURSING DIAGNOSIS: KNOWLEDGE DEFICIT RELATED TO KS DISEASE AND TREATMENT

ASSESSMENT

Signs and symptoms that may alert the nurse to potential and actual knowledge deficits include: new KS diagnosis, institution of new treatment, failure to report new suspicious lesions, and altered coping skills.

OUTCOME CRITERIA

- Patient will verbalize correct knowledge of illness and treatments.
- Patient will report suspicious lesions.
- Patient will exhibit adequate coping skills.

INTERVENTION

- Assess patient knowledge and learning patterns.
- Provide a variety of educational resources including videos, printed materials, one-on-one instruction.
- Explain all procedures and treatments to patient.
- Encourage patient and family to ask questions.

increases in the population and as HIV infected individuals survive for longer periods of time.[10]

The epidemiology data indicate a disproportionate number of cases among HIV infected patients with rates nearly twice those of non-HIV infected patients. In certain areas of the country with high rates of HIV infection, the incidence of NHL is now five times greater than the highest pre-epidemic rate.

The median age of diagnosis in HIV related NHL ranges from 26 to 40 years; the median age among HIV negative patients is 56. Clearly, immune suppression as a result of HIV infection is a risk factor in the development of NHL.

Etiology and Risk Factors

The etiology of lymphoid neoplasia in the setting of HIV infection remains unclear. Lack of similarity in the molecular characteristics of these tumors suggest several different mechanisms may be responsible for the development of lymphoma in HIV infected individuals. Pathogenesis of many of these lymphomas has been linked to latent infection of B lymphocytes with the Epstein-Barr virus (EBV). EBV does seem to be present in approximately 50% of the tumors with monoclonal origins but not in those of polyclonal origin. In both EBV positive and negative tumors, however, the onset of disease appears related to the degree of immune suppression in the patient created by the original HIV infection.

Prevention, Screening, and Detection

Currently, there is no known way to prevent or screen for NHL. Clinicians should be suspicious toward a NHL diagnosis in any HIV infected patient who presents with a history of a lump or other mass. Laboratory evaluation is difficult to evaluate in this patient population. A complete blood count is usually normal, although anemia may be present and lymphopenia can occur in as many as 50% of cases. Erythrocyte sedimentation rate and lactic acid dehydrogenase may be elevated, although these elevations may also be attributable to HIV diseases or opportunistic infection.

Classification

NHL in HIV infected patients are classified similarly to those occurring in noninfected patients. Rappaport introduced a classification system for the various histologic types of NHL in the late 1950s. This classification system has been formalized and is now commonly referred to as the Working Formulation.

In the Working Formulation classification scheme, the HIV-associated NHL are generally placed in the intermediate and high-grade categories. Diffuse large cell lymphoma, especially the high-grade immunoblastic type, is the most commonly diagnosed NHL.

The majority of cases of HIV-related NHL consist of high-grade NHL with B phenotype. The most represented histologies are Burkitt's lymphomas, immunoblastic lymphoma, and the otherwise nonspecified "undifferentiated" lymphoma. Diffuse large cell lymphoma, particularly of the high-grade immunoblastic type, is the most commonly diagnosed HIV related NHL.[10]

Clinical Features

Patients presenting with HIV associated NHL are a heterogeneous group. The most common symptom of NHL is painless lymphadenopathy that may involve the abdominal nodes. One third of patients with NHL have had preceding persistent generalized lymphadenopathy (PGL). Patients may present with systemic B symptoms such as fever, chills, and weight loss, although these symptoms may be difficult to differentiate from those associated with HIV infection and related opportunistic infections. Since extranodal sites such as the gastrointestinal tract, bone marrow, spleen, and liver may be affected, patients may present with symptoms of vague abdominal discomfort, back pain, gastrointestinal complaints, or ascites.

Diagnosis and Staging

The findings of lymphadenopathy, splenomegaly, or hepatomegaly is suggestive of lymphoma, but NHL may also present as an abdominal mass or as a discrete lesion of the lung or central nervous system. A complete physical examination is essential. In addition, routine tests, including a complete blood count and chemistries, should be obtained. Abnormal liver function tests may suggest involvement of the hepatic sytem and liver biopsy may be indicated. Bone marrow involvement is common in HIV-associated NHL and bone marrow aspiration and biopsy should be performed early in the diagnostic work-up. Chest x-ray evaluation may reveal mediastinal, hilar, or parenchymal involvement and more sophisticated nuclear medicine studies such as the CAT scan and MRI can be used to scan the liver and spleen. The clinical value of the staging laparotomy has yet to be demonstrated and bone marrow evaluation may provide adequate information.

The Ann Arbor Staging Classification is used to categorize the extent of disease, although its prognostic significance is unknown:

Stage I   Involvement of a single lymph node region or of a single extralymphatic organ or site

Stage II   Involvement of two or more lymph node regions on the same side of the diaphragm

Stage III   Involvement of lymph node regions on both sides of the diaphragm

Stage IV   Disseminated involvement of one or more extralymphatic organs or tissues

Metastasis

Few patients present with stage I or II disease. In fact, most patients present with stage IV disease, which is further complicated by frequent involvement of the bone marrow and the central nervous system. In addition, the immunodeficiency and possible history of previous opportunistic infections may potentiate the aggressive course of the disease. Widely disseminated disease is diagnosed at the time of initial presentation in greater than two thirds of patients. Also common to this population is occurrence of unusual sites of lymphomatous disease including the myocardium, adrenals, ear lobes, maxillae, gall bladder, orbit, and rectum.[6]

Treatment Modalities

Treatment of patients with HIV-related NHL is often complicated by their underlying immunodeficiency. As a group, these patients generally do not respond well to treatment. Those patients more likely to tolerate intensive therapy and to do relatively well are those without a prior history of profound immune deficiency or opportunistic infections. Unfortunately, most patients have significant immunodeficiency at presentation. In addition, the majority of patients have advanced stage IV disease of a high grade type with possible involvement of the bone marrow and/ or CNS. The leukopenia commonly seen in this patient population secondary to the HIV infection further complicates the use of conventional multiagent chemotherapy regimens.

Recent approaches to treatment have focused on variations in the dosing of the standard chemotherapeutic agents. Hematopoietic growth factors have also been used to alleviate the myeloid toxicity associated with chemotherapy. These trials have demonstrated that hematologic toxicity can be reduced by using reduced dosages of chemotherapy and by using myeloid growth factors with standard doses. It is still unclear, however, which of these treatment approaches will be associated with improved response and survival.[10]

In general, standard chemotherapy doses should be given to patients with T4 helper counts greater than 200. Growth factor support is also recommended in this population. For patients with more compromised immune function (with T4 helper cell counts below 200), reduced dosage chemotherapy regimens are advised since these patients are less likely to tolerate cytotoxic therapy. The most commonly used regimen is that of mBACOD, which includes methotrexate, bleomycin, doxorubicin, cyclophosphamide, vincristine, dexamethasone, and folinic acid. For patients

---

NON-HODGKIN'S LYMPHOMA DISEASE AND TREATMENT RELATED COMPLICATIONS

Disease Related Complications
  Pain secondary to lymphadenopathy and associated dysfunction
  Mental status changes secondary to CNS involvement
  Abdominal pain secondary to hepatic, splenic, or GI involvement
  Fatigue secondary to constitutional symptoms of fever, chills, and weight loss
Treatment Related Complications
  Infection related to myelotoxicity of chemotherapy
  Fatigue related to myelotoxicity of chemotherapy
  Altered nutrition secondary to emetigenic potential of chemotherapy, mucositis, stomatitis
  Pain related to mucositis associated with chemotherapy
  Pain and self-care deficit secondary to peripheral neuropathy related to chemotherapy
  Altered respiratory function related to chemotherapy

---

who are profoundly ill with significantly compromised immune status, the option of only palliative therapy should be considered.

Non-Hodgkin's lymphoma has potential disease and treatment related complications. See box above.

Prognosis

The prognosis for patients with HIV-associated NHL is poor. Median survival for patients with peripheral NHL treated with a variety of standard chemotherapeutic regimens ranges from 4 to 7 months. For those with CNS involvement, the prognosis is even poorer, with median survival of approximately 2.5 months. Treatment for these patients, however, has a significant impact on survival, since the anticipated survival for untreated patients would be on the order of weeks.

A small percentage of patients will be expected to live a median of 1 or 2 years in complete remission. These patients are more likely to tolerate intensive therapy, because they present without prior history of opportunistic infection and with higher performance status.

OTHER HIV RELATED MALIGNANCIES

In addition to the more common HIV related malignancies such as Kaposi's sarcoma and non-Hodgkin's lymphoma, a variety of other malignancies are also becoming evident. Unfortunately, it is becoming apparent that as patients live longer with HIV disease, more malignancies will become clinically significant.

Nursing Management

NURSING DIAGNOSIS: POTENTIAL FOR INFECTION

The risk of infection may be related to the disease process itself, particularly when bone marrow involvement is present. Infection potential may also be related to the immune suppression from the underlying HIV disease or the treatment regimens for NHL.

ASSESSMENT

A variety of signs and symptoms may alert the nurse to an impending or current infection: neutropenia, decreased T4 helper cell count, fever, shortness of breath/cough, mental status change, and nausea, vomiting, or diarrhea.

OUTCOME CRITERIA

* The patient will remain free of infection.
* Infections will be identified early and treatment initiated quickly.

INTERVENTIONS

* Carefully monitor vital signs and laboratory results for signs of possible infection.
* Institute a low microbial diet for patients with an absolute neutrophil count below 500 cell/cm³.
* Perform appropriate physical assessment including careful examination of skin integrity, respiratory and gastrointestinal status.
* Perform appropriate mental status examinations.
* Maintain asepsis when caring for patient, including appropriate handwashing, limiting of infectious visitors.
* Educate patient in protective strategies such as handwashing, diet precautions, and pet care precautions.

NURSING DIAGNOSIS: ALTERATION IN NUTRITION (LESS THAN BODY REQUIREMENTS)

A compromised nutritional status may be related to anorexia secondary to chemotherapy or chronic infection; nausea, vomiting, or diarrhea secondary to opportunistic infection or treatment; impaired swallowing related to mucositis secondary to infection or treatment; or knowledge deficit.

ASSESSMENT

People with HIV infection in general are at risk for the development of malnutrition. The nutrition of these patients is further compromised when treatments for NHL are instituted. In addition, these treatment modalities may further compromise the immune status, resulting in GI opportunistic infections, which may further deplete the nutritional status. Signs and symptoms of altered nutritional status include weight loss, anorexia/nausea/vomiting, dehydration, and mucositis.

OUTCOME CRITERIA

* The patient will achieve or maintain body weight.

INTERVENTIONS

* Monitor at least weekly weights, daily intake and output.
* Assess for signs and symptoms of malnutrition such as weight loss, weakness, fatigue, and decreased intake.
* Monitor laboratory data such as serum protein, albumin, and electrolytes.
* Minimize anorexia, nausea, and vomiting by administering antiemetics, offering small frequent meals of cool or room temperature; avoid spicy foods.
* Assist with good oral hygiene.
* Consult dietician.
* Educate patient in nutritional needs and ways to reduce nausea, anorexia, and pain.

Primary CNS Lymphoma

Primary CNS lymphoma is of B-cell origin in the majority of reported cases. It is not simply a manifestation of systemic NHL but instead is a discrete entity. HIV infected individuals demonstrate an increased frequency of primary CNS lymphoma, and it is now estimated that its incidence is approaching 6% of all cases of AIDS.

It is difficult to diagnose CNS lymphoma in the setting of HIV disease because the differential diagnoses include a variety of opportunistic infections involving the CNS. Presenting signs and symptoms may include confusion, lethargy, memory loss, hemiparesis or dysphasia, seizures, or headaches.

Computer assisted tomographic brain scanning is usually nonspecific for CNS lymphoma and lumbar puncture is rarely diagnostic. Open brain biopsy is technically required to confirm the diagnosis. The current treatment approach includes combination radiation therapy and corticosteroids. The prognosis for these individuals remains poor, with long-term survival of only a few months.[17]

Cervical Cancer

The gynecologic problems associated with HIV infection includes a variety of sexually transmitted diseases, pelvic inflammatory disease, genital ulcers, vaginal candidiasis, and cervical neoplasia, which can be a precursor to cervical cancer. The most common neoplasia of the cervix, squamous cell neoplasia, has been linked to early age at first sexual intercourse, multiple sexual partners, and infection with the human papillomavirus (HPV). HPV is also thought to be the causative agent for most condylomata acuminata (genital warts).

Genital warts in HIV infected women may exist as multiple small lesions or as unusually large and profuse lesions. External warts often extend to adjacent, moist epithelium, including the vagina, cervix, urethra, and rectum. Cervical dysplasia, the premalignant changes noted on Pap smear screening, can result from HPV infection and can progress to cervical cancer. Cervical dysplasia occurs at an unusually high rate in HIV infected women at 5 to 10 times the expected rate. Cervical cancer caused by HPV is potentially fatal and is the most serious gynecologic disease for HIV infected women. In addition, cervical dysplasia and cancer may be more aggressive and persistent among HIV positive women than among uninfected women.[13]

Recently, the adequacy of the Pap smear as a screening device has been questioned. Nearly 80% of HIV infected women had normal Pap smears, but nearly half of these women were later found to have histologic evidence of cervical intraepithelial neoplasia when they underwent colposcopy. Colposcopy evaluation should be considered for all HIV positive women.[2]

The presence and severity of cervical neoplasia correlates with both absolute number and function of T4 helper cells. Women with more profound immunodeficiency are more likely to have high-grade lesions than are asymptomatic HIV-positive women. Lymph node involvement is common, although markedly enlarged nodes may also result from HIV disease. Women with HIV disease also have higher recurrence and death rates with shorter intervals to recurrence.

For patients with early disease, radical hysterectomy and pelvic lymphadenectomy may be performed safely. In patients with advanced or systemic disease, chemotherapy may be used along with radiation therapy, although careful monitoring of hematologic toxicities must be performed. Drugs that are relatively sparing of the bone marrow, such as cisplatin, bleomycin, and vincristine may be used.[19]

Anal Carcinoma

Anal carcinoma in HIV infected men is similar to cervical carcinoma in HIV infected women. Increasing numbers of men with concurrent HIV and HPV infection are now showing signs of intra-anal cytologic abnormalities. Greater than 50% of patients with abnormal anal cytology have been shown to have HPV DNA on specimen. The prevalence of these abnormalities seems to increase with time in serial follow up.[1]

Anal intraepithelial neoplasia (AIN), like CIN, can develop into a malignant process. Among HIV-negative men, AIN is relatively uncommon. Approximately 15% of symptomatic HIV positive men, however, have been shown to have AIN and this number increases to about 30% over longitudinal follow up. The risk appears to increase with advancing immune suppression.[16] Since anal cancer may take several years to develop from AIN, it seems likely that the rate of anal cancer will continue to increase as immunosuppressed individuals live longer.

Patients with anal carcinoma have a much higher incidence of venereal warts when compared to patients with carcinoma of the colon or rectum.[17] What role HIV plays in the pathogenesis of this malignancy has yet to be defined. It is possible that HIV promotes the development of papillomavirus-related malignancies or allows a broadened expression of the latent HPV.

AIN and early stages of anal cancer usually are not associated with any symptoms. Some individuals may notice rapid growth of an external anal lesion or may develop new onset of anal pruritus or other change in bowel habits. In advanced disease, anal cancer may be associated with weight loss, pelvic pain, and even obstruction of the anal canal.

The natural history of AIN is currently under study. It is not yet known what percentage of those with AIN will go on to develop anal cancer if left untreated. It seems likely, however, that treatment of AIN will prevent the development of anal cancer. It therefore seems reasonable to perform an anal Pap test and anoscopy on any HIV positive patient with new onset signs or symptoms related to anal carcinoma as well as on those who have a history of venereal warts. Although the optimal forms of treatment have not yet been identified, fulguration or cryotherapy of anal lesions through the use of a proctoscope or sigmoidoscope seems reasonable. If the lesion has progressed to anal carcinoma, chemotherapy and possibly radiation therapy may be considered.

Other Malignancies

While only a handful of cases of malignant melanoma have been reported in HIV positive patients, it is possible that this incidence will increase as survival length of immunosuppression are extended. The incidence of malignant melanoma in renal transplant patients, a group with iatrogenic immune suppression, is reported to be approximately four times that of the general population. Since this is in all likelihood related to immune suppression, it is possible that we will see the same increase in occurrence in the HIV infected population. The possibility of an increased incidence of hepatocellular carcinoma also seems likely in HIV infected patients who are concurrently infected with chronic Hepatitis B.

CONCLUSION

HIV disease has quickly become an overwhelming epidemic, claiming the lives of hundreds of thousands of people throughout the world and threatening to defeat our current health care delivery systems. It is a sexually transmitted, blood borne viral infection that destroys the host's immune system, resulting in life-threatening opportunistic infections and a variety of malignant processes.

HIV disease is now the fifth leading cause of death among American women of childbearing ages and the second leading cause of death of young American men. There are approximately 1.5 million people currently infected in the United States with a new infection occurring approximately every 54 seconds. It is estimated that as many as 110 million people world wide will be infected by the end of this decade.

As the number of infected individuals continues to grow and as scientific advances are made in this disease, extending the life span of those infected, our health care system will be burdened even more with the ever increasing load of patients requiring comprehensive, extended care. Caring for the patient with HIV disease is a complex issue given the life-threatening nature of the disease, the relative youth of the affected population, and the sociopolitical issues surrounding the epidemic. Nurses have played critical roles in defining the need for comprehensive, compassionate care of patients with HIV disease.

Patient teaching priorities are given in the box on this page.

BIBLIOGRAPHY

1. Abrams DI: Acquired immunodeficiency syndrome and related malignancies: A topical overview, Semin Oncol 18(5):41-45, 1991.
2. ACOG: Human immunodeficiency virus infections, ACOG Tech Bull 165:1-11, 1992.
3. American Foundation for AIDS Research: Statistics, AIDS Clin Care 4(6):1, 1992.
4. Centers for disease control: The HIV/AIDS epidemic: The first 10 years, Morbid Mortal Weekly Report 40(22):357-375, 1991.
5. Centers for Disease Control: Update: Acquired immunodeficiency syndrome: United States, 1991, Morbid Mortal Weekly Report 41(16):308-309, 1993.
6. Errante D and others: Management of AIDS and its neoplastic complications, Eur J Cancer 27(3):389-399, 1991.
7. Food and Drug Administration: Trials sanctioned for study of potential therapeutic use of new AIDS vaccine in HIV infected individuals, Communication: March 12, 1990.
8. Friedland G: AIDS: The first decade, AIDS Clin Care 3(6):41-47, 1991.
9. Gee G: AIDS: Concepts in nursing practice, Baltimore, 1988, Williams & Wilkins.
10. Kaplan L: HIV-associated lymphoma, AIDS File 6(1):6-8, 1992.
11. Lucey D: The first decade of human retroviruses: A nomenclature for the clinician, Military Med 156(10):555-557, 1991.
12. Lusso P and Gallo R: Pathogenesis of AIDS, J Pharmaceut Pharmacol 44(suppl 1):160-164, 1992.
13. Marte C and Allen M: HIV-related gynecologic conditions: Overlooked complications. Focus: A Guide to AIDS Research and Counseling 7(1):1-4, 1991.
14. McPhedran P: Using hematopoietic hormones in HIV disease, AIDS Clin Care 4(6):43-44, 1992.
15. Northfelt D: AIDS-associated Kaposi's sarcoma, AIDS File 6(1):1-4, 1992.
16. Palefsky J: Anal cancer among HIV-positive men, AIDS File 6(1):9-10, 1992.
17. Schwartz J, Dias B, and Safai B: HIV-related malignancies, Dermatol Clin 9(3):503-515, 1991.
18. Thompson D: Invincible AIDS, Time August 3:30-37, 1992.

PATIENT TEACHING PRIORITIES

- Risk Reduction Techniques: Minimize the number of sexual partners and engage in a mutually monogamous sexual relationship
- Safe Sex Counseling: Any exchange of blood, semen, or vaginal secretions can potentially put an individual at risk for HIV disease.
- Intravenous Risk Reduction: The use of contaminated needles for any injection represents a serious risk for HIV infection.
- Signs and Symptoms of Infectious Process: These include fever, chills, shortness of breath, cough, pain, diarrhea, nausea, vomiting, skin breakdown, weight loss, and a sense of mental confusion.
- Self-Help Care Strategies: Know where and when to seek medical, psychosocial, and financial assistance.

19. Tinkle M, Amaya M, and Tamayo O: HIV disease and pregnancy, JOGNN 21(2):86-92, 1992.

20. Torres G: Update on vaccine development, Treatment Iss 5(6):3-5, 1991.

21. Volberding P: Management of HIV infection: Treatment team workshop handbook, New York, 1991, World Health Communications.

22. Wright M: Guide to opportunistic infections, Project Inform Perspective Oct:11-13, 1991.

CHAPTER 14

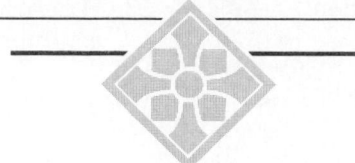

Leukemia

Linda Meili

The leukemias are a complex collection of diseases that were first described in 1845 by Virchow. He described a condition in which the relationship between red and colorless corpuscles was the reverse of normal. He coined the term *weisses blut* or *white blood*.[46]

There are two major classifications of leukemia: acute and chronic. These two types of leukemia are similar in that they are the product of a dysfunctional bone marrow, but they differ dramatically in disease presentation, treatment, and prognosis. Additionally, the two types of acute and chronic leukemia can be characterized by the cell line of origin—myeloid or lymphoid.

An understanding of any leukemia must begin with a knowledge of normal bone marrow function. The first section of this chapter, Pathophysiology, describes this function. The chapter is then divided into three major sections: acute leukemias, chronic leukemias, and nursing management of the patient with leukemia.

Much of the scientific knowledge of adult leukemia is derived from the studies done in pediatric leukemia. Although pediatric leukemia is referred to in this chapter, especially in the acute lymphoblastic leukemia section, the focus of this chapter is the adult patient with leukemia.

PATHOPHYSIOLOGY

Leukemia is a malignant hematologic disorder characterized by a proliferation of abnormal blood cells that infiltrate the bone marrow, peripheral blood, and other organs. Leukemia may present as an acute or chronic disease process.

Elements of the blood are formed in the bone marrow, vertebrae, clavicle, scapula, sternum, ribs, skull, proximal ends of long bones, and pelvis. The body can be imagined to have three pools of blood cells. The first pool of cells are the pluripotent stem cells of the bone marrow, the most primitive form of blood cell from which all blood cells originate. The stem cell pool is responsible for the generation of new cells to meet the body requirements throughout the person's lifetime. The pleuripotent stem cell can proliferate or differentiate. The decision is based on the current needs of the body. With every stem cell division, one daughter cell remains in the stem cell pool, so the life-time pool of stem cells is never depleted. An injury to the stem cell pool, such as a lethal dose of radiation, prevents the production of blood cells and results in marrow aplasia. The stem cell pool cannot be assessed by a routine bone marrow examination. Studies of the stem cell population are called "colony forming assays" and are performed by in vitro culturing. In the bone marrow blood cells mature within a framework of supportive cells and blood vessels that supply nutrition and growth factors for proliferation and differentiation.[24]

Proliferation of stem cells is mediated by specific colony-stimulating factors acting on progenitor cells to give rise to granulocytes, erythrocytes, macrophages, and megakaryocytes.[2]

The second pool of cells are precursor cells for red blood cells, platelets, granulocytes, and lymphocytes. A stem cell becomes committed to a certain blood cell line when it leaves the stem cell pool. In the second pool, the cells differentiate and mature. Figure 14-1 illustrates the steps of cell differentiation and maturation. The second pool cells at the blast phase of development cannot function as mature blood cells, but they can undergo mitosis. At this stage of development, the blasts may be responsive to specific colony stimulating factors. As the cells divide, they dif-

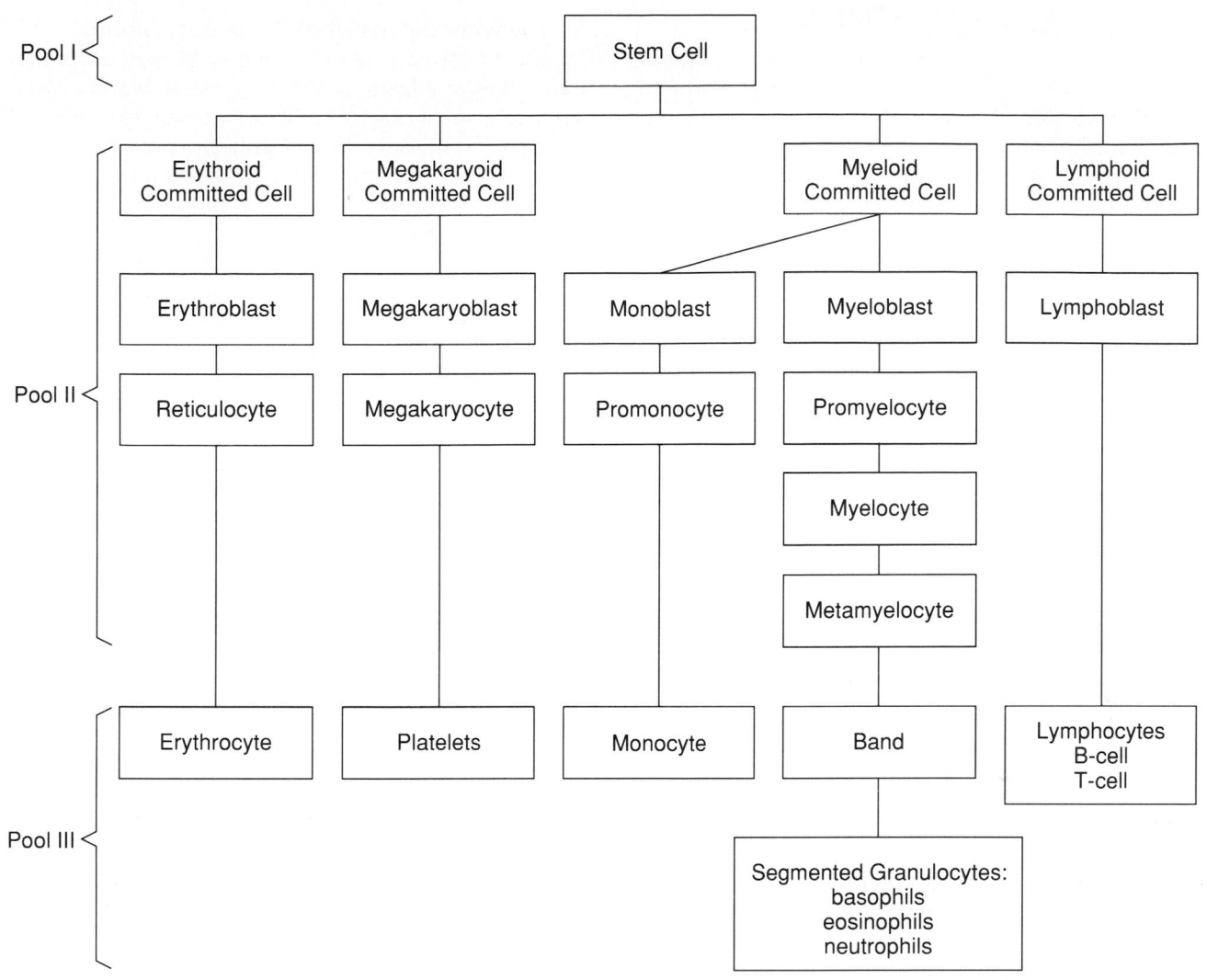

Pool I

Pool II

Pool III

Stem Cell

Erythroid Committed Cell | Megakaryoid Committed Cell | Myeloid Committed Cell | Lymphoid Committed Cell

Erythroblast | Megakaryoblast | Monoblast | Myeloblast | Lymphoblast

Reticulocyte | Megakaryocyte | Promonocyte | Promyelocyte

Myelocyte

Metamyelocyte

Erythrocyte | Platelets | Monocyte | Band | Lymphocytes B-cell T-cell

Segmented Granulocytes: basophils eosinophils neutrophils

Figure 14–1 The maturation process of various blood cell lines originating from the stem cell.

ferentiate, enabling them to carry out only specific functions, and they lose their proliferative response to CSFs.

When the precursor cells of the second pool are mature, they are released into the peripheral circulation, the third pool. Each mature blood cell performs a specific function (red blood cells—oxygen transport; granulocytes—phagocytosis; platelets—clotting). The mature circulating cells cannot undergo mitosis and must be replaced at the end of their life span (red blood cells—120 days; granulocytes—6 to 8 hours, platelets—8 to 10 days). Mature blood cells are released from the bone marrow responding to the body's need.

In leukemia, the control factors regulating the orderly differentiation and maturation of the blood cells are absent. This lack of regulatory control results in the arrest of the maturation process of a specific cell line. The involved immature cell form proliferates and

accumulates in the bone marrow, resulting in crowding of the normal marrow cells. This marrow crowding impairs the production and function of normal cell lines; ultimately, the marrow is replaced by leukemic cells, which are released into the circulating blood. The leukemic cells may also invade body organs.

Research may eventually define the cause of malignant transformation in the blood-forming process, but the currently accepted theory is that leukemias develop from a single malignant clone. The specific type of leukemia depends on which stem cell line is affected (myeloid or lymphoid) and the point of maturation at which growth is arrested. Acute leukemias result from arrest of immature blood cells, chronic leukemias involve more mature blood cells. Leukemic cells actually generate more slowly than normal white cells, but the mechanisms controlling cellular division are errant, allowing more cells to be capable of division at any point in time.

ACUTE LEUKEMIAS

Acute leukemia is a severe and aggressive disease characterized by rapid onset and a rapidly terminal course if untreated. There are two types of acute leukemia: lymphocytic (ALL) and myeloid (AML).

In acute leukemia, the leukemic or "blast" cells function abnormally and accumulate in the peripheral blood, bone marrow, reticuloendothelial system, and possibly the central nervous system. The overproduction of leukemic cells in the bone marrow impairs normal hematopoiesis, resulting in anemia, granulocytopenia, and thrombocytopenia.

Acute Lymphocytic Leukemia

EPIDEMIOLOGY AND ETIOLOGY

The exact etiology of ALL is unknown. Radiation, chemicals, drugs, viruses, and genetic abnormalities have been implicated in the etiology of this disease. A causal relationship between the human T-cell leukemia virus-I (HTLV-I) and T-cell leukemias and lymphoma is suspected, but not proven.[65]

ALL or leukemia in adults usually occurs in the third decade of life. This disease is seen less often in adults than acute myelocytic leukemia. ALL is more common in children; 85% of all cases of ALL occur in children. This disease comprises 20% of adult leukemia.

CLINICAL FEATURES

The patient with ALL has complaints and physical findings related to the rapidly expanding leukemic cell population.

The most common complaint is fatigue persisting over several weeks. Anorexia, shortness of breath on exertion, malaise, and weight loss may be reported. One third of patients may have minor bleeding problems. Patients with ALL frequently present with signs of infection. Neurologic symptoms, such as headache or visual disturbances, may be identified. Up to 10% of ALL patients may display no symptoms.[84]

Minimal to moderate lymph node enlargement, especially in the cervical region is common in ALL. More than 50% of patients also have some degree of splenomegaly.[84] In addition patients may present with hepatomegaly and bone or joint pain.

DIAGNOSIS

The diagnosis of ALL is often indicated by the peripheral blood smear; however, a bone marrow evaluation is essential to finalize the diagnosis and provide specimens for further subclassification studies.

The peripheral blood smear must be evaluated by an experienced clinician.[16] The diagnosis of ALL is usually made without difficulty when there is marked increase in immature lymphs (lymphoblasts) associated with anemia and thrombocytopenia.

The white blood cell (WBC) count is normal to high in the majority of ALL patients. Nearly all patients have lymphoblasts in the peripheral blood. Platelet counts in most cases of ALL are normal to moderately decreased and only 30% of patients present with less than 50,000/mm^3 platelets. Most patients will have hematocrits in the 30% to 35% range.[84]

The bone marrow aspirate is used to obtain the "differential" count. The differential quantitates the percentage of each of the hematologic components in the marrow. Lymphoblasts comprise at least 50% of the marrow cells in ALL.[84]

Smears of the bone marrow aspirate are specially stained to define the specific subtype of ALL. A portion of the bone marrow aspirate is heparinized for cytogenetic analysis. These studies may reveal certain patterns of gene translocations or rearrangements that are prognostically significant.

A core biopsy of the bone is obtained during the bone marrow procedure. This specimen is used to determine the marrow "cellularity." Cellularity refers to the ratio of hematopoietic tissue to adipose tissue in the marrow. The amount of blood-forming or "red" marrow decreases with the aging process and is replaced by fat or "yellow" marrow. "Normocellular" marrow for an adult is 30% to 40% cellularity. These age-related changes are reflected in defining marrow cellularity. Normocellular marrow has normal proportions of the hematopoietic cells and adipose cells, hypocellular marrow has a reduced number of hematopoietic cells and an increase in adipose elements, and hypercellular marrow has an increased number of hematopoietic cells and a decreased amount of adipose tissue.[45] A bone marrow report in a newly diagnosed ALL patient is usually hypercellular with increased lymphoblasts (for example, cellularity = 90%; lymphoblasts = 80%).

Infiltration of the cerebrospinal fluid (CSF) by leukemic cells is most common in children with acute lymphocytic leukemia, but may be present in 5% to 10% of adult ALL patients.[16]

The CSF specimen is centrifuged and stained to determine the presence of leukemic cells. A low glucose level or a high protein level may indicate either leukemic infiltration or an infectious process. Platelet transfusions may be required before the procedure in thrombocytopenic patients to decrease the potential risk of bleeding.

Table 14-1 presents the physical findings, lab values, bone marrow, and CSF results in ALL and AML patients.

CLASSIFICATION

Classification of leukemias at diagnosis is necessary to determine prognosis and select therapy. The French-American-British (FAB) classification system,

Table 14–1 Physical Examination Findings, Laboratory Results, Bone Marrow, and CSF Evaluation in ALL and AML Patients

History/Physical Exam	Acute Lymphoblastic Leukemia	Acute Myeloid Leukemia
Infection	Frequently present	30% have serious infections
Bleeding	Mild in 30%	30% have significant bleeding or petechiae
		75% have intracutaneous bleeding
Adenopathy	Minimal to moderate cervical adenopathy	Rare
Splenomegaly	Minimal to moderate	Occurs in 25%
Gingival hypertrophy	Rare	Present with monocytic element
Neurologic	Headaches, visual disturbances	Rare
LABORATORY FINDINGS		
WBC	85% normal to high	30% decreased
	25% WBC > 50,000/mm³	30% normal
	15% neutropenic	30% increased
	All patients have blasts	>50,000/mm³ in 25%
	Two thirds have > 50% blasts	10% have no blasts
Platelets	<50,000/mm³ in 30%	<20,000/mm³ common
Uric acid	Increased	Increased in 50%
LDH	Increased	Commonly elevated
BONE MARROW		
Cellularity	Hypercellular	Hypercellular
Blasts	50% or greater	50% or greater
Erythroid elements	Decreased	Increased
Morphology	Normal	Bizarre granulation of mature granulocytes
CEREBROSPINAL FLUID		
Cytology	5%-10% + at presentation	<5% occurrence; greater risk in M₄ and M₅, greater risk with WBC >100,000

developed in 1976, based on cellular morphology and histochemical staining of blast cells, is universally accepted.[16] Acute lymphocytic leukemias are also subclassified according to their immunophenotypic features. Cytogenetic analysis further defines the specific clonal abnormalities found in acute leukemia. Information about the role of molecular genetic techniques and the relationship of retroviruses and oncogenes is increasing the knowledge of the nature of acute leukemia.

The three FAB classes of acute lymphocytic leukemia are L_1, L_2, and L_3.[4] The L_1 classification is most common in childhood leukemias. Morphologically, the leukemia cells are small, homogeneous, and nongranular with scanty cytoplasm. The common adult form of ALL is the L_2 classification.[49] Microscopically, these blasts appear larger and are heterogeneous. The L_3 classification is very rare and resembles Burkitt's lymphoma.[49] Morphologically the L_3 blasts are large and homogeneous with moderately abundant cytoplasm.

It is also important to perform cell surface marker studies on the blast cells of a patient with ALL to identify leukemia associated antigens. Originally three groups of ALL were identified by these methods: B-ALL, T-ALL, and non-B, non-T, ALL. New monoclonal antibodies developed against a host of leukemia-associated antigens have allowed for the subdivision of non-B, non-T ALL into four phenotypes based on the predominance of cells that are either B-cell or T-cell precursors. These groups are: common ALL (CALLA), pre-B ALL, pre-T ALL, and null cell ALL.[84]

PROGNOSIS

Approximately 75% of adults treated for acute lymphocytic leukemia will achieve complete remission, and 40% wil be cured.[16] These figures do not reflect the poorer prognosis B-cell or null-cell ALL. Patients who do not achieve complete remission have a median survival of less than 6 months.

A reasonable interpretation of currently available data is that adults with T-cell ALL have the best prognosis, those with common ALL have an intermediate prognosis, and those with null-cell ALL have a slightly inferior prognosis.[49] Patients with hybrid leukemias and adults with B-cell ALL have the least favorable prognosis.[49]

AGE.   Age has a greater impact on length of remission and overall survival than on attaining an initial complete remission.[50] It is generally believed patients under the age of 35 have the best prognosis.

WHITE BLOOD COUNT.   A high initial white blood cell count (WBC) is a poor prognostic indicator and

```
┌─────────────────────────────────────────────────────┐
│              PROGNOSTIC INDICATORS IN ALL             │
│                                                       │
│   Good                      Poor                      │
│   L₁, L₂                    L₃                        │
│   T-cell, CALLA posi-       B-cell, null-cell         │
│     tive                                              │
│   Age < 35                  Age > 35                  │
│   Female                    Male                      │
│   WBC < 30,000/mm³          WBC > 30,000/mm³          │
│     at diagnosis              at diagnosis            │
│   CR < 4 weeks              CR > 4 weeks              │
│   Normal karyotype          Cytogenetic abnormalities │
│                             CNS involvement           │
└─────────────────────────────────────────────────────┘
```

PROGNOSTIC INDICATORS IN ALL	
Good	**Poor**
L_1, L_2	L_3
T-cell, CALLA positive	B-cell, null-cell
Age < 35	Age > 35
Female	Male
WBC < 30,000/mm³ at diagnosis	WBC > 30,000/mm³ at diagnosis
CR < 4 weeks	CR > 4 weeks
Normal karyotype	Cytogenetic abnormalities
	CNS involvement

has an adverse effect on remission duration.[40] A patient with a WBC below 30,000/mm³ and less than 80% circulating blasts has a better chance of attaining a durable complete remission.

TIME TO RESPONSE.   The factor of time to response strongly determines the length of remission. In one study of 365 patients, median remission duration was 31 months in the 214 patients achieving complete remission (CR) within 4 weeks compared to only 12 months in 54 patients requiring more than 4 weeks to achieve CR.[43]

CYTOGENETICS.   Patients with a normal cytogenetic karyotype achieve complete remission twice as often as those with abnormal karyotypes.[30] The 9, 22 translocation is the most common abnormality in adults and is an adverse risk factor independent of age, immunophenotype, and initial WBC.[18]

SEX.   Males have an inferior long-term survival rate in both adult and pediatric populations.[18] Testicular relapses may account for the poorer survival of male children with ALL.[40]

OTHER RISK FACTORS.   Central nervous system leukemia occurs in 10% of adults, and when diagnosed is a poor risk factor, especially when associated with the L_3 or B-cell subset.[18] Splenomegaly, hepatomegaly, thrombocytopenia, low LDH, increased SGOT, and weight loss have been shown to be poor prognostic indicators in single studies and require confirmation.[49]

The box above lists the factors affecting prognosis in ALL.

TREATMENT MODALITIES

The treatment goal in ALL is to achieve a cure. Standard treatment regimens in this disease consist of two parts, induction therapy and postremission therapy. Prophylactic treatment to prevent central nervous system disease is incorporated into both parts of treatment.

The purpose of induction therapy is to induce a complete response (CR). A CR is documented by a bone marrow aspirate containing <5% lymphoblasts and the elimination of extramedullary disease. Postremission therapy is administered over a 2- to 3-year period after CR to eradicate completely any remaining clinically undetectable leukemia cells that may potentially cause disease relapse.

Induction Therapy

The primary chemotherapeutic agents used to induce remission are vincristine and prednisone. Vincristine is administered weekly for 3 to 5 weeks, and prednisone is given daily for 3 to 5 weeks. These agents alone induce remission in 36% to 67% of patients.[50] The addition of daunorubicin to the induction regimen increases the remission rate to 80%.[49] Some induction regimens use additional drugs (L-asparaginase, cyclophosphamide, methotrexate, 6-mercaptopurine, cytosine arabinoside), but these do not appear to increase response rates.[49]

Central Nervous System Treatment

The central nervous system (CNS) may serve as a "sanctuary" site for leukemia cells. Leukemic involvement in the CSF at the time of diagnosis is more common in children than in adults, where it is detected 5% to 10% of the time.[16] However, if the CNS is not treated, up to 40% of adults will develop CNS involvement.[16] Repeated treatments with intrathecal methotrexate is the standard preventive therapy.

An Ommaya reservoir may be inserted in patients at high risk for developing CNS leukemia (high initial WBC, T-cell subtype). The advantages of drug administration through an Ommaya include ease of access to CSF and higher and more predictable levels of the drug in ventricular CSF than when administered by lumbar puncture. The role of CNS prophylaxis in adult ALL has not been determined, and its full impact may not be obvious until more effective systemic therapy is developed.

Postremission Therapy

ALL will almost certainly recur without some form of postremission therapy. The optimal form of this therapy remains controversial, but the two most widely used types of therapy are consolidation/intensification therapy or maintenance therapy.

CONSOLIDATION/INTENSIFICATION   THERAPY. There are limited data concerning the role of this therapy in adults. The regimens may include high-dose chemotherapy or may repeat the drugs used in induction therapy. Some consolidation/intensification programs increase the duration of remission to 2 years,[16] but neither the optimal drugs nor the optimal duration of treatment is known.[49]

MAINTENANCE THERAPY
An extended program of low-dose maintenance therapy using weekly 6-mercaptopurine and methotrex-

ate is effective in preventing relapse and improving survival in children. There are, however, no large prospective study results in adults to confirm the most effective maintenance regimen.

Recurrent Disease Therapy

Most ALL relapses occur within the first 2 years of remission. Up to half of relapsed patients may achieve a second remission by repeating their original induction regimen.[85] Patients who relapse after completing maintenance therapy have a better chance of attaining second remission than those patients who relapse while on therapy.[49]

Patients with resistant disease who fail to achieve a first remission may respond to treatment with intermediate to high-dose methotrexate and leukovorin rescue or 1-asparaginase.

Bone marrow transplantation may allow long-term survival for up to 50% of patients after second relapse and 10% to 20% of patients after third relapse.[50] These survival rates in advanced disease may exceed those of conventional or experimental agents. The bone marrow transplantation process is discussed in Chapter 24.

Acute Myelogenous Leukemia

EPIDEMIOLOGY AND ETIOLOGY

Specific risk factors have been identified in acute myelogenous leukemia (AML). People with certain genetic disorders, such as Down's syndrome (trisomy 21), Bloom's syndrome, Klinefelter's syndrome, and Fanconi's anemia, are at increased risk to develop AML.[48] Exposure to the hydrocarbon benzene also increases the risk of disease development. Benzene is an aromatic solvent and is present in unleaded gasoline, rubber cement, and cleaning solvents.[70] Leukemia has been associated with exposure to ionizing radiation from nuclear reactions and from exposure to therapeutic and occupational radiation.[48] Because some RNA tumor viruses (retroviruses) cause myeloid leukemias in rodents, felines, and avians, a viral etiology of AML has been suspected in humans.[38]

Improvements in multimodality therapy over the past decade have resulted in increased survival and potential cure for patients with a variety of cancers. Long-term survival now allows evaluation of late effects of cancer therapy. The incidence of secondary malignancies related to cytotoxic therapy and especially therapy-related acute nonlymphocytic leukemias (T-AML) has increased dramatically over the past decade. The median interval of occurrence of T-AML is 4 to 6 years after the original cancer treatment and is usually preceded by a preleukemic state detectable for 6 months.[23]

Alkylating agents, especially prolonged use of melphalan in ovarian cancer,[28] multiple myeloma[6] and breast cancer[67] and nitrogen mustard for Hodgkin's disease[64] are strongly implicated. The risk of leukemia rises with increasing doses of alkylating agents so that the rise is directly related to the total dose received. Chlorambucil, busulfan, and thiotepa are also associated with an increased risk of developing a later malignancy.

The incidence of AML is 3 cases per 100,000 population with approximately 6500 new cases each year in the United States.[3] The median age at diagnosis is about 50 years.

CLINICAL FEATURES

As with ALL, AML symptoms are related to the rapidly expanding leukemic cell population. Symptoms of anemia are also found in AML patients at presentation. In addition, a very common finding is that of recurrent infections unresponsive to standard oral antibiotics. Reports of easy bruisability, epistaxis, or gingival bleeding reflect thrombocytopenia. Unlike ALL patients, virtually all AML patients are symptomatic at presentation.

Abnormal findings on physical examination are related to leukemic infiltration of an organ, granulocytopenia, or thrombocytopenia. A thorough and systematic physical examination confirms many of the patient's complaints and is an integral part of the diagnosis. Table 14-2 lists possible physical exam manifestations of both ALL and AML.

DIAGNOSIS

A diagnosis of AML is highly suspect when the examination of peripheral blood smears shows an increased number of immature blast cells associated with anemia and thrombocytopenia. The presence of Auer bodies (rods) suggests a diagnosis of AML before other diagnostic results are available.

The total white blood cell count in AML may be normal, decreased, or increased. A small percentage of AML patients may present without peripheral blast cells. Platelet counts of less than 20,000/mm^3 are common in AML.

As with ALL, the marrow aspirate is used to obtain the differential count, and the biopsy is used to establish the percentage cellularity. Myeloblasts comprise at least 50% of the nucleated cells in AML, and the marrow is hypercellular. It is not uncommon in AML to observe a "packed" bone marrow with cellularity of 90% to 100%.

A small sample of marrow aspirate is used for cytogenetics; the FAB stains and flow cytometry techniques are used to establish the specific subclassification.

Table 14-1 compares physical examination findings, laboratory findings, bone marrow, and cerebrospinal fluid results of ALL and AML.

Table 14-2   Clinical Features in Acute Leukemias

System	Manifestation	Cause
HEENT	Retinal capillary hemorrhage	Infiltration of leukemic cells
	Fundic leukemic infiltration	Infiltration of leukemic cells
	Papilledema	Infiltration of leukemic cells
	Oropharyngeal infections	Secondary to immunocompromise
	Periodontal infections	Secondary to immunocompromise
	Gingival hypertrophy (AML)	Leukemic infiltration
	Dry mucous membranes	Overall systemic illness
	Dysphagia	Possible leukemic infiltration
	Cervical adenopathy	Leukemic infiltration
	Epistaxis	Thrombocytopenia
	Gingival bleeding	
Cardiovascular/Pulmonary	Possible tachycardia, tachypnea	Anemia or infection
	Conduction defects	Leukemic infiltration of bundle of His,
	Murmurs	valves, pericardium or myocardium
	Pericarditis	(rare)
	Congestive heart failure	
	Abnormal lung sounds	Possible bacterial pneumonia
Abdomen	Splenomegaly (ALL)	Leukemic infiltration
	Enlarged, tender kidneys (more common in pediatric ALL)	Leukemic infiltration
	Hepatomegaly	Leukemic infiltration
	Menorrhagia	Thrombocytopenia
Genitourinary	Renal failure or anuria	Uric acid nephropathy
Rectal	Perirectal abscesses	Decreased infection-fighting capabilities
Extremities	Skin pallor	Anemia
	Ecchymosis, petechiae	Thrombocytopenia
	Leukemic skin infiltrates: small, raised, pinkish nodules	Leukemic infiltration
	Swollen joints or tenderness (most common in pediatric ALL)	
Neurologic	Headache, vomiting	Possible infiltration of CNS
	Visual disturbances	Possible CNS hemorrhage
	Cranial nerve VI, VII palsy	Infiltration of nerve sheath
Musculoskeletal	Bone or joint pain	Leukemic infiltration
	Swelling	
	Osteolytic lesions	

CLASSIFICATION

AML is classified morphologically according to the FAB criteria by the degree of differentiation along different cell lines and the extent of cell maturation.[4] Familiarity with this system is helpful for nurses caring for AML patients because it identifies the unique features of each subtype. The FAB classification for AML is described in Table 14-3.

PROGNOSIS

Oncology nurses should understand the factors affecting the prognosis of the patient with AML. In this disease, certain prognostic factors influence the rate of remission; other factors affect the duration of response.

Patients over the age of 70 are less likely to survive the rigors of induction therapy, but those who do achieve remission generally survive as long as younger patients.

Patients presenting with a WBC count >100,000/mm³ have significantly more deaths during the first week of therapy, die more frequently of CNS hemorrhage, and have shorter overall remissions and survival than those presenting with lower white cell counts.[26] Perhaps the worst prognostic factor in AML patients is prior treatment with chemotherapy or radiation therapy. This group includes patients with a treatment-related secondary leukemia and AML patients with recurring or resistant disease.

A preexisting hematologic disorder, serious infec-

Table 14–3 Classification of Acute Myelogenous Leukemias, French-American-British System (FAB)

FAB Type	Bone Marrow Morphology	Clinical Features/Prognosis
M_0	Myeloid lineage cannot be determined by conventional morphologic or cytochemical analysis; can be identified by immunophenotyping	
M_1: Myeloblastic	Without maturation >90% blasts Auer bodies present	M_1, M_2 are the most common adult AML diagnoses
M_2: Myeloblastic	With maturation Blasts + promyelocytes > 50% Auer bodies and/or granules	
M_3: Promyelocytic (APL)	Majority of cells are abnormal promyelocytes Cells filled with large granules; may be microgranular Nucleus varies in size and shape Bundles of Auer bodies 15:17 chromosome translocation	10% of adult AML, disseminated intravascular coagulation present in 80% of patients: May occur after treatment initiation Granules are released as blasts die and initiate coagulation cascade Good duration of remission
M_3 variant (M_3V)	Granules detected only on electron microscopy (microgranular varient)	
M_4: Myelomonocytic	Promonoblasts and monoblasts > 20%, myeloblasts plus promyelocytes > 20% of cells	Organomegaly Lymphadenopathy Gingival hyperplasias Soft tissue infiltration CNS leukemia
M_4E	Variable number of morphologically abnormal eosinophils present; associated abnormalities of chromosome 16	
M_5: Monocytic *Subtype A*—poorly differentiated: all monoblasts *Subtype B*—differentiated: promonocytes predominant	Monocytic cells exceed 80% Granulocytic component rarely exceeds 10% Few cells may have Auer bodies	Organomegaly Lymphadenopathy Gingival hyperplasia Soft tissue infiltration CNS leukemia
M_6: Erythroleukemia (Di Guglielmo syndrome)	Erythropoietic component exceeds 50% of marrow cells Blasts have bizarre morphology Myeloblasts and promyelocytes > 30% of erythroid cells	Occurs in < 5% AML Prolonged prodromal period May present with rheumatic disorder; 75% have positive Coombs' test; 30% have rheumatoid factor Almost always progresses to M_1, M_2, M_4
M_7: Megakaryocytic	Reticulin and collagen fibrosis; blasts resemble immature megakaryocytes or may be quite undifferentiated	Rare variant Marrow difficult to aspirate Increased LDH Intense myelofibrosis Very poor prognosis

tion at diagnosis, CNS leukemia, organomegaly, and lymphadenopathy are clinical features indicative of poor prognosis.[38] Laboratory findings predictive of poor response include anemia, high peripheral blast count, thrombocytopenia, elevated BUN and creatinine, increased LDH, or increased fibrinogen.[38] Specific chromosomal abnormalities are also associated with a poorer prognosis.

TREATMENT MODALITIES

The treatment goal of AML, as in ALL, is cure. Treatment is divided into two phases: induction and postremission therapy. Currently, maintenance therapy is not recommended in the treatment of AML. More recent studies utilize "consolidation" therapy with drug regimens almost as intensive as induction therapy. Consolidation is given over a period of months following the attainment of a complete remission. Both allogeneic and autologous bone marrow transplant are potential consolidation therapies for patients in remission.

A complete remission in AML is defined as less than 5% marrow blasts and less than 5% progranulocytes in a normocellular marrow. Peripheral blood counts must return to normal, and preexisting adenopathy or organomegaly must be absent.[16]

Induction Chemotherapy

Successful treatment of AML requires the control of bone marrow and systemic disease, and specific treatment of CNS disease, if present. Cytarabine with an anthracycline, either daunorubicin or doxorubicin, are the most effective induction agents, and result in complete remission 65% of the time.[16] Daunorubicin and doxorubicin are equally effective, but daunorubicin is usually preferred because it is less cardiotoxic and produces fewer gastrointestinal symptoms.[16] A newer anthracycline, Mitoxantrone, was approved by the FDA in 1989 for the treatment of AML.[60] Idarubicin, another anthracycline, is undergoing clinical trials to compare efficacy and cardiotoxicity to standard anthracyclines.[7] A common dosing schedule for induction is as follows:

- Ara-C, 100 to 200 mg/m^2 continuous IV infusion for 7 days
- Daunorubicin, 45 to 70 mg/m^2 IV on days 5, 6, and 7[16]

Patients over the age of 60 receive the lower dose of daunorubicin. It is not clear if the addition of vincristine, corticosteroids, or 6-thioguanine increases response rates.[16]

A bone marrow examination is repeated the second week after treatment to assess for antileukemic response. A positive response is indicated by a hypocellular, aplastic marrow. Peripheral blood studies reflect marrow aplasia with profound neutropenia and thrombocytopenia at the 14-day nadir. The marrow examination is repeated as the peripheral counts begin to recover. If evidence of leukemia persists 3 to 4 weeks after the start of induction and the marrow cellularity is recovered, the patient is reinduced with the same drugs and doses.

Current induction regimens produce CR in 65% to 80% of patients of whom 15% to 30% may be cured. The age-related CR rates are:

- <20 years old—70% to 85% CR
- 20-40 years old—60% to 75% CR
- 40-60 years old—49% to 50% CR
- >60 years old—25% to 40% CR[16]

Seventy-five percent of CRs occur after one induction course. Twenty percent of the remaining patients achieve CR on reinduction, but these remissions are less durable.[16]

Postremission Therapy

If further chemotherapy is not administered to the AML patient in remission, the survival time is much shorter and most patients will experience disease relapse within 6 to 8 months.[10,12] The most effective postremission therapy and optimal length of the postremission program are not known. Recent studies have shown no benefit from maintenance therapy over the shorter, more intense consolidation therapies.[68,80] Other studies, however, found benefit when comparing maintenance therapy to historical controls.[14,27] Because this conflicting information exists, patients should be entered on randomized clinical trials.

Bone Marrow Transplant

Bone marrow transplant may be the treatment of choice in certain AML patients in first remission. Bone marrow for the transplant may be harvested from the patient (autologous transplant) or from a histocompatible donor (allogeneic transplant). See Chapter 24 for more information on transplant options in AML patients.

Recurrent Disease Therapy

Achieving remission after relapse is difficult, and these remissions rarely last more than a year. Retreatment with ara-C and daunorubicin in patients treated with this regimen initially have a 30% to 50% chance of attaining a second remission.[39] High-dose ara-C with or without daunorubicin, L-asparaginase, amsacrine, or mitoxantrone has been used with some success in resistant AML. High-dose ara-C (2 to 3 g/m^2) may be associated with considerable toxicity, most notably cerebellar dysfunction ranging in severity from mild incoordination to coma. Neurologic symptoms occur more frequently in patients over 50 years old, but, when diagnosed early, symptoms may be reversible with discontinuation of therapy.[21]

CHRONIC LEUKEMIA
Chronic Myelogenous Leukemia

Chronic myelogenous leukemia (CML) is a myeloproliferative disorder characterized by proliferation of the granulocyte cell series. Chronic leukemias differ from acute leukemias in that the malignant white cells are mature-appearing and well-differentiated. These white cells do not function normally, however. A second unique difference is the progression of CML through three stages: chronic phase, accelerated phase, and blastic transformation or blast crisis.

EPIDEMIOLOGY AND ETIOLOGY

The incidence of CML increases with exposure to radiation but is not clearly associated with alkylating agents or hereditary factors.[44] The chemical benzene is also associated with chronic myelogenous leukemia. The annual incidence of CML is 1.4 per 100,000[44]; chronic myelogenous leukemia is less common than chronic lymphocytic leukemia and is one fourth as common as acute leukemia. This disease is most frequently encountered between the ages of 20 and 60 with the peak incidence between 50 and 60 years.[44] Some studies report a slightly higher incidence of CML in males.[77]

Significant advances have been made in understanding the biology of CML, and therapeutic improvements have increased the length of the chronic phase.

Philadelphia Chromosome

The hallmark of CML is the presence of a Philadelphia chromosome (Ph[1]). Nowell and Hungerford[63] identified this unusually small chromosome occurring in CML patients in 1960 at the University of Pennsylvania and named the chromosome for its city of origin. Chromosome 22 is missing part of its long arm, which is translocated to the long arm of chromosome 9. Although this translocation is identified in nearly 95% of CML patients, controversy exists whether all malignant cells are Ph[1]-positive, or if the acquisition of the Ph[1] chromosome is the initial oncogenic event.[77] Research in the field of oncogenes may eventually answer this question.

Apart from serving as a valuable diagnostic marker, the significance of the Ph[1] chromosome remains speculative. It is clear, however, that most of the Ph[1]-negative CML patients follow a considerably different clinical course and have a poorer prognosis.

CLINICAL FEATURES AND DIAGNOSIS
Chronic Phase

The presenting symptoms of chronic phase CML are related to expansion of the granulocytic mass. Other symptoms may include fatigue, pallor, dyspnea, anemia, anorexia, weight loss, and sternal tenderness. The most common finding on physical exam at diagnosis is splenomegaly. The spleen may be only minimally enlarged or it may be greatly enlarged, filling most of the abdomen.

The majority of patients are diagnosed during the chronic phase, which has a median duration of 3 to 5 years. Chronic phase is the initial indolent form of CML. The presenting symptoms resolve as the patient responds to therapy. Patients usually feel well and are ambulatory during this period. Presenting complaints may include symptoms related to massive splenomegaly caused by infiltration of white cells, left upper quadrant abdominal pain, early satiety, and abdominal fullness.

A very high WBC count can cause leukostatic lesion development in the microvasculature of the lungs or central nervous system. Leukostasis may lead to thromboembolic episodes and pulmonary or CNS bleeding. Presentation with an excessively high white count is a medical emergency, and the white count must be reduced rapidly with hydroxyurea and/or leukapheresis.

Diagnosis of CML is established by hematologic evaluation. The following results on a complete blood cell count are characteristic of CML:

- WBC $> 100,000/mm^3$
- Mature and immature granulocytes; segmented neutrophils predominate
- Myelocytes $>$ metamyelocytes
- Increased eosinophils
- Increased basophils
- Normal or increased platelets

A bone marrow evaluation is required to assess cellularity, detect fibrosis, and to obtain a specimen for cytogenetic analysis.

In addition to the presence of the Ph[1] chromosome in 95% of CML patients, the marrow is extremely hypercellular and may be devoid of fat. Myeloid elements are increased, and megakaryocytes may be excessive.[18] Cytogenetic studies to detect the Ph[1] chromosome may be performed on peripheral blood if the white cell count is sufficiently elevated.

Accelerated Stage

The term *accelerated stage* is generally used to refer to patients who have been under treatment for some time and have shown a variety of signs of disease progression but who do not meet the criteria for blastic disease.[66] Progression to accelerated phase is characteristic of all patients with CML. The time of progression to accelerated phase is variable and greatly impacts length of survival. The leukocyte doubling time (LDT) shortens to 20 days or less during this stage. The first evidence of accelerated stage may be failure to respond to drugs effective during the chronic stage.[17]

Physical examination reveals increased fatigue, increasing anemia, recurrence of splenomegaly, and thrombocytopenia; occasionally fever of unknown origin, lymphadenopathy, hepatomegaly, thrombocytosis, and basophilia are also noted. The patient may exhibit signs of hypermetabolism including night sweats, decreased appetite, and weight loss. Perios-

---

COMPARISON OF CLINICAL FEATURES IN CHRONIC PHASE CML AND ACCELERATED PHASE/BLASTIC TRANSFORMATION

Chronic phase	Accelerated phase/blastic transformation
Fatigue	Increased fatigue
Pallor	Increasing anemia
Dyspnea	Recurrence of splenomegaly
Anemia	Thrombocytopenia
Anorexia	Fever of unknown origin
Weight loss	Lymphadenopathy
Sternal tenderness	Hepatomegaly
Splenomegaly	Thrombocytosis/thrombocytopenia

---

teal infiltrates and lytic lesions may cause bony pain in addition to sternal pain.

Blood and bone marrow evaluation reveals increased promyelocytes and blasts. The onset of accelerated phase is difficult to distinguish, and the diagnosis may be made retrospectively. The box above differentiates the clinical features in chronic phase, accelerated phase, and blastic transformation.

Survival for patients in accelerated phase is difficult to describe because of disease heterogeneity but can be estimated at about a year.[73] Research efforts are in progress to identify early progression of the disease, before it enters the accelerated phase. Aggressive treatment at this point may offer the best chance to reestablish the chronic phase.

Blastic Phase

Patients with CML inevitably enter the blastic stage, an aggressive, rapidly terminal phase, which is refractory to treatment. The International CML Prognosis Study Group uses any one of the following criteria to define the blastic stage[53]:

- Blasts > 20% in peripheral blood or marrow
- Blasts plus promyelocytes > 30% in peripheral blood
- Blasts plus promyelocytes > 50% in marrow
- Extramedullary blastic infiltrates
- Leukemic tumor masses

Two thirds of patients have cells with predominantly myeloblastic characteristics; one third exhibit lymphoblastic features.[17] It is important to distinguish between myeloid or lymphoid transformation because lymphoid disease patients respond better to treatment (with vincristine and prednisone) and live longer. The presence of the enzyme deoxynucleotidyltranferase (Tdt) in blasts identifies the presence of lymphoblastic disease. The blastic stage resembles a disease similar to acute myelogenous leukemia or acute lymphocytic leukemia.

Median survival after blastic transformation is usually less than 6 months.[76] At least 85% of patients die during the blast phase with complications such as bleeding, infections, and cerebral or pulmonary hemorrhages.[79]

TREATMENT MODALITIES

Treatment of CML is usually initiated when the diagnosis is established. At this stage patients under the age of 50 should be considered for bone marrow transplant, the only curative treatment for this disease. When appropriate family donors are not available the National Marrow Donor registry may help find a nonrelated donor.

Chemotherapy

Busulfan is an oral alkylating agent. Its use is well documented in the treatment of chronic phase CML. This agent is active against the primitive hematopoietic stem cells and thus has a prolonged duration of myelosuppressive effect.

- Usual dose: 4 to 8 mg orally daily or in 2-week courses
- Dose decreased by one half as WBC decreases by one half
- CBC and dose adjustment monitored weekly
- Treatment is discontinued when WBC drops to <25,000/mm^3
- Patient is followed at monthly intervals during remission
- Treatment is reinstituted when WBC reaches 50,000/mm^3
- Long-term side effects: pulmonary fibrosis, dryness of mucous membranes, cataracts, irreversible gonadal failure in both sexes, prolonged marrow suppression, and second malignancies

Remissions are shorter with successive reinductions because the regrowth of the leukemic cell population is faster. Use of larger doses of busulfan given at 2- to 6-week intervals has been evaluated, but there is no evidence that it prolongs the duration of the chronic phase.[25]

Hydroxyurea (Hydrea) is a ribonucleotide reductase inhibitor of DNA synthesis discovered in 1960. Its activity against CML was reported in 1965. Hydrea is cytotoxic to cycling cells and acts partially by inhibiting ribonucleotide reductase.

- Usual dose: 1.0 to 3.0 orally daily in a single dose on an empty stomach.
- Dose decreased by one half as WBC decreases by one half
- Treatment is discontinued when WBC reaches 10,000 to 15,000/mm^3
- Provides rapid disease control, but shorter remissions
- Can be used after busulfan failure
- Survival equivalent to busulfan

- Does not produce prolonged marrow suppression or other long-term side effects
- Drug of choice for potential transplant candidates

While treatment during chronic phase with busulfan or hydroxyurea will improve marrow cellularity and decrease splenomegaly, it does not eliminate the Philadelphia chromosome. Thus, even though the disease is controlled by these agents for an average of 3 years, all patients will progress to accelerated and blastic phases.

Intensive combination chemotherapy has been developed with the goal of reducing or eradicating the Ph-positive clones to delay the onset of blast crisis and to prolong survival. Regimens appropriate for the treatment of acute myeloblastic leukemia have been evaluated in a number of small studies. The results showed conversion to a Ph[1]-negative state in up to 25% of patients. This conversion, along with the duration of normal hematopoiesis, was transient, however, and no cures were achieved.[44]

Intensive multidrug regimens are the treatment of choice for the blastic transformation phase of CML in patients who are not BMT candidates. These regimens include ara-C, programs with anthracyclines, amsacrine (m-AMSA), 6-thioguanine (6TG), and hydroxyurea. More recently high doses of ara-C (2 g/m^2) with anthracyclines and mitoxantrone have been studied. Overall response rates are low, ranging from 10% to 30%.[78] Patients with lymphoid blast crisis, however, have a 40% to 70% response rate with acute lymphocytic leukemia regimens based on vincristine and prednisone.[78]

Interferon

Interferon has been studied in the treatment of CML since 1981. Encouraging results have been observed in previously untreated CML patients.[1] Interferon is also capable of slowing the leukocyte doubling time and prolonging busulfan-induced remissions.[78] Findings suggest that alpha-2b interferon can partially suppress the expression of Ph[1]; however, a number of patients still progressed from chronic to blastic phase in spite of interferon.[5] (See Chapter 23 for a complete discussion of interferon and its side effects.)

Bone Marrow Transplantation

Bone marrow transplantation following high-dose chemotherapy and radiation is the only potentially curative treatment for CML.[62] Best results occur when the transplant is performed early in the chronic phase of the disease.[61] The 5-year survival for chronic phase patients is 60%, compared to 22% in accelerated phase, and 13% in blast phase.[81]

All patients less than 50 years old with identical twin or with HLA-matched siblings should be considered for bone marrow transplantation early in the chronic phase. Many BMT centers will now transplant patients with CML up to the age of 60.

It is not yet certain how many patients are cured by bone marrow transplantation, as many of the survivors have persistent Ph-positive cells in the marrow, and it is possible late relapses will occur.[81]

Future Treatments

The inevitably fatal outcome with conventional approaches in spite of the chronic nature of CML has stimulated an increased readiness to test unique treatment approaches in the chronic phase of the disease. Biologic response modifiers and growth factors including interleukins, tumor necrosis factor, and colony-stimulating factors are under investigation. They could ultimately be used in optimal combinations to control the disease and allow normal stem cell growth. Combinations of chemotherapy and biologic response modifiers have to be tested for the optimal treatment form. Because of the limitations of allogeneic marrow transplant in relation to patient age, donor compatibility, and graft-versus-host complications, alternative marrow ablative regimens with reinfusion of autologous peripheral or marrow stem cells are needed. Interferon may play a role in relapse therapy following bone marrow transplantation or as maintenance therapy to decrease or prevent CML relapse.[79]

Chronic Lymphocytic Leukemia

Chronic lymphocytic leukemia (CLL) is a malignant hematologic disorder characterized by proliferation and accumulation of relatively normal appearing lymphocytes. The majority of cases (95%) are B-cell lymphoproliferative disorders with a single clone of B-cell lymphocytes undergoing malignant transformation. The remaining 5% of cases are T-cell lymphoproliferative disorders.[17]

Technological developments in the areas of immunology, virology, cytochemistry, electron microscopy, and molecular genetics now allow a more precise diagnosis.

EPIDEMIOLOGY AND ETIOLOGY

The development of CLL is more a result of genetic predisposition than environmental influences. A familial tendency has been suggested, as well as concordance in several identical twins, but no pattern of inheritance has been reported.[20] There is a strong correlation between CLL and autoimmune diseases such as systemic lupus erythematosus, Sjögren's syndrome, and autoimmune hemolytic anemia.

CLL is the most common leukemia in the United States, accounting for 30% of all newly diagnosed leukemias. The median age of CLL patients is 60 years. The disease affects twice as many males as females.[17]

The clinical course and prognosis of B-cell CLL is quite variable and depends on the disease stage at the time of diagnosis. Patients with early stage disease may live 10 years or longer without treatment; patients with a more aggressive, advanced stage at diagnosis usually die within 2 years.[35]

CLINICAL FEATURES

Chronic lymphocytic leukemia is discovered on routine physical examination or routine laboratory work in the 25% of patients who are asymptomatic. Because CLL is a disease of immunoglobulin-secreting cells, recurrent skin and respiratory infections may be elicited from the patient history.

Nearly 50% of the bone marrow is infiltrated before peripheral blood counts are compromised. Progressive accumulation of the abnormal lymphocytes into nodal structures and the advancing marrow involvement yield symptoms of malaise, anorexia, fatigue, and lymphadenopathy in the patient with advanced disease. Gastrointestinal and genitourinary complaints are related to enlarging abdominal lymph nodes. Splenomegaly may cause abdominal discomfort or early satiety.

Physical examination findings may be negative or positive only for splenomegaly in the early stage patient. Advanced patients with anemia and thrombocytopenia display the typical findings of anemia and bruising or petechiae. Lymph node enlargement may be present on physical examination. Hepatomegaly may be present in addition to splenomegaly if there is portal obstruction related to abdominal adenopathy.

DIAGNOSIS AND STAGING

The diagnosis of CLL is suspected in the presence of unexplained lymphocytosis on the peripheral blood examination. Monoclonal antibodies directed at specific heavy and light chains of immunoglobulins or gene rearrangement studies define the clonal nature of the disease, thus establishing the diagnosis. A bone marrow or lymph node biopsy is rarely required to establish the diagnosis but, for patients on research studies, may provide valuable information about treatment response, cytogenetics, and molecular biology.

In the diagnostic evaluation of CLL, lymphocytosis is the most consistent finding. The peripheral WBC count may exceed 50,000/mm³ with greater than 90% mature lymphocytes.

The bone marrow is hypercellular with a diffuse infiltration of small and medium lymphocytes with mature morphologic features. Myeloid elements of the marrow have normal morphology and maturation.

Lymph node biopsy shows a histopathologic pattern of diffuse lymphoma with small, noncleaved lymphocytes. Immunologic studies and cytogenetics further define the disease process.

In 1975, Rai and others[69] proposed a clinical staging system based on lymphocytes, lymphadenopathy, splenomegaly, hepatomegaly, anemia, and thrombocytopenia.

RAI CLINICAL STAGING SYSTEM

Stage 0	Lymphocytosis only, in blood (>15,000/mm³) and bone marrow (>40%). Median survival = 12+ years.
Stage I	Lymphocytosis with lymphadenopathy. Median survival = 8+ years.
Stage II	Lymphocytosis + splenomegaly ± hepatomegaly. Median survival = 6 years.
Stage III	Lymphocytosis + anemia (Hbg <11 g%). Median survival = 1.5 years.
Stage IV	Lymphocytosis + thrombocytopenia (platelets <100,000/mm³). Survival = 1.5 years.

Other staging systems have widespread acceptance, but the Rai system is most commonly used.

TREATMENT MODALITIES
Indications for Treatment

One of the most difficult decisions in CLL is when to initiate treatment.[35] Most patients fall into the intermediate stages of disease and do reasonably well for several years without therapy, but they eventually require specific treatment.[34] Treatment does not prolong survival in early stage patients. Patients should be observed for 3 to 6 months, if possible, to assess the clinical aggressiveness of the disease.

Cheson defines indications for therapy as the following.[17]

- *Disease related symptoms:* fevers, sweats, weight loss, fatigue, or mechanical problems related to lymphadenopathy or organomegaly
- *Progressive cytopenias:* symptomatic anemias or progressive thrombocytopenia with transfusion requirements
- *Repeated infections:* systemic or disseminated bacterial, viral, or fungal infections requiring antibiotics or localized infections poorly responsive to conventional antibiotic therapy

Treatment is discouraged for stable Stage I and II patients because the chemotherapeutic agents all have serious side effects. Of important note is that a high WBC count alone is not an indication for treatment.

Single-Agent Chemotherapy

Chlorambucil, an alkylating agent, is the most commonly used and best tolerated treatment. It is given orally in 6-mg to 14-mg doses. The dose is reduced once the disease is controlled. Several months of treatment are required to obtain a complete response. A response rate of 60% is common with 10% to 20% complete remissions.[35] Studies also show comparable responses and decreased toxicity using a pulse program with a high drug dose administered once every 2 to 4 weeks.[54]

Cyclophosphamide is as effective as chlorambucil, and its non–cross-resistance makes it useful in treating patients unresponsive to chlorambucil.[34]

Prednisone has been used to control leukocytosis and to treat immune-mediated hemolytic anemia and thrombocytopenia. Patients with extensive disease are often treated with steroids before initiating chemotherapy.[35]

Fludarabine is a new drug that was approved by the FDA in 1992 for patients with refractory B-cell CLL.

Combination Chemotherapy

The precise role of combination chemotherapy in CLL is controversial.[35] A study of 96 patients with Stages III and IV disease compared prednisone alone to prednisone plus daily chlorambucil to prednisone plus monthly chlorambucil. Response rates for prednisone alone were 11%, 37% for daily chlorambucil and prednisone, and 47% for monthly chlorambucil and prednisone. Responders lived longer than nonresponders in each group, but there was not substantial difference in median survival among the groups.[47]

Combination chemotherapy with cyclophosphamide, vincristine, and prednisone (CVP) has been used in patients with advanced disease.[34] The addition of doxorubicin to this regimen (CHOP) resulted in a survival advantage.[37] This observation requires confirmation in a randomized trial, however, before it can be accepted as standard treatment.

Currently there is little evidence of a role for maintenance chemotherapy in CLL once a response has been obtained.[34]

Splenectomy

Splenectomy has no influence on survival in CLL but may be indicated for autoimmune anemia or thrombocytopenia refractory to systemic therapy, or persistent symptomatic splenomegaly in a patient responding to chemotherapy.[17]

Radiation Therapy

- A total of 300 to 800 cGy in 150-cGy fractions may benefit cases of hypersplenism, progressive splenomegaly, or lymphocytosis. Splenic radiation alone results in a partial remission rate of 70%, but the resulting neutropenia, thrombocytopenia, and short remission duration limit the utility of this treatment.[75]
- Nodal radiation may be employed to palliate

symptoms or relieve organ dysfunction caused by abdominal adenopathy, such as biliary tract or urinary tract obstruction.[35]
- Total body radiation is infrequently used because it is less effective at controlling disease than chlorambucil and induces more profound cytopenias.

Future Treatments

There is hope that biologic therapies such as gamma interferon and monoclonal antibodies, possibly linked to drugs, toxins, or isotopes, will prove useful in the treatment of CLL. New chemotherapy agents and new combinations of drugs, possibly including biologic therapies, may improve the treatment of this disease.

HAIRY-CELL LEUKEMIA

EPIDEMIOLOGY AND ETIOLOGY

Hairy cell leukemia (HCL) is a rare chronic lymphoproliferative disorder of unknown etiology.[77] There does not seem to be an association with ionizing radiation or other environmental factors. The disease is usually diagnosed in middle-aged patients and is quite rare, representing less than 2% of adult leukemia.[82]

CLINICAL FEATURES

Clinical manifestations of this disease are related to excessive infiltration of the bone marrow and/or spleen with "hairy cells." This results in underproduction or excessive peripheral sequestration of circulating cells manifested as granulocytopenia, anemia, or thrombocytopenia.[9] The presenting complaints in more than half of patients are constitutional symptoms of weakness, lethargy, or fatigue. Up to one fourth of patients are diagnosed incidentally when a routine complete blood cell count reveals abnormalities. Physical findings are limited to splenomegaly, which is seen in up to 90% of patients.[82]

DIAGNOSIS

The hallmark of HCL is the presence in the blood, bone marrow, and reticuloendothelial organs of the peculiar hairy cell. This cell is characterized morphologically by its hair-like projections. Cytochemical stains demonstrate the presence of tartrate-resistant acid phosphatase (TRAP). Patients are diagnosed based on the presence of cytopenias, hairy cells in the peripheral blood, splenomegaly, and bone marrow aspiration and biopsy. The bone marrow is frequently fibrotic and may not be aspirable.

CLASSIFICATION

There is generally no accepted staging system that is useful both for prognosis and therapy. For the purpose of treatment decisions, it is best to consider this disease in two broad categories: untreated and progressive.

TREATMENT

Hairy cell leukemia is a highly treatable and sometimes curable disease. Patients who are asymptomatic with acceptable blood counts can be observed until the disease progresses and requires treatment. Treatment is required when cytopenias become symptomatic, splenomgaly increases, or infectious complications exist.

The standard therapy for HCL was originally splenectomy. This procedure normalizes the peripheral blood in most patients, but there is virtually no change in the bone marrow and all patients have progressive disease in 12 to 18 months.[71]

Alpha-interferon in low, well-tolerated doses is effective in hairy cell leukemia.[41,56,71,72,77] The interferon is administered subcutaneously three times a week for 1 year and yields a 10% complete remission rate and an 80% overall response rate.[41] This treatment is not curative, however, and retreatment is necessary in most patients whose therapy is stopped.[74] Reinitiation of interferon therapy is capable of inducing second responses in at least some patients.[77]

Deoxycoformycin (dCF), also called Pentostatin, was first reported to have activity in HCL in 1984. This drug is given as a short infusion every other week for 3 to 6 months and produces a 57% complete response rate and an overall 83% response rate. Complete remissions are of substantial duration and some patients appear to be cured by this agent.[13,41] Currently, dCF is the treatment of choice for hairy cell leukemia.

A new agent available is Leustatin [2-chlorodeoxyadenosine (2-CdA)]. The drug is given IV daily for 1 week and produces a CR rate of 80% and an overall response rate of 95%.[29] Responses are durable and a fraction of patients appear to be cured with this short course of treatment.[71]

MYELODYSPLASTIC SYNDROMES
EPIDEMIOLOGY AND ETIOLOGY

The myelodysplastic syndromes (MDS) are a heterogeneous group of disorders previously referred to as oligoblastic leukemia, smoldering acute leukemia, or preleukemia.[15] The syndrome is classified into five distinct pathologic entities: (1) refractory anemia (RA), (2) refractory anemia with ringed sideroblasts (RARS), (3) chronic myelomonocytic leukemia (CMML), (4) refractory anemia with excess blasts (RAEB), and (5) refractory anemia with excess blasts in transition (RAEB-T). These disorders vary from relatively indolent hematologic disorders to conditions indistinguishable from acute leukemia.

Myelodysplasia is a disease of the elderly and most commonly affects people over 60 years of age and is rarely seen in people under the age of 30.

Although the etiology of MDS is unclear, its manifestations result from neoplastic transformation at the level of the pleuripotent stem cell.[11] Some studies have implicated exposure to benzene, radiation, chemotherapy, and alkylating agents in particular as initiating factors in the development of myelodysplasia.[58]

CLINICAL FEATURES

Patients with MDS usually present with severe cytopenias or pancytopenia.[22] Infections, particularly respiratory or gram-negative septicemias, are frequently the presenting symptom. Bleeding may be present as a result of either thrombocytopenia or poorly-functioning circulating platelets.[11]

DIAGNOSIS

The diagnosis is established by bone marrow aspiration and biopsy. Particular morphologic changes can be seen in both the marrow and peripheral blood. Chromosomal studies are also performed as approximately half of all MDS patients display karyotypic abnormalities.[22]

CLASSIFICATION

The FAB classification system developed in 1982 is used to classify the myelodysplastic syndromes into the five groups previously listed.

TREATMENT

Patients with only refractory anemia may have an indolent disease course and can be supported by transfusion therapy for many years. The patients with the excess blasts conditions (RAEB, RAEB-T, CMML) may be candidates for differentiating agents. The induction of differentiation can transform nonfunctional immature blasts and promyeloblasts into functional mature granulocytes.[11] Various agents have been studied including retinoic acids, low dose cytarabine, tretinoin, alpha interferon, and hexamethamelamine bisacetamide. So far, none of these agents have achieved a measure of success large enough to consider differentiating agents to be standard therapy for MDS.

Chemotherapy for the myelodysplastic syndromes has ranged from single agent to low doses of multi-agent regimens, to conventional antileukemia programs. Many patients die during treatment with complications related to marrow hypoplasia and a significant number show clinical drug resistence.[15] Allogeneic bone marrow transplantation is the only curative approach currently available, but unfortunately this disease most commonly occurs in people too old for transplantation.

Hematologic growth factors are currently being studied in this disease, but since the growth factors can stimulate proliferation of leukemic blasts in vitro, there is concern that the factors may accelerate development of acute leukemia rather than selectively induce cellular differentiation.[15] Multipotent hema-

topoietins such as I1-3 and I1-1 may have applications to MDS and are currently under investigation. Future clinical trials should incorporate recombinant growth factors with agents that preferentially suppress the malignant clone and thereby halt progression of the neoplastic clone.[58]

Text continued on p. 298.

Nursing Management

The medical and nursing management of lymphocytic and nonlymphocytic patients is similar and is detailed here.

Supportive care of the leukemic patient is a major contributor to increased survival and improved quality of life. The talents and resources of all members of the interdisciplinary team are required to support the patient and family through the phases of this disease process. The nurse, relying on a strong knowledge of the disease and the potential complications, uses systematic assessments to monitor physiologic homeostasis. For the person experiencing leukemia, medical and nursing support is required in three areas: (1) to prevent or correct expected side effects of the disease and treatment, (2) to anticipate and treat unexpected or potential complications, and (3) to facilitate psychosocial adaptation of the patient and family.[51]

NURSING DIAGNOSIS

- Knowledge deficit related to new leukemia diagnosis, disease process, treatment plan, and side effects.

INTERVENTIONS

- Review disease process, treatment regimen, and goals of treatment.
- Assess patient's preferred style of learning; identify any existing barriers to learning; teach in short sessions; involve family members and significant others in teaching sessions; question patient to evaluate understanding of new information; continue to reinforce information.
- Participate in informed consent process if patient is eligible for a clinical trial (see Chapter 25).
- Assess and discuss patient's desired level of information. Explain common terminology.
- Orient patient and family to hospital unit and services (e.g., parking, accommodations, meals).
- Explain role of multidisciplinary team members and how to access their services.
- Provide information about insertion of venous access devices and promote self-care of line following insertion.
- Explain purpose of baseline testing.
- Provide a calendar of planned treatments and tests (see Figure 14-2).

NURSING DIAGNOSIS

- Anxiety related to new diagnosis, uncertain outcome of potentially fatal disease, loss of control in hospital environment, alteration in body image, alteration in interpersonal relationships.

INTERVENTIONS

- Perform psychosocial assessment of patient, family; identify strengths, weaknesses, coping skills.
- Recognize increased anxiety levels that may occur while awaiting an official diagnosis, before painful or frightening procedures, before major treatments, upon learning of relapse, and on anniversery dates.[55]
- Administer antianxiety medications as ordered, assess effectiveness.
- Use guided imagery, relaxation training, and cognitive distraction to alleviate anxiety before painful or stressful procedures.[55]
- Assist patient and family to set realistic goals concerning level of activity, work schedule, and self-care activities.[55]
- Encourage patient/family to verbalize questions, fears, concerns.
- Involve chaplaincy services, social workers, support volunteers as needed.
- Inform patient/family of available community resources: Leukemia Society of America and American Cancer Society.

PREINDUCTION PHASE

The nurse caring for the patient with leukemia must have a thorough knowledge of the medical management of treatment-related toxicities and potential disease complications to provide effective nursing care.

The following assessments and medical interventions are performed before initiating antileukemia therapy. The nurse must incorporate the rationale for these studies into the patient teaching plan to help orient the patient and family to the plan of care.

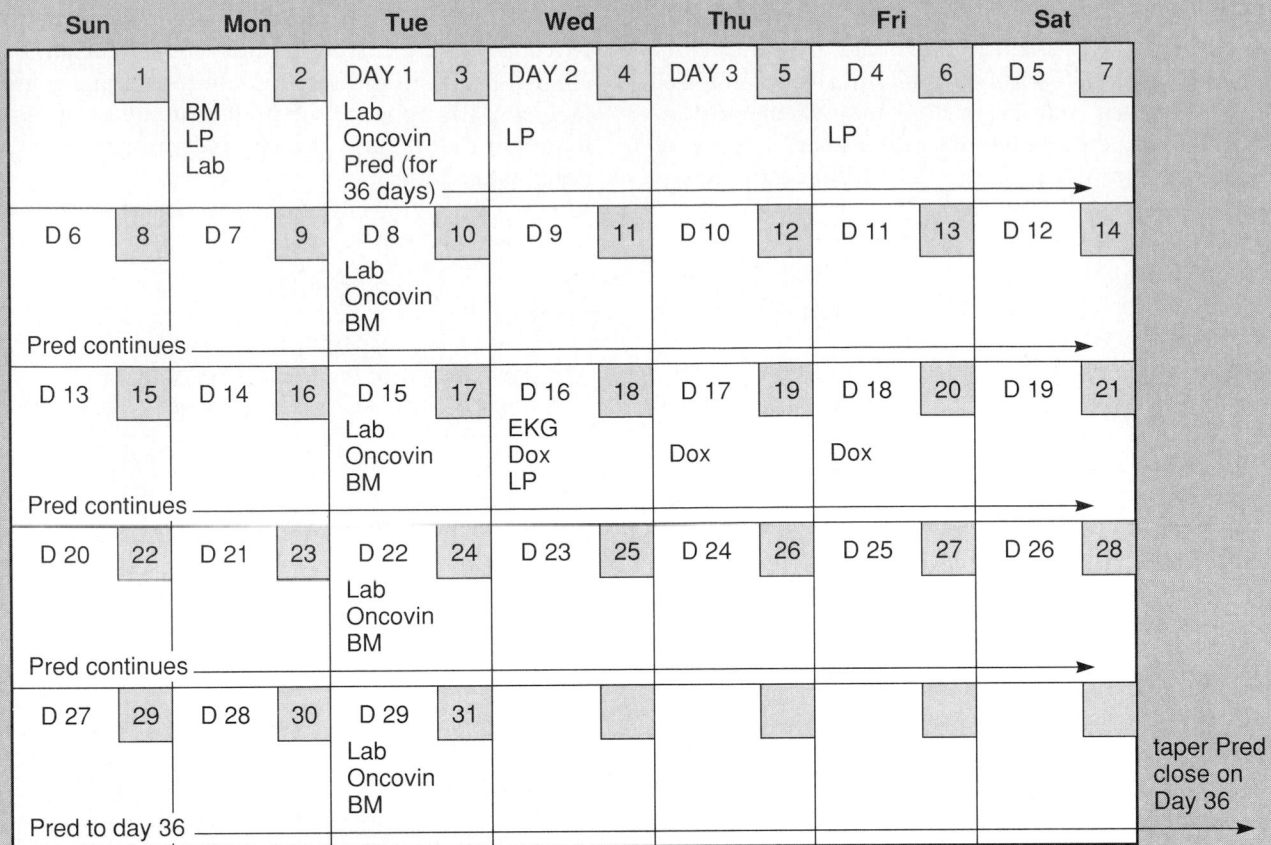

Sun		Mon		Tue		Wed		Thu		Fri		Sat	
	1		2	DAY 1	3	DAY 2	4	DAY 3	5	D 4	6	D 5	7
		BM LP Lab		Lab Oncovin Pred (for 36 days) —————→		LP				LP			
D 6	8	D 7	9	D 8	10	D 9	11	D 10	12	D 11	13	D 12	14
				Lab Oncovin BM									
Pred continues ——————————————————————→													
D 13	15	D 14	16	D 15	17	D 16	18	D 17	19	D 18	20	D 19	21
				Lab Oncovin BM		EKG Dox LP		Dox		Dox			
Pred continues ——————————————————————→													
D 20	22	D 21	23	D 22	24	D 23	25	D 24	26	D 25	27	D 26	28
				Lab Oncovin BM									
Pred continues ——————————————————————→													
D 27	29	D 28	30	D 29	31								
				Lab Oncovin BM								taper Pred close on Day 36	
Pred to day 36 ——————————————————————→													

D = day of treament
BM = bone marrow biopsy
LP = lumbar puncture or spinal tap
Lab = blood counts and/or blood chemistries
Pred = prednisone
Dox = Doxorubicin

Figure 14–2 Example of a patient teaching calendar outlining a common induction regimen for acute lymphocytic leukemia.

- Assessment of serum chemistries
  Renal function: an elevated creatinine may limit the use of aminoglycoside antibiotics.
  Hepatic function: doses of anthracyclines or vincristine may require reduction for elevated liver enzymes.
  Electrolytes: normal electrolytes may minimize the risk of certain drug side effects.
- Blood typing should be performed to ensure the availability of red cell and platelet transfusions.
- HLA typing should be performed on admission for patients who are possible transplantation candidates.
- A baseline coagulation profile should be performed on patients with acute promyelocytic leukemia. These patients have an increased incidence of disseminated intravascular coagulation (DIC). (Chapter 19 discusses DIC in detail). Patients with DIC may require heparinization or fresh-frozen plasma and platelet support before treatment initiation.
- A baseline chest film eliminates later confusion and assesses presence of possible pulmonary complications prior to treatment.
- Radionucleotide ventriculogram ensuring an adequate left ventricular ejection fraction before treatment requiring anthracyclines is important in patients with a questionable cardiac history.
- It is important to establish central venous access, preferably with a multiple-lumen catheter before treatment. If the patient is thrombocytopenic at diagnosis, platelet transfusion may be required before the invasive procedure to reduce the risk of bleeding. The catheter site must be monitored closely for postoperative bleeding.
- The decision to delay chemotherapy initiation to resolve an infection is determined by the status of

leukemia, severity of infection, and the number of circulating granulocytes.

- Acute tumor lysis syndrome occurs more commonly in L_2 and L_3 ALL. Patients at risk should receive high doses of allopurinol before treatment and urinary alkalinization with sodium bicarbonate added to intravenous solutions.
- Although uncommon, uric acid deposits in the urinary tract may occur in patients with very high white blood cell counts. Again, allopurinol, 300 mg orally daily, should be instituted before starting treatment.

By monitoring the results of these studies, the nurse can assess potential patient complications. For example, an abnormal coagulation profile in a patient with acute promyelocytic (M_3) leukemia should signal the nurse to incorporate bleeding precautions and assessment for shocklike symptoms into the patient care and teaching plan.

CHEMOTHERAPY SIDE EFFECTS

Regardless of the chemotherapy regimen chosen, infection and bleeding are the most common side effects of acute leukemia therapy. Induction chemotherapy not only kills the malignant clone of leukemia cells in the marrow but suppresses the production of normal hematologic elements. Thus, as the platelets, white cells, and, to a lesser extent, red cells in the peripheral blood die, there are no new cells to replace them. The patient is severely immunocompromised until the normal marrow components begin to regenerate.

One of the most important considerations in the care of the leukopenic patient is the lack of the normal host responses to infection. (Chapter 29 discusses the care of the immunosuppressed patient.) An increased temperature may be the only indication of an infectious process. Astute nursing assessment is required to monitor potential sites of infection and provide appropriate interventions. The primary nurse, caring for the leukemic patient on a daily basis, is also in the best position to detect subtle changes that may be the earliest indicators of impending septic shock.

With the availability of platelet transfusion support, hemorrhage is less of a problem than in past years. Prophylactic transfusions are usually administered in asymptomatic patients when the platelet count is below 10,000 to 20,000/mm³. Platelet counts should be checked 1 hour after transfusion to assess the increment of platelet increase. This also enables evaluation of possible alloimmunization and the need for a different platelet product.

Transfusion of packed red cells may be required to control anemia. Patients are usually transfused when their hemoglobin falls below 7 to 8 g/dl because hemorrhage is more likely to occur in the severely anemic patient.

NURSING DIAGNOSIS

- Infection, potential for, related to alteration in immune function secondary to leukemia and immunosuppressive chemotherapy.

INTERVENTIONS

- Teach patient/family the purpose and importance of neutropenic precautions.
- If appropriate, encourage patient to keep a chart of daily blood counts.
- Monitor temperature and vital signs every shift. Assess for changes in blood pressure, urine output, mental status that may be early signs of septic shock.
- Avoid fresh fruits and vegetables.
- No fresh flowers in patient's room.
- No rectal manipulation.
- Consistent handwashing by all people entering patient's room.
- Limit number of visitors to two at a time. No visitors with colds, influenza, herpes, or recent vaccinations.
- Avoid trauma to skin and mucous membranes.

NURSING DIAGNOSIS

- Injury, potential for bleeding related to alteration in clotting factors, thrombocytopenia secondary to leukemia and/or treatment.

INTERVENTIONS

- Teach patient/family the significance of platelet function, bleeding precautions.
- Check platelet count at least every other day during immunosuppressive leukemia therapies.
- Monitor results of coagulation studies; assess for signs and symptoms of disseminated intravascular coagulation.
- Assess for petechiae, bruising, epistaxis, hematuria, hematochezia, oral, rectal, or vaginal bleeding.
- Monitor platelet transfusions.
- Apply pressure on bone marrow or venipuncture sites for 3 to 5 minutes.
- No intramuscular or subcutaneous injections or rectal manipulation
- Use Water-pik® on lowest setting or toothettes for oral care.
- No aspirin-containing medications.
- Ensure safe environment: no sharp objects, bed rails up, ambulate with assistance.
- Prevent trauma to skin and mucous membranes.

NURSING DIAGNOSIS

- Alteration in nutrition: less than body requirements, related to treatment induced nausea, vomiting, stomatitis, anorexia.

INTERVENTIONS

- Monitor weights.
- Record intake and output every shift.
- Record calorie counts.
- Administer antiemetics for nausea and assess effectiveness.
- Assess for diarrhea and medicate as needed.
- Daily assessment of lips and oral mucosa.
- Teach patient the purpose of oral care protocol and evaluate technique.
- Evaluate and document compliance to oral care protocol.
- Use topical analgesics in mouth and on lips if open ulcers are present.
- Encourage small, frequent meals with high calorie, high protein foods.

DISEASE-RELATED COMPLICATIONS
Leukostasis

Patients with exceptionally high circulating blast counts are at risk to develop leukostasis. This syndrome is caused by leukemic blasts aggregating and invading capillary walls, causing rupture and bleeding. This occurs most commonly in the brain because of its vascularity and limited space. Intrapulmonary bleeding can also result from this "sludging syndrome." These complications are associated with significant morbidity and mortality, and this medical emergency necessitates immediate reduction of the circulating leukocytes. High doses of hydroxyurea or high-dose chemotherapy may be instituted, or leukapheresis with a filtered continuous flow cell separator may help reduce the cell burden. Once the danger of leukostasis is eliminated, definitive antileukemia therapy is initiated.

INTERVENTIONS

- Monitor for changes in level of consciousness; perform neurologic examinations as ordered.
- Monitor respiratory status.
- Administer high-dose chemotherapy as ordered.
- Monitor leukapheresis process.
- Monitor absolute blast counts after interventions.

$$\text{Absolute blast count} = \frac{\text{Total WBC} \times \text{blasts}}{100}$$

Disseminated Intravascular Coagulation

Diffuse or disseminated intravascular coagulation is a complex syndrome characterized by the activation of coagulation and formation of fibrin within the general circulation (see Chapter 19). Patients with promyelocytic leukemia (M_3) are at high risk of developing DIC after the initiation of chemotherapy as the granules from the promyelocytes are released and initiate the coagulation cascade.

INTERVENTIONS

- Ensure systematic assessment for occult, overt, or sudden massive bleeding.
- Initiate antileukemia therapy to correct the underlying disease pathology.
- Administer antibiotics for sepsis.
- Administer blood products (platelets, fresh-frozen plasma) as ordered.
- Apply pressure to venipuncture sites.
- Administer heparin if ordered.

Treatment for DIC must focus on eliminating the underlying cause and supportive therapy with the appropriate blood products.

Typhlitis

Typhlitis, or inflammation of the cecum, is thought to be related to *Clostridia* sepsis or other bacteria including *Pseudomonas*, *Escherichia coli*, or *Klebsiella*. This diagnosis should be considered in the neutropenic patient who develops severe abdominal pain. Bloody diarrhea, absence of bowel sounds, rebound tenderness, and fever may accompany the pain. An abdominal x-ray may reveal a right lower quadrant soft-tissue mass, dilated colon, or pericecal edema. The pathologic diagnosis is established by stool culture, and the identified pathogen is treated with appropriate antibiotics.

INTERVENTIONS

- Put patient on bedrest.
- Maintain intravenous fluids.
- Assess fluid and electrolyte balance.
- Ensure patient has no oral intake.
- Administer and evaluate analgesics.

Renal Failure

Renal failure in leukemia patients may result from urate nephropathy, aminoglycoside toxicity, sepsis, or leukemic infiltration of the kidneys.

INTERVENTIONS

- Monitor BUN and creatinine values.
- Record accurate intake and output.
- Monitor vital signs, mental status.
- Assess for signs of alteration in tissue perfusion.

PATIENT AND FAMILY TEACHING

As with other types of cancer care, the teaching of leukemic patients should begin at the time of diagnosis and continue throughout the disease course. In acute leukemia, teaching is required in both the inpatient setting during the induction phase and intensive supportive care period and in the outpatient setting during continuation therapy and long-term follow-up.

A leukemia diagnosis may be a shock to patients experiencing few if any symptoms at the time of di-

Table 14–4   Patient/Family Teaching Topics

Topic	Pretreatment Phase	Treatment Phase	Outpatient/Follow-up Care
DISEASE DESCRIPTION	X	X	
Disease-related symptoms	X	X	
Potential disease-related complications	X	X	
TREATMENT DESCRIPTION	X	X	
Goals of treatment	X	X	
Duration of treatment	X	X	
Treatment schedule	X	X	
Chemotherapeutic agents	X	X	
TREATMENT-RELATED SIDE EFFECTS	X	X	
Immunosuppression	X	X	
Thrombocytopenia	X	X	
Nausea and vomiting	X	X	
Stomatitis	X	X	
Alopecia	X	X	
Fatigue	X	X	
Anorexia	X	X	
MULTIPLE-LUMEN TUNNELED CATHETER	X	X	
Surgical procedure	X	X	
Catheter care	X	X	
SUPPORTIVE CARE		X	
Infection precautions		X	
Bleeding precautions		X	
Red cell transfusions		X	
Platelet transfusions		X	
Antibiotics		X	
DISEASE-RELATED COMPLICATIONS AND TREATMENT		X	
Sepsis		X	
DIC		X	
Tumor lysis syndrome		X	
SELF-CARE		X	
Oral care		X	
Nutrition		X	
Care of tunneled catheter		X	
DETERMINATION OF RESPONSE		X	
Meaning of remission		X	
Continuation therapy		X	
Possible preparation for discharge		X	
PSYCHOSOCIAL ADJUSTMENT	X	X	X
Coping strategies	X	X	X
Referral to social services, psychologist/psychiatrist	X	X	X
Identification of community resources (family support groups, Leukemia Society of America, American Cancer Society)	X	X	X
Schedule for lab work			X
Schedule for office visits			X
Outpatient medications			X
Diet			X
Exercise			X
Return to work			X
Sexuality			X
Long-term side effects of treatment			X
Surveillance bone marrow biopsies			X

agnosis. Some patients experiencing an acute illness or a lengthy period of medical evaluation before the discovery of the diagnosis may feel a sense of relief to know finally a definitive diagnosis. Certainly the diagnosis of any potentially fatal disease is a time of crisis for the entire family.

Teaching topics in the pretreatment period, treatment period, and follow-up period are listed in Table 14-4. See also the boxes on this page.

To provide effective care, the nurse must always be sensitive to the patient's feelings of isolation and loss of control. The patient may display the need to regain control especially during lengthy hospitalizations. Addressing this need for control early in the hospitalization is important. Control issues can be divided into three areas as follows:

PATIENT CONTROLLED	NO CONTROL
Antibiotic skin care regimen	Disease process
Choosing the time to bathe	Administration of blood
Time for dressing change	products
Performing oral care	X-rays
Dietary choices	Laboratory work
Analgesia	
Visiting times	

NURSE CONTROLLED	
Scheduled medications	Weights
Vital signs	Meal times

The main point to remember is that many things in nursing care can be flexible, and items such as when the patient will bathe can be negotiated.

GERIATRIC CONSIDERATIONS

- Cardiovascular evaluation including radionucleotide ventriculogram to assess left ventricular ejection fraction.
- Modify doses of daunorubicin and high-dose cytosine arabinoside for patients over 60 years old.
- Monitor for signs and symptoms of fluid overload.
- Maintain a safe environment: bed rails, call light within reach, assistance with ambulation.
- Assess potential barriers to learning: decreased visual acuity, poor hearing, decreased concentration.

PATIENT TEACHING PRIORITIES

- Normal hematopoiesis, purpose of red blood cells, white blood cells, and platelets.
- Pathophysiology of leukemia.
- Goals of planned treatment.
- Treatment schedule and method of administration.
- Expected side effects and related interventions.
- Plan for symptom management.
- Neutropenia and bleeding precautions.
- Plan for patient/family participation in treatment and shared decision-making.

CONCLUSION

Great progress has been made in the knowledge of the biologic nature and treatment of leukemia in the past decade. Advances in supportive care of the immunosuppressed patient have dramatically improved survival in leukemia patients. Much research is still required to define more effective therapies to increase disease-free survival and decrease relapse rates.

The challenges and opportunities for nurses are numerous in the field of leukemia. The patient care acuity for those with leukemia depends on the disease variables and practice setting. Hospital-based nurses provide care for the leukemic patient who is acutely ill. The intensity and complexity of the nursing care required for many of these patients rival those of intensive care units. Other patients with leukemia, such as in chronic phase CML, early CLL, AML, or ALL in remission or on milder continuation therapy are seen in the clinic or outpatient setting.

Another practice setting is the bone marrow transplantation unit where intensive acute care as well as ambulatory care are required. Historically, the majority of leukemia patients were transferred to major metropolitan centers for treatment. However, in recent years with improved mechanisms to transfer medical technology into the community, more patients are being cared for locally.

The National Cancer Institute's Cooperative Group Outreach Program (CGOP) and, since 1983, the Community Clinical Oncology Program (CCOP) provide the capability to enroll leukemia patients in cooperative group clinical trials. The number of institutions performing bone marrow transplantation has also increased dramatically and will continue to increase over the next decades as BMT becomes a promising treatment option for many types of cancer.

The nurse in clinical practice may easily feel overwhelmed by the complexity and intensity of both learning about the disease of leukemia and providing care to the patient with leukemia. A useful strategy for learning this information and integrating it into one's nursing practice is to focus on one type of leukemia at a time. The nurse should select a patient newly diagnosed with leukemia, review the individual patient's presenting symptoms, results of the diagnostic evaluation, prognostic indicators, and treatment plan. The nurse should monitor this treatment plan, the selected drug regimen, blood counts, marrow results, and the potential side effects experienced by the patient as a result of the disease or treatment. These concepts should be incorporated into an individualized nursing plan of care. Depending on the practice setting, the nurse may wish to collaborate with another inpatient or outpatient nursing colleague to follow the progress of the patient. After completing this exercise a few times, the nurse will gain confidence in the knowledge of the leukemias and their treatment and thereby improve clinical practice expertise in caring for patients with leukemia.

The intensity and complexity of caring for leukemic patients are both rewarding and frustrating. Providing direct care to an acutely ill patient in a life-threatening situation fosters very close relationships with both the patient and the members of their support system. These relationships can be intensely rewarding. At the same time, the intensity of care can lead to frustration and exhaustion when the patient does not respond to therapy or dies. Sudden and unexpected medical crisis and death are not uncommon in this population of patients. Nurses caring for patients with leukemia must be cognizant of their own feelings and needs. The most valuable support system oncology nurses have is the support and understanding of their peers. These are the people who experience the same joys, fears, pain, and frustration of caring for the acutely ill patient. The oncology unit psychologist or psychiatrist is not only available to the patient and family, but also to the nursing staff. The most important self-care aspect of the nurse caring for the patient with leukemia is recognizing the level of investment and acknowledging the emotional peaks and valleys that accompany this investment.

BIBLIOGRAPHY

1. Alimena G and others: Treatment of Ph¹-positive chronic myelogenous leukemia (CML) with recombinant interferon alpha-2b (Intron A), Cancer Treat Rev 15(suppl A):21, 1988.
2. Alkire K and Collingwood J: Physiology of blood and bone marrow, Semin Oncol Nurs 6:99, 1990.
3. American Cancer Society: Facts and figures 1993, Atlanta, 1993, American Cancer Society.
4. Bennett JM and others: Proposals for the classification of the acute leukemias, Br J Haematol 33:451, 1976.
5. Bergsagel DE: Interferon alfa-2b in the manage-
ment of chronic granulocytic leukemia, Cancer Treat Rev 15(suppl A):15, 1988.
6. Bergsagel DE, Bailey MB, and Langley GR: The chemotherapy of plasma-cell myeloma and the incidence of acute leukemia, N Engl J Med 301:743, 1979.
7. Berman E and others: Results of a randomized trial comparing idarubicin and cytosine arabinoside with daunorubicin and cytosine arabinoside in adult patients with newly diagnosed acute myelogenous leukemia, Blood 77:1666, 1991.
8. Bishop JF and others: Etoposide in acute nonlymphocytic leukemia, Blood 75:27, 1990.
9. Bouroncle BA: Leukemic reticuloendotheliosis, Blood 53:412, 1979.
10. Buchner T and others: Intensified induction and consolidation with or without maintenance chemotherapy for AML: two multicenter studies of the German AML Cooperative Group, J Clin Oncol 3:1583, 1985.
11. Cain J and others: Myelodysplastic syndromes: a review for nurses, Oncol Nurs Forum 18(1):113, 1991.
12. Cassileth PA and others: Maintenance chemotherapy protocols remission duration in adult acute nonlymphocytic leukemia, J Clin Oncol 6:583, 1988.
13. Cassileth PA and others: Pentostatin induces durable remissions in HCL, J Clin Oncol 9:243, 1991.
14. Champlain R and others: Postremission chemotherapy for adults with acute myelogenous leukemia: improved survival with high-dose cytarabine and daunorubicin consolidation treatment, J Clin Oncol 8:1199, 1990.
15. Cheson BD: The myelodysplastic syndromes: current approaches to therapy, Ann Intern Med 112:932, 1990.
16. Cheson BD: The acute leukemias. In Wittes RE, editor: Manual of oncology therapeutics, Philadelphia, 1989/1990, JB Lippincott Co.
17. Cheson BD: Chronic leukemias. In Wittes RE, editor: Manual of oncology therapeutics, Philadelphia, 1989/1990, JB Lippincott Co.
18. Clarkson B and others: Acute lymphoblastic leukemia in adults, Semin Oncol 12:160, 1985.
19. Clarkson B: The chronic leukemias. In Wyngaarden JB and Smith LJ, editors: Cecil textbook of medicine, ed 18, Philadelphia, 1988, WB Saunders.
20. Conley CL, Misiti J, and Laster AJ: Genetic factors predisposing to chronic lymphocytic leukemia and to autoimmune disease, Medicine 5:323, 1980.
21. Conrad KJ: Cerebellar toxicities associated with cytosine arabinoside: a nursing perspective. Oncol Nurs Forum 3:57, 1986.

22. Dang CV: Myelodysplastic syndrome, JAMA 267(15):2077, 1992.

23. DeGramont A and others: Preleukemic changes in cases of non-lymphocytic leukemia secondary to cytotoxic therapy: analysis of 105 cases, Cancer 58:630, 1986.

24. DiJulio J: Hematopoiesis: An overview, Oncol Nurs Forum 18(suppl):3, 1991.

25. Douglas IDC and Wiltshaw E: Remission induction in chronic granulocytic leukemia using intermittent high dose busulfan, Br J Haematol 40:59, 1978.

26. Dutcher JP, Schiffer CA, and Wiernik PH: Hyperleukocytosis in adult nonlymphocytic leukemia: impact on remission rate, duration, and survival, J Clin Oncol 5:1364, 1987.

27. Dutcher JP and others: Intensive maintenance therapy improves survival in adult nonlymphocytic leukemia: An eight-year follow-up, Leukemia 2:413, 1988.

28. Einhorn N: Acute leukemia after chemotherapy (Melphalan), Cancer 41:444, 1978.

29. Estey EH and others: Treatment of hairy cell leukemia with 2-chlorodeoxyadenosine (2-CdA), Blood 79:882, 1992.

30. Fenaux P and others: Cytogenetics and their prognostic value in childhood and adult acute leukemia, Hematol-Oncol 7:307, 1989.

31. Fialkow PJ and Singer JW: Chronic leukemias. In DeVita VT, Hellman S, and Rosenberg SA, editors: Cancer: principles and practice of oncology, New York, 1989, JB Lippincott Co.

32. Fialkow PJ and others: Evidence for a multistep pathogenesis of chronic myelogenous leukemia, Blood 58:158, 1981.

33. Foon FA and Todd RF: Immunologic classification of leukemia and lymphoma, Blood 68:1, 1986.

34. Foon KA and Gale RP: Biology of chronic lymphocytic leukemia, Semin Hematol 24(4):209, 1987.

35. Foon KA and Gale RP: Staging and therapy of chronic lymphocytic leukemia, Semin Hematol 24(4):264, 1987.

36. Fraser MC and Tucker MA: Second malignancies following cancer therapy, Semin Oncol Nurs 5:43, 1989.

37. French Cooperative Group on Chronic Lymphocytic Leukemia: Effectiveness of "CHOP" regimen in advanced untreated chronic lymphocytic leukemia, Lancet 1:1346, 1986.

38. Gale RP and Foon KA: Acute myelogenous leukemia. In Gale RP, editor: Acute leukemia, Boston, 1986, Blackwell Scientific Publications.

39. Gale RP and Foon KA: Therapy of acute myelogenous leukemia, Semin Hematol 24(1):40, 1987.

40. Giona F and others: Adult acute lymphoblastic leukemia: description and analysis of long-term survivors. A retrospective study, Haematologica 74:475, 1989.

41. Golomb HM and Ellis E: Treatment options for hairy cell leukemia, Semin Oncol 18(suppl 7):1991.

42. Goodman M: Managing the side effects of chemotherapy. Semin Oncol Nurs 5(suppl):29, 1989.

43. Green MH and others: Evidence of a treatment dose response in non-lymphocytic leukemia which occur after therapy of non-Hodgkin's lymphoma, Cancer Res 43:1891, 1983.

44. Griffin JD: Management of chronic myelogenous leukemia, Semin Hematol 23(suppl):20, 1986.

45. Gulati GL, Ashton JK, and Hyun BH: Structure and function of the bone marrow and hematopoiesis, Hematol Oncol Clin North Am 2(4):495, 1988.

46. Gunz FW: Leukemia in the pase. In Gunz FW, editor: Leukemia, Orlando, FL, 1983, Grune & Stratton.

47. Han T and others: Chlorambucil vs. combined chlorambucil-corticosteroid therapy in chronic lymphocytic leukemia, Cancer 31:502, 1973.

48. Heath CW: Epidemiology and heredity aspects of acute leukemia. In Wiernik P, editor: Neoplastic diseases of the blood, New York, 1985, Churchill Livingstone.

49. Hoezler D and Gale RP: Acute lymphoblastic leukemia in adults: recent progress, future directions, Semin Hematol 24(1):27, 1987.

50. Jacobs AD and Gale RP: Acute lymphoblastic leukemia in adults. In Gale RP, editor: Acute leukemia, Boston, 1986, Blackwell Scientific Publications.

51. Johnson BL: Leukemias. In Groenwald SL, editor: Cancer nursing: practice and principles, Boston, 1987, Jones & Bartlett Publishers, Inc.

52. Kantarjian HM, Schachner J, and Keating MJ: Fludarabine therapy in hairy cell leukemia, Cancer 67:1291, 1991.

53. Karanas A and Silver RT: Characteristics of the terminal phase of chronic granulocytic leukemia, Blood 32:445, 1968.

54. Knospe WH, Loeb V Jr, and Huguley CM Jr: Biweekly chlorambucil treatment of chronic lymphocytic leukemia, Cancer 33:555, 1974.

55. Levenson JA and Lesko LM: Psychiatric aspects of adult leukemia, Semin Oncol Nurs 6:76, 1990.

56. Lill MC and Golde DW: Treatment of hairy cell leukemia, Blood-Rev 4:238, 1990.

57. Linos A and others: Low-dose radiation and leukemia, N Engl J Med 202:1101, 1980.

58. List AF and others: The myelodysplastic syndromes: biology and implications for management. J Clin Oncol S: 1424, 1990.

59. MacDonald JS and others: Subacute and chronic toxicities associated with nitrosurea therapy. In Prestayko AW and others, editors: Nitrosureas: current status and new developments, New York, 1981, Academic Press.

60. Maguire-Eisen M: Diagnosis and treatment of adult acute leukemia, Semin Oncol Nurs 6:17, 1990.

61. Martin PJ and others: HLA-identical marrow transplantation during accelerated-phase chronic myelogenous leukemia: analysis of survival and remission duration, Blood 72(6):1978, 1988.

62. McGlave P and others: Therapy of chronic myelogenous leukemia with allogeneic bone marrow transplantation, J Clin Oncol 5:1033, 1987.

63. Nowell PC and Hungerford DA: A minute chromosome in human granulocytic leukemia, Science 132:1497, 1960.

64. Papa G and others: Acute leukemia in patients treated for Hodgkin's disease, Br J Haematol 309:1079, 1984.

65. Pape LH: Therapy-related acute leukemia, Cancer Nurs 11(5):295, 1988.

66. Parkman R: Current status of bone marrow transplantation in pediatric oncology, CA 58:569, 1986.

67. Portugal MA and others: Acute leukemia as a complication of advanced breast cancer, Cancer Treat Rep 63:177, 1979.

68. Preisler H and others: Comparison of three remission induction regimens and two postinduction strategies for the treatment of acute nonlymphocytic leukemia: a Cancer and Leukemia Group B study, Blood 69:1441, 1987.

69. Rai KR and Montserrat E: Prognostic factors in chronic lymphocytic leukemia. Semin Hematol 24(4):252, 1987.

70. Rinsky RA and others: Benzene and leukemia, N Engl J Med 316:1044, 1987.

71. Saven A and Piro LD: Treatment of hairy cell leukemia, Blood 79:1111, 1992.

72. Schiffer CA: Interferon studies in the treatment of patients with leukemia, Semin Oncol 18(suppl 7):1, 1991.

73. Silver RT: Chronic myeloid leukemia: a perspective of the clinical and biologic issues of the chronic phase, Hematol Oncol Clin N Am 4:319, 1990.

74. Smith JW and others: Prolonged continuous treatment of hairy cell leukemia patients with recombinant interferon-alpha 2a, Blood 78:1664, 1991.

75. Smith RE: Leukemia. In Thorup OA, editor: Fundamentals of clinical hematology, Philadelphia, 1987, WB Saunders Co.

76. Sokal JE and others: Staging and prognosis in chronic myelogenous leukemia, Semin Hematol 25(1):49, 1988.

77. Steis RG and Longo DL: Update on the treatment of hairy cell leukemia, In DeVita VT, Hellman S, and Rosenberg SA, editors: Cancer principles and practice, ed 3, Philadelphia, 1989, JB Lippincott Co.

78. Talpaz M: Clinical studies of alpha-interferons in chronic myelogenous leukemia, Cancer Treat Rev 15(suppl A):49, 1988.

79. Talpaz M and others: Therapy of chronic myelogenous leukemia: Chemotherapy and interferons, Semin Hematol 25(1):62, 1988.

80. The Toronto Leukemia Study Group: Survival in acute myeloblastic leukemia is not prolonged by remission maintenance or early reinduction chemotherapy, Leuk Res 12(3):195, 1988.

81. Thomas ED: Marrow transplantation for chronic myelogenous leukemia. In Gale RP and Champlin R, editors: Bone marrow transplantation: current controversies, San Diego, 1988, Academic Press.

82. Westbrook CA and Golomb HM: Hairy cell leukemia, Curr Concepts Oncol Winter, 1984.

83. Winston DJ and others: Prevention and treatment of infection in leukemia patients. In Gale RP, editor: Leukemia therapy, Boston, 1986, Blackwell Scientific Publications.

84. Wiernik PH: Acute leukemia. In DeVita VT, Hellman S, and Rosenberg SA, editors: Cancer principles and practice, ed 3, Philadelphia, 1989, JB Lippincott Co.

85. Woodruff RK and others: Combination chemotherapy for hematological relapse in adult lymphoblastic leukemia, Am J Hematol 4:1973, 1978.

86. Wujcik D: Options for postremission therapy in acute leukemia, Semin Oncol Nurs 6:25, 1990.

CHAPTER 15

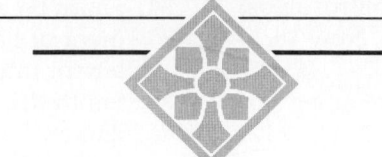

Lung Cancer

Susan Penny Schmidt
Judith A. Shell

Lung cancer is the leading cause of cancer-related deaths in men 35 years of age and older and in women 55 to 74 years of age.[15] While lung cancer mortality continues to rise among American men, the incidence of lung cancer among males has leveled off or slightly declined for the first time.[94] Despite research and public education efforts, however, lung cancer incidence and mortality continue to rise among American women.

Most patients present with metastatic disease, which ultimately leads to death. Clinical trials using multimodality therapies or new agents are trying to reverse this trend. In the meantime, smoking prevention remains the key to reducing lung cancer deaths and is a major focus for nursing intervention. Patients with lung cancer must learn to deal not only with the physiologic and economic effects of cancer and its treatment, but also with fears about the disease, its treatment, and dying. Compassionate and knowledgeable nursing care of the patient with lung cancer is essential and a particular challenge for the nurse.

EPIDEMIOLOGY

It is estimated that there will be 170,000 new cases of lung cancer in the United States in 1993 and 149,000 deaths.[2] More men than women develop lung cancer, but the gap is narrowing. Lung cancer mortality among women has skyrocketed over 400% during the past 30 years.[2]

The authors wish to gratefully acknowledge the work and effort put forth on this chapter by Christy Riner. We also wish to recognize Ace Allen, MD, Kansas University Medical Center, Kansas City, Kansas, for his support.

In 1987, lung cancer surpassed breast cancer as the leading cause of cancer deaths in women.[85] Although not the most common cancer in either sex, lung cancer will continue to be the leading cause of cancer death for both men (34%) and women (22%) in 1993.[15]

ETIOLOGY AND RISK FACTORS
Smoking

Death from lung cancer was relatively rare until this century. In 1912, Adler found only 374 cases of lung cancer described in world literature, and questioned the value of writing about such an insignificant problem.[115] Little did he expect the abrupt increase in deaths related to lung cancer beginning around 1935 (4300 deaths) and continuing until now (149,000 deaths estimated in 1993).[2] The increased incidence in men in the 1930s and in women in the 1960s followed the pattern of increased acceptance of smoking behavior, first in men and then in women. A prospective study by Hammond[55] in 1954 first demonstrated the relationship between smoking and the risk of developing lung cancer. Observers note that lung cancer mortality rates in people who have smoked two packs per day for 10 years (20 pack years) are 15 to 25 times higher than in nonsmokers.[134] It is estimated that 85% of lung cancer deaths are related to smoking.[18,85] The latency period between initiation of smoking and the development of lung cancer is about 15 to 20 years.

Air Pollution

Air pollutants have been incriminated in the etiology of lung cancer (e.g., sulfur dioxide). Nevertheless, although high rates of lung cancer occur in Los Angeles, where high levels of air pollution are a problem, no definite correlation to lung cancer incidence has been proven.[18,101]

Race and Socioeconomics

Among black males of all ages in the United States, there has been a decreased incidence of lung cancer since 1980, and this may be associated with a corresponding drop in mortality rates.[14] Smoking prevalence among blacks is also on the decline (from 41% in the mid-1970s to 34% in 1987).[14] Nevertheless, cancer mortality is higher among nonwhites than whites and may be related to the increased smoking and use of nonfilter cigarettes by blacks.[101] Socioeconomic factors (e.g., workplace conditions, poor nutrition, and so forth) might contribute to this difference, but this is only speculation. Unconfirmed studies suggest, however, that there is an increased risk of squamous cell and small cell lung cancers in men with diets low in vitamin A.[101]

Geography

Geographic clustering of lung cancer among males has been noted along the Gulf of Mexico and the southeastern Atlantic coast.[77] Whether this is related to industrial asbestos exposure from industries such as shipbuilding is not known. Mortality rates are lowest in farming areas and lower in rural versus urban counties.[127]

Industry

Industrial exposure to the following agents is believed to place persons at greater risk of lung cancer: mustard gas, radon, asbestos, radioisotopes, polycyclic aromatic hydrocarbons (present in crude petroleum, coal, tars, combustion products of most organic materials), nickel, chromium, haloethers, iron ore, inorganic arsenic, wood dust, and isopropyl oil.[18,101] Certain occupational groups at risk because of potential exposure to the above agents have been identified (see box on this page).

Family and Health History

The risk of lung cancer is increased in persons with a prior history of lung disease or a family history of lung cancer.[149] Recent research supports the idea that lung cancer risk is an inherited trait. A specific gene that predisposes to early age onset of lung cancer may account for up to 47% of cases by age 60.[120] In a recent analysis of 337 lung cancer families, a mendelian codominant inheritance that predisposed those exposed to smoking to the development of lung cancer was the best explanation of the data.[121] If this genetic predisposition proves true, it could mean that lung cancers occur uniquely among gene carriers,[121] and helps explain why all smokers don't develop lung cancer. This would have a major impact on approaches to

OCCUPATIONAL GROUPS AT RISK FOR LUNG CANCER
Atomic energy workers
Automobile maintenance
Asbestos workers
Chemical workers
Chloromethyl ethyl workers
Copper smelter workers
Gas workers
Glass, pottery, linoleum workers
Foundry workers
Insecticide workers
Insulation workers
Nickel workers
Metal material workers
Petroleum workers
Shipyard workers
Spray painters
Steel workers
Uranium miners

Modified from Oleske DM: The epidemiology of lung cancer: an overview, Semin Oncol Nurs 3:3, 1987.

lung cancer prevention, screening, and early detection.

PREVENTION, SCREENING, AND DETECTION
Primary Prevention

SMOKING.   Of the 526,000 estimated cancer deaths in 1993, 149,000 (28% of all cancer deaths) will be due to lung cancer. The majority (at least 85%) of lung cancer deaths are smoking-related and thus preventable. If smoking did not exist, the number of people dying from all cancer would be reduced by one third. Smoking has been implicated in up to 40% of all cancer deaths[107] and one sixth of deaths from all causes.[96] Up to one third of heavy smokers ($\geq$25 cigarettes/day) who are 35 years old will experience premature death from a smoking-related disease.[96]

Primary lung cancer prevention focuses on decreasing the number of new smokers and helping present smokers to quit. It may involve decreasing the hazards of smoking through use of low tar and filtered cigarettes for those who continue to smoke. The risk of developing and dying from lung cancer correlates directly with the number of cigarettes smoked, and lung cancer incidence can be reduced by as much as 20% by use of low tar and filter cigarettes assuming no increase in number of cigarettes smoked.[101]

Studies show that the spouse of a smoker can have an increased risk of developing lung cancer (1.3 to 3.4 times) depending on the exposure time and number of cigarettes smoked.[101] This is called *passive smoking;* side-stream smoke contains as many, if not more, carcinogens than inhaled smoke. Many work sites where extensive smoking occurs (e.g., bars and restaurants) may also place people at risk. In a population-based case control study of cancer risk secondary to passive smoking, the only individuals found to be at increased risk (twice the risk of an unexposed nonsmoker) were those exposed during childhood and/or adolescence to the secondary smoke of more than one smoker in the home.[69]

The cost of cancer research in the United States exceeds $1 billion annually.[115] For many cancers, research money and time is aimed at discovering etiologies in hope of suggesting preventive interventions. The irony is that lung cancer is one cancer for which the primary cause is known. The inability to curb its epidemic growth has been due to human choice to smoke because of: (1) the pleasure and addictiveness of tobacco and (2) a denial of personal vulnerability. Although much is being learned about the biology of lung cancer through research, the failure to impact mortality rates has not been due to lack of knowledge about the primary etiology. Lung cancer research money and time is spent on a disease that is, for the most part, preventable. There are other societal costs due to smoking, not mentioning the obvious human suffering and loss associated with lung cancer. The annual U.S. cost for health care and lost productivity due to smoking-related illness is greater than $65 billion.[95]

While smokers are encouraged to stop smoking, a smoker's risk of developing lung cancer may never equal that of one who has never smoked (perhaps due to the prolonged lag time in the development of lung cancer). One study found no benefit from smoking cessation at 10 years,[100] while others found lung cancer risk dropping to 5.9 times by 10 years.[134] Smokers who quit at least 15 years may still have twice the risk of developing lung cancer as those who never smoked.[134] It may take 20 years before the risks are similar.

Smoking and Advertising.   Those who begin or persist in smoking have not been helped by the tobacco industry's advertising campaign and political lobby. It was estimated in 1989 that the smoking industry would need to recruit about 1000 new smokers per day to fill the ranks of those who quit or die. The tobacco industry spent $4 billion on advertising and promotion in 1990.[68] Magazines in which cigarettes are advertised are less likely to publish articles on the hazards of smoking.[143] This makes magazines targeted at women, teenagers, blue-collar workers, and minorities a particular concern, because studies and literature note the influence of cigarette advertising campaigns on specific audiences.[23] While smoking prevalence has decreased among both U.S. men and women since 1965, women are not quitting as rapidly as men. If the current trends continue, women smokers will outnumber men smokers, perhaps in this de-

cade.[50] There are more blue-collar smokers than white-collar smokers, and more blacks than whites who smoke. More high school drop outs smoke than do students who remain in school.[68] Public education must focus on these high risk groups.

Smoking Cessation and Public Education.   The overall prevalence of smoking among high school seniors has decreased from 27% when programs were instituted in the 1970s, but has now leveled off at about 18% of students. By age 18, 75% of smokers have tried their first cigarette, and 50% are regular smokers.[95] The trend toward recruitment of smokers in adolescence, especially among teenage girls, needs to be broken. Programs found most successful in preventing initiation of smoking among youth are school-based, using peer leaders and role playing.[107] Because over half of female smokers begin smoking before age 13, prevention efforts must be aimed at the junior high age group or younger.

Among adults, many avenues are available to encourage smoking cessation, but 95% of smokers who quit do not seek outside help, preferring methods that can be done on their own.[107] Nurses need to set an example in smoking cessation; their rate (23.6%) exceeds that of the general female population (21.5%).[107] Factors that distinguish those smokers who quit from those who do not include a strong motivation to quit, use of behavioral techniques, and good social support to quit. Physician advice, even if only minimal, fosters quitting, particularly when the patient is experiencing increased symptoms or a new smoking-related illness, such as emphysema. (For an excellent review of smoking cessation methods, see Risser[107] and National Cancer Institute.[96])

Public Policy and Smoking.   Reduction of exposure to carcinogens and cocarcinogens in the workplace is occurring. Hospitals and public offices have smoking bans. Airline flights within the United States are smoke-free. While some private businesses have smoking bans, public education and pressure are needed to make this trend more universal. Health advocates encourage increasing sales tax on cigarettes as an incentive to smoking cessation. Tax on a pack of cigarettes in the United States is among the lowest worldwide. Some states, however, have passed or are considering special cigarette tax laws.[68] Such taxes may especially change smoking habits among youth and the poor, and could be a means to raise revenue to cover smoking-related health care costs. Unfortunately, the effects of current smoking cessation efforts and policies on lung cancer mortality figures may not be appreciated for another 20 years.

RADON.   Identification of risk groups helps to establish safety guidelines. Much media coverage has been given to the risk of lung cancer resulting from radon or asbestos exposure. Radon has been implicated as a significant cause of lung cancer.[29,140] However, even in uranium miners with high cumulative radon exposure, most lung cancers can be attributed to synergism between radon and cigarette smoking.[30,118,146] Extrapolating risks from high-level, industrial radon exposure (uranium mining) to low-level, nonindustrial (home/worksite) exposure is met with conflicting opinions. A recent review of published studies found inconsistencies in results and methodology leaving the correlation between residential radon exposure and lung cancer weak at best.[99] There is some agreement, however, that most lung cancers attributed to indoor radon probably occur among smokers; only about 2,000 of the 13,000 estimated annual lung cancer deaths attributed to nonindustrial radon exposure occur in nonsmokers.[29,73,119]

ASBESTOS. Before the establishment of the 1971 Occupational Safety and Health Administration (OSHA) asbestos exposure guidelines, studies done on workers in the asbestos industry (e.g., automobile maintenance, insulation, and shipyard workers) showed clearly that lung cancer was vastly increased if workers also smoked. Numerous studies have shown a strong synergism between smoking and asbestos exposure in the development of lung cancer.[55,86] Asbestos workers who did not smoke had a risk of lung cancer about five times that of nonsmokers who worked in other industries. This compared to a ten times greater risk for smokers not working in the asbestos industry, and an 87 times greater risk for asbestos workers who were smokers. Again, extrapolating the risk from industrial to low-level (school/worksite) asbestos exposure is controversial. It appears that the risk of lung cancer related to exposure to the levels of asbestos left intact in public buildings is very small.[64] If primary prevention priorities are based on the numbers of persons expected to die of lung cancer caused by environmental exposure, then efforts should focus on elimination of passive smoking, which results in about 4000 lung cancer deaths per year in Americans, rather than on reducing low-level radon (which is associated with the deaths of about 2000 nonsmokers per year) or low-level asbestos exposure (which causes far fewer deaths).[38,64]

Secondary Prevention

Secondary prevention is aimed at early diagnosis of lung cancer in populations at high risk. Populations considered at high risk generally include persons more than 45 years of age who have smoked heavily, that is, one or more packs per day. Patients who claim to be nonsmokers need to be queried as to past smoking history.

The National Cancer Institute (NCI) sponsored three large randomized, controlled trials beginning in the early 1970s to examine the benefit of radiologic exams and sputum cytology as lung cancer screening tools in asymptomatic, high-risk individuals. The initial results of these studies completed at Johns Hopkins, the Memorial Sloan-Kettering Cancer Center, and the Mayo Clinic were impressive, demonstrating an increase in the discovery of early stage lung cancer, and an improved 5-year survival in the Mayo group for those receiving intense screening.[46] However, none of the studies showed a difference in the lung cancer mortality rates among screened versus control groups. It is possible that patients who undergo regular screening eventually die of their lung cancer at the same rate as others, having only been diagnosed earlier in the natural history of their disease (lead time bias).[107] The problem with rejecting any efforts at early detection is that, apart from prevention, the surest guarantee of curing lung cancer has been via complete resection of early stage I disease. To address this apparent contradiction, Fontano and co-workers[46] noted that these studies did not compare screening to no screening, but rather intense screening to less intense (perhaps yearly chest x-rays) screening in high-risk individuals. There were additional problems noted (poor compliance in both screened and control groups) that reduced the study's ability to detect significant differences.[46] The National Cancer Institute began a large scale study in late 1992 at 15 U.S. centers and will continue over 16 years to assess the value of screening in reducing mortality in prostate, lung, and colorectal cancers.[26] There will be 37,000 men in both the screened and control groups. Hopefully, this study will at last answer the important questions about lung cancer screening. Current practice varies based on physician-client preference, but there is no support to date for broad scale lung cancer screening (due to lack of survival benefit) even in high-risk individuals. Early detection and screening is not without monetary concern or personal risks.[58] Prevention and early detection teaching priorities are listed in the box on p. 306.

In persons presenting with symptoms, a history of lung disease, a family history of lung cancer, and/or a heavy smoking history, chest x-ray and sputum cytology are the primary tools used to screen for lung cancer. Monoclonal antibodies may prove to be a valuable tool in the detection of early lung cancer by sputum cytology. Early findings showed that cells in sputum specimens that stained positive with anti-lung cancer antibodies were 91% predictive of the development of lung cancer within 2 years.[138] No useful tumor markers are currently available for screening. Carcinoembryonic antigen (CEA), elevated in only 50% of lung cancer patients, may be useful in postoperative followup,[18] but it is not useful in lung cancer screening or for prognostic purposes.

LUNG CANCER: PREVENTION AND EARLY DETECTION TEACHING PRIORITIES

1. Avoid use of tobacco
- Risks increase according to number of cigarettes/day, number of years smoking, tar and nicotine content of cigarettes.
- Passive smoking increases the risk of lung cancer in nonsmokers, especially children and adolescents.
- Parental smoking habits influence children.
- Pipe or cigar smoking or smokeless tobacco is not an acceptable alternative.
- Smoking cessation clinics/programs and medications are available to help those who desire to quit.
- Women, youth, blacks, and the uneducated should be the focus of smoking cessation efforts.

2. Know environmental carcinogens that increase risk
- High-risk occupations have been identified that expose persons to high levels of carcinogens.
- Certain toxic substances increase risk (see Oleske[101]).
- The synergistic effects of environmental carcinogens (especially radon or asbestos) and cigarette smoking increase risk.

3. Personal and family history are important risk factors
- Lung cancer risk may be inherited and is greater in those with a history of lung disease.
- Lung cancer is difficult to detect early and symptoms do not appear until disease is advanced. Best advice is to *quit smoking now.*
- There are currently no special tools for detecting cancer early enough to improve cure rates, even in high-risk populations.

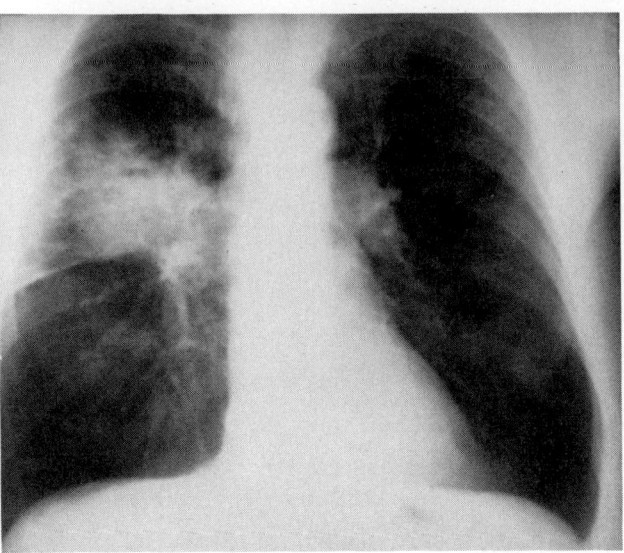

Figure 15–1 Patient with small cell lung cancer in which large tumor mass is centrally located, adjacent pleura is thickened. There is fluid in fissure and possible postobstructive signs of atelectasis. (Courtesy of Dr. Norman Martin, Diagnostic Radiology, University of Kansas Medical Center.)

CLASSIFICATION

The World Health Organization (WHO) has identified numerous categories of lung tumors or lesions, but the overwhelming majority (90%) consist of one of five types.[57,89] Technological advances in immunohistochemistry are helping to clarify pathologic subtypes of these five main categories and may help explain variations in treatment responses for the same histologic diagnoses. Relative incidence of the major histologic types varies depending on the series and the method of obtaining tissue. Squamous cell carcinoma is still cited as the most common type (30% to 64% of all lung cancers), but some authors suggest adenocarcinoma is becoming the most common.[57,148] Other literature still notes adenocarcinoma as the second most common lung cancer (16% to 30%) and as the most common type in females.[87] The incidence of small cell carcinoma is rising among women.[56,93] Small cell anaplastic carcinoma (19% to 25%), large cell carcinoma (9% to 20%), and all other types (1% to 3%) occur less often. Some 2% to 4% may be an adenosquamous hybrid.[18,89]

Although the histology of a lung cancer is often suggested by the clinical signs and symptoms at presentation, adequate tissue for cytologic or pathologic examination is essential for diagnosis. The following will describe some of the clinical and histologic features of the five main types of lung cancer. It is now believed that all lung cancers arise out of a common stem cell gone awry.[18]

Small Cell Lung Cancer

Small cell anaplastic carcinoma behaves biologically and clinically so differently from all other cell types that the latter are referred to as non–small cell lung cancers (NSCLC). Although usually metastatic at the time of diagnosis (more than two thirds of the time) because of its rapid growth and aggressive nature, small cell lung cancer (SCLC) is the most sensitive of all lung cancers to chemotherapy and radiation therapy. It is thought to arise from the basal cell lining of the bronchial mucosa called a Kulchitsky-type cell. Because it most often arises in the central part of the chest, postobstructive pneumonia and atelectasis are common (Figure 15-1). Frequent sites of distant metastasis are brain, liver, and bone marrow. SCLC has sometimes been referred to as *oat cell* carcinoma due to its microscopic resemblance to oats.

Paraneoplastic syndromes in SCLC patients include Eaton-Lambert syndrome (proximal muscle weakness), syndrome of inappropriate antidiuretic hormone or SIADH (from ectopic arginine vasopressin [AVP]), and Cushing's syndrome (from ectopic adrenocorticotropic hormone [ACTH]). Cushing's syndrome in conjunction with SCLC may be a poor prognostic sign. While the incidence of ectopic ACTH production and Cushing's in association with SCLC may be low (4.5% in one series), its appearance has been associated with a poor response to chemotherapy, a shortened survival time, and an increase in therapy-related complications.[125] Other hormones produced by SCLCs include calcitonin and gastrin-releasing peptide (GRP) or bombesin.[57,80] That SCLC cells contain neurosecretory granules and are capable of hormone production was once thought to be due to neural crest embryologic origin.[57] The term *dispersed neuroendocrine cells* is now used to describe the variety of cells (carcinoid, some large cell, and small cell undifferentiated carcinomas) that share similar morphologic and immunohistochemical features (see Biology of Lung Cancer and Clinical Significance below) and are capable of peptide hormone production.[57] SCLC cells share antigens common to neural cells, and it has been hypothesized that the body's formation of antibodies to these antigens shared with neural tissues is the cause for such paraneoplastic neurologic syndromes as cerebellar degeneration.[18] SCLC patients have a deficiency of major histocompatibility antigens (MCH class I and II antigens), which help the immune system recognize foreign and malignant cells.[18] This perhaps explains the highly metastatic nature of SCLC. Interferons can reverse this type of deficit and theoretically could be useful in treatment where tumor burden is low.

Non-Small Cell Lung Cancer

Squamous cell carcinoma may be described as well, moderately, or poorly differentiated. These cells differentiate toward stratified columnar (squamous) epithelium lining the airway and have receptors for epidermal growth factor, which stimulates the growth of epidermal tissues and is perhaps critical to malignant cell growth.[18] It may not be visualized easily on chest x-ray because it tends to arise in the central (medial) portion of the lung. This may delay diagnosis (Figure 15-2). Squamous cell is the most likely lung cancer to present as a Pancoast's tumor, which is high in the lung apex with extension to the chest wall and causing a classic shoulder pain that radiates down the ulnar nerve distribution (Figure 15-3). It is often associated with sudden onset of hypercalcemia resulting from the production of a parathyroid hormone-like substance, not associated with the presence of bone metastases.

Adenocarcinoma is increasing in frequency, perhaps as a result of the increasing incidence of women with

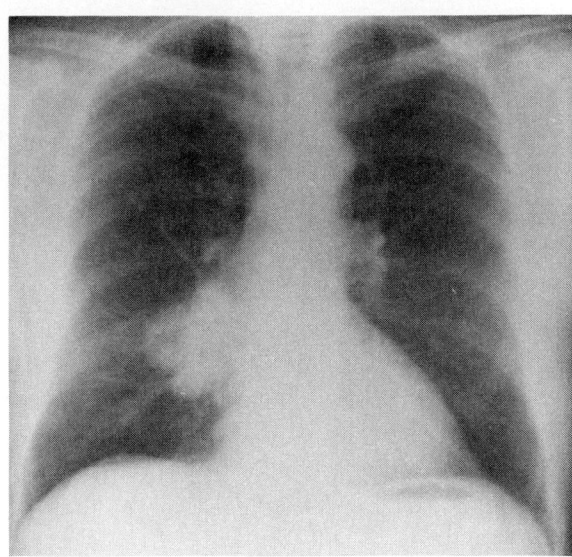

Figure 15-2 Patient with squamous cell carcinoma that developed centrally (RML) with left hilar prominence showing regional lymph node spread. (Courtesy of Dr. Norman Martin, Diagnostic Radiology, University of Kansas Medical Center.)

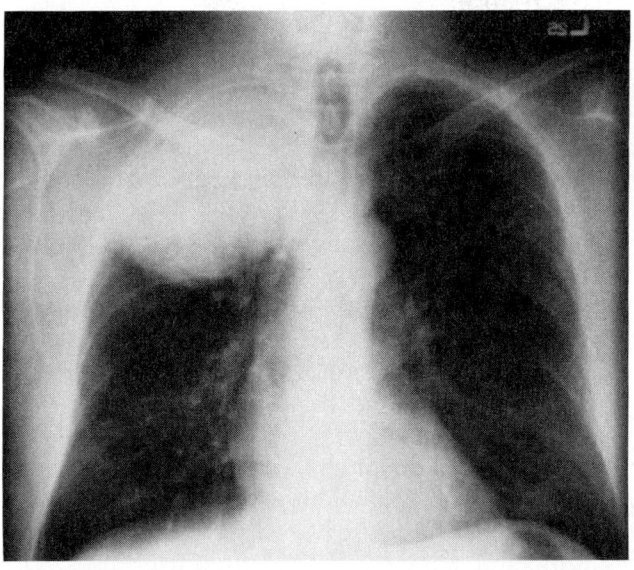

Figure 15-3 Classic Pancoast's tumor in patient with squamous cell carcinoma of lung. Large right upper apex mass with nearly complete right first rib bony destruction and right supraclavicular fullness. (Courtesy of Dr. Norman Martin, Diagnostic Radiology, University of Kansas Medical Center.)

lung cancer. This type is often recognized microscopically by its glandular appearance and mucin production, and includes acinar, papillary, solid, and bronchioalveolar types.[57] Along with large cell carcinoma, it is easily seen on chest x-ray because it usually arises in radiographically visualized, peripheral lung tissue (Figure 15-4). Because of adenocarcinoma's highly metastatic nature, patients may present with

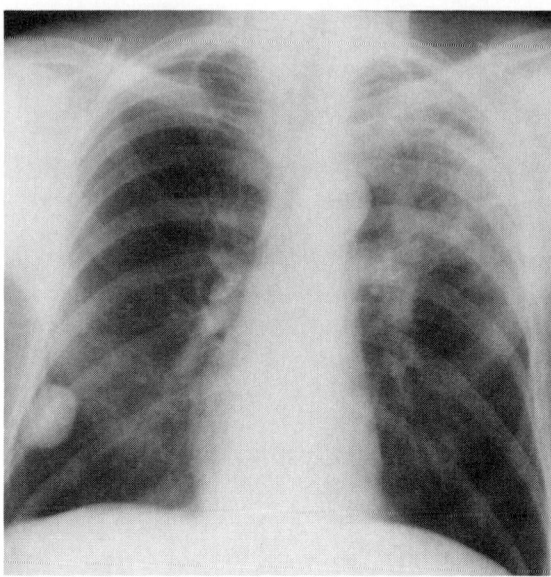

Figure 15–4 Adenocarcinomas can present as clearly defined peripheral lesions. Patient with right lower lobe lesion. (Courtesy of Dr. Norman Martin, Diagnostic Radiology, University of Kansas Medical Center.)

or develop brain, liver, adrenal, or bone metastasis. Paraneoplastic syndromes commonly associated with adenocarcinomas are hypercoagulability syndromes (marantic endocarditis, disseminated intravascular coagulation [DIC], migratory thrombophlebitis) and clubbing of the fingers with hypertrophic pulmonary osteoarthropathy.[18]

Large cell anaplastic carcinoma is so named because it appears microscopically as large cells lacking any distinguishing features.[57] Clinical signs and symptoms are similar to those seen in adenocarcinoma, such as pain from pleural or chest wall invasion and lung abscesses, but this lesion is less likely to spread beyond the chest cavity.[18]

Mixed cell types comprise the final major lung cancer category. The idea that all lung cancers have the same stem cell origin helps explain the existence of mixed cell tumors. In a review of 100 lung cancer cases, 45% showed two different major histologic cell types.[58] Multiple cell lines are seen in 10% to 20% of specimens.[21] In a given patient, any combination of cell types is possible within a single lesion or specimen, while the predominant cell type in different metastatic lesions may vary.[18]

BIOLOGY OF LUNG CANCER AND CLINICAL SIGNIFICANCE

Multiple genetic lesions and events may be necessary in the development of lung cancer.[121] Chromosomal mutations or deletions that appear to play a role in malignant transformation and growth involve both the activation of "up-regulating" genes (proto-onco-

genes) and the inactivation or deletion of "down-regulating," suppressor genes (anti-oncogenes).[80] Recent research demonstrates a deletion in the 3p chromosome region of 100% of SCLCs and up to 74% of NSCLCs.[18,21] This chromosome region has become the focus of intense research to determine the exact gene and its function. Whether or not the deletion is the same in both SCLC and NSCLC is not known. Other chromosomal deletions common in lung cancer are in the regions of 11p, 17p (p53 gene), and the retinoblastoma (Rb) gene.[18,21] The p53 gene is frequently mutated or inactivated in all types of lung cancer.[21] Reincorporation of some of these genes in malignant cell cultures has halted cell growth,[18,21] suggesting these genes control or down-regulate cellular growth.

In contrast, products of the myc-oncogenes are important in SCLC proliferation. Patients whose tumors show c-myc-oncogene overexpression have a poorer prognosis than others with extensive disease,[21] indicating this may be a late event or its activation correlates with aggressive SCLC behavior as seen at relapse. While not present in SCLC, ras gene point mutations (especially K-ras codon 12) are found in about 35% of adenocarcinomas of the lung.[21] In one series of patients with "completely resected" adenocarcinoma of the lung, the presence of K-ras point mutations correlated with a significantly decreased overall and disease-free survival regardless of age, sex, or evidence of disease.[129] Among 280 human lung cancer specimens, 30% of adenocarcinomas from smokers had point mutations in codon 12 of K-ras, while only 5% of those from nonsmokers did, implying that K-ras mutations may be directly caused by exposure to tobacco carcinogens.[108] The K-ras positive tumors were less differentiated. Correlating such findings with outcomes can eventually assist in treatment decisions.

A wide variety of neuroendocrine properties have been found in association with 50% to 90% of SCLCs and up to 40% of NSCLCs.[18] These properties include the cell's ability to produce proteins and peptides or the presence of cell surface receptors for neuropeptides (including GRP, somatostatin, insulin-like growth factor-1 [ILGF-1], transferrin, and neural cell adhesion molecule).[18,21] GRP and other neuropeptides appear to be autocrine growth factors (factors that stimulate self-replication).[21,122] When receptors are present on SCLC for GRP, GRP secretion triggers DNA synthesis and cellular proliferation. The discovery of these and other growth factors suggest interventions to block or otherwise interfere with their pathways in causing cell growth or spread.[122] Monoclonal antibodies to these cell markers are being used in research to purge bone marrow, discover bone metastases, or direct tumor-specific cytotoxic therapy.[18,21] Monoclonal antibodies may eventually be used to dis-

---

**DISEASE-RELATED COMPLICATIONS
LUNG CANCER**

Direct spread or metastases
    Bone marrow involvement (pancytopenia)
    Bone metastasis (pain, pathologic fractures)
    Brain metastasis
    Spinal cord compression (paralysis)
    Superior vena cava syndrome (respiratory
      distress)
    Pleural effusion
    Pericardial effusion (tamponade, arrhythmias)
    Endobronchial lesion (cough, hemoptysis)
    Postobstructive atelectasis and/or pneumonia
    Liver metastasis
    Regional spread (see Clinical Features)
Indirect effects or paraneoplastic syndromes
    Inappropriate ADH (small cell) and hypona-
      tremia
    Hypercalcemia (squamous cell)
    Cushing's syndrome and ectopic ACTH
    Anorexia, taste changes, weight loss, cachexia
    Degenerative neuropathies
    Fever of unknown origin (multiple cultures
      and work-ups)
    Disseminated intravascular coagulopathies
      (bleeding, DVTs)
    Clubbing and hypertrophic osteoarthropathy
    Anemia
    Granulocytosis, thrombocytosis

**CLINICAL FEATURES
LUNG CANCER**

Most common symptoms at presentation
- A change in cough (most have a chronic smoker's cough)
- Chest pain
- Recurrent bronchitis or pneumonia unresponsive to antibiotics
- Shortness of breath or wheezes
- Hemoptysis
- Weight loss
- Fatigue
- Dysphagia

Symptoms of regional tumor spread
- Superior vena cava syndrome (SVCS; see Chapter 19)
- Hoarseness as a result of recurrent laryngeal nerve paralysis
- Phrenic nerve paralysis with an elevated hemidiaphragm and dyspnea
- Horner's syndrome (unilateral ptosis, miosis, loss of facial sweat)
- Pancoast's syndrome (shoulder pain radiating down an arm along ulnar nerve distribution)
- Tracheal or esophageal obstruction
- Pericardial effusion and tamponade (see Chapter 19)
- Pleural effusion
- Hypoxia and dyspnea related to lymphangitic spread

Evidence of metastatic disease or a paraneoplastic syndrome
- Headaches, mental status changes, or other neurologic findings due to brain metastasis or SIADH with hyponatremia (see Chapter 19)
- Abdominal discomfort, elevated liver function tests, enlarged liver and/or nausea and vomiting owing to liver involvement
- Bone pain related to bone involvement [18]
- Pancytopenia secondary to bone marrow involvement
- Other paraneoplastic syndromes

Modified from Bunn PA: Lung cancer: current understanding of biology, diagnosis, and treatment. A monograph of Bristol-Myers, Evansville, 1988.

tinguish SCLC from NSCLC. There is research suggesting that NSCLCs that have neuroendocrine features will be more likely to respond to chemotherapy, and that completely resected stage I and II patients with these features may need adjuvant chemotherapy.[18] Some of the neuroendocrine factors may someday be useful as tumor markers in screening and early detection or as means of assessing response to therapy, but currently lack adequate sensitivity to be applied clinically.

The disease-related complications of lung cancer are listed in the box above.

DIAGNOSIS

The search for a lung cancer diagnosis is undertaken only after a good preliminary evaluation including:

1. A history and physical exam (see box at upper right for clinical features common in lung cancer)
2. A chest x-ray (anterior/posterior and lateral), which may reveal peripheral lesions at least 1 cm in size, a widened mediastinum, or hilar adenopathy
3. A complete blood count with differential and platelet count, and blood chemistries

Histologic diagnosis, which may be as simple as collecting early morning sputum 3 days in a row (80% of the time, this will be diagnostic), is most valuable

in squamous cell carcinoma.[107] However, bronchoscopy is commonly used today because it expedites diagnosis, provides a better specimen for histologic evaluation, and aids in staging. Efforts to obtain adequate tissue for diagnosis become increasingly more invasive and can involve:

- Fiberoptic bronchoscopy with biopsy or bronchial brushings or washings for cytology (90% efficient)[18]
- Percutaneous transthoracic needle aspiration or biopsy under fluoroscopy and/or computed tomography (CT) guidance for peripheral lung lesions
- Biopsy of supraclavicular or scalene lymph nodes
- Mediastinoscopy (or mediastinotomy, if left up-

per chest lesions) to biopsy nodes or tissues, which aids in staging
- Biopsy of accessible metastatic sites (e.g., bone)
- Thoracentesis for cytology or pleural biopsy
- Thoracotomy as a last resort

STAGING

Obtaining a tissue diagnosis may involve use of staging procedures. The histology (SCLC versus NSCLC) will then determine how to proceed with staging. Histology and stage of disease help dictate prognosis and treatment options. When discussing treatment options with the patient, prognosis is an important consideration because risks/toxicities associated with the treatment must be balanced against potential survival benefits. Prognostic factors in lung cancer are discussed later in this chapter.

In general, a CT scan or magnetic resonance imaging (MRI) of the chest down through the adrenal glands must be done in addition to the studies listed above for either SCLC or NSCLC. Some argue that further staging in asymptomatic patients is unwarranted because it rarely reveals metastatic disease.[18,93] The incidence of "silent" metastases in asymptomatic patients who appear to be clinically stage I or II disease is low; incidence of metastases to the brain (2.7%), to bone (3.4%), and to the liver (9.3%).[93] Others note that 46% of patients with NSCLC have metastatic disease, and because of inadequate staging up to one fourth of patients who undergo so-called "curative" therapy will eventually die as a result of metastatic disease.[58] In many cases, nonresectability will, nonetheless, be demonstrated by the time the above studies are done.[18] If NSCLC patients have evidence of bone pain, weight loss, abnormal liver function or calcium levels, further work-up might require the following:
- Bone scan
- CT scan of the abdomen or liver
- CT or MRI study of the head
- Liver or bone marrow biopsy
- Plain films of bone

One of the greatest current controversies in the treatment of NSCLC is the resectability of stage IIIA disease (based upon mediastinal lymph node involvement) with curative intent. Therefore, preoperative staging of these patients has become more critical. CT scans and MRI are often inadequate in diagnosing chest wall and mediastinal involvement,[88] essential determinants of resectability and likelihood of cure. While CT or MRI scans guide decisions regarding the necessity of invasive procedures and which procedure to perform, mediastinoscopy, mediastinotomy, and/or thoracotomy will frequently be required after the scans (at least in the study setting) to document involvement histologically.[93]

Table 15–1 Stage Grouping

Occult carcinoma	T_x	N_0	M_0
Stage 0	T_{is}	N_0	M_0
Stage I	T_1	N_0	M_0
	T_2	N_0	M_0
Stage II	T_1	N_1	M_0
	T_2	N_1	M_0
Stage IIIA	T_1	N_2	M_0
	T_2	N_2	M_0
	T_3	N_0, N_1, N_2	M_0
Stage IIIB	Any T	N_3	M_0
	T_4	Any N	M_0
Stage IV	Any T	Any N	M_1

From Beahrs OH and others, editors: Manual for staging of cancer, ed 4, Philadelphia, 1992, JB Lippincott Co.

If the cancer is deemed resectable, pulmonary function and blood gas studies are required to determine if the patient is able to undergo pneumonectomy or pulmonary resection.

Because two thirds of SCLC patients have metastatic disease, initial staging will routinely include:
- Bone scan
- CT scan of the abdomen
- Bone marrow biopsy
- CT or MRI study of the head
- +/− Liver biopsy[18,27]

The American Joint Committee for Staging's Tumor, Node, Metastasis (TNM) cancer staging system has been useful in prognosis and planning treatment for NSCLC. The TNM system classifies cancers according to the following staging designations[7] (see Table 15-1):

PRIMARY TUMOR (T)*

T_x Primary tumor cannot be assessed, or tumor proven by the presence of malignant cells in sputum or bronchial washings but not visualized by imaging or bronchoscopy

T_0 No evidence of primary tumor

T_{is} Carcinoma in situ

T_1 Tumor 3 cm or less in greatest dimension, surrounded by lung or visceral pleura, without bronchoscopic evidence of invasion more proximal than the lobar bronchus (i.e., not in the main bronchus)

T_2 Tumor with any of the following features of size or extent:
- More than 3 cm in greatest dimension
- Involvement of main bronchus 2 cm or more distal to the carina
- Invasion of the visceral pleura
- Associated with atelectasis or obstructive pneumonitis that extends to the hilar region but does not involve the entire lung

*Reprinted with permission from Beahrs O and others, editors: Manual for staging of cancer, ed 4, Philadelphia, 1992, JB Lippincott Co.

T_3 Tumor of any size that directly invades any of the following: chest wall (including superior sulcus tumors), diaphragm, mediastinal pleura, parietal pericardium; or tumor in the main bronchus less than 2 cm distal to the carina; or associated atelectasis or obstructive pneumonitis of the entire lung

T_4 Tumor of any size that invades any of the following: mediastinum, heart, great vessels, trachea, esophagus, vertebral body, carina; or tumor with a malignant pleural effusion

REGIONAL LYMPH NODES (N)

N_x Regional lymph nodes cannot be assessed

N_0 No regional lymph node metastasis

N_1 Metastasis in ipsilateral peribronchial and/or ipsilateral hilar lymph nodes, including direct extension

N_2 Metastasis in ipsilateral mediastinal and/or subcarinal lymph node(s)

N_3 Metastasis in contralateral mediastinal, contralateral hilar, ipsilateral or contralateral scalene, or supraclavicular lymph node(s)

DISTANT METASTASIS (M)

M_x Presence of distant metastasis cannot be assessed

M_0 No distant metastasis

M_1 Distant metastasis

For the most part, the TNM system is not useful in SCLC. TNM only takes on clinical significance when surgery for stage I SCLC is a consideration. The Veterans Administration Lung Cancer Study Group's two-stage system is commonly used for SCLC because it correlates with prognosis. There is controversy regarding what constitutes limited versus extensive disease. A 1989 international workshop on SCLC reached the following consensus regarding staging[136]:

Limited—Disease restricted to one hemithorax with regional lymph node metastases including hilar, ipsilateral and contralateral mediastinal and/or supraclavicular nodes, and including ipsilateral pleural effusion regardless of cytology.

Extensive—Disease beyond the above definition and may involve metastasis to liver, bone, bone marrow, brain, adrenals, and lymph nodes.

Other authors maintain that limited disease is that which is confined to one hemithorax and can be encompassed in a single radiation port.[18] They therefore continue to assign pleural effusions to the extensive stage category because of the large volume of tissue requiring radiation to treat the pleural surface. Because pleural effusions are a poor prognostic factor, variations in staging SCLC can make comparisons of treatment response rates and survival data by stage confusing and possibly misleading.

METASTASIS

Metastasis to any site, as a consequence of lung cancer, can seriously interfere with the patient's ability to accomplish simple activities of daily living. Depending on where the metastatic lesion is located, clinical manifestations can lead to critical oncologic emergencies. Cancers of the lung find many distant sanctuaries including bone marrow, pericardium and heart, kidney, and adrenal gland. The most common sites of metastasis of lung cancer are to the other lung and pleura, brain, bone, liver, and lymph nodes. These sites are also the most common for metastasis of other types of cancer.

Because of its relevance to staging of NSCLC, only intrathoracic spread will be addressed here. Other sites of metastasis will be discussed later in conjunction with their treatment.

Intrathoracic Spread

As previously reviewed, various methods are employed to assess lymph node involvement. In patients with SCLC, if there is a definite diagnosis, further invasive procedures to determine lymph node involvement are usually not done. Work-up will continue to ascertain brain, bone, and liver metastasis.[31] Even in limited disease, local thoracic extension may account for chest pain, wheeze, hemoptysis, dysphagia, and hoarseness. If there is a pleural effusion or an abnormal LDH, long-term survival is not likely.[1]

The usual consensus is that a primary NSCLC tumor is incurable if nodes (high paratracheal, subcarinal, or contralateral) are replaced with tumor.

When evaluating NSCLC for mediastinal involvement, some literature notes that on CT scan: (1) nodes less than 1 cm are considered normal; (2) nodes from 1 to 1.5 cm in diameter are considered suspicious; and (3) nodes greater than 1.5 cm in diameter are considered abnormal. Nodes considered normal may harbor disease, and nodes considered abnormal may just be reactive to pneumonia or other disease.[49,61]

There is controversy over what constitutes a "normal" node. Study results conflict on the accuracy of CT or MRI staging. Of patients with a negative CT, 10% to 20% will prove to have positive mediastinal lymph nodes at the time of thoracotomy, while 30% of those with enlarged nodes on CT will be negative on biopsy.[137] Mountain recommends mediastinoscopy and/or mediastinotomy for patients who might otherwise be denied curative resection based on the radiologist's interpretation.[93] Based upon examination of the mediastinum by mediastinoscopy, Mountain cites the following criteria for incurable and unresectable NSCLC: (1) tumor involvement of "contralateral paratracheal lymph nodes or ipsilateral paratracheal lymph nodes in the upper half of the intrathoracic trachea"; (2) direct invasion of the trachea; and (3) evidence of gross perinodal disease.[93] If surgery is to be performed for NSCLC, Watanabe and others recommend extensive nodal dissection for accurate postoperative staging.[72] Obvious clinical contralateral lymph node involvement is associated with a much poorer 5-year survival than when only microscopic nodal involvement is discovered.[137] Resection may be possible, however, and radiation therapy may be added.[31]

TREATMENT MODALITIES
Non-small Cell Lung Cancer

SURGERY. Surgery is the treatment of choice for stages I and II NSCLC, representing 25% of all lung cancers, and the primary hope for cure.[93] Some selected stage IIIA patients may benefit from surgical resection in terms of improved survival.[58,93] Stage IIIB patients are not surgical candidates.[137] Pneumonectomy for stage II and some stage I patients may be required unless precluded by preexisting cardiopulmonary disease. Some surgeons advocate wedge or segmental resection for small, peripheral lung lesions; others find the incidence of local recurrence too high with this limited procedure when a more aggressive approach could be curative. At the very least, lobectomy with regional lymph node dissection is most optimal for early stage disease whenever possible.[58] Criteria for nonresectability include: T4, N3, M1 lesions (stages IIIB and IV), the presence of small cell histology, or inability of the patient to tolerate the procedure clinically.[18] A "complete" resection should mean: (1) the surgeon is certain the operation removed all known disease; (2) the proximal margins of the resected specimen are microscopically free of tumor; (3) the most distant lymph nodes within each lymphatic drainage area are microscopically free of tumor; and (4) the resected lymph node capsules are intact.[93]

Squamous cell cancer patients have the best survival rates, perhaps as a result of earlier diagnosis and because the disease exhibits less of a tendency to metastasize and a slower growth rate.[58] Over 70% of patients relapse after "curative" surgery because of distant metastases rather than local lesions (less than 25%). This argues for improved methods of early detection and/or good systemic adjuvant therapy. Five-year survival after curative therapy is excellent for stage I patients (60% to 80%) but drops dramatically to 28% for the best stage IIIA patients.[93] Thus, the potential benefit of surgery must be weighed against the risks of operative morbidity and mortality. Operative mortality for patients undergoing lung resection as reported by the Lung Cancer Study Group (LCSG) ranges from 1.4% for segmentectomy or wedge resection to 7.7% for pneumonectomy.[52] However, it may reach 15% for high risk resections (chest wall and extrapleural pneumonectomy).[93] The incidence of lung resection complications increases with age (over 70 years of age). However, age alone is not a contraindication to surgery as age may not reflect other important risk factors (coexisting diseases, low forced

> **SURGERY TREATMENT-RELATED COMPLICATIONS OF LUNG CANCER**
>
> Fever, sepsis (antibiotics, empyema, fistula formation)
> Bleeding (hypotension, cardiogenic shock)
> Cardiac arrhythmias, CHF, fluid overload
> Airway obstruction, dyspnea, hypoxemia, respiratory failure
> Pneumothorax
> Pulmonary embolus
> Pneumonia
> Prolonged hospitalization, ICU psychosis
> Death

expiratory volume, weight loss, disease stage, and extent of resection).[93] Surgery for palliation of NSCLC metastases can help maintain a decent quality of life in cases of rapidly progressing or recurrent spinal cord compression[89] or for solitary brain metastasis.[58] Surgery treatment-related complications of lung cancer are listed in the box above.

LASER. Lung cancer patients may experience distressful symptoms or complications due to endobronchial lesions including postobstructive atelectasis and/or pneumonia, hemoptysis, irritating and uncontrolled cough, and hypoxemia and self-care deficit. If the endobronchial lesions involve the trachea or mainstem bronchii, laser therapy may be successfully used with palliative intent. Laser is less effective in treating obstructions of smaller airways. Treatment may be repeated and can be done entirely on an outpatient basis.[111] The procedure has been associated with a 75% success rate in advanced lung cancer.[110] Effectiveness of the procedure is independent of other modes of therapy, patient's age, or performance status. Patients whose airway is obstructed by an exophytic lesion of squamous cell origin may derive the greatest benefit.[110]

RADIATION THERAPY. Optimal doses of external beam radiation for NSCLC are now believed to be around 60 Gy. Best tumor control occurs with five fractions (treatments) per week over 6 to 7 weeks without interruption (no midtherapy "rests" as in treatment known as a split course).[11] Hyperfractionation schedules (more than one treatment per day) are currently under study, and preliminary findings suggest these achieve better responses than standard schedules.[18,58] A hyperfractionated dose-response relationship to survival appears to plateau at 69.9 Gy. Since doses in this range can be delivered by standard radiation with comparable survival, studies are now comparing hyperfractionated to standard schedules to answer the question of superior method.[11] However, tumors of greater than 6 cm are not effectively destroyed by external beam therapy, while tumor size less than 3 cm is associated with a favorable prognosis.[11]

BRACHYTHERAPY. Local recurrences develop in up to 60% of patients within 15 months of standard radiation therapy to the chest primary.[104] Brachytherapy, based upon the known dose-response relationship to tumor control, is being used to treat these relapses. It is also indicated for the patient who cannot undergo resection because of the location of the tumor, medical contraindications, or refusal of surgery. In the last two cases, patients with otherwise resectable NSCLC could be offered radiation therapy with curative intent; 5-year survival rates may be as high as 23%.[18] In some cases, brachytherapy radiation implants with iodine-125 are used to sterilize tumors 7 to 8 cm in size by delivering doses of 160 to 250 Gy to the tumor without significant damage to surrounding tissue.[58] These treatments require hospitalization while the radioactive implants are in place. More recently, high dose-rate (HDR) brachytherapy is used, often in combination with laser, to treat recurrent and obstructing lung lesions. This technology allows for careful placement of catheters close to the tumor. Then, via computerized, remote control, HDR iridium (^{192}Ir) is introduced into the catheter. Within a few minutes, while caregivers are safe from exposure, a very high dose of radiation (5 to 10 Gy/session) can be delivered to select tissue without injury to adjacent healthy tissue, especially critical at this anatomic site.[71] Sessions may be repeated every 1 to 2 weeks for a cumulative dose in the range of 20 to 43.6 Gy.[11,71,74] Symptoms (cough, hemoptysis, and dyspnea) can be relieved 30% to 80% of the time with minimal risk in properly selected patients.[11,71] This is experimental palliative therapy, but the role of HDR brachytherapy in primary treatment is being explored via randomized comparisons with external beam.[11,71]

For inoperable, locally advanced NSCLC in poor prognostic patients, radiation alone is usually reserved for palliation of symptoms such as painful bone metastases, superior vena cava syndrome, or those previously mentioned. Symptoms will be relieved in 24% to 100% of these patients.[11,18] Some studies have shown comparable symptom relief with lower than standard radiation doses at considerably less cost and inconvenience for these terminal patients.[11]

The use of definitive radiotherapy in unresectable early stage (stages I to IIIA) remains controversial.[67] Some recognize improved median or 5-year survival in the clinical setting.[53,67] The median survival in stage IIIA or IIIB NSCLC treated with radiation alone is less than 1 year.[54] Results of trials comparing chemotherapy plus radiation to radiation alone in unresected, locally advanced NSCLC have been contradictory. One author notes a modest survival benefit if the chemotherapy regimen is cisplatin-based and no difference in survival if it is not.[18] An important Eastern Cooperative Group/Radiation Therapy Oncology Group (ECOG/RTOG) study addresses the issue of superior modality. The study randomizes patients to cisplatin-velban followed by chest radiation versus standard radiation alone (60 Gy) versus hyperfractionated chest irradiation alone.[54] No randomized clinical trial has shown a survival advantage to either preoperative or postoperative radiation therapy in resected NSCLC, although it may reduce local recurrence in N1 or N2 disease.[11]

CHEMOTHERAPY. As many as 80% of all lung cancers are NSCLC, half of which (46%) have metastatic disease.[58] Even in the best of cases involving surgical resection (stage I), some 20% to 40% will relapse.[18] Relapse occurs in 70% of patients with more advanced disease.[18,58] Thus, the majority of lung cancer patients have frank or occult metastatic NSCLC and could benefit from effective systemic therapy. Response rates with single agents have been notoriously low (9% to 27%).[18] The most active single agents in NSCLC include mitomycin-C, vindesine, vinblastine, etoposide, ifosfamide, cisplatin, carboplatin,[18] cyclophosphamide, vincristine, doxorubicin, and bleomycin.[111] Among newer single agents showing promise is epirubicin (56% response rate in previously untreated and unresectable NSCLC).[54] Two phase II trials using different doses of Taxol in previously untreated NSCLC patients were recently reported to show response rates of 21% and 24%, but median survival is still pending.[26] ECOG is planning a phase III, three-arm trial comparing two doses of Taxol with or without cisplatin and/or granulocyte colony-stimulating factor (G-CSF).[26] Severe myelosuppression has been a dose-limiting toxicity of Taxol. What role Taxol will play in the treatment of NSCLC is unclear. However, in a phase I trial of Taxol in combination with cisplatin, one patient with a large (18 cm) primary NSCLC had a pathologic complete response (CR) systemically, although she developed CNS metastasis.[113]

Current combination chemotherapy regimens are producing the following response rates in advanced NSCLC: stage III (34%), select stage IIIA or IIIB (50% to 70%), and stage IV (22% to 28%).[12,54] Many of these trials use cisplatin-based regimens in combination with one or two other active agents. A cisplatin-based regimen was a favorable prognostic indicator in a review of Southwest Oncology Group (SWOG) studies, and the highest 1-year survival rate (25%) has been seen with etoposide-cisplatinum (EP) combinations.[12] Since no regimen has proven superior to EP in stage IV NSCLC and toxicity is acceptable, some advocate its use in nonprotocol patients.[12] The MIP regimen (mitomycin-C, ifosfamide, and cisplatin) has been associated with a 60.7% response rate in advanced

NSCLC.[6] Although high-dose cisplatin-based regimens are associated with improved responses, they have also proven highly toxic (myelosuppression, cumulative peripheral neuropathies), which limits the number of courses patients can tolerate. Since their attempt to substitute carboplatin for cisplatin in combination with etoposide was met with a disappointing response rate and severe toxicity (myelosuppression, septic death) in advanced disease, the CALGB does not plan to study the combination further in this group of patients.[79] Others report decreased toxicity and comparable responses when carboplatin is substituted in this combination.[18] These variations may be due to carboplatin dose and patient performance status in the different studies. Performance status has become a major factor in deciding who should undergo chemotherapy. A SWOG study (9015) is comparing upfront surgical resection to preoperative chemotherapy in NSCLC stages IB to IIIA. Patients are pathologically staged prior to therapy if mediastinal nodes are greater than 1 cm on CT. Another SWOG study (9019) will assess the role and necessity of surgery in select stage IIIA and IIIB patients when concurrent preoperative chemotherapy and radiation therapy are compared to chemotherapy and radiation alone. Outside a protocol setting, some will recommend chemotherapy to patients with NSCLC only if the patient: is informed of the limitations of therapy; is clearly incurable by surgery or radiation; has no significant symptoms that radiation could palliate; has a good performance status; and has measurable disease to assess any response so that treatment can be discontinued appropriately.[67]

More optimistically, Bunn summarized the findings of six randomized trials comparing best supportive care to various cisplatin-based chemotherapy regimens in patients with advanced NSCLC.[18] On the average, survival benefit in favor of the treated group was 11 weeks. This represents the first significant evidence of survival advantage with combination chemotherapy in these patients.[18] Clearly, quality of life studies must be used to corroborate the benefit of modest 3 to 4 month gains in survival for the patient with advanced disease. An encouraging corollary to these findings is that if micrometastases respond equally well to current chemotherapy regimens, more cures may be expected in "completely resected" stages I to IIIA NSCLC, where micrometastases are the only harbinger to failure.

COMBINATION CHEMOTHERAPY AND RADIATION THERAPY. For inoperable, locally-advanced NSCLC, cisplatin-based regimens in combination with radiotherapy may improve median but not long-term survival.[18] Postoperative cisplatin-based regimens plus radiotherapy in incompletely[18] or fully resected[54] stage II and IIIA patients is associated with

improved median survival and a decrease in distant relapses (except for brain), but has not reduced mortality rates. Because of an apparent synergism when cisplatin is combined with radiation, studies continue to investigate this combination to achieve improved cure rates. There are three trials in North America currently evaluating the role of adjuvant chemotherapy in fully resected NSCLC.[54]

The best inroads seem to be occurring in the treatment of stage IIIA NSCLC with preoperative adjuvant (also known as protoadjuvant or neoadjuvant) chemotherapy with or without radiation therapy. Although results are difficult to compare due to inconsistencies in staging (lack of pretreatment pathologic staging) and absence of multi-institutional trials, preliminary findings indicate a prolonged survival for patients receiving adjuvant therapy. Preoperative chemotherapy alone or in combination with radiotherapy is apparently rendering some patients pathologic CRs at thoracotomy (9% to 11% in one series).[18,93,109] Three-year survival rates ranged from 26% to 45%. The Cancer and Leukemia Group B (CALGB) has designed a study to address prior inconsistencies. Patients will be surgically staged prior to treatment with preoperative chemotherapy. After a thoracotomy in patients responding to or stable on chemotherapy, additional chemotherapy followed by radiation will be given. Unresectable patients will receive radiation alone.[11] At issue will be the ability of patients to tolerate intense chemotherapy in the postoperative period.[54] Although findings provide hope, preoperative chemotherapy in stage IIIA NSCLC is still investigational and is appropriate only in a clinical trial setting.[137] Patients should be informed of this option. If recent and upcoming trials demonstrate a survival advantage to preoperative chemotherapy and radiotherapy, those most likely to benefit are the 20% of patients having a normal CT, but who are found to have positive mediastinal nodes after biopsy.

FUTURE CONCERNS. New, more effective chemotherapy agents and combinations are needed, especially if they are associated with a low toxicity profile. Randomized phase III trials should only be carried out in clearly defined patient groups (pathologic staging, performance status, etc.).[133] Immunohistochemical analysis may help to identify that subgroup of NSCLCs with neuroendocrine features that may benefit from adjuvant chemotherapy. Examination of chromosomes for K-ras mutations may also delineate patients with adenocarcinoma of the lung who may benefit by either more aggressive treatment or else should not be subjected to treatment because of the aggressive nature of their disease and guaranteed short survival. There is on-going biotherapy research, but thus far the trial results have been disappointing.

Small Cell Lung Cancer

SURGERY.   In the 1960s and 1970s, most surgical attempts to treat small cell lung cancer (stages I and II) met with dismal results, with less than 1% surviving at 5 years.[18] The Veterans Administration and Armed Forces Cooperative Group found an amazing 36% 5-year survival among SCLC patients who had an unknown diagnosis and a single pulmonary lesion preoperatively.[62] However, less than 5% of SCLC patients are diagnosed in the early stages of disease when it is resectable, and the chest is still the most common site of relapse.[4,18,27] Adjuvant chemotherapy after surgical resection for stage I disease results in about a 45% 5-year survival.[75] Current recommended treatment of SCLC presenting as a single pulmonary nodule is surgery followed by adjuvant chemotherapy and prophylactic cranial irradiation with or without radiation to the chest.[75] The Lung Cancer Study Group (LCSG) and ECOG just completed a prospective randomized study to examine the benefit of surgery in patients with stage I to IIIA SCLC.[76] Patients were randomized to receive either preoperative chemotherapy plus surgery and radiotherapy or chemotherapy and radiation therapy alone. Preliminary results show no survival benefit to surgery. Unless randomized trials can demonstrate an advantage to chemotherapy plus surgery in early stage disease, the exact role of surgery will remain unclear. There does appear, however, to be a small group of SCLC patients (less than 1%) with true stage I disease who may be cured by surgery with or without chemotherapy.[18,62,90]

RADIATION THERAPY.   In limited disease (LD) SCLC, trials combining chest radiation and chemotherapy have now shown improved long-term survival rates (24% to 54% at 2 years; 7% to 20% at 4 years) and a decrease in local recurrences.[1,25,70,139] Upfront concurrent radiotherapy with chemotherapy[1] or alternating chemotherapy with radiotherapy every other week seem to produce the best results.[139] It is too early to know whether long-term survival will translate to cures. Prior to etoposide-cisplatin (EP) regimens, organ toxicities from combined modality approaches were too severe (congestive heart failure, dyspnea, etc.) and without survival benefit. Toxicities noted with EP plus radiation were myelosuppression, esophagitis, and some report of pulmonary toxicity (possibly due to the radiation port size), but none were life-threatening.[139] Use of CT guidance in radiation treatment planning, individually designed blocks, and a shrinking field help protect surrounding healthy lung, esophagus, and spinal cord tissues from unwanted radiation.

With the combined modality approach, the most common site of failure is the chest[4] in about 30% of LD SCLCs.[139] When chemotherapy is given alone in LD SCLC, however, the incidence of local chest relapse is 80%.[25] Some note that the intensity of the first chemotherapy dose may predict survival.[25] Current trials are examining the role of dose intensity and timing of modalities in preventing local recurrences and in improving long-term survival.

In extensive SCLC, there is no advantage to combining radiation therapy with chemotherapy; it only adds toxicity.[18] The main role for radiation therapy in these patients is palliation of symptoms, as was described for NSCLC patients with metastatic disease.

The brain is a frequent site of metastasis, and the effect of most systemic chemotherapy on the CNS is extremely limited. Whole brain irradiation (WBI) is often necessary. If brain metastasis has occurred, 40 Gy are needed to prevent relapse.[139]

Unlike treatment in NSCLC, prophylactic cranial irradiation (PCI) has often been done to prevent CNS failure. PCI can reduce the incidence of CNS relapse from 25% to 6%, and has generally been reserved for patients achieving a complete systemic response (CR) to chemotherapy. PCI may be used during systemic therapy in a clinical trial involving a potential cure. However, authors are questioning the value of PCI due to the high incidence and severity of CNS toxicities.[45] Late toxicities from PCI in long-term survivors are only now being realized and may be underreported in some studies because of only incidental and retrospective reporting. Among the 7% of patients surviving beyond 5 years in one retrospective review, 22% were found to have developed probable CNS toxicity that surfaced 2 to 5 years after combination chemotherapy and radiotherapy.[1] Patients had neurologic complaints, abnormal neurologic findings, and/or abnormal CT scans. In some cases, progressive clinical deterioration due to neurologic deficits required lifestyle changes or extended care.[1] Because of late toxicities, PCI is usually limited to no more than 30 Gy and is not given concurrently with chemotherapy to avoid synergistic injury to brain tissue. Many still reserve PCI until treatment of the primary is completed.[34,139]

Radiation to other common sites of metastasis (e.g., liver or spine) will not prevent tumor spreading to those sites. Prompt therapy (chemotherapy or radiation) for known meningeal carcinomatosis and spinal metastases is useful and necessary, but there is no preventive therapy for these complications.

Extensive disease (ED) patients who present with superior vena cava syndrome should be spared radiation as they will respond, in most cases, adequately to chemotherapy.[18,56]

CHEMOTHERAPY.   Before chemotherapy, half of SCLC patients with limited disease died within 12 to 14 weeks, and half of those with extensive disease died within 6 weeks without treatment.[27] Combination chemotherapy became the cornerstone of treatment in the 1980s for SCLC with overall responses of up to 90% and complete responses of 40% to 50%.[18,56] Long-term survival depends on achieving a CR, usually within the first months of treatment.

Single agents capable of producing overall responses greater than 20% with response duration of 2 to 4 months include cyclophosphamide, doxorubicin, vincristine, methotrexate, nitrogen mustard, and hexamethylmelamine. Lomustine (CCNU) will often be used in combination with other agents in spite of low activity (only 14% response rates) because it is associated with prolonged survival. There is slight activity with vindesine and procarbazine. One of the most active single agents is etoposide (VP-16) with responses ranging from 20% to 58%.[70] Its relative, teniposide (VM-26), showed a high response rate (90%) in a small study of previously untreated ED SCLC patients compared to only an 18% response rate in previously treated patients.[16,56] Reports are conflicting as to whether these agents are crossresistant (tumor resistance to one agent means tumor resistance to the other agent). Etoposide does appear to produce a very dose-dependent and schedule-dependent response. There are improved response rates in SCLC when etoposide is given in multiple daily IV doses (for 3 to 5 days) rather than as a single bolus.[130] A study has demonstrated excellent response rates and minimal toxicities (primarily mild myelosuppression) when etoposide is given as a daily oral dose (50 mg/m²) for 5 to 21 consecutive days every 4 weeks.[70] The optimal schedule and dose, however, have yet to be defined in SCLC. New active agents whose role in the treatment of SCLC is being studied include carboplatin, ifosfamide, and epirubicin. As single agents, response rates in previously untreated patients were 70% for ifosfamide and 49% for epirubicin.[18] The response rate to carboplatin is only 22%. However, this should not discourage its use in combination regimens, since cisplatin demonstrated only a 15% response rate as a single agent. In combination with other agents like etoposide, cisplatin has become an important part of induction regimens due to apparent synergism. ECOG recently completed a trial of Taxol in previously untreated SCLC patients.[26] Preliminary results suggest a 25% to 30% response rate.

Combination chemotherapy appears to be improving survival statistics in SCLC.[18] Before the advent of etoposide-cisplatin regimens, the best responses to chemotherapy were obtained with either lomustine, methotrexate, and cyclophosphamide or cyclophosphamide, doxorubicin, and vincristine (CAV) combination regimens. Results were as follows:

	CRs	MEDIAN SURVIVAL	2-YEAR DISEASE FREE
Limited disease	50%	14 months	15% to 35%
Extensive disease	20%	10 months	1% to 5%

Etoposide plus cisplatin has proven superior to CAV regimens for both limited and extensive disease in regard to responses, survival, and reduced toxicities.[18] Large cooperative group and single institution studies found improved median survival (18 to 19 months) in limited disease patients receiving regimens containing VP-16 plus cisplatin with or without radiation therapy to the primary tumor.[18]

Current practice is to give intense chemotherapy of short duration (<6 cycles) with active agents.[56] Restaging should include bronchoscopy and all initial staging studies to determine response. No study has shown a survival benefit for prolonged (1 to 2 year) maintenance chemotherapy in patients achieving a CR with induction therapy. In limited disease patients, late dose intensification after a CR was achieved during induction therapy proved a superior treatment to maintenance therapy. The only current maintenance studies are those evaluating the role of biologicals.

Overall, 80% to 90% of SCLCs will respond to chemotherapy.[56] Of patients who respond to chemotherapy, 50% will begin to relapse within 10 to 12 months.[56] From 30% to 64% of SCLCs that relapse after an initial response will subsequently respond to either the same or another type (second-line) of chemotherapy.[3] Some 20% to 25% of ED patients will achieve a CR with combination chemotherapy usually without radiation therapy.[18,56] Trials using combination chemotherapy regimens have reported survival rates of 23% at 1 year and 4% at 2 years in ED SCLC.[1] Perhaps 1% of ED patients survive beyond 5 years and may be cured, although relapse is possible beyond 5 years.[18,135] Current clinical trials using combinations of new and active agents are underway to try to improve long-term survival and reduce toxicity. A German phase II trial using carboplatin-etoposide-vincristine (CEV) in 121 previously untreated SCLC patients was associated with impressive response rates in both LD (56%) and ED (35%).[51] While median survival was only 13 months for LD and 9.5 months for ED, survival rates at greater than 2 years were impressive (29% for LD, 9% for ED). The major toxicity, myelosuppression, was considered well tolerated. A SWOG trial using intense, weekly multidrug therapy in extensive SCLC has early evidence of improving survival rates (42% at 1 year and 19% at 2 years), but final results are pending.[1] A pilot study (14 subjects) using another intense weekly chemotherapy regimen in ED SCLC met with significant toxicity (anemia, neurotoxicity, 21% septic deaths) and no improvement in median survival (9.3 months) over less toxic regimens.[142] Efforts to overcome drug resistance by use of alternating noncrossresistant regimens or high-dose regimens with or without autologous bone marrow transplant in ED have not generally improved disease-free survival, although initial

CRs are impressive.[27,56] Aggressive chemotherapy is currently not warranted outside a protocol setting for these poor prognosis SCLC patients. Most patients, however, can achieve some quality time by means of chemotherapy regimens with mild toxicities before eventual death as a result of their disease.

DELAYED EFFECTS OF TREATMENT.   Only now are there sufficient numbers of SCLC survivors to appreciate the late effects of treatment. The late toxicity of PCI with or without chemotherapy depends on total dose of radiation, port size, and concurrent therapies. Findings include cerebral atrophy, dementia, confusion, and personality changes. Efforts to decrease these effects are already in place and research is focused on whether late toxicity from PCI is worth any survival benefit.[1,45,133]

Secondary leukemias (AML) can occur, presumably resulting from chemotherapy.[56] This problem may be resolved by avoiding maintenance regimens and alkylating agents. Patients cured of SCLC who continue to smoke tobacco have a greater risk of developing a second primary lesion than of experiencing a relapse from SCLC.[18] These people need to be so advised and encouraged to stop smoking.

FUTURE CONCERNS.   Controversial issues that need to be addressed focus on the best schedule and dose of etoposide, and the role of radiation therapy in the long-term survival of limited disease SCLC patients. Whether or not chemotherapy dose intensification will lead to improved long-term survival or if the survival benefit of PCI is worth the toxicities remain to be seen. Insights gained through genetic engineering and the discovery of genetic variations unique to SCLC (i.e., myc-oncogene amplification and gene deletions in chromosome 3p) may lead to improved early detection or treatment by genetic manipulation. Two trials (SWOG 8991 and an Intergroup study) will correlate survival data with variant versus classic SCLC subtypes to assess the prognostic significance of these histologies. Use of granulocyte-macrophage colony-stimulating factor (GM-CSF) or granulocyte colony-stimulating factor (G-CSF) to prevent the frequent dose-limiting side effect of neutropenic sepsis with chemotherapy is being tested in clinical trials. Preliminary results of a SWOG study (8812) in LD SCLC suggest that patients randomized to the combined chemotherapy-radiotherapy plus GM-CSF arm had more severe toxicity (infection, thrombocytopenia) than did those who did not receive GM-CSF.

TREATMENT OF METASTASIS
Brain Metastasis

Distant metastasis rather than local chest recurrence is the most common reason for failure after curative surgery for NSCLC, and the predominant site of metastasis is the brain.[93] According to a recent Radiation Therapy Oncology Group (RTOG) study, 60% of all metastatic brain tumors come from lung cancers. Therefore, even the most vague CNS symptoms suggest the need for follow-up with CT scan.[147] Wright and Delaney report that ≥53% of lesions will be multifocal[147] (Figure 15-5). Increased intracranial pressure and cerebrospinal fluid obstruction will cause generalized symptoms such as change in level of consciousness (LOC), pupillary changes and papilledema, headache and seizures, vomiting, and change in vital signs (wide pulse pressure, increased blood pressure, bradycardia, or irregular pulse).[147] Local compression or destruction of tissue from edema or encroachment of the mass can cause a multitude of problems depending on location. "Aphasia (inability to express or understand verbal symbols), agnosia (inability to recognize objects), and apraxia (inability to execute purposeful movements)" result from pressure on the right parietal lobe.[117] A tumor in the left parietal lobe can cause difficulty with the simplest of tasks such as reading or adding up the grocery bill. Other subtle mental changes, such as recent memory loss, can occur if the limbic system is involved.

Treatment should be palliative to correct the patient's neurologic deficits, which in turn enhances quality of life.[9] For acute management of increased intracranial pressure, large doses of corticosteroids (Decadron or Medrol) can be administered, followed by radiation therapy to the whole brain (20 to 40 Gy).[10] Certain patients can benefit from surgical resection of solitary lesions followed by a course of radiation therapy, although some clinicians are questioning the value and necessity of radiation due to its late debilitating neurologic effects. A SWOG study (9021) is prospectively evaluating the benefit of postoperative radiation (in terms of both survival and quality of life) in patients with single brain metastasis via a randomized trial. The following factors must be considered in choosing the type of local treatment*:

- Number of lesions
- Location of the lesion(s)
- Type of primary tumor (whether or not it is lung cancer)
- Patient's age and performance status
- Status of other metastatic disease and the primary tumor
- Relative responsiveness to and ability to be controlled by radiotherapy
- Interval between treatment of the primary tumor and the development of brain metastasis

Coping with this very devastating complication

---

*Modified from Kornblith P and others: Treatment of metastatic cancer. In DeVita V and others, editors: Cancer: principles and practices of oncology, Philadelphia, 1985, JB Lippincott Co.

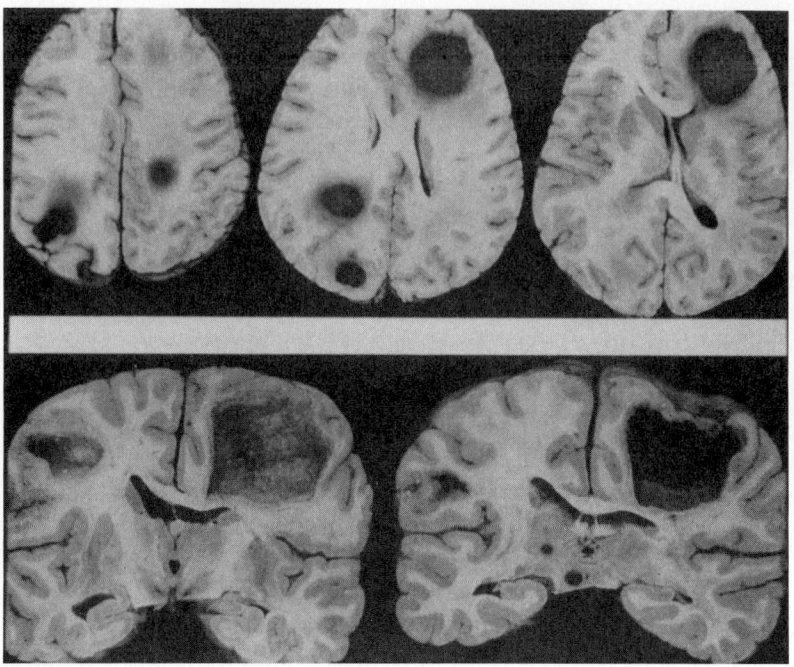

Figure 15–5 Brain metastases. (Top) Gross specimens show metastic deposits of an undifferentiated large cell lung carcinoma. The metastases form essentially necrotic masses with peripheral enhancement and peritumoral edema. (Bottom) Occasionally, extensive necrosis transforms metastases into cysts lined by only a thin rim of viable tumor.

poses a dilemma for both patient and family. The goal of treatment is to control the neurologic deficits and promote optimal lifestyle.

The following interventions may be helpful for patients with alterations in thought processes. The nurse can orient the patient through the following measures:

- Introduce self and face patient while speaking.
- Inform the patient of date, day, and time upon awakening and as needed.
- Decrease noise level and refrain from talking to other people over the patient.
- Keep patient's bed side rails up and avoid restraints unless necessary for patient safety.
- Supervise activities but allow as much autonomy as possible.
- Provide simple, step-by-step instructions for tasks.
- Provide positive reinforcement for accomplished tasks (bath, self-care, eating).
- Allow patient to sleep in clothing/shoes if no injury will occur.
- Provide for rest/naps; reduce mental activity late in day.
- Check on patient at least every hour.
- Include significant other (SO) in teaching and management of patient and refer to community resources and social services as needed.
- Encourage SO to verbalize fears and concerns, and provide support for SO.

Bone Metastasis

Characteristically, pain that becomes progressively worse over weeks or months is frequently associated with bone metastasis in the patient with lung cancer. Although this complication is rarely life-threatening, it can be disabling if pathologic fractures occur or extradural spine disease results in spinal cord compression. Malawer and Delaney report that 32.5% of all lung cancer patients will develop osseus metastasis; therefore, careful evaluation with x-rays and bone scan is required if symptoms are present.[81] Some nonspecific chemical markers may also be used, including serum alkaline phosphatase and urine hydroxyproline secretion. When bone destruction occurs, such as from metastasis, there is an elevation of alkaline phosphatase. As osteoblasts then remake new bone, hydroxypraline is released into the blood and is, in turn, secreted in the urine.

Skeletal metastasis usually occurs in the vertebra (69%), pelvis (41%), femur (25%), and skull (14%).[81] Appearance on x-ray can differ markedly. Osteolytic lesions have ragged margins and can infiltrate an entire bone. Osteoblastic lesions are sclerotic metastatic foci characterized by increased radiographic density (Figure 15-6). Occasionally, both sclerotic and lytic patterns emerge.

Patients with widespread bony metastasis, compared to a single bony lesion, usually have decreased survival time. Management for this problem is aimed at patient comfort and prevention of additional effects

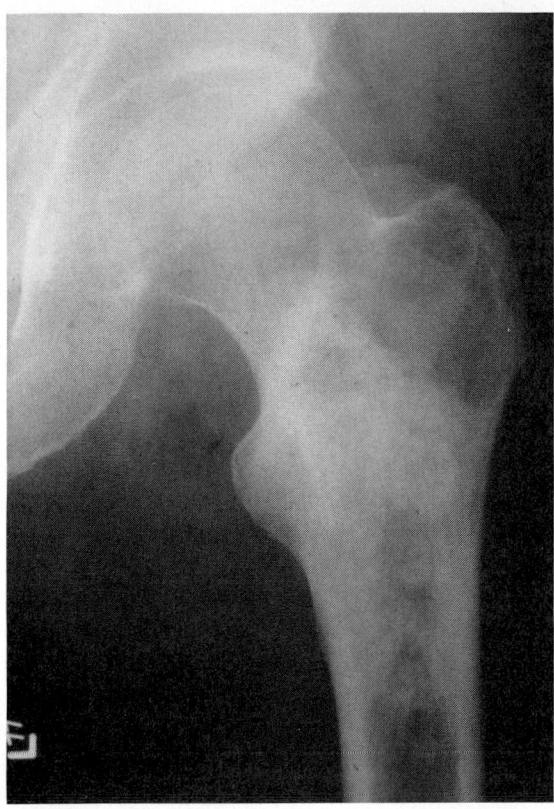

Figure 15–6 An osteoblastic metastatic lesion to the hip from adenocarcinoma of the lung.

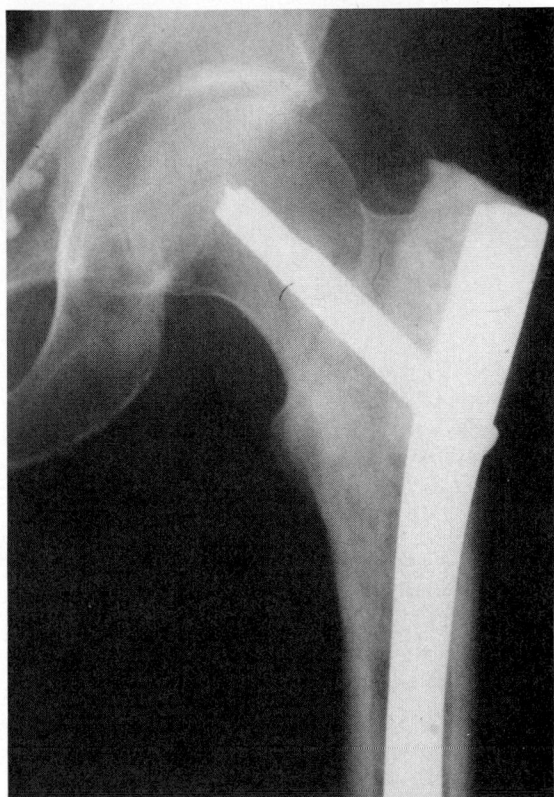

Figure 15–7 An example of a prophylactic zickel hip nailing from metastatic adenocarcinoma of the lung.

such as motor paresis and sensory loss. Narcotic medications, local nonsteroidal antiinflammatory drugs, and radiation therapy are commonly and successfully used to promote comfort and increase ambulation and mobility. Orthopedic management can be attempted to promote spinal stabilization and prevent cord compression. Prophylactic fixation of metastatic lesions in the long bones with rods (Enders) or implants (Zickel, Moore, bipolar, or total hip) can prevent pathologic fractures and ensure ambulation or upper extremity control (see Figures 15-6 and 15-7). Combination chemotherapy may also help alleviate or modify this painful process. Management for patients with bone metastasis, according to Carpenito's nursing diagnosis, includes surgical treatment and pain management.[22] The major problems for this patient are discomfort related to metastatic bone disease and impaired physical mobility resulting from surgical fixation to prevent or repair pathologic fracture.

Although most lung cancer patients will not experience prolonged survival, control of painful bony metastasis remains essential.

Liver Metastasis

For the patient with lung cancer, the added diagnosis of liver metastasis is a poor prognostic sign. Current methods of treatment with systemic or intraarterial chemotherapy or radiotherapy have little to offer in terms of prolonged survival for the patient with liver metastasis from any primary tumor site.[72] Through improved radiologic methods, however, liver anatomy and number and location of metastasis are better appreciated by the surgeon, which leads to improved resection. Also, more refined surgical techniques have somewhat improved this patient's prognosis from a surgical standpoint.

Patients with solitary metastatic sites generally survive longer than those with widespread liver metastasis.[72] Elevated liver function tests characteristic of metastatic involvement include alkaline phosphatase, gamma-glutamyl transpeptidase (GGTP), serum glutaminoxaloacetic transamine (SGOT), and lactate dehydrogenase. Hepatomegaly and liver pain denote massive end-stage liver disease.

Prophylactic treatment of liver metastasis is virtually nonexistent; palliative therapy is available through radiation or chemotherapy. Once again, in patients with lung cancer, radiation to the liver or intraarterial therapy is rarely, if ever, used. Systemic chemotherapy may be somewhat effective for a brief period of symptom control, however liver metastasis is part of the malignant process that often leads to early death.[72] If liver metastasis produces no symptoms, many clinicians believe no treatment should be initiated. Patients with painful liver involvement can usually be made comfortable with narcotics and celiac plexus blocks.

Cardiac Metastasis

Malignant involvement of the cardiac muscle produces pericardial effusion; if enough fluid accumulates in the pericardium to obstruct blood flow to the ventricle, cardiac tamponade will result.[24] The symptoms induced by pericardial effusion often mimic the cancer's overall systemic effects and include dyspnea and cyanosis, orthopnea, venous distention, leg edema, and cardiac enlargement.[102] The nurse may also observe cough, hiccups, and pain. Tamponade may develop slowly or quickly, and the severity of onset of symptoms depends on how rapidly the fluid accumulates. The nursing diagnosis would be alteration in cardiac output: decreased.[22] Treatment is generally conservative and consists of pericardiocentesis, systemic chemotherapy, or intrapericardial administration of various other agents. (See Chapter 19 for a more in-depth explanation.) If the patient's mean life expectancy is from 9 to 13 months, active treatment should be pursued. Treatment may also be undertaken for comfort reasons. Cardiac tamponade can be treated successfully and easily with a cardiac window done under local anesthesia. This is done for palliative purposes and can improve the quality of the patient's remaining life.

PLEURAL EFFUSIONS AND CHEST TUBES

The pleural cavity consists of the space between the parietal pleura and the visceral pleura. The parietal pleura lines the chest, and the visceral pleura covers the lung. The two pleura, lubricated by a thin layer of fluid, glide over each other during inspiration and expiration. A vacuum is created by the fluid and causes the surfaces to adhere to each other. In the normal lung, no true space exists between the two pleura, and, if one develops, it alters respiratory function and the lungs can no longer expand properly.[39] A pleural effusion has been created.

Lung cancer is one of the most common causes of malignant pleural effusions. About 12% of lung cancer patients present with a pleural effusion that is usually tumor related.[93] Pleural fluid can accumulate as a result of obstructed lymphatic drainage and increased capillary permeability.[24] Lung expansion is impaired with poor gas exchange, and respiratory embarrassment is the outcome. Other consequences include atelectasis and recurrent infections.[83] Many months of productive life may be possible and repeated thoracentesis may be avoided if the effusion is properly treated.

Various methods of treatment for pleural effusion are available, including repeated thoracentesis, intrapleural instillation of chemotherapy, intracavitary radioactive colloids, and pleurectomy.[102] Because these patients already have a limited life expectancy, treatment should be as fast and painless as possible to control symptoms. Instillation of a sclerosing agent—either antibiotic, antineoplastic, or radioactive—for pleural sclerosis can prevent repeated hospitalization and affords the patient good palliation.

The pleural effusion patient to be sclerosed has a chest tube, and caring for patients with chest tubes in place is always cause for concern. Assessment of the function of the chest tube should be done frequently and skillfully by the nurse.

When a chest tube is inserted, placement depends on whether it is to drain air only, such as pneumothorax (second or third intercostal space) or if it is to drain fluid, such as effusion (fourth or sixth intercostal space). Because air rises, placement will be higher for pneumothorax.

Once the chest tube has been inserted and sutured in place, it will be connected to underwater seal drainage (i.e., Pleur-evac; Figure 15-8). The principle is to keep the chest tube under sterile fluid (usually water) to prevent air from going back up the tube into the pleural cavity. If a pleural effusion is present, suction will remove the fluid from the pleural space. However, as the lung contracts during expiration, it is important to prevent air and the effusion fluid from returning to the chest cavity. This will not happen because the tube is sealed under water.

When a commercial drainage system like the Pleur-evac is used, three separate chambers (formerly bottles) are usually visible. The first compartment collects the fluid from the chest, the second compartment is the water seal chamber, and the third compartment is the suction control chamber. It maintains proper suction and limits the negative pressure applied to the pleura. This is usually set at 20 cm of water, negative pressure for adults.[39,40] If the flow rate is increased by turning up the suction regulator, more vigorous bubbling will occur in the suction control chamber, and air or fluid will be pulled more quickly from the chest. But, because the water level is set at 20 cm H_2O, there will be no increase in the negative pressure applied to the pleural cavity.

There are a few specifics to assess once the chest-tube system is in place. If the patient has a pleural effusion rather than a pneumothorax, bubbling in the water-seal chamber could indicate a leak in the system. The nurse should clamp the drainage tube near the patient with a padded hemostat, and, if the bubbling stops, there is probably a leak at the insertion site or inside the pleural cavity. If the bubbling does not stop when the tube is clamped, a leak is present in the system itself. The most likely place is the link between the chest tube and the drainage system. This must always be secured with adhesive tape to reduce the risk of air leakage.

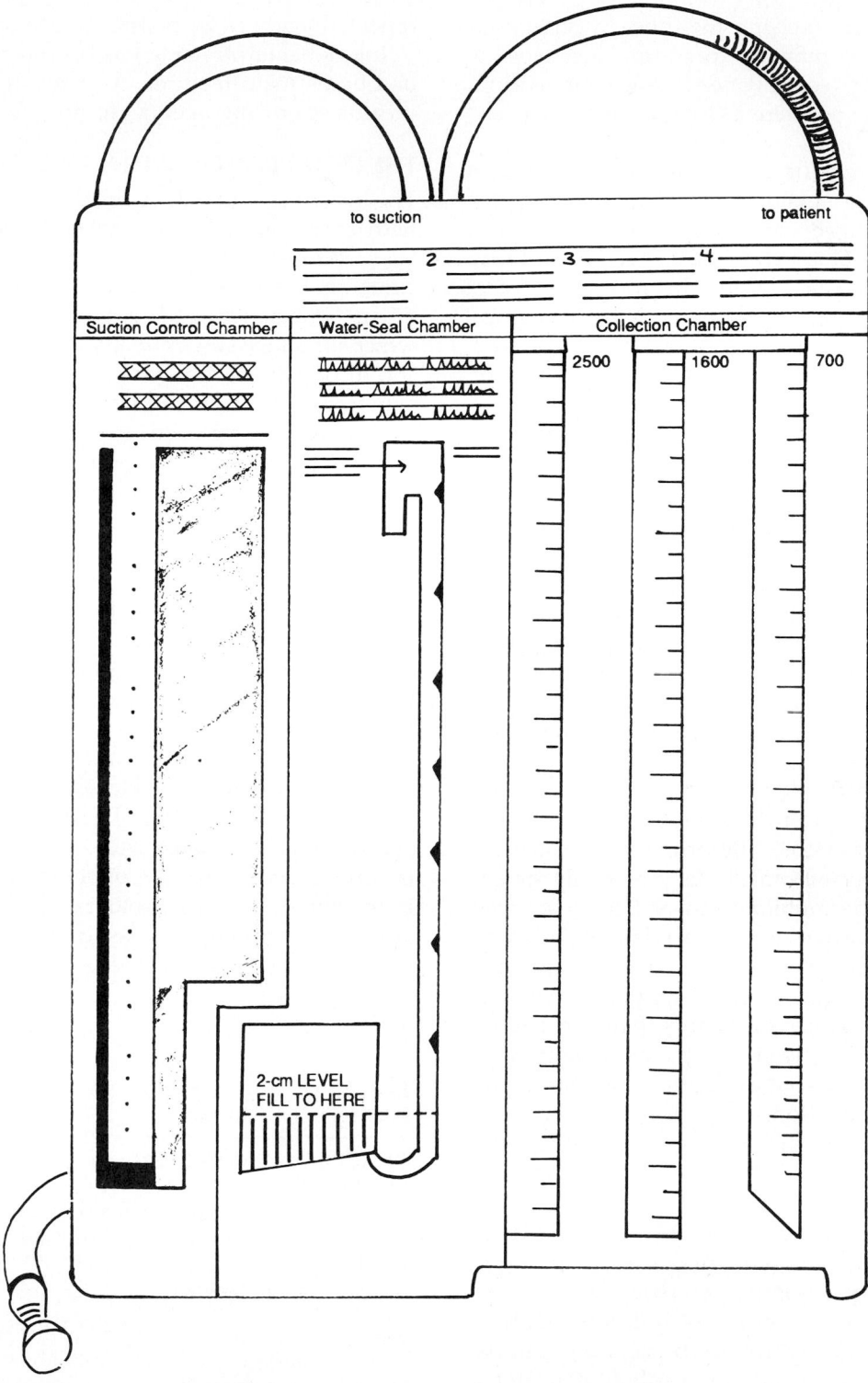

to suction

to patient

Suction Control Chamber	Water-Seal Chamber	Collection Chamber

2500   1600   700

2-cm LEVEL
FILL TO HERE

Figure 15—8 Example of Pleur-evac underwater seal drainage system. Drawing by Julie Beets.

Great *caution* must be exercised when using clamps on a chest tube. If air or fluid can no longer come out of the pleural space, but is still entering the space through the lung, a tension pneumothorax can ensue. This situation is serious because, with increased tension in the pleural space, the mediastinum is shifted to the opposite side and blood return to the

heart is dangerously impaired. If there is no blood available for cardiac output, the blood pressure is unobtainable and the patient will be in respiratory distress.[39,40]

It is rarely necessary to clamp a chest tube. Even if the chest tube becomes disconnected from the system, it is easier to reconnect it than to clamp the tube, reconnect, and then unclamp the tube. In certain instances, the clamp may be forgotten and tension pneumothorax may result. Patients can be moved and ambulated with no problem as long as the water seal is kept intact.

Stripping and milking the chest tube can also be dangerous because suction is created affecting the pleural space. This procedure may be done if the tube is obstructed by a blood clot or other material. Pressure as "high as 350 cm H_2O has been recorded with stripping. . . . Milking is a more gentle form of stripping; both forms use manual compression between the chest tube and drainage system."[40] To prevent obstruction, the nurse must ensure that there is good gravity drainage from the patient to the unit. Any dependent loop of tubing or tubing laid on the bed can create back pressure.

Unless fluid is within the drainage tube, raising the system above the chest causes no problem. Even if drained fluid is within the tubing, the only harm would be fluid returning to the pleural space. This may not be pleasant, but it is not an emergency. Other minor problems can develop, but usually these are not life-threatening. (For an in-depth and excellent chart on troubleshooting chest drainage problems, see references 39 and 40.)

Because malignant pleural effusion carries a poor prognosis in lung cancer (two thirds of patients will be dead within 3 months), the primary management goal is to control symptoms.[102] As previously stated, an agent such as the antibiotic tetracycline can be used to sclerose the patient's lung with relatively good results. Although more expensive, some physicians prefer to use bleomycin as a sclerosing agent, because there is little or no pain associated with its instillation. More important than any antineoplastic activity is the sclerosis of the pleura that the agent produces to prevent fluid reaccumulation.

Sclerosing is accomplished by instilling the tetracycline through a thoracostomy tube.[24] Closed-tube thoracostomy attached to a water seal drainage with gentle suction (usually 20 cm of H_2O) should be in place 24 to 48 hours before pleural sclerosing to promote chest drainage. Sclerosis is usually done when the total chest tube output for 24 hours is less than 100 ml. Since this procedure can be very painful, patients are usually given morphine sulfate, 5 to 10 mg IVP, 30 minutes before the procedure. Lidocaine (150 mg) is added to the tetracycline medium and the solution is instilled through the chest tube to sclerose the pleura. The chest tube is then clamped for 2 hours, and the patient is turned side to side, onto the stomach, and in Trendelenburg's and reverse Trendelenburg's position every 15 minutes to ensure equal distribution of the tetracycline. The tube is then unclamped, left to drain for 12 to 24 hours, and removed if chest tube drainage is minimal. Sclerosing can be repeated again in 24 hours, if necessary.

Injectable tetracycline has been recently discontinued by its manufacturer. As a result alternative efficacious sclerosing agents are now needed.

THE OLDER PERSON WITH LUNG CANCER

The incidence and risk of developing cancer increases with age because of several related factors that include ". . . accumulation of, or repeated contact with, carcinogens, decreased immunological resistance, hormonal imbalance and age-related cell alterations which influence susceptibility to cancer."[128] Lung cancer, in particular, may be ignored because the vague symptoms can be linked with the aging process such as fatigue, a decreased appetite, nonspecific aches and pains, and even a cough.[32]

Treatment modalities associated with lung cancer can be devastating to an older person, especially if they are already debilitated. Chemotherapy not only suppresses already tired bone marrow, but it also causes severe compromise to the patient's nutritional status (see Table 15-2). Many clinicians automatically reduce chemotherapy doses based on a patient's age. Others examine factors like the physiologic rather than the chronologic age and the likelihood of cure in decisions about doses. Intensity of chemotherapy and quality of life in the elderly have become a focus for research, particularly because of the shortened survival time associated with a lung cancer diagnosis. In a retrospective review of chemotherapy for SCLC in the elderly (age 70 or older), intensive chemotherapy (CAV regimen) was associated with more severe toxicities and deaths compared to less intensive ther-

Table 15–2 The Impact of Cancer, Cancer Treatment, and Aging on Nutrition

CANCER AND CANCER TREATMENT	
Tumor/host competition	Impaired taste
Increased requirements	Decreased salivation
Malabsorption/obstruction	Slowing of digestive process
Taste alteration (dysgeusia)	Mastication difficulties
Anorexia	Coexisting pathology
Nausea/vomiting	Altered hormonal secretions
Mucositis/oesophagitis	
Depression/fatigue	**INCREASED RISK OF**
Early satiety	Weight loss
Fluid and electrolyte imbalance	Malnutrition
	Cachexia
AGING	Muscle wasting
Impaired ability to plan/prepare meals	Impaired wound healing
Psychological/social/sensory-motor factors	Increased susceptibility to infection
	Depression, apathy
	Impaired tolerance to treatment
	Poor prognosis

From Sims S: Cancer and aging, Nursing Times 84:29, 1988.

apy (single agent, radiation alone).[43] The more intensely treated survived about 5 months longer than those less intensely treated. Authors concluded that the small survival advantage did not justify the severe toxicities of intense chemotherapy. Johnson cites two reports using single agent etoposide, which was well tolerated in the elderly.[70] One of the trials used oral etoposide (160 mg/m²) days 1 to 5 every 4 weeks in previously untreated SCLC patients age 70 and older.[131] There was a 71% response rate among 35 patients, and median survival (16 months in LD and 9 months in ED) was comparable to that achieved with combination regimens. No patient required hospitalization for neutropenia and fever, and toxicities were mild. Clearly, more research is needed in defining who among elderly lung cancer patients might benefit from treatment.

Radiation therapy is notorious for causing increased fatigue, which can cause increased problems in patients who, likely, have other chronic diseases. One important related consequence of lung cancer in the elderly is decreased comfort, not only physical, but psychological. The attitude held by many caregivers may compromise the level of comfort afforded to the elderly. Engelking gives an example of a 70-year-old lung cancer patient and states ". . . the caregiver who automatically anticipates reduced breathing capacity subsequent to the patient's age might underdose the patient with narcotic analgesics or hold back sleep medications because of concern about respiratory compromise."[37] Psychosocially, the patient may be anxious about learning how to care for themselves at home and/or obtaining assistance with this care, the increased costs of treatment and decreased insurance coverage, and, in addition, there may be an ill spouse that the patient has been caring for in the home.[48]

Many of these issues encompass all patients with cancer, however, the concern with the patient with lung cancer is their usually limited survival time after diagnosis. For the elderly, adjustments to change often come with greater difficulty, and the adjustment to lung cancer and its treatments must be made rapidly. Consequently, the nurse must be alerted to these particular problems so he or she can provide timely interventions for this patient's rapidly increasing nursing care needs.

REHABILITATION
Activity Maintenance

Little has been written on long-term survival of patients with lung cancer. Those who survive and complete their course of treatment may experience problems with radiation pneumonitis and pulmonary fibrosis, second malignancies, and neurologic complications (such as memory loss, confusion, ataxia, vision loss, and dysphagia) from prophylactic cranial irradiation. It is important to encourage patients and family members with supportive counseling, but the nurse must also offer some concrete suggestions for maintaining activities of daily living in the face of an altered life-style (see box below).

PULMONARY PROGRAM.   Patients with pulmonary fibrosis may experience exacerbation of dyspnea, which can be frightening for both the patient and family member. If this can be anticipated and measures made available to help control the physical sensations, fear and anxiety will be reduced.

Family members or significant others must be aware of what to expect and what to do if breathing difficulties ensue. Most people become agitated, diaphoretic, and pale, and they gasp for breath. They may speak with short staccato words and have a frozen appearance with large staring eyes.[59]

Patients must be educated in strategies for managing dyspnea (see box on p. 324). A grading scale for dyspnea may be helpful for the patient to describe the severity of current symptoms. If instructed to grade the dyspnea on a scale from 0 to 10 with 0 being no difficulty and 10 being unable to breathe, patients can more accurately relate the problem.[47]

Critical nursing assessment and identification of specific management techniques can prevent a crisis. The patient and caregiver will feel more comfortable knowing that, although dyspnea may occur, a program is in place to manage it.

EXERCISE AND RELAXATION TECHNIQUES.   Most patients who have been successfully treated for lung

---

MODIFICATIONS OF ACTIVITIES OF DAILY LIVING FOR PATIENT/FAMILY EXPERIENCING LUNG CANCER

Do not treat patient as an invalid just because his or her activity tolerance has decreased.

Encourage the spouse/children to include the patient in family decision making.

Help the patient establish a new daily routine with realistic goals.

• Patient can assist with small tasks (e.g., make lunches, fold clothes, help kids with homework, pay bills if mentally alert).

• Patient should try to accomplish one large task every day, every other day, or every week.

Have some small activity to look forward to (e.g., visit from a friend, ride in the car, church prayer meeting, eat out at a restaurant, call a friend long distance, participate in a support group [patient can help others as well as himself or herself], enjoy nature).

If larger scale activities are possible, encourage them but caution patient to use moderation (e.g., take a trip [there is an oncology nurse to whom the patient can be referred in almost every U.S. city], participate in an activity you have always wanted to do, such as hot air balloon ride, take a class).

STRATEGIES FOR MANAGING DYSPNEA

Breathing

Teach new breathing pattern.

Take slow, deep breaths.
Use diaphragm.
Exhale through pursed lips.
Exhale longer than inhale.

Positioning

Have patient assume comfortable position.

Sit on bedside, fold arms over pillow on bedside table.
Sit on chair, feet wide apart, elbows resting on knees.
Lean on wall, feet apart, shoulders relaxed and bent forward.
Elevate head of bed.

Emotional support

Do not leave patient in distress alone.

Observe patient frequently.
Place frequent phone call to patient on home care.
Teach coaching and support to family or caregiver.

Relaxation

Relaxation conserves oxygen.

Place hands on patient's shoulders and press downward.
Dangle arms and rotate shoulders.

Planned activity

Have patient conserve energy and get adequate rest.

Assess normal life-style and activities of daily living.
Plan chores around rest period.
Establish support for household activities, recreation.

Oxygen therapy

Provide oxygen supply and implement safety precautions.

Provide instructions regarding smoking, storage, heat, and use of equipment.

Pharmacologic agents

Some agents relieve dyspnea, especially in patients who are terminally ill.

Sedatives, narcotics, steroids, scopolamine.

Reprinted with permission from Haylock P: Breathing difficulty: changes in respiratory function, Semin Oncol Nurs 3:293, 1987.

cancer or are presently going through treatment realize intellectually that they must begin exercise gradually, but many do not comply. Exercise is a positive reinforcer for patients, in that it helps them feel good and increases their activity tolerance, but the nurse must caution the patient against too much exercise and activity too soon.

An assessment should be made of anticipated activities and activity tolerance. Foote explains that the assessment should include "patient responsibilities, normal routine of activities, support systems, recreational activities, and tolerance to activity."[47] The patient's overall state of health will dictate level of functioning and ability to maintain an exercise program (see box on p. 323 for modifications of activities of daily living).

The effective management of short- and long-term side effects from lung cancer treatment is essential for patient rehabilitation. The aforementioned activities foster hope in patients with lung cancer and assure

them that they are not forgotten or abandoned. However, Bernhard and Ganz explain that although there is a high incidence of lung cancer, we know very little about the varied psychosocial issues related to this disease[8,9] (see Table 15-3). Increasing our knowledge base relative to the psychosocial impact of lung cancer will assist the nurse in planning appropriate intervention programs and promote optimal use of resources. Overcoming as many treatment barriers as possible will motivate the patient and family toward achieving increased and sustained independence.

HOME HEALTH AND HOSPICE

The majority of lung cancer patients will experience progressive disease with increasing symptoms and consequently increased dependency on others for self-care needs. Inherent in such a downhill trajectory is the need for frequent interventions and/or hospitalizations. In one study, the most common reasons for hospital admissions of lung cancer patients were:

Table 15–3 Currently Available Database on Disease and Treatment—Related Psychosocial Issues in Lung Cancer

Symptoms	Data Availability
Psychosocial impact of surgery	Partly available
Acute side effects of chemotherapy	Well documented
Late side effects of chemotherapy	Partly available
Side effects of radiotherapy	Not available
Pain	Partly available
Dyspnea	Well documented
Cognitive changes	Well documented
Sleep disorders	Not available
Psychologic distress	Partly available
Social interaction	Partly available
Consequences for patient's next of kin	Not available
Multidisciplinary interventions in regard to:	
Anticipatory nausea and vomiting	Partly available
Learned food aversions	Partly available
Self-care of dyspnea	Not available
Pain management	Not available
Management of sleep disorders	Not available

Adapted with permission from Bernhard J and Ganz P: Psychosocial issues in lung cancer patients (Part 2), Chest 99:480-485, 1991.

cancer therapy (the primary reason), respiratory problems, gastrointestinal symptoms, pain, anemia, and thrombocytopenia.[82] At issue is how to maintain the best quality of life for these patients. Because DRGs and cost-containment have relegated so much care to the outpatient setting, early referral to home health is often indicated, preferably to an agency that allows patients to convert to hospice care when appropriate. A nursing study found that early referral (within 2 months of diagnosis) of patients eligible for home health care compared to routine follow-up through a doctor's office was associated with a 6-week delay in symptom distress, a longer period of independence, and a more realistic perception of declining health.[82] In addition, patients referred to specialized oncology home care versus standard home care or routine doctor's office follow-up, spent fewer days hospitalized. This finding, although not statistically significant, is of economic significance, and suggests that oncology specialization among RNs contributes to improved symptom management at home and reduction of hospitalized days.

Nurses caring for lung cancer patients in the home setting today may be involved in their actual therapy via chemotherapy administration and management of side effects. The nurse's knowledge base must include use of newer technology (care of various central venous or arterial access devices, patient-controlled an-

algesia pumps, and epidural catheters). Nursing expertise to assist patients in understanding chronic pain management (use of scheduled versus PRN narcotics, oral dosing in preference to use of pumps when appropriate, prophylactic bowel regimens to prevent constipation) may obviate trips to the emergency room or hospitalizations. Patient and family may need assistance to understand the important role of low dose morphine (2.5 mg to 5 mg every 4 hours) as it acts centrally in the brain to relieve severe dyspnea and "air hunger" associated with end-stage respiratory compromise, crucial comfort measures. Compassionate nursing can assist families to know what to expect and how to deal with these events, particularly when death may be that event. Death from fatal hemoptysis, though sometimes feared, is rare; only 3.3% of patients in one large series died of exsanguination from tumor eroding through a major pulmonary vessel.[74] Historically, 60% of lung cancer patients die from tumor causing airway obstruction, postobstructive pneumonia, and sepsis.[71] Caring and knowledgable home health and hospice nurses can do much to reduce the suffering associated with lung cancer.

PROGNOSIS
Prognostic Factors

Three factors play a major role in the prognosis of lung cancer: extent of disease, cell type, and performance status. The survival rate for patients with localized disease is 37%, however, survival at 5 years is 13% for all patients regardless of stage at diagnosis.[2] This represents a slight improvement in overall survival since the early 1970s.[15] Prognosis is best for patients with well-differentiated squamous cell lung cancer, and those with small cell cancer have the poorest survival rate. Performance status is critical in determining the patient's treatment regimen and, therefore, the prognosis. Patients who are ambulatory tolerate treatment better than those who are not fully ambulatory but are out of bed 50% of the time. Prognosis continues to decline as the patient becomes more debilitated.

Age, sex, weight loss, and immune status will also affect the patient's response to treatment.[27] Physiologic rather than chronologic age is the important assessment factor when making treatment decisions, and age may influence treatment options and prognosis in the elderly (see earlier in this chapter).

Adenocarcinoma is more predominant in female lung cancer patients, whereas squamous cancer is more prevalent in male patients. Overall, women with lung cancer survive longer than their male counterparts in the United States.[89] In addition to the previous prognostic factors, weight loss of greater than 10 pounds in 6 months is not a favorable sign. Patients with an intact immune system, as evidenced by a normal reaction to an immunologic challenge, will respond better.[89] Patients with SCLC have an immune deficit that may contribute to the rapid growth of this cancer.[18] Because any lung cancer patient will be exposed to multimodality treatment, it is important to be able to predict tolerance to such intense therapy.

Correlation with Histologic Cell Type and Stage

NON-SMALL CELL LUNG CANCER (NSCLC). The American Joint Committee on Cancer (AJCC) classification system and new international staging system are used to determine the best therapy modalities for NSCLC. Successful treatment with surgery or radiation therapy is possible in a majority of patients with stage I disease; however, only 25% to 30% of patients present with stage I and II NSCLC.[89,93] Adjuvant chemotherapy is currently being investigated for use in patients with early stage disease.[10] For patients who present with widespread advanced disease, the administration of new combinations of chemotherapy has shown only a slight survival benefit.

Even with new treatment combinations, benefits and cure rates are modest. Five-year survival rates following resection for NSCLC are reasonably good and have continued to improve as the result of stricter patient selection and progressive nursing support.[58] Few patients are eligible for resection, however, and Mountain reports that one half of one group of patients died from recurrent or metastatic disease after apparent complete resection.[92]

Patients with squamous cell cancer survive longer than do those with adenocarcinoma and large cell undifferentiated carcinoma. Also, those patients with stage I squamous cell cancer do significantly better than those with stage II and III tumors.[89] Table 15-4 depicts the overall 5-year postoperative survival of both squamous cell and adenocarcinoma lung cancer patients.

Depending on the TNM status and cell type of stage IIIa patients, survival ranges from 18% to 40%. The outlook for stage IIIb and IV patients remains bleak, but therapeutic strategies including biologic response modifiers and monoclonal antibodies are continually being pursued.[89] More successful treatments for NSCLC are being discovered, albeit slowly.

SMALL CELL LUNG CANCER (SCLC). Given the great biologic and clinical difference from other lung cancer types, SCLC is also staged differently. The two-stage (limited and extensive) classification system is a useful prognostic tool. Limited stage disease is present in about 30% of all SCLC patients. Patients with limited stage disease who are treated with combination chemotherapy experience a 12 to 16 month median survival time, and a 15% to 20%, 2-year disease free survival rate.[89] Recent combined radiation-che-

Table 15-4 Five-Year Postoperative Survival by TNM Groups Based on Data From Lung Cancer Study Group Trials

Classification	*Percent Surviving Squamous Cell Carcinoma* (n = 549)	*Percent Surviving Adenocarcinoma* (n = 572)
Stage I		
T1N0	83	69 (P = 0.02)
T2N0	64	57
Stage II		
T1N1	75	52 (P = 0.04)
T2N1	53	25 (P ≤ 0.01)
Stage IIIA		
T1-2N2	46	35
T3N0	37	21

From Carmack Holmes E: Staging Non-Small Cell Lung Cancer, Bristol-Meyers Squibb Co.

motherapy approaches show 24% to 54% survival at 2 years in LD.[1,25,70,139] Unfortunately, patients with SCLC may still relapse 5 years after treatment.[135] Without treatment, SCLC results in death in about 3 months.[65]

The best approach for long-term survival in limited stage SCLC appears to be combination chemotherapy and radiation therapy to the chest. Researchers advocate alternating chemotherapy treatment cycles to prevent resistance to the drugs,[41] however, clinical trials have failed to demonstrate improved survival by this technique, perhaps due to the inability to define truly non-crossresistant regimens.[56]

In limited stage I and II disease, patients without mediastinal node involvement who underwent surgical resection and received combination chemotherapy following surgery had a 5-year survival rate of 35%.[5] These patients represent less than 5% of SCLC patients. For patients with stage III disease, preoperative chemotherapy followed by surgery was attempted without dramatic results. Many randomized prospective studies have incorporated all the treatment modalities both alone and in combination. Although investigations continue to look for the best combination, preliminary data suggest benefit from combined therapy in limited SCLC if full doses of chemotherapy and radiation therapy are given.[1,25]

The majority of patients (70%) with SCLC have extensive disease, and the outlook for their survival is dismal. Seven to 20% of these patients will be alive 2 years after diagnosis.[1] In one study from The National Cancer Institute of Canada, median survival was 8.1 months in patients treated with Carboplatin and etoposide.[42] Radiation plays a major role in local control and in symptom management to limit or modify cranial and bone metastasis and superior vena cava syndrome. Many patients with extensive disease respond to therapy involving a combination of drugs and achieve notable palliation.

In a review of SWOG trials, one versus multiple metastatic sites was a predictor of survival.[1] In patients with a single site, median survival was 12 months versus only 7 months in those with multiple metastatic sites. Other factors predictive of survival are a normal LDH and absence of a pleural effusion.[1]

Patients with extensive disease who experience a complete remission will usually survive beyond the median timeframe.[27] Although initial responses can be dramatic for both limited and extensive SCLC, long-term survival is worse than that seen with NSCLC. SCLC overall survival rate at 2 years is less than 10%.[25,56] It is obvious that more knowledge of this disease and new agents or treatment combinations are needed to obtain better outcomes.

Text continued on p. 335.

Nursing Management

Nursing diagnoses related to lung cancer listed below are followed by nursing interventions for various treatments and rehabilitation.

PRINCIPAL NURSING DIAGNOSES

- Knowledge deficit related to prevention of lung cancer (see p. 303 for suggested educational guidelines)
- Ineffective breathing pattern related to loss of adequate ventilation (actual or potential)
- Impaired gas exchange related to decreased passage of gases between the alveoli of the lungs and the vascular system (actual or potential)
- Knowledge deficit related to a new medical condition, new treatments, surgical procedures (preoperative and postoperative), and medications
- Alteration in nutrition: less than body requirements related to anorexia
- Alteration in comfort related to liver and/or bone metastasis (actual or potential)
- Alteration in thought processes related to brain metastasis (actual or potential)
- Fatigue related to treatment and treatment sequelae

SECONDARY NURSING DIAGNOSES

- Anxiety related to dyspnea
- Powerlessness related to hospitalization and feelings of lack of control
- Noncompliance (potential) related to negative side effects of prescribed treatments
- Grieving related to loss of function of body system
- Disturbance in self-concept related to loss of body functions
- Sexual dysfunction related to change of body part/physiologic limitations
- Coping, ineffective individual/family related to rapidly progressive disease process

SURGERY

Surgical nursing care begins during the diagnostic period for those patients requiring mediastinoscopy (a small suprasternal incision) or mediastinotomy (a small parasternal incision that allows direct visualization of lymph nodes or through which left mediastinal lymph nodes or even a lung primary may be biopsied) for tissue diagnosis and/or staging purposes.[90] Monitoring blood pressure, pulse, respirations, and observing dressings for indication of internal or external bleeding are necessary in the immediate postoperative period. Fever can indicate mediastinitis; crepitus can indicate air leakage into subcutaneous tissues; and the development of dyspnea, cyanosis, or decreased breath sounds can be signs of pneumothorax.[77] Postoperative, local pain will require analgesics. See box on p. 312.

In patients who undergo thoracotomy for wedge resection, lobectomy, or pneumonectomy, nursing care is more complex. Standard nursing concerns in these patients are the same as for other cancer surgeries (e.g., adequate nutritional state, coping mechanisms, and risk of postoperative emboli) and are addressed in depth in Chapter 27. Some of these concerns will be addressed here.

Malnutrition, hypoalbuminemia, smoking history, and chronic obstructive pulmonary disease (COPD) place lung cancer patients at higher risk of postoperative complication such as pneumonia, fistula formation, and respiratory or congestive heart failure.[83] Preoperative or postoperative total parenteral nutrition may be necessary to improve nutritional status and promote recovery from thoracotomy. If there is a delay in surgery, smokers should be advised to stop smoking at least a few weeks before surgery. Although preoperative pulmonary function studies should predict the patients' ability to undergo surgery, patients need to know before thoracotomy that they may be placed on a ventilator and will have one or more chest tubes after the procedure.

The most common postoperative complication is cardiac dysrhythmia. Often asymptomatic, it is responsive to appropriate drugs.[89] The nature of drainage from chest tubes placed after partial pulmonary resection can reveal bleeding complications or development of empyema. In patients who become agitated, confused, then dyspneic and hypoxic, serious alterations in ventilation and respiration are likely, and monitoring vital signs, breath sounds, and blood gases is important. Diligent aspiration of the tracheobronchial tree with frequent deep breathing and coughing can prevent mechanical obstruction and pneumonia resulting from the accumulation of secretion. However, deep suctioning that could cause trauma to the suture line is to be avoided.[77]

The need for good pulmonary toilet cannot be overemphasized. Patients may have a lot of fear and discomfort associated with chest tubes or a ventilator, for which medication may be required. Good pain management, a major nursing concern after thoracotomy, can enhance mobility, coughing, and deep breathing. An epidural catheter to control pain may be placed during surgery; this enables the patient to recover more comfortably. Some patients may need narcotic analgesics for several months after the operation to ease persistent pain. For prolonged postoperative pain, nerve blocks or other interventions should be considered. Depending, of course, on the amount of healthy lung tissue remaining after surgery, most patients will not experience severe respiratory compromise affecting life-style activities.[83] See the box on this page for important patient teaching priorities related to surgical procedures.

RADIATION THERAPY
Radiation to the Chest

Side effects experienced during or after radiation therapy will vary depending on (1) the organ systems or normal tissue within the radiation port (field), (2) the amount and duration of radiation, and (3) the type of concurrent or recent chemotherapy. When radiation is given to the primary tumor in the chest, portions of normal lung tissue, heart, skin, and contents of the mediastinum (major vessels, trachea, esophagus) may also receive radiation, although the dose will be much lower. By noting the tattoos or marks delineating the radiation port on the patient's chest, the nurse can make some assumptions about the effects of radiation on normal tissues. Although efforts are made to block vital organs, some side effects are unavoidable. Nursing interventions focus on avoidance, relief, or management of side effects. See box on p. 329.

Skin alterations related to radiation are much less severe than in the past. Equipment has been improved so it can deliver the radiation beneath the surface of the skin and more directly to the desired depth and location. Nursing assessment of skin integrity, the patient's complaints, and knowledge of anticipated side effects form the basis of interventions. Skin damage may be only mild erythema or can progress to dry and then moist desquamation. If moist desquamation occurs, radiation treatments will likely be interrupted.[36] Therefore, teaching should highlight pre-

---

PATIENT TEACHING PRIORITIES
SURGERY

Preoperative
- Have patient relate knowledge of reason for surgery preoperatively.
- Describe the type of procedure to be done (wedge resection, lobectomy, pneumonectomy).
- Discuss the need for optimal ventilation (stop smoking, cough, and take deep breaths immediately after surgery).
- Explain the need for leg and arm exercises. Shoulder on the affected side will be very sore and must be moved to prevent frozen shoulder.[8]
- Discuss different methods of pain relief (IM, IV, epidural) with the patient. Encourage the patient to ask for medication when needed. This promotes coughing and deep breathing.
- Explain the postoperative routine and that the patient will most likely have a chest tube in place.

Postoperative
- Reinforce the need for early ambulation despite the chest tube, and also the need to cough and deep breathe.
- Reinforce all postoperative routines previously taught.
- Review surgical results with the patient and ensure proper follow-up.
- Explore with the patient the implications of altered body image:
  Changes in lifestyle
  Verbalization of fear of rejection and reaction of others
  Changes in relationships
  Problems with sexuality

---

ventive care: avoid constrictive clothing over irradiated areas; avoid tape, perfume, deodorants, iodine, talcum, or other irritating substances on irradiated skin; wear soft cotton clothing over skin; and avoid heat, cold, or sunlight on these areas. The skin should be kept dry and open to the air when possible. For tender or dry skin, use water-based ointments (e.g., A & D Ointment, hydrous lanolin) rather than oil-based creams or ointments, which may contain heavy metals. Vigorous scrubbing or rubbing is to be avoided, but use of gentle soaps (Aveeno, Dove) is usually allowed.[60,124] If moist desquamation occurs, the area may be cleansed with half-strength hydrogen peroxide and normal saline, rinsed gently with saline, and patted dry.[124] Areas of skin break-down should be monitored for infection. Moisture-vapor-permeable dressings (Op-site, Tegaderm) could offer protection to these areas.[123] Most patients have skin reactions by their last week of therapy.[60] Administration of certain chemotherapeutic drugs (e.g., dactinomycin and doxorubicin) during or close to the time radiation ther-

---

PATIENT TEACHING PRIORITIES
RADIATION THERAPY

General side effects of radiation therapy

- Explain measures to limit, as necessary, the patient's activities during treatment to conserve energy.
- Discuss measures to maintain adequate nutritional intake.
- Explain measures to control radiodermatitis if necessary.
- Describe rationale and measures to take following a decrease in hematopoietic function.
- Discuss reasons for and measures to deal with sexuality concerns.

Site-specific side effects

- Describe signs and symptoms of pneumonitis, esophagitis, and cough.
- Discuss measures to maintain adequate oxygenation.
- Consider forcing fluids to loosen thick secretions.
- Administer antiemetics for nausea/vomiting.
- Caution patient to avoid tobacco and alcohol.
- Note availability of patient information booklets.

Emotional support

- Educate patient/family regarding radiation therapy procedures to decrease anxiety.
- Explain that side effects may last for 2 to 4 weeks after treatment completion.
- Ensure understanding of anxiety or grief process because of illness and reassure patient that this is normal response.

---

apy starts can lead to radiation recall, and erythema or skin break-down may occur.[36,60]

Sore throat resulting from esophagitis can develop by the third week of radiation.[36,60] If the pain is severe, food and fluid intake may be decreased because of difficulty swallowing. Patients should be advised that, if this occurs, they should contact the nurse or doctor. Not only can nutrition be impaired, but esophagitis may become a source for infection. If signs of candidiasis (white, adherent plaques) are present in the oral cavity, an antifungal agent should be prescribed (Mycelex Troches, nystatin, or ketoconazole). A soft, bland diet (noncitrus) and nutritional supplements (e.g., Ensure, Instant Breakfast) can be beneficial.[124] If weight loss resulting from esophagitis occurs, the patient should be weighed daily and evaluated for dehydration. A mixture of diphenhydramine elixir, viscous lidocaine, and Mylanta or Amphojel (depending on the consistency of the patient's stools) in a 1:1:1 ratio can be administered as a swish and swallow remedy when esophagitis is painful (5 ml before meals and as needed). Systemic analgesics may be required.

Nutritional status can be further compromised by anorexia, which occurs in the majority of patients by the fourth week of treatment.[36,60] Anorexic patients should be encouraged to eat small amounts frequently. The book *Eating Hints* by the NCI may aid patients and their families in discovering types of food more tolerable to these patients. Good nutrition is essential to repair and heal normal tissues during radiation therapy.

Fatigue is a major problem in over 90% of patients by the third week of treatment.[60] Patients should be so warned and guided into planning any activities with scheduled rest periods. Symptoms may persist 3 months after completion of radiation therapy (in 46% of patients in one study).[84]

If more than 25% of active bone marrow is in the radiation port, myelosuppression may occur.[84] Complete blood counts should be done weekly during therapy. Neutropenia and thrombocytopenia precede a drop in hemoglobin. Packed red cells may be transfused if the latter drops below 10 g, because effective radiation treatment depends on an adequate oxygen supply to the tumor.[124] If the white blood cell count (WBC) drops to below 3000 or the platelets drop below 40,000, radiation therapy may be temporarily discontinued.

Radiation pneumonitis is uncommon but is dose-limiting, should it occur during radiation treatments. Being dose-dependent, it can occur 3 to 24 weeks after therapy.[84] In acute radiation pneumonitis, a hacking cough or mild chest pain might be the first sign. Symptoms include dyspnea and hypoxia, fever, night sweats, there will be evidence of interstitial or alveolar infiltrates on chest x-ray, and the sputum will be negative for pathogens.[141] The severity of symptoms correlates with the dose and lung volume irradiated. In severe cases, pneumonitis may be associated with hemoptysis, fever, chills, or abscess, and may even result in death.[84] Usually, doses of 45 Gy or less will not lead to severe toxicity, and pneumonitis will resolve, often within 3 to 4 weeks.[141] Patients may require temporary hospitalization for administration of oxygen, steroids, antibiotics, sedatives, and cough suppressants. Cultures are obtained to rule out infection, but antibiotics may be given empirically. Steroids are the cornerstone of therapy for radiation pneumonitis. At the start of therapy, patients should be given at least 60 mg of prednisone per day. Tapering is carried out very gradually, and the patients must be watched for any recurrence of symptoms.

Coping strategies for dyspnea are often self-taught, but may include position changes, moving slowly, and planning in advance for activities.[145] If pneumonitis leads to subsequent scarring and tissue changes (pulmonary fibrosis), chest auscultation will reveal muffled and diminished vesicular sounds, rhonchi, and wheezes from air flow across narrowed airways. Late fibrotic changes resemble severe chronic obstructive pulmonary disease and can lead to anxiety and fear with dyspnea.[59]

Cardiac toxicities, albeit minimal today because of blocking techniques, can include pericarditis, the classic symptom for which is chest pain, or a pericardial effusion and tamponade, which involves increased central venous pressure noted by jugular venous distention that is followed by tachycardia, dyspnea, and cough (see Chapter 19). Cardiac toxicities usually depend on delivery of at least 40 Gy to the heart.

Radiation to the Brain

Radiation to the brain can lead to hair loss, but the severity of hair loss is usually dose-dependent. At doses of 15 to 30 Gy, the degree of hair loss is variable. At a dose of 45 Gy or more, permanent loss is likely.[84] Because PCI in SCLC is usually no more than 30 Gy, hair will begin to regrow about 3 to 4 weeks after the completion of radiation. However, hair loss after PCI will be temporarily complete, including the eyebrows.[84] Resources and ways to deal with hair loss are discussed later in Chapter 31.

During brain irradiation, patients are placed on dexamethasone to reduce resultant edema of brain tissue. However, symptoms of neurologic impairment related to edema should be monitored and could include irritability, confusion, restlessness, headaches, memory loss, a change in personality or mental status, nausea, unequal or decreased pupil reactivity to light, elevated blood pressure, sensory or motor changes, or a drop in pulse rate. Cerebral edema can lead to obstruction of the eustachian tube with resultant local ear pain or infection.[84]

Late effects of whole brain irradiation (WBI) in long-term survivors may be even more severe when it is given concurrently with chemotherapy. Findings reflecting neurologic injury can include memory loss, problems in judgment, parkinsonian symptoms, weakness, confusion, depression, dizziness, organic brain syndrome, abnormal gait, ataxia, intention tremors, inability to concentrate, and cerebral atrophy.[1,18] Symptoms have become so severe that one patient had to quit work while another was placed in an extended care facility.[1] Any sequelae such as these should be documented, and the physician should be notified for possible CT or MRI evaluation. Any such changes could also herald a CNS relapse. Potential radiation treatment-related complications of lung cancer are listed in the box on this page.

Radiation Implant

Implants may be used to treat large and otherwise inaccessible tumor masses in the lung. Nursing care of these patients follows guidelines discussed on p. 329. For an excellent high dose-rate brachytherapy

---

RADIATION TREATMENT-RELATED COMPLICATIONS OF LUNG CANCER

Radiation (or radiation plus chemotherapy-induced)*

From radiation to the chest
- Skin erythema to wet desquamation
- Esophagitis, dysphagia, strictures, weight loss
- Acute pneumonitis or pulmonary fibrosis (dyspnea, hypoxemia, chronic or temporary oxygen and steroid-dependency)
- Pericarditis, arrhythmias, pericardial effusion, CHF
- Myelosuppression (sepsis, bleeding, fatigue)
- Fatigue

From radiation to the brain
- Early and usually temporary effects: hair loss, skin erythema, nausea
- Signs of cerebral edema that need immediate attention during radiation: irritability, confusion, restlessness, headaches, nausea, change in personality, sensory or motor changes
- Late and permanent effects: memory loss, problems in judgment, parkinsonian symptoms, weakness, confusion, depression, dizziness, organic brain syndrome, abnormal gait, intention tremor, inability to concentrate, loss of self-care or work capability, cerebral atrophy

*Concurrent chemotherapy and radiation can augment all these effects.

---

guide regarding nursing care and patient educational material, the reader is referred to Jordan.[71]

Patient teaching related to radiation therapy should include the information given in the box on p. 329.

Combined Radiation and Chemotherapy

Normal radiation therapy toxicities on organ systems are increased to varying degrees by concomitant or consecutive (within weeks of) administration of certain chemotherapy drugs. The severity of the toxicity depends on the drug and its dose, the radiation dose, and the timing of each in relation to the other. Damage to the target organ may be short-term, permanent and life-changing, or fatal. Because radiation therapy ports for lung cancer patients can involve the heart, the lungs, the brain, and other contents of the mediastinum, the potential severity of any synergistic drug-radiation toxicity is great. Specifically, esophagitis can lead to a stricture, CNS damage can include leukoencephalopathy or necrosis, or fatal interstitial fibrosis of large lung volumes can occur.[43] Nursing knowledge of these agents can help prevent toxicities resulting from their concomitant administration during radiation therapy. Combination chemotherapy regimens involving any of the drugs listed in the left-hand box on p. 331 may enhance and broaden the spectrum of usual organ system toxicities. Neither intrathecal therapy nor systemic chemotherapy with these

DRUGS POTENTIATING RADIATION TOXICITY AND TARGET ORGAN	
Bleomycin*	Lung,* skin, mucosa
Doxorubicin*	Lung,* heart,* skin, mucosa, esophagus
Etoposide (VP-16)	Heart
5-Fluorouracil	Lung, heart, skin, mucosa
Hydroxyurea	Lung, skin, mucosa, esophagus
Methotrexate*	CNS,* lung, skin, mucosa, bone/soft tissue
Mitomycin	Lung, heart
Procarbazine	Esophagus
Vinblastine	Esophagus
Vincristine	CNS

*Drugs/organ systems with potential for fatal toxicity if chemotherapy given in combination with radiation.
Modified from McNaull F: Radiation therapy for lung cancer: nursing considerations, Semin Oncol Nurs 3:194, 1987.

CHEMOTHERAPY TREATMENT-RELATED COMPLICATIONS OF LUNG CANCER

Myelosuppression (sepsis, bleeding, weakness, fatigue)
Nephrotoxicity (compromised renal function, Mg + wasting)
Hemorrhagic cystitis
Neurotoxicity
  Peripheral neuropathies (paresthesias, jaw pain, sensory loss, motor weakness, constipation or ileus, tinnitus, permanent hearing loss)
  CNS toxicity (confusion, hallucinations, somnolence, coma)
Cardiac (myopathy, arrhythmia, CHF, MI)
Pneumonitis or pulmonary fibrosis
Nausea and vomiting (dehydration, weight loss)
Taste changes (anorexia, weight loss)
Mucositis (pain, difficulty swallowing, weight loss, diarrhea)
Anaphylaxis (death) or hypotension
Alopecia
Tissue damage and pain if vesicant extravasates
SIADH and hyponatremia

agents should be given during radiation to the associated target organ unless part of a specific protocol or investigational study, in which the rationale for combined radiation and chemotherapy is clearly stated and the patient understands the risks before therapy is begun.

Chemotherapy

Patients with lung cancer, especially small cell carcinoma, may receive a number of chemotherapy drugs having multiple potential toxicities and, in some cases, synergistic toxicities because two or more treatment modalities are being used sequentially or simultaneously (see box at upper right). These toxicities include myelosuppression, nausea and vomiting, renal damage, cardiac insult, pneumonitis/fibrosis, hemorrhagic cystitis, neurotoxicities, stomatitis, extravasation, and phlebitis.

Because Taxol is becoming more available[26] and has shown activity in lung cancer in phase I and II clinical trials, it warrants some discussion. After reconstitution in cremophor and further dilution in normal saline or D5W, Taxol must be infused through a 0.2 micron in-line filter using non-polyvinyl chloride tubing. While the major and dose-limiting side effect is neutropenia (nadir day 8 to 10), others include:

1. Thrombocytopenia and anemia
2. Cumulative peripheral neuropathies (most often glove-and-stocking distribution)
3. Reversible anaphylactoid hypersensitivity reaction due to the cremophor vehicle and usually avoided by slowing the rate of IV infusion (3- to 24-hour infusions rather than bolus) and pretreatment with steroids and antihistamines (diphenhydramine and cimetidine)
4. A 30% incidence of asymptomatic or symptomatic cardiac arrhythmias (bradycardia, A-V

block, bundle branch block, ventricular tachycardia) or acute myocardial infarction
5. Complete and sudden alopecia (all body hair)
6. Stomatitis (can be severe)
7. Rare nausea and vomiting
8. Also: arthralgias or myalgias (2 to 3 days after treatment, can require narcotic analgesics); occasional phlebitis; brawny induration if extravasation occurs; fatigue; hepatic dysfunction[35,78,112,113]

The significance of the cardiac arrhythmias is still unclear, but is the focus of current research. For the present, Rowinsky recently recommended a conservative approach (use of cardiac monitoring) when Taxol is given with cisplatin or for patients receiving only Taxol but having known cardiac disease.[114]

Nursing assessment and management of these toxicities can help to greatly improve the quality of life for the patient and are discussed in depth in Chapter 22. For an excellent nursing process approach to managing side effects of chemotherapy, the reader is referred to Burke.[19]

Some of the newer or investigational regimens used in small cell and non-small cell lung cancer are listed in Tables 15-5 and 15-6. Some of these have been associated with significant toxicity. For doses and schedules of common chemotherapeutic regimens, see Tables 15-7 and 15-8. These tables are not intended to be a comprehensive summary of all available regimens, but merely a sample of current therapies.

Patient teaching priorities related to chemotherapy are listed in the box on p. 334.

Table 15–5   New or Investigational Chemotherapy Regimens in Nonsmall Cell Lung Cancer[17,26,113]

Drug Regimen	Dose	Schedule
ICE		
Ifosfamide (+Mesna)	4 gm/m² IV day 1	Every 4 weeks
Cisplatin	25 mg/m² IV days 1-3	Every 4 weeks
Etoposide (VP-16)	100 mg/m² IV days 1-4	Every 4 weeks
or		
Ifosfamide (+Mesna)	5 gm/m² IV over 24 hour day 1	Every 4 weeks
Carboplatin	300 mg/m² IV day 1	Every 4 weeks
Etoposide (VP-16)	120 mg/m² IV days 1-2 and 240 mg/m² PO day 3	Every 4 weeks
MIP		
Mitomycin-C	6 mg/m² IVP day 1	Every 3-4 weeks
Ifosfamide (+Mesna)	4 gm/m² IV day 1	Every 3-4 weeks
Cisplatin	100 mg/m² IV day 2	Every 3-4 weeks
or		
Mitomycin-C	6 mg/m² IVP day 1	Every 4 weeks
Ifosfamide (+Mesna)	3 gm/m² IV day 1	Every 4 weeks
Cisplatin	50 mg/m² IV day 1	Every 4 weeks
TAXOL		
Taxol	200-250 mg/m² IV over 24 hour day 1	Every 3 weeks
TAXOL-CISPLATIN		
Taxol	135-170 mg/m² IV over 6 hour day 1 followed by	Every 3 weeks
Cisplatin	75 mg/m² IV day 1	Every 3 weeks

PO = oral; IVP = IV push.

Table 15–6   New or Investigational Chemotherapy Regimens in Small Cell Lung Cancer[17,44,51,70]

Drug Regimen	Dose	Schedule
CEV		
Carboplatin	300 mg/m² IV day 1	Every 4 weeks
Etoposide	140 mg/m² IV days 1-3	Every 4 weeks
Vincristine	1.4 mg/m² IVP days 1, 8, 15	Every 4 weeks
VIP		
Etoposide (VP-16)	75 mg/m² IV days 1-4	Every 3 weeks
Ifosfamide (+Mesna)	1.2 gm/m² IV days 1-4	Every 3 weeks
Cisplatin	20 mg/m² IV days 1-4	Every 3 weeks for 4 cycles
IFEX/VP-16		
Ifosfamide (+Mesna)	5 gm/m² IV over 24 hour day 1	Every 3 weeks
Etoposide (VP-16)	120 mg/m² IV days 1-2 and 240 mg/m² PO day 3	Every 3 weeks
ICE		
Ifosfamide (+Mesna)	5 gm/m² IV over 24 hour day 1	Every 4 weeks
Carboplatin	300-400 mg/m² IV day 1	Every 4 weeks
Etoposide	100 mg/m² IV days 1-3	Every 4 weeks

PO = oral; IVP = IV push.

Table 15-7   Common Chemotherapy Regimens in Advanced Non-Small Cell Lung Cancer[17,18,28,44]

Drug Regimen	Dose	Schedule
CAMP		
Cyclophosphamide	300 mg/m^2 IV days 1 and 8	Every 4 weeks
Doxorubicin	20 mg/m^2 IV days 1 and 8	Every 4 weeks
Methotrexate	15 mg/m^2 IV days 1 and 8	Every 4 weeks
Procarbazine	100 mg/m^2 PO days 2-11	Every 4 weeks
CAP		
Cyclophosphamide	400 mg/m^2 IV day 1	Every 3-4 weeks
Doxorubicin	40 mg/m^2 IV day 1	Every 3-4 weeks
Cisplatin	40 mg/m^2 IV day 1	Every 3-4 weeks
CBP		
Cyclophosphamide	500 mg/m^2 IV days 1 and 8	Every 4 weeks
Bleomycin	20 mg/m^2 IV days 1 and 8	Every 4 weeks
Cisplatin	30 mg/m^2 IV days 1 and 8	Every 4 weeks
FOMi		
5FU	1000 mg/m^2 IV CI days 1-4	Every 3 weeks
	or 200 mg/m^2 IV CI	
	or 300 mg/m^2 IVP days 1, 8, 15	Every 3 weeks
Vincristine	2 mg IV day 1	Every 3 weeks
Mitomycin-C	10 mg/m^2 IV days 1, 21, 42	Every 6 weeks
EP		
Etoposide (VP-16)	80-120 mg/m^2 IV days 1-3	Every 3-4 weeks
Cisplatin	60-120 mg/m^2 IV day 2	Every 3-4 weeks
MVbP		
Mitomycin-C	10 mg/m^2 IV day 1	Every 6-12 weeks
Vinblastine	6 mg/m^2 IV day 1	Every 2-3 weeks
Cisplatin	40-100 mg/m^2 IV day 1	Every 3-6 weeks
VbP		
Vinblastine	4 mg/m^2 IV days 1 and 2	Every 3 weeks
Cisplatin	20 mg/m^2 IV days 1-3	Every 3 weeks
VdP		
Vindesine	3 mg/m^2 IV q week ×5	Every other week
Cisplatin	120 mg/m^2 IV days 1 and 29	Every 6 weeks

PO = oral; CI = continuous infusion; IVP = IV push.

Table 15–8 Common Chemotherapy Regimens in Small Cell Lung Cancer*

Drug Regimen	Dose	Schedule
CAV (OR CHO)		
Cyclophosphamide	750-1500 mg/m² IV day 1	Every 3 weeks
Doxorubicin	40-50 mg/m² IV day 1	Every 3 weeks
Vincristine	2 mg IV day 1	Every 3 weeks
CAE		
Cyclophosphamide	1000 mg/m² IV day 1	Every 3 weeks
Doxorubicin	45 mg/m² IV day 1	Every 3 weeks
Etoposide	50 mg/m² IV days 1-5	Every 3 weeks
CEV		
Cyclophosphamide	1000 mg/m² IV day 1	Every 3 weeks
Etoposide (VP-16)	50 mg/m² IV day 1	Every 3 weeks
Etoposide	100 mg/m² PO days 2-5	Every 3 weeks
Vincristine	2 mg IV day 1	Every 3 weeks
EVAC		
Etoposide (VP-16)	150 mg/m² IV days 1 and 8	Every 3-4 weeks
Vincristine	1 mg/m² IV days 1 and 8	Every 3-4 weeks
Doxorubicin	40 mg/m² IV day 1	Every 3-4 weeks
Cyclophosphamide	200 mg/m² PO days 3-6	Every 3-4 weeks
HANSEN'S		
Cyclophosphamide	700 mg/m² IV day 1	Every 4 weeks
Lomustine	70 mg/m² PO day 1 HS	Every 4 weeks
Vincristine	1 mg IV weekly ×4, then day 1 only	Every 4 weeks
Methotrexate	20 mg/m² PO days 18 and 21	Every 4 weeks
HANSEN'S VP		
Cyclophosphamide	1000 mg/m² IV day 1	Every 4 weeks
Lomustine	70 mg/m² PO HS day 1	Every 4 weeks
Vincristine	1 mg IV weekly ×4, then day 1 only	Every 4 weeks
Etoposide	70 mg/m² PO days 3-6	Every 4 weeks
EP		
Etoposide	80-120 mg/m² IV days 1-3	Every 3-4 weeks
Cisplatin	60-100 mg/m² IV day 1	Every 3-4 weeks

*References 17, 18, 28, 44, 56, 70.

PATIENT TEACHING PRIORITIES: CHEMOTHERAPY

Chemotherapeutic agents
- Review patient knowledge of chemotherapy and explain the therapeutic effects.
- Provide patient/family with written information regarding all chemotherapeutic agents used.
- Explain immediate and late (7 to 14 days) side effects of specific drug regimen.
- Note availability of patient information booklets and community resources.

General side effects
- Provide information for patient/family on self-management of stomatitis, nausea/vomiting, diarrhea and constipation, alopecia, myelosuppression, fatigue, and sexuality concerns.
- Discuss which side effects must be reported to the physician/nurse immediately.

Specific side effects
- Discuss specific side effects with patient/family according to prescribed drug regimen.

- Explain which side effects are reversible.
- Explain which medications/foods are to be avoided, if any.
- Review how patient makes contact with appropriate health-care team member should side effects occur that cannot be handled at home.
- Review community resources available to patient.

Emotional support
- Encourage patient/family to verbalize needs and questions concerning chemotherapy and its side effects.
- Encourage patient to maintain activities and relationships to promote self-worth.
- Encourage patient to verbalize feelings, frustrations, anger, and thoughts regarding their changed life-style.
- Teach patient/family problem-solving techniques.
- Discuss methods of handling/addressing stress and coping with family/friends.

CONCLUSION

Lung cancer remains the most common cause of cancer death for both women and men, and most patients will present with metastatic disease at the time of diagnosis. Their overall 5-year survival is 13%.[2] Smoking prevention remains the key to reducing lung cancer disease and death. Because of the many complications such as brain, bone, liver, and cardiac metastases and pleural effusions, nursing care can be very challenging. Compassionate and knowledgeable nursing care is of great importance to the patient with lung cancer and the family.

BIBLIOGRAPHY

1. Albain KS, Crowley JJ, and Livingston RB: Long-term survival and toxicity in small cell lung cancer: expanded southwest oncology group experience, Chest 99:1425, 1991.
2. American Cancer Society: Cancer facts & figures—1993, Atlanta, GA, 1993.
3. Andersen M, Kristjansen PE, and Hansen H: Second-line chemotherapy in small cell lung cancer, Cancer Treat Rev 17:427, 1990.
4. Arrigado R and others: Competing events determining relapse-free survival in limited small cell lung cancer, J Clin Oncol 10:447, 1992.
5. Baker R and others: The role of surgery in the management of selected patients with small cell cancer of the lung, J Clin Oncol 5:697, 1987.
6. Baron MG and others: Non-small cell lung cancer (NSCLC): chemotherapy in advanced disease, Am J Clin Oncol 15:23, 1992.
7. Beahrs OH and others, editors: Manual for staging of cancer, ed 4, Philadelphia, 1992, JB Lippincott Co.
8. Bernhard J and Ganz P: Psychosocial issues in lung cancer patients (Part I), Chest 90:216, 1991.
9. Bernhard J and Ganz P: Psychosocial issues in lung cancer patients (Part II), Chest 90:480, 1991.
10. Bitram J and others, editors: Lung cancer: a comprehensive treatise, Orlando, FL, 1988, Grune & Stratton.
11. Bleenhen NM: The current role of radiotherapy in the treatment of non-small cell lung cancer. Educa Session, Proc Am Soc Clin Oncol, May, 1992.
12. Bonomi P: Recent advances in etoposide therapy for non-small cell lung cancer, Cancer 67:254, 1991.
13. Borgelt B and others: The palliation of brain metastasis: final results of the first two studies by the radiation oncology study group, Int J Radiat Oncol Biol Phys 6:1, 1980.
14. Boring CC, Squires TS, and Heath CW: Cancer statistics for african americans, CA 42:7, 1992.
15. Boring CC, Squires TS, and Tong T: Cancer Statistics, 1992, CA 42:19, 1992.
16. Bork E and others: Teniposide (VM-26): an overlooked highly active agent in small cell lung cancer: results of a phase II trial in untreated patients, J Clin Oncol 4:524, 1986.
17. Bristol-Myers Squibb Co: Ifex, mesna: clinical guidelines and applications, Evansville, 1991.
18. Bunn P: Lung cancer: current understanding of the biology, diagnosis, staging, and treatment. A monograph of Bristol-Myers, Princeton, 1992.
19. Burke MB and others: Cancer chemotherapy: a nursing process approach, Boston, 1991, Jones and Bartlett Publishers.
20. Carney DN: The biology of lung cancer, Acta Oncol 28:1, 1989.
21. Carney DN: Lung cancer biology, Eur J Cancer 27:366, 1991.
22. Carpenito L: Nursing diagnosis: application to clinical practice, Philadelphia, 1987, JB Lippincott Co.
23. Centers for Disease Control. Comparison of the cigarette brand preferences of adult and teenaged smokers: United States, 1989, and 10 U.S. communities, 1988 and 1990, Morbid Mortal Weekly 41:169, 1992.
24. Chernecky C and Krech R: Complications of advanced disease. In Baird S, McCorkle R, and Grant M, editors: Cancer nursing: a comprehensive textbook, Philadelphia, 1991, WB Saunders Co.
25. Chevalier TL, Arriagada R, and Tubiana M: Combined chemotherapy and radiotherapy in small cell lung cancer. In Muggia FM, editor: New drugs, concepts, and results in cancer chemotherapy, Boston, 1992, Kluwer Academic Publishers.
26. Clinical Cancer Letter 15:9, 1, Washington, DC, 1992.
27. Comis R and Marstin G: Small cell carcinoma of the lung: an overview, Semin Oncol Nurs 3:174, 1987.
28. Coughenour M: Common chemotherapeutic treatments for cancer at the University of Kansas, unpublished pamphlet, 1988.
29. Council on Scientific Affairs: Radon in homes: council report, JAMA 258:5, 1987.
30. Damber L and Larsson S: Combined effects of mining and smoking in the causation of lung carcinoma, Acta Radiol Oncol 21:305, 1982.
31. Delarve N and Eschapasse H: Lung cancer: international trends in general thoracic surgery, vol 1, Philadelphia, 1985, WB Saunders Co.
32. Dellefield M: Informational needs and approaches for early cancer detection in the elderly, Semin Oncol Nurs 4:156, 1988.

33. Devesa SS, Blot WJ, and Fraumeni JF: Declining lung cancer rates among young men and women in the United States: a cohort analysis, J Natl Cancer Inst 81:1568, 1989.

34. Diggs CH and others: Small cell carcinoma of the lung: treatment in the community, Cancer 69:2075, 1992.

35. Donehower RC and others: Phase I trial of Taxol in patients with advanced cancer, Cancer Treat Reports 71:1171, 1987.

36. Dow K and Hilderly L: Nursing care in radiation oncology, Philadelphia, 1992, WB Saunders Co.

37. Engelking C: Comfort issues in geriatric oncology, Semin Oncol Nurs 4:198, 1988.

38. Eriksen M, Lemaistre C, and Newell GR: Health hazards of passive smoking, Ann Rev Public Health 9:47, 1988.

39. Erickson R: Mastering the in's and out's of chest drainage (Part I), Nursing '89 19:36, 1989.

40. Erickson R: Mastering the in's and out's of chest drainage (Part 2), Nursing '89 19:46, 1989.

41. Evans W and others: Superiority of alternating non-cross-resistant chemotherapy in extensive small cell lung cancer: a multicenter, randomized clinical trial by the NCI of Canada, Ann Intern Med 107:451, 1987.

42. Evans W and others: VP-16 and carboplatin in previously untreated patients with extensive small cell lung cancer: a study of the National Cancer Institute of Canada Clinical Trials Group, Br J Cancer 58:464, 1988.

43. Findlay MP and others: Retrospective review of chemotherapy for small cell lung cancer in the elderly: does the end justify the means? Eur J Cancer 27:1597, 1991.

44. Fischer DS and Knobf MT: The cancer chemotherapy handbook, ed 3, St Louis, 1993, Mosby.

45. Fleck JF and others: Is prophylactic cranial irradiation indicated in small cell lung cancer? J Clin Oncol 8:209, 1990.

46. Fontana RS and others: Screening for lung cancer: a critique of the Mayo Lung Project, Cancer 67:1155, 1991.

47. Foote M and others: Dyspnea: a distressing sensation in lung cancer, Oncol Nurs Forum 13:25, 1986.

48. Frank-Stromborg M: Future projected trends in the care of the elderly individual with cancer, and implications for nursing, J Oncol Nursing 4:224, 1988.

49. Friedman P: Lung cancer: update on staging classifications, Am J Radiol 150:261, 1988.

50. Garfinkel L and Silverberg E: Lung cancer and smoking trends in the United States over the past 25 years, CA 41:137, 1991.

51. Gatzemeir U and others: Combination chemotherapy with carboplatin, etoposide, and vincristine as first-line treatment in small cell lung cancer, J Clin Oncol 10:818, 1992.

52. Ginsberg RJ and others: Modern thirty-day operative mortality for surgical resections in lung cancer, J Thorac Cardiovasc Surg 86:654, 1983.

53. Gradishar WJ and others: The impact on survival by adjuvant chemotherapy and radiation therapy in stage II non-small cell lung cancer, Am J Clin Oncol 15:405, 1992.

54. Green MR: New directions in chemotherapy for non-small cell lung cancer, Educa Session, Proc Am Soc Clin Oncol May, 1992.

55. Hammond E, Selikoff I, and Seidman H: Asbestos exposure, cigarette smoking and death rates, Ann NY Acad Sci 330:473, 1979.

56. Hansen HH and Kristjansen PE: Chemotherapy of small cell lung cancer, Eur J Cancer 27:342, 1991.

57. Haque AK: Pathology of carcinoma of the lung: an update on current concepts. J Thorac Imaging 7:9, 1991.

58. Harwood K: Non-small cell lung cancer: issues in diagnosis, staging, and treatment, Semin Oncol Nurs 3:183, 1987.

59. Haylock P: Breathing difficulty: changes in respiratory function, Semin Oncol Nurs 3:293, 1987.

60. Haylock P: Radiation therapy, Am J Nurs 87:1441, 1987.

61. Heitzman E: The role of computed tomography in the diagnosis and management of lung cancer, Chest 89:237, 1986.

62. Higgins GA, Shields TW, and Keehn RJ: The solitary pulmonary nodule: ten-year follow-up of veterans administration armed forces cooperative study, Arch Surg 110:570, 1975.

63. Hilderly L and Dow K: Radiation oncology. In Baird S, McCorkle R, and Grant M, editors: Cancer nursing: a comprehensive textbook, Philadelphia, 1991, WB Saunders Co.

64. Hughes J and Weill H: Asbestos exposure—quantitative assessment of risk, Am Rev Respir Dis 133:5, 1986.

65. Iannuzzi M and Scoggin C: Small cell lung cancer, Am Rev Respir Dis 134:593, 1986.

66. Ihde DC and Minna JD: Non-small cell lung cancer: Part I: biology, diagnosis and staging, Curr Prob Cancer 15:61, 1991.

67. Ihde DC and Minna JD: Non-small cell lung cancer, Part II: treatment, Curr Prob Cancer 15:105, 1991.

68. Jackson DZ: Tax Big Tobacco till it chokes, Wilmington Morning Star (editorial), Wilmington, NC, October 5, 1992.

69. Janerich DT and others: Lung cancer and ex-

posure to tobacco smoke in the household, N Engl J Med 323:632, 1990.

70. Johnson DH, Hainsworth JD, Hande K, and Greco FA: Current status of etoposide in the management of small cell lung cancer, Cancer 67:231, 1991.

71. Jordan LN and Mantravadi RVP: Nursing care of the patient receiving high dose rate brachytherapy, Oncol Nurs Forum 18:1167, 1991.

72. Kemeny N and Sugarbaker P: Treatment of metastatic cancer to liver. In DeVita V and others, editors: Cancer: principles and practice of oncology, Philadelphia, 1992, JB Lippincott Co.

73. Kerr RA: Indoor radon: the deadliest pollutant, Science 240:606, 1988.

74. Khanavkar B, Stern P, Alberti W, and Nakhosteen JA: Complications associated with brachytherapy alone or with laser in lung cancer, Chest 99:1062, 1991.

75. Kreisman H, Wolkove N, and Quoix E: Small cell lung cancer presenting as a solitary pulmonary nodule, Chest 101:225, 1992.

76. Lad T, Thomas P, and Piantadosi S: Surgical resection of small cell lung cancer: a prospective randomized evaluation, Proc Am Soc Clin Oncol 10:244, 1991.

77. Lind J: Lung cancer. In Clark JC and McGee RF, editors: Core curriculum for oncology nursing, Philadelphia, 1992, WB Saunders Co.

78. Lobert S and Correia JJ: Antimitotics in cancer chemotherapy, Cancer Nurs 15:22, 1992.

79. Lyss AP and others: Intensive etoposide and carboplatin chemotherapy for advanced non-small cell lung cancer: a phase II trial of the cancer and leukemia group b, Am J Clin Oncol 15: 399, 1992.

80. Makela TP, Mattson K, and Alitalo K: Tumor markers and oncogenes in lung cancer, Eur J Cancer 27:1323, 1991.

81. Malawer M and Delaney T: Treatment of metastatic cancer to bone. In DeVita V and others, editors: Cancer: principles and practice of oncology, ed 3, Philadelphia, 1989, JB Lippincott Co.

82. McCorkle R and others: A randomized clinical trial of home nursing care for lung cancer patients, Cancer 64:1375, 1989.

83. McIntire S and Cioppa A, editors: Cancer nursing: a developmental approach, New York, 1984, John Wiley & Sons.

84. McNaull F: Radiation therapy for lung cancer: nursing considerations, Semin Oncol Nurs 3:134, 1987.

85. McNaull F: Lung cancer: what are the odds? Am J Nurs 87:1428, 1987.

86. Meurman L: Combined effect of asbestos exposure and tobacco smoking on Finnish anthophyllite miners and millers, Ann NY Acad Sci 330:491, 1979.

87. Miaskowski C: Knowledge deficit related to surgery. In McNally J and others, editors: Guidelines for cancer nursing practice, ed 2, Philadelphia, 1991, WB Saunders Co.

88. Miller JD, Gorenstein LA, and Patterson GA: Staging: the key to rational management of lung cancer, Ann Thorac Surg 53:170, 1992.

89. Minna J and others: Cancer of the lung. In DeVita V and others, editors: Cancer: principles and practice of oncology, ed 3, Philadelphia, 1989, JB Lippincott Co.

90. Moran J: Personal communication, 1989.

91. Moseley J: Nursing management of toxicities associated with chemotherapy for lung cancer, Semin Oncol Nurs 3:202, 1987.

92. Mountain C: A new international staging system for lung cancer, Chest 89:225, 1986.

93. Mountain CF: Surgical treatment of lung cancer, Crit Rev Oncol Hematol 11:179, 1991.

94. National Cancer Institute: Gloeckler-Ries LA, Hanky BF, and Edwards BK, editors: Cancer Statistics Review: 1973-87, Bethesda, MD: US Department of Health and Human Services, 1990, NIH Pub. No. 90-2789.

95. National Cancer Institute: School programs to prevent smoking: the national cancer institute guide to strategies that succeed, Bethesda, MD: US Department of Health and Human Services. 1990, NIH Pub. No. 90-5000.

96. National Cancer Institute: Self-guided strategies for smoking cessation: a program planner's guide, Bethesda, MD: US Department of Health and Human Services, 1990, NIH Pub. No. 91-3104.

97. National Research Council: Environmental tobacco smoke: measuring exposures and assessing health effects, Washington, DC, 1986, National Academy Press.

98. NCI conducting four epidemiology studies on residential radon threat, Cancer Letter 14:5, 1988.

99. Neuberger JS: Residential radon exposure and lung cancer: an overview of published studies, Cancer Detect Prev 15:435, 1991.

100. Ockene JK, Kuller LH, Svendsen KH, and Meilahn E: The relationship of smoking cessation to coronary heart disease and lung cancer in the multiple risk factor intervention trial, Am J Pub Health 80:954, 1990.

101. Oleske D: The epidemiology of lung cancer: an overview, Semin Oncol Nurs 3:165, 1987.

102. Pass H: Treatment of malignant pericardial ef-

fusions. In DeVita V and others, editors: Cancer: principles and practice of oncology, Philadelphia, 1989, JB Lippincott Co.

103. Pearson F: Lung cancer: the past twenty-five years, Chest 89:200, 1986.

104. Perez CA and others: A prospective randomized study of various irradiation doses and fractionation schedules in the treatment of inoperable non-oat cell carcinoma of the lung, Cancer 45:2744, 1980.

105. Poplin E and others: Small cell carcinoma of the lung: influence of age on treatment outcome, Cancer Treat Rep 71:291, 1987.

106. Raju P, Maruama Y, DeSimone P, and others: Treatment of liver metastasis with a combination of chemotherapy and hyperfractionated external radiation therapy, Am J Clin Oncol 10:41, 1987.

107. Risser N: The key to prevention of lung cancer: stop smoking, Semin Oncol Nurs 3:228, 1987.

108. Rodenhuis S and Slebos RJ: Clinical significance of ras oncogene activation in human lung cancer, Cancer Res 52:2665s, 1992.

109. Rose LJ: Neoadjuvant and adjuvant therapy of non-small cell lung cancer, Semin Oncol 18:536, 1991.

110. Ross DJ, Mohsenifar Z, and Koerner SK: Survival characteristics after neodymium: YAG laser photoresection in advanced stage lung cancer, Chest 98:581, 1990.

111. Rostad M: Advances in nursing management of patients with lung cancer, Nurs Clin N Am 25:393, 1990.

112. Rowinsky EK, Cazenave LA, and Donehower RC: Taxol: a novel investigational antimicrotubule agent, J Natl Cancer Inst 82:1247, 1990.

113. Rowinsky EK and others: Sequences of taxol and cisplatin: a phase I and pharmacologic study, J Clin Oncol 9:1692, 1991.

114. Rowinsky EK and others: Cardiac disturbances during the administration of taxol, J Clin Oncol 9:1704, 1991.

115. Rubin SA: Lung cancer: past, present, and future, J Thorac Imaging 7:1, 1991.

116. Ruchdeschel JC: Etoposide in the management of non-small cell lung cancer, Cancer 67:250, 1991.

117. Ryan L: Lung cancer: psychosocial implications, Semin Oncol Nurs 3:222, 1987.

118. Saccomanno G and others: Relationship of radioactive radon daughters and cigarette smoking in the genesis of lung cancer in uranium miners, Cancer 62:1402, 1988.

119. Samet J and Nero A: Indoor radon and lung cancer, N Engl J Med 320:591, 1989.

120. Sellers TA and others: Evidence for mendelian inheritance in the pathogenesis of lung cancer, J Natl Cancer Inst 82:1272, 1990.

121. Sellers TA and others: Lung cancer detection and prevention: evidence for an interaction between smoking and genetic predisposition, Cancer Res 52(suppl):2694s, 1992.

122. Sethi T and others: Growth of small cell lung cancer cells: stimulation by multiple neuropeptides and inhibition by broad spectrum antagonists in vitro and in vivo, Cancer Res 52:2737s, 1992.

123. Shell J, Stanutz F, and Grimm J: Comparison of moisture vapor permeable (MPV) dressings to conventional dressings for management of radiation skin reactions, Onc Nurs Forum 13:11, 1986.

124. Shell J: Knowledge deficit related to radiation therapy. In McNally J, Sommerville E, Miaskowski C, and Rostad M, editors: Guidelines for cancer nursing practice, ed 2, Philadelphia, 1991, WB Saunders Co.

125. Shepherd FA, Laskey J, Evans WK, and others: Cushing's syndrome associated with ectopic corticotropin production and small cell lung cancer, J Clin Oncol 10:21, 1992.

126. Shields TW: Screening, staging, and diagnostic investigation of non-small cell lung cancer patients, Curr Opin Oncol 3:297, 1991.

127. Silverberg B and Lubera J: Cancer statistics, Cancer 39:3, 1989.

128. Sims S: Cancer and aging, Nurs Times 84:29, 1988.

129. Slebos RJ and others: K-ras oncogene activation as a prognostic marker in adenocarcinoma of the lung, N Engl J Med 323:561, 1990.

130. Slevin ML and others: A randomized trial to evaluate the effect of schedule on the activity of etoposide in small cell lung cancer, J Clin Oncol 7:1333, 1989.

131. Smit EF and others: A phase II study of oral etoposide in elderly patients with small cell lung cancer, Thorax 44:631, 1989.

132. Sommerville E: Knowledge deficit related to chemotherapy. In McNally F, Sommerville E, Miaskowski C, and Rostad M, editors: Guidelines for cancer nursing practice, ed 2, Philadelphia, 1991, WB Saunders Co.

133. Splinter TA: Management of non-small cell and small cell lung cancer, Curr Opin Oncol 3:312, 1991.

134. Sridhar KS and Raub WA: Present and past smoking history and other predisposing factors in 100 lung cancer patients, Chest 101:19, 1992.

135. Stahel RA: Diagnosis, staging, and prognostic factors of small cell lung cancer, Curr Opin Oncol 3:306, 1991.

136. Stahel RA and others: Staging and prognostic factors in small cell carcinoma of the lung. Con-

sensus report, Lung Cancer 5:119, 1989.

137. Sugarbaker DJ: Non-small cell lung cancer: surgical approach to staging and therapy, Educational Session: Proc Am Soc Clin Oncol May, 1992.

138. Tockman M and others: Sensitive and specific monoclonal antibody recognition of human lung cancer antigen on preserved sputum cells: a new approach to early lung cancer detection, J Clin Oncol 6:1685, 1988.

139. Turrisi AT: The integration of platinum and radiotherapy in the treatment of lung cancer, Semin Oncol 18:81, 1991.

140. US Environmental Protection Agency: A citizen's guide to radon: what it is and what to do about it, Washington, DC, 1986, USDHHS Office of Air and Radiation (OPA-86-004).

141. Varricchio C and Jassah P: Acute pulmonary disorders associated with lung cancer, Semin Oncol Nurs 1:269, 1985.

142. Wampler GL, Ahlgren JD, and Schulof RS: A pilot study of intensive weekly chemotherapy for extensive disease small cell lung carcinoma, Cancer Invest 10:97, 1992.

143. Warner K, Goldenhar L, and McLaughlin C: Cigarette advertising and magazine coverage of the hazards of smoking: a statistical analysis, N Engl J Med 326:305, 1992.

144. Watanabe Y and others: Mediastinal spread of metastatic lymph nodes in bronchogenic carcinoma, Chest 97:1059, 1990.

145. White E: Home care of the patient with advanced lung cancer, Semin Oncol Nurs 3:216, 1987.

146. Whittemore A and McMillan A: Lung cancer mortality among U.S. uranium miners: a reappraisal, J Natl Cancer Inst 71:489, 1983.

147. Wright D and Delaney T: Treatment of metastatic cancer to the brain. In DeVita V and others, editors: Cancer: principles and practice of oncology, ed 3, Philadelphia, 1989, JB Lippincott Co.

148. Wu A and others: Secular trends in histologic types of lung cancer, J Natl Cancer Inst 77:53, 1986.

149. Wu AH and others: Personal and family history of lung disease as risk factors for adenocarcinoma of the lung, Cancer Res 48:7279, 1988.

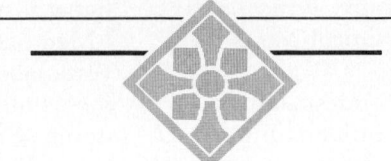

CHAPTER 16

Malignant Lymphoma

Jill Grodecki Moore

Malignant lymphoma is a diverse group of neoplasms that originate in the lymphatic system. Included in this system are organs and tissues such as the thymus, lymph nodes, spleen, bone marrow, blood, and lymph. Lymph is derived from interstitial fluid and flows through lymphatic vessels so that it is eventually returned to the circulatory system by way of the thoracic duct. Along its course, lymph is filtered of particulate through lymph nodes, which are small, encapsulated organs located along the lymphatic vessels (Figure 16-1). Lymph nodes have a very specific architecture (Figure 16-2) that allows for areas of lymphocyte maturation and differentiation. Lymphocytes are the predominant cell present in lymph nodes and are the cellular element involved in malignant lymphoma.

Lymphocytes originate in the bone marrow and, through the process of maturation and differentiation, develop into several different types of mature lymphocytes (Figure 16-3). At any stage of this maturation and differentiation, the normal cell may transform into a malignant cell, giving rise to a malignancy that is specific to the stage in which the cell became transformed.

Based on the characteristics of the malignant lymphocytes, malignant lymphomas are divided into two major subgroups—Hodgkin's disease and non-Hodgkin's lymphoma. This chapter discusses the incidence, etiology, classifications, clinical manifestations, diagnosis, and treatment of Hodgkin's disease and non-Hodgkin's lymphoma, and also provides guidelines for care of patients with malignant lymphoma.

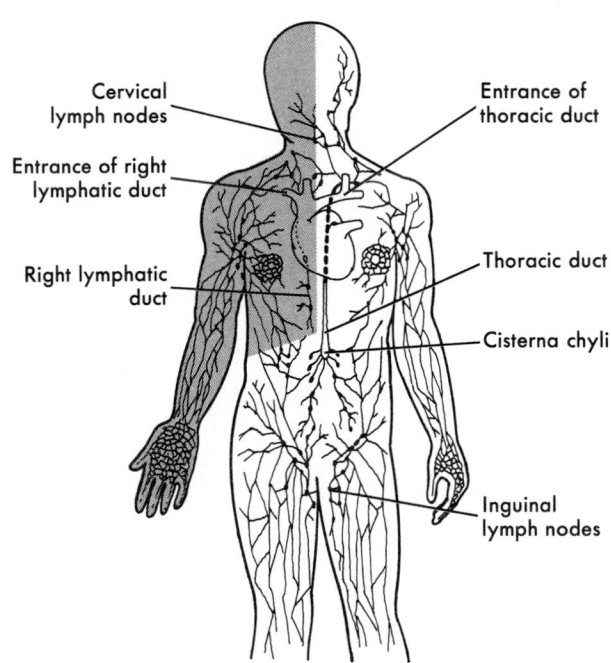

Figure 16–1 The lymphatic system. (From Beare P and Myers J: Principles and practice of adult health nursing, St. Louis, 1990, Mosby.)

HODGKIN'S DISEASE

HISTORICAL BACKGROUND

In 1832, Thomas Hodgkin described a progressively fatal disease characterized by lymphadenopathy with eventual spread to the lungs, liver, spleen, bone marrow, and other organs. Characteristic cells involved in this disease were identified microscopically by Sternberg and Reed in 1898 and 1902, respectively.

Afferent lymph vessel
PLF
OC
PC
SLF
Valves
Sinus
Nodal blood vessels
Efferent lymph vessel

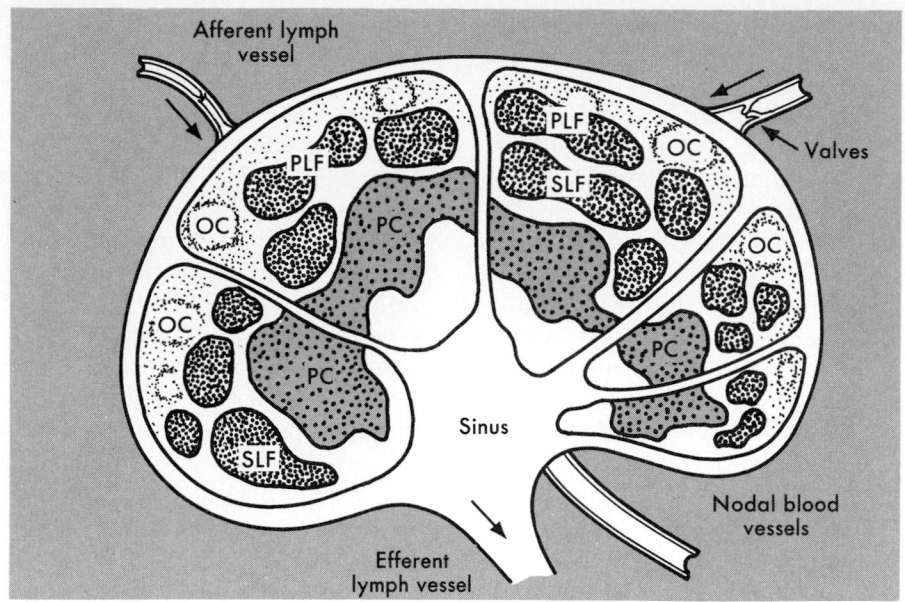

Figure 16–2 Cross-section of a lymph node (PLF = primary lymphoid follicles; SLF = secondary lymphoid follicles; OC = outer cortex; PC = paracortical area). (From Powers: Diagnostic hematology, St. Louis, 1989, Mosby.)

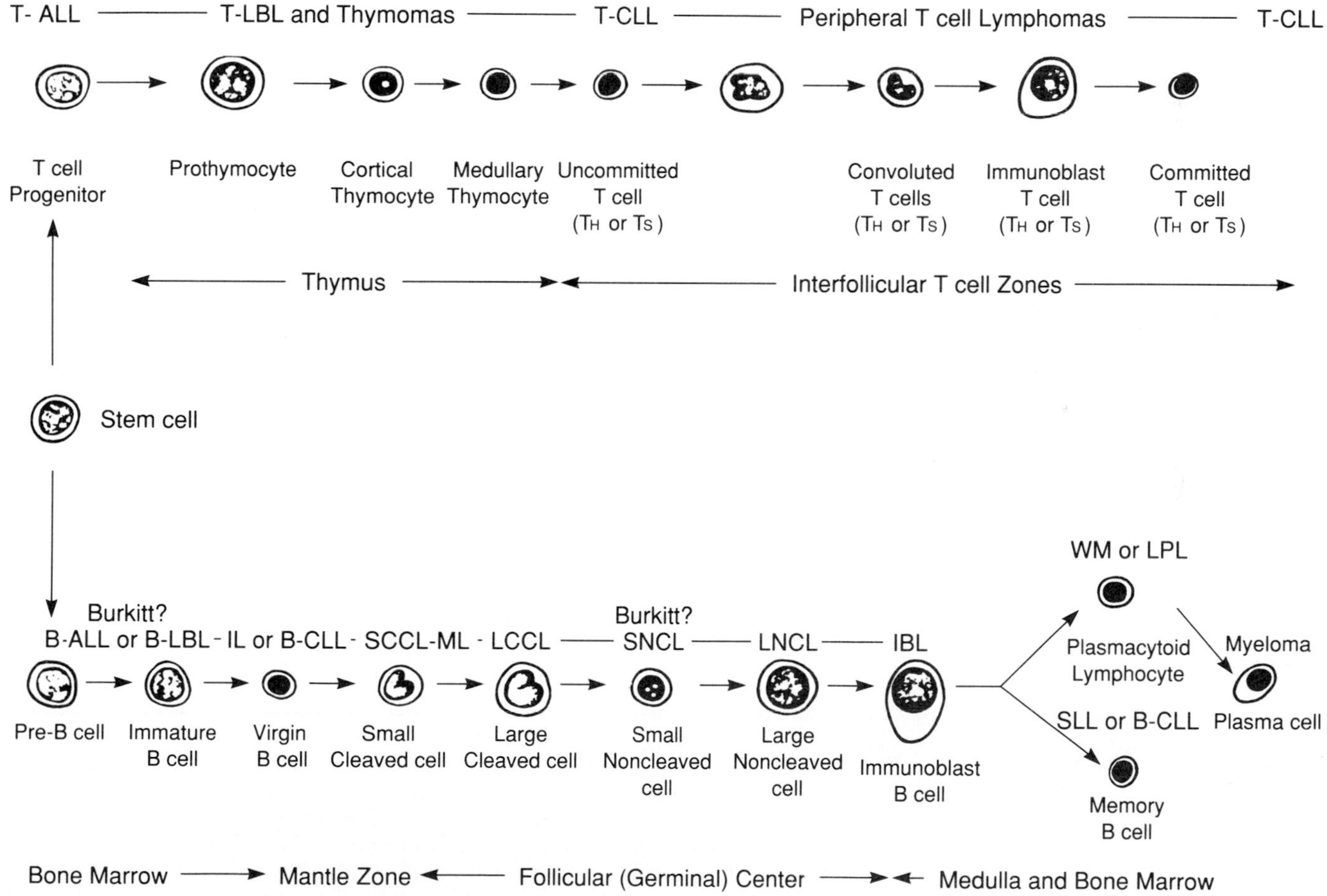

T- ALL
T-LBL and Thymomas
T-CLL
Peripheral T cell Lymphomas
T-CLL
T cell Progenitor
Prothymocyte
Cortical Thymocyte
Medullary Thymocyte
Uncommitted T cell (TH or TS)
Convoluted T cells (TH or TS)
Immunoblast T cell (TH or TS)
Committed T cell (TH or TS)
Thymus
Interfollicular T cell Zones
Stem cell
WM or LPL
Burkitt?
B-ALL or B-LBL - IL or B-CLL - SCCL-ML - LCCL
Burkitt?
SNCL
LNCL
IBL
Plasmacytoid Lymphocyte
Myeloma
Pre-B cell
Immature B cell
Virgin B cell
Small Cleaved cell
Large Cleaved cell
Small Noncleaved cell
Large Noncleaved cell
Immunoblast B cell
SLL or B-CLL
Plasma cell
Memory B cell
Bone Marrow
Mantle Zone
Follicular (Germinal) Center
Medulla and Bone Marrow

Figure 16–3 Lymphocyte differentiation. Immunologic classification of non-Hodgkin's lymphomas. This schema is based on a correlation between the immunologic phenotyping and morphologic appearance of a large number of non-Hodgkin's lymphomas. *T-ALL,* T cell acute lymphoblastic leukemia; *T-LBL,* T cell lymphoblastic lymphoma; *T-CLL,* T cell chronic lymphocytic leukemia; *TH,* helper T cell; *Ts,* suppressor T cell; *B-ALL,* B cell acute lymphoblastic leukemia; *B-LBL,* B cell lymphoblastic lymphoma; *IL,* intermediate (mantle zone) lymphoma; *B-CLL,* B cell chronic lymphocytic leukemia; *SCCL,* small cleaved cell (poorly differentiated lymphocytic) lymphoma; *ML,* mixed small cleaved and large cell (mixed lymphocytic-histiocytic) lymphoma; *LCCL,* large cleaved cell (histiocytic) lymphoma; *SNCL,* small noncleaved cell (undifferentiated) lymphoma, Burkitt's and non-Burkitt's subtypes; *LNCL,* large noncleaved cell (histiocytic) lymphoma; *IBL,* immunoblastic lymphoma; *WM,* Waldenström's macroglobulinemia; *LPL,* lymphoplasmacytoid lymphoma; *SSL,* small lymphocytic (well-differentiated lymphocytic) lymphoma. (Adapted from Thorup O: Fundamentals of clinical hematology, ed 5, Philadelphia, 1987, WB Saunders.)

The identification of these cells (now known as Reed-Sternberg cells) allowed for the initial classification of Hodgkin's disease. Tissues that have Reed-Sternberg cells are classified as Hodgkin's disease.

The potential curability of Hodgkin's disease was first recognized in 1939 when patients with localized tumors treated with high-dose radiation were shown to have long-term disease-free survival.[33] Because of the responsiveness of localized disease, research focused on ways to define the extent of disease before treatment. In 1969, researchers at Stanford University developed an extensive systematic way of staging and subsequently treating Hodgkin's disease based on the stage.[33] In 1970, the National Cancer Institute reported that patients with advanced Hodgkin's disease could attain complete remission and long-term survival using a combination chemotherapy of nitrogen mustard, Oncovin (vincristine), procarbazine, and prednisone, known as MOPP.[33] These advances resulted in a standard approach to the diagnosis and treatment of Hodgkin's disease. Since the mid-1970s, development and research efforts have focused on more accurate ways of staging, initial therapies for various stages, treatment of resistance and relapsed disease, and the long-term effects of treatment regimens.

EPIDEMIOLOGY AND ETIOLOGY

Each year, there are an estimated 7400 new cases of Hodgkin's disease and an estimated 1600 deaths.[2] This represents an incidence of less than 1% of all cancers. However, Hodgkin's disease is the most common cancer of young adults. Incidence peaks in the second and third decades, then gradually declines until age 45. A gradual increase in incidence is noted after age 45, with a second peak occurring in the sixth and seventh decades. Hodgkin's disease is also slightly more common in males, who may have a poorer prognosis.

The cause of Hodgkin's disease remains elusive. No strong evidence for specific etiologic factors exists. However, clinical manifestations and epidemiologic studies have suggested a viral etiology or disturbance of the immune system. The infectious agent most frequently implicated is the Epstein-Barr virus (EBV).[33,37] Epidemiologic studies of clusters of Hodgkin's disease cases suggest the possibility that the disease occurs as a rare consequence of EBV infection. No conclusive evidence for a relationship between the Epstein-Barr virus and Hodgkin's disease exists.[23,29,33]

Genetic and occupational predispositions for Hodgkin's disease may also exist. Epidemiologic studies have identified an increased risk of disease among siblings of persons with Hodgkin's disease and among persons in the occupation of woodworking.[16,17] Evidence to support these ideas is inconclusive.

PREVENTION, SCREENING, AND DETECTION

Prevention of Hodgkin's disease is not applicable because there are no identified preventable risks. Early detection is important but may be hampered by the vagueness of the common symptoms. Patients should be encouraged to seek medical attention for persistent common signs and symptoms.

CLASSIFICATION

Since the identification of Reed-Sternberg cells (giant multinucleated transformed lymphocytes) as the diagnostic hallmark of Hodgkin's disease, histologic subtypes have been recognized. The Rye histopathologic classification identifies four subtypes of Hodgkin's disease based primarily on the microscopic features of the involved tissues. The identified characteristics help to distinguish Hodgkin's disease from other disorders. The characteristics of the four subtypes are listed in Table 16-1. Although these subtypes predict prognosis of the natural history of the disease,

Table 16-1   Rye Histopathologic Classification

Type	Cases (%)	Characteristics
Lymphocyte predominance	5–10	Most favorable prognosis Reed-Sternberg cells are difficult to locate Often early stage at presentation
Nodular sclerosing	40–70	More aggressive than lymphocyte predominate type Fibrosis divides lymph tissue into nodules Often associated with mediastinal involvement
Mixed cellularity	20–40	More aggressive than lymphocyte predominant and nodular sclerosing types Reed-Sternberg cells are frequent and plasma cells and eosinophils infiltrate tissue Often associated with abdominal disease
Lymphocyte depleted	<5	Most unfavorable prognosis Reed-Sternberg cells are abundant with decreased lymphocytes Often advanced stage at presentation

Data from Thorup CA: Fundamentals of clinical hematology, ed 5, Philadelphia, 1987, WB Saunders Co.

they are poor predictors of prognosis when the disease is treated. Age, stage of disease, and adequacy of treatment are more important than histologic subtype in determining prognosis.

CLINICAL FEATURES

The most common signs and symptoms of Hodgkin's disease are lymphadenopathy, fever, night sweats, weight loss, pruritus, and alcohol-induced pain. Painless lymphadenopathy is evident in 70% to 90% of cases and is usually the symptom that causes patients to seek medical attention. The enlarged nodes are usually nontender, discrete, have a rubbery texture, and have been present for several weeks. Fever, night sweats, and weight loss of greater than 10% of baseline weight usually signify advanced disease. Therefore, noting the presence or absence of these symptoms is important. All or only one of these symptoms may occur, and their presence generally denotes a poor prognosis. Generalized pruritus without skin lesions occurs in 10% to 15% of cases and is usually associated with mediastinal or abdominal masses. Pain in the enlarged nodes following the ingestion of alcohol occurs in about 20% of cases. Neither pruritus nor alcohol-induced pain has any pathologic or prognostic significance. See box below.

Less common presentations are cough, chest pain, superior vena cava syndrome, ascites, abdominal pain or fullness, jaundice, and gastrointestinal or genitourinary problems. Almost all of these signs and symptoms can be attributed to enlarged nodes or lymph tissue impinging on other structures. Respiratory symptoms or superior vena cava syndrome indicates intrathoracic involvement, usually mediastinal. These symptoms are more common in women because they have a higher incidence of mediastinal involvement. The abdominal-related symptoms are generally indicative of retroperitoneal node, liver, or spleen involvement.

There are no specific laboratory values indicative of Hodgkin's disease. Complete blood counts and routine chemistry evaluations are generally within normal limits. The exceptions to this are usually seen in advanced disease. Anemia is identified in approximately 10% of cases, and increased granulocytes are noted in about 25% of cases. Decreased lymphocytes occur about 20% of the time and are a poor prognostic sign. The only laboratory study that may be a nonspecific indicator of Hodgkin's disease is the erythrocyte sedimentation rate (ESR). ESR is elevated in about 50% of cases with advanced disease. When a complete remission is obtained, ESR returns to normal. A subsequent rise in ESR predicts relapse 90% of the time.[33,37]

DIAGNOSIS AND STAGING

When a patient presents with clinical manifestations suggestive of Hodgkin's disease, a thorough history and physical examination must be performed. A biopsy of the enlarged node is necessary for diagnosis. However, if there is evidence of a recent infectious process a lymph node biopsy may be delayed a short period of time to observe the clinical course. When feasible, the most accessible and most abnormal node should be biopsied. The entire node should be removed to ensure adequate histologic examination.

After a tissue diagnosis of Hodgkin's disease has been established, the extent of disease involvement must be determined. This process is referred to as staging and is very important because it influences treatment decisions. The Ann Arbor Staging Classification is used to categorize the extent of disease into four stages[10,33,37]:

Stage I   Involvement of a single lymph node region or of a single extralymphatic organ or site
Stage II   Involvement of two or more lymph node regions on the same side of the diaphragm
Stage III   Involvement of lymph node regions on both sides of the diaphragm
Stage IV   Disseminated involvement of one or more extralymphatic organs or tissues

Because Hodgkin's disease spreads in an organized contiguous manner from one node region to another, this system of staging clearly identifies the extent of the disease. The presence or absence of fever, night sweats, or weight loss is also noted in the staging. The suffix "A" denotes the absence of these symptoms; the suffix "B" denotes the presence of these symptoms.

To stage the extent of the disease accurately, it is recommended that the following procedures be initiated as soon as possible after a definitive diagnosis of Hodgkin's disease[10,33,37]:

1. Detailed history and physical examination with emphasis on history of fever, night sweats, weight loss, and pruritus, and examination of lymph node regions, liver, and spleen
2. Laboratory work-up including complete blood count, differential, platelet count, ESR, liver, renal function, and cytogenetic studies
3. Radiology work-up including a chest x-ray, CT

CLINICAL FEATURES

Hodgkin's disease
Painless lymphadenopathy, fever, night sweats, weight loss, pruritus, and alcohol induced pain.

Non-Hodgkin's lymphoma
Generalized painless lymphadenopathy, vague abdominal discomfort, back pain, gastrointestinal complaints.

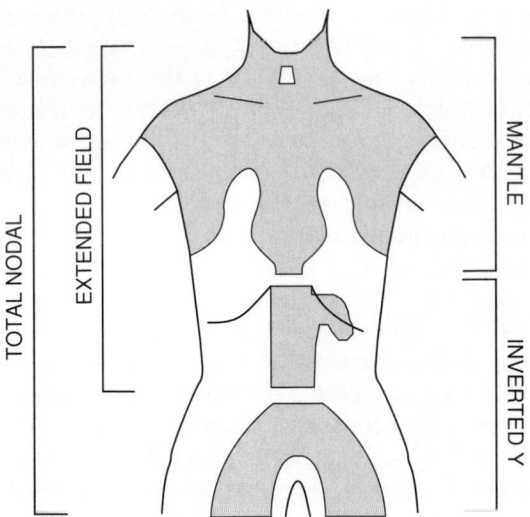

Figure 16–4 Standard radiation fields for Hodgkin's disease. *Mantle*, from mandible to diaphragm. Lungs, heart, spinal cord and humeral heads are shielded. *Inverted Y*, from diaphragm to ischial tuberosities, including the spleen if not removed; spinal cord, kidneys, bladder, rectum and gonads are shielded. *Extended field*, involves mantle zone and uppermost inverted Y zone, does not include the pelvic, inguinal, or femoral nodes. *Total nodal*, mantle zone and complete inverted Y zone.

COMMON CHEMOTHERAPY REGIMENS FOR HODGKIN'S DISEASE		
MOPP		
Nitrogen Mustard	6 mg/m² IV days 1 and 8	
Oncovin (vincristine)	1.4 mg/m² IV days 1 and 8	
Procarbazine	100 mg/m² PO days 1-14	
Prednisone	40 mg/m² PO days 1-14	
ABVD		
Adriamycin	25 mg/m² IV days 1 and 15	
Bleomycin	10 mg/m² IV days 1 and 15	
Vinblastine	6 mg/m² IV days 1 and 15	
Dacarbazine	375 mg/m² IV days 1 and 15	

scans or MRI of the chest, abdomen, and pelvis, and a bilateral lower extremity lymphangiogram
4. Bilateral bone marrow biopsy and aspirate
5. Skeletal survey if bone tenderness is noted on history and physical
6. Percutaneous liver biopsy if liver abnormalities are present on laboratory and radiology work-ups and no other abdominal disease is detected
7. Exploratory laparotomy and splenectomy if other studies do not prove abdominal disease and identification of abdominal disease will affect treatment decisions

During and after treatment, many of the same staging procedures will be repeated to document response to treatment and then to document complete remission. When recurrence is suspected, the diagnostic and staging process is repeated. It is important to document disease recurrence by node biopsy and to determine the site and extent of recurrence. All of these factors are as important for effective treatment of recurrence as they are for the management of new diagnoses.

METASTASIS

Involvement of retroperitoneal nodes, liver, spleen, and bone marrow usually occurs after the disease is generalized. Mesenteric lymph nodes and any organ can be involved in advanced disease cases.

TREATMENT MODALITIES

The appropriate use of radiotherapy and chemotherapy is required for effective treatment of Hodgkin's disease. Radiation therapy is generally given to nodal areas (Figure 16-4). A total dose of 4000 to 4400 cGy (rads) to the involved nodal areas is usually well tolerated and curative. The most common chemotherapy regimens are MOPP and ABVD (see box above). Both regimens are given in 28-day cycles for a minimum of six cycles. Chemotherapy is generally continued for two cycles after complete remission is achieved.

Initial Therapy

Because a high percentage of patients may be cured with initial therapy, it is important to select the initial therapy carefully. Proper staging, prognostic indicators, and knowledge of the toxicities of the treatment regimens are important factors considered in the selection of therapy.[6,20] Staging is the most important factor in determining if radiotherapy alone, chemotherapy alone, or a combination of both is the treatment of choice (Table 16-2). Unfavorable prognostic factors such as number of disease sites, bulk of tumor mass, presence of "B" symptoms, age greater than 60, male sex, and lymphocyte-depleted histology also influence treatment choice. Finally, the long-term toxicities of treatment, such as secondary malignancy, sterility, cardiomyopathy, pneumonitis, and opportunistic infections, are considered when therapy is chosen.

When poor prognostic factors are present, the treatment regimen chosen is generally more aggressive. For example, a patient with stage IIA disease without a bulky mass will receive radiation alone; a patient with stage IIA disease with a bulky mass will receive a combination of radiation and chemotherapy. However, aggressive therapy must be chosen with care. The more aggressive the treatment regimen, the more severe the immediate and long-term toxicities. Aggressive therapy may decrease the chances of retreating the patient because of toxic damage to major organs.

Table 16–2   Treatment for Hodgkin's Disease

Stage	Common Treatment	Prognosis
IA and IIA without bulky disease	Radiation to nodal areas of known and suspected disease	70%-85% 10-year DFS*
IB and IIB without bulky disease	Radiation to nodal areas of known and suspected disease; no clear evidence that addition of chemotherapy increases DFS	40% 10-year DFS
IIA and B with bulky disease	Chemotherapy followed by radiation to bulky disease	75% 10-year DFS
IIIA and B	Optimal treatment unresolved Possibilities: Chemotherapy alone Chemotherapy with radiation to bulky disease Chemotherapy with total nodal radiation	No long-term results available
IVA and B	Chemotherapy (MOPP alternating with ABVD)	70% 8-year DFS

*DFS, disease free survival.
Data from Bonadonna G and others: Treatment strategies for Hodgkin's disease, Semin Hematol 25(suppl 2):51, 1988.

Recurrent Disease Therapy

Following initial therapy, 20% to 50% of patients will have residual or recurrent disease.[35] The optimal treatment regimen for these patients continues to be controversial.[35] Patients who relapse following radiation alone are generally treated with chemotherapy and, if technically feasible, with further radiation therapy. For patients relapsing after chemotherapy, several treatment approaches have been used, with varying degrees of success.[35]

When relapse occurs after chemotherapy, the length of disease-free survival is important. Patients experiencing relapse less than 12 months after initial therapy are less likely to achieve a complete remission.[35] ABVD is the most common salvage regimen used in this population. Other regimens have been developed and used, but none are any more effective than ABVD.[35] Overall, approximately 50% of patients will achieve a complete remission and 5% to 10% will have long-term disease-free survival. Patients who experience relapse greater than 12 months after initial therapy can be retreated with the same regimen, usually MOPP. Although 70% to 80% of these patients will achieve a complete remission, only 10% to 20% will experience long-term disease-free survival.

High dose therapy and bone marrow transplantation is another salvage regimen that has gained increased support in the treatment of Hodgkin's disease. Trials of allogeneic, autologous, and peripheral stem-cell transplants have shown effectiveness as a treatment modality.[35] Patients who have been transplanted in early relapse and who have not been treated with multiple chemotherapy regimens have the best results.[35] (See Chapter 24 for further information.)

PROGNOSIS

Patients who achieve remission after second-line therapy have a wide range of reported long-term survival—20% to 80%. Patients who have residual disease or who relapse after second-line therapy have diseases that are difficult to control.[20] Most oncologists do not believe these patients can be cured.

Complications from curative therapy for Hodgkin's disease can occur years after diagnosis and treatment. The major long-term complications of Hodgkin's disease and its treatment are second malignancies and gonadal dysfunction.[3] The most common second malignancies are acute nonlymphocytic leukemia, non-Hodgkin's lymphoma, osteosarcoma, and epithelial tumors. Acute nonlymphocytic leukemia is the most common second malignancy to occur, and it generally occurs anytime within the first decade after treatment. The treatment regimen most often implicated as the risk factor for developing secondary acute nonlymphocytic leukemia is combined modality therapy.[22] The incidence of non-Hodgkin's lymphoma as a secondary malignancy is slightly less than that of acute nonlymphocytic leukemia and it is usually not observed until more than 4 years after treatment.[7,21] Osteosarcoma is more common among survivors of childhood Hodgkin's disease, and the epithelial tumors (e.g., lung or colon) are more common among survivors of adult-onset Hodgkin's disease.[22] The solid tumors are generally not observed until 10 or 20 years after treatment. See the boxes on p. 346.

Gonadal dysfunction and sterility are common long-term effects from the treatment of Hodgkin's disease.[3] In men, chemotherapy (MOPP in particular) is the major cause of infertility. Radiation scatter from pelvic radiation can also significantly affect testicular function. Patients should be made aware of these possible effects before treatment, and sperm banking should be discussed. The testicles should be shielded during pelvic radiation.[7] In women, reproductive dysfunction after radiation or chemotherapy is usually related to primary ovarian failure. Approximately 50% of all female Hodgkin's disease patients will experi-

---

DISEASE RELATED COMPLICATIONS

Hodgkin's disease
Secondary disease development: childhood—osteosarcoma; adult-onset—epithelial (lung and colon).

Non-Hodgkin's lymphoma
Superior vena cava syndrome, central nervous system involvement, spinal cord involvement.

TREATMENT RELATED COMPLICATIONS

Chemotherapy: Secondary malignancies: acute nonlymphocytic leukemia, epithelial tumor
Gonadal dysfunction: sterility, infertility
Radiation therapy: Gonadal dysfunction: sterility, infertility; pneumonitis
Cranial radiation: confusion, headache, nausea, vomiting, seizure, slurred speech, vision changes, changes in mental status, and motor function disabilities.

---

ence some ovarian dysfunction, and 20% to 30% will experience permanent amenorrhea.[7] Women older than 25 years of age and those who are treated with chemotherapy and pelvic radiation have the highest incidence of ovarian failure. These possible effects should be discussed with patients, and, when feasible, the ovaries should be shielded during pelvic radiation. (See Chapter 31 for further information.)

NON-HODGKIN'S LYMPHOMA

EPIDEMIOLOGY AND ETIOLOGY

As a group of neoplasms, non-Hodgkin's lymphoma (NHL) is morphologically and clinically different from Hodgkin's disease. After the Reed-Sternberg cell was identified as the characteristic cell of Hodgkin's disease, all other lymphomas were classified as non-Hodgkin's. Basically, NHL became a term to identify diseases with similarities to Hodgkin's but without the characteristic Reed-Sternberg cell.

In 1993, there were an estimated 43,000 new cases of NHL and 20,500 deaths attributed to NHL.[2] Men are at slightly higher risk than women, and whites are at higher risk than blacks. There is a preadolescent peak of incidence, then a later teenage drop off followed by a steady increase of incidence with age.

The etiology of NHL remains unknown. However, several etiologic factors have been suggested. The most plausible one is immune abnormality.[33,37] The theory suggests that chronic stimulation of the immune system combined with other factors leads to the uncontrolled proliferation of the abnormal lymphocytes that occur in NHL. In support of this theory

is the increased incidence of NHL that occurs with age, in patients on long-term immunosuppression (e.g., organ transplant recipients), and in patients with autoimmune diseases, primary immunodeficiency, or acquired immunodeficiency.[37] Patients who are HIV positive have a four times greater risk of developing NHL.[32] Viruses may also be etiologic factors by virtue of contributing to the chronic stimulation of the immune system. Two viruses linked to NHL are the Epstein-Barr virus and the human T-cell leukemia virus-I (HTLV-I). EBV is most commonly associated with the Burkitt's NHL; HTLV-I is implicated in the etiology of adult T-cell NHL.[12,37]

Exposure to some drugs has also been associated with an increased incidence of NHL. NHL has occurred as a secondary malignancy following chemotherapeutic treatment of acute leukemia and Hodgkin's disease.[33,37] There have also been anecdotal reports of NHL occurring secondary to treatment with diphenylhydantoin.[37]

PREVENTION, SCREENING, AND DETECTION

Prevention of NHL is not applicable because there are no identified preventable risks. Early detection is important but may be hampered by the vagueness of the common symptoms. Patients should be encouraged to seek medical attention for persistent common signs and symptoms.

CLASSIFICATION

Non-Hodgkin's lymphoma is a group of diseases with diverse histologies. Over the years, it was noted that the histology of the tumor has a significant influence on treatment and prognosis of the disease. In the late 1950s, Rappaport introduced a classification system for the various histologic types of NHL that used cell morphology, cytology, and the possible origin of the cell to categorize the diseases.[37] This system was widely accepted and used throughout the United States as a prognostic indicator.[12] As knowledge of the immune and lymphatic systems has increased over the years, the Rappaport classification has undergone alterations. These alterations were formalized into the Working Formulation.[12]

The Working Formulation divides the lymphomas into histologic grades based on the aggressiveness of the cell type and the observed growth pattern.[37] The histologic grades—low, intermediate, and high—generally correspond with the expected clinical course. For example, diseases with a low-grade histology are the least aggressive, and survival is measured in years. There are problems with the Working Formulation in terms of omitted disease entities and exceptions to the prognostic categories.[12] Recently, the National Cancer Institute developed a new clinical schema for NHL that closely mirrors the Working For-

---

NATIONAL CANCER INSTITUTE CLINICAL SCHEMA FOR LYMPHOCYTIC LYMPHOMAS BASED ON NATURAL HISTORY OF UNTREATED OR PALLIATIVELY TREATED PATIENTS

Indolent (median survival measured in years)
Small lymphocytic
Follicular, small cleaved cell
Follicular, mixed
Diffuse, small cleaved cells*
Diffuse, intermediately differentiated (or mantle zone)†
Cutaneous T-cell†

Aggressive (median survival measured in months)
Follicular, large cell
Diffuse mixed
Diffuse large cell
Diffuse immunoblastic‡

Highly aggressive (median survival measured in weeks)
Diffuse small noncleaved cell (Burkitt's)
Diffuse small noncleaved cell (non-Burkitt's)
Lymphoblastic
Adult T-cell leukemia/lymphoma†

---

*Working Formulation intermediate-grade tumor with an indolent natural history.
†Omitted from the Working Formulation.
‡Working Formulation high-grade tumor with an aggressive natural history.
From DeVita VT, Hellman S, and Rosenberg SA: Cancer: Principles and practice of oncology, ed 3, Philadelphia, 1989, JB Lippincott Co.

mulation but addresses its inadequacies (see box above).

CLINICAL FEATURES

The most common symptom of NHL unrelated to AIDS is a painless, enlarged, discrete lymph node in the neck (lymphadenopathy) similar to that of Hodgkin's disease. However, the lymphadenopathy of NHL tends to be more generalized and more commonly involves abdominal nodes and extranodal sites such as the gastrointestinal tract, bone marrow, and liver. Therefore, symptoms of vague abdominal discomfort, back pain, gastrointestinal complaints, and ascites may be present and are usually indicative of abdominal node or gastrointestinal involvement.[12,33] The "B" symptoms (fever, night sweats, and weight loss) occur 20% to 30% of the time, and, although their presence signifies advanced disease, it is not as predictive of prognosis as in Hodgkin's disease (see box on p. 343).

Other possible signs and symptoms depend on the location and extent of involvement. Cough, dyspnea, and chest pain occur about 20% of the time and are indicative of lung involvement.[33] Superior vena cava syndrome may occur, but it is rare because medias-

tinal involvement occurs in less than 20% of cases and is primarily seen in adult T-cell lymphoma.[12] Skin lesions that appear as isolated nodules or papules and frequently ulcerate occur in about 20% of cases and are most common in diseases of a T-cell origin, specifically cutaneous T-cell lymphoma.[12,33] Central nervous system involvement may be primary (mass lesions) or secondary (meningeal involvement). It is most commonly an aggressive type of NHL and is the most common extra-nodal site in HIV positive patients.[32] Manifestations of central nervous system involvement, such as headache, mental changes, confusion, lethargy, seizures, visual defects, cranial nerve palsies, or acute spinal cord compression, depend on the site of involvement.[12,33]

As in Hodgkin's disease, there are no specific laboratory studies indicative of NHL. A complete blood count is normal most of the time, even if bone marrow involvement is present. Unexplained anemia may be present in about 20% of cases, and lymphopenia can occur in as many as 50% of cases. ESR may be elevated as occurs in Hodgkin's disease.[33] Increased uric acid and calcium are frequent at diagnosis, and alkaline phosphatase is usually elevated when the liver is involved.[33] When the lactic acid dehydrogenase (LDH) is elevated there is generally a large tumor burden. The lymphocytes may show chromosomal abnormalities; however, the diagnostic value of such abnormalities is not known.[33]

DIAGNOSIS AND STAGING

A biopsy of an abnormal lymph node or mass is necessary to diagnose NHL. Following a diagnosis of NHL, the clinical stage of the disease must be determined. Although only 15% to 20% of cases have localized disease, a staging process is necessary to identify the extent of the disease and the bulk of the tumor mass. The Ann Arbor Staging Classification is used to identify the extent of disease in NHL, although it is not as prognostically important as in Hodgkin's disease.[12]

The recommended staging procedures for NHL are as follows[10,12,33,37]:

1. Detailed history and complete physical examination with close examination of all peripheral node regions
2. Laboratory work-up including complete blood count, differential, platelet count, ESR, liver function tests, renal function tests, uric acid, calcium, alkaline phosphatase, LDH, serum immunoglobulins, and serologic tests
3. Radiology work-up including a chest x-ray and CT scan or MRI of the abdomen and pelvis if presenting signs and symptoms indicate
4. Bilateral posterior iliac crest bone marrow aspirate and biopsy

5. Diagnostic lumbar puncture, if central nervous system symptoms are present or if bone marrow is involved
6. Endoscopy or gastroscopy if gastrointestinal lymphoma is suspected
7. Diagnostic thoracentesis or paracentesis if pleural or ascitic fluid is present
8. Lymphangiogram, liver biopsy, or laparotomy are rarely necessary but may be done if the treatment plan would be altered by outcome

METASTASIS

The metastatic process varies with the type of lymphoma: Follicular has bone marrow involvement and diffuse disseminates rapidly and involves areas such as the central nervous system, bone, and gastrointestinal tract.

TREATMENT MODALITIES AND PROGNOSIS

The histologic type, the extent of the disease, and the patient's performance status are the most important factors in determining the treatment approach to NHL.[12,33] The histologic type as identified by the classification systems is the best indicator of the natural history of the disease. Indolent (low-grade) lymphomas have a natural history that can be measured in years, aggressive (intermediate-grade) lymphomas' natural history is measured in months, and highly aggressive (high-grade) lymphomas' natural history can be measured in weeks. Thus, the treatment approach is logically dictated by the aggressiveness of the histologic type.[12]

The extent of disease is considered in conjunction with the histologic type in the determination of treatment.[5] However, histologic type is the more important factor. As previously mentioned, the Ann Arbor staging system is of limited use in staging NHL because, according to this system, most patients with NHL have widely disseminated disease at diagnosis. Although staging is considered when determining treatment, the staging for NHL needs to be modified according to histologic type to be of significant use.[12]

Performance status of the patient is important in determining treatment regimens because of the toxicities of the regimens. The patient's physical status, age, and underlying medical problems may affect the choice of therapy.[12] It is important for long-term survival that adequate treatment is given from the beginning. Therefore, the extent of disease and patient performance status need to be addressed so that treatment regimens can be modified, if necessary (e.g., a patient with underlying chronic obstructive pulmonary disease should not receive regimens containing bleomycin).

The treatment of primary lymphoma in extra-nodal sites is the exception to determining treatment by histologic type. The gastrointestinal tract and the central nervous system are the most common extra-nodal sites affected by NHL. Involvement of the gastrointestinal tract accounts for about 10% of all cases of NHL.[15,30] Surgery, chemotherapy, and radiation therapy may all be used to treat primary lymphoma involving the gastrointestinal tract. Surgery alone is curative only in patients with truly localized disease. The addition of either radiation or chemotherapy postoperatively has improved survival.[24] However, controlled trials and longer follow-up periods are necessary.

The incidence of primary central nervous system lymphoma is increasing and survival for these patients is short.[28] Cranial radiation, commonly done in conjunction with surgery, has prolonged survival, but with few long-term survivors. Due to the blood-brain barrier, systemic chemotherapy is only modestly effective in these patients.[28] Regimens providing high-dose methotrexate have shown the best results. However, these results are transient with few long-term survivors.[28] For chemotherapy to be more effective, the drugs must be able to be delivered across the blood-brain barrier. Some current trials are investigating means of improving the drug delivery across the blood-brain barrier.[28]

Indolent Non-Hodgkin's Lymphoma

There is controversy whether treatment of indolent or low-grade NHL can induce long-term disease-free survival and actually alter the natural history of the disease.[12,38] Because the natural history of indolent lymphomas is such that most patients live with disease and eventually die of their disease in spite of treatment, the controversy is understandable. With treatment, patients will experience several episodes of remission and subsequent relapse, and the question remains whether the benefit of multiple remissions outweigh the toxicities of the treatment.

Localized (stage I or II) indolent NHL is rare and easily treated. Radiation therapy to the involved field or total nodal radiation produces 60% to 80% 5-year disease-free survival.[12] The role of chemotherapy in the treatment of localized indolent lymphoma has not been greatly explored and is, therefore, unclear.

Most patients with indolent NHL have disseminated (stage III or IV) disease at diagnosis. As discussed above, the optimal treatment regimen for these patients is controversial. Treatment may be deferred until symptoms become bothersome or the disease has evolved into a more aggressive type of lymphoma.[12] Patients whose histology converts to an aggressive type are then treated with curative therapy appropriate for the more aggressive histology. Patients who receive radiation tend to relapse in unirradiated sites, and those who receive chemotherapy tend to relapse in previous disease sites. Hence, the question arises as to the efficacy of combined modality (chemotherapy and radiation) therapy. Current clinical trials are exploring the options of deferred treatment, combination chemotherapy, and combined modality therapy.

Aggressive Non-Hodgkin's Lymphoma

The aggressive lymphomas constitute about 60% of all NHL.[12] Hence, more is known and more treatments have been tried for this group of lymphomas. In the treatment of the aggressive lymphomas, the relationship of tumor burden and bulk to prognosis is well-documented. As tumor burden and bulk increase, prognosis declines. The prognostic features that signal increased tumor burden and bulk are poor performance status, more than one mass that is greater than 10 cm in diameter, presence of disease in multiple extranodal sites, presence of "B" symptoms, and elevation in LDH (greater than 500 IU/ml).[5,12] These prognostic features are important considerations in the choice of treatment regimens.

Localized disease occurs in less than 20% of aggressive lymphomas.[12] Radiation to the site of disease is the treatment of choice. However, the addition of chemotherapy to radiation regimens seems to improve results because it decreases the risk of relapse in unirradiated sites. There is little information available on the effect of chemotherapy alone in the treatment of localized aggressive NHL.

Patients with disseminated disease and those with local disease that have one or more poor prognostic features are considered to have advanced aggressive lymphoma. Combination chemotherapy is the treatment of choice (Table 16-3). Patients with advanced aggressive lymphoma are more readily cured than those with indolent lymphomas, and more than 60% of these patients are being cured.[12] The achievement of a first complete remission is a must in achieving prolonged survival.

A variety of chemotherapy regimens have been shown to be successful in the treatment of advanced aggressive lymphomas (Table 16-3). The drawback to these regimens is the toxicity, particularly myelotoxicity, that may cause doses to be modified or courses to be delayed. When this occurs, patients are not receiving the optimal therapy and chances of achieving a complete remission are decreased. Regimen schedules have been developed to stagger myelotoxic and nonmyelotoxic agents so that optimal doses can be given with decreased toxicity.[12]

This patient population is also at risk for central nervous system relapse following successful systemic therapy. The central nervous system is a sanctuary site for lymphomas. To minimize the risk of central nervous system relapse, high-dose methotrexate, which crosses the blood-brain barrier, or intrathecal chemotherapy agents have been added to the regimens.[12] See the boxes on p. 346.

Highly Aggressive Non-Hodgkin's Lymphoma

Highly aggressive lymphomas are almost always disseminated. Therefore, staging is of questionable value.[12] The treatment of highly aggressive lymphomas requires an intense chemotherapy regimen similar to those used to treat acute leukemia.[12] The treatment regimen should include induction, consolidation, and maintenance phases and provide prophylactic treatment to the central nervous system. If complete remission is not achieved with initial therapy, the chance of any significant disease-free survival is dismal. Following aggressive treatment, as many

Table 16–3 Chemotherapy Regimens for Aggressive Lymphomas

ProMACE-MOPP Flexitherapy	Day 1	Day 8	Day 15	Days 16-28
				No therapy
Cyclophosphamide 650 mg/m² IV	x	x		
Doxorubicin 25 mg/m² IV	x	x		
Etoposide 120 mg/m² IV	x	x		
Methotrexate 1.5 mg/m² IV			x with leucovorin rescue	
Prednisone 60 mg/m² PO	x..................................... x			

Flexible number of cycles until complete response or decreased rate of response, then switch to:

	Day 1	Day 8	Day 14	Days 15-28
				No therapy
Nitrogen mustard 6 mg/m² IV	x	x		
Vincristine 1.4 mg/m² IV	x	x		
Procarbazine 100 mg/m² PO	x..................................... x			
Prednisone 60 mg/m² PO	x..................................... x			

Same number of cycles as ProMACE, then restart ProMACE.

Continued.

Table 16–3 Chemotherapy Regimens for Aggressive Lymphomas—cont'd

m-BACOD	Day 1	Day 8	Day 15	Days 16-21
				No therapy
Cyclophosphamide 600 mg/m² IV	x			
Doxorubicin 45 mg/m² IV	x			
Vincristine 1 mg/m² IV	x			
Bleomycin 4 mg/m² IV	x			
Methotrexate 200 mg/m² IV		x rescue x with leucovorin rescue		
Dexamethasone 6 mg/m² PO	xxxxx			

COP-BLAM	Day 1	Day 10	Day 14	Days 15-21
				No therapy
Cyclophosphamide 400 mg/m² IV	x			
Doxorubicin 40 mg/m² IV	x			
Vincristine 1 mg/m² IV	x			
Procarbazine 100 mg/m² PO	x.................... x			
Prednisone 40 mg/m²	x.................... x			
Bleomycin 15 mg IV			x	

COP-BLAM III	Day 1	Day 2	Day 3	Day 4	Day 5
Cycle A					
Vincristine 1 mg/m²/day IV infusion	x................ x				
Bleomycin 7.5 mg/m² IV bolus, then 7.5 mg/m²/day IV infusion	x... x				
Cyclophosphamide 350 mg/m² IV	x				
Doxorubicin 35 mg/m² IV	x				
Prednisone 40 mg/m² PO	x	x	x	x	x
Procarbazine 100 mg/m² PO	x	x	x	x	x

Cycle B
Like Cycle A without bleomycin and without day 2 of vincristine infusion

Week	1	3	7	10	13	16	19	22	25	28	31	34
Cycle	A	B	A	B	A	B	A	B	A	B	A	B

CAP-BOP	Day 1	Day 7	Day 8	Day 21
Cyclophosphamide 650 mg/m² IV	x			
Doxorubicin 50 mg/m² IV	x			
Procarbazine 100 mg/m² PO	x.................... x			
Vincristine 1.4 mg/m²			x	
Bleomycin 10 U/m² SC			x	
Prednisone 100 mg PO			x................. x	

Cycles repeated every 3-4 weeks

ProMACE-CytaBOM	Day 1	Day 8	Day 14	Days 15-21
				No therapy
Cyclophosphamide 650 mg/m² IV	x			
Doxorubicin 25 mg/m² IV	x			
Etoposide 120 mg/m² IV	x			
Cytarabine 300 mg/m² IV		x		
Bleomycin 5 mg/m² IV		x		
Vincristine 1.4 mg/m² IV		x		
Methotrexate 120 mg/m² IV		x with leucovorin rescue		
Prednisone 60 mg/m² PO	x x			
Cotrimoxazole 2 PO bid throughout 6 cycles of therapy				

MACOP-B Week	1	2	3	4	5	6	7	8	9	10	11	12
Cyclophosphamide 350 mg/m² IV	x		x		x		x		x		x	
Doxorubicin 50 mg/m² IV	x		x		x		x		x		x	
Vincristine 1.4 mg/m² IV		x		x		x		x		x		x
*Methotrexate 400 mg/m² IV		x				x				x		
Bleomycin 10 mg/m² IV				x				x				x
Prednisone 75 mg/m² PO od	x... taper											
Cotrimoxazole 2 PO bid	x... x											

*With leucovorin rescue.
From DeVita VT, Hellman S, and Rosenberg SA: Cancer: Principles and practice of oncology, ed 3, Philadelphia, 1989, JB Lippincott Co.

as 94% of patients with good prognostic features (LDH < 300 IU/ml and no bone marrow involvement) can experience a 5-year relapse-free survival. More recently, clinical trials are investigating the use of bone marrow transplantation as a consolidation therapy for this group of patients.

Recurrent Disease Therapy

Effective treatment regimens for residual or relapsed NHL are being investigated. Patients with indolent lymphoma who relapse usually receive symptomatic treatment. High dose therapy followed by bone marrow transplantation holds the most promise for recurrent aggressive lymphoma. Allogeneic, autologous, and peripheral stem-cell transplants are being investigated to determine their efficacy as a standard treatment modality for NHL. (See Chapter 24 for further information.)

Nursing Management

Patients with malignant lymphona can experience a broad range of physical conditions, from being mildly symptomatic to being acutely ill. Patients with localized or indolent disease may be relatively asymptomatic from the disease and treatment. The majority of these patients are treated as outpatients, and the side effects from their treatments are generally not severe. Patients with extensive or aggressive disease are more often acutely ill and at risk for potentially severe side effects of therapy.

There are several potential complications specific to patients with malignant lymphoma that nurses need to monitor so nursing care can be planned appropriately and nursing interventions can be implemented promptly. These potential complications are lymphadenopathy, myelosuppression, and central nervous system involvement.

Lymphadenopathy is the primary symptom of malignant lymphoma. Most of the time, the enlarged nodes are nontender. However, they can cause pain or dysfunction by compressing neighboring tissues or organs. Lymphadenopathy can also cause a decrease in lymph and venous return to the heart. The flow of lymph through the affected lymph nodes is blocked because the disease process has destroyed the architecture of the nodes. Because the lymphatic system is in close proximity to the venous system, enlarged nodes may mechanically obstruct venous blood flow. The blockage of lymph and venous flow creates lymphedema in the tissues distal to the affected node region. When assessing a patient with lymphadenopathy, it is important to note the function of the surrounding tissues and organs and the presence of lymphedema. A plan must be implemented that provides for optimal mobility and drainage of the affected limb.

Myelosuppression is a common complication of cancer treatment. Patients experiencing myelosuppression are at increased risk for infection, bleeding, and anemia. As in the leukemias, myelosuppression in lymphoma can be caused by the disease as well as by the treatment regimens. This is significant in this population because patients may experience marked and prolonged myelosuppression that results in increased morbidity. Patients who have compromised bone marrow function before treatment will experience a more rapid and generally prolonged myelosuppressive period. Patients who are myelosuppressed must be monitored closely for signs and symptoms of infection, bleeding, and anemia. Thorough assessment and prompt treatment are essential to decreasing the morbidity and mortality of the myelosuppressed patient.

The degree and length of myelosuppression may also affect the treatment plan. Treatment may be delayed until bone marrow function recovers and future chemotherapy doses may be decreased to prevent severe myelosuppression. In both instances, optimal treatment is being compromised and may affect disease response. In addition to protecting patients from infection, bleeding, and anemia, nurses must assist patients in coping with possible changes in their treatment plans.

Lymphomatous involvement of the central nervous system is another potential complication of malignant lymphoma. It is more common in the aggressive and highly aggressive types of NHL. The involvement can occur as a space-occupying lesion in the brain or spinal cord or as an infiltration of the cerebral spinal fluid that causes irritation to the meninges. Cord compression, seizures, altered mental status, or cranial nerve palsies can occur as a result. Nurses, therefore, must be alert to subtle changes in patients' neurologic functioning. Nursing care must include assessment of mobility, sensory deficits or enhancements, cognitive abilities, and self-care abilities. Interventions must be appropriate to the patient's level of functioning. The ultimate goal is to assist the patient to achieve optimal functioning.

More than 50% of patients diagnosed with malignant lymphoma today will be alive in 5 years. However, complications can occur years after diagnosis and successful treatment and can have a significant impact on psychosocial functioning. Patients generally have an increased sense of vulnerability, fear of recurrence, and distress over changes in physical condition. Patients may have no apparent body changes secondary to disease and treatment but may feel less adequate, physically damaged, and less in control.

Patients and families all bring their past history, experiences, and preconceived ideas into new situations. For teaching to be effective, these things need to be identified and incorporated into the teaching plan. Because the malignant lymphomas are such a diverse group of diseases, they are often confusing. This is also a stressful time for patients and families, and it can be difficult for them to understand the abstract concepts of the disease and treatment. Consistent repetition and varying ways of providing information generally increase the ability to understand new concepts. Community resources often provide educational, emotional, or financial support and assistance. An assessment of patients' support systems, resources, and ability to communicate needs and feelings is important for nurses to be able to assist patients in maintaining or re-establishing roles and identities in school, work, and interpersonal relationships. Patient teaching priorities and geriatric considerations are given in the boxes at right.

Examples of nursing care plans for malignant lymphoma follow.

PATIENT TEACHING PRIORITIES

Signs and symptoms of disease: fever, night sweats, weight loss, painless lymphadenopathy, generalized vague gastrointestinal discomfort, and back pain.

Signs and symptoms of infection: fever, chills, cough, erythema, and malaise.

Sexual dysfunction: infertility, sterility, discuss options for contraception and ovary and sperm banking.

Discuss treatment options: chemotherapy, radiation therapy, surgery, bone marrow transplant: purpose, schedule, simulation plan for radiation therapy, monitoring weekly blood counts, chemotherapy drug side effects and schedule, bone marrow transplant types (allogenic/autologus) pre-during-post transplant care components.

GERIATRIC CONSIDERATIONS

Chemotherapy dose and schedule may be altered related to compromised cardiac, hepatic, renal, respiratory, and or neuromuscular function.

Radiation therapy side effects: skin-excessive dryness, and early skin reactions; increased fatigue; medication dose adjustment to minimize side effects; consider facilitation with transportation.

Financial considerations: Fixed income—consider consultation with social services regarding housing, meals on wheels, medication prescriptions, self-care needs.

NURSING DIAGNOSES

• Coping, ineffective, individual:
    Related to new diagnosis
    Related to potential life-style changes

INTERVENTIONS

• Assess patient's level of distress and anxiety related to:
    Uncertainty of future
    Bothersome symptoms
    Changes in self-concept
    Effect of past experiences
• Assess for signs of maladaptive or risky behaviors that interfere with responsible health practices:
    Missed appointments
    Failure to attend to symptoms
    Chronic attention to symptoms
    Loss of future orientation
• Identify patient's support system, resources, and communication patterns.
• Assess patient's problem solving capabilities.
• Assess patient's level of knowledge regarding recurrence, development of secondary malignancy, and long-term effects of treatment.
• Listen attentively and provide support.
• Encourage verbalization of fears and concerns.
• Assist patient to recognize stressors and assist with problem solving.
• Provide reassurance that anxiety or distress about health are common feelings among cancer survivors.
• Initiate referrals to social work, psychology, or community resources, as appropriate.

NURSING DIAGNOSES — cont'd

- Coping, compromised, family:
    Related to new diagnosis

- Infection, potential for:
    Related to myelosuppression

- Knowledge deficit:
    Related to disease process
    Related to treatment
    Related to complications

- Physical mobility, impaired, potential for:
    Related to CNS involvement
    Related to lymphadenopathy

INTERVENTIONS — cont'd

- Assess past family relationships and coping patterns.
- Provide opportunities for expression of feelings.
- Include family/significant other in teaching sessions.
- Assist family/significant other in meeting adaptations and changes in activities and roles, as needed.
- Initiate referrals to social work, psychology, or community resources, as appropriate.
- Assess for presence of risk factors:
    Bone marrow involvement
    Decreased WBC
- Assess for signs and symptoms of infection:
    Fever
    Cough
    Erythema
- Institute measures to prevent exposure to potential sources of infection:
    Meticulous hand washing
    Meticulous hygiene
    Avoid people with colds, flu
    Good oral hygiene after meals
- Monitor laboratory values:
    Blood counts
    Electrolytes
    Liver enzymes
- Minimize invasive procedures.
- Reassure patient and family that increased susceptibility to infections is temporary.
- Evaluate patient and family readiness to learn.
- Identify barriers to learning, such as language, physical deficiencies, psychologic deficiencies, intellectual development.
- Determine patient and family level of knowledge of:
    Function of lymph system
    Signs and symptoms of lymphoma
    Chemotherapy and radiation therapy
    Side effects of treatment
- Review information patient and family have already been given. Reinforce and clarify misconceptions.
- Explain basic anatomy and physiology of lymphatic system and of specific body systems affected by location of disease.
- Review and reinforce information regarding recurrence, secondary malignancy, and long-term effects of treatment.
- Individualize information for subtype of lymphoma and extent of disease.
- Explain symptoms of potential complications.
- Explain radiation therapy fields and possible side effects (see Chapter 21).
- Explain principles of chemotherapy, names of specific agents, and possible side effects (see Chapter 22).
- Provide written materials to reinforce teaching.
- Encourage verbalization of questions, fears, and concerns.
- Listen attentively and provide support.
- Initiate referrals to other health care professionals and community resources as needed.
- Assess range of motion, strength of hands, arms, and legs.
- Assess mobility for ambulation and for self-care activities.
- Take steps to reduce environmental hazards.
- Encourage patient to perform active range of motion, moderate exercise, and adequate rest.
- Assist patient with ambulation as needed.

NURSING DIAGNOSES — cont'd
- Self-care deficit, potential for:
    Related to CNS involvement
    Related to disease progression

- Sensory alteration, potential for:
    Related to CNS involvement

- Sexuality patterns, altered:
    Related to disease process
    Related to treatment

- Tissue perfusion, alteration, potential for:
    Related to lymphadenopathy

INTERVENTIONS — cont'd
- Assess patient's abilities for
    Self-feeding
    Self-bathing and grooming
    Self-dressing
- Assess patient's motivation and endurance for self-care.
- Promote patient's maximum involvement in self-care activities.
- Provide assistance with self-care activities as appropriate to patient's level of functioning.
- Assess patient for level of orientation and level of activity.
- Orient patient to all three spheres as needed.
- Provide meaningful sensory input (e.g., clock, calendar, familiar objects).
- Explain all activities and request patient's perception of situation.
- If patient becomes confused, direct back to reality.
- Assess for physical symptoms that may affect libido:
    Fatigue
    Nausea and vomiting
    Anorexia
    Pain
- Assess for fear, anxiety, depression, and diminished self-concept.
- Promote open communication about sexual issues by bringing up the subject.
- Discuss possible effects of disease and treatment regimen on libido and sexual functioning (see Chapter 31).
- Assess for signs and symptoms of lymphedema
    Redness
    Warmth
    Swelling
- Assess function of surrounding tissues and organs.
- Encourage mobility of affected limb.
- Elevate affected limb.
- Assess for infection secondary to lymphedema.

CONCLUSION

To provide the best patient care, nurses must be knowledgeable of the disease process and the principles of chemotherapy and radiation therapy. Nurses need to be able to provide patients and families with information regarding the disease process, treatment options, possible side effects of treatment, and consequences of treatment. This information is necessary for patients and families to make informed choices and to monitor signs and symptoms on a routine basis. Providing consistent repetition of information can help patients and families understand the abstract concepts of the disease and treatment regimen.

Psychosocial issues, such as coping, sexuality, and survivorship, also must be addressed. Malignant lymphomas, particularly Hodgkin's disease, have peak incidences in young to middle adulthood, affecting most patients at a very productive, goal-oriented time of life. Caring for lymphoma patients offers the nurse varied and exciting challenges.

BIBLIOGRAPHY

1. Acker B and others: Histologic conversion in the non-Hodgkin's lymphomas, J Clin Oncol 1:11, 1983.
2. American Cancer Society: Cancer facts and figures—1993, Atlanta, 1993, American Cancer Society.
3. Bakemeier RF: Recent advances in the management of Hodgkin's disease, Curr Concepts Oncol Fall:2, 1984.
4. Bierman P and Armitage JO: Salvage therapy for patients with relapsed or refractory aggressive non-Hodgkin's lymphoma, Oncology 1:11, 1987.
5. Bonadonna G and Jotti GS: Prognostic factors and response to treatment in non-Hodgkin's lymphoma (review), Anticancer Res 7:685, 1987.
6. Bonadonna G and others: Treatment strategies for Hodgkin's disease, Semin Hematol 25(Suppl 2):51, 1988.
7. Bookman MA and Longo DL: Concomitant illness in patients treated for Hodgkin's disease, Cancer Treat Rev 13:17, 1986.

8. Canellos GP, Nadler L, and Takvorian T: Autologous bone marrow transplantation in the treatment of malignant lymphomas and Hodgkin's disease, Semin Hematol 25(Suppl 2):58, 1988.

9. Carella AM and others: High-dose chemotherapy with autologous bone marrow transplantation in 50 advanced resistant Hodgkin's disease patients: An Italian study group report, J Clin Oncol 6:1411, 1988.

10. Casciato DA and Lowitz BB: Manual of bedside oncology, Boston, 1983, Little, Brown & Co.

11. Cohen DG: Metabolic complications of induction therapy for leukemia and lymphoma, Cancer Nurs 6:307, 1983.

12. DeVita VT, Hellman S, and Rosenberg SA: Cancer: Principles and practice of oncology, ed 3, Philadelphia, 1989, JB Lippincott Co.

13. DeVita VT and others: The role of chemotherapy in diffuse aggressive lymphomas, Semin Hematol 25:2, 1988.

14. Eddy JL, Selgas-Cordes R, and Curran M: Cutaneous T-cell lymphoma, Am J Nurs 84:202, 1984.

15. Gospodarowicz MK and others: Outcome analysis of localized gastrointestinal lymphoma treated with surgery and postoperative irradiation, Int J Radiation Oncology Biol Phys 19:1351, 1990.

16. Grufferman S and others: Hodgkin's disease in siblings, N Engl J Med 296:248, 1977.

17. Grufferman S, Duong T, and Cole P: Brief communication: occupation and Hodgkin's disease, J Natl Cancer Inst 57:1193, 1976.

18. Guyton AC: Textbook of medical physiology, ed 7, Philadelphia, 1986, WB Saunders Co.

19. Jagannath S and others: Prognostic factors for response and survival after high-dose cyclophosphamide, carmustine, and etoposide with autologous bone marrow transplantation for relapsed Hodgkin's disease, J Clin Oncol 7:179, 1989.

20. Jotti GS and Bonadonna G: Prognostic factors in Hodgkin's disease: implications for modern treatment (review), Anticancer Res 8:749, 1988.

21. Koletsky AJ and others: Second neoplasms in patients with Hodgkin's disease following combined modality therapy—the Yale experience, J Clin Oncol 4:311, 1986.

22. Kushner BH, Zauber A, and Tan CTC: Second malignancies after childhood Hodgkin's disease, Cancer 62:1364, 1988.

23. Lacher MJ: Hodgkin's disease and infectious mononucleosis: is there a causal association? CA 31:359, 1981.

24. Liang R and others: Chemotherapy for early-stage gastrointestinal lymphoma, Cancer Chemother Pharmacol 27:385, 1991.

25. List AF and others: Non-Hodgkin's lymphoma of the gastrointestinal tract: an analysis of clinical and pathologic features affecting outcome, J Clin Oncol 6:1125, 1988.

26. McNally JC, Miaskowski C, Rostad M, Somerville ET, editors: Guidelines for oncology nursing practice, Philadelphia, ed 2, 1991, WB Saunders.

27. Miller TP and others: Southwest Oncology Group clinical trials for intermediate- and high-grade non-Hodgkin's lymphomas, Semin Hematol 25(suppl 2):17, 1988.

28. Neuwelt EA and others: Primary CNS lymphoma treated with osmotic blood-brain barrier disruption: Prolonged survival and prevention of cognitive function, J Clin Oncol 9:1580, 1991.

29. Paffenbarger RS, Wing AL, and Hyde RT: Brief communication: characteristics in youth indicative of adult-onset Hodgkin's disease, J Natl Cancer Inst 58:1489, 1977.

30. Sharma S and others: Primary gastric lymphoma: A prospective analysis of 12 cases and review of the literature, J Surgical Oncol 43:231, 1990.

31. Silverberg E, Boring CC, and Squiries TS: Cancer statistics, 1990, CA 40:1, 1990.

32. Stanley H, Fluetsch-Bloom M, and Bunce-Clyma M: HIV-related non-Hodgkin's lymphoma, Oncol Nurs Forum 18:875, 1991.

33. Thorup OA: Fundamentals of clinical hematology, ed 5, Philadelphia, 1987, WB Saunders Co.

34. Velasquez WS and others: Effective salvage therapy for lymphoma with cisplatin in combination with high-dose Ara-C and dexamethasone (DHAP), Blood 71:117, 1988.

35. Vose JM, Bierman PJ, and Armitage JO: Hodgkin's disease: The role of bone marrow transplantation, Semin Oncol 17:749, 1990.

36. Wasserman AL and others: The psychological status of survivors of childhood/adolescent Hodgkin's disease, Am J Dis Child 141:626, 1987.

37. Williams WJ and others: Hematology, ed 3, New York, 1983, McGraw-Hill.

38. Young RC and others: The treatment of indolent lymphomas: watchful waiting V aggressive combined modality treatment, Semin Hematol 25(suppl 2):11, 1988.

CHAPTER 17

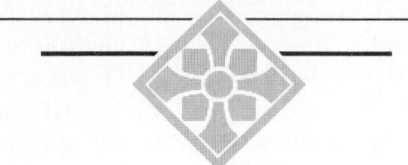

Multiple Myeloma

Jane C. Clark

EPIDEMIOLOGY

Multiple myeloma is a rare malignancy of plasma cells that accounts for only 1% of all hematologic malignancies diagnosed in the United States.[1] The disease accounts for an estimated 12,800 new cases and 9400 deaths each year.[1] An increase in the incidence rate over the past decades is partially attributable to an improvement in diagnostic techniques.

Multiple myeloma is diagnosed in an equal number of men and women and occurs 14 times more frequently in blacks than whites. Multiple myeloma is diagnosed primarily in individuals over 40 years of age with a peak incidence at about 60 years of age.[3]

ETIOLOGY AND RISK FACTORS

The etiology of multiple myeloma is not completely understood. Basic research in animal models has identified cellular factors such as chromosome abnormalities, host-genetic factors, chronic antigenic stimulation, viruses, and growth factors as possible contributors to the development of plasma cell dyscrasias. Other host factors, such as increasing age, race, and occupational exposure to petroleum products, asbestos, and radiation, may contribute to increasing risk for the disease.[3,5,11]

PREVENTION, SCREENING, AND DETECTION

No recommendations exist for the prevention or screening of asymptomatic individuals for multiple myeloma.[1,3] Detection of multiple myeloma in symptomatic individuals is based on a thorough history, physical examination, laboratory and radiographic studies.

CLINICAL FEATURES

Although some individuals may be asymptomatic, the majority of individuals present to the clinician with a history of weakness, anorexia, weight loss, and fatigue. Symptoms of more advanced disease include bone pain, particularly in the back, and anemia. Depending on the sites of involvement, additional symptoms may include recurrent infection, changes in urinary patterns, and cognitive, sensory, or motor changes.[2,5,8,11] Findings on physical examination are related to the sites of involvement. Fever, redness, swelling, tenderness, and pus formation associated with bacterial infections may be present. Peripheral neuropathies may be noted. The skin may be pale and petechiae and/or ecchymoses may be present (Figure 17-1). The box on p. 357 gives the clinical features and disease and treatment related complications of multiple myeloma.

DIAGNOSIS AND STAGING

The diagnosis of multiple myeloma is based on findings obtained from laboratory and radiographic studies. Serum and urine electrophoretic and immunologic studies will reveal elevations in IgG, IgA, and/or light chain levels. Additional laboratory studies may demonstrate anemia, thrombocytopenia, and leukopenia in the presence of bone marrow involvement, hypercalcemia in the presence of lytic bone lesions, and proteinuria, hyperuricemia, azotemia, elevated BUN, creatinine, and Bence-Jones urine protein levels with renal involvement. Radiographic studies commonly include skeletal x-rays, bone surveys, and magnetic resonance imaging (MRI) to detect the presence of osteoporosis, osteolytic lesions, or pathologic fractures.[2,3,5,11] For a diagnosis of multiple myeloma to be made, one or more of the following criteria must be met: (1) plasma cell infiltration of the bone marrow of at least 10%, (2) a monoclonal spike on serum or urine electrophoresis, (3) radiographic confirmation of osteoporosis and osteolytic lesions, and (4) soft tissue plasma cell tumors.

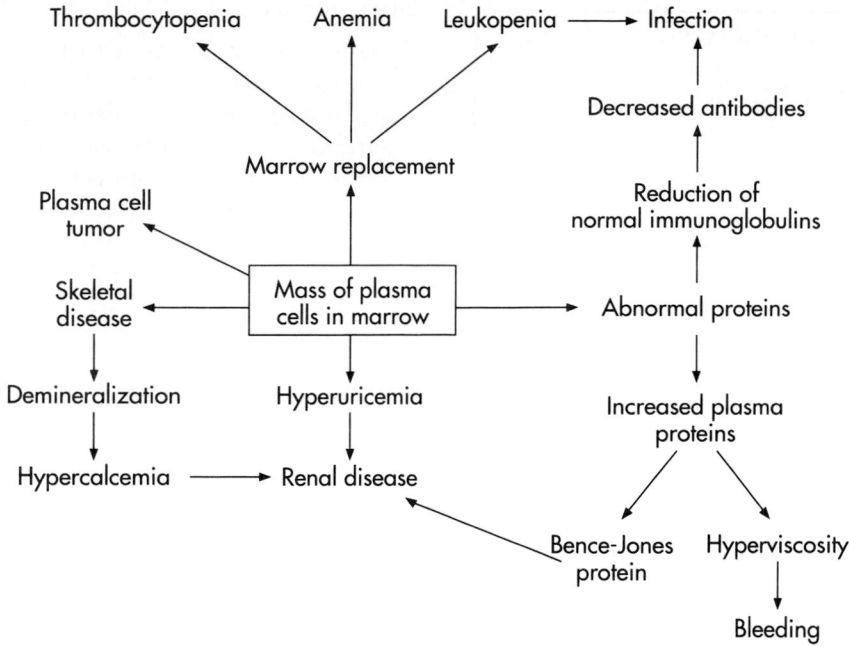

Figure 17–1   Pathogenesis of multiple myeloma. (From Megliola B: Multiple myeloma, Cancer Nursing 3(3):221, 1980.)

> **MULTIPLE MYELOMA**
>
> *Clinical features*
> Anorexia, fatigue, weight loss; back and bone pain; recurrent infections; changes in cognitive, sensory, and motor function, and urinary pattern
>
> *Disease-related complications*
> Thrombocytopenia, severe anemia, leukopenia and renal failure, spinal cord compression, hypercalcemia and dehydration
>
> *Treatment-related complications*
> Myelosuppression, renal insufficiency, mental status changes, neuropathy, cardiopulmonary toxicities

No universal staging system for multiple myeloma exists currently. One example of a commonly used staging system based on tumor burden is presented in the box on p. 358.

TREATMENT MODALITIES

Treatment of multiple myeloma in the early stages of the disease consists of observation if patients are asymptomatic. Patients are monitored with interval clinical examinations, laboratory, and radiographic studies for signs of progressive disease such as severe anemia, thrombocytopenia and leukopenia, bone pain, osteolysis, or renal failure. Once progression of disease is documented, active treatment with antineoplastic agents or radiation therapy is initiated.

Chemotherapy

Chemotherapy most commonly consists of intermittent melphalan and prednisone and results in a 60% response rate. Responses are generally short-term and most patients will experience progression of the disease. Clinicians have used combinations of prednisone, high-dose melphalan, vincristine, BCNU, cyclophosphamide, and doxorubicin as salvage therapy with limited success.[2,3,5,11] The use of biologic therapy, alpha interferon and interleukin-2, has shown some potential when used in combination with antineoplastic agents.

Radiation Therapy

Radiation therapy may be used to treat patients with chemotherapy-resistant disease, to relieve bone pain, and to treat spinal cord compression. Although radiation therapy can markedly improve the quality of life for patients with multiple myeloma, length of survival is not enhanced.[3]

Bone Marrow Transplantation

Recently, the role of autologous bone marrow transplantation in the treatment of patients with multiple myeloma has been explored. Success has been limited by the inability to eradicate the malignant plasma cell clone. However, researchers continue to evaluate the effectiveness of high-dose antineoplastic therapy followed by autologous transplant with marrow that has been purged with an antibody specific for plasma cells.[3]

```
┌─────────────────────────────────────────────┐
│              MYELOMA STAGING SYSTEM           │
│                                               │
```

A. Multiple myeloma
   Major criteria
   I. Plasmacytoma on tissue biopsy
   II. Bone marrow plasmacytosis with > 30% plasma cells
   III. Monoclonal globulin spike on serum electrophoresis exceeding 3.5 g/dl for G peaks or 2.0 g/dl for A peaks, ≥ 1.0 g/24 h of κ- or λ-light chain excretion on urine electrophoresis in the presence of amyloidosis
   Minor criteria
   a. Bone marrow plasmacytosis 10% to 30% plasma cells
   b. Monoclonal globulin spike present, but less than the level defined above
   c. Lytic bone lesions
   d. Residual normal IgM < 50 mg/dl, IgA < 100 mg/dl, or IgG < 600 mg/dl
      Diagnosis will be confirmed when any of the following features are documented in symptomatic patients with clearly progressive disease. The diagnosis of myeloma requires a minimum of one major + one minor criterion or three minor criteria that must include a + b, i.e.:
      1. I + b, I + c, I + d (I + a not sufficient)
      2. II + b, II + c, II + d
      3. III + a, III + c, III + d
      4. a + b + c, a + b + d
B. Indolent myeloma (same as myeloma except)
   I. No bone lesions or only limited bone lesions (≤3 lytic lesions); no compression fractures
   II. M-component levels: (a) IgG < 7 g/dl; (b) IgA < 5/dl
   III. No symptoms or associated disease features, i.e.:
      a. Performance status > 70%
      b. Hemoglobin > 10 g/dl
      c. Serum calcium normal
      d. Serum creatinine < 2.0 mg/dl
      e. No infections
C. Smoldering myeloma (same as indolent myeloma except)
   I. No bone lesions
   II. Bone marrow plasma cells ≤ 30%
D. MGUS
   I. Monoclonal gammopathy
   II. M-component level
      IgG ≤ 3.5 g/dl
      IgA ≤ 2.0 g/dl
      BJ protein ≤ 1.0 g/24 h
   III. Bone marrow plasma cells < 10%
   IV. No bone lesions
   V. No symptoms

IgA, immunoglobulin A; IgG, immunoglobulin G; IgM, immunoglobulin M; BJ, Bence Jones light chain.
From Salmon SE & Cassady JR: Plasma cell neoplasms. In DeVita VT Jr, Hellman S, Rosenberg SA, editors, Cancer: Principles & practice of oncology, ed 3, Philadelphia, 1989, JB Lippincott Co., p. 1864.

PROGNOSIS

Prognosis for patients with multiple myeloma is determined by the severity of organ involvement at the time of diagnosis and response to active treatment. Asymptomatic patients may live with the disease for months to years without active treatment. For symptomatic patients requiring treatment, a pattern of response has been described. During the initial 2 to 3 years of treatment, patients respond well to antineoplastic therapy. A plateau phase follows when the disease remains stable but does not respond as well as in the initial phase. During the third phase, the disease becomes resistant to the antineoplastic therapy and progresses at a rapid rate.[3,5] A statistically significant improvement in the relative 5-year survival rate (26%) occurred from the 1970s to 1980s.[1]

CONCLUSIONS

The patient with multiple myeloma will present many challenges to the health care team during the course of the disease. As no cure for the disease is available and the course of disease is protracted over several years for most patients, the focus of the team is to plan with the patient and significant others care that will maintain as much independence in activities or daily living, provide as safe a living and treatment environment, and preserve an acceptable level of patient comfort. The care demands cooperation and support from significant others as well as members of the health care team in the acute care and community settings.

Table 17–1 Nursing Assessments for Complications of Multiple Myeloma

Complication	Nursing Assessments
Renal Insufficiency	• Monitor BUN, creatinine, uric acid, calcium, potassium, glucose, and phosphorus levels as ordered by the physician. • Assess for changes in the character of the urine: volume, color, and odor.
Hyperviscosity Syndrome	• Monitor for intermittent claudication and changes in the skin color of the extremities. • Assess for neurologic changes such as headache or visual disturbances. • Monitor for changes in mental status such as irritability, drowsiness, confusion, or coma. • Assess for signs and symptoms of congestive heart failure.[5]
Dehydration	• Monitor intake and output every 8 hours. • Assess skin turgor each day. • Evaluate subjective symptoms by patient such as thirst, dryness of skin.

Nursing Management

Nursing care for the patient with multiple myeloma centers on educating the patient and significant others about the disease and treatment, teaching self-care skills to minimize threats to quality of life, monitoring for signs and symptoms of complications of the disease and/or treatment, and coordinating implementation of an interdisciplinary plan of care that addresses complications of the disease and/or treatment. The teaching plan for patients with multiple myeloma and their significant others includes information about the chronic nature of the disease, rationale for observation in patients without symptoms, and health-enhancing strategies such as maintaining an adequate fluid intake of 3000 cc each day, maintaining mobility to decrease the risk of bone destruction from inactivity, and safety precautions to minimize the risk of injury from thrombocytopenia, anemia, and leukopenia. Specific nursing interventions to address common nursing diagnoses among patients with multiple myeloma are presented in other chapters in this text (i.e., Chapter 28 and Chapter 29).

As bony destruction is a common effect of multiple myeloma and pathological fractures can alter the quality of life significantly, safety precautions are stressed in developing a long-term plan of care.

NURSING DIAGNOSES: POTENTIAL FOR INJURY RELATED TO BONY DESTRUCTION BY PLASMA CELL TUMORS

Assessment

- Identify personal risk factors for injury (extent and sites of bony involvement, muscle strength of extremities, changes in sensation, difficulty in ambulating, type of shoes worn when ambulating, knowledge of proper body mechanics, mental status).
- Identify environmental risk factors for injury (crowded rooms, area rugs, proximity of needed articles or bathroom).
- Assess perceived threats to safety from the patient's perspective.

Interventions

- Consult physical therapy for instruction in proper body mechanics, transfer techniques, positioning, and use of assistive devices, for development of an exercise program to maintain muscle strength and range of motion without jeopardizing risk of pathologic fractures.

- Arrange the hospital room environment to decrease the risks to safety: Phone, call light, and personal articles within easy reach, clear pathway to the bathroom.
- Refer to home health agency to evaluate home environment for safety risk factors and recommended modifications prior to discharge.
- Encourage the patient to ask for assistance from health care team or significant others, as needed, with ambulation or activities of daily living.[4,8,10]

The nurse also assumes responsibility for monitoring the patient with multiple myeloma for signs and symptoms of complications of the disease and/or treatment such as hypercalcemia, pain, spinal cord compression, renal insufficiency, hyperviscosity syndrome, and dehydration. Often early recognition and treatment of these complications will result in improvement in the ability of the patient to tolerate treatment as well as in quality of life. Specific nursing assessments and interventions for patients at risk for or experiencing hypercalcemia, spinal cord compression, and pain are detailed in Chapters 19 and 29. Nursing assessments to monitor for renal insufficiency, dehydration, and hyperviscosity syndrome are presented in detail in this chapter (Table 17-1). Presence of any of the signs and symptoms should be reported to the physician.

The boxes below list patient teaching priorities and geriatric considerations.

PATIENT TEACHING PRIORITIES

Signs and symptoms of infection (fever, chills, pain, erythema, swelling, and pus formation); monitoring fluid intake and output, self-care measures: potential for injury (walking, changes in sensation, muscle strength) and chronic nature of the disease

---

GERIATRIC CONSIDERATIONS

Peak incidence of disease 60 years of age
Issues regarding occupation and potential for early retirement
Social and recreational activities may need adjustment to conserve energy and minimize injury risks
Potential for mental status changes
Consider environmental safety factors and abilities to meet self-care needs for hygiene, nutrition, elimination, and comfort

---

REFERENCES

1. American Cancer Society: Cancer facts and figures—1993. Atlanta, 1993, American Cancer Society.
2. Anderson MG: The lymphomas and multiple myeloma. In Baird SB, Donehower MG, Stalsbroten VL, and Ades TB, editors: A cancer source book for nurses, ed 6, Atlanta, 1991, American Cancer Society.
3. Bubley GJ and Schnipper LE: Multiple myeloma. In Holleb AI, Fink DJ, and Murphy GP, editors: American Cancer Society textbook of clinical oncology, Atlanta, 1991, American Cancer Society.
4. Clark JC, McGee RF, and Preston R: Nursing management of responses to the cancer experience. In Clark JC and McGee RF, editors: Core curriculum for oncology nursing, ed 2, Philadelphia, 1992, WB Saunders Co.
5. Cook MB: Multiple myeloma. In Groenwald SL, Frogge MH, Goodman M, and Yarbro CH, editors: Cancer nursing: Principles and practice, ed 2, 1990, Boston, Jones and Bartlett Publishers.
6. Finley JP: Nursing care of patients with metabolic and physiological oncological emergencies. In Clark JC and McGee RF, editors: Core curriculum for oncology nursing, ed 2, Philadelphia, 1992, WB Saunders Co.
7. Fleck A: Mobility, impaired physical, related to disease process and treatment. In McNally JC, Stair JC, and Somerville ET, editors: Guidelines for cancer nursing practice, Orlando, FL, 1985, Grune & Stratton, Inc.
8. Megliola B: Multiple myeloma, Cancer Nursing 3(3):209-218, 1980.
9. North Central New Jersey Local Chapter. Body fluid composition, alteration in hypercalcemia. In McNally JC, Stair JC, and Somerville ET, editors: Guidelines for cancer nursing practice, Orlando, FL, 1985, Grune & Stratton, Inc.
10. North Central New Jersey Local Chapter. Mobility, impaired physical, related to primary bone malignancy or metastatic bone disease. In McNally JC, Stair JC, and Somerville ET, editors: Guidelines for cancer nursing practice, Orlando, FL, 1985, Grune & Stratton, Inc.
11. Salmon SE and Cassady JR: Plasma cell neoplasms. In DeVita VT Jr., Hellman S, Rosenberg SA, editors: Cancer: Principles & practice of oncology, ed 3, Philadelphia, 1989, JB Lippincott Co.
12. Schnipper L, Wagner H, and McCaffrey R: Multiple myeloma and plasma cell dyscrasias. In Cady B, editor: Cancer manual, Boston, 1986, American Cancer Society.
13. Sporn J and McIntyre O: Chemotherapy of previously untreated multiple myeloma patients: An analysis of recent treatment results, Semin Oncol 13(3):318-325, 1986.
14. Willoughby S: Pain. In McNally JC, Stair JC, and Somerville ET, editors: Guidelines for cancer nursing practice, Orlando, FL, 1985, Grune & Stratton, Inc.

CHAPTER 18

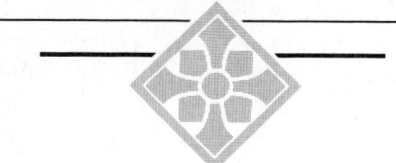

Skin Cancers

Shirley E. Otto

Skin cancers are classified into two basic groups: nonmelanoma and malignant melanoma. The two major cancers in the nonmelanoma group are basal cell and squamous cell carcinomas. Basal and squamous cell carcinomas combined account for more than one third of the 1.8 million new cases of cancer reported each year in the United States.[1,12]

Malignant melanoma is an increasingly common cutaneous malignancy. The incidence has doubled every decade since 1930. Unlike many other forms of cancer that disproportionately affect older individuals, melanoma frequently affects young people. The median age is in the early 40s. Survival of patients with malignant melanoma is directly related to early detection and prompt medical intervention.[11,13,15]

NONMELANOMA SKIN CANCERS
Basal Cell Carcinoma

EPIDEMIOLOGY
Basal cell carcinoma is the most commonly occurring skin cancer and malignant tumor found in humans. This tumor most frequently affects whites and rarely occurs in dark-skinned persons. Basal cell carcinoma is two times more common in men than women and is usually seen in persons after the age of 40.[12] Sun-exposed areas of the body, primarily the head and neck region, are frequent sites of basal cell carcinoma. Numerous types of basal cell carcinoma exist: including nodular, superficial, morpheaform, pigmented, and keratonic basal cell carcinoma syndrome. The most common form is the nodular type. This type of basal cell carcinoma frequently occurs on the face, especially the cheeks, forehead, eyelids, and nasolabial folds.[1,12]

ETIOLOGY AND RISK FACTORS
Environmental factors play an important role in the development of basal cell carcinoma. Ultraviolet radiation, primarily chronic exposure to the sun, appears to be the most important environmental risk factor.[9,10,12] Other environmental factors in basal cell carcinoma may include exposure to coal tar, pitch, creosote, and arsenic and chronic ingestion of inorganic arsenicals.[1,2,9] Genetic factors such as basal cell nevus syndrome, fair skin, and light-colored hair have been associated with the development of basal cell carcinoma. A persons' medical history is also important. An increased risk of developing basal cell carcinoma is present in persons who have received a deep burn or have been exposed to x-rays, especially during the first half of this century.[2,3,12,34]

PREVENTION, SCREENING, AND DETECTION
The primary cause of skin cancers is solar exposure. Ultraviolet (UV) radiation is divided into three different wavelengths: UVA, UVB, and UVC. UVA waves are longer and penetrate more deeply into the dermis than UVB waves. As a result of the deeper level of penetration, UVA radiation causes changes in blood vessels and premature aging, and is linked with carcinogenesis.[12] In contrast, UVB waves are shorter (penetrating into the epidermis) than UVA waves. UVB radiation produces the most damage to the skin in the form of sunburns and premature aging. Exposure to UVB radiation is associated with development of malignant melanoma.[7,13] UVC waves are the shortest and rarely reach the surface of the earth because of the blocking effect of the ozone layer and offer little threat.[22]

Most tanning booths emit UVA radiation. Indoor

tanning with UVA radiation is frequently promoted as providing protection against UVB sunburns. The deeper penetration of UVA waves into the dermis causes melanin production; however, the melanosomes are not transferred to the superficial layer of the skin known as the epidermis.[15,34] Persons with a UVA tan who are exposed to UVB radiation receive skin damage in the form of sunburns. The erythema associated with the sunburn is not visible because of the masking effect of the UVA suntan. Exposure to ultraviolet radiation from tanning beds should be avoided.[15,24,35]

While it has been shown that UVB radiation is related to carcinogenesis of both melanoma and nonmelanoma skin cancer, it has not definitively been shown that stratospheric ozone depletion is translating into increasing penetrating ultraviolet radiation. The ozone depletion issue is very controversial and complex. Studies will need to continue to determine the varying effects the ozone depletion has on skin cancer development and trends.[2]

Some experts recommend that "When you reach for the sunglasses, reach for the sunscreen."[20]

Protecting the cutaneous surfaces from excess solar exposure would greatly decrease the incidence of skin cancers. Solar exposure may be decreased without adversely affecting outdoor activities by employing a few simple measures. Intense sunlight should be avoided between 10:00 A.M. and 3:00 P.M. when ultraviolet rays are the strongest. Outdoor activities, such as walking, gardening, and other hobbies, should be planned for the early morning or late afternoon to minimize exposure. Protective clothing, such as hats and long-sleeved shirts, helps to minimize sun exposure.

The use of sunscreens with sun protection factor (SPF) ratings of 15 or higher are preferred over those with low ratings (less than 10). Sunscreens should be applied 15 to 30 minutes before exposure and every 2 to 3 hours during exposure. Sunscreens may need to be applied more often because heat, humidity, and sweat combine to decrease the effectiveness of the sunscreens. Sunscreens should be applied liberally to sun-exposed areas of the body, especially the head and neck region, which are frequent sites of occurrence of basal cell carcinoma. Special attention should be paid to the nose, rim of the ears, cheeks, and forehead.[6,24,27]

CLASSIFICATION AND CLINICAL FEATURES

Basal cell carcinoma often presents as a single, small, firm, dome-shaped, flesh-colored nodule with raised edges and pearly white borders. Telangiectatic vessels are usually prominent and easily recognizable through the thin epidermis. The center of the lesion frequently ulcerates and bleeds and may resemble a

---

CLINICAL FEATURES
BASAL CELL CARCINOMA

Nodular basal cell carcinoma

Bulky, nodular growth due to lack of keratinization

Characteristics include a thinning epidermis, producing a shiny translucent, pearly hue over the lesion

Early stages resemble a smooth pimple that fails to heal

As the tumor enlarges, the border edge raises and the center becomes necrotic

Lesion bleeds easily from mild injury and doubles in size every 6 to 12 months[3,10] at the rate of 5 millimeters per year[34]

Superficial basal cell carcinoma

Tends to develop in multiple sites, growing peripherally across the skin surface, becoming as large as 10 to 15 centimeters

Appears most frequently on the trunk as a well-demarcated, erythematous, scaly, patch with[3,9] discreet nodules

Often confused with psoriasis[34]

Pigmented basal carcinoma

Contains melanin in the epidermis, dermis, and within the tumor itself

Often mistaken clinically as melanoma

Colors include: blue, black, brown appearance with a raised pearly border

Found in dark-complexioned persons such as Latin Americans or Japanese (not blacks)[36]

Morpheaform or sclerotic basal cell carcinoma

A more aggressive lesion that appears as a flat, depressed scar-like plaque, pale yellow or white in color

Margins are indistinct with nodules, ulcerations, or bleeding occurring within the plaque

Often undetected or misdiagnosed and has a lower cure rate than nodular BCC[3,9,34]

Keratonic basal cell carcinoma

Appears clinically similar to nodular ulcerative

Located in the preauricular and postauricular sulcus

Aggressive in its growth

Often recurs locally

Type most likely to metastasize[3,9,34]

---

pimple that has failed to heal. Examination of all skin surfaces once a month is imperative for those persons at risk of developing new lesions or recurrences of old lesions.[34] Basal cell carcinoma is classified according to clinical and histologic differences (see box above).

DIAGNOSIS AND STAGING

Clinical diagnosis of skin cancers must be confirmed by histologic studies. A shave biopsy (top of lesion into depth of middermis) is performed using local anesthesia. Punch biopsy (sharp, small circular "punch" similar to a cookie cutter approach) is used if the tumor is suspected to be in the deeper layers of the skin. The tissue sample is examined to determine the clinical diagnosis and identifying features of the various classifications.

Upon determination of the clinical diagnosis, classification, and histopathologic grading, specific treatment modalities are recommended.[3,4,12,34]

The American Joint Committee on Cancer recommends the following stage grouping:

CLINICAL STAGING FOR NONMELANOMA SKIN CANCER (BASAL AND SQUAMOUS)*

Stage 0 (T_{is}, N_0, M_0)
1. Carcinoma in situ
2. No evidence of regional lymph node or distant metastasis

Stage I (T_1, N_0, M_0)
1. Primary tumor is superficial and is 2 cm or less at largest dimension
2. No evidence of regional lymph node or distant metastasis

Stage II (T_2, N_0, M_0; or T_3, N_0, M_0)
1. Primary tumor is greater than 2 cm but no larger than 5 cm in largest dimension, *or* primary tumor is greater than 5 cm in largest dimension
2. No evidence of regional lymph node or distant metastasis

Stage III (T_4, N_0, M_0; or any T, N_1, M_0)
1. Primary tumor invades deep extradermal structures such as cartilage, skeletal muscle, or bone, *or* any tumor size with evidence of regional lymph node metastasis
2. No evidence of distant metastasis

Stage IV (any T, any N, M_1)
1. Presence of distant metastasis regardless of tumor size or nodal involvement

Histopathologic grading for basal and squamous cell carcinomas is similar to the grading system for other cancers. G_1 signifies well-differentiated tumor cells, G_2 equals moderately well-differentiated cells, G_3 signifies poorly differentiated cells, and G_4 signifies undifferentiated cells. Confirmation of the extent of disease by biopsy of the suspected cutaneous or subcutaneous spread is imperative.[3,4,34]

METASTASIS

Basal cell cancer metastasizes via the lymphatics or blood and is a rare occurrence. The most common predisposing factors are size of primary tumor and response to surgery and radiotherapy. Recurrence of the disease varies with the size of the tumor and length of follow-up. Recurrence rates vary; less than one third occur in the first year; 50% occur in 2 years; and nearly 66% within the first 3 years; 18% occur in the fifth and tenth year following treatment.[34]

TREATMENT MODALITIES

Treatment for both basal and squamous cell carcinomas depends on many factors: the size and location of the lesion, the histologic type of cancer, extension into nearby structures, presence of metastases, previous treatment, anticipated cosmetic results, and the age and condition of the patient. Multiple modalities exist for the treatment of basal cell carcinoma: surgery, radiation therapy, chemotherapy, and biotherapy.†

Surgery

Surgical intervention is used to treat about 90% of basal cell carcinoma. The goal is the complete removal of the tumor. Most of the procedures require local anesthesia, minimal equipment, and can be performed in an ambulatory setting. The various surgical methods are listed below.[3,34,36]

EXCISIONAL SURGERY. Excisional surgery is usually performed with a 4 mm margin. This is the treatment of choice in large tumors or those with poorly defined margins on cheeks, forehead, trunk, and legs. Surgical excision may also be indicated when metastasis is present.[9,17,34]

CRYOSURGERY. Cryosurgery involves tissue destruction by freezing. Liquid nitrogen is administered by a spray or the use of cryoprobes. Rapid freezing results in intracellular and extracellular ice crystallization. Cell destruction is potentiated by a rapid freeze and slow thaw cycle. This method is useful in small to large nodular and superficial basal cell carcinomas, but is *not* indicated for deeply invasive tumors.[9,17]

ELECTRODESICCATION AND CURETTAGE. This surgical method uses heat to destroy tissue. After the tumor is marked and anesthetized, a debulking process is used to scrape away abnormal tissue within 1 to 2 mm. The base of tumor is then electrodesiccated. Curettage of the base is performed using a large and tiny curet to track any extension of the tumor. The procedure is repeated as necessary until a normal plane of tissue is reached. These interventions are useful with small (<2 cm) to medium nodular and superficial basal cell carcinomas with well-defined margins. Basal cell carcinomas larger than 2 cm in diameter, those located in zones at high risk for recurrence, and all high-risk squamous cell carcinoma are best treated by other methods.[3,9,34]

MOHS CHEMOSURGERY. Mohs chemosurgery in-

---

*Adapted from Beahrs OH and Myers MH, editors: Manual for staging of cancer, ed 4, Philadelphia, 1992, JB Lippincott.

†References 3, 9, 10, 33, 34.

volves surgical removal of the tumor layer by layer until all margins are free of the tumor on microscopic examination. This is the treatment of choice for invasive squamous cell and primary basal cell carcinomas that are larger than 2 cm in diameter, have indistinct clinical margins, are located on zones of the face, with a known high recurrence rate, occurring in a cosmetic or functional area, such as the nose or eyelid, or are aggressive, such as morpheaform basal cell carcinoma.[3,17,34]

Regardless of the surgical treatment used, the cure rate for basal cell carcinoma following surgical intervention is nearly 95%.

Radiation Therapy

Radiation therapy is a viable and effective alternative when surgical interventions are contraindicated and in elderly or debilitated persons who are unable to tolerate a surgical procedure. Tissue conservation is a benefit of radiation therapy, especially when dealing with lesions on the nose, eyelid, or lips. Cosmetic results are good with this type of treatment because surgical scars and skin grafting are eliminated. A combined approach of preoperative and postoperative radiation and surgery may be indicated for extensive tumors. Disadvantages of this treatment method are related to the administration schedule. Radiation is fractionated over multiple treatment sessions (usually 450 Gy/3 weeks in 300 cGy daily fractions) to reduce radiation-induced side effects. This schedule may pose problems for patients and their families who must travel a distance to reach the treatment center.[9,34]

Radiation therapy is not recommended for tumors located on the trunk, extremities, dorsum of the hands, tumors of the scalp, those arising in sweat and sebaceous glands and for morpheaform basal cell, verrucous squamous cell, tumors over 8 cm in size, and/or those tumors located on the upper lip growing into the nostril.[19,34]

Chemotherapy

Topical 5-fluorouracil (5-FU) may be used in nevoid basal cell carcinoma syndrome but is contraindicated in treating any of the other types of basal cell carcinoma. 5-FU will destroy the surface tumor without affecting deeper cells, thus allowing invasion to continue at the base of the tumor.

The lack of an established systemic therapy for recurrent or advanced local, regional, or metastatic disease has led to the use of biologic response modifiers (BRM), especially α-interferon. Systemic α-interferon has produced a 50% objective response rate in clinical testing. Intralesional α-interferon has produced an even greater response rate of 77%.[3] Other agents, specifically retinoids, have also shown some activity against basal cell carcinoma. Topical retinoid therapy and systemic retinoid therapy have both produced objective response rates greater than 50% in both basal and squamous cell carcinomas.[9,34]

PROGNOSIS

Metastatic disease is rarely seen with basal cell carcinoma, even though it tends to be a locally aggressive tumor. If left untreated, the tumor will locally invade vital structures such as blood vessels, lymph nodes, nerve sheaths, cartilage, bone, lungs, and the dura mater.[9,29,30]

Basal cell carcinoma is highly curable with early detection and treatment. Cure rates are close to 100% in persons with lesions less than 1 cm. The overall 5-year survival rate is approximately 95% when surgical intervention or radiation therapy is used.[9,30]

It is adamant that patients with basal cell carcinoma continue defined scheduled follow-up examinations by a physician. Follow-up examinations should be performed at 6-month intervals during the first 2 years and then yearly for 5 years to detect the recurrence of previously treated or new primary basal cell carcinomas, while they are small enough to remove without significant cosmetic loss.[29,30]

Squamous Cell Carcinoma

EPIDEMIOLOGY

Squamous cell carcinoma is less common than basal cell carcinoma. Squamous cell carcinoma occurs more frequently in persons with light complexions. Squamous cell carcinoma is also more common in men, and the incidence increases with advancing age. The average age of onset for squamous cell carcinoma is approximately 60 years. Unlike basal cell carcinoma, this tumor frequency occurs on the hands and forearms as well as on the head and neck region,[12] especially the ears, lower lip, scalp, and upper face.[1,15,34]

ETIOLOGY AND RISK FACTORS

Squamous cell carcinoma is most often found in sun-damaged skin previously affected by actinic keratoses. All of the predisposing risk factors mentioned in regards to basal cell carcinoma have also been associated with the development of squamous cell carcinoma.[24]

PREVENTION, SCREENING, AND DETECTION

Prevention and detection methods are similar for both squamous cell and basal cell carcinoma. The avoidance of ultraviolet light and the use of sunscreens and protective clothing are important. In addition to the head and neck area, sunscreens should also be liberally applied to the hands and forearms.[22,24]

CLINICAL FEATURES
SQUAMOUS CELL CARCINOMA

General characteristics

Occurs anywhere on sun-damaged skin and/or on mucous membrane with squamous epithelium

Appears as a round to irregular shape, with a plaque-like or nodular character covered by a warty scale, indistinct margins, firm erythematous dome shaped nodule with a corelike center that ulcerates

Dull red in color

Grows by expansion and infiltration as well as by tracking along various tissue planes

Invades below the level of the sweat gland and has a higher degree of malignant potential[9,22,34]

Ischemic ulceration

Occurs in varicose ulcers, chronic ulcers, poorly healed fistulas/tracks with old scars

Accompanied by increased drainage, pain, and bleeding

Bowen's disease

Associated with arsenic ingestion

Occurs on sun-exposed and non-sun-exposed areas of the skin including mucous membrane of vulva, vagina, nose, and conjunctiva

Nodular reddish-brown plaque with areas of scales and crusts[9,34]

Actinic chelitis

Rapidly growing progressive invasive lesion that occurs on the lip often as the result of smoking

Lower lip is the primary site in 95% of the cases

Early appearance is a local thickening, progressing to a firm nodular lesion with destructive ulceration

Diagnosis is frequently missed (2 years after onset) and is usually 1 to 2 cm in diameter at initial biopsy[22,34]

Verrucous

A well-differentiated lesion frequently seen on the glans penis, vulva, scrotum, sole, back, or buttock and appears as a slowly growing, warty lesion[22,34]

CLASSIFICATION AND CLINICAL FEATURES

Squamous cell carcinoma has a more indiscriminate method of classification. Because of the varying general characteristics and the source of tissue presentation, it is classified by presenting symptoms, tissue source, and histologic difference (see box above).

DIAGNOSIS AND STAGING

Diagnosis and staging for squamous cell carcinoma are the same as for basal cell described earlier in this chapter.[3,4]

METASTASIS

Overall, 2% to 3% of all patients with squamous cell of the skin develop metastatic disease, with death resulting in 75% of these patients. The occurrence and degree varies according to morphologic characteristics, and size and depth of penetration of the tumor. Metastasis occurs late via the lymphatics (within 2 years) after the tumor has invaded the subcutaneous lymph nodes and the lymphatics of the deeper structure.[5,9,10,34]

TREATMENT MODALITIES
Surgery

Squamous cell carcinoma can be treated by procedures similar to those used with basal cell carcinoma. Some exceptions exist; for example, a slightly larger excisional margin should be performed surgically. In addition, it is important to examine the regional lymph nodes for the presence of tumor.

The treatment of high risk squamous cell with no palpable nodes may involve local control alone, regional control with prophylactic lymph node dissection, radiation to draining nodes, or combined therapy. Metastatic squamous cell in lymph nodes is treated surgically, with adjuvant radiation therapy given preoperatively or postoperatively.[5,9,34]

Chemotherapy

Topical 5-FU is recommended for treatment of premalignant actinic keratosis. In advanced squamous cell carcinoma, systemic retinoids have produced response rates greater than 70%.[9]

Radiation Therapy

Radiation therapy is used for primary squamous cell using a variety of fractionation regimens ranging from 22 Gy in a single fraction to 70 Gy in multiple fractions.

PROGNOSIS

Of the two nonmelanoma skin cancers, metastasis is seen more often in squamous cell carcinoma. Ordinarily, primary squamous cell carcinoma localized to the skin has an incidence of metastasis of approximately 3%. The ability of the lesion to metastasize depends on the size, the degree of differentiation, and the depth of invasion. Squamous cell carcinoma may metastasize to the regional lymph nodes or to the lung. Primary lesions of the lip metastasize more frequently at a rate greater than 10%.

Squamous cell carcinoma also has high cure rates (75% to 80%) when either surgery or radiation therapy is used. Because this lesion has the ability to metastasize as well as recur, it is generally considered a higher risk skin cancer. Most of the deaths resulting from nonmelanoma forms of skin cancer can be attributed to squamous cell carcinoma.

As in basal cell carcinoma, regularly scheduled follow-up is adamant for patients with squamous cell carcinoma. The recommended schedule is 6-month intervals during the first 2 years and then yearly for 5 years.[3,9,29,30]

Nursing Management

Nursing diagnoses for basal cell and squamous carcinoma are similar. Some variations may be necessary depending on type and location of skin cancer and method of treatment.

NURSING DIAGNOSES
- Knowledge deficit related to prevention and early detection of skin cancer
- Knowledge deficit related to disease process
- Knowledge deficit regarding method of treating disease (surgery, radiation therapy, and chemical therapy)
- Knowledge deficit regarding home care management of surgical wound
- Skin integrity, impaired, related to skin cancer and surgical treatment
- Infection, potential for, related to surgical wound
- Impaired physical mobility, potential for, related to surgical treatment and possible skin graft
- Self-concept, disturbance in, related to location and surgical treatment for skin cancer
- Social interaction, potential for impairment, related to location and surgical treatment of skin cancer
- Anxiety, potential for, related to diagnosis of cancer, fear of recurrence, death, pain, disfigurement, and changes in life-style

Nursing assessment and intervention should focus on prevention, detection, and treatment methods. The nursing history should include a thorough skin assessment, which consists of information regarding patient risk factors, and a complete skin examination. Patient teaching should include the prevention and detection methods discussed in this chapter (see box at right). Geriatric considerations are listed in the left-hand box on p. 367.

Postsurgical interventions include instructing patients and families on the management of a surgical wound. Keeping the area clean and dry, and observing for signs and symptoms of infection are imperative. If skin grafting is required, patients and their families should be instructed to keep the graft immobile to prevent stress on the edges of the wound. Limbs should be elevated to minimize edema. Mineral oil or lanolin may be used to remove superficial crusts, moisten the site of the skin graft, and stimulate circulation. Treatment and disease related side effects are listed in the right-hand box on p. 367. Nursing man-

agement of side effects of other treatment methods such as radiation therapy, chemotherapy, and biotherapy are discussed in detail in Chapters 21, 22, and 23, respectively.

The importance of early detection should be stressed with both patients and families. Basal cell

---

PATIENT TEACHING PRIORITIES

Risk factors for the development of malignant melanoma

Family history of malignant melanoma
Presence of blond or red hair
Presence of marked freckling on the upper back
History of three or more blistering sunburns prior to age 20
History of 3 or more years of an outdoor summer job as a teenager
Presence of actinic keratosis[6,12,13,24]

Prevention of skin cancer measures

Avoid excessive sun exposure, particularly the hours between 10:00 AM and 3:00 PM
Wear sunscreens and lip balm with a sun protection factor of 15 or greater
Use available shade
Wear protective clothing
Refrain from using manufactured tanning devices[11,20,24]

Skin cancer screening and detection

Perform monthly self-examination of skin and/or with use of a buddy or other person
With good lighting, use two mirrors to visualize the abdomen, perineal area, and back
Use blow hairdryer and mirror to visualize the scalp
Observe each body part carefully, especially hidden areas such as between the toes and folds of skin
Use of body chart will facilitate documentation of changes and suspected lesions to report
Persons with two or more family members with a history of malignant melanoma should be examined by a dermatologist every 6 months
Recognize and report symptoms or changes in skin characteristics promptly to the physician such as:
   A = Asymmetry of shape
   B = Border irregularity
   C = Color variegation (black, brown, white, (blue, and red)
   D = Diameter larger than 5 mm[6,8,14,19,20,24]

carcinoma is almost always curable. Recurrent lesions or new lesions can be successfully treated when detected early for basal and squamous cell carcinoma.

Patients and family members should be instructed on the procedure and the importance of periodic skin self-examination. Patients should be encouraged to keep appointments for regular follow-up examina-

tions with their physician. Methods of prevention should also be taught, primarily the importance of avoiding intense sunlight and using protective sunscreens and clothing.[6,7,14,22]

GERIATRIC CONSIDERATIONS[11,18,22,27]

Geriatric population has the greatest incidence of precancerous and cancerous skin lesions

Average age of onset for squamous cell, lentigo malignant melanoma, and acral lentiginous melanoma is 60 years

Age-related sensory and muscle deficits require assistance of buddy for monthly self-skin examination

Age-related changes in skin characteristics include fair skin, easily bruised superficial tissue

Limited access to health care system, and limited health care resources that may inhibit preventive health care

Target senior citizen centers to reach those who participate in organized activities

---

TREATMENT-RELATED COMPLICATIONS FOR SKIN CANCERS

Surgery and radiation therapy[18]

Scarring of affected tissue, skin discoloration, alterations in cosmetic appearance, chronic skin ulcerations, limited use of limb if extensive treatment

Chemotherapy and biotherapy[18,21,22]

Nausea and vomiting, flu-like syndrome, myelosuppression, paresthesia, necrotic tissue as result of drug extravasation, pulmonary fibrosis, renal damage, hot flashes, hypersensitivity, ototoxicity, alopecia, and allergic reaction

General

Alteration in cosmetic appearance and body image, loss of functional use of extremity, scarring and skin discoloration, metastatic disease process resulting in invasive treatment and potential ultimate death

---

MALIGNANT MELANOMA

EPIDEMIOLOGY

Melanoma, a relatively uncommon tumor, affects approximately 32,000 persons in the United States each year.[1] The incidence of melanoma is increasing at the rate of 4% annually.[1] Estimates are that, by the year 2000, 1 in 100 persons will develop a primary malignant melanoma during their lifetime.[12] The increase in incidence has been greater in men than women. White males have increased 5.1% each year, 93.3% overall, while females have increased only 3.8% per year, 67.7% overall.

Similar to the nonmelanoma skin cancers, malignant melanoma most frequently affects whites. The most common site of occurrence in dark-skinned persons are palms, soles, nailbeds, fingers, toes, and mucous membranes. Unlike basal and squamous cell carcinomas, melanoma may occur in persons in their teens and early twenties and thirties.[12] The highest incidence rates occur in persons over the age of 60.[15] In men, the upper back and trunk are the most common sites of occurrence; the back and lower extremities are the most common sites in women (Figure 18-1).

ETIOLOGY AND RISK FACTORS

Two important environmental factors are sun exposure and geographic latitude. Intense, intermittent

exposure to the sun, especially during childhood and adolescence, increases the risk for melanoma in later life.[1,12] A latitude gradient for melanoma also exists in countries with areas of high solar exposure also being the areas of highest melanoma incidence. For every 1000 feet above sea level, there is a compounded 4% increase in UVR exposure.[12,13] In short, the closer one lives to the equator, the higher the risk for developing melanoma.[15,25]

Genetic risk factors, such as fair complexion and blond or red hair color, are similar for the development of both nonmelanoma skin cancers and malignant melanoma. A person's ability to tan seems to be a factor; persons who burn easily and are poor tanners have an increased risk.[1,2] Persons who experience intermittent heavy sun exposure are also at higher risk. In addition, a personal or family history of melanoma, dysplastic nevus syndrome, or congenital nevi also increases one's risk. First-degree relatives of patients with melanoma are roughly two to eight times more likely than the general public to be diagnosed with melanoma.[14,25,28]

PREVENTION, SCREENING, AND DETECTION

Prevention methods for nonmelanoma skin cancers and malignant melanoma are similar. The avoidance of intense sun exposure and the use of protective clothing and sunscreens are important. Children

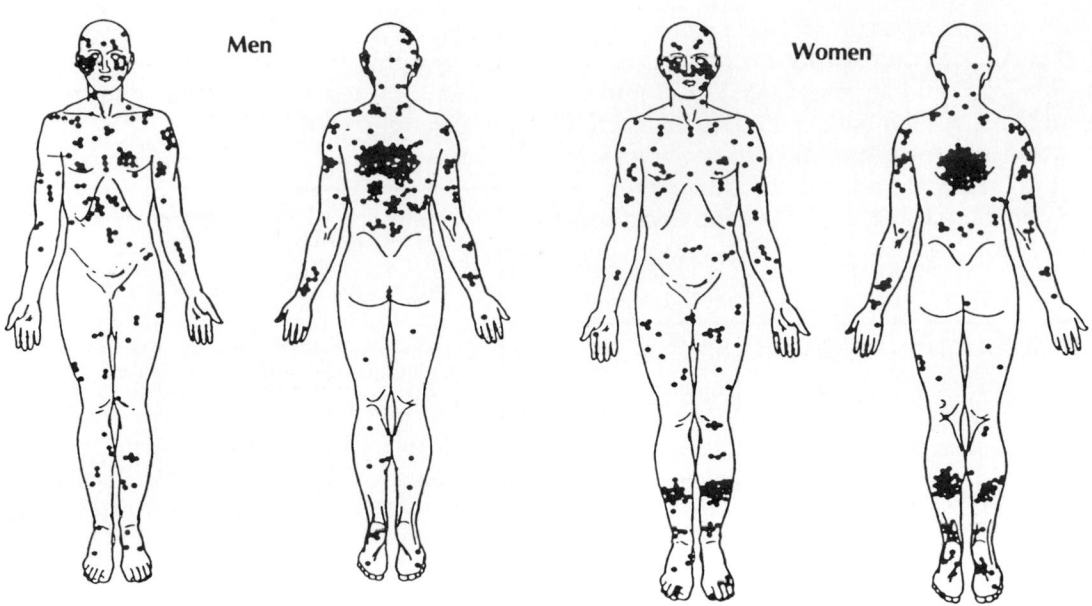

Figure 18–1   Anatomic distribution of malignant melanoma in men and women. (From Becker J, Goldberg L, and Tschen J: Differential diagnosis of malignant melanoma, Am Fam Physician 39(5), 1989.)

should also be protected from sunburns because there is an increased risk of melanoma in persons who have experienced traumatic sunburns as children.

Early detection and prompt treatment are essential. Warning signs of melanoma are: any unusual skin condition; scaliness, oozing, and/or bleeding of a mole or other pigmented growth; a change in color or size of a mole or any other pigmented growth or spot; a spread of the pigment beyond the normal border; a change in sensation, itchiness, tenderness, or pain; and the development of a new nodule.[1,11,13]

The early warning signs of malignant melanoma can be easily remembered by thinking of the acronym ABCD: *A*symmetry, *B*order, *C*olor, and *D*iameter. Malignant melanomas are usually asymmetrical (i.e., one half of the mole does not match the other half). Early malignant melanomas tend to have irregular borders. The edges may be ragged, notched, or blurred, unlike benign lesions, which usually have regular, smooth margins. Pigmentation in malignant melanomas is not uniform. Colors may range from various hues of tan and brown to black, with red and white intermingled. Malignant melanomas are often greater than 5 mm when first identified. A sudden or continued increase in the size of a mole should be reported.[1,13]

Examination of the skin once a month by inspecting all skin surfaces for any of the above changes is imperative for those persons at risk of developing malignant melanoma (see box on p. 366). Persons previously diagnosed with malignant melanoma should also perform skin self-examination once a month because of the increased likelihood for recurrence.[6,7,13]

The educated patient or family member is often the first person to detect changes in skin conditions. Koh and others reported that approximately one half (53%) of 216 incident cases of melanoma in Massachusetts were self-discovered, whereas the remaining cases were detected by medical providers (26%), family members (17%), and others (3%). Compared with men, women were more likely to discover their own lesions and those of their spouses.[19,20,25]

CLASSIFICATION AND CLINICAL FEATURES

Malignant melanomas may arise from three types of moles or nevi: the common acquired nevi (CAN), dysplastic nevi (DN), or congenital melanocytic nevi. The most frequently encountered benign pigmented lesion is the common acquired nevi, better known as the "normal" mole. CAN are absent at birth. Nevus production begins in childhood with increased development during puberty. Production begins to taper at about 35 to 40 years of age. Most adults have about 20 to 40 nevi on their bodies. CAN are usually small (<5 mm), exhibiting uniformity in color, surface, symmetry, and regularity of borders.[28] The risk that any one CAN will develop into a malignant melanoma is small. See box on p. 369 for characteristics and clinical features of common benign pigmented lesions.

Dysplastic nevi (DN) are acquired pigmented lesions. These nevi are considered to be precursors of cancer as well as markers of persons at risk for development of malignant melanoma. Dysplastic nevus syndrome (DNS) usually manifests itself during young adulthood. Persons with DNS develop nevi throughout their lifetime and may have more than 100 nevi on their bodies.[5,11,28] Clinical characteristics

Table 18–1   Comparison of Common Acquired Nevus and Dysplastic Nevus

Characteristic	Common Acquired Nevus	Dysplastic Nevus
Color	Uniformly tan or brown; one mole looks much like another	Variegated, mottled, mixture of tan, red/pink, brown, within a single nevus; nevi look very different from each other
Shape	Round; sharp, clear-cut borders between nevus and surrounding skin; may be flat or elevated	Irregular, notched border; borders may fade off into surrounding skin; always have a macular or flat component
Size	Usually <5 mm diameter (smaller than the size of a pencil)	Usually >5 mm diameter
Number	Average adult has 20 to 40 scattered over body	Typically 100, although some people may have only a few nevi
Location	Usually on sun-exposed surfaces of body above waist; scalp, breast, buttocks rarely involved	Back is most common site; may occur below waist and on scalp, breast, buttocks, genitals

Modified from Lawler PE and Schreiber S: Cutaneous malignant melanoma; nursing's role in prevention and early detection, Oncol Nurs Forum 16(3):348, 1989.

**CLINICAL FEATURES
COMMON BENIGN PIGMENTED LESIONS**

Simple lentigo

Small 1-5 mm macular, pigmented lesion
Precursor to common mole
Sharply defined, round
Smooth or jagged edges that may appear on the surface of the skin
More concentrated on sun-exposed areas

Junctional nevi

Small, less than 6 mm, well-circumscribed pigmented lesion with a smooth surface
Relatively uniform pigmentation that ranges very dark brown to black

Compound nevus

Well circumscribed, less than 6 mm raised papule
Uniform in pigmentation
Skin colored tan to various shades of brown

Solar lentigo

Small to somewhat larger macule known as a "liver spot"
Found on sun-exposed people with significant sun damage: face, chest, back, dorsa of hands
Uniform tan to brown

Seborrheic keratosis

Sharply demarcated purple that ranges in diameter
Few millimeter to several centimeter
Verrucous, round, ovid, variably raised
Surface "dull" or "warty"
Common on face, neck, trunk
Variably raised
Light brown to dark brown

---

of DN are compared and contrasted with CAN in Table 18-1. Basically, DN are larger with irregular borders and variegated colors. DN can occur anywhere on the body but are more commonly found on the trunk, back, breasts, buttocks, genitals, and scalp.[5,11,28]

DNS may be classified as familial or sporadic. Familial DNS is an inherited autosomal dominant trait. Persons with DN who have two or more first-degree relatives with melanoma have almost a 100% chance of developing melanoma.

Sporadic DNS is seen in persons with no family history of DN or melanoma. The risk of developing melanoma for these persons is anywhere from 5% to 26% greater than the general population.[3,5,9,10]

Congenital melanocytic nevi appear as raised, dark brown to black, oval or round macules that may contain coarse hairs. Congenital nevi are present at birth and are classified by size in diameter as small (<1.5 cm), medium (1.5 to 19.9 cm), and large (>19.9 cm). Most congenital nevi are small or medium. The risk of developing malignant melanoma from congenital nevi is controversial with estimates as high as 22 times. Persons with congenital nevi larger than 3 to 5 cm are thought to be at even greater risk of developing malignant melanoma.*

Four types of malignant melanoma exist: superficial spreading, nodular, lentigo maligna, and acral lentiginous (see box on p. 370 for clinical features). Superficial spreading malignant melanoma is the most common form. About 70% of all cutaneous melanomas are of the superficial spreading type. Superficial spreading melanoma occurs more frequently in women than men and is usually seen in persons in the 40- to 50-year-old age group.[21,31] Common sites of occurrence of this lesion are the lower extremities and back in women, and the back in men.

Nodular malignant melanoma is the next most frequently occurring melanoma. This lesion occurs twice as often in men than in women and tends to affect

---

*References 3, 5, 9, 10, 13.

**CLINICAL FEATURES
MALIGNANT MELANOMA PIGMENTED LESIONS**

Superficial spreading melanoma
Variegated in color with areas appearing blue, black, gray, white, or pink
Irregular pigmented plaque with areas of regression and notched borders
May appear scaly, crusty and itch

Nodular melanoma
Often resembles a "blood blister"
Appears as a symmetrical, raised dome-shaped lesion
Blue-black in color
Can be amelanotic

Lentigo malignant melanoma
Appears as a large, flat, irregular lesion resembling a stain
Variegated in color ranging from tan to black with areas of regression

Acral lentiginous melanoma
Usually flat, irregular, with an average diameter of 3 cm
Blue or black discoloration or a tan and brown stain

---

persons in their fifties and sixties. Nodular melanoma may occur anywhere on the body; however, common sites of occurrence are the head, neck, and trunk regions.

Lentigo maligna melanoma is a rare lesion accounting for 5% to 10% of melanomas. This lesion primarily occurs after the age of 60. Most lesions affect the face, but they may also occur on any sun-exposed area of the body, such as lower legs and hands.[3,5,9,12]

Acral lentiginous melanoma is the least common, accounting for less than 10% of all melanomas. This lesion tends to occur on the palms, soles, nailbeds, fingers, toes, and mucous membranes. Acral lentiginous melanoma is the most common type of melanoma among blacks, Orientals, and Hispanics.[21,31]

DIAGNOSIS AND STAGING

When a lesion is suspected to be melanoma, a biopsy should be performed. The technique of choice is a total excisional biopsy with narrow margins. The biopsy procedure is accompanied by a thorough history and a complete physical examination. The skin should be carefully inspected and palpated for intracutaneous metastasis. Further diagnostic evaluation includes routine laboratory tests (CBC, LDH, BUN, PTT), liver enzyme studies, urine analysis, serum creatinine, blood chemistries, and a chest x-ray. Other essential studies are guided by the symptomatology reported by the patient and outcome of above tests. If lymphadenopathy is present at diagnosis and the

index of metastasis is high, definitive nodal dissection may be performed without a biopsy. Radiographic studies to define the direction of the lymphatic drainage will be performed before the nodal dissection.[18,21,31]

The most important prognostic factors in melanoma are depth of invasion (Clark's levels) and thickness of the tumor. Both of these factors determine the T classification and, ultimately, the stage grouping. If the depth of invasion (Clark's level) and the thickness of the tumor do not match, the tumor is assigned to the higher T classification (Figure 18-2).[18,26,31]

CLINICAL AND MICROSTAGING CLASSIFICATIONS FOR MELANOMA OF THE SKIN*

Stage IA (T_1, N_0, M_0; Clark's level II)
1. Primary tumor invades the papillary dermis
2. Primary tumor is 0.75 mm or less in thickness
3. No evidence of regional lymph node or distant metastasis

Stage IB (T_2, N_0, M_0; Clark's level III)
1. Primary tumor fills the papillary dermis but does not penetrate the reticular dermis
2. Primary tumor is 0.76 to 1.5 mm thick
3. No evidence of regional lymph node or distant metastasis

Stage II (T_3, N_0, M_0; Clark's level IV)
1. Primary tumor invades the reticular dermis but does not invade subcutaneous tissue
2. Primary tumor is 1.51 to 4.0 mm thick
3. No evidence of regional lymph node or distant metastasis

Stage IIIA (T_4, N_0, M_0; Clark's level V)
1. Primary tumor invades reticular dermis extending into subcutaneous tissue, and/or the presence of satellite(s) within 2 cm of primary tumor)
2. Primary tumor is greater than 4.0 mm thick
3. No evidence of regional lymph node or distant metastasis

Stage IIIB (any T, N_1, or N_2, M_0)
1. Primary tumor invades any depth
2. Evidence of regional lymph node metastasis and/or in-transit metastasis
3. No evidence of distant metastasis

Stage IV (any T, any N, M_1)
1. Evidence of distant metastasis regardless of tumor depth or thickness or nodal metastasis

Histopathologic grading for melanoma is identical to the grading system used for basal and squamous cell carcinoma.

METASTASIS

Malignant melanoma may spread to any organ or remote viscera. Common sites for disseminated disease

---

*Adapted from Beahrs OH and Myers MH, editors: Manual for staging of cancer, ed 4, Philadelphia, 1992, JB Lippincott.

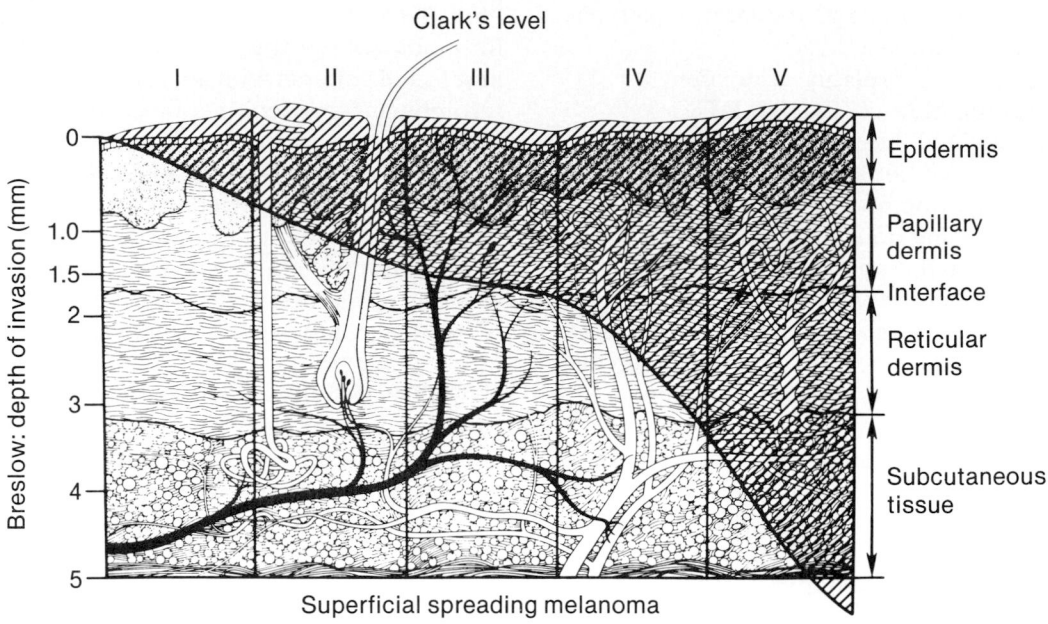

Clark's level

I   II   III   IV   V

Epidermis

Papillary dermis

Interface

Reticular dermis

Subcutaneous tissue

Breslow: depth of invasion (mm)

Superficial spreading melanoma

Figure 18–2   Anatomic landmarks and Clark's level of invasion. (From DiSaia P: Clinical gynecological oncology, ed 3, 1989, Mosby.)

are the skin (intracutaneous or subcutaneous metastasis), bone, brain, liver, and lung.[18,21]

Malignant melanomas may grow radially or vertically. All melanomas except the nodular type have an initial radial growth phase, which may last more than a decade. During this phase, the melanoma cells remain confined to the epidermis. The lesion expands horizontally with only a slight increase in the depth of the tumor.

The vertical phase is characterized by dermal penetration and invasion of the dermis and subcutaneous tissue by the melanoma cells. The lesion may then metastasize by way of vascular or lymphatic channels. The melanoma cells then spread rapidly to other parts of the body. Nodular malignant melanoma has no radial growth phase. These lesions are usually convex and are palpable because of the growth elevation above the level of the normal skin.[3,10,18,21]

TREATMENT MODALITIES
Surgery

Surgical excision of the primary growth is the preferred treatment method. The shave biopsy technique should not be used. For lesions less than 1.5 mm thick, the surgeon usually makes a wide excision (approximately 2 cm), removing more normal tissue than with other skin cancer surgeries. For lesions that are greater than 1.5 mm thick, most surgeons excise margins of 5 cm including the underlying fascia.[18,36]

ELECTIVE REGIONAL NODE DISSECTION (ERLAND). The rationale for performing ERLAND is based on the hypothesis that melanoma metastasize sequentially first to the regional lymph nodes and later from the nodes to distant sites. ERLAND improves survival rates for intermediate thickness (1.5 to 4 mm); for melanoma 0.76 to 1.5 mm thick there is no significant difference in survival; and ERLAND has no advantage for patients with melanoma less than 0.75 mm or more than 4.0 mm in thickness.[18,21,36]

Cutaneous melanoma spreads to four main lymph node basins; intraparotid, cervical, axillary, and illoguinal. If metastatic disease appears first in intraparotid nodes, superficial parotidectomy in conjunction with nodal dissection is usually performed. If cervical nodes are extensively affected, a radical neck dissection is the operation of choice. Axillary node dissection with an enbloc removal of pectoralis minor muscle is the standard procedure.[17,18,31]

Radiation Therapy

Melanoma has traditionally been considered relatively radioresistant. Experimental radiation therapy endeavors include radiosensitizers such as Misonidiazole, and the use of fast neutrons. The energy released by the neutrons destroys the melanoma cells while the surrounding normal tissue are spared. Radiation therapy is useful, however, in alleviating symptoms from metastasis to the bone, brain, and other organs.[8,21,31]

Chemotherapy

Dacarbazine (DTIC) is the most extensively studied and regarded as the most effective single agent. The most common dosage schedule has been 250 mg/m² daily for 5 days every 4 weeks. The major side effects are severe nausea and vomiting and flu-like symptoms. Other cytotoxic agents reported to demonstrate some efficacy include carmustine (BCNU), semustine (methyl CCNU), vindesine, and cisplatin. Combination chemotherapy includes:

DBPT: DTIC, BCNU, cisplatin, tamoxifen
BELD: Bleomycin, eldesin, CCNU, DTIC
BOLD: DTIC, CCNU, bleomycin, vincristine

Responses to these regimens range from 40% to 50% with predominantly lung and or soft tissue metastasis. Although most remissions were partial and short-lived, some have lasted several years.[18,21]

High-dose chemotherapy followed by autologous bone marrow transplant is another option for patients being explored in clinical studies. This regimen requires intensive hospitalization and is associated with significant morbidity.[18,21]

New investigational drugs such as: Amonafide, Didemnin-B, Merberone, Piroxantrone, and Taxol have been developed and have shown promise in early clinical trials.[18]

HYPERTHERMIC REGIONAL PERFUSION

Hyperthermic regional perfusion or isolated limb perfusion is being used for intransit metastasis and as an adjuvant therapy. This form of therapy allows a large dose of chemotherapy to be delivered to a malignant melanoma affected extremity with minimal systemic toxicity. The limb is usually perfused for 1 hour with a high concentration of melphalan at 39 to 41° C with a perfusion pump and extracorporeal circulator. The hyperthermia enhances the cytotoxic effect so that the total dose of drug may be reduced. This procedure should only be performed by experts. Complications include arterial and venous thrombosis, tissue necrosis, nerve and muscle damage, and, rarely, loss of the extremity.[18,21]

Biotherapy

Recombinant interferons have shown some response in selected patients with advanced disease. High-dose recombinant interleukin-2 has been used to treat distant metastasis with some success. This treatment is associated with a severe, toxic, vascular, hypermeability syndrome and requires intensive hospitalization.

BCG, a form of a nonspecific immune stimulation, was one of the first agents used. It has shown tumor regression when injected intralesionally.[18,21]

Hormonal Therapy

Estrogen and progesterone receptors found on melanoma cells signify a relationships between hormones and malignant melanoma.

Hormonal therapy for malignant melanoma is under investigation. Currently tamoxifen and diethylstibesterol are being explored.[18,21]

PROGNOSIS

Several factors affecting prognosis are the clinical stage location and depth and thickness of the lesion. Currently, thickness of malignant melanoma (with local disease) is the best independent predictor of survival.[18] The overall 5-year survival rate for melanoma is 80%. The prognosis for persons with thin lesions less than 0.76 mm thick is excellent, with 5-year survival 98%. The difference in 5-year survival rates of localized (90%) versus regional disease (50%), and distant (14%) validates the importance of early diagnosis and prompt treatment to ensure high cure rates.[13,18]

Nursing Management

Nursing diagnosis, assessment, and interventions are similar for both nonmelanoma and malignant melanoma. Some variations may be necessary depending on type and location of skin cancer and method of treatment. A complete nursing history includes information regarding risk factors, previous treatment, and a thorough skin examination focusing on all moles for any suspicious changes. Nursing management of side effects of treatment methods are discussed in detail in Chapters 20 to 23. Skin grafting is common after surgical treatment of melanoma.

Postsurgical interventions include instructing patients and families on the management of a surgical wound. Keeping the area clean and dry, and observing for signs and symptoms of infection are imperative. If skin grafting is required, patients and their families should be instructed to keep the graft immobile to prevent stress on the edges of the wound.

Limbs should be elevated to minimize edema. Mineral oil or lanolin may be used to remove superficial crusts, moisten the site of the skin graft, and stimulate circulation.

The results of treatment of both nonmelanoma and malignant melanoma may lead to rehabilitation problems. Disfigurement may occur as a result of surgical interventions. Nonmelanoma skin cancers tend to occur in sun-exposed areas of the body, especially the head and neck regions. Surgical interventions to this area of the body may affect a person's body image and self-esteem. Assisting patients to cope with alterations in body image is a prime responsibility of the nurse.

Immobility may also occur as a result of surgical interventions. The wider margins necessary in malignant melanoma coupled with skin grafting may lead to problems of immobility. Assisting patients to maintain their level of functioning is also an important responsibility of the nurse.

Patient/family teaching for malignant melanoma is similar to the teaching for nonmelanoma skin cancers. The importance of early detection should be emphasized with both patients and family members. Patients and family members should be instructed on the importance of monthly, systematic skin self-examination. Individuals should be instructed to check the entire skin surface, paying special attention to all moles for suspicious changes. Family members can be taught to assist patients by checking the scalp and back region. Patients diagnosed with melanoma and those at risk of developing melanoma should be encouraged to keep regularly scheduled appointments with their physician.

Methods of prevention, primarily the importance of avoiding intense sunlight and the use of protective clothing and sunscreens, should also be taught. Parents should be instructed on the above mentioned prevention measures for their children. Both patient and family members should be instructed about the ABCD rules for remembering the warning signs of melanoma.[6,7,14,22]

NURSING DIAGNOSIS

- Knowledge deficit related to prevention and early detection of skin cancer

INTERVENTIONS

- Define and describe risk factors: fair complexion, sunburn easily, red or blond hair, reside in geographic region that receives high levels of ultraviolet radiation, history of nonmelanoma/melanoma skin cancer[24]
- Describe and discuss methods to minimize sun exposure: wear lip balm/sunscreen with SPF of 15 or more, avoid exposure to sun between hours of 10:00 A.M. and 3:00 P.M.; wear protective clothing, maximize use of available shade, keep infants and children out of the sun, and teach and practice sun protection measures early in children's growth and developmental process
- Discuss importance of and procedure for routine skin self-examination: cover entire skin in a methodic fashion, use good lighting, use mirrors, blow hairdryer, and a buddy system to examine difficult-to-see areas (scalp, perineum, back), document and report promptly any changes and or new conditions

NURSING DIAGNOSIS

- Knowledge deficit related to disease process

INTERVENTIONS

- Discuss signs and symptoms related to expectations for basal cell, squamous cell, and malignant melanoma (see boxes on pp. 362, 365, and 370).[24]

- Discuss potential diagnostic related procedures to be used in diagnosis and treatment of the specific skin cancer.
- Discuss symptoms to report to physician regarding disease process and/or a change in recovery; e.g., pain, fever, redness, swelling, drainage at the biopsy/treatment site.

NURSING DIAGNOSIS

- Knowledge deficit regarding method of treating disease (surgery, radiation therapy, chemical therapy, chemotherapy, biotherapy, isolated limb perfusion)

INTERVENTIONS

- Discuss schedule of specific therapy
- Discuss treatment-related side effects
- Discuss signs and symptoms related to complications from the various therapies
- Discuss resources/alternative plans to facilitate compliance in the treatment of the disease (travel to/from physician/radiation therapy, dressings, supplies, home care assistance)
- Provide written materials explaining disease and treatment of disease[3,5]

NURSING DIAGNOSIS

- Knowledge deficit regarding home care management of surgical wound

INTERVENTIONS

- Demonstrate dressing change with return demonstration of procedure, patient/family states place for purchase of supplies, resource to contact for assistance and/or to report symptoms, signs and symptoms that may indicate infection, knows procedure and can demonstrate proper body mechanics for mobility purposes, limitations and/or restrictions for elevation of extremity and/or general hygiene[18,21]

NURSING DIAGNOSIS

- Skin integrity, impaired, related to skin cancer and surgical treatment

INTERVENTIONS

- Discuss/demonstrate hygiene (wash affected area with tepid water and pat dry); avoid pressure and/or irritating clothing
- Discuss nutrition and hydration needs
- Explain need to avoid exposure to infection

NURSING DIAGNOSIS

- Infection, potential for, related to skin cancer and surgical treatment

INTERVENTIONS

- Discussion of signs and symptoms of infection: pain, redness, swelling, drainage, fever 38° C; patient/family identifies when, where, and who to report information regarding infection potential
- Provide prescribed therapies (antibiotics, analgesics, dressings)[20,21]
- Implement measures to protect skin and/or affected area from trauma and bleeding

NURSING DIAGNOSIS

- Impaired physical mobility, potential for, related to surgical treatment and possible skin graft

INTERVENTIONS

- Discuss and teach proper body mechanics when transferring to/from bed/chair/commode; and/or walking
- Discuss and demonstrate restrictions and limitations for affected extremity.
- Discuss/demonstrate rationale for body position changes if immobilized in bed.
- Discuss/demonstrate body mechanics for daily hygiene; any restrictions on shower/tub bath.[20,21,24]

NURSING DIAGNOSIS

- Self-concept, disturbance in, related to location and surgical treatment for skin cancer

INTERVENTIONS

- Encourage patient to share feelings with physician/nurse/family regarding changes in body image.
- Arrange and/or consult with professional/lay resources (cancer survivor) if requested by patient/family.
- Provide materials and pictorial images regarding invasive procedures and reconstruction process.

- Discuss/arrange cosmetic resources to enhance positive feelings about body image changes.[20,24]

NURSING DIAGNOSIS

- Social interaction, potential for impairment, related to location and surgical treatment of skin cancer

INTERVENTIONS

- Discuss and plan selected enjoyment activities patient can pursue; e.g., music, movies, reading, hobbies, crafts
- Discuss and plan with family/significant other/home care agency resources to utilize in the community (meals on wheels, social contacts appropriate to age and developmental needs)
- Discuss/arrange for rehabilitation resources (physical therapy, occupational therapy)[22,24]

NURSING DIAGNOSIS

- Anxiety, potential for, related to diagnosis of cancer, fear of recurrence, death, pain, disfigurement, and changes in life-style

INTERVENTIONS

- Discuss feelings and concerns related to these topics and ask what do these experiences mean to the patient.
- Identify patient's previous/present coping strategies when encountering difficult situations.
- Identify specific concerns and fears patient may be experiencing
- Encourage patient to share feelings with family/friends/health care team
- Demonstrate and encourage patient to use relaxation/distraction/meditation exercises to aid in other coping strategies.[22,24]

CONCLUSION

There are over 700,000 new cases of skin cancer per year, the vast majority of which are highly curable basal cell or squamous cell cancers. Malignant melanoma is the most serious skin cancer and is increasing at the rate of 4% per year.[1] In the year 2000, malignant melanoma is expected to occur in 1 of every 100 persons.[1] Excessive exposure to the sun remains the primary risk factor for all skin cancers. Prevention, early detection, and prompt treatment are essential to effect a cure or improve survival. Nurses have a major role on the health-care team in all aspects of care for the patient with skin cancer.

According to the American Cancer Society,[1] deaths related to skin cancer total 8800 each year. Of those 8800, malignant melanoma accounts for 6800, while

other skin cancers account for the remaining 2000.

Progress coupled with prompt surgical removal, the current death rate from malignant melanoma can be reduced to nearly zero through early detection. Clearly if every American were completely examined yearly for malignant melanoma, death from this disease would be a rare event. The cost-benefit ratio of skin cancer screening as well as the feasibility of screening 250 million Americans for skin cancer, however, need to be resolved.[13,14,33]

BIBLIOGRAPHY

1. American Cancer Society: Cancer facts and figures—1993, Atlanta, 1993, American Cancer Society.
2. Amron DM and Moy RL: Stratospheric ozone de-

pletion and its relationship to skin cancer, J Dermatol Surg Oncol 17:370, 1991.

3. Arnold HL and others: Epidermal nevi, neoplasms, and cysts. In Arnold HL, Odom RB, and James WD, editors: Andrew's diseases of the skin, clinical dermatology, ed 8, Philadelphia, 1990, WB Saunders Co.

4. Beahrs OH, Henson DE, Hutter RP, and Myers MH, editors: Manual for staging of cancer: American Joint Committee on Cancer, ed 4, Philadelphia, 1992, JB Lippincott.

5. Becker JK, Goldberg LH, and Tschen JA: Differential diagnosis of malignant melanoma, Am Fam Physician 39(5):203, 1989.

6. Berwick M and others: The role of the nurse in skin cancer prevention, screening, and early detection, Semin Oncol Nurs 7(1):64, 1991.

7. Bolognia JL and others: Complete follow-up and evaluation of a skin cancer screening in Connecticut. J Am Acad Dermatol 23:1098, 1990.

8. Buller DB and Buller MK: Approach to communication preventive behaviours, Semin Oncol Nurs 7(1):53, 1991.

9. Caro WA and Bronstein BR: Tumors of the skin. In Moschella SL and Hurley HJ, editors: Dermatology, ed 2, Philadelphia, 1985, WB Saunders Co.

10. Crijins MB and others: Dysplastic nevi occurrence in first- and second-degree relatives of patients with 'sporadic' dysplastic nevus syndrome, Arch Dermatol 127(9):1346, 1991.

11. Crutcher WA and Cohen PJ: Dysplastic nevi and malignant melanoma, Am Fam Phy 42(2):372, 1990.

12. Fraser MC and others: Melanoma and nonmelanoma skin cancer: epidemiology and risk factors, Semin Oncol Nurs 7(1):2, 1991.

13. Friedman RJ and others: Malignant melanoma in the 1990s: the continued importance of early detection and the role of the physician examination and self-examination of the skin, CA 41(4):201, 1991.

14. Geller AC and others: Practices and beliefs concerning screening family members of patients with melanoma. J Am Acad Dermatol 26(3):419, 1992.

15. Glass AG and Hoover RN: The emerging epidemic of melanoma and squamous cell skin cancer, JAMA 262:2097, 1989.

16. Greenwald P: Principles of cancer prevention: diet and nutrition. In DeVita VT, Hellman S, Rosenberg SA, editors: Cancer principles and practice of oncology, ed 3, Philadelphia, 1989, JB Lippincott Co.

17. Hall VL and others: Treatment of basal cell carcinoma comparison of radiotherapy and cryotherapy, Clin Radiol 37:33, 1986.

18. Ho VC and Sober AJ: Therapy for cutaneous melanoma: an update, J Am Acad Dermatol 22:159, 1990.

19. Koh HK and others: Who discovers melanoma? Patterns from a population-based survey, J Am Acad Dermatol 26(6):914, 1982.

20. Lawler PE and Schreiber S: Cutaneous malignant melanoma: nursing's role in prevention and early detection, Oncol Nurs Forum 16(3):345, 1989.

21. Lawler PE: Cutaneous malignant melanoma, Semin Oncol Nurs 7(1):26, 1991.

22. Loescher LJ and Booth A: Skin cancer. In Groenwald SL, Frogge MH, Goodman M, and Yarbro CH, editors: Cancer nursing principles and practice, Boston, 1990, Jones and Bartleet.

23. Loescher LJ and Meyskens FL, Jr: Chemoprevention of human skin cancers, Semin Oncol Nurs 7(1):45, 1991.

24. Longman A: Skin cancer. In Clark JC and McGee RF, editors: Core curriculum for oncology nursing, ed 2, Philadelphia, 1992, WB Saunders Co.

25. Mackie RM and others: Personal risk-factor chart for cutaneous melanoma, Lancet 2:487, 1989.

26. McFadden ME: Cutaneous T-cell lymphoma, Semin Oncol Nurs 7(1):36, 1991.

27. Pollack SV: Skin cancer in the elderly, Clin Geriatr Med 3(4):715, 1987.

28. Rigel DS and others: Dysplastic nevi- markers for increases risk for melanoma, Cancer 63:386, 1989.

29. Robinson JK: What are adequate treatment and follow-up care for nonmelanoma cutaneous cancer, Arch Dermatol 123:331, 1987.

30. Rowe DE and others: Long-term recurrence rates in previously untreated (primary) basal cell carcinoma: implications for patient follow-up, J Dermatol Surg Oncol 15:315, 1989.

31. Shapiro PE: Malignant melanoma. In Schein PS, editor: Decision making in oncology, Philadelphia, 1989, BC Decker.

32. Shimm DS and Wilder RB: Radiation therapy for squamous cell carcinoma, Am J Clin Oncol 14(5):383, 1991.

33. Sober AJ: Cutaneous melanoma: opportunity for cure, guest editorial, CA 41(4):197, 1991.

34. Vargo NL: Basal and squamous cell carcinomas: an overview, Semin Oncol Nurs 7(1):13, 1991.

35. Volker DL: Standards of oncology practice and standards of oncology education; patient, family, and public. In Clark JC and McGee RF, editors: Core curriculum for oncology nursing, ed 2, Philadelphia, 1992, WB Saunders Co.

36. Wolf DJ and Zitelli JA: Surgical margins for basal cell carcinomas, Arch Dermatol 123:340, 1987.

CHAPTER 19

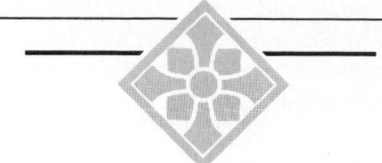

Oncologic Complications

Sandra Lee Schafer

Cancer involves a multiplicity of tissues in a wide range of locations with metabolic diversities and various metastatic potentials that can result in a wide variety of oncologic complications.[12] The complex nature of the disease, together with the fact that patients with cancer are living longer because of improvements in the diagnosis and treatment of cancer and its sequelae, result in an increase in the frequency of cancer-related complications. This trend will probably continue, since cancer is the second leading cause of death in the United States. Most patients with cancer die of metastatic disease and related complications of the disease, which can occur at any time during the course of the disease. Therefore, prevention, early recognition, adequate decision-making, and prompt treatment of oncologic complications are of paramount importance when delivering care to patients with cancer.

Once the oncologic complication is analyzed, the decision whether to treat or not and to what degree to treat can be made. Treatment may be aggressive where there is potential for a cure or prolonged survival. On the other hand, in advanced disease the treatment may be given to palliate symptoms and restore functional status. Finally, withholding treatment and providing supportive care may be the most appropriate decision in the presence of disseminated metastatic disease.[12,55,100] Quality of life should always be the driving force in any decision regarding care of the patient with cancer. The overall goal is to prevent, reverse, or minimize life-threatening oncologic complications through prophylactic measures, early detection, and effective management.

Management of an oncologic complication is dependent upon many important factors related to the patient and the underlying disease (see box on p. 377).

These factors must be given thorough consideration before the initiation of treatment.

Nursing care of the patient with a potential for or an actual oncologic complication is multifaceted and challenging. The patient status may be anywhere along a continuum from being at high risk for the development of a problem through manifestations of it in various degrees (mild, moderate, or severe). There are striking similarities among these patients in spite of the extreme individual differences.

Those common nursing care threads are not addressed in this chapter. Instead the focus is on selected nursing diagnoses related to specific problems. However, it is important to review these similarities for purposes of comprehensive care planning. Common nursing diagnoses for patients with oncologic complications include the following:
- Alteration in comfort: pain
- Alteration in nutrition: less than body requirement
- Anxiety
- Knowledge deficit
- Potential for ineffective individual coping
- Potential for ineffective family coping

These diagnoses, along with those listed for specific problems, will assist in the nursing management of these patients. See Chapters 27, 28, and 30.

Assessment is of the essence, since a change in the patient's condition may be subtle or dramatic. Two key concepts when caring for people with cancer are first, the identification of patients at risk for developing an oncologic complication and secondly, the involvement of the family and significant other(s). The patient and family require considerable education and support. Time limits are the greatest enemy, creating a great deal of anxiety. Explanations of tests and

---

MANAGEMENT FACTORS IN THE EVALUATION AND TREATMENT OF AN ONCOLOGIC EMERGENCY

Symptoms and signs
1. Are the symptoms and signs due to the tumor or to complications of treatment?
2. How quickly are the symptoms of the oncologic emergency progressing?

Natural history of the primary tumor
1. Is there a previous diagnosis of malignancy?
2. What is the disease-free interval between the diagnosis of the primary and the onset of the emergency?
3. Has the emergency developed in the setting of terminal disease?

Efficacy of available treatment
1. No prior therapy vs. extensive pretreatment
2. Should treatment be directed at the underlying malignancy and/or the urgent complication?
3. Will the patient's general medical condition influence the ability to administer effective treatment?

Treatment and goals
1. Potential for cure
2. Is prompt palliation required to prevent further debilitation?
3. What is the risk vs. benefit ratio of treatment?
4. Should treatment be withheld if the patient is terminal with minimal chance of response to available antitumor therapies?

From Glover D and Glick JH: Oncologic emergencies. In Holleb AI, Fink DJ, and Murphy GP, editors: American Cancer Society textbook of clinical oncology, Atlanta, 1991, American Cancer Society.

procedures and the rationale for changes in patient care or setting must be kept simple. Treatment options and goals of therapy must be explained and discussed. This is especially important when the realistic outcome is palliation. Anticipatory guidance and discharge planning may be necessary because some therapies may last several weeks or longer.

DISSEMINATED INTRAVASCULAR COAGULATION

DEFINITION

Disseminated intravascular coagulation (DIC) is considered to be a bleeding disorder. In the past it was referred to as a "consumptive coagulopathy." Bleeding disorders are classified as congenital or acquired. DIC is one of the acquired disorders. It is not a disease entity but rather an event that can accompany various disease processes. DIC is an alteration in the blood clotting mechanism, with abnormal acceleration of the coagulation cascade in which both thrombosis and hemorrhage may occur simultaneously.[58,126,133,161]

ETIOLOGY AND RISK FACTORS

DIC is not a primary independent disorder. An underlying pathology, benign or malignant, is responsible for DIC. The pathology creates the triggering mechanism or initiating event necessary for the activation of thrombin, which is responsible for the cascade of blood clot formation and clot dissolution, thus producing DIC.* A variety of pathologies involve a triggering event, which can cause either endothelial tissue injury or blood vessel injury.

Endothelial injuries include the following:
Shock or trauma—head injury, burns
Infections—aspergillosis, gram-positive or gram-negative sepsis
Obstetric complications—abruptio placenta, amniotic fluid embolism
Malignancies—acute promyelocytic myelogenous leukemia (APML), acute myelogenous leukemia (AML), melanoma, cancers of the lung, colon, breast, stomach, pancreas, ovary, and prostate
Blood vessel injuries include the following:
Infectious vasculitis—Rocky Mountain Spotted Fever, certain viral infections, severe glomerulonephritis
Vascular disorders—aortic aneurysm, giant hemangioma, angiography
Intravascular hemolysis—hemolytic transfusion reaction, multiple whole blood transfusions, massive trauma, extracorporeal circulation devices (cardiopulmonary bypass machine, aortic balloon pump), heatstroke, peritonovenous shunting
Miscellaneous—pancreatitis, liver disease (obstructive jaundice, acute hepatic failure), snakebite

In patients with cancer the incidence of DIC is less than 10% to 15%. It is usually related to the disease process and/or the treatment of the cancer, and it often occurs concomitantly with sepsis.[38,45,105]

PATHOPHYSIOLOGY

Body hemostasis is dependent upon an intricate balance between blood clot formation and blood clot dissolution. The fibrin blood clot is the end product of the blood-clotting mechanism.[155,161] Normally this mechanism is initiated when tissues sustain an injury. Disruption of the vascular endothelium exposes collagen fibers to blood. Smooth muscle spasm then occurs, releasing serotonin. Vasoconstriction follows, which slows the flow of blood and causes circulating platelets to change shape and adhere to the rough surface of injured vessels within 1 to 2 seconds.[133] More platelets aggregate and form a loose plug at the site of injury, creating a seal on the vessel wall to control bleeding. The injured vascular tissue also re-

---

*References 3, 38, 100, 101, 126, 133.

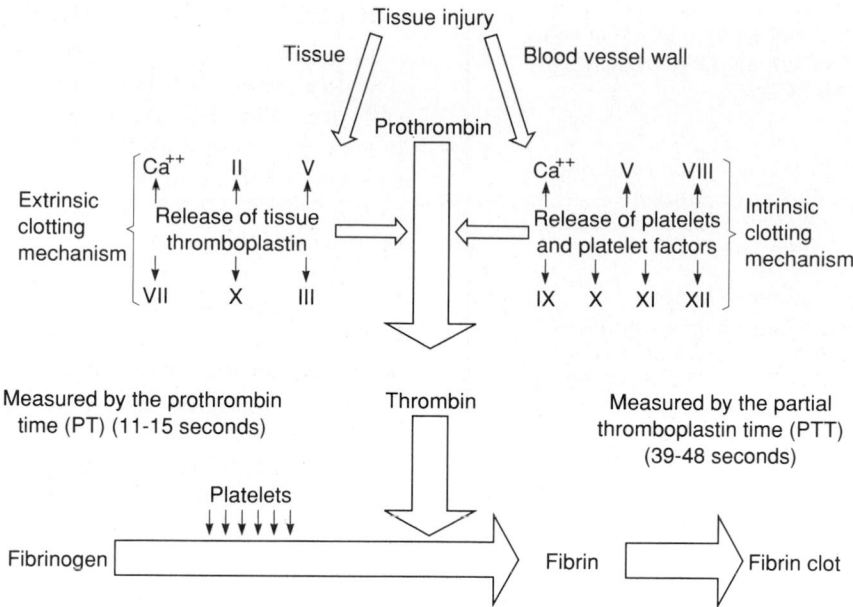

Figure 19-1 Formation of a blood clot. (From Yasko JM and Schafer SL: Disseminated intravascular coagulation. In Yasko JM, editor: Guidelines for cancer care: symptom management, Reston, Va, 1983, Reston Publishing Co.)

leases a phospholipid called thromboplastin, which initiates the clotting reaction.[1,29,72,107,161]

The fibrin blood clot is formed through a series of sequential reactions that are protein activated (Figure 19-1). This protein activation occurs through two different cascades of reactions known as the intrinsic and extrinsic pathways, which operate jointly to form the blood clot. The intrinsic pathway is activated by injury to the blood vessel wall. Activation of the extrinsic pathway occurs following tissue injury. Central to each pathway is the conversion of prothrombin to thrombin through a series of reactions involving various blood factors (phospholipids, proteins, and calcium). The thrombin then acts as a catalyst to convert fibrinogen (monomer) to fibrin (polymer).[161] The fibrin polymers form a mesh of fibrin strands, which trap platelets, red blood cells, and leukocytes, making an occlusive clot.

The series of reactions that forms the clot is balanced by a series of reactions that limits the size of the clot and later dissolves it. Therefore, clot dissolution occurs in conjunction with clot formation. When the clot is no longer needed, it is converted from a polymer back to a monomer by fibrinolysin (plasmin). Fibrinolysin is formed in the presence of thrombin during coagulation when preactivators come in contact with a tissue enzyme known as kinase.[161] Fibrinogen and fibrin are broken down by fibrinolysis, resulting in fibrin degradation products (FDPs) or fibrin split products (FSPs). As these fragments circulate, they interfere with the formation of fibrin and coat the platelets, thus decreasing their

adhesive ability. The result is anticoagulation along with the process of fibrinolysis; the body forms antithrombins, natural anticoagulants that also interfere with thrombin (clotting) activity. Hemostasis is therefore balanced between fibrin clot formation (coagulation) and clot dissolution by fibrinolysis (anticoagulation).[72,161]

DIC is a disruption of body hemostasis. One of the triggering mechanisms from the underlying pathology initiates the process (Figure 19-2), which results in the formation of thrombin and fibrinolysin (plasmin). Thrombin acts to convert fibrinogen to fibrin to form clots. At the same time fibrinolysin degrades some of the fibrin into a soluble monomer form; this initiates clot dissolution. The remaining portion of fibrin is an insoluble polymer, which continues to form clots. These clots may be deposited in the extremities or in organs such as the lungs, kidneys, and brain. Capillary clots slow the blood flow resulting in tissue ischemia, hypoxia, and necrosis.[161] The clots also trap circulating platelets in the microvasculature, which results in the thrombocytopenia. As the fibrinolysin continues to degrade fibrin, the byproducts FDPs are produced. These FDPs disrupt the conversion of fibrin to a polymer; coat platelets, decreasing their adherence; and degrade factors V, VIII, and X, which leads to capillary hemorrhage.[13,126]

If the underlying pathology with its triggering mechanism is not treated or otherwise eliminated, it will promote further coagulopathy. The term *consumptive coagulopathy* has been used to describe this increased use (consumption) of platelets and clotting

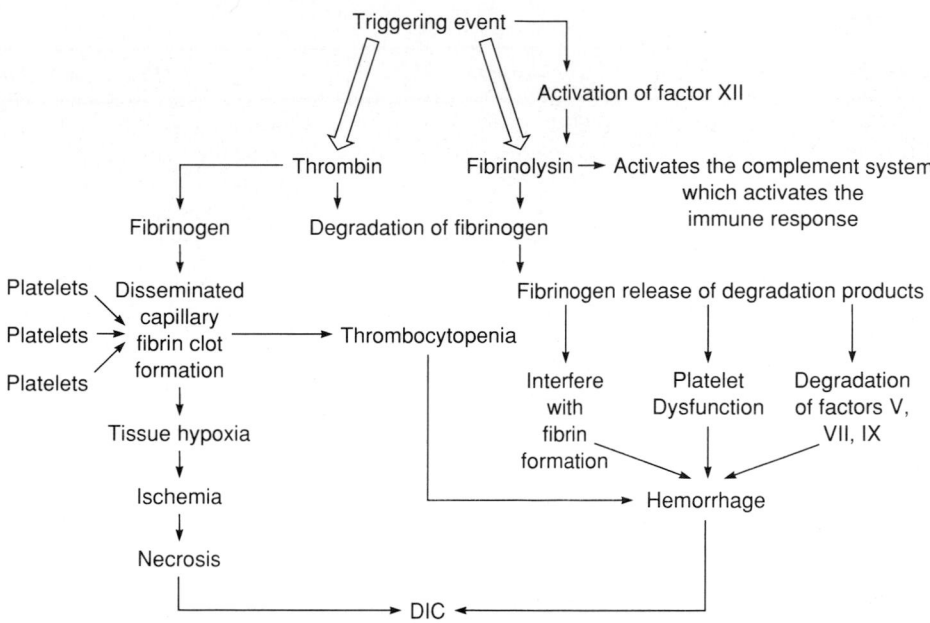

Figure 19-2   Pathophysiology of disseminated intravascular coagulation. (From Yasko JM and Schafer SL: Disseminated intravascular coagulation. In Yasko JM, editor: Guidelines for cancer care: symptom management, Reston, Va, 1983, Reston Publishing Co.)

factors, leading to a continuation of thrombocytopenia and a further decrease of clotting factors and resulting in bleeding. Thus the abnormal activation of thrombin in DIC results in a cyclical paradox of thrombosis or hemorrhage or both (Figure 19-2).

CLINICAL FEATURES

The onset of DIC may be acute, chronic, or somewhere in between. The clinical manifestations and laboratory findings are dependent upon the triggering event and the body tissues involved. The presenting signs and symptoms result from disseminated clotting and bleeding, which may be overt or occult. Bleeding usually predominates.[142]

Signs of bleeding are multiple and may be seen from any body orifice. Bleeding may range from oozing to frank bleeding or hemorrhage. Patients may have overt oozing from venipuncture sites, mucous membranes, needle puncture sites, or incisions. Petechiae ecchymoses, purpura, or hematomas may be evident. Profound menstrual or gastrointestinal bleeding may occur, as well as epistaxis or hemoptysis.

Less dramatic but equally critical is the possibility of occult internal or intracerebral bleeding. Abdominal distention, blood in stools, blood in urine or skin, and scleral changes may be observed. Other signs of occult bleeding may be mental status changes, orthopnea, and tachycardia.

Clotting as a result of fibrin deposits in the microcirculation will impede blood flow and can cause severe tissue ischemia and lead to tissue necrosis. Mul-

tiple system changes may be observed. Observation of the skin may show acrocyanosis, also known as Raynaud's sign (generalized sweating with symmetrical mottling of the nose, fingers, toes, and genitalia), and other ischemic changes, which can lead to superficial gangrene. Pulmonary signs such as severe, sudden dyspnea at rest with tachypnea and progressive rales and rhonchi are similar to those observed with adult respiratory distress syndrome (ARDS).[1] The gastrointestinal tract may have ischemic insult appearing as ulceration, and tubular necrosis of the kidney may lead to renal failure. If microcoagulation occurs in the brain, multifocal strokes, mental change, delirium, and coma may result.[5] The associated symptoms of bleeding or clotting will vary depending upon the system sustaining the ischemic insult or bleeding. Complaints include malaise, weakness, air-hunger, altered sensorium, visual changes, and headaches. The presence and magnitude of these disturbances will depend on the extent of the clotting and bleeding.

A major concern for a person experiencing DIC is the possibility of a life-threatening syndrome known as multiple systems organ failure (MSOF). This is a phenomenon described as a progressive, sequential deterioration of two or more organ systems occurring over a brief period of time. Tissue injury or illness produces intravascular inflammation. This triggers a nonspecific systemic response mediated by a number of cellular, humoral, and biochemical reactions. This response is usually seen in conjunction with a septic focus that is considered essential for the occurrence of MSOF.[100,101]

Table 19–1   DIC Laboratory Profile

Diagnostic Test	Normal Value	Expected Value in DIC
Prothrombin time	10-13 sec	Prolonged
Partial thromboplastin time	39-48 sec	Usually prolonged
Thrombin time	10-13 sec	Usually prolonged
Fibrinogen level	200-400 mg/100 ml	Decreased
Platelet level	150,000-400,000/mm³	Decreased
Factor assay (II, V, VII, VIII, IX, X, XI, XII)		Decreased levels of factors VI, VIII, and IX
Fibrinogen/fibrin degradation products	<10	Increased
Protamine sulfate test (soluble fibrin monomer)	Negative	Strongly positive
Antithrombin III levels (AT-III) (used to monitor response to therapy)	89%-120%	Decreased

From Yasko JM and Schafer SL: Disseminated intravascular coagulation. In Yasko JM, editor: Guidelines for cancer care: symptom management, Reston, Va, 1983, Reston Publishing Co, p 327.

DIAGNOSIS

Laboratory findings substantiate a diagnosis of DIC (Table 19-1). There is no single blood test that can confirm or exclude a diagnosis of DIC; instead, a classic triad of screening tests is used, which includes platelet count, prothrombin time (PT), and fibrinogen level. The abnormal results of these tests reflect the consumption of clotting factors and the occurrence of fibrinolysis resulting in the production of FDPs or FSPs that further interfere with clotting[1,126]:

- Platelet count is decreased. This indicates thrombocytopenia, which is the cardinal laboratory finding. Over 90% of patients with DIC have abnormal platelet count and PT.[1] In about 50% of these patients, the platelet count is less than 50,000/mm³ (normal: 150,000 to 400,000 mm³).
- PT is prolonged (normal: 10 to 13 seconds). This evaluates the extrinsic coagulation system, reflecting decreased levels of clotting factors II, V, and X and of fibrinogen.
- Fibrinogen level is decreased (normal: 200 to 400 mg/100 ml). This results from the consumption of fibrinogen by thrombin-induced clotting and excessive fibrinolysis.[58] Fibrinogen levels of less than 150 mg/100 ml are found in 70% of patients with DIC.[142]

Other laboratory indicators for DIC are the following:

- Partial thromboplastin time (PTT) is prolonged (normal: 39 to 48 seconds). This evaluates the intrinsic coagulation system. However, during DIC, PTT is less sensitive than PT.
- Thrombin time is usually prolonged, indicating depression of clotting factors (normal: 10 to 13 seconds).
- Fibrin degradation products (FDPs or FSPs) are increased (normal: <10). A D-Dimer test is a recent (1988) semiquantitative analysis for FDPs. Although this study has extreme sensitivity, it is not exclusive for DIC.

- Factor assays, especially V and VIII, are decreased.
- Protamine sulphate precipitation test (thrombin activation test) is strongly positive (normal: negative).
- Antithrombin III levels are decreased (normal: 89% to 120%).

Laboratory tests for DIC can be complicated by underlying conditions. Patients with liver disease have abnormal clotting studies and often thrombocytopenia. Laboratory findings in these patients show prolonged PT and decreased fibrinogen levels. Fibrinogen levels, usually elevated in the presence of sepsis, pregnancy, or malignancy, may fall within the normal range if DIC is present concurrently. Finally, multiple transfusions may cause alteration in the levels of clotting factors or platelets.

TREATMENT MODALITIES

There is no specific medical treatment for DIC. Instead, the goal of therapy is to eliminate or alter the triggering event. Common examples are the treatment of sepsis with antibiotics and treatment of cancer with surgery, chemotherapy, and radiation therapy. If the DIC is chronic, only supportive measures may be necessary until the DIC is resolved. Dependent upon the progression of the DIC and the success of treating the triggering event and the predominant signs and symptoms, therapy will be directed at stopping the intravascular clotting process and controlling the bleeding.

When bleeding is severe, blood component therapy is necessary to achieve hemostasis. It is used to correct the clotting deficiencies caused by the consumption of blood components during the DIC process. Common blood products used in treating DIC are as follows:

- Platelets contain platelet factor III, which strengthens the endothelium, prevents petechial hemorrhage, facilitates the conversion of prothrombin to thrombin, and functions as a mechanical plug by adhering to the vessel wall.[126] The amount and frequency of platelet replacement are dependent upon the patient's platelet count and physical condition. Spontaneous hemorrhage is of concern especially when the platelet count falls below 20,000. Usually 8 to 10 U are given once or twice a day. One unit of infused platelets should increase the platelet count by 5000 to 8000 mm^3.

- Fresh frozen plasma (FFP) is used for volume expansion. It contains clotting factors V, VIII, XIII, and antithrombin III. Usually 2 to 4 units of FFP are given once or twice a day. Each unit of infused FFP raises each clotting factor by 5%.
- Packed red blood cells (PRBCs) are used to increase red blood cells and clotting factors. Packed cells are used instead of whole blood to reduce the development of antibodies and fluid overload. Usually 2 U are given when the hematocrit drops below 28%. Each unit of RBCs should raise the hemoglobin count by 1.
- Cryoprecipitate contains fibrinogen (approximately 200 mg/unit) and factor VIII.[133] It is used for patients with severe hypofibrinogenemia. Usually 2 U of cryoprecipitate are given every 6 hours when the fibrinogen level is below 50 mg/100 ml. A total of 10 U of cryoprecipitate are administered. Each unit of cryoprecipitate increases the level of fibrinogen and factor VIII by 2%.

Heparin therapy, which inhibits thrombin formation, has met with controversy for the treatment of DIC. Research is lacking to support its utilization or withholding.[142] The anticoagulation effects of heparin result from its prevention of the platelet aggregation that initiates the intrinsic pathway of the coagulation cascade.[133] Heparin interferes with thrombin and stops the conversion of fibrinogen to fibrin, which prevents clot formation. It does not lyse those clots that are already formed; that requires thrombin to activate fibrinogen.

Usual doses of heparin are from 2500 to 5000 U subcutaneously every 8 to 12 hours, 50 U/kg by IV bolus every 4 to 6 hours, or 100 to 200 U/kg every 24 hours by IV infusion. Effective heparin therapy produces cessation of clot formation, a rise in platelet count and fibrinogen levels, and a decrease in the level of FSPs. Partial thromboplastin time (PTT) is monitored to assess patient response to heparin. A therapeutic level is reached when the patient's PTT is 1.5 to 2 times normal level.

Failure to respond to heparin therapy has been attributed to a depletion of antithrombin III (AT-III). AT-III is a blood component factor that inhibits the competitive action of thrombin during heparin therapy.[133] Therefore, in cases where AT-III levels are low and there is no response to heparin therapy, AT-III is administered along with heparin. The usual dose is 1500 to 1725 U in 50 m of distilled water infused over 10 hours concurrently with 500 to 1500 U of heparin/hour by IV. This form of therapy is still considered experimental.[161]

Finally, in addition to the control of clotting, medical attention is given to the control of bleeding. Usually heparin therapy produces anticoagulation and at the same time controls fibrinolysis. However, in 5% of the cases, fibrinolysis continues and uncontrolled bleeding results.[133] In those instances, antifibrinolytic therapy may be administered, using a drug called epsilon-amino-caproic acid (EACA). EACA interferes with the intrinsic fibrinolytic process, which can lead to further clot formation. Therefore, EACA is used only in instances where heparin is effectively controlling intravascular clotting. The usual dose is 5 to 10 g given by IV slow bolus followed by 2 to 4 g every 1 to 2 hours for 24 hours or until bleeding stops. Patients receiving EACA must be closely monitored for hypotension, hypokalemia, cardiac arrhythmias, and increased intravascular coagulation.[38] This drug is used rarely and is considered controversial.

PROGNOSIS

The prognosis of DIC is dependent upon the underlying cause, the degree of disruption of the coagulation system, and the effects of bleeding and clotting.[1] Most patients with cancer who develop DIC experience hemorrhage. A smaller number demonstrate thromboembolism. The estimated mortality rate for DIC is 54% to 68%. Increasing age, severity of laboratory abnormalities, and number of clinical manifestations increase the mortality from DIC.[29,133] In the DIC patient, a minor injury can have a fatal consequence. See pp. 382-383 for nursing management of DIC.

HYPERCALCEMIA

DEFINITION

A metabolic condition referred to as hypercalcemia occurs when the serum calcium level rises above the normal level of 9 to 11 mg/100 ml. Hypercalcemia is a frequent complication of certain types of malignancies and metastatic disease. It is a potentially life-threatening problem because the onset is variable and often goes unnoticed until the problem becomes severe. With prompt recognition and adequate treatment, this condition can be reversed.

ETIOLOGY AND RISK FACTORS

A variety of conditions can cause hypercalcemia. The common malignancies associated with this condition include cancers of the breast and kidney, squamous cell cancers of the lung, head, neck, or esophagus, lymphoma, leukemia, and multiple myeloma. Patients with metastatic cancers being treated with estrogens or antiestrogens may experience progression

Nursing Management

The nursing management for DIC, like the condition itself, is extremely complex. Depending upon the onset and severity of DIC, the nurse's role may vary from watchful waiting to intensive participation in treatment.[142] Nursing care is focused on minimizing the multitude of potentially life-threatening problems associated with DIC. Therefore, care must be directed toward astute and ongoing assessment to detect bleeding (overt or occult) or thrombosis, the provision of care for bleeding and thrombosis, the prevention of further complications, and the support of other needs.

NURSING DIAGNOSIS
* Potential for injury (bleeding and/or thrombosis) related to:
    Fibrous clot formation in the microcirculation
    Clotting factor consumption and decreased platelets
    Fibrinolysis or clot dissolution

INTERVENTIONS
Observation for signs of bleeding and thrombosis
* Assess organ systems for evidence of bleeding and thrombosis:
    Integumentary — observe skin for evidence of bleeding (petechiae, ecchymosis, purpura, pallor, frank blood or oozing). Closely examine the mouth (include the mucous membranes of the palate and gums), sclera, nose, ears, urethra, vagina, and rectum. Check all venipuncture and puncture or wound sites.
    Pulmonary — auscultate lungs for crackles, wheezes, or stridor. Observe for dyspnea, tachypnea, cyanosis, hemoptysis or chest pain.
    Cardiovascular — monitor for tachycardia, hypotension, or changes in peripheral pulse. Assess for palpitations or angina.
    Renal — measure intake and output. Observe for peripheral edema and oliguria.
    Gastrointestinal — palpate abdomen for pain. Measure abdominal girth daily.
    Neurologic — observe for irritability or changes in mental status. Assess frequently for headache, blurred vision, and vertigo.
* Monitor vital signs (temperature, pulse, blood pressure, and respirations) every 4 hours.
* Test all excreta (urine, stool, sputum, and vomitus) for blood.
* Assess for fatigue, lethargy, muscle weakness, and pain.
* Monitor laboratory values closely for abnormalities indicative of bleeding or infection. This should include complete blood count, platelet count, prothrombin time, and fibrinogen level.

Measures to prevent further tissue trauma
* Prevent further bleeding.
* Prevent skin breakdown.
* Institute safety measures:
    Keep bed rails up at night.
    Pad bed rails and any sharp objects.
    Instruct patient to ambulate with assistance.
* Perform activities that decrease risk of bleeding:
    Provide adequate hydration and soft diet.
    Avoid administration of aspirin or products that contain aspirin.
    Discourage activities that increase intracranial pressure or intraabdominal pressure (Valsalva's maneuver).
    Administer stool softeners as ordered.
* Prevent further clotting:
    Provide adequate hydration.
    Avoid constrictive clothing and devices.
    Use prescribed elastic support hose.
    Discourage dangling of legs, sitting for long periods of time, and crossing legs.
    Elevate legs at intermittent intervals to prevent venous stasis when sitting or lying.
    Perform range of motion exercises for legs.
    Encourage deep breathing and coughing.
    Administer heparin therapy as ordered using an infusion-controlling device.

NURSING DIAGNOSIS
* Impaired skin integrity

INTERVENTIONS
* Observe skin and mucous membranes for changes in integrity, color, and moisture
* Provide meticulous skin care and lubrication
* Maintain skin and mucosal integrity
    Limit venipunctures and, when necessary, use small-gauge needles.
    Avoid subcutaneous and intramuscular injections.
    Apply pressure to puncture sites for 5 minutes.
    Administer medications orally or intravenously.
    Avoid rectal manipulation (rectal suppositories, thermometers, digital exams).
    Use electric razors instead of straight-edged razors.
    Avoid indwelling catheters and, when necessary, keep them well lubricated and without tension.
    Avoid vaginal manipulation (tampons, douches).

Use paper tape instead of adhesive tape and remove gently.
Use Montgomery straps on wound dressings.
Suction with care.
- Perform frequent gentle oral hygiene:
Use soft bristled toothbrush or sponge toothettes.
Avoid mouthwashes with high alcohol content.
Lubricate mucous membranes and lips.

NURSING DIAGNOSIS
- Potential or actual fluid volume deficit related to bleeding

INTERVENTIONS
- Observe for signs of active bleeding, hypocalcemia, and hypoxia (decreased blood pressure, tachypnea, tachycardia, restlessness, irritability, confusion, dizziness, decreased urine output).
- Measure intake and output.
- Administer fluids, blood, and blood products as ordered.

NURSING DIAGNOSIS
- Alteration in tissue perfusion related to bleeding or thrombosis

INTERVENTIONS
- Assess organ systems for malfunctions due to ischemia.
- Monitor laboratory values closely.
- Measure intake and output.
- Provide oxygen therapy as prescribed.
- Administer vasoactive drugs as ordered.
- Administer pain medications as ordered.

The management of a patient with DIC is complex and difficult. The experience is often terrifying for the patient and family and frustrating for the nurse. The patient's condition can change rapidly. Everyone must be alert to, and prepared for, all possible sequelae of DIC.

of hypercalcemia, possibly from hormonal stimulation of the tumor.[5,43] Bony metastasis from any malignant primary tumor may also be a causative condition. Nonmalignant conditions that can induce or worsen hypercalcemia include primary hyperparathyroidism, thyrotoxicosis, prolonged immobilization, vitamin A and D intoxication, renal failure, and diuretic therapy with thiazide preparations.[39,124,143] Dehydration, volume depletion, and hypoalbuminemia may contribute to or aggravate hypercalcemia.[150]

Hypercalcemia is considered the most frequent complication in oncology, occurring in 10% to 20% of patients with cancer.* With advanced breast cancer, the frequency of hypercalcemia may be as high as 30% to 50%.[31,43,143] Any patient with cortical bony metastatic disease is particularly at risk for the development of this condition. However, 10% to 15% of patients with cancer and hypercalcemia have no known bone metastasis.[86]

PATHOPHYSIOLOGY
Calcium is an essential inorganic element in the body. Most of it (99%) is found in skeletal tissue providing strength and durability. The remaining 1% is in the serum. One half of the serum calcium (0.5%) is ionized and one half (0.5%) is bound to circulating albumin. Laboratory reports reflect the total serum calcium level, which includes both the ionized portion and the protein-bound portion.[5] Under normal conditions the ionized calcium is in equilibrium with the

protein-bound calcium. Changes in serum albumin level directly affect serum calcium levels.

Serum calcium levels in the presence of hypoalbuminemia may not be representative of the true value for ionized calcium. Reduction of serum albumin, which is often seen in very ill patients or in the elderly, may result in a greater proportion of ionized calcium due to the unavailability of albumin for binding. Therefore, the severity of hypercalcemia in a patient with hypoalbuminemia may be underestimated.[5,24,164] A formula to correct for decreased serum albumin is given in the box below.

It is the ionized portion of calcium that is capable of physiologic function. Calcium is responsible for bone and tooth formation, normal clotting mechanism, and cellular permeability. Calcium ion concentration regulates the contractility of the cardiac, smooth, and skeletal muscles and the excitability of nerve tissue.[86]

Normal serum calcium levels are maintained in a

*References 14, 43, 97, 114, 122, 143.

CALCULATION OF ESTIMATED IONIZED SERUM CALCIUM

Formulas to correct for changes in serum albumin concentrations (allow 0.8 mg/dL for each g/dL change in serum albumin):
1. Corrected serum calcium = measured total serum calcium value (mg/dL) + [4.0 − serum albumin value (g/dL)] × 0.8.
2. Corrected serum calcium = measured total serum calcium value (mg/dL) − serum albumin value (g/dL) + 4.0.

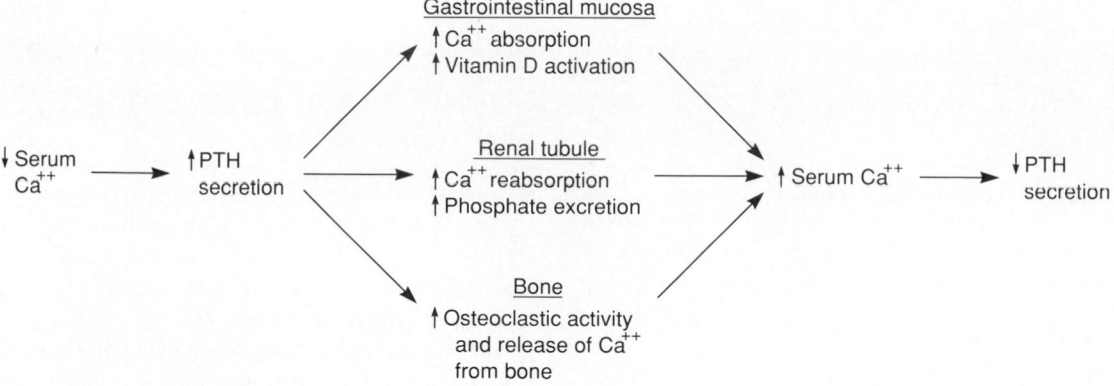

Figure 19-3 Effects of parathyroid hormone on serum calcium levels.

state of equilibrium through a dynamic relationship among all three forms of calcium (stored, ionized, and albumin-bound) with a constant shifting from one form to another.[150] Homeostasis is maintained through several body processes: gastrointestinal calcium absorption, renal calcium reabsorption, and a balance of bone resorption (absorption or removal) of calcium and deposition of calcium through new bone formation.[31,43] Metabolism of calcium is controlled by a negative feedback mechanism between calcium ion concentration and three hormones: parathyroid hormone, activated vitamin D, and calcitonin.

A decrease in serum calcium stimulates an increase in parathyroid hormone (PTH) secretion (Figure 19-3). PTH enhances calcium absorption from the gastrointestinal tract and renal tubular reabsorption of calcium with increased excretion of phosphorus. Calcium ions and phosphorus ions have a directly inverse relationship: when the amount of one is increased, the amount of the other is decreased. Parathyroid hormone also promotes osteoclastic activity. Osteoclasts are multinucleated bone cells, which function to remove damaged bone tissue. This results in the destruction of bones, releasing calcium into the bloodstream.

Vitamin D is activated by PTH and increases calcium absorption from the gastrointestinal mucosa. Calcitonin is released by the thyroid gland in response to an increased serum calcium level and inhibits bone resorption of calcium. The effect of calcitonin is short-lived.[150] In general, hypercalcemia is the result of increased bone resorption of calcium, which exceeds renal ability to excrete the calcium overload. Hypercalcemia resulting from malignancies occurs through several different mechanisms, depending upon the location and action of the cancer cells, as follows[86,143]:
- Direct bony destruction by tumor cells, which causes osteoclastic activity resulting in the release of calcium from the bone into the serum.

- Prolonged immobilization, which increases osteoclastic activity.
- Ectopic parathyroid hormone (PTH) production by tumor cells, which enhances calcium resorption. Secretion continues in spite of an elevated serum calcium level.
- Metabolic substances produced by the tumor, such as osteoclastic activating factor (OAF), prostaglandin or prostaglandin-like substances, all of which enhance osteoclastic activity.[20,43]

Other contributing conditions include the following:
- Dehydration or volume depletion or both
- Hypervitaminosis of A and D (excessive use of vitamin A and D supplements)
- Excessive use of calcium supplements
- Hyperparathyroidism
- Prolonged use of thiazide diuretics

CLINICAL FEATURES

Hypercalcemia disrupts normal cellular functions and adversely affects various organs. Clinical manifestations vary tremendously depending upon the level of serum calcium, the rate of onset, the underlying cause, and the patient's general condition. Patients may be asymptomatic, mildly symptomatic, or have severe problems (Table 19-2). Onset may be insidious or acute. Diagnosis is often difficult because of multisystem involvement making it resemble other disorders.[90,100,101] Clinical features of hypercalcemia are listed in the box on p. 385.

Signs and symptoms are directly related to cellular activity of the involved body system (Table 19-2). Normal cell membranes are lined with calcium ions, which control the permeability of the cell. This gating mechanism allows sodium ions to enter the cell and depolarization to occur. Increased calcium ions decrease cellular permeability and subsequently alter cellular function. This decreases neuron permeability, resulting in a depressive effect on the central and

Table 19–2   Degrees of Hypercalcemia: Signs and Symptoms*

Body System Affected	Mild (Less Than 12 mg/dl)	Moderate (12-15 mg/dl)	Severe (Above 15 mg/dl)
Gastrointestinal	Anorexia, nausea, vomiting, vague abdominal pain	Constipation, increased abdominal pain, abdominal distension	Atonic ileus, obstipation
Neurologic	Restlessness, difficulty in concentrating, depression, apathy, lethargy, clouding of consciousness	Confusion, psychoses, somnolence	Coma→death
Muscular	Easily fatigued, muscle weakness (generalized or involving shoulders and hips), hyporeflexia	Increased muscular weakness, bone pain	Profound muscular weakness, ataxia, pathologic fractures
Renal	Nocturia, polyuria, polydipsia	Renal tubular acidosis, renal calculi	Oliguric renal failure, renal insufficiency, azotemia
Cardiovascular	Hypertension (may or may not be present)	Cardiac dysrhythmias, ECG abnormalities (shortening of QT interval on ECG, coving of ST-T wave, widening of T wave)	Cardiac arrest→death

*Signs and symptoms regardless of serum calcium levels may vary from person to person.
From Poe CM and Radford AI: The challenge of hypercalcemia in cancer, Oncol Nurs Forum 12(6):29, 1985.

CLINICAL FEATURES OF HYPERCALCEMIA

Clinical signs	*Symptoms*
Lethargy	Anxiety
Change in mental status (restlessness, confusion, stupor, coma)	Fatigue and weakness
	Anorexia
Vomiting	Nausea
Arrhythmias	Polydipsia
Polyuria	Constipation
ECG changes	
Renal calculi	
Renal failure	

---

peripheral nervous system.[150,164] Symptoms may include restlessness, agitation, lethargy, and confusion and may lead to coma. Skeletal muscles become hypotonic with decreased or absent deep tendon reflexes, ataxia, and fatigue. The smooth muscle action of the gastrointestinal system slows, leading to decreased motility, anorexia, nausea, vomiting, constipation, possible abdominal distention, and later ileus. Impaired cardiac muscle conduction and contractility can result in arrhythmias or even cardiac arrest.

Compensatory renal mechanisms increase urinary calcium reabsorption, leading to an inability to concentrate urine. This causes a syndrome similar to nephrogenic diabetes insipidus manifested by polyuria and polydipsia.[31,90] The polyuria and hypercalciuria result in dehydration and a decrease in glomerular filtration rate (GFR). Dehydration from this event or from nausea and vomiting produces a further decline in the GFR of the kidney. The lowered GFR in turn increases reabsorption of sodium in the proximal tubules in an attempt to retain water. Since sodium and calcium work closely, calcium is also reabsorbed. This can further potentiate the hypercalcemia. Elevation of serum calcium levels produces a supersaturation of calcium and then precipitation. Precipitation in the kidneys can lead to calcium renal stones and possible renal failure as evidenced by an elevated BUN and creatinine.[90]

The clinical syndrome of hypercalcemia is complex because of the extreme variability in its manifestation of signs and symptoms. In addition, the symptomatology does not always correlate with serum calcium levels. These must be closely correlated with an in-depth history, physical examination, and laboratory profile. Diagnosis can be confusing, but because of its frequency in patients with cancer, hypercalcemia of malignancy should be one of the first differential diagnoses in patients who develop a change in mental status.

DIAGNOSIS

The diagnostic workup for hypercalcemia begins with laboratory determination of the serum calcium level. Normal values are 9 to 11 mg/100 ml. The procedure for obtaining a serum calcium level should include the following measures:

- Two determinations to ensure accuracy
- A fasting specimen to avoid postprandial changes
- Removal of tourniquet before 2 minutes because of a possible 10% elevation in level thought to be

caused by oxidation of fluid from increased venous pressure.[15,122]

Urinary calcium should be measured. Hypercalciuria may be detected before an elevation in serum calcium.[5] Other serum laboratory testing should include phosphorous, alkaline phosphatase, BUN, creatinine, electrolytes, and PTH. Patients with no bony involvement (i.e., squamous cell cancer of the head and neck) whose tumor is producing PTH-like substances may have a normal serum phosphorous. Hypercalcemia resulting from direct bony involvement (breast cancer, myeloma, renal cell carcinoma) often results in increased serum phosphorous levels. Furthermore, within this subset of patients, only those with breast cancer and bone metastasis usually have an elevated alkaline phosphatase. Serum albumin should be tested, since patients may be more hypercalcemic than serum levels indicate, as a result of hypoalbuminemia as discussed earlier.[90]

Radiographic examinations can be helpful in differential diagnosis. A chest x-ray may suggest tumor, sarcoidosis, or bony changes associated with hyperparathyroidism.[124] Plain x-rays or a radioisotope bone scan may demonstrate bone metastases or multiple myeloma. Electrocardiograms may show tachycardia, increased PR segment, shortened QT interval, and widening of the T wave. However, these changes may be subtle and difficult to detect.[43]

TREATMENT MODALITIES

Decisions concerning whether and how to treat hypercalcemia caused by malignancy are dependent upon the clinical situation.[31,86] The degree of serum calcium elevation, the symptomatology, the condition of the patient, and the ability to treat the underlying disease are determining factors in the decision-making process. Untreated cancer-induced hypercalcemia is usually progressive, and death is usually inevitable. Death from hypercalcemia may be a reasonable way to die for the patient with advanced cancer, since most people become comatose and do not experience pain.[114] However, death may not be rapid, and unpleasant symptoms may occur. Patients with advanced disease must be evaluated carefully, since the only effective long-term treatment for hypercalcemia is antineoplastic therapy directed at the underlying malignancy.[31] The choice of treatment for the patient whose cancer cannot be eradicated is therefore a difficult one. If quality of life will not be improved, the decision may be to provide no treatment.

When a decision is made to treat the hypercalcemia, the medical treatment is based upon two principles: reduction of bone resorption of calcium and promotion of urinary excretion of calcium.[43]

Hydration

Adequate hydration is usually the primary treatment for hypercalcemia. Increased fluids by mouth and/or intravenously rehydrate the patient and dilute the urine, which prevents supersaturation with calcium ions.[150] Large volumes of isotonic saline (Table 19-3) restores plasma volume and promotes urinary calcium excretion through sodium diuresis. Calcium loss follows sodium loss. Fluid volume in the range of about 5 to 8 L/day is common for the first 24 hours followed by 3 L/day thereafter. Infusions of large volumes of fluids may necessitate central venous pressure monitoring to avoid fluid overload. Accurate recordings of intake, output, and weight and laboratory studies should be done to prevent hyponatremia, hypomagnesemia, and hypokalemia.

Mobilization

Immobilization should be avoided since it will increase resorption of calcium from the bones. Activity should be appropriate for the physical condition of the patient. Weight-bearing through standing and ambulation produces physical stress at the ends of long bones resulting in osteoblastic activity. Osteoblasts synthesize the collagen and glycoproteins to form a matrix and develop into osteocytes, which are mature bone cells.[20] Muscle activity produces acid end products needed to assist in the production of acid urine.[150] Physical therapy may be helpful to establish a program of active exercises with resistance. A pain management program may be necessary to support activities.

Dialysis

Patients who are in renal failure secondary to hypercalcemia but who have a relatively good prognosis with their malignancy could benefit from renal dialysis.[31,43] Dialysis will remove both excess calcium and phosphate. Serum phosphate levels should be measured and phosphates replaced as necessary.[31,143]

Dietary Manipulation

Little attention is given to dietary restriction of calcium since the increase in calcium is due to resorption from the bones rather than gastrointestinal absorption of calcium.[31] However, excessive volumes of milk and dairy products should be discouraged. Furthermore, a diet low in calcium may also lack phosphate, which would promote an increase in serum calcium.[122]

Pharmacologic Therapy

The first pharmacologic consideration in the treatment of increased serum calcium is the discontinuation of any medications known to precipitate hyper-

Table 19–3   Therapy for Hypercalcemia of Malignancy

Therapy	Dosage	Comments
Saline; add loop diuretics such as furosemide.	5-8 L IV during the first 24 hr, then 3 L/day of normal saline. Diuretic dose 20 mg q 4-6 hr. Calciuretic dose 80-100 mg q 1-2 hr.	Restores plasma volume, increases glomerular filtration rate and promotes renal calcium excretion. Loop diuretics block calcium reabsorption in the loop of Henle. Especially important when hypercalcemia is severe and the patient is dehydrated. Should not be used as sole therapy.
Pamidronate disodium (Aredia)	60-90 mg IV infusion over 4-24 hours for 1 day	Interferes with osteoclast activity by absorbing to calcium crystals in bone blocking dissolution of calcium. This inhibits bone resorption. Safe in patients with renal failure.
Gallium nitrate (Gallium)	200 mg/m²/d IV 24 hr infusion for 4-5 days	Inhibits bone resorption without compromising bone strength. Nephrotoxicity is a potential toxicity. Discontinue this drug if serum creatinine exceeds 2.5 mg/dL.
Etidronate (Didronel, Didronel IV)	7.5 mg/kg/day IV infusion over 2 hours for 4-5 days, then 10 mg/kg/day orally for up to 3 mo	Inhibits bone resorption. Limits calcium absorption from gut. Promotes soft tissue and skeletal calcification. Returns serum calcium level to normal within 3 to 5 days. Contraindicated in patients with renal failure. Given with saline hydration.
Calcitonin-salmon* (Calcimar, Miacalcin) plus a glucocorticoid	Calcitonin-salmon, 200 MRC U every 12 hr subcutaneously; hydrocortisone, 100 mg IV every 6 hr	Impairs bone resorption and increases renal calcium excretion. Especially effective in patients with hematologic malignancies. Safe in patients with renal or cardiac failure.
Plicamycin (Mithracin)	15-25 ug/kg/day by slow IV infusion over 4 hr for 1 day	Inhibits bone resorption by direct injury to osteoclasts. Calcium-lowering effects not seen for 24-48 hr. Potentially dangerous in patients with renal or hepatic failure.
Phosphate	Up to 0.5 g orally 4 times daily	Reciprocal relationship between calcium and phosphorus. Useful when hypercalcemia is associated with low serum phosphorus level. Diarrhea may be a problem. Contraindicated in patients with renal failure or serum phosphorus levels >3.8 mg/dL. Often used as maintenance therapy.

*Calcitonin-human (Cibacalcin) has not yet been approved for use in hypercalcemia but is expected to be as effective as calcitonin-salmon for this condition.
Adapted from Mundy G: Options for correcting hypercalcemia of malignancy, Hospital Therapy, Feb 1988; and Zimberg M and Mahon S: Understanding delirium: an impediment to quality of life, Qualify of Life—A Nursing Challenge 1(1).

calcemia, such as estrogens, antiestrogens, thiazide diuretics, high doses of vitamin A and D, and calcium supplements.

The second measure involving medications is the administration of chemotherapy to treat patients with underlying hematologic malignancies such as multiple myeloma or lymphoma. In patients with breast cancer, chemotherapy or hormonal therapy may produce a remission. However, the initial use of hormonal therapy, especially tamoxifen (Nolvadex), may worsen the hypercalcemia. Some patients receiving hormonal therapy for breast cancer metastatic to the bone may experience episodes of increased serum cal-

cium. This is often referred to as a "flare" that is indicative of tumor response to the hormone. These patients need to be monitored closely.

Diuretics have been given in addition to saline infusions to increase calcium excretion. Furosemide (Lasix) and ethacrynic acid (Edecrin) are frequently used since their mechanism of action on the kidney decreases reabsorption of calcium and sodium.[43,143] During diuresis, serum levels of potassium and magnesium should be monitored closely and cardiac medication given cautiously.

The use of oral phosphates (Table 19-3) is somewhat limited. It has been shown that patients with renal failure or patients with serum phosphorus levels > 3.8 mg/L will not benefit from the use of phosphates.[114] However, patients with low serum phosphorus levels may benefit from oral phosphorus administered in doses of 0.5 g 4 times a day. The mechanism of action, although uncertain, appears to be the reduction of bone resorption of calcium and impairment of the absorption of calcium from the intestine. Diarrhea, which can result at these high oral doses, may hamper the use of oral phosphorus. Large intravenous doses may cause precipitation of calcium in the heart, lung, or soft tissues, which can lead to renal failure; therefore they are rarely indicated.

Glucocorticoids have been used to treat hypercalcemia associated with breast cancer, myeloma, and lymphoma. Prednisone (40 to 60 mg/day) has been given. Steroids may have some direct effect on the tumor itself, but the exact mechanism is unknown. Increasing the dose of the steroids does not increase their effectiveness.[3,43,55,86] The effect of steroids may be delayed by a week, and chronic use enhances immune suppression, which can result in osteolytic activity. Steroids are not recommended for long-term maintenance in view of the possible toxicities associated with chronic administration.[5]

Nonsteroidal anti-inflammatory drugs (NSAIDs) such as indomethacin (Indocin) or aspirin appear to inhibit prostaglandin synthesis and thus mediate bone resorption. Although their role in treating hypercalcemia may be minor, they may be of value in patients with refractory hypercalcemia who are unable to tolerate other agents and/or if NSAIDs are part of a regimen for cancer pain control. The usual dose of indomethacin is 75 to 100 mg/day in divided doses. Gastric upset is a frequent side effect of this drug.[5]

Recently, cisplatin, a widely used antineoplastic agent with broad spectrum of anti-tumor activity, has demonstrated efficacy in reducing serum calcium levels. The calcium lowering effect was delayed (10 days) and prolonged (mean duration 38 days) and independent of anti-tumor activity because the decrease in calcium levels occurred in patients for whom there was no tumor regression. The toxicities (gastrointestinal, renal, and neurological) associated with cisplatin may limit its consideration for antihypercalcemic therapy.[5]

Currently, five parenteral medications with similar mechanisms of action are used to treat hypercalcemia (Table 19-3). Each drug impairs bone resorption and increases renal calcium excretion. Calcitonin-salmon appears to have a transient effect in lowering serum calcium.[43,114,143] A usual dose is 200 MRC given intramuscularly or subcutaneously every 12 hours. One benefit of this drug is its safety in patients with renal failure. The addition of a glucocorticoid to calcitonin

has prolonged its effect in lowering serum calcium. The current recommendation is hydrocortisone sodium succinate (100 mg IV every 6 hours). The combination of calcitonin and a glucocorticoid has been especially efficacious in patients with hematologic malignancies.[43,114] Plicamycin (Mithramycin) has calcium-lowering effects that may not appear for 24 to 48 hours.[43,86,114,143] The usual dosage is a slow infusion of 15 to 25 µg/kg/day. Disadvantages of plicamycin are its venous irritation, myelosuppressive effects, liver toxicity, and potential danger in patients with renal failure. Etidronate (Didronel) has shown efficacy in more than 80% of patients with cancer-induced hypercalcemia. Lowered serum calcium is seen in 3 to 5 days following a regimen of 7.5 mg/kg/day intravenously for 4 to 5 days. The daily dose of etidronate is diluted in 250 ml of normal saline and administered over a period of at least 2 hours. Intravenous administration can be followed with oral doses of 10 mg/kg/day for 7 to 10 days, which may be continued for up to 3 months. However, the oral efficacy of this agent is still under study. Etidronate is contraindicated in patients with a serum creatinine > 5 or those with renal failure.[14,114] Hyperphosphatemia may result from etidronate therapy.[5]

Gallium nitrate is an antineoplastic agent noted to have hypocalcemia effects by directly inhibiting bone resorption without causing toxicity to bone cells. It is administered over 24 hours daily for 5 days at a dose of 100 to 200 mg/m^2 mixed in 1 liter of 0.9% normal saline or 5% dextrose in water. Adequate hydration must be maintained throughout the treatment period. Nephrotoxicity is the major side effect of gallium nitrate. The requirement of continuous infusion potentially limits its usefulness, especially in the outpatient setting.[5] Pamidronate is a highly effective second generation bisphosphonate derivative. Dosage is not based on body surface area, but on the severity of the hypercalcemia. The recommended dosage of pamidronate in moderate hypercalcemia (corrected serum calcium 12 to 13.5 mg/dL) is 60 to 90 mg given as a single IV infusion over 24 hours. For patients with severe hypercalcemia (corrected serum calcium greater than 13.5 mg/dL) 90 mg should be given as the initial treatment. The drug is usually mixed in 1 liter of 0.45% or 0.9% normal saline or 5% dextrose in water and infused over 4 to 24 hours. Adequate hydration is necessary during treatment. Hypocalcemia and hypophosphatemia have occurred following therapy. However, nephrotoxicity does not appear to be a problem. Current studies of multiple low doses (15 mg/d) and single doses (5 to 90 mg) have shown significant activity and the possibility of a dose-response relationship. Oral preparations are also being tested.[61]

The choice of therapy for hypercalcemia depends

on how fast a response is desired, the functional status of the renal system and other major organ systems, the potential for side effects, ease of administration, and the cost of therapy.[14,114,143] Response to treatment, a decrease in serum calcium, is usually seen within 24 hours peaking at 48 hours.[55] Consideration must also be given to long-term therapy, since it is easier to lower the serum calcium level than to keep it low.

PROGNOSIS

Cancer-induced hypercalcemia is a common complication of certain cancers and has the potential to be life-threatening. Clinical manifestation and onset vary greatly, but the course is usually progressive and can worsen quickly. Hypercalcemia is reversible in 80% of episodes if it is recognized and prompt aggressive therapy is initiated. It has been shown that the more severe the hypercalcemia, the poorer the prognosis and vice versa.[22] Without prompt treatment, it is associated with a 50% mortality rate.[20,38,97]

Nursing Management

Nursing care of the patient with hypercalcemia is directed at early detection and support through treatment. A thorough nursing assessment should include a history of the patient's cancer and cancer treatment and a review of all medications. Drugs that may cause or potentiate hypercalcemia such as lithium carbonate, thiazide diuretics, vitamins A and D, and large doses of calcium supplements should be reported and discontinued. Notation should also be made of drugs whose action may be altered by high serum calcium, such as digitalis and some antihypertensive agents.

Physical examination results should be correlated with potential symptomatology of hypercalcemia.[49,90,97] This is often difficult because of the varying possibilities and degrees of clinical manifestations. However, the initial assessment will dictate the intensity of nursing care.

NURSING DIAGNOSES

- Potential for fluid volume deficit related to:
    Effects of the disease (impending renal failure with increased polyuria; fluid loss related to nausea and vomiting)
    Effects of treatment (increased urine output secondary to diuretic therapy; fluid loss related to diarrhea)
- Potential for fluid volume excess related to effects of treatment (hydration)

INTERVENTIONS

- Assess for signs and symptoms of alterations in fluid volume:
    Excess—rales, shortness of breath, neck vein distention, weight gain, edema of sacrum and/or lower extremities
    Deficit—dry mucous membranes, poor skin turgor, weight loss, rapid thready pulse, orthostatic hypotension, restlessness
- Auscultate lungs for breath sounds every 4 hours.

- Monitor intake and output closely:
    Encourage oral fluids.
    Maintain intravenous fluids as per physician orders (usually 6 to 8 L/day of saline).
    Monitor intravenous infusions carefully using flow regulator.
    Accurately measure urine output (maintain output at least at 50 ml/hour).
- Obtain daily weight.
- Monitor laboratory values (serum BUN, creatinine, sodium, and potassium).
- Administer diuretics as ordered. Thiazide diuretics are contraindicated because they inhibit urinary excretion of calcium and therefore may potentiate hypercalcemia.
- Obtain urine pH. An acidic urine should be maintained to prevent calcium precipitation, which can lead to renal calculi.

NURSING DIAGNOSES

- Impaired physical mobility related to bone breakdown secondary to metastasis.
- Potential for injury or trauma related to bone destruction.

INTERVENTIONS

- Assess patient for presence of spinal cord compression (signs and symptoms: pain, sensory loss or paresthesia, motor weakness or dysfunction, changes in patterns of elimination).
- Establish activity and exercise regimen according to patient's physical ability and physician order. Change patient's position every 2 hours. Stand patient at bedside for short periods of time (several minutes) at least 4 to 6 times a day:
    Use isometric exercises each hour while awake.
    Institute passive range of motion exercises if patient is on bedrest.
- Provide a footboard for bedridden patients and use a tilt table several times a day.

- Check for evidence of venous thrombosis in lower extremities due to immobilization (redness, swelling, warmth, positive Homan's sign, pain, or dorsiflexion).
- Monitor skin integrity and provide skin care.
- Promote and assist with regulation of elimination.
- Provide pain control as needed.
- Obtain consultation with physical therapy and occupational therapy for evaluation and assistance.
- Discuss and teach the use of assistive and supportive devices as needed.
- Use safety precautions:
    Move patients with care (use lift sheets and support joints).
    Assist patient with transfer and ambulation as needed.
    Place all articles within patient's reach.
    Pad bed rails.
    Modify bed surface with approved pressure-reducing mattress.
    Use bed rails at night.
    Closely monitor restless, anxious, or confused patients.
    Employ restraints as necessary.

NURSING DIAGNOSIS

- Potential for altered thought processes

INTERVENTIONS

- Assess level of consciousness changes in mentation and/or behavior.
- Closely observe for restlessness or anxiety.
- Orient patient frequently to time and place.
- Allow time for verbalization of feelings regarding condition.
- Teach patient and family about changes caused by hypercalcemia and the potential for its recurrence and appropriate measures to be taken.

NURSING DIAGNOSIS

- Potential for alteration in cardiac output related to changes in serum calcium and electrolytes

INTERVENTIONS

- Assess for changes in cardiac function:
    Monitor for presence of arrhythmias, bradycardia, tachycardia.
    Observe ECG for shortened QT intervals or prolonged PR intervals.
    Take pulse and blood pressure every 4 hours.
- Monitor serum calcium and electrolytes.
- Administer oral potassium as ordered (hypokalemia frequently occurs in the presence of hypercalcemia).
- Monitor effects of digitalis and digoxin, if given to patient, since hypercalcemia potentiates their action. The dose is usually reduced in the presence of hypercalcemia.

NURSING DIAGNOSIS

- Alteration in elimination; diarrhea related to treatment for hypercalcemia

INTERVENTIONS

- Monitor status of bowel elimination every day (color, texture, frequency of stools).
- Assess the abdomen daily:
    Observe for distention.
    Auscultate for the presence of bowel sounds.
    Palpate to determine any painful areas.
- Provide perianal hygiene and skin care (use anesthesia and lubricants as ordered).
- Monitor perianal skin integrity.
- Avoid administration of antidiarrheal agents since calcium is excreted via stool.
- Provide explanation of diarrhea to patient and family.

Hypercalcemia is one of the most common oncologic problems seen in patients with cancer. Therefore, nurses practicing in all areas of cancer care should be educated regarding this problem. Nursing assessment of patients with cancer, especially those cancers commonly associated with hypercalcemia (breast, lung, head and neck, lymphoma, and myeloma, and any patient with bony metastases), should focus on the potential manifestations of this problem.

MALIGNANT PLEURAL EFFUSION

DEFINITION

Pleural effusion, the abnormal accumulation of fluid in the pleural cavity, is a common complication of malignancy. Effusions in any body cavity are a potential problem with cancer, and the pleural space is the most frequent site, followed by the pericardial and the peritoneal spaces. Abnormal fluid accumulation results when there is an alteration in the balance between secretion and reabsorption. Malignant pleural effusion is debilitating and life-threatening because the increased pleural fluid affects respiratory function by restricting lung expansion, decreasing lung volume, and altering gas exchange.[110,145,147]

ETIOLOGY AND RISK FACTORS

Abnormal fluid accumulation in the pleural space may be the result of a benign or neoplastic process. Benign causes of pleural effusion include congestive heart failure, pericarditis, respiratory infections (pneumonia, tuberculosis), superior vena cava syndrome, mediastinal irradiation, ascites, hypoalbuminemia, and nephrosis. Patients with cancer often develop pleural effusions in the course of their disease, especially if their disease involves primary or secondary intrathoracic malignancies. This may be the first sign of their cancer, a complication of existing disease, or a late manifestation in metastatic disease, or it may be related to a nonmalignant process.[56] Regardless of etiology, malignant pleural effusion causes alterations in ventilation and perfusion, hypoxia, pain, and hemorrhage and may lead to atelectasis, infection and death.[163] The reported incidence of malignant pleural effusion varies tremendously from 25% to 53%. The true incidence remains unknown, since there has been no recent report on the incidence in the general hospital population.[116,136]

At least one third to one half of all pleural effusions are thought to be caused by cancer.[112,135] Exudative pleural effusion in patients over the age of 60 years is caused by malignancy.[112] Malignant pleural effusion is the result of metastatic disease of the pleura or mediastinal lymph nodes. Approximately one half of patients with lung cancer or breast cancer will develop pleural effusions at some point during the course of their disease. In the early 1980s, breast cancer was the leading malignancy associated with pleural effusion, but more recent studies report that lung cancer is the most common primary site to develop pulmonary metastases.[64,116] This probably reflects the increased incidence and death rate from lung cancer in this decade. Lung cancer is followed by breast cancer, lymphomas and leukemias, and ovarian cancer as causes of pleural effusions. Less frequent causes include malignant mesothelioma (primary pleural tumor), gastrointestinal malignancies, genitourinary cancers, and sarcomas. Of interest is the finding that many malignant pleural effusions are caused by pulmonary adenocarcinomas of unknown primary origin.[110] In essence, all types of cancer have the potential to cause malignant pleural effusion.

PATHOPHYSIOLOGY

The pleura is a thin serosal membrane that envelops the lungs and lines the interior of the thoracic cavity (Figure 19-4). There are two portions of the pleura, a visceral surface and a parietal surface lined by two thin layers of mesothelial cells. The visceral pleura adheres to the lung, encases each lobe, and extends within the interlobar fissures. Capillaries of the visceral pleura originate from the bronchial circulation. Lymphatic channels are present and coincide with the capillary bed. No nerve endings for pain are present. The parietal pleura lines the mediastinum, diaphragm, and chest wall. Capillaries of the parietal pleura are supplied by the intercostal arteries. Nerve endings for pain are present and, when stimulated, produce referred pain to the adjacent chest wall, shoulder, or abdomen.[98] The right and left pleura have no communication.[135,138]

There is a potential space between the two layers of pleural membrane, which is referred to as the pleural space or pleural cavity. Within the pleural space is a small amount of relatively protein-free transudative fluid produced by the mesothelial cells of the pleura, which flows across, from one pleura to the other, lubricating, moistening, and cushioning the pleural surfaces during respiration, providing lung movement without friction. Normally, there are 5 to 10 ml of fluid present in the pleural space. Fluid is continuously produced and shunted to the pleural space from the systemic capillaries of the parietal pleura. Approximately 80% to 90% of the fluid is then reabsorbed by the pulmonary capillaries of the visceral pleura. The remaining 10% to 20% of the pleural fluid, which contains large molecular substances, proteins, and erythrocytes, is reabsorbed through the lymphatic channels of the visceral pleura.[127,135,138]

Equilibrium of pleural fluid movement is regulated by five dynamic forces (Figure 19-4): capillary permeability, hydrostatic pressure (capillary and interstitial), colloidal osmotic pressure (plasma protein and interstitial protein), negative intrapleural pressure, and lymphatic drainage. The Starling hypothesis of fluid movement from intravascular to extravascular space also applies to formation and removal of pleural fluid.[116,135,138] The lymphatic channels regulate fluid and protein reabsorption. It is estimated that 5 to 10 L of fluid pass through the pleural space in 24 hours, yet only 5 to 10 ml remain in the space at any given time.[56] Abnormal fluid accumulation occurs when there is a disruption of the regulating forces, causing excessive fluid production or decreased fluid reabsorption.

Cancer will disrupt one or more of the five processes that are relative to the dynamics of fluid exchange in the pleural space, causing excess fluid accumulation. Malignant pleural effusions will result by several different mechanisms: pleural implants, tumor cell suspensions, lymphatic metastasis with blockage, venous obstruction, necrotic malignant cell shedding, and obstruction with tear of the thoracic duct.[56,116] Malignant tumors may produce pleural implants, which are tumor cells found in either the parietal or visceral pleura. These implants are caused by

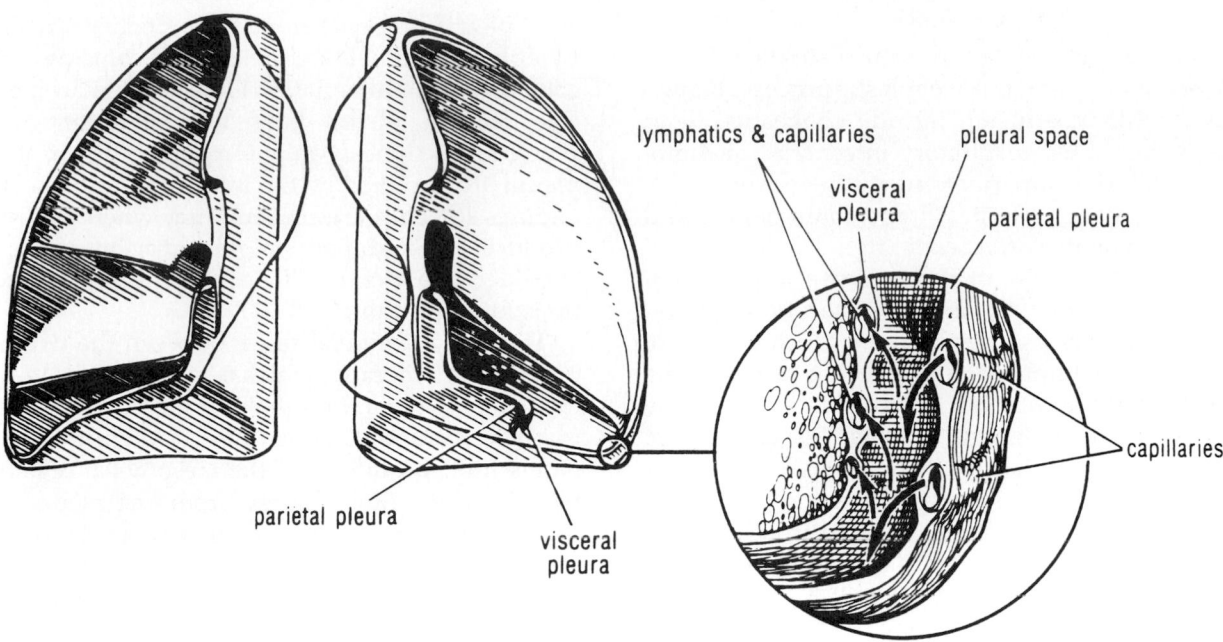

lymphatics & capillaries

pleural space

visceral pleura

parietal pleura

capillaries

parietal pleura

visceral pleura

Figure 19-4 Right and left pleural membranes. Inset shows fluid movement from parietal pleura across pleural space to visceral pleura. (From Miller SE and Campbell DB: Pleural effusions in malignant disease. In Polomano RC and Miller SE, editors: Understanding and managing oncologic emergencies, Monograph, Columbus, Ohio, 1987, Adria Laboratories.)

seeding of the primary tumor by direct extension or by metastasis via the pulmonary artery. This is a common finding with lung cancer and mesothelioma.[64] The presence of implants causes irritation and an inflammation that makes the capillaries more permeable to fluid and protein and leads to increased fluid in the pleural space.

Malignant cells shed from the pleura and may grow freely in the pleural space, forming tumor cell suspensions. These collections of malignant cells are similar to pleural implants in origin and nature of growth. The difference between a tumor cell suspension and an implant is the greater number of cells found on cytologic examination. A tumor cell suspension may have cell counts higher than 4000 cells/ml, which is more than an implant. Ovarian cancer and lung cancer are often associated with tumor cell suspension.[56,127]

Lymphatic blockage or venous obstruction interfere with drainage of fluid and large molecules from the pleural space, resulting in an overaccumulation of fluid. Lymphatic blockage is seen with lymphoma and metastasis from breast or lung cancer. Disruption of the capillary endothelium changes hydrostatic pressure gradients and allows fluid and protein to leak into the pleural space.

Necrotic malignant cells may shed into the pleural space, which raises its colloid osmotic pressure, thus reducing absorption of fluid by the visceral pleural

capillaries. This is common in patients with lung or breast cancer. Obstruction and tear of the thoracic duct may produce a true chylous pleural effusion as seen with lymphoma.[116]

Finally, other pathologies may contribute to the development of malignant pleural effusion. These include superior vena cava syndrome, postobstructive pneumonitis, pericardial effusion, bronchial obstruction with atelectasis, hypoalbuminemia, and congestive heart failure. Any condition in which fluid formation in the pleural space exceeds fluid removal will lead to fluid accumulation. The space between the two pleural surfaces will then expand to accommodate the fluid (pleural effusion). Expansion of the pleural space leads to compression or collapse of the lung with decreased lung volume.

CLINICAL FEATURES

Alterations in pulmonary function by a pleural effusion produce clinical signs and symptoms related to impairment of lung expansion and hypoxia. The onset of a malignant pleural effusion may be slow or rapid. Insidiously developing effusions can produce a moderate to large amount of fluid overaccumulation before diagnosis.[163] Thus, 25% of patients may be asymptomatic upon presentation.[56,112,137]

Physical examination will disclose abnormal findings if more than 300 ml of fluid has accumulated in the pleural space.[56] Pleural effusion commonly causes

---

CLINICAL FEATURES
MALIGNANT PLEURAL EFFUSION

Clinical signs

Labored breathing

Tachypnea

Restricted chest wall expansion

Decreased tactile fremitus on palpation

Dullness or flatness to percussion on the affected side

Decreased diaphragmatic excursion with percussion

Diminished or absent breath sounds over the affected area during auscultation

Pleuritic rub over the affected area during auscultation

Egophony (change in transmitted sound) with auscultation just above the level of effusion: the letter *E* spoken by the patient becomes higher pitched and sounds like an *A*[47]

If the effusion is large, additional signs could include:

> Bulging of the intercostal spaces on the affected side
>
> Splinting of the chest on the affected side
>
> Cyanosis
>
> Chest tenderness
>
> Shift in the point of maximum intensity (PMI) to the left if the effusion is on the right
>
> Tracheal deviation to the unaffected side[135]

Symptoms

Dyspnea on exertion or at rest

Dry, nonproductive cough

Shortness of breath

Chest pain often described as a "heaviness" or dull and aching rather than pleuritic[135]

Desire to lie on the affected side[135]

Malaise

Weight loss

Anxiety, fear of suffocation

---

atelectasis, which predisposes the patient to respiratory infection. This would present signs of infection such as fever, chills, and night sweats.

Symptoms expressed by a patient with malignant pleural effusion are related to alterations in pulmonary function, which are due to impairment from the effusion, and baseline respiratory status. The degree of symptomatology is dependent upon the rapidity of fluid accumulation rather than the amount of fluid present.[163] Clinical features of malignant pleural effusion are listed in the box above.

Physical findings of a pleural effusion are often not enough to make a differential diagnosis from a pleural or pulmonary mass or to determine a malignant versus benign underlying process. Further workup is necessary to confirm a diagnosis of pleural effusion.

DIAGNOSIS

Pleural effusion is usually detected by chest x-ray. The lateral and decubitus views are most helpful and reveal as little as 100 ml of pleural fluid. Accumulation must be about 300 ml to be seen in the upright anterior-posterior position on chest x-ray, where they appear as opacity in the lower lung field or hemithorax on the affected side.[47] Additional radiographic studies could include an ultrasound of the chest or a computerized tomography (CT) scan of the thorax. These two tests, as well as serial chest x-rays, are especially helpful in identifying a site for thoracentesis and demonstrating the mobility of fluid and absence of loculation that mean the fluid is separated into cavities by adhesions.[47,110]

Confirmation of a pleural effusion in a patient with cancer does not necessarily indicate a malignant process. Aspiration and cytologic examination of the pleural fluid are required to identify the nature of the effusion. The mechanism of fluid accumulation should be ascertained since it will guide treatment decisions.

Thoracentesis is a procedure in which a needle is introduced into the pleural space and fluid is aspirated. This procedure is indicated for diagnostic and therapeutic reasons. It is performed at the bedside. The patient is placed in the upright position with neck and dorsal spine flexed and arms extended and raised, usually over a bedside table. In this position, fluid will shift down into the dependent portion of the pleural space and the intercostal spaces will widen. A needle puncture is made, under local anesthesia, through the second intercostal space below the scapula on the affected side. The needle is directed inferiorly to avoid the neurovascular bundles located beneath and along the lower borders of the ribs.[110] Fluid is removed by a syringe or vacuum drainage collection, depending on the amount present. A minimum of 25 to 50 ml of fluid is needed for laboratory examination, but usually more than 250 ml is sent for analysis. Several puncture sites may be necessary if the fluid is loculated.

Initially, large volumes of fluid can be removed rapidly. However, this should not exceed 1500 ml because it could result in hypotension, circulatory collapse, or pulmonary edema. The effusion should never be tapped dry. Leaving a small amount of fluid facilitates the placement of a chest tube.[47] Although thoracentesis is a relatively safe procedure, other potential complications include pneumothorax, if the lung is lacerated; hemorrhage, if a blood vessel is lacerated; vasovagal symptoms; and infection.[110] To rule out complications, a chest x-ray is done after the thoracentesis.

Thoracentesis alone will not prevent fluid reaccumulation. Recurrence of pleural effusion is seen within a few days in as many as 87% of patients.[64] Repeated therapeutic thoracenteses for symptom relief may be warranted, but they are expensive and painful. In addition, they place the patient at risk for electrolyte imbalance, hypoproteinemia, pneumothorax, fluid loculation, and infection and may damage underlying lung parenchyma.[32,127,163]

Pleural fluid analysis helps establish the underlying mechanism of fluid accumulation. Normal pleural fluid is straw colored. Fluid from an effusion will be either a transudate or an exudate. A transudate fluid is a clear fluid usually attributed to an increased leakage of water. It is found in diseases characterized by sodium and water imbalances, such as congestive heart failure, cirrhosis, nephrotic syndrome, peritoneal dialysis hypoalbuminemia, and constrictive pericarditis.[138] Although most diseases associated with transudate fluid are benign, it is also seen in some patients with lymphoma whose lymph nodes are obstructed because of adenopathy rather than pleural surface involvement by the lymphoma.[56] An exudate fluid usually occurs when there is an excessive accumulation of protein in the pleural space. This is commonly seen when the pleural surface is irritated or seeded with tumor. Although an exudate fluid does not specify neoplastic involvement in the pleural space, the most common cause is a malignancy. Other causes of an exudative effusion are tuberculosis, pneumonia, systemic lupus erythematosus, pancreatitis, chylothorax, sarcoidosis, Meig's syndrome, prior radiation therapy, and mesothelioma. Most malignant effusions are exudative. The color of the pleural fluid can further define the type of exudate, as follows[56,116,138]:

Purulent fluid—emphysema or infection (tuberculosis or pneumonia)

Chylous fluid (milky)—blockage of the thoracic duct where there is involvement of the mesenteric or retroperitoneal lymph nodes (lymphoma or benign disease process)

Bloody fluid (more than 100,000 erythrocytes/mm³)—usually indicates malignancy. A pleural fluid hematocrit higher than 50% than that of the blood characterizes hemothorax.

Malignant pleural effusions are always classified as an exudate. They usually have a bloody color and, in addition, meet one of the following conditions: lactic dehydrogenase (LDH) level greater than 200 U; ratio of pleural fluid LDH level to serum LDH level greater than 0.6; ratio of pleural fluid protein to serum protein greater than 0.5.[127]

Other less sensitive markers in the fluid that indicate a malignant effusion are the following:

White blood cell count greater than 1000/mm
Red blood cell count greater than 100,000/mm
Low ph
Low glucose
High specific gravity
High amylase
Carcinoembryonic antigen (CEA) level greater than 12 ng/ml[127]

Cytologic examination, which determines cell count and cell composition of fluid, is considered the most specific test for malignancy. Malignant cells tend to exfoliate more readily than normal cells. Approximately 60% to 80% of pleural specimens have been positive for malignant cells.[47,110,112] A negative cytology does not exclude malignancy as the cause of the effusion.[47] Repeated negative cytology is more common with lymphoma and warrants a pleural biopsy. In general, though, the patient with a malignant effusion will have other convincing evidence of cancer. Therefore, a pleural biopsy may not be required.[47]

However, in situations with a false negative finding, other procedures can be done to make a differential diagnosis if necessary and if the patient can tolerate the workup. Testing would include bronchoscopy, mediastinoscopy, thoracoscopy, transcutaneous needle biopsy, open lung biopsy, or thoracotomy. Future techniques that may prove to be beneficial in identifying malignant cells are those involving monoclonal antibodies and various types of chromosomal analysis.[12]

TREATMENT MODALITIES

Once a diagnosis of malignant pleural effusion has been confirmed and the cause established, therapy will be determined by the underlying cancer (Figure 19-5). The goal of treatment will be related to the patient's overall medical condition, the degree of respiratory impairment and underlying pulmonary status, the extent and nature of the malignancy, the cause of the pleural effusion, prior or concurrent tumor therapy, and the patient's life expectancy.[124] Treatment may be focused on systemic therapy, local therapy, a combination of both systemic and local, or no therapy.

Systemic Therapy—Chemotherapy

If the underlying cancer is treatable, therapy is directed at the primary malignancy and not the effusion. Following diagnostic thoracentesis and lung reexpansion, systemic chemotherapy is initiated to prevent fluid reaccumulation. If the patient has a new diagnosis of lung cancer, a pleural effusion does not rule out surgery unless the cytology is positive. In that instance the tumor would be inoperable and therapy would be determined by the responsiveness of the tumor. Treatment options (Figure 19-5) could be chest tube drainage with or without sclerosis, local radiation therapy, systemic chemotherapy, or any combination of these.[110]

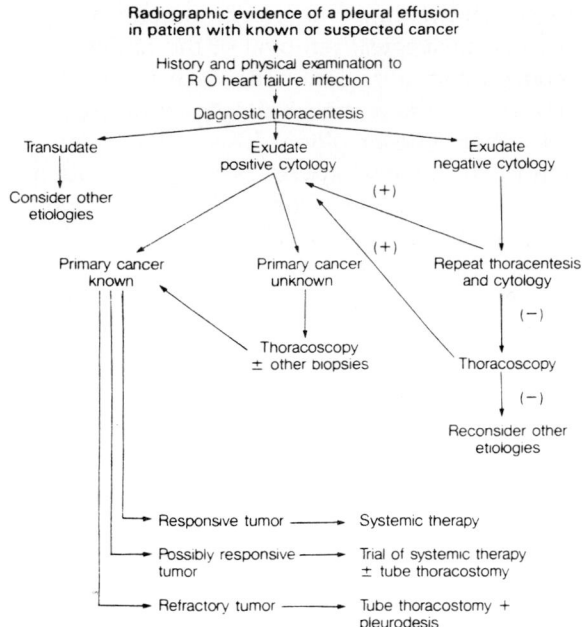

Figure 19-5 Clinical algorithm for prompt diagnosis and management of malignant pleural effusions. R-O, rule out; (+), positive; (−), negative. (From Ruckdeschel JC: Management of malignant pleural effusion: an overview, Semin Oncol 15[suppl 3]:27, 1988.)

Local Therapy—Radiation Therapy

Local radiation therapy may be used to treat malignant pleural effusions when the cause is a lymphoma. It may also be indicated in certain types of lung cancer. Radiation therapy in these two diseases may be the primary treatment or it may be combined with other types of treatment such as chest tube drainage, pleurodesis, or systemic chemotherapy.

Chest tube drainage is considered a more appropriate means of controlling pleural effusion than repeated thoracenteses, which can lead to complications. A thoracostomy tube inserted into the pleural space will not prevent fluid recurrence, but it will facilitate drainage and then pleural sclerosing. The procedure can be performed at the patient's bedside. The patient should be premedicated with a systemic analgesic such as meperidine or morphine sulfate.

Under local anesthesia, the chest tube is inserted through the fifth intercostal space on the anterior or lateral chest wall. These sites are usually chosen for patient comfort when lying and to prevent occlusion or kinking of the tube. Following insertion, the tube is connected to a water seal drainage system under suction. This restores negative pressure in the pleural space, removes the fluid, and allows the lung to reexpand.[110] A chest x-ray is done immediately following insertion of the chest tube to confirm its placement and to rule out a pneumothorax. Drainage usually requires 2 to 3 days, and subsequent chest films will be done, usually daily, to monitor fluid level and sta-

tus of the lungs. Patients often complain of a cough as the lung reexpands.

Chest tube insertion may cause complications similar to those from thoracentesis. These include pneumothorax, hemorrhage, infection, and damage to the lung parenchyma. An additional problem may be subcutaneous emphysema, or air under the subcutaneous tissues, although this is unusual unless the lung was injured.[110] Fluid or air may leak around the insertion site, which would require future stitching at the insertion site and/or a more occlusive vaseline gauze dressing. Malfunctions of the drainage system are possible, so frequent monitoring of the drainage system for patency is required.

Pleurodesis (Chemical Sclerosing)

Needle thoracentesis and chest tube drainage can successfully remove fluid from the pleural cavity. However, neither procedure can consistently prevent recurrence of fluid accumulation. Therefore, chest tube drainage is usually followed by pleurodesis (Figure 19-5), which is the chemical sclerosing of the two pleural membranes. The goal is to obliterate the pleural space by instilling an irritating chemical into the space, causing the formation of adhesions that prevent fluid accumulation around the lung. These chemical agents damage the alveolar membrane and permeability, allowing clotting proteins like fibrinogen to leak into the pleural space. Fibrinogen converts to fibrin, which accumulates and forms a lattice. Fibroblasts deposit collagen on the lattice and create the pleural adhesions.[48] Pleurodesis can be done at the bedside after the effusion has been drained by the chest tube producing less than 100 ml of fluid in 24 hours. Drainage of the effusion is confirmed by chest x-ray showing lung reexpansion. If larger quantities of fluid continue to drain, pleurodesis may be less effective and require a repeated procedure.

Pleurodesis is initiated by selecting the sclerosing agent. Many different agents have been used, including talcum powder, an antimalarial agent called quinacrine, radioisotopes of gold or phosphorus, antineoplastic agents, and antibiotics. The antineoplastic agents were employed with the hope that there would be a cytotoxic effect, as well as sclerosing effect. Findings show that the effectiveness of neoplastic agents when used as sclerosants depends on the ability to cause irritation and not on their antineoplastic activity. Thiotepa, 5-FU, nitrogen mustard, adriamycin, and bleomycin were researched with varying results.[37,118,138] Continued research with bleomycin as a sclerosant have shown it to be as effective as or superior to tetracycline for pleurodesis. There are many studies that demonstrate an overall response rate of 50% to 85%. The major disadvantage is the high cost. Problems of systemic absorption, bone marrow suppression, and other toxicities have limited the use of most of these agents.[47,112,135,138]

Tetracycline has been the most commonly used sclerosing agent to date, with 80% being its highest reported response rate.[124] A bulb syringe is prepared with a concentrated solution of tetracycline (500 mg in 50 ml of normal saline to 2 g/200 ml of normal saline) with lidocaine HCl 1% (15 to 30 ml).[127] However, injectable tetracycline was recently discontinued by its manufacturer and as a result alternative efficacious and safe sclerosing agents are now needed.[48] Minocycline and doxycycline may be alternatives to tetracycline because there are analogues putting them in the same drug class; they all have a similar pH in solution, are readily available, do not cause bone marrow suppression, and are inexpensive. Currently there has not been enough research on the use of minocycline and doxycycline for pleurodesis. The studies have been too few, too small, and have had varying results. It is clear though that doxycycline requires multiple instillations and that bleomycin may be cost prohibitive. Ongoing research is needed.[48,112,136,138]

Because the sclerosing agents work by irritation of the pleura, patient preparation for pleurodesis may involve sedation with an intravenous sedative (diazepam) or narcotic analgesic (meperidine or morphine sulfate). Even with intrapleural lidocaine the pain may be quite severe. Therefore, bleomycin, which is far less painful and better tolerated, has gained popularity as a sclerosant. Doses vary from 60 U in 100 ml of 5% dextrose in water to 120 or 150 U in normal saline.[137]

The chest tube is unclamped by the physician, who then slowly injects the prepared sclerosing mixture into the pleural cavity. The chest tube is clamped, and the patient is asked or helped to turn from side to side to allow contact between the sclerosing agent and the entire surface of the pleura. Repositioning is continued every 15 to 30 minutes for 2 to 6 hours. The chest tube is then opened to drainage and the amount of drainage is monitored. The drainage of pleural fluid usually decreases over a period of a few days, and when the amount is less than 50 ml in an 8-hour period, the chest tube is removed.[110] A chest x-ray is repeated to evaluate the success of the pleurodesis and to rule out a pneumothorax following chest tube removal.

Surgery

PLEURECTOMY (MECHANICAL PLEURODESIS). Surgical intervention for the management of pleural effusion is usually reserved for those situations when other treatment options fail to resolve the accumulation of fluid in the pleural cavity (Figure 19-5) and the patient has a life expectancy that makes the pro-

cedure worth the time and energy expenditure. Pleurectomy is the surgical removal of the parietal pleura with concomitant abrasion of the visceral pleura. Thus it is referred to as a mechanical pleurodesis.[110] The goal of either type of pleurodesis is the same, obliteration of the pleural space. Both require adequate lung expansion to meet the chest wall. Therefore, drainage of the pleural space by a chest tube is done preoperatively.

Removal of the parietal pleura involves the same considerations as for any other thoracotomy procedure. It is done in the operating room under general anesthesia. A thoracotomy incision is established, and the parietal pleura is separated and removed from the chest wall. The visceral pleura, on the lung, is then swabbed with dry gauze, which causes granulation and the formation of adhesions. Chest tubes are inserted and kept in place initially during the postoperative period to allow effective sclerosing. In certain cases of chylous effusions caused by neoplastic obstruction of the mediastinal lymphatics, the surgical procedure may include ligation of the thoracic duct at the level of the diaphragm.[110]

Pleurectomy has produced excellent results; however, it has been accompanied by a morbidity rate of 20% or more and a 10% mortality rate.[56] Complications include air leaks, bleeding, and infection (pneumonia and empyema). Surgical removal of the pleura is a radical procedure usually reserved for patients in good physical condition and with a good life expectancy.

PLEUROPERITONEAL SHUNTS. Another surgical treatment is available for intractable effusions when chemical pleurodesis is not feasible or has failed or when pleurectomy is not a viable option. The procedure involves the shunting of fluid from the pleural cavity into the abdominal cavity (Figure 19-6). Under local anesthesia in the operating room, a commercially available device with one-way valved tubing is placed subcutaneously on the lateral chest wall. One end is inserted into the pleural cavity and the other into the abdominal cavity.

Early shunting devices were manually operated and required manual activation of the pump approximately 50 times a day.[64] More recent devices drain spontaneously by positive pressure in the pleural cavity created by the effusion. This can be supplemented manually by applying pressure on the subcutaneous device (Figure 19-6). Patients are often taught to activate the device themselves.[110] Success of the device will depend upon the amount and rate of fluid accumulation and proper pump function.

LONG-TERM THORACOTOMY ACCESS AND DRAINAGE. A final alternative for the control of pleural effusion is long-term thoracotomy access and drainage. This approach is used for palliation. Patient se-

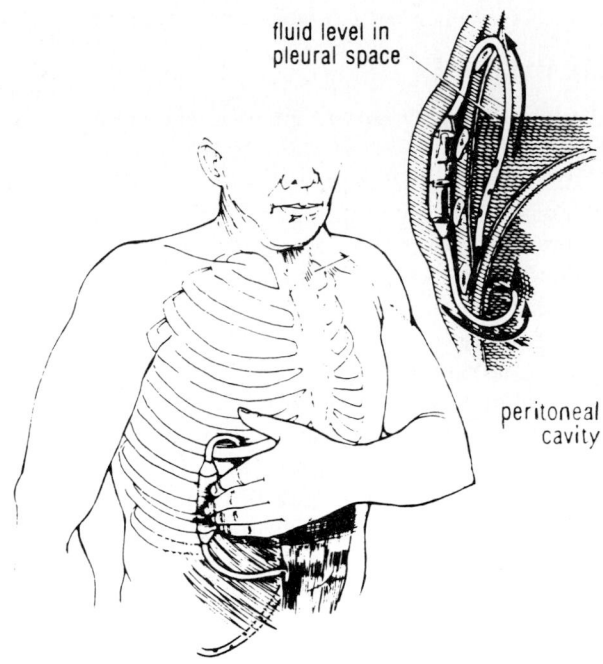

fluid level in
pleural space

peritoneal
cavity

Figure 19-6 Operation of pleuroperitoneal shunt. Inset shows position of device on rib cage. Arrows indicate direction of flow. (From Miller SE and Campbell DB: Pleural effusions in malignant disease. In Polomano RC and Miller SE, editors: Understanding and managing oncologic emergencies, Monograph, Columbus, Ohio, 1987, Adria Laboratories.)

lection is based on patient performance status and degree of disability, general health condition with attention to past and present pulmonary status, extent of underlying malignancy, and estimated life expectancy.[64,124] Eligible patients include those with debilitating symptoms who have been unsuccessfully treated for pleural effusion by thoracentesis, chest tube drainage, pleurodesis, radiation therapy, or chemotherapy and those patients who are not candidates for surgery.

Access to the pleural cavity is accomplished by either a long-term access device, such as an implantable subcutaneous port, or by a chest tube. The subcutaneous port, with attached catheter or drainage tube, is placed into the pleural cavity by surgical implantation. The port is accessed through the usual subcutaneous method and fluid is withdrawn intermittently. This can be done as often as deemed necessary but in most cases it is done twice a week.[64] Complications include infection, bleeding, occlusion, and device malfunctions.

Continuous long-term drainage can be accomplished by using either a standard chest tube or a small bore catheter such as a Foley catheter placed into the pleural space. The smaller catheters are less traumatic to insert, may be sewn in place onto the skin, and will not cause splinting of the ribs, which is sometimes a complication with larger tubes.[32] The

principles and procedures of long-term drainage represent modifications of those for the standard short-term chest tube drainage system.[64] The two necessary components of a long-term drainage system include the drainage tube and the collection equipment. Options are available and choices depend on the patient's status. The following comparisons may help the decision process:

STANDARD CHEST TUBE	SMALL-BORE CATHETER
Drainage Tube	
Large, allows view of fluid	Small, may or may not give view of fluid
Rigid, uncomfortable	Flexible, more comfortable
Anchored by sutures only	An inflatable bulb is available in addition to sutures
Collection Equipment	
Drainage under water seal	Drainage without water seal (continuous urinary drainage bag or system may be used)
Large and cumbersome	Smaller and easier to handle
Expensive	Less expensive
May or may not be portable	Usually portable
Noisy, requires suction	Quiet, drains by gravity

A one-way valve (Heimlich valve) may or may not be used between the drainage tube and collection equipment. It is usually indicated when there is a risk of pneumothorax since it allows the drainage of fluid and escape of air from the thorax but prevents their return. An advantage of the one-way valve is that the collection equipment can be kept at any level below or above the chest without adverse effects. However, if the one-way valve is not used, all collection equipment must be at or below the chest tube insertion site for adequate drainage and to prevent complications.[64,145]

Long-term thoracotomy access drainage provides an important alternative method for managing intractable pleural effusions. It can reduce cost by decreasing the number of procedures and hospitalizations. Many patients can be managed at home using this method. This long-term treatment can provide comfort through relief of respiratory distress and control of associated symptoms. Most importantly, it can improve quality of life, the primary goal of any treatment.

PROGNOSIS

Patients with pleural effusion have a variable prognosis depending on the extent of the effusion and the success of treatment for the underlying disease. Malignant pleural effusion is usually an indication of

Nursing Management

Nursing care of a patient with pleural effusion is dependent on the extent of the effusion, the underlying disease, and the patient's overall condition. The problem is serious, and nursing care will be diverse, as with other oncologic complications. However, pleural effusions usually have a more gradual and detectable onset. This fact, coupled with a high recurrence rate, places great emphasis on the assessment skills of the nurse. Objective and subjective data must be collected systematically.[68,84,139,144,151]

NURSING DIAGNOSES

- Ineffective breathing patterns related to limited lung expansion secondary to pleural effusion
- Potential for impaired gas exchange related to ineffective breathing patterns and pleural effusion

INTERVENTIONS

- Determine current respiratory status:
    Observe for signs and symptoms of respiratory difficulty (dyspnea, shortness of breath, tachypnea, increased sputum production, change in color of sputum, hemoptysis, persistent cough, decreased activity tolerance, chest, arm, or shoulder pain, headache).
    Assess lungs. Observe ventilatory movements (rate and depth), patency of the airway, use of accessory muscles, clubbing of fingernails, discoloration of nail beds or mucous membranes. Palpate chest for fremitus, crepitance, deviation of trachea, or nonsymmetrical chest expansion. Percuss chest for density or consolidation and displacement of organs. Auscultate chest for breath sounds.
    Monitor laboratory and other respiratory function tests: CBC, electrolytes, arterial blood gases, chest x-ray, pulmonary function studies, scans.
- Assist with breathing and pulmonary toilet:
    Positioning for comfort and enhanced chest expansion
    Deep breathing and coughing every 2 hours
    Pursed-lip breathing
    Postural drainage
    Mouth care frequently
    Suctioning if necessary
- Provide oxygen therapy as indicated.
- Consult with physician regarding need for more aggressive pulmonary toilet measures (incentive spirometry, ultrasonic nebulizer, chest physical therapy).
- Administer respiratory medications as ordered.
- Provide mechanical ventilation if necessary.

- Teach measures to maintain optimal respiratory abilities:
    Use of oxygen therapy
    Pursed-lip breathing
    Breathing exercises
    Scheduled rest periods
    Humidification
    Adequate hydration and nutrition
    Use of incentive spirometry and/or inhalers
    Smoking cessation if indicated
    Measures to decrease anxiety and stress (environmental manipulation, relaxation techniques, antianxiety medications)
- Make referrals to other health care professionals in the hospital and community as needed.
- Monitor chest tube drainage if indicated, as outlined in hospital procedure.
- Assist with pleurodesis if ordered, as outlined in hospital procedure.

NURSING DIAGNOSIS

- Potential for alteration in tissue perfusion related to impaired gas exchange due to pleural effusion

INTERVENTIONS

- Assess organ systems for malfunction related to ischemia.
- Evaluate skin color of extremities.
- Note any change in mental status.
- Monitor laboratory values closely.
- Measure intake and output.
- Provide oxygen therapy as prescribed.
- Administer vasoactive drugs as ordered.

If the treatment used is surgery, the usual postoperative nursing care is implemented. The goal is to prevent or minimize complications. Patient assessment, pain management, oral hygiene, skin care, nutrition, and passive/active exercising are all important aspects of surgical nursing care planning. When the patient is undergoing chemotherapy or radiation therapy, the nurse will manage any side effects that may occur, such as fatigue, skin changes, alopecia, nausea, vomiting, diarrhea, and bone marrow suppression.

Discharge planning for patients treated for pleural effusion is dependent on their status following treatment. Some patients may go home symptom-free and need only follow-up care to monitor for recurrence. Some patients may need support at home for intermittent or continuous pleural drainage. Other patients may require a hospice or extended care facility to continue management of the pleural effusion. The nurse is responsible for the transition from the hospital setting. (See Chapter 26.)

advanced disease. Survival rates vary from 3 months to 4 years, with the longest survival in patients with lymphoma.[32,110] Results from several studies indicate that mean survival from time of diagnosis of the effusion is about 6 months in lung cancer and 1 year in breast cancer.[32] Treatment efforts must be aimed at the underlying disease; however, they are always accompanied by measures to improve the patient's quality of life. With improving technology, earlier diagnosis and better interventions may increase survival rates.

NEOPLASTIC CARDIAC TAMPONADE

DEFINITION

Neoplastic cardiac tamponade is the compression of the cardiac muscle by pathologic fluid accumulation under pressure within the pericardial sac. Fluid accumulates because the pericardium is constricted by a tumor or by the presence of postirradiation pericarditis.[163] Compression of the myocardium interferes with dilatation of the heart chambers, which prevents adequate cardiac filling during diastole. This in turn reduces blood flow to the ventricles and reduces stroke volume, which results in decreased cardiac output. Other pressures are then affected including an elevated central venous pressure and a lowered left atrial pressure (Figure 19-7). Two compensatory mechanisms that attempt to counteract these pressures are an increase in heart rate (tachycardia) and peripheral vasoconstriction, which maintains arterial pressure and venous return.[38] If cardiac output is not increased by compensatory mechanisms, this can cause circulatory collapse, which if untreated is fatal.[7,55]

ETIOLOGY AND RISK FACTORS

A variety of conditions can be responsible for the development of cardiac tamponade. These may be nonmalignant or malignant. Nonmalignant causes include the following[110,147]:

- Cardiovascular causes: heart surgery, chest trauma, aneurysm, rupture of the great vessel, cardiac procedures (angiography, insertion or removal of pacer wires), insertion of central venous catheter
- Infectious pericarditis; bacterial, fungal, viral, or tubercular infections
- Connective tissue disorders: systemic lupus erythematosus, scleroderma, rheumatoid disease
- Myxedema
- Uremia
- Pharmacologic therapy; anthracyclines (adriamycin, daunomycin), anticoagulants (heparin, Coumadin), hydralazine (Apresoline), procainamide (Procan/Pronestyl)

Malignant causes include the following[110,163]:

- Neoplastic pericarditis with effusion: primary tumors of the pericardium (mesotheliomas and sarcomas); and metastatic tumors of the pericardium (lung, breast, leukemia, lymphoma, melanoma, sarcomas)
- Neoplastic constrictive pericarditis (metastatic tumor infiltration)
- Radiation pericarditis (exposure of the heart to 400 Gy or more)

INCIDENCE/RISK FACTORS

Pericardial effusion with tamponade is a life-threatening problem whether the cause is malignant or nonmalignant. Open heart surgery is the leading cause of cardiac tamponade, which occurs postoperatively in approximately 3% to 8% of patients.[7,32] Malignant pericardial tamponade occurs in approximately 10% to 20% of patients with a neoplasm that involves the heart. The high estimates of this complication are based on compilations of autopsy data regarding cardiac (including pericardial) metastasis, which range from 0.1% to 21%.[32] The majority of these patients were asymptomatic, only 10% to 25% showing clinical evidence of cardiac disease before death.[32]

The majority of cases of neoplastic cardiac tamponade represent metastatic invasion of the pericardium. Pericardial metastasis is unusual without documentation of other metastases. Only rarely is the cause primary disease of the myocardium (mesothelioma, angiosarcoma, fibrosarcoma, malignant teratoma).[70] Any cancer has the potential for metastatic spread to the pericardium via direct tumor extension, lymphatic invasion, or hematogenous dissemination. Patients with pericardial effusions are at risk for tamponade. Pericardial effusions due to metastatic disease are present in 5% to 50% of patients with cancer.[32] However, cancers at greatest risk for the development of neoplastic cardiac tamponade include breast cancer, lung cancer, lymphoma, leukemia, and melanoma. Approximately 5% of patients who receive radiation therapy to the mediastinum (400 Gy or more) develop acute pericarditis with or without pericardial effusion during treatment or chronic constrictive pericarditis up to 20 years after treatment.[81,116] More than 90% of the cases occur in the first year after radiation treatment.[118]

PATHOPHYSIOLOGY

The heart and a portion of the great vessels are encased in a thin, tough, double-layered fibrous sac called the pericardium, which contains little elastic tissue. The inner layer, or sheath, is known as the visceral pericardium. It is a delicate serous membrane that lines the interior of the fibrous sac and is continuous with the surface of the heart.[135] The outer layer

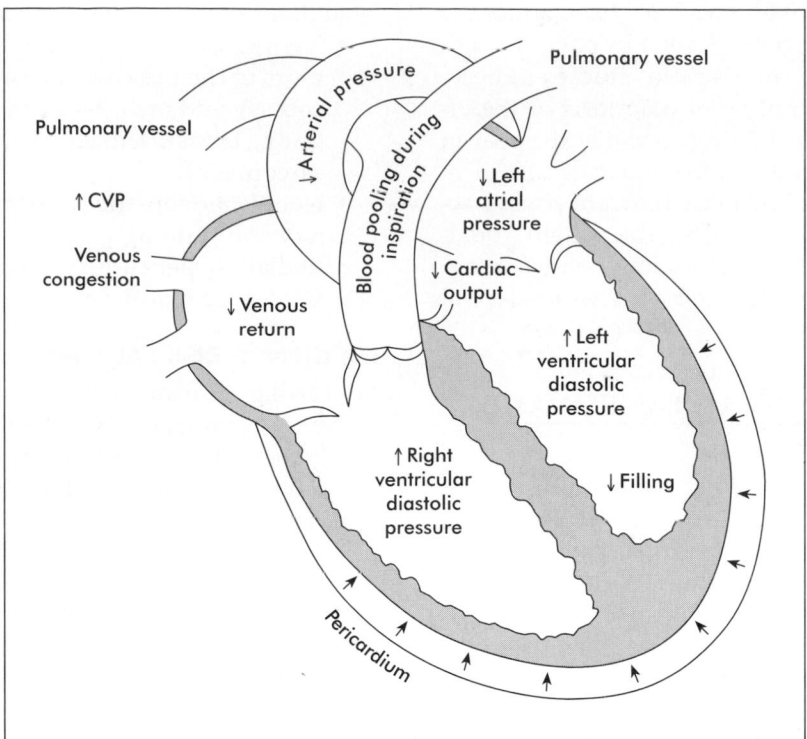

Figure 19-7 Cardiovascular effects of increased intrapleural pressure. Intraventricular diastolic pressure rises as a result of higher intrapericardial pressure. This prevents adequate filling of the ventricle, causing venous congestion, decreased cardiac output, lowered left atrial pressure, and elevated central venous pressure. ↑, Increased; ↓, decreased. (From Dietz KA and Flaherty AM: Oncologic emergencies. In Groenwald SL and others, editors: Cancer nursing: principles and practice, ed 2, 1990, Jones and Bartlett.)

of the pericardium is called the parietal pericardium. This sheath is fibrous and provides strength and protection. The left sternal portion is in direct contact with the chest wall. Between the two layers of the pericardium is a cavity that contains 10 to 20 ml of a clear serous lubricating fluid, originating from the lymphatic channels surrounding the heart and serves to cushion the myocardium.

The pathophysiology of pericardial tamponade is a progressive accumulation of fluid in the pericardial sac (Figure 19-8), which leads to compression of the heart, hampering dilatation of its chambers and thus limiting diastolic atrial filling: intrapericardial pressure rises and bilateral ventricular stroke volume decreases. Initially, the sac will stretch to accommodate increases in fluid, and compensatory mechanisms—an increased heart rate (tachycardia) and increased peripheral vascular tone (peripheral vasoconstriction)—will maintain adequate cardiac output. However, as these temporary adaptive responses begin to fail, a vicious cycle of increased fluid with decreased atrial pressure, decreased cardiac output, and decreased venous return will progress to circulatory collapse and, if untreated, to shock, cardiac arrest, and death.

The severity of cardiac tamponade depends on the amount of fluid in the pericardium, the rate of accumulation, and the degree of pericardial and organic compromise. Usually there will be no change in cardiac activity with the addition of 50 ml or less of fluid in the pericardial space. Gradual fluid accumulation permits the pericardium to stretch and accommodate. As much as 2 L or more can accumulate without producing signs of cardiac compromise.[55,56,70,91,110] However, 100 to 200 ml of fluid may cause severe cardiac impairment if the accumulation occurs rapidly.[147] Whether gradual or acute, the fluid accumulation that leads to cardiac tamponade in the presence of malignant disease is the result of one of the following mechanisms:

- Direct tumor (primary or metastatic) extension and blockage of the lymphatic drainage
- Malignant lymphatic engorgement and impairment of drainage
- Tumor (primary or metastatic) implantation in or around the pericardium with inflammation and fluid production
- Radiation-induced pericarditis of the pericardium with fluid accumulation

Retrograde lymphatic dissemination is thought to be the main pathway of pericardial metastasis creating fluid seepage through the visceral pericardium and

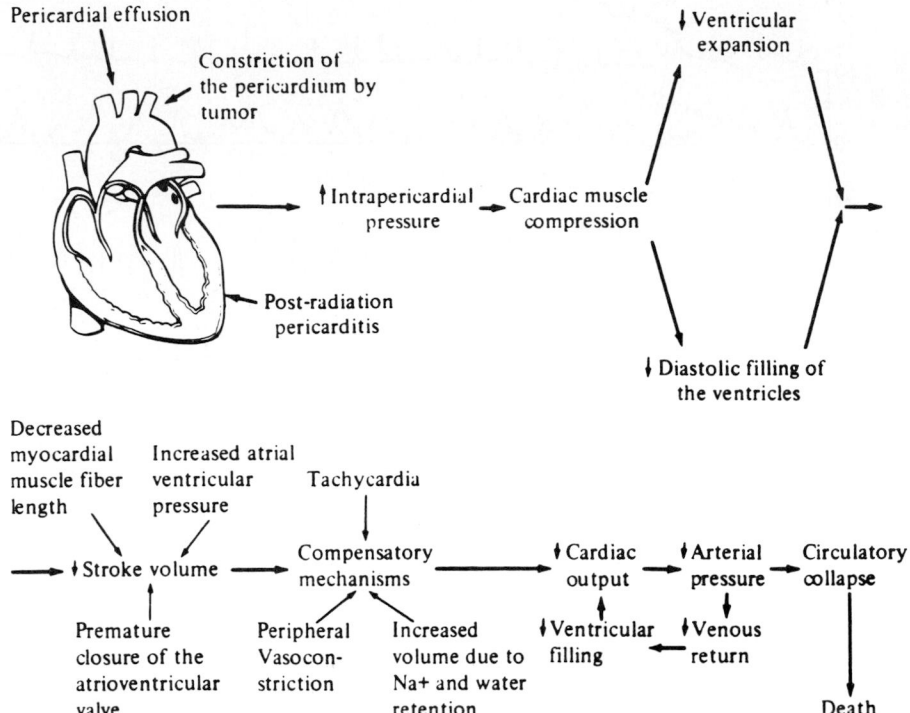

Figure 19-8 Development of neoplastic pericardial tamponade. (From Yasko JM and Schafer SL: Neoplastic pericardial tamponade. In Yasko JM, editor: Guidelines for cancer care: symptom management, Reston, Va, 1983, Reston Publishing Co.)

into the pericardial space.[91] Neoplastic cardiac tamponade related to malignant pericardial effusion, whether resulting from a constricting tumor, lymphatic dissemination, or postirradiation pericarditis, is a medical emergency and must be recognized and treated promptly.

CLINICAL FEATURES

Patients with neoplastic cardiac tamponade manifest a wide variety of clinical signs and symptoms, directly related to the degree of fluid accumulation (amount and rapidity of onset) and subsequent disruption of normal hemodynamics. Clinical features and the related stages of a progressive pericardial effusion are listed in the box at right and Figure 19-8.

Identification of neoplastic cardiac tamponade is greatly dependent upon a clinical diagnosis based on a detailed history and thorough physical examination. The presence or absence of any of the signs and symptoms will depend on the stage of cardiac tamponade. Notation should be made of a current or past history of cancer and cancer treatments. Occasionally neoplastic cardiac tamponade is the first sign of a malignancy.

Beck's triad has been considered a hallmark of cardiac tamponade. These three signs include an elevated CVP, distant heart sound, and arterial hypotension. However, these signs may not be found in all patients, and their appearance usually marks an advanced stage of tamponade. Therefore, Beck's triad

---

**CLINICAL FEATURES
NEOPLASTIC CARDIAC TAMPONADE**

Clinical signs

Tachycardia
Low systolic blood pressure
Tachypnea with normal breath sounds
Vasoconstriction
Thready diminished pulse pressure or pulsus paradoxus
Increased central venous pressure (CVP)
Arterial hypotension
Cardiomegaly
Precordial dullness to percussion
Distant weak heart sounds
Pericardial friction rub
Engorged neck veins
Ascites
Hepatomegaly
Hepatojugular reflux
Peripheral edema
Cool, clammy extremities or peripheral cyanosis
Oliguria secondary to decreased renal perfusion
Apprehension, anxiety
Clouded sensorium or impaired consciousness

Symptoms

Dyspnea or shortness of breath
Retrosternal chest pain
Diaphoresis
Anxiety
Cough
Hoarseness, hiccups
Nausea, vomiting
Abdominal pain

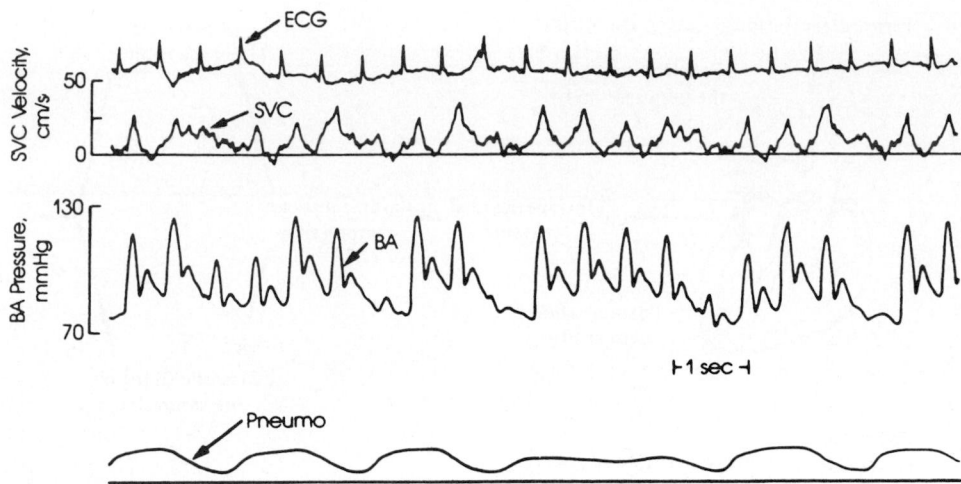

Figure 19-9 Simultaneous recording of electrocardiogram *(ECG)*, blood flow velocity in the superior vena cava *(SVC)*, brachial arterial pressure *(BA)*, and the pneumogram *(Pneumo)* in a patient with cardiac compression and paradoxical pulse. A downward deflection of the pneumogram denotes inspiration, when SVC blood velocity rises and arterial pressure falls (paradoxical pulse). Arterial pressure is maintained during prolonged expiratory pause. (From Braunwald E: Pericardial disease. In Braunwald E and others, editors: Harrison's principles of internal medicine, ed 11, New York, 1987, McGraw-Hill Book Co.)

is not a sufficient clinical indicator of cardiac tamponade.[154]

DIAGNOSIS

A differential diagnosis of neoplastic cardiac tamponade is often difficult; in a patient with cancer it becomes even more complex. With no known history of cancer, other possible diagnoses must be ruled out, such as right ventricular heart failure, hydropericardium, rapid blood volume expansion, congestive heart failure, and pulmonary edema.[8,56]

Patients with cancer present a challenge for differential diagnosis because of the different malignant and nonmalignant pathophysiologic processes that can cause pericarditis and result in cardiac tamponade.[110,139] Patients who have received radiation therapy to the mediastinal area may develop cardiac tamponade secondary to pericardial constriction. This process is more difficult to diagnose than malignant tumor invasion and requires a different treatment. Cardiac function may also be affected without fluid accumulation by cancer-related or treatment-related processes such as radiation fibrosis, heart muscle metastasis, coronary artery occlusion, or drug-induced congestive heart failure.[135]

Two clinical findings that are classic features of cardiac tamponade are pulsus paradoxus and hepatojugular reflux. Testing for these two manifestations can be performed at the bedside. Pulsus paradoxus (Figure 19-9) is an abnormal finding of a weaker pulse during inspiration, resulting from a greater than normal (10 mm Hg) decrease in systolic blood pressure during the inspiratory phase of normal respiration.

Cardiac tamponade constricts the myocardium, and during inspiration the diaphragm exerts additional pressure on the pericardial sac. The left ventricle receives less blood, and stroke volume is decreased, which is seen as a decrease in systolic blood pressure during inspiration. The arterial pulse may also be absent during inspiration.[56,70,91,110,139]

Pulsus paradoxus can be determined in one of two ways (Figure 19-9): patients with an indwelling arterial catheter can have their blood pressure monitored during inspiration. Patients without invasive equipment can have their blood pressure evaluated by routine sphygmomanometry. A blood pressure cuff is placed around the arm and inflated to greater than 20 mm Hg above systolic pressure. The cuff is deflated slowly until the first systolic sound (Korotkoff sound) is auscultated and the reading is noted. This will be during expiration, and the sounds will disappear during inspiration. The cuff is further deflated until sounds can be heard throughout the respiratory cycle (expiration and inspiration). This reading is also noted. The difference in mm Hg between the two readings is the value of the paradox. If there is a difference of more than 10 mm Hg between the two readings, pulsus paradoxus is present.[47,79,91,139]

Inaccurate results may occur when assessing for pulsus paradoxus. Mechanical ventilation can artificially mimic pulsus paradoxus.[56] If hypotension is present, pulsus paradoxus may not be found by auscultation. In this situation the inspiratory decline in blood pressure can be noted by close examination of the carotid or femoral pulse. Pulsus paradoxus may disappear during extreme tamponade when the systolic pressure may decrease below 50 mm Hg. Finally, other conditions may be manifested with pulsus paradoxus. These include obesity, severe obstructive respiratory disease, acute cor pulmonale, right ventricular infarction, and hypovolemic shock.[44,47,56,91]

Hepatojugular reflex is an elevation in jugular venous pressure by 1 cm or more. Testing for this abnormal condition is accomplished by placing the patient in the supine position with the head of the bed elevated to a level where jugular venous pulsations are visible. Pressure is then exerted continuously over the right upper quadrant of the abdomen for 30 to 60 seconds and jugular pressure is observed. An increase in the pressure represents a positive reflex arising from venous congestion associated with a prolonged elevation of the CVP.[56,91,139]

Tests ordered by the physician will include a chest x-ray, ECG, and an echocardiogram. A routine chest x-ray is not a specific diagnostic tool since it cannot differentiate among possible causes of an enlarged heart shadow. Fluid accumulation of 100 ml will not change the cardiac silhouette on x-ray, yet this amount of fluid can produce tamponade if onset is rapid. More than 250 ml of fluid within the pericardial sac will enlarge the cardiac silhouette. A "water bottle heart" is seen on the x-ray as a result of the disappearance of the normal contours between the great vessels and the cardiac chambers.[47,91,139] More than half of the patients with cardiac tamponade have cardiac enlargement, mediastinal widening, or hilar adenopathy.[71] Lung fields on chest x-ray are usually normal since pulmonary bed capacity has not been impaired.

The electrocardiogram provides a limited amount of useful information. Elevated ST segments, nonspecific T wave changes, decreased QRS voltage and sinus tachycardia may be seen.[91,110,147] Electrical alternans, which is the alternation of amplitude and direction of the P wave and QRS complexes on every other beat, is a common abnormality in patients with neoplastic cardiac tamponade. This heart block, appearing at every other beat, is thought to result from variations in cardiac position at the time of electrical depolarization.[8,47,70,91,139]

Echocardiography, both M-mode (motion mode) and two-dimensional, is the most specific and sensitive technique for establishing the presence of pericardial effusion. This noninvasive, reliable test should always be done when cardiac tamponade is suspected. The presence, location, and approximate quantity of fluid can be determined by the cardiac ultrasound. Normal findings on the echocardiogram show the posterior left ventricular wall in contact with the posterior pericardium and pleura and the anterior right ventricular wall in close approximation to the chest wall.[135] In tamponade, echo-free spaces that separate the moving walls from the immobile pericardium indicate the presence of fluid.[47,139] The spaces appear first posteriorly and then anteriorly. The absence of pericardial fluid usually rules out cardiac tamponade. Although an echocardiogram cannot determine the cause of the pericardial fluid, it is extremely helpful in the evaluation of an effusion, as well as in site selection for pericardiocentesis.

Recent advances in echocardiography have added new dimensions to diagnostic testing. Transesophageal Echo, StressEcho, and Intraarterial Echo are such examples. Transesophageal Echo (TEE) has been used in critically ill patients as a diagnostic tool in hypotensive crisis. Pericardial tamponade has been correctly diagnosed in this type of patient. The esophagus is the closest structure to the heart. Positioning the TEE scope with its transducer in that location permits high resolution images of the cardiac structure. The TEE scope is a modification of the endoscope, and its tip can be moved antigrade, retrograde, and/or laterally to obtain tomographic views of cardiac structures using a biplane or omniplane transducer. This procedure can be done at the bedside, in the operating room, or as an outpatient procedure.[11,77]

Other testing that may be performed during a diagnostic workup for neoplastic cardiac tamponade includes cardiac catheterization, various types of scanning, and laboratory blood work. Catheterization of the heart can confirm a diagnosis of tamponade and determine the size and exact location of the pericardial fluid. In the presence of tamponade, there will be an increased intracardiac pressure and an abnormal near equality of diastolic pressures in all chambers of the heart (10 to 25 mm Hg) as measured during catheterization.

Recent improvements in technology have assisted in the diagnosis of cardiac tamponade. CT and magnetic resonance imaging (MRI) have been useful in the assessment of a thickened pericardium and the diagnosis of constrictive pericarditis with effusion versus radiation fibrosis. These specific differential diagnoses are crucial since treatment will differ in each situation.

Laboratory blood tests ordered during the diagnostic workup for neoplastic cardiac tamponade may include hematocrit, potassium (K^+), calcium (Ca^{++}), and arterial blood gases (ABGs). These tests are not conclusive for cardiac tamponade, but they can support a differential diagnosis.

Testing for neoplastic cardiac tamponade will vary greatly in scope and depth as determined by the clinical appearance of the patient, including patient tolerance for various procedures. Time is of the essence. Clinically evident neoplastic effusions are usually large enough to be evaluated by echocardiography.[139,147]

TREATMENT MODALITIES

Neoplastic cardiac tamponade is a life-threatening situation that requires immediate medical intervention as soon as the diagnosis is confirmed. The immediate goal of treatment is the removal of pericardial fluid to relieve impending circulatory collapse. Following symptomatic relief of tamponade, the longer-range goal is management of the underlying disease.

Pharmacologic Therapy

Mild neoplastic cardiac tamponade may be treated with drug therapy using corticosteroids and diuretics. Supportive measures during cardiac tamponade are aimed at maintaining blood pressure and cardiac functioning.[70] Common prescriptions include prednisone (40 to 60 mg/day) with furosemide (Lasix) (40 mg/day) or Aldactazide (25 to 200 mg/day). Radiation pericarditis is often effectively treated with high-dose steroid or NSAIDs. However, when these drugs are discontinued, the pericarditis often recurs.[118,163] If an effusion recurs or tamponade becomes acute, more aggressive treatment is indicated.[47,139] Infusions of blood products and intravenous fluids will increase ventricular filling pressures. Vasoactive drugs may be useful. Isoproterenol can increase heart rate and contractility, and low-dose dopamine may improve contractility. However, alpha-adrenergic medications will likely increase afterload and adversely affect cardiac output. The use of diuretics at this point will decrease volume and further impair ventricular filling.[70]

Pericardiocentesis

Pericardiocentesis, which is a percutaneous needle pericardiotomy with aspiration, is done for both therapeutic and diagnostic reasons. Indications for this approach include a slow leak, diagnostic confirmation, rapid relief of acute tamponade, or symptomatic relief when deterioration of the patient's condition is evidenced by cyanosis, dyspnea, changes in mental status, or shock.[56,71,139] Another indicator for an aggressive approach to relieve tamponade is the "rule of 20," or a decrease in pulse pressure of more than 20 mm Hg, pulsus paradoxus greater than 20 mm Hg, and CVP greater than 20 cm H_2O before pericardiocentesis.

When there is a delay in aspiration, treatment may be initiated along with pharmacologic measures to improve hemodynamic status. Temporary interventions include the administration of volume expanders such as plasma blood or other colloid solutions that help to increase ventricular filling pressure. Vasoactive drugs such as isoproterenol, epinephrine, and dopamine are used in efforts to improve cardiac contractility and filling. Oxygen therapy may also be given. These combined measures are often continued during the pericardiocentesis.

The technique most commonly used for pericardiocentesis is the introduction of a large-bore needle into the pericardial space through a small stab incision by a subxiphoid approach. The needle is angled toward the left shoulder.[135] The safety of this procedure depends upon attention to the underlying disease and the amount and exact location of the fluid present. An echocardiogram done before pericardiocentesis can be of great assistance in site selection. There is less risk with larger volumes of fluid accumulation because of the increased distance between the pericardium and the surface of the heart. To reduce the risks associated with pericardiocentesis, the procedure is performed with continuous monitoring of CVP and ECG using the V-lead directly attached to the metal hub, or shaft, of the needle.[135]

Possible complications of pericardiocentesis include puncture of the right atrium or ventricle, laceration of the coronary artery, accidental introduction of air into the chambers of the heart, arrhythmias, vasovagal reaction with bradycardia, and infection. Although the subxiphoid approach avoids the pleural space, pneumothorax or other injury to the lungs can occur.[47,139] Throughout the procedure, equipment must be available for emergency surgery and cardiopulmonary resuscitation.

Successful penetration of the pericardial sac during pericardiocentesis is often confirmed by a palpable "pop."[135] This is accompanied by an increase in the QRS complex voltage on the ECG, resulting when the pericardium is touched. If there is an acute elevation of the ST and PR segments, premature atrial contractions (PACs), or premature ventricular contractions (PVCs), there has been contact between the needle and the myocardium, and the needle should be withdrawn.[56] Following confirmation of needle location, fluid is aspirated slowly over 10 to 30 minutes. Although there is dramatic improvement in the patient with the removal of 25 to 50 ml of fluid, as much of the fluid as possible should be removed.[8,147]

Fluid return from the pericardium is normally clear and straw colored. In the presence of a malignancy, it is often bloody. This fluid should be immediately tested for hematocrit and fibrinogen to distinguish between a bloody effusion and penetration of the heart. Bloody effusions have lower levels of hematocrit and fibrinogen than circulating blood.[147]

Malignant effusions are usually serosanguinous; however, clear fluid does not rule out a neoplastic disease. Fluid studies include specific gravity, protein, cell count, stains, cultures, and cytologic analysis. Cytologic examination of pericardial fluid is essential to assist with diagnosis. With metastatic cancer, the cytologic identification is 80% to 90% accurate, with essentially no false positive. The results with lymphomas, sarcomas, and primary mesotheliomas of the

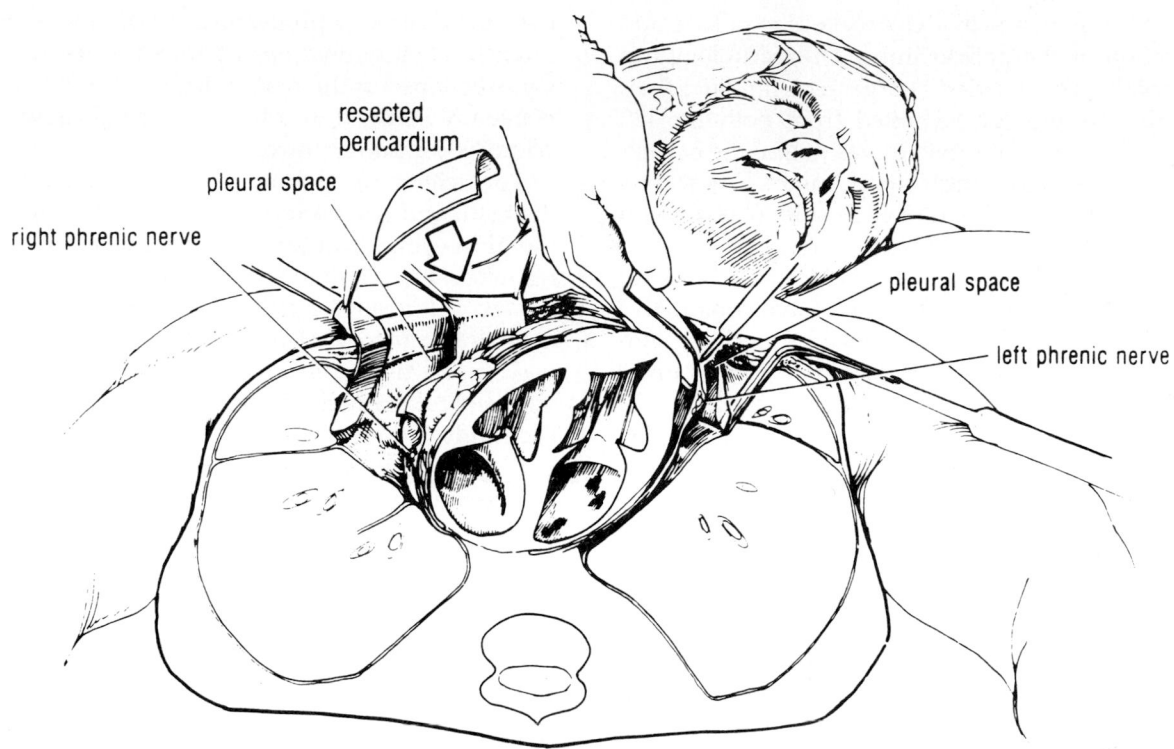

Figure 19-10 Pericardiectomy through a median sternotomy approach. (From Miller SE and Campbell DB: Malignant pericardial effusions. In Polomano RC and Miller SE, editors: Understanding and managing oncologic emergencies, Monograph, Columbus, Ohio, 1987, Adria Laboratories.)

pericardium are much less sensitive. Although a positive cytology may define the histopathology of the neoplastic disease, it may not identify the primary site.[139,147]

Pericardiocentesis is usually effective in relieving signs and symptoms of neoplastic cardiac tamponade, but fluid generally reaccumulates in 24 to 48 hours. In some instances the elevated venous pressure associated with cardiac tamponade may remain in spite of pericardiocentesis. This situation may be due to superior vena cava syndrome, congestive heart failure, or effusive-constrictive pericardial disease resulting from radiation therapy (400 Gy or more), tuberculosis, or extensive malignancy. This condition can be confirmed by measuring simultaneous pressures in the pericardial sac and the right atrium.[110,147] Therefore, further local and/or systemic therapy is required following any pericardiocentesis. The choice of treatment depends upon the etiology and extent of the underlying disease and the overall condition of the patient.

Multiple taps, or the placement of an indwelling catheter, have been helpful in controlling fluid accumulation. These measures, though, are temporary. Long-term catheter placement is contraindicated because of the high risk of infection. A short-term indwelling pericardial catheter with multiple holes for drainage can be easily inserted with an introducer over a flexible guide wire. Once it is in place, a stopcock is placed at the distal end of the catheter. The catheter is drained each shift and may be irrigated daily with a small volume (5 to 10 ml) of saline or heparinized saline (100 U/cc). Irrigation may be useful if the tamponade is caused by a coagulopathy. In the presence of neoplastic fluid, it is probably not necessary, since fibrinogen levels of the fluid are low.

Surgery

Surgical procedures can provide prolonged palliation of recurrent neoplastic cardiac tamponade. The type and extent of the surgery depends on the amount and cytology of the pericardial fluid and the overall condition of the patient. A pericardial "window" (partial pericardiectomy) is created by means of a small left anterior thoracotomy. Through this subxiphoid approach, a piece of the pericardium measuring several square centimeters is removed. The open window permits drainage of the pericardial fluid into the pleural space.[110,139]

A more extensive surgical procedure is a total pericardiectomy (Figure 19-10), in which most of the visceral pericardium is removed. A median sternotomy is performed, which provides excellent exposure and visualization of the pericardium. The pathology can be observed and biopsied. Large rectangular pieces of the pericardium are removed from both the left and right sides. The phrenic nerves define the boundaries of the operation and remain intact. For several days, a chest tube is placed in each side to assist with drainage.[135]

Total pericardiectomy is the treatment of choice for patients with radiation-induced effusive-constrictive pericardial disease, or fibrosis, and also for those with pericardial mesothelioma. It is usually contraindicated in patients with extensive metastatic disease.[139,147]

These surgical procedures are usually effective in controlling pericardial effusions by allowing the pericardial fluid to drain into the pleural cavity, which provides greater surface area for reabsorption. It is rare that pericardial effusions or tamponade recur following these surgical procedures. However, in some instances the windows have closed. There are several potential complications of these operations, which include the usual risks associated with general anesthesia and the possibility of arrhythmias, bleeding, infection, and hemothorax. Pulmonary edema can occur with postoperative diuresis in patients who were heavily hydrated before surgery.[135]

Radiation Therapy

Radiation therapy may be the treatment of choice for neoplastic cardiac tamponade of gradual onset caused by a radiosensitive tumor of the lung or breast or a hematopoietic malignancy. Generally, external beam radiation therapy (200 to 400 Gy) is delivered to a port that includes the heart and pericardial structures and the lower mediastinum. Careful assessment of any previous radiation therapy is important to establish tissue tolerance. Cardiac tolerance is 350 to 400 Gy, beyond which a complication of pericarditis may develop.[109] External beam radiotherapy is most commonly employed, but internal radiation therapy has been done using radioactive phosphorus, yttrium, or gold instilled into the pericardial space.[163]

Chemotherapy

The use of local or systemic chemicals to treat neoplastic cardiac tamponade has had varying degrees of success. Local treatment with chemotherapy involves the instillation of antineoplastic agents or sclerosing substances into the pericardial space through an indwelling pericardial catheter following drainage. Chemotherapeutic agents used include bleomycin, nitrogen mustard, 5-FU, methotrexate, and thiotepa. Tetracycline and quinacrine have also been instilled

for their sclerosing properties. All of these substances cause local inflammation and then fibrosis, which prevents collapse of the pericardial sac.[110,139,163] Lidocaine is usually instilled into the pericardial cavity prior to sclerosis for pain control.

The sclerosing technique used the most involved the instillation of tetracycline (500 to 1000 mg) through the indwelling catheter. This is followed by a flush of normal saline. The procedure is repeated every 2 to 3 days. Sclerosis is considered successful when there is no drainage for a 24-hour period. Response to tetracycline sclerosing has not proven to be as effective as such obliterative treatment for pleural effusions.[135,139] Currently, injectable tetracycline has been discontinued by its manufacturer. Other sclerosing agents such as bleomycin, minocycline, and doxycycline have been used to treat malignant pleural effusion. However, few studies have been published regarding pericardial effusions. Recent reports have shown effective pericardial sclerosing with one instillation of bleomycin (30 to 60 mg) through a pericardial catheter 24 hours after the fluid has been evacuated. The tube is then clamped for 10 minutes and then withdrawn. No major side effects were noted except transient temperature elevation. Severe fibrous of the pericardial sac was not reported or found at autopsy.[48,55,136]

Systemic chemotherapy may be given to responsive tumors such as lymphoma, breast cancer, or small (oat) cell carcinoma of the lung. This may be the initial treatment of a pericardial effusion when it is slow and the patient is asymptomatic. However, in acute neoplastic cardiac tamponade, systemic chemotherapy is done when the patient is clinically stable following pericardiocentesis.

PROGNOSIS

Survival of the patient with neoplastic cardiac tamponade depends upon the cause of the primary malignancy, the stage of cancer at the time of intervention, tumor responsiveness to radiation therapy or chemotherapy, the hemodynamic significance of the tamponade, the effectiveness of therapy, and the general medical condition of the patient. Response rate with local therapies is 50%, with duration of remission approximately 4 to 6 months.[110,147] Average survival, regardless of neoplastic cause, is reported at 16 months. Patients with breast cancer or Hodgkin's disease may survive for more than 2 years.[135] Patients with effusions and tamponade related to radiation therapy may survive longer than any others. Although the overall prognosis of the patient may be poor, the spectacular response that is usually seen with the removal of pericardial fluid warrants aggressive action.

Nursing Management

Nursing interventions for the patient with neoplastic cardiac tamponade are multifaceted and highly variable, depending on the acuteness of the patient's condition. Onset of tamponade may be impending and insidious, or it may be rapid and life-threatening. Knowledge of the patient's current and past history, coupled with astute physical assessment skills, is necessary.

Patients may be in a routine hospital unit or in the critical care area. Close monitoring of vital signs is of paramount importance. Nursing care is directed at maintaining optimal cardiopulmonary function and preventing circulatory collapse through immediate identifications and treatment of neoplastic cardiac tamponade.*

NURSING DIAGNOSES

- Decreased cardiac output related to diastolic filling of the ventricles due to compression of the heart
- Alteration in tissue perfusion related to decreased cardiac output

INTERVENTIONS

- Assess hemodynamic status.

Cardiovascular

Monitor blood pressure, pulse, CVP, and cardiac output.

Observe cardiac rhythm continuously (note abnormalities associated with cardiac tamponade: ST segment elevation, T-wave inversion, and electrical alterations).

Heart sounds.

Assess extremities for color, temperature, and pulses.

Respiratory

Observe breathing patterns (note abnormalities associated with cardiac tamponade: pulsus paradoxus, respiratory alkalosis, Kussmaul's sign, and hypoxemia).

Auscultate lungs for breath sounds.

Integumentary

Observe skin temperature, color, and turgor.

Genitourinary

Monitor intake and output.

Gastrointestinal

Measure abdominal girth and note any ascites.

Determine positive hepatojugular reflux.

Neurologic

Determine orientation to person and place.

Assess responses to verbal and tactile stimuli and report any changes in level of consciousness.

- Monitor laboratory values and test results:

Electrolytes, with attention to Ca^+ and K^+ because of the risk of cardiac arrhythmias

ECG for changes

Echocardiogram

Chest x-ray

- Reposition patient to enhance circulation. This must be done slowly to allow compensation for decreased cardiac output.
- Perform measures to reduce the work load of the heart:

Assist with all activities.

Schedule rest periods.

Use comfort measures (analgesics, repositioning, relaxation techniques, antianxiety medications).

- Administer vasoactive drugs as ordered.
- Be prepared for cardiac arrest and emergency resuscitation.

NURSING DIAGNOSIS

- Potential for impaired gas exchange related to decreased circulation and pulmonary congestion

INTERVENTIONS

- Monitor respiratory status:

Observe for signs and symptoms of respiratory difficulty (dyspnea, tachypnea, Kussmaul's sign, shortness of breath, air hunger).

Auscultate chest for breath sounds.

Monitor laboratory values (arterial blood gases, electrolytes, chest x-ray).

- Assist with breathing and pulmonary toilet:

Position for comfort and enhanced chest expansion

Deep breathing and coughing every 2 hours

Frequent mouth care

Suctioning if needed

- Administer oxygen therapy and mechanical ventilation as prescribed.

---

*References 69, 76, 84, 107, 110, 139, 144, 145, 151.

NURSING DIAGNOSIS
- Potential for injury: trauma related to invasive procedures/surgery

INTERVENTIONS
- Assess patient for complications: bleeding, infection, atelectasis, pneumothorax, pleural effusion.
- Check vital signs every 15 minutes for the first hour after procedure or surgery and continue frequently as indicated.
- Monitor respiratory status closely.
  Observe respirations for rate, rhythm, and depth and note any difficulties.
  Auscultate chest for breath sounds and expansion.
- Observe monitoring equipment frequently for changes.
- Assess all catheters for patency and drainage and observe site for signs of infection.
- Assess patient with care but encourage as much independence as possible.

SEPTIC SHOCK

DEFINITION
Shock comprises a group of diverse life-threatening syndromes that result from different pathophysiologic circumstances (decreased cardiac function, hemorrhage, trauma, antigen/antibody reaction, and sepsis). There are three major classifications of shock: hypovolemic, cardiogenic, and distributive or vasogenic. Hypovolemic shock is a result of decreased intravascular volume. Cardiogenic shock results from the impaired ability of the heart to adequately pump blood. Distributive or vasogenic shock is the result of an abnormality in the vascular system. Included under distributive shock is neurogenic, anaphylactic, and septic shock.[128] The progression of septic shock produces a severe maldistribution of blood flow in the microcirculation. This leads to inadequate tissue perfusion, cellular ischemia, cellular hypoxia, and organ or system failure.[119,128] If not immediately treated and reversed, shock will result in death.[9,128,152,159]

Septic shock is a shock syndrome in response to sepsis. Septicemia is usually the result of a gram-negative bacterial infection or toxins produced by the bacteria.[62,85,88,159] It is accompanied by a disseminated inflammatory response unrelated to the causative organism.[88] Infection and sepsis are common causes of morbidity and the leading causes of death in patients with cancer.[74]

ETIOLOGY AND RISK FACTORS
Septic shock as a consequence of gram-negative bacteremia has been documented extensively in the literature.[9,62,85] It is estimated that septic shock strikes 200,000 patients per year with 20% to 40% being gram-negative bacteremias and that 50% of these are nosocomial.[44,62,103] However, a wider variety of microorganisms is responsible for the invasion of the bloodstream leading to sepsis and septic shock. The most predominant pathogens in patients with cancer are three gram-negative bacilli (*Escherichia coli*, *Klebsiella pneumoniae*, and *Pseudomonas aeruginosa*). Other bacteria (*Staphylococcus aureus* and *S. epidermidis*), viruses, fungi, protozoa, and rickettsia are all potential pathogens for septicemia.

Mortality from septic shock has been estimated at 25% to 60% of reported cases of septicemia.[62,88] Among patients with cancer, the rate is between 30% and 80%.[9,44,62,152] Infectious processes are the cause of death in at least 50% of patients with solid tumors.[44,152] In patients with uncontrolled leukemia and lymphoma who develop septic shock, death almost always follows in 80% of the cases.[44,103]

Patients with cancer are at increased risk of developing infection and subsequent septicemia because of the profound suppression of their normal body defense mechanisms. This suppression is due to both host-related and cancer treatment-related factors.[9,74,85] A decrease in host resistance permits tissue invasion by endogenous or exogenous flora.[4,25] Gram-negative bacteria, which are the most common infective microorganisms, are normally found in the mouth and gastrointestinal tract, vagina, feces, and on the skin.[13]

Patterns of bacterial infections have changed over the years because of improved antibiotic therapy. Beta-lactamase-resistant penicillins provided highly effective therapy against *Staphylococcus aureus*, a gram-positive organism most commonly identified in immunocompromised patients in the 1950s and 1960s. Today the use of empiric combination antibiotic therapy including third-generation cephalosporins has greatly reduced the number of gram-negative infections. A recent resurgence of gram-positive infections is thought to be related to a prevalence of methicillin-resistant strains of *Staphylococcus*.

A particular infectious life-threatening condition seen in patients with cancer is neutropenic enterocolitis, also called typhilitis, an inflammation of the small intestine or colon. The exact pathologic etiology is unclear. However, it is proposed to be initiated by direct cytotoxic damage from chemotherapy, radiation therapy, or neoplastic infiltration. Disruption of mucosal integrity, alteration of normal gut flora, and lack of neutrophil response lead to invasion of the gastrointestinal tract by bacteria, viruses, and fungi. The implicated organisms include gram-negative bacilli such as *Klebsiella, Pseudomonas, Escherichia coli, Candida,* and *Clostridium septicum.* Although *Clostridium septicum* is not a flora, which is normally found in the gut, it may appear following the use of multiple antibiotics, which alter the normal gut flora. Neutropenic enterocolitis can lead to septic shock. Mortality rates have been estimated to be greater than 50%.[146]

The factors that predispose a patient with cancer to infection and sepsis can be categorized according to the precipitating event, site of infection, and pathogen (see Table 19-4 and the box on p. 411).[60,62,74] Each of the events that may initiate an infection leading to septic shock is a consequence of the underlying cancer and/or its treatment. All four treatment modalities (surgery, radiation therapy, chemotherapy, and biotherapy) can result in profound suppression of host defense mechanisms. Monitoring the patient for effects of tumor growth and side effects of therapy is crucial to preventing septic shock.

PATHOPHYSIOLOGY

Septic shock is a complex interaction of hemodynamic, humoral, cellular, and metabolic abnormalities.[9,111] This is a result of the effects of the proliferation of gram-negative bacteria and/or the release of endotoxins by those bacteria (Figure 19-11). Endotoxin is a component of the cellular wall of gram-negative bacteria and, when released, it activates the coagulation complement and kinin systems.[9,62,159] This toxin-induced reaction activates the humoral cellular and immunologic defense mechanisms leading to a generalized inflammatory response.[44,62,88] Evidence of this response is the production of various chemical mediators such as prostaglandins, endorphins, and kinins, which modulate the variety of multisystem alterations seen in septic shock.[62,88,103]

The abnormalities seen in septic shock (Figure 19-12) can be summarized as follows.[9,44,88,159]

Hemodynamic Instability

Abnormal coagulation occurs through a variety of processes initiated by the gram-negative bacteria. It damages the endothelial lining of the capillaries, which is the site of thrombus formation. The bacteria attach to the erythrocytes (RBCs) producing an antigen/antibody reaction. Hemolysis results, and microhemorrhagic lesions appear in major organs. Clotting factor XII (Hageman factor) is activated by the bacteria. This initiates the clotting mechanisms, causing the formation of microthrombi and, at the same time, fibrinolysis for clot dissolution. The result is consumption of clotting factors (consumptive coagulopathy) and platelets (thrombocytopenia). The final outcome of all of these processes is disseminated intravascular coagulation (DIC)—simultaneous hemorrhage and thrombosis.[103]

Cardiovascular alteration is present during shock in two different patterns. Initially, cardiac output (CO) is higher than normal yet still inadequate to supply the peripheral blood vessels because of massive vasodilatation. Later the CO is low, accompanied by severe vasoconstriction.[62]

Table 19—4 Factors Predisposing Cancer Patients to Infection

Precipitating Event	*Common Site of Infection*	*Common Organism*
Local effects of tumor growth or treatment		
Skin or mucous membrane breakdown	Cancer or treatment of skin, head and neck, gastrointestinal tract, female genital tract	Locally colonizing organisms
Obstruction of natural passages (obstructive phenomenon)	Solid tumors or treatment of cancer (especially pulmonary, biliary, and urinary tracts)	Locally colonizing organisms
Alterations in microbial flora	All cancer sites or treatment of cancer (especially pulmonary, gastrointestinal)	Locally colonizing organisms
Stasis of blood and body fluids secondary to obstruction or inactivity	All cancer sites or treatment of cancer	Locally colonizing organisms
Central nervous system dysfunction (brain tumors, spinal cord tumors, metabolic abnormalities)	Pulmonary (aspiration pneumonia) Urinary tract	Locally colonizing organisms

Continued.

Table 19—4 Factors Predisposing Cancer Patients to Infection—cont'd

Precipitating Event	Common Site of Infection	Common Organism
Hyposplenism secondary to neoplastic infiltration or splenectomy	Disseminated	Bacteria: *Streptococcus pneumoniae*, *Neisseria meningitidis*, *Escherichia coli*, *Hemophilus influenzae*, *Clostridium difficile*, Staphylococcus spp
Granulocytopenia (neutropenia) prevalent with acute leukemia	Skin lesions, thrombophlebitis, pulmonary (pneumonia), peridontinum, sinuses, pharynx, esophagus, colon, perianal	Gram-negative bacilli: *Escherichia coli*, *Pseudomonas aeruginosa*, *Klebsiella pneumoniae*, *Staphylococcus aureus* Yeasts: Candida Filamentous fungi: Aspergillus sp, agents of mycomycosis
Cellular immune dysfunction (T-cell immune alteration) prevalent with lymphoma	Disseminated	Bacteria: *Listeria monocytogenes*, Salmonella sp, Mycobacterium sp, *Nocardia asteroides*, Legionella Fungi: *Cryptococcus neoformans*, *Histoplasma capsulatum*, *Coccidioides immitis* Viruses: *Varicella zoster*, cytomegalovirus, herpes simplex Protozoa: *Pneumocystis carinii*, *Toxoplasma gondii*, Cryptosporidium Helminths: *Strongyloides stercoralis*
Humoral immune dysfunction (B cell immune alteration) prevalent with multiple myeloma	Disseminated	*Streptococcus pneumoniae*, *Hemophilus influenzae*
Iatrogenic factors (invasive procedures, devices, and equipment) Diagnostic procedures (barium enema, endoscopies), urinary catheterization Genitourinary tract manipulations Bone marrow aspirations Biopsies Placement of shunts, stents, and tubes Venipuncture Long-term venous access devices Respiratory-assist devices	Skin Mucous membranes	*Staphylococcus epidermis* Locally colonizing organisms
Nosocomial sources Air	Pulmonary	Aspergillus sp
Surface contact	Skin and mucous membranes	*Staphylococcus aureus*
Food (fresh fruits and vegetables)		Bacteria, fungi
Water (humidifiers, respiratory devices, flowers, water pitchers, faucet aerators, skin drains, shower heads, ice machines)	Disseminated	*Pseudomonas aeruginosa*, *Serratia marcescens*
Medical personnel (illness, organism transmission or cross-contamination, poor hand washing)	Various	Locally colonizing organisms
Extended prophylactic use of broad-spectrum antibiotic therapy (superinfection secondary to overgrowth of resistant strains)	Disseminated	Bacteria

---

FACTORS PREDISPOSING TO INFECTION IN PATIENTS WITH CANCER

Granulocytopenia (e.g., acute leukemia)

Sites of infection
 Pneumonia
 Perianal lesions
 Pharyngitis
 Skin lesions
 Esophagitis
Most common pathogens
Gram-negative bacilli
 Escherichia coli
 Pseudomonas aeruginosa
 Klebsiella pneumoniae
 Staphylococcus aureus
Yeasts
 Candida
Filamentous fungi
 Aspergillus sp
 Agents of mucormycosis

Cellular immune dysfunction (e.g., lymphoma)

Common organisms
Bacteria
 Listeria monocytogenes
 Salmonella sp
 Mycobacterium sp
 Nocardia asteroids
 Legionella
Fungi
 Cryptococcus neoformans
 Histoplasma capsulatum
 Coccidioides immitis
Viruses
 Varicella zoster
 Cytomegalovirus
 Herpes simplex
Protozoa
 Pneumocystis carinii
 Toxoplasma gondii
 Cryptosporidium
Helminths
 Strongyloides stercoralis

Humoral immune dysfunction (e.g., multiple myeloma)

Common organisms
 Streptococcus pneumoniae
 Hemophilus influenzae

Obstructive phenomena (e.g., solid tumors)
Common sites
 Respiratory tract
 Biliary tract
 Urinary tract
Common organisms
 Locally colonizing

Central nervous system dysfunction (e.g., brain tumors)
Common sites
 Pneumonitis
 Urinary tract infection
Common organisms
Locally colonizing

Iatrogenic procedures
Disruption or bypassing of anatomic barriers
Indwelling venous or arterial catheters
 Bacteremia
Indwelling urinary catheters
 Urinary tract infection
Respiratory-assist devices
 Pneumonia
 Immune suppression
 Chemotherapy, surgery, radiation

Alterations in microbial flora
Underlying illness
Stasis
Antibiotics

Acquisition of potential pathogens
Air
 Aspergillus sp
Water
 Pseudomonas aeruginosa
 Serratia marcescens
Contact
 Staphylococcus aureus

From Joshi J: Epidemiology of infections in cancer patients, Mediguide to Infectious Diseases 9(2):2, 1989.

Humoral/Cellular Alterations

The microcirculation is grossly altered through a variety of mechanisms attributed to the production of several vasoactive mediators: bradykinin, histamine, and serotonin (Figure 19-11). The bacterial endotoxin is responsible for the activation of Factor XII, which in turn initiates the release of bradykinin, a potent vasodilator. The complement system is also activated by the endotoxin, which causes the release of hista-mine and serotonin. These substances produce vasodilatation or vasoconstriction depending on the status of the circulation.[19,111,159]

Changes in the microcirculation occur as the arterioles dilate and the venules constrict, resulting in increased vascular permeability. In response to this, the internal cellular sodium-potassium pump is hampered and water accumulates in the cells causing them to swell. Secretion of antidiuretic hormone (ADH) and

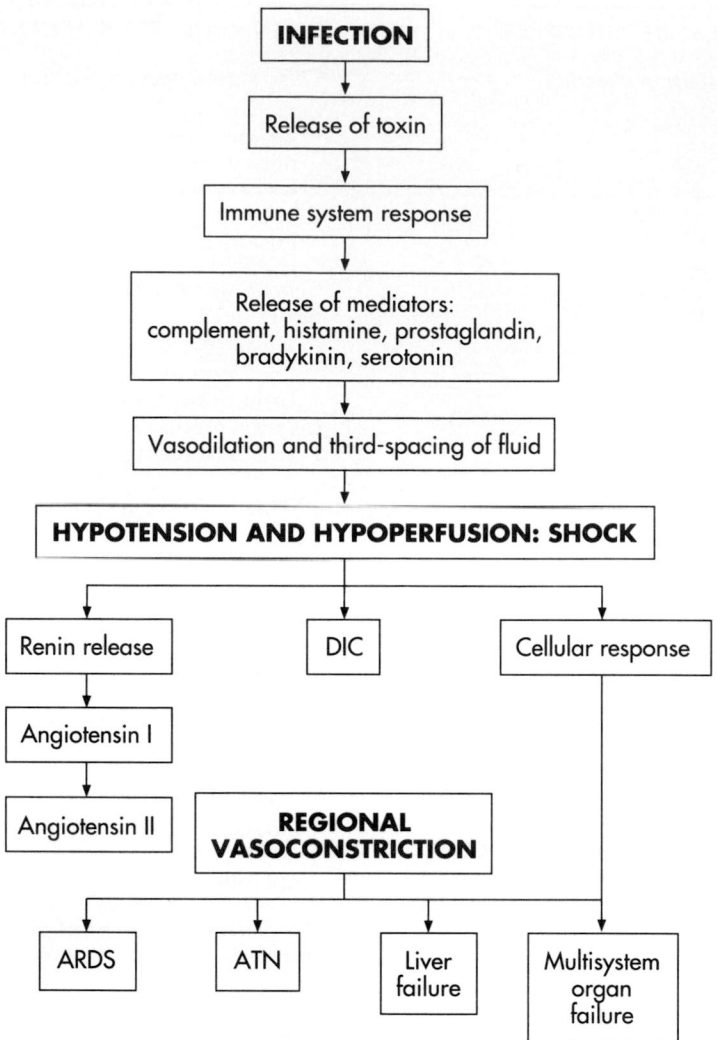

Figure 19-11 The pathophysiology of septic shock. (From McMorrow ME and Cooney-Daniello M: When to support septic shock, RN 54[10]:32, 1991.)

aldosterone increases sodium and water retention. Capillary pressure increases, and plasma oncotic pressure changes and allows intravascular fluid to leak to the extravascular space. This fluid shift into the interstitial spaces occurs throughout the body.

Insufficient blood perfusion to peripheral tissues results from the impaired microcirculation. This leads to cellular hypoxia and death. The lungs are a target organ for dysfunction because of the fluid shifts and cellular hypoxia. There will be marked changes in lung compliance and impaired gas exchange. Consequently patients in septic shock may develop pulmonary edema and adult respiratory distress syndrome (ARDS).

Metabolic Dysfunction

A variety of metabolic alterations take place during septic shock (Figure 19-12). There is a mobilization of energy stores producing a conversion of carbohydrate

(glucose), fat, and protein to energy. Gluconeogenesis (endogenous production of glucose) occurs, but there is a progressive inability to utilize the energy stores. Protein catabolism leads to a negative nitrogen balance. Tissues are unable to receive oxygen or nutrients because of impaired blood flow. There is a shift from oxidative metabolism to anaerobic metabolism. Lactic acid accumulates in the blood and leads to metabolic acidosis. To compensate, hyperventilation occurs, leading to respiratory alkalosis. The depletion of cellular energy and inhibition of protein synthesis lead to cellular death and major organ failure.[88,111,159]

Septic shock results from a maldistribution of blood flow. Microcirculatory alterations are caused by endotoxin produced by the invading pathogen, which is usually gram-negative bacteria. As shock progresses, there is inadequate tissue perfusion of somatic cells of major systems or organs. System malfunction can result in DIC, ARDS, and acute tubular necrosis

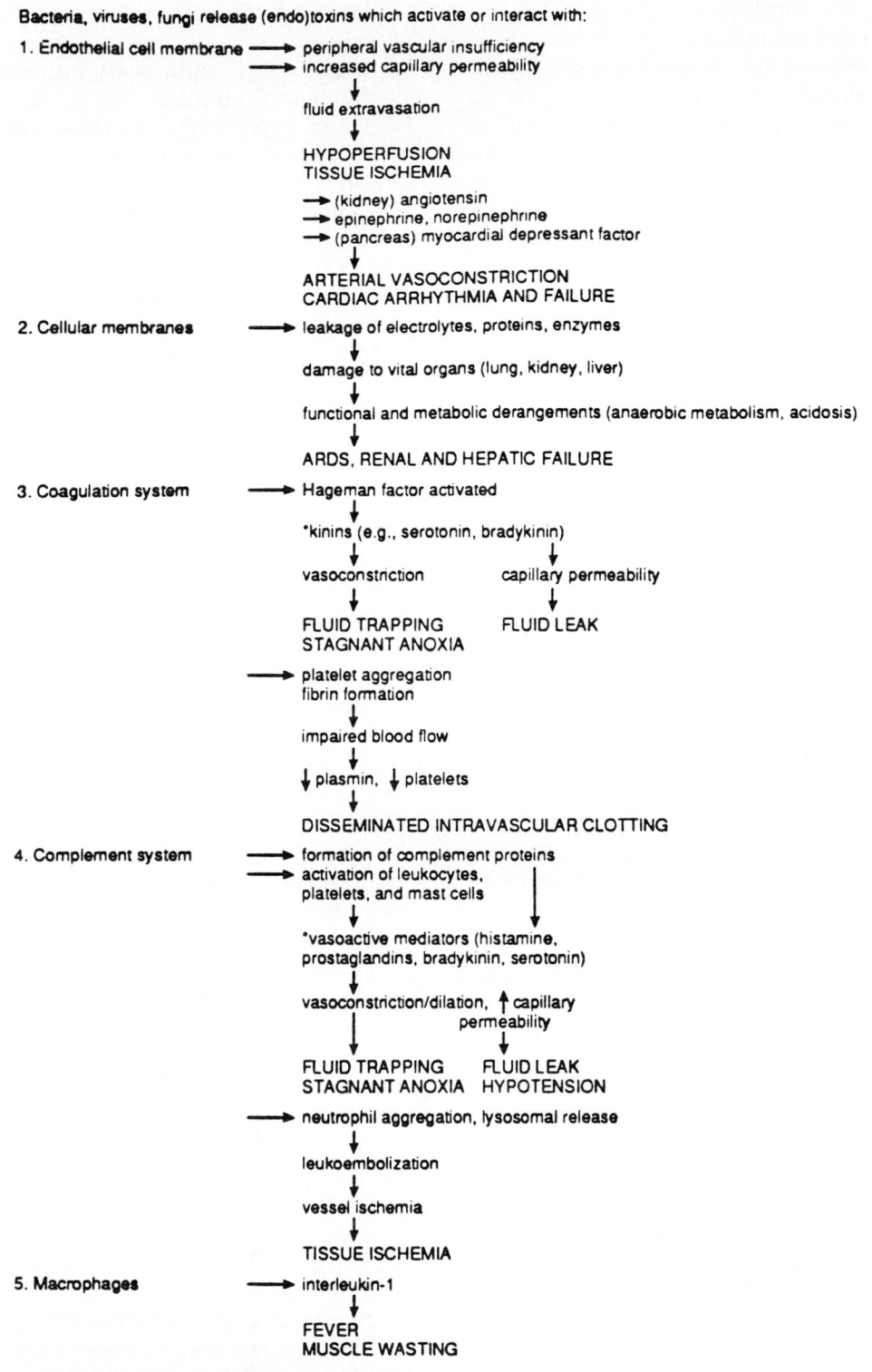

Bacteria, viruses, fungi release (endo)toxins which activate or interact with:

1. Endothelial cell membrane ⟶ peripheral vascular insufficiency
          ⟶ increased capillary permeability
            ↓
           fluid extravasation
            ↓
           HYPOPERFUSION
           TISSUE ISCHEMIA

           ⟶ (kidney) angiotensin
           ⟶ epinephrine, norepinephrine
           ⟶ (pancreas) myocardial depressant factor

           ARTERIAL VASOCONSTRICTION
           CARDIAC ARRHYTHMIA AND FAILURE

2. Cellular membranes ⟶ leakage of electrolytes, proteins, enzymes

           damage to vital organs (lung, kidney, liver)

           functional and metabolic derangements (anaerobic metabolism, acidosis)

           ARDS, RENAL AND HEPATIC FAILURE

3. Coagulation system ⟶ Hageman factor activated

           *kinins (e.g., serotonin, bradykinin)

           vasoconstriction   capillary permeability

           FLUID TRAPPING   FLUID LEAK
           STAGNANT ANOXIA

           ⟶ platelet aggregation
           fibrin formation

           impaired blood flow

           ↓ plasmin, ↓ platelets

           DISSEMINATED INTRAVASCULAR CLOTTING

4. Complement system ⟶ formation of complement proteins
          ⟶ activation of leukocytes,
           platelets, and mast cells

           *vasoactive mediators (histamine,
           prostaglandins, bradykinin, serotonin)

           vasoconstriction/dilation, ↑ capillary
                  permeability

           FLUID TRAPPING   FLUID LEAK
           STAGNANT ANOXIA   HYPOTENSION

           ⟶ neutrophil aggregation, lysosomal release

           leukoembolization

           vessel ischemia

           TISSUE ISCHEMIA

5. Macrophages ⟶ interleukin-1

           FEVER
           MUSCLE WASTING

*During a septic shock episode, shock mediators may be activated by more than one pathway.

Figure 19-12 The pathophysiology of septic shock. (From Harnett S: Septic shock in the oncology patient, Cancer Nurs 12[4], 1989.)

(ATN). When capillary occlusion occurs for longer than 2 hours, the cells in that area do not receive adequate nutrition or oxygen, and cellular death results.[119] Cellular death causes organ failure and is ultimately fatal.

The process of septic shock is complex and its progress can be rapid (Figure 19-12). The progression of shock depends on several factors[49,119]:

- The patient's physical condition before the onset of the incident

- Duration of the shock state
- Effectiveness of treatment
- Correction of reversible causes (in septic shock it would be infection and sepsis)

Although sepsis is a triggering process that can lead to shock, attention should be given to several other treatable causes of shock: hemorrhage, trauma, or a reduction in cardiac function. Consideration should also be given to other situations that are frequently overlooked as possible causes of shock[99,119]:

- Inadequate infusion of fluids
- Inadequate ventilation
- Unrecognized pneumothorax
- Pulmonary emboli
- Previous prolonged treatment with antihypertensive drugs
- Cardiac tamponade
- Acid-base abnormalities
- Adrenal insufficiency
- Hypothermia

CLINICAL FEATURES

The signs and symptoms of septic shock vary with the stage of shock manifested by the patient. Some patients progress from early to late shock; others appear in late shock initially.[1,2,38] Complications and major organ failure may be prevented if shock is detected early and treated immediately.

There are several ways to classify the stages of shock. A three-stage classification is particularly useful.[159] The clinical findings associated with each stage are listed in the box on p. 415.

Once a patient has entered Stage Three shock, there will be no response to treatment. Multiple organ failure occurs, leading to death.

DIAGNOSIS

The diagnosis of septic shock is critically dependent upon astute observations of the patient. Sepsis may or may not have been confirmed. An initial finding could be a subtle patient complaint of "just not feeling right." Physical assessment of all systems is crucial and should be correlated with a brief recent history highlighting any changes and noting any possible sources of infection. Continuous assessment and monitoring of the patient is essential. This includes taking vital signs, observing tissue perfusion, watching for signs of bleeding, checking mental status, and assessing heart, lung, and kidney function.[19,62,88]

Initial testing includes a chest x-ray, 12-lead ECG, and blood work (complete blood count and chemistry panel). Other laboratory tests should include coagulation studies, cardiac and liver enzymes, urinalysis, arterial blood gases, and various culture and sensitivity testing (blood, urine, sputum, wound, etc). The following findings could assist in the diagnosis of sepsis:

Chest x-ray—pulmonary infiltrates

ECG—arrhythmias

Urine—glycosuria, elevated specific gravity, increased urine sodium

WBC count—low (leukopenia)

Platelet count—low (thrombocytopenia)

Coagulation profile—fibrinogen levels decreased, FDPs elevated, prothrombin time and partial prothrombin time prolonged

Serum glucose—elevated

Serum lactate—elevated

Careful evaluation of the febrile patient is important. Fever is classically the telltale sign of infection. Contrary to popular myth, fever is present in immunocompromised and neutropenic patients, including those with cancer. Elevated temperature is produced in the body by the monocytes, not neutrophils. Some monocytes migrate into body tissue where they become macrophages. The monocyte secretes an endogenous pyrogen that affects the thalamus, which houses the body's temperature control, resulting in a rise in temperature.[60,159]

Patients with neutropenia who have an infection or sepsis will have fever, but they may not have other signs of inflammation, such as ulceration, fissure, and exudate. These signs are markedly diminished since there are little to no granulocytes (white blood cells) to produce the inflammatory process. Erythema and pain will be present if the infection is localized. However, fever is the most important clinical sign of infection in a patient with neutropenia.[60]

Febrile episodes in the patient with granulocytopenia or neutropenia are indicative of infection 60% to 80% of the time.[60,74,85] In patients with cancer whose granulocyte counts are normal, fever is usually due to causes other than infection. These include tumor-associated fever (hepatoma, renal cell carcinoma, and childhood sarcoma); chemotherapeutic agents (bleomycin, cytosine arabinoside (Ara-C), and high-dose methotrexate); and blood product transfusions.[60]

TREATMENT MODALITIES

The identified stage of septic shock will dictate the necessary medical interventions. Prompt medical treatment is essential to prevent progression of shock syndrome to the irreversible stage and subsequent death. Most patients in septic shock are transferred to the intensive care unit for close observation and invasive hemodynamic monitoring. Recognition of the signs and symptoms of shock and the determination of sepsis are the first medical interventions. Following this, antibiotic therapy should be initiated within 1 hour of the appearance of the signs and

---

STAGES OF SHOCK

Stage One: hyperdynamic stage (early shock, warm shock)
Decreased tissue perfusion—10% reduction in blood volume
Usually lasts less than 24 hours
- Feelings of anxiety, apprehension, nervousness
- Complaints of nausea
- Altered mental status, restlessness, irritability, disorientation, or inappropriate euphoria
- Temperature normal, below normal, or above normal
- Skin warm and flushed because of arteriole dilatation
- Peripheral cyanosis
- Tachycardia and bounding peripheral pulses
- Normal or slightly elevated blood pressure with a widening pulse pressure
- Tachypnea and/or hyperventilation
- Rales and decreased breath sounds
- Respiratory alkalosis—decreased PO_2
- Renal output normal or elevated (polyuria)
- BUN and creatinine may be slowly increasing
- Hyperglycemia
- Urine may test positive for sugar (glycosuria)
- Urine specific gravity normal
- No signs of bleeding
- Coagulation profile normal

Stage Two: normodynamic stage (intermediate shock, cool shock)
Decreased tissue perfusion—15% to 20% reduction in blood volume
Usually lasts a few hours
- Complains of thirst
- Altered mental status—lethargy, confusion
- Skin pale, cool, and clammy because of peripheral vasoconstriction and diversion of blood to vital organs
- Peripheral edema may be present because of increased secretion of ADH and aldosterone leading to sodium and water retention
- Temperature normal or subnormal
- Tachycardia continues
- Blood pressure decreases with a narrow pulse pressure because of decrease in cardiac output
- Respirations slow and shallow
- Respiratory acidosis
- Renal output decreased (oliguria)
- Urine specific gravity elevated
- Abdominal distention because of air swallowing and decreased peristalsis
- Hemorrhagic lesions may be apparent

Stage Three: hypodynamic stage (late shock, refractory shock, irreversible shock, cold shock, "classic" shock)
Decreased cardiac output, decrease in blood volume
- Altered mental status, stupor, coma
- Skin cold, possible cyanosis of digits and mottling
- Temperature subnormal
- Tachycardia
- Weak or absent pulses because of decreased myocardial contractility—"pump failure"
- Hypotension
- Respiratory depression
- Pulmonary edema, or "shock lung," because of decreased PO_2 and decreased pulmonary microcirculatory ARDS
- Metabolic acidosis because of anaerobic metabolism and increased levels of lactic acid
- Hypoglycemia
- No renal output (anuria)
- Renal failure—ATN
- Hemorrhagic lesions

---

symptoms of shock.[62,85,159] Broad-spectrum antibiotics (cephalosporins, gentamicin, aminoglycosides) are the drugs of choice until the specific pathogens responsible can be identified, which usually takes at least 24 hours.

Additional blood work is ordered depending on the stage of shock. The first stage of shock would indicate testing for elevated catecholamine and cortisol levels. Later stages would indicate screening for the coagulopathies related to DIC.

Restoration of hemodynamic status is a major challenge in the treatment of septic shock.[4,9] Blood volume replacement is achieved through the use of intravenous fluids and plasma expanders. Blood transfusions may be warranted. Blood pressure and cardiac output are restored with the administration of vasoactive drugs and inotropic agents. The progress of therapy is determined by clinical aspects of the patient's status, through intensive observation and monitoring.

The provision of optimal oxygenation often requires respiratory assistance.[62,159] Oxygen and respiratory therapy may be ordered. Mechanical ventilation may be necessary. These measures will manage the metabolic acidosis seen in septic shock. The blood gas level of pH should be 7.35 to 7.45, and the Po_2 should be kept at 80 to 100 mm Hg.

The underlying infection, if determined, should be treated. Initial antibiotic therapy is tailored to the specific organisms identified in the culture and sensitivity reports. Various procedures including surgery may also be indicated to treat the infection.

Fluid and electrolyte balance must be maintained and any metabolic abnormalities corrected. Urinary output should be at least 50 ml/hour. Serum chemistry levels are done at least daily to evaluate renal function. Aminoglycoside antibiotics and various chemotherapeutic agents can compromise renal function, warranting a potential change in therapy.[4,25]

Steroid therapy is often administered to the patient in septic shock. The doses are extremely high, and it is important to observe the patient closely for potential side effects, especially those of gastrointestinal bleeding and mental changes. The steroids are given to decrease the inflammatory response, neutralize the endotoxin, protect the cell membrane and structure from the endotoxin, increase cardiac contractility, and enhance cellular glucose metabolism.[159]

The administration of hematopoietic growth factors, which mediate the production, maturation, regulation, and activation of various blood cells (granulocytes, monocytes, macrophages, lymphocytes, erythrocytes, and platelets), may help to prevent septicemia. These growth factors are commonly referred to as colony stimulating factors (CSFs) because they stimulate the growth of colonies of maturing blood cells from these hematopoietic precursors. Classified as cytokines, the CSFs are a group of naturally occurring glycoproteins. Each CSF affects a major cell lineage and has been given the following respective name:

- Granulocyte—macrophage colony stimulating factor (GM-CSF)
- Granulocyte colony stimulating factor (G-CSF)
- Macrophage colony stimulating factor (M-CSF)
- Pleuripoietin interleukin-3 (IL-3) or multicolony stimulating factor (multi-CSF)

- Erythrocyte colony stimulating factor (erythropoietin)

The exact mechanism of action of the CSFs is unknown. However, there appears to be a crossover of the effects of one factor on the others. The growth factors hold a promising future in the treatment of immunosuppression, anemia, and thrombocytopenia that result from disease states (neoplasia, myelodysplasia, congenital neutropenia, and AIDS) and/or treatment-induced states (high dose chemotherapy and/or radiation therapy). Improving bone marrow recovery may decrease infection-related morbidity and mortality. Dosage, route, and schedule for the administration of the CSFs are being investigated. See chapter 23 for more information.[22,35,78]

The use of investigational agents such as naloxone (an opiate antagonist), human antiserum, and endotoxin has been reported.[60] However, results are preliminary. More research is needed on these agents and on the role of shock mediators such as prostaglandins, complement, and tumor necrosis factor.[62]

The mainstay of treatment for septic shock is antibiotic therapy. Additional treatment for septic shock has been summarized by the acronym VIP. V = ventilate (provide oxygen); I = infuse (administer solutions to maintain an adequate blood pressure); P = perfuse (administer vasopressor therapy to improve cardiac output).[107] In the late stages of shock, additional management measures are aimed at the treatment of DIC, ARDS, and ATN.

PROGNOSIS

Mortality from septic shock is as high as 75% in spite of advanced technology and new treatment modalities.[9,25,49,88] Survival is contingent upon preventing or reversing the process of shock and on the status of the underlying disease (nonfatal, ultimately fatal, rapidly fatal). Remarkably, 60% of all patients survive warm shock, and 40% survive cool or cold shock.[62] Prompt recognition and treatment of septic shock can mean the difference between life and death.

SPINAL CORD COMPRESSION

DEFINITION

A malignant tumor in the epidural space can encroach upon the spinal cord or cauda equina and result in spinal cord compression (SCC). SCC is a medical emergency requiring early detection and prompt treatment. Although it is rarely fatal, it can result in permanent neurologic deficits or other complications that increase mortality.

ETIOLOGY AND RISK FACTORS

Bone metastases in patients with cancer are extremely common; they are second only to pulmonary metas-

Nursing Management

The nursing care of a patient with sepsis varies with the identified stage of septic shock. Infection and sepsis have a high correlation in the patient with neutropenia.[4,25,62] Patients at highest risk are those whose neutrophil count is less than 100/mm³ for more than 3 weeks.[4,46] Therefore, the first nursing goal in the management of septic shock is prevention of infection. The following general measures outline the nursing care for the patient with neutropenia. Complete reverse isolation, although it reduces exogenous colonization, is no longer recommended for patients with neutropenia since endogenous flora are the major source of infection. Thus, current practice is to use protective isolation.

NURSING DIAGNOSIS[44,49,69,128-131]

- Potential for injury (infection/sepsis) related to neutropenia

INTERVENTIONS

Observation for signs and symptoms of infection

- Monitor vital signs at least every shift. An elevated temperature and/or changes in blood pressure, pulse, and respiration may be the only sign of an impending infection since neutropenia patients have a diminished inflammatory response.[4,25]
- Observe for other general signs and symptoms of infection/sepsis: nausea, abdominal discomfort, changes in renal status, irritability, or changes in mental status.
- Assess blood counts daily, or every other day, to determine the onset of infection, the recovery of the bone marrow, the status of renal function, and the possible need to change antibiotic regimen. This should include complete blood count with differential, platelet count, and chemistry panel.[4,25]

Prevention of cross-contamination

- Place patient in a disinfected private room.
- Provide care first to patients with neutropenia before caring for other patients.
- Do not care for both patients with neutropenia and patients with infection.
- Wash hands consistently and thoroughly with each patient contact.

Prevention of disease transmission

- Educate patient, staff, and visitors in all aspects of infection prophylaxis.
- Screen personnel and visitors. The patient should not be exposed to anyone with an infection, recent vaccination, or recent exposure to a communicable disease (bacterial infections, herpes, colds, influenza, chicken pox, or measles).[4,25]
- Limit the number of visitors.

Elimination of possible sources of infection

- Provide a neutropenic diet (microbiotic diet) that eliminates unpared fresh fruits and raw vegetables. Food items should all be cooked.
- Avoid the placement of fresh fruits, flowers, or plants in the patient's room.
- Change water to prevent stagnation (denture cups, water pitchers, humidifiers, respiratory equipment, and irrigation containers).

Maintenance of integrity of the skin and mucous membranes

- Inspect the body daily with attention to the mouth, all orifices, all skin folds, and any site of an intravenous catheter insertion, a tube insertion, or a wound. Change dressings at least every other day using occlusive materials.
- Instruct patient and provide assistance in meticulous skin and mouth care. Provide lubrications to prevent dryness and cracking. Female patients should also keep the vaginal area clean and lubricated.
- Prevent trauma to the skin and mucous membranes by avoiding intramuscular or subcutaneous injections whenever possible; rectal manipulations, as with enemas, suppositories, or thermometers; urinary catheterization; douching and using tampons with the female patient. If urinary catheterization is necessary, maintain a closed sterile drainage system.
- Avoid rectal trauma by preventing constipation with dietary measures or stool softeners.

Respiratory status assessment

- Auscultate lungs at least every shift.
- Encourage mobility and frequent deep breathing and coughing.

Nutrition

- Assess patient's food preferences.
- Administer nutrition (oral, tube feeding, or parenteral) to meet increased nutritional demands.
- Encourage and provide high-calorie, high-protein food items.
- Obtain dietician consult.
- Measure weight every day.
- Monitor laboratory values to assess for protein wasting, with particular attention to serum albumin level. Encourage fluids to 3000 ml/day.
- Conserve energy.

NURSING DIAGNOSES

- Alteration in tissue perfusion related to the response to the release of endotoxins
- Alteration in cardiac output (decreased) related to decreased cardiac function

INTERVENTIONS

- Monitor vital signs (temperature, pulse, blood pressure, and respirations) every 4 hours.
- If hypotension is present, place patient flat in bed or in Trendelenburg position.
- Assess skin color, temperature, and moisture every 4 hours.
- Assess organ systems for malfunctions due to ischemia.
- Monitor ECG for evidence of arrhythmias.
- Monitor laboratory values closely.
- Obtain specimens for culture and sensitivities as ordered:
     Blood samples are usually taken two times, 4 hours apart.
     Urine, stool, throat, and sputum or any draining wound, intravenous catheter, or tube insertion site.
- Administer antibiotics as ordered. Observe patient closely for possible toxicities (nephrotoxicity and neurotoxicities are prevalent with the use of aminoglycosides such as tobramycin and gentamicin).
- Provide oxygen therapy as prescribed.
- Administer vasopressive drugs as ordered.
- Administer pain medication as ordered.
- Control fever.
     Administer antipyretic medications such as acetaminophen.
     Lower room temperature.
     Use sponge bath with tepid water.
     Utilize hypothermia blanket.
- Monitor laboratory values with attention to K^+, BUN, and creatinine.

NURSING DIAGNOSES

- Ineffective breathing patterns related to pulmonary edema and metabolic acidosis

- Impaired gas exchange related to circulatory collapse and pulmonary edema

INTERVENTIONS

- Observe ventilatory function for difficulties: shallow respirations, tachypnea, dyspnea, frothy secretions, and jugular vein distention.
- Auscultate lungs for evidence of impairment: rales, chronic and diminished breath sounds.
- Monitor intake and output.
- Measure CVP.
- Obtain or assist with measurement of arterial blood gases.
- Adjust position accordingly:
     High Fowler's position enhances lung expansion.
     Turn patient every 1 to 2 hours to mobilize secretions and prevent atelectasis, but keep most congested lung up to prevent further ventilation/perfusion problems.
- Administer humidified oxygen therapy by mask if ordered.
- Administer diuretics and decrease fluid intake as ordered.
- Suction nasopharynx and lungs as ordered.

NURSING DIAGNOSIS

- Fluid volume deficit related to capillary dilatation or leakage leading to third spacing of fluid

INTERVENTIONS

- Monitor intake and output every 30 to 60 minutes.
- Measure urine specific gravity.
- Insert indwelling urinary catheter as ordered.
- Measure CVP.
- Monitor blood pressure every 30 to 60 minutes.
- Administer crystalloids, colloids, and blood products as ordered to maintain circulating fluid volume.

The nursing management of a patient with septic shock is extremely complex and challenging. It requires astute assessment and often quick decision-making. Since septicemia is the triggering event, infection prophylaxis is crucial.

tases in frequency of occurrence.[132] The overall incidence of bony metastases is approximately 85%.[23] Cancers of the lung, breast, and prostate account for most skeletal involvement. Following closely are renal carcinoma, lymphoma, and myeloma.

Although lymphoma has a high incidence of SCC, it has declined over the past decade. This is due to the use of aggressive radiation therapy early in the treatment of lymphoma. Lymphomas compress the cord by direct extension through the intervertebral foramina which is the target area for radiotherapy.[38]

Metastatic bony lesions most frequently involve the thoracic and lumbar spine. The location of epidural metastasis and cord compression is related to the origin of the primary cancer and influenced by vascular supply and venous drainage.[36,38] The ribs, sternum, humerus, femur, and skull are also common areas of disease spread.[6] It has been noted that in 35% of all cases of SCC, this complication was the first evidence of cancer.[132]

The frequency of SCC in patients with systemic cancer is approximately 5% to 10%.[124] This figure may be rising because of the prolongation of life and the increased incidence of the cancers responsible for its occurrence. Primary lung cancer is the most common cause of SCC in men; in women it is breast cancer. Therefore, those at risk for SCC are those with a known bone metastasis or with a cancer that has a greater potential for skeletal involvement (lung, breast, prostate, kidney, lymphoma, and myeloma). However, SCC can occur at any time, even during active treatment for cancer.

PATHOPHYSIOLOGY

The adult human vertebral column, or backbone, is a versatile arrangement of 26 separate bony segments joined in series and supported by ligaments. The 26 vertebrae include 7 cervical, 12 thoracic, 5 lumbar, 1 sacral, and 1 coccyx. The vertebrae support the body by strength and rigidity while also providing flexibility and mobility. In addition, the column surrounds and protects the spinal cord, which is enlarged in the cervical and lumbar areas. The cord itself is covered by three protective meninges or membranes.

These meninges originate as coverings for the brain and extend downward over the spinal cord. The outermost membrane is the dura mater (hard mother), which is made up of dense fibrous connective tissue. The space between the walls of the vertebral column and the outer surface of the dura mater is referred to as the epidural, or extra dural, space. Within that space can be found blood vessels and connective and adipose tissue. No lymph nodes are located within this space.[132] The subdural space follows next, between the inner surface of the dura mater and the underlying arachnoid membrane. Below the arachnoid membrane is the subarachnoid space. It lies between the arachnoid membrane and the innermost membrane, the pia mater (gentle mother), which is closely attached to the spinal cord. The subarachnoid space contains liquid referred to as spinal fluid. However, it is more accurately called cerebrospinal fluid since the subarachnoid space begins in the brain and follows down the cord. Prevertebral lymph nodes are also located in this space.[132]

Bone metastasis involves the vertebral column and invades the epidural space (Figure 19-13). It is estimated that 95% of SCC are due to tumor in the epidural space or outside the spinal cord.[38,59] The destruction taking place in the bone is one of two types: osteolytic or osteoblastic. The more common osteolytic lesions cause bone destruction as tumor cells stimulate bone reabsorption by the osteoclasts (cells developing bone that absorb bony tissue). Stimulation of the osteoblasts (cells that develop into bone or secrete substances producing bony tissue) by the tumor cells causes formation of new bone, resulting in the less common osteoblastic lesions. Both processes are problematic. They can be differentiated by radiographic studies.[6]

The epidural space is invaded by tumor by one of three mechanisms[38,55,59,155]:

- Direct extension of the tumor into the space following bony erosion of the vertebral body. Carcinoma of the lung, breast, and prostate are mostly responsible for this mechanism, and it occurs with the greatest frequency.
- Lymph node growth through the foramina into the epidural space by adjacent prevertebral lymph nodes. Lymphomas usually grow in this manner.
- Hematogenous spread by means of an embolic process through the paravertebral and extradural venous plexus. Intramedullary metastases are one such process resulting from vascular dissemination, but they are rare, with an occurrence of 1% to 3%.[132]

Neurologic deficits result from these three mechanisms of metastases by three different processes:

- Direct compression of the spinal cord or cauda equina by the tumor itself.
- Interruption of the vascular supply to neural structure by the tumor.
- Compression due to vertebral collapse resulting from pathologic fracture or dislocation. The bone may extrude onto the cord and produce pressure that compresses the nerve roots.

The severity of the compression can increase in the presence of edema from obstruction of the venous plexus, which supplies the spinal cord.

CLINICAL FEATURES

The clinical presentation of SCC is similar in all patients, regardless of the origin of the tumor. Symptomatology is directly related to the location of the compression. The distribution of spinal metastases with SCC correlates with the number of vertebrae and size of the epidural space in each segment, with 10% in the cervical area, 70% in the thoracic, and 20% in the lumbosacral.[36,68,75,115,156]

The cardinal signs and associated symptoms of SCC are well documented and usually follow an established pattern of appearance, which includes pain, motor weakness, sensory loss, and finally autonomic dysfunction. See box on p. 420.

Back pain is the presenting complaint in 97% of patients.* It is related to SCC and may occur weeks or months before the compression takes place. It is

---

*References 36, 38, 42, 59, 68, 75.

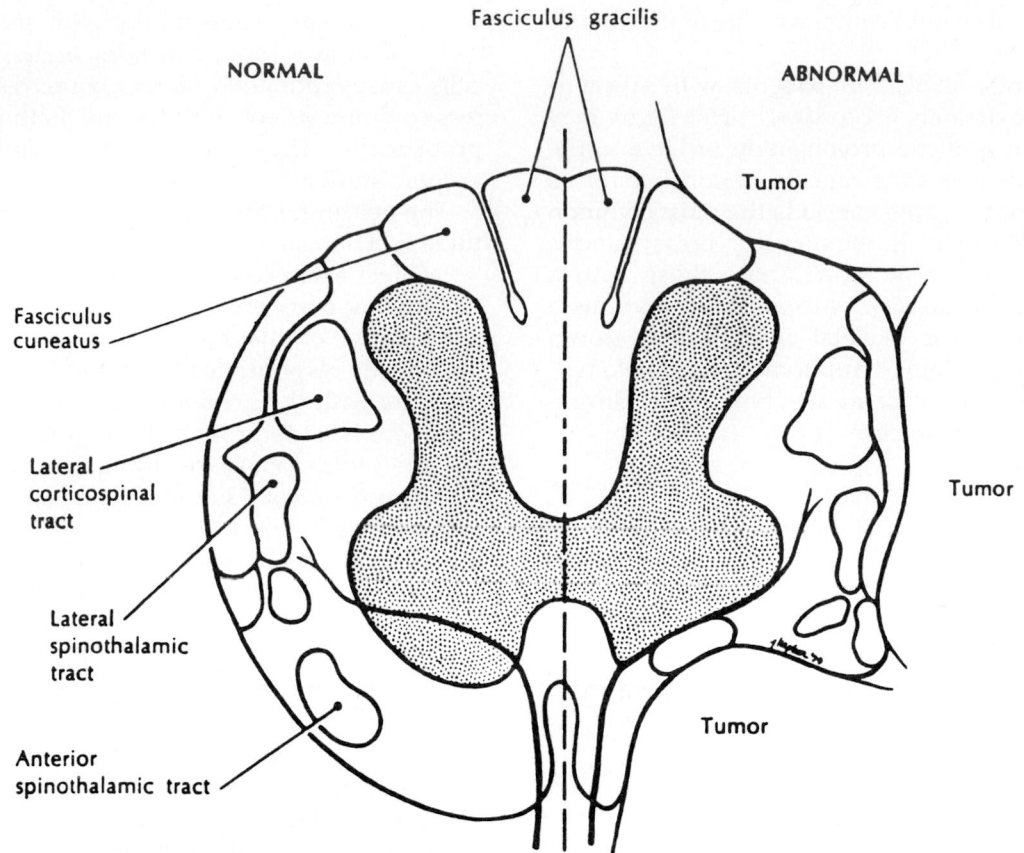

Figure 19-13 View of spinal cord at thoracic level with effects of epidural tumor shown in several locations. (From Nissenblatt M: Oncologic emergencies, Am Fam Phys 20[2], 1979.)

CLINICAL FEATURES: SCC

Clinical signs

Muscle weakness (unsteadiness, foot drop, paralysis)
Sensory impairment (paralysis, loss of bowel and bladder control, paraplegia)

Symptoms

Pain
Tingling and/or numbness in extremities
Diminished pain and temperature sensation
Sexual dysfunction

---

either localized or radicular. Localized pain is classically the initial symptom and results from stretching of the periosteum of the afflicted bone or from vertebral collapse. Pain that is radicular in nature is due to nerve root compression caused by pathologic fracture and compression of the vertebrae (Figure 19-13). The distribution of radicular pain depends on the level of spinal involvement. It may move along the dermatomal distribution and is aggravated by movement such as coughing, sneezing, straining as with Valsalva's maneuver, or straight leg raising. Thoracic radic-

ular pain, which is most common, radiates in a band around the chest or abdomen.[3,75]

The pain associated with SCC is usually intense, persistent, and progressive, although thoracic compression is often felt as a constriction.[3,55,156] Any pain of SCC may be accompanied by vertebral tenderness upon percussion at or near the level of compression. It is often unilateral when the compression is in the cervical or lumbosacral area and usually bilateral in the thoracic region. The pain is usually worse at night because the spine lengthens when recumbent. A key to early detection is a detailed assessment for any changes in pain. Patients may have been suffering with pain due to bony metastasis for a period of time. With the onset of SCC, the pain often changes its location and/or intensity.

The development of pain is followed by motor weakness. The time frame is quite variable, from hours to days, weeks, or months.[6,55,75,156] Common patient complaints include stiffness and heaviness of the affected extremity. It may manifest itself as an unsteady gait or ataxia with a favoring or dragging of the affected extremity or extremities.

Sensory loss usually follows motor weakness but precedes actual motor loss. Symptoms of sensory loss

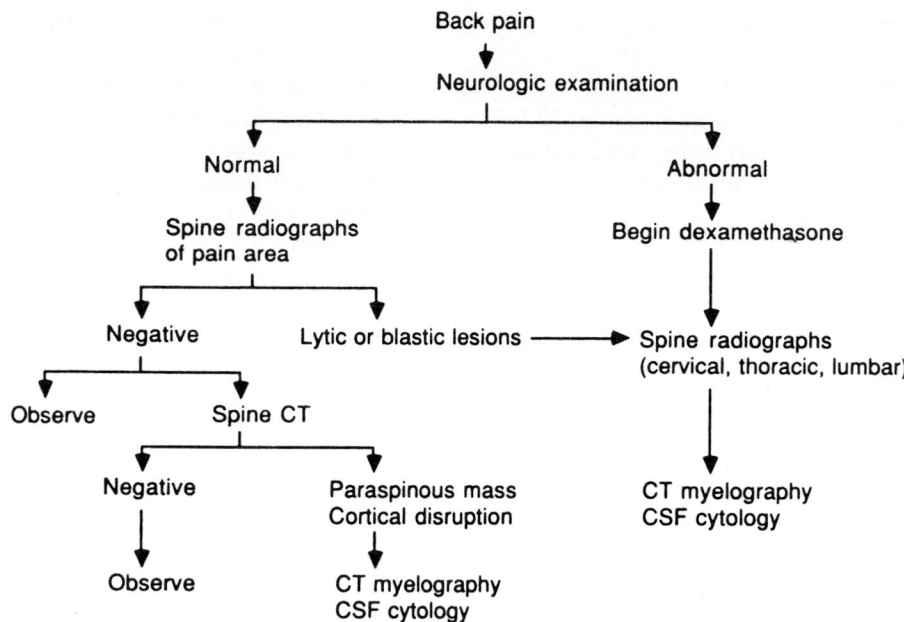

Figure 19-14 Algorithm of epidural spinal cord compression. (From Gilbert MR: Epidural spinal cord compression and carcinomectous meningitis. In Johnson RT, editor: Current therapy in neurologic disease, 3rd ed, St Louis, 1990, Mosby.)

include numbness, tingling, paresthesia, and feelings of coldness in the affected area. Loss of sensation to light touch first, then loss of pain, followed by loss of thermal sensation occurs in 80% of patients.[39] Concurrent loss of proprioception, deep pressure, vibratory and position sense indicates a severe compression. If the motor weakness and sensory loss progress rapidly to motor loss, the prognosis is poor.

Autonomic dysfunction will appear if the compression progresses. Urinary disturbances include hesitancy and retention, followed by overflow and incontinence. Early changes may be as subtle as an increased postvoid residual volume.[75] Lack of urge to defecate and inability to bear down are initial bowel disturbances, which may led to constipation, obstipation, and finally incontinence. Loss of sphincter control is a later sign and is associated with a poorer prognosis. Sexual dysfunction may be manifested as impotence.[132,156]

DIAGNOSIS

When SCC is suspected in any patient, a diagnosis should be confirmed immediately because of the potential for rapid progression and possible permanent neurologic dysfunction. Figure 19-14 provides an algorithm for evaluating possible epidural metastasis.[52,59] A good history and physical examination should be accompanied by thorough neurologic testing. Physical findings include percussion tenderness at the level of compression. If radicular pain is pres-

ent, it will increase with spinal movement on straight leg raises. Motor and sensory involvement is manifested by hyperactive reflexes, positive Babinski signs, variable spastic weakness, and bilateral sensory loss below the level of the compression. Absence of sweating below the level of involvement may be noted.[126] Bowel and bladder dysfunction may also be detected. Corresponding subjective data should be elicited because differences could be significant.

Testing for a patient with suspected SCC begins with plain x-ray films and a radioisotope bone scan. Both are positive in 85% of patients with SCC.[55,132] X-ray findings reveal osteolytic lesions with loss of a pedicle, vertebral body destruction, or collapse of vertebral body. A problem with plain x-rays is that if the tumor grows paraspinally, with invasion of the epidural space through the foramina, the bone film may be normal. This is common with lung tumors and lymphoma. Another concern is that a tumor can be present for 6 months without x-ray changes. A bone scan is often more sensitive and may be positive 6 months before plain films.[75] Osteoblastic lesions show new bone formation that may extend into the epidural space.[6,156]

A lumbar puncture may be performed; however, examination of the cerebrospinal fluid (CSF) may be helpful but is not diagnostic. CSF protein elevations greater than 100 mg/ml have been noted in most patients with SCC. Glucose is normal, cell count is unremarkable, and cytology is usually negative.[124] Progression of symptomatology has been reported following lumbar puncture, and it may interfere with the performance of myelography.[132]

Computerized tomography may identify early destructive lesions not seen on plain films, differentiate tumor from osteoporosis, and define paraspinal tumors that may extend epidurally.[75,156]

Myelography is often considered the most definitive diagnostic procedure for SCC. In 85% of patients, the blockage revealed on myelography corresponds to the site of known vertebral involvement by physical exam or x-ray findings.[53,55,65] The flow of the contrast material injected at the lumbar region will be partially or completely obstructed at the level of compression. If a complete blockage is demonstrated, additional contrast material will be injected into the cisterna magna to locate the upper margin of the obstruction.[55,132] Accurate visualization of the location, extent of compression, and upper and lower borders of a block are crucial for planning treatment by either decompressive laminectomy or radiation therapy. The usual contrast material used for these myelograms is pantopaque because of its ability to be left in the subarachnoid space for repeat fluoroscopy to evaluate response to therapy or recurrence at another site. A cerebrospinal fluid sample can be obtained during the procedure.

New imaging technology such as MRI is gaining increasing use for the evaluation of neurologic problems. Today, MRI is chosen over CT scan as a diagnostic procedure for spinal diseases.[23,36,55,59] The definitive role for MRI in SCC will be established with further clinical studies comparing MRI with myelography in terms of sensitivity, specificity, and accuracy. Current practice utilizes them in a complimentary manner. The major benefits of MRI are[23,36,55,59]:

- Its sensitivity to neurologic tissue.
- It is noninvasive.
- It is helpful in patients with severe contrast allergies.
- It images the entire spine providing various views.
- It is helpful in patients with brain metastasis.
- It may show multiple epidural deposits of tumor that may not be obvious on initial myelogram.
- It avoids the risk of neurologic deterioration after lumbar puncture, which occurs in as many as 14% of patients with complete block.[36]

The disadvantages of MRI are:

- The need for the patient to lie still in one position, which may be difficult for someone with central back pain.
- Claustrophobia has been a common problem.

TREATMENT MODALITIES

The choice of treatment for patients with SCC is dependent on the primary tumor, the rapidity of onset of the compression, and the level, severity, and duration of the blockage. The two most frequent treatment modalities for SCC are surgery and radiation therapy. The goal of therapy is symptom relief from metastatic disease and improvement of quality of life.

Patients are initially treated nonsurgically except in three situations that would warrant a decompressive laminectomy:

- Prior maximum-tolerance radiation at the site of compression precludes further irradiation.
- The cause for SCC is questionable or there is no known primary malignancy.
- Neurologic deterioration occurs during radiation therapy. In most other situations, radiation therapy is the initial treatment.[75,124,156]

Laminectomy with decompression of the spinal cord and nerve roots will relieve compression and improve symptoms, but it rarely achieves complete removal of the tumor. Surgery affords diagnostic and therapeutic benefits. It may provide a diagnosis for a patient with no known history of cancer. As a treatment modality it allows tumor debulking, decompression of the spinal cord, and possibly bone grafting at the location of erosion.[39,42]

In select patients, surgery may be done to remove a tumor or bone from the area of compression, followed by stabilization with hardware and methyl methacrylate placed into the space. However, the surgical technique is difficult and poses a potential risk of major complications.[23,36,42]

Technical difficulties can arise because the surgical approach may be posterior and most tumors present in the vertebral body and invade the epidural space anteriorly. Therefore, in addition to incomplete tumor removal, the removal of the posterior elements of the vertebrae can produce an unstable spine necessitating postoperative therapy and back braces.[6,42]

Following surgery, postoperative radiation therapy is administered to treat the remaining tumor. Portal size depends on residual tumor and extends one to two vertebrae above and below the level of involvement to assure an adequate dosage and field. Irradiation may be initiated a few days after surgery and continues for 2 weeks, with total dose approximately 270 to 300 Gy.[53,75] Caution should be used during and after radiation therapy since normal osteocytes will be destroyed along with tumor cells. This disrupts the balance of osteoblastic (formation) and osteoclastic (absorption) processes. Wound separation may occur, and delay in healing is possible. Therefore, complete normal bone repair is rare, and support to the spine may be necessary until radiation therapy is completed.[6,42]

Radiation therapy alone as primary treatment for SCC has been gaining increased attention. Studies comparing surgery with radiation therapy to radiation therapy alone have shown them to have equal efficacy.[6] However, response may depend on the radiosensitivity of the tumor.[75] When radiation therapy is the treatment choice, it should begin immediately following definitive diagnosis. The total dose given is 270 to 300 Gy over a 2-week period; margins are generous (two spinal segments above and below the lesion).[38,75] Neurologic examinations should be done frequently to assess patient response.

The use of steroids in the management of SCC is advocated to decrease edema, relieve symptoms, and control pain. Pain relief in the majority of patients will occur within a few hours.[23,66,75] However, the presence of edema related to compression is not well substantiated. Most evidence is clinical at diagnosis of SCC or during administration of radiation therapy. Current recommendations vary among clinicians. The drug most frequently ordered is Decadron, but the dosage is either high (100 mg by IV push, initial dose) with tapering, or low conventional (16 to 24 mg/day) with tapering.[66,75,132]

Chemotherapy has a role as adjuvant therapy in the treatment of SCC. In most instances alkylating agents alone or combined with radiation therapy are used to treat cord compression resulting from lymphoma.[38,55,132] Chemotherapy may be given concomitantly or following radiation therapy as systemic treatment for the primary underlying malignancy.

PROGNOSIS

Response to therapy for SCC depends on the severity and rapidity of onset of symptoms more than on their duration.[21] Patients with intramedullary metastasis usually have a rapid progression of dysfunction and therefore a poorer prognosis.[18] Surgical intervention results in 5% mortality.[30] The amount of functional recovery following radiation therapy is often predictable when one half of the total dose is delivered.[6] If patients are ambulatory at the initiation of therapy, 80% will retain the ability to walk after treatment, whereas only 30% to 40% of patients with pretreatment motor dysfunction are ambulatory after treatment.[38,131] If the underlying malignancy is lymphoma, chances for continued ambulation are 80% as compared to 60% in patients with carcinomas since these patients often experience late SCC.[55,124] Patients who are paraplegic before therapy have a 5% to 7% chance to become ambulatory.[132] This statistical picture of response emphasizes the crucial role of early detection of SCC.

Nursing Management

Spinal cord compression is a true oncologic emergency requiring immediate attention. The primary aspect of nursing care is early detection since response to therapy is directly related to the patient's functional status at diagnosis. An in-depth history and data collection are essential in those patients who are at risk for SCC. Nursing assessment should focus on pain, motor and sensory status, and bowel and bladder functions. The nursing care of these patients is extremely variable, depending on the presence and severity of the compression and the medical treatment. Very subtle changes in patient status are significant and should be reported.[6,21,23,65,107]

NURSING DIAGNOSIS

• Impaired physical mobility related to spinal cord compression

INTERVENTIONS •

• Assess patient's level of function/mobility:
  Check for the presence of sensory loss and paresthesia by noting sensation and deep tendon reflexes in extremities.
  Monitor serum calcium level for potential increase due to immobility.
  Determine motor weakness and dysfunction by checking gait, range of motion, and coordination.
  Determine bowel, bladder, and sexual function.
• Check for evidence of venous thrombosis due to immobilization:
  Determine the presence of redness, swelling, warmth, positive Homan's sign (pain on dorsiflexion), and venous streaking and erythema.
  Use antiembolic stockings as ordered.
  Measure calves each day and note any edema.
• Implement pain management program as indicated.
• Establish activity regimen according to patient's physical status and physician order:
  Institute passive range of motion exercises as ordered.
  Assist patients with transfer and ambulation as needed.
  Provide back brace for patients with unstable spines as ordered.
  Move bedridden patients with extreme care and maintain proper body alignment. Use lift sheets and assistive devices (e.g., trapeze, Hoyer lift). Support joints. Turn patient by log-rolling method.
• Obtain consultations with physical and occupational therapy for evaluation and assistance.

- Implement safety measures as appropriate:
  Place all articles within patient's reach.
  Keep bed rails up and pad them if necessary.
  Assist patient with all movements or encourage use of assistive devices.
- Encourage and assist patient to perform self-care when possible.
- Discuss and teach the use of assistive and supportive devices.
- Arrange consultation or referral to rehabilitative services as needed.

NURSING DIAGNOSIS

- Potential/actual ineffective breathing patterns related to the level of compression and/or immobility

INTERVENTIONS

- Assess respiratory status:
  Observe breathing for distress (respiratory rate, rhythm, and amplitude).
  Auscultate lungs for breath sounds every shift.
  Obtain arterial blood gases as ordered.
- Encourage and assist patient with pulmonary hygiene every 2 hours:
  Reposition every 2 hours.
  Facilitate deep breathing and coughing.
- Consult with physician regarding need for more aggressive pulmonary measures (incentive spirometry, ultrasonic nebulizer, chest physical therapy).
- Provide mechanical respiratory support if necessary.

NURSING DIAGNOSIS

- Potential/actual impairment of skin integrity related to immobility

INTERVENTIONS

- Assess skin integrity with special attention to areas over bony prominences (note any redness, discoloration, swelling, or breakdown).
- Culture any suspicious drainage.
- Institute skin care protocol specific to assessment.
- Modify bed surface with approved pressure-reducing mattress.
- Change patient's position every 2 hours and massage pressure areas.

NURSING DIAGNOSIS

- Alteration in bowel elmination, contipation related to decreased activity or immobility

INTERVENTIONS

- Obtain history of bowel elimination including laxative use and other aids for elimination.
- Assess abdomen each day (observe for distention, auscultate for bowel sounds, perform rectal examine for impaction).
- Monitor bowel movements (frequency, amount, odor, consistency).
- Encourage fluids as appropriate.
- Increase bulk and fiber in diet as indicated.
- Administer stool softeners, laxatives, bulk products, and lubricants as ordered.
- Initiate bowel training program as necessary and encourage compliance.

NURSING DIAGNOSIS

- Potential/actual alteration in pattern of urinary elimination related to neurogenic bladder/loss of voluntary control of micturation

INTERVENTIONS

- Obtain history of bladder elimination patterns.
- Assess abdomen (observe for distention, percuss area above symphysis pubis).
- Monitor urinary output (frequency, amount, odor, color).
- Check for residual after each voiding as ordered.
- Monitor laboratory values (urinalysis, serum BUN, and creatinine).
- Assess for signs and symptoms of a urinary tract infection (elevated temperature, changes in odor or color of urine, frequency and dysuria, complaints of burning and/or urgency).
- Culture urine as ordered.
- Observe for presence of hyperreflexia (reaction that occurs with blocks at T_6 or above in which there is increased production of norepinephrine in an attempt to cause evacuation of the bowel or bladder). Signs and symptoms include increased blood pressure, pounding headache, vasodilatation, flushing, increased temperature, profuse sweating, chest pain, bradycardia, nausea).[27,51]
- Obtain order for indwelling urinary catheter if repeated catheterization is necessary to relieve distention or continued urinary residual.
- Initiate bladder training program as necessary and encourage compliance.

NURSING DIAGNOSIS

- Alteration in sexual dysfunction related to disease process and treatment

INTERVENTIONS

- Examine own attitudes, knowledge, and skills in the area of sexuality, sexual function, and sexual counseling.
- Provide a therapeutic environment that demonstrates acceptance of sexual behavior and allows patient to feel comfortable to discuss sexual concerns.
- Elicit a sexual history as appropriate.
- Be respectful of social, cultural, and religious factors that may influence patient perceptions of sexuality,

sexual function and identity, and assure confidentiality.
- Utilize the Plissit model to develop relevant nursing interventions.[67] Use levels with which you feel comfortable:
    - P = Permission: convey permission to have (or not have) sexual thoughts, concerns, feelings (assure patient that concerns regarding sexual function after cancer diagnosis are legitimate).
    - LI = Limited Information: provide limited information relative to patient's problem while acknowledging that other individuals experience similar concerns (e.g., many individuals have concerns about type of birth control recommended while receiving chemotherapy).
    - SS = Specific Suggestions: offer specific suggestions relevant to patient's problems (e.g., use of pillows and coital positions that minimize or allay threat of pathologic fractures).
    - IT = Intensive Therapy: refer to appropriate resource for longer-term therapy or rehabilitation (e.g., sex therapist for continued erectile dysfunction, surgeon for reconstructive surgery).
- Discuss the potential impact of disease and/or treatment on sexuality and/or sexual function.
- Identify available resources and make referrals as appropriate.

NURSING DIAGNOSIS
- Alteration in self-concept: disturbance in body image and/or role performance related to physical dysfunction related to disease process and/or immobility

INTERVENTIONS
- Assess patient's past and present coping abilities through interview, observation of physical and verbal participation in self-care, and discussion.
- Promote and observe interaction with family, friends, and staff.
- Encourage verbalization of feelings and concerns.
- Assist and support the establishment of goals and adaptive coping mechanisms.
- Make referrals as appropriate for counseling and rehabilitative services.

Nursing care of a patient with SCC is complex and challenging, reflecting the extreme variability among patients. Situations exist along a continuum from early detection and alarm through emergency and rehabilitation. The role of the nurse in coordinating care is crucial.

SUPERIOR VENA CAVA SYNDROME

DEFINITION

The superior vena cava is a major venous vessel that returns blood to the right atrium of the heart from the head, upper thorax, and upper extremities. Obstruction of the venous flow through this vessel results in impaired venous drainage with engorgement of the vessels from the head and upper body torso. As the venous pressure rises in the superior vena cava, blood is shunted to collateral venous pathways to facilitate return to the right atrium. The result is a characteristic constellation of physical findings known as superior vena cava syndrome (SVCS).[38,40,89]

ETIOLOGY AND RISK FACTORS

The causes ascribed to SVCS have changed over the years as information has increased regarding the cancer process. SVCS was first described by William Hunter in 1757 in a patient with a syphilitic aneurysm.[89] Over the years, benign conditions such as aortic aneurysms, thyroid goiter, tuberculous mediastinitis, and infectious diseases were most frequently considered to be the cause of SVCS. Today only 3% of the cases of SVCS have a benign cause; cancer is responsible for more than 97% of all cases. Any tumor, primary or metastatic, can block the blood flow of the superior vena cava. Three fourths of all malignant cases of SVCS are caused by bronchogenic cancer, particularly oat cell carcinoma of the lung. Lymphomas account for approximatley 15% to 20% of SVCS cases.[55,134,158] This includes both Hodgkin's disease and non-Hodgkin's lymphoma. Most frequent in the latter group is diffuse histiocytic lymphoma. Other malignancies associated with SVCS have been Kaposi's sarcoma, adenocarcinoma of the breast, thymomas, and primary or metastatic seminoma and other germ cell tumors.[108] SVCS may be present in cases where there is no known diagnosis of cancer.[55,118,158]

Innovations in therapeutic interventions for cancer have added two new causes. Venous thrombosis related to indwelling central venous catheters has been observed in patients with SVCS. Several authorities ascribe this to be the most common nonmalignant cause of SVC obstruction.[38,55,140] Radiation-induced fibrosis can result in the narrowing of the superior vena cava and produce the same clinical picture.

SVCS occurs in approximately 3% to 4% of patients

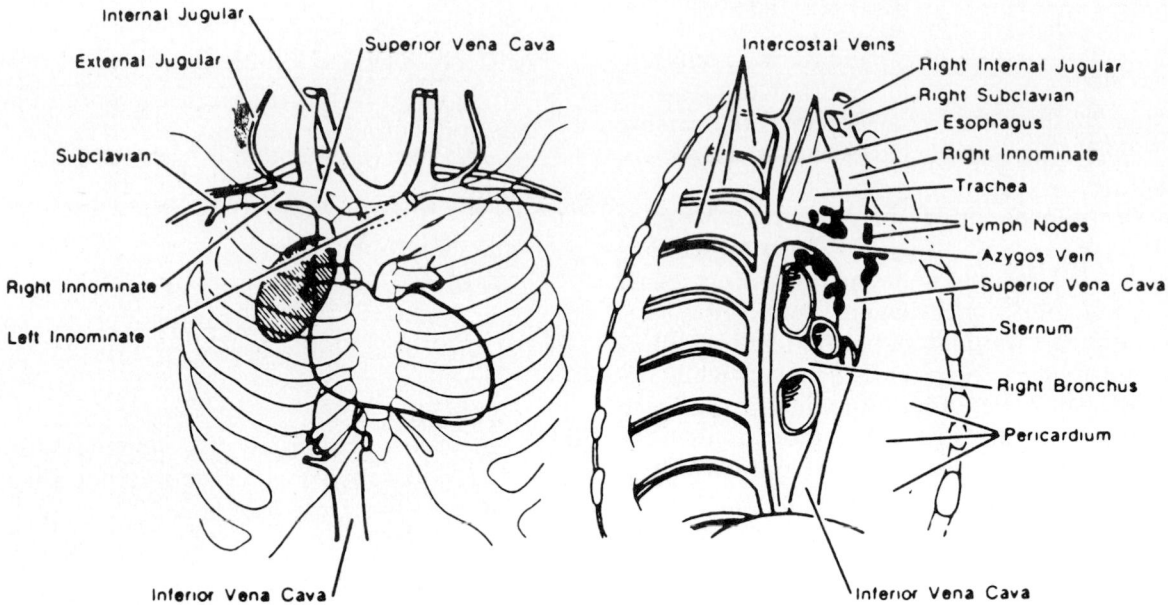

Figure 19-15 Schematic representation of the thorax, frontal and lateral views. Shaded areas indicate typical site of obstruction. (From Lockich J and Goodman R: Superior vena cava syndrome, JAMA 231[1], 1975.)

with cancer.[40] The majority of patients with SVCS are in the fourth to seventh decade of life. The ratio of men to women is approximately 3:1.[117] However, as lung cancer incidence and death rates change, especially among women, so too will the incidence and age and sex distribution of SVCS.

PATHOPHYSIOLOGY

The superior vena cava is a thin-walled, low-pressure vessel about 7 cm in length (Figure 19-15). It extends from the junction of the right and left innominate veins to the right atrium. Location in the thorax is to the right of the arteries of the trachea and right mainstem bronchus and posterior to the sternum. The thorax is a rigid anatomic compartment with little ability for expansion. In its space within the thorax, the superior vena cava is extremely vulnerable to displacement and compression because it has a thin wall, low venous pressure, and is surrounded by the rigid structures of the sternum, trachea, vertebrae, lymph nodes, the aorta, the pulmonary artery, and the right bronchus.[68] Therefore, obstruction of the superior vena cava can be a consequence of three physiologic events.[77,107,108]

- External compression by an extrinsic mass, solid tumor, or enlarged lymph node
- Intravascular obstruction by tumor or thrombosis
- Intraluminal reaction to tumor invasion or inflammation

Impedance of venous flow through the superior vena cava and subsequent development of SVCS depends on several factors: the degree and location of the blockage, growth rate of the tumor, patency of the azygos vein, and proliferation of collateral circulation. The azygos vein (Figure 19-15) plays a pivotal role in the flow of blood through the superior vena cava, entering it just above the pericardial reflection and making it a major tributary. There are three places where the superior vena cava may be obstructed relative to the azygos vein[158]:

- Above the azygos vein, allowing patency of the proximal vena cava. In this situation, venous return from the upper body continues through the subclavian vein to the azygos, on to the proximal vena cava, and finally into the right atrium. Obstruction above the azygos vein is the least serious.
- Proximal to the entrance of the azygos vein. Venous return is accomplished through blood shunting to the inferior vena cava by way of the azygos vein.[140]
- At the junction of the azygos vein with the superior vena cava. All blood flow through the superior vena cava is blocked. This necessitates rerouting of the blood flow to the inferior vena cava by way of the azygos vein. Blockage at the junction of the azygos vein is the most complex.

Impairment of the venous circulation through the superior vena cava reduces blood flow to the right atrium, which results in venous hypertension with venous stasis and a decrease in cardiac output. If untreated, the progression is from vascular congestion to thrombosis, cerebral edema, pulmonary complications, and death.

CLINICAL FEATURES: SVCS

Clinical signs

Edema of the face, neck, upper thorax and breasts and upper extremities

Periorbital edema and/or edema of the conjunctivae, with or without protrusion of the eye

Horner's syndrome (sinking of eye with ptosis of eyelid)

Plethora of the face

Increased pressure of the jugular veins

Dilatation and prominence of collateral vessels in upper thorax and neck

Telangiectasis (capillary dilatation)

Compensatory tachycardia

Symptoms

Respiratory compromise (dyspnea, shortness of breath, tachypnea, cough, orthopnea)

Feeling of facial fullness

Headache

Visual disturbances

Dizziness

Hoarseness

Chest pain

Stokes' sign (tightness of shirt collar)

Swelling of fingers (difficulty removing rings)

CLINICAL FEATURES

The clinical picture seen in SVCS is directly related to obstruction of venous drainage in the upper body (Figure 19-15). Onset is usually insidious, but when fully developed it requires immediate attention. The onset and severity of signs and symptoms vary directly with the underlying disease and related pathophysiology. Compression of intrathoracic structures, vascular congestion, and venous hypertension present remarkable clinical features. The presentation may be unilateral or bilateral. Since pressures in the head are higher in the supine than in the standing position, a person with early SVCS may initially have signs and symptoms only in the morning. Symptomatology will also vary greatly depending upon the underlying pathophysiology. Early detection of SVCS hinges on a careful in-depth history and physical assessment. See the box above for clinical features of SVCS.[38,55,68,154]

Progression of symptoms may lead to severe respiratory obstruction, paralyzed vocal cord, cyanosis of the upper torso, "wet brain syndrome" (manifested by drowsiness, stupor, unconsciousness, and seizures), and possible coma.[140]

DIAGNOSIS

The diagnostic evaluation of a patient with SVCS is highly dependent on the patient's physical condition. If SVCS onset is insidious, the diagnostic workup can proceed slowly and treatment will not be initiated until a diagnosis is confirmed. However, if the onset is rapid and symptoms are acute, a definitive diagnosis may be deferred and treatment (usually radiation therapy) is begun immediately, especially where there is a known diagnosis of cancer. SVCS may be considered one of the rare occasions when treatment can be started even before a tissue diagnosis is confirmed. In this life-threatening situation, chest radiography, the results of which rarely appear normal, and clinical presentation are considered diagnostic. A tissue biopsy to determine a primary lesion and further workup for metastases can proceed during the course of treatment.

Chest films are abnormal in 80% of the cases of SVCS.[124,158] Most common findings are a lung or mediastinal mass, most frequently on the right side since the superior vena cava enters from the right. Also seen may be mediastinal widening and pleural effusion.[158]

CT scan and MRI may further define the lesion and its location. Important information obtained by radiographic findings includes more detailed information about the SVC and its tributaries as well as the source, size, and exact location of the mass in relation to the azygos vein.[158]

Further diagnostic procedures must be evaluated for their risk versus benefit to the patient. Biopsy of palpable superficial lymph nodes, sputum for cytology, and bone marrow biopsy are associated with low risk and may provide information about the primary tumor. Invasive procedures such as bronchoscopy, mediastinoscopy, thoracotomy, or supraclavicular lymph node biopsy may be necessary but are associated with significant morbidity and the risk of fatal thrombosis or bleeding as a result of increased venous pressure. On the other hand, immediate radiation therapy may impede later tissue biopsy because of radiation-induced tissue changes.

Bronchoscopy has established a diagnosis in approximately 70% of patients.[108] Percutaneous needle biopsy, mediastinoscopy, and thoracotomy are associated with increased risk of bleeding and, if necessary, should be deferred until venous pressure is reduced. Superior venacavography is infrequently done. However, it can be most helpful in determining location and degree of obstruction, measuring venous pressure through the catheter, distinguishing between vascular and nonvascular lesions, evaluating collateral circulation, and assessing operability.[158] To establish the extent of obstruction and determine the hemodynamics of the vessel, venacavography has also been used in early diagnosis when SVCS is only suspected. New technology and improved methodology in diagnosing SVCS presents a challenge to clinicians, who must assess each patient carefully to determine the timing and appropriateness of the diagnostic evaluation.

TREATMENT MODALITIES

There are four therapeutic modalities to be considered in the treatment of SVCS: radiation therapy, chemotherapy, surgery, and pharmacologic therapy. The goals are relief of symptoms and reduction of the obstructing lesion. Cure may be the goal when the primary diagnosis is small cell lung cancer, non-Hodgkin's lymphoma, or a germ cell tumor, which account for nearly half of the malignant causes of SVCS.[158]

The choice of treatment depends on the rate of onset, the causative process (benign or malignant), and the type of mass (intraluminal or extraluminal).

Radiation Therapy

Radiation therapy has been the treatment of choice for SVCS because of its local therapeutic response and minimal toxicities. Treatment is begun immediately in acute and life-threatening situations. The total dose, dose fractionation, and size and type of field depend on tumor histology, patient condition, radiologic response, and symptom relief. Delivery of radiation begins initially with high doses of 4 Gy/day for the first 3 days, followed by a reduction of the daily dose to 1.5 to 2 Gy/day, for a total dose of 500 to 600 Gy in 5 to 7 weeks.[40,108,118] The higher initial doses are favored because of an apparently more rapid tumor response. Patients with lymphoma require a lower total dose of 300 to 400 Gy, unless bulky masses are present, which may necessitate a total dose of 500 Gy.[38,55,118,158]

Tumor reduction usually occurs with radiation therapy, especially in patients with lymphoma and small (oat) cell lung cancer. Less tumor response is seen in patients with nonsmall cell lung cancer (epidermoid, adenocarcinoma, and large cell). Subjective improvement has been noted in 3 to 4 days in 75% of patients, regardless of tumor histology. Within 7 days, 91% obtain relief.[113] Objective response, with decrease in facial swelling and plethora, reduction of venous engorgement, and shrinkage of tumor mass, is evident within 7 to 14 days.[113,117]

Chemotherapy

The use of chemotherapy to treat SVCS has come to the forefront of the treatment regimen. It is an effective primary treatment when the cause of SVCS is small cell lung cancer lymphoma or a germ cell tumor.[158] Chemotherapy may be used alone if the mediastinal area has received a maximum of radiation or when reduction of tumor mass will provide a smaller radiation treatment field.

The choice of chemotherapeutic agents is based on the malignant cause of SVCS. Following the selection of agents, consideration must be given to intravenous administration. Edema and dilatation of the veins in the upper extremities lead to impaired circulation. Limited venous access, poor drug distribution, and increased risk of venous irritation and/or extravasation of medications may contraindicate use of the upper extremities for therapy. In some situations, the lower extremities may be used to administer chemotherapy by a central intravenous catheter placed in the femoral vein; however, this practice is highly controversial.

Surgery

Specific surgical approaches to SVCS include superior vena cava bypass or stent placement. These approaches are used very judicially since postoperative morbidity is high. Bypass surgery is indicated when the tumor could be completely removed if the superior vena cava were excised with it; where venous return is inadequate in spite of collateral circulation; and when the obstruction is due to venous thrombosis or fibrosis. This operative procedure is delicate, precise, and dependent upon the same factors as in arterial grafts. The graft may be constructed using a synthetic dacron prothesis or the patient's own saphenous vein. The graft creates a new vessel, which rechannels blood flow around the obstruction. One end of the graft is sutured to the right atrium, and the other is sutured to either the internal jugular or innominate vein.[10,158]

Patency of the bypass graft depends on the size of the anastomotic site, internal venous pressure, and blood flow. External rigidity of the graft is helpful to prevent collapse but is not required. Postoperatively, patients usually receive anticoagulation therapy and aspirin for an indefinite period of time to assist with graft patency.[2,108,148] When patency is maintained for several weeks, it increases the likelihood of long-term function. Reports demonstrate patency beyond a year.

The placement of a wire stent offers an alternative for the palliation of symptoms in patients with SVCS. Use of a stent may be indicated when other treatments for SVCS are unusable or ineffective. The most common situation is recurrence of SVCS following maximum-tolerance radiation. The stainless steel stent was designed by Gianturco and is usually referred to as the Gianturco expandable wire stent (GEWS).[148]

The stent is placed using a small balloon catheter inserted percutaneously with fluoroscopy under local anesthesia. The catheter is introduced into the vessel with the stent in a compressed form. When the stent is released, it expands and dilates the narrowed venous lumen. If the expansion is insufficient, the balloon is used to enlarge the stent to the desired diameter. A period of about 4 weeks is necessary for the stent to become incorporated into the endothelium of the venous wall.[148] The stent may remain patent for long periods of time because of its relatively low thrombogenicity.

One study has indicated some prognostic factors for longer-term palliation using the stent. It was found that patients with postirradiation fibrosis or slowly progressive pressure from a recurrent extrinsic tumor had longer relief of symptoms than patients whose symptoms resulted from direct tumor invasion.[125] The use of GEWS looks promising, but further clinical studies using the stent are necessary to define its role in the treatment of SVCS.

Pharmacologic Therapy

Thrombus formation in patients with SVCS has gained increasing attention over the years. Autopsy reports have demonstrated thrombosis of the superior vena cava in patients who died during treatment of SVCS.

The increased use of indwelling central venous catheters has contributed to a rise in the incidence of SVCS.[38,55,140] Whatever the cause, irritation and inflammation of the superior vena cava related to an intraluminal or extraluminal lesion produce platelet aggregation leading to clot formation. Fibrinolytic therapy with streptokinase or urokinase has been used to treat intraluminal thrombosis.*

Recent research has demonstrated that fibrinolytic therapy is most likely to succeed in patients with SVCS due to a central venous catheter of urokinase is used and if therapy is initiated within five days of the onset of symptoms.[57]

Anticoagulation therapy is indicated for SVCS because of venous stasis. It may be used alone to resolve thrombus obstruction secondary to a central venous catheter or following initial fibrinolytic therapy. It is also used as a maintenance treatment to reduce the extent of the thrombus and prevent its progression. Removal of the central venous catheter should also be followed by anticoagulation to avoid embolization.[55,158]

During the administration of radiation therapy or chemotherapy, anticoagulants may be given concomitantly as a preventive treatment.

Other medical interventions may be instituted as adjunctive therapy for SVCS. Diuretics may be given to reduce edema of the head and neck, which could improve cerebration and breathing. Caution should be used when giving diuretics because venous return

---

*References 12, 16, 57, 77, 108, 140, 158.

to the heart is low and hypovolemia resulting from diuresis may induce shock. Steroids may be administered during active treatment to reduce inflammation related to the obstruction, to radiation, or to chemotherapy and resulting tumor necrosis.[155] Oxygen therapy may be necessary for the management of respiratory complications.

PROGNOSIS

Patients usually respond to treatment for SVCS, showing regression of the tumor.

The prognosis of patients with SVCS strongly correlates with the prognosis of the underlying disease.[38,158] In some instances there has been no response to treatment. This has been attributed to poor general condition, presence of thrombosis in the superior vena cava, and metastatic disease.[140] Overall, patient survival is not good, since most patients are diagnosed in an advanced stage and die from metastatic disease. Recurrence is not a problem in general, but this is probably because of the relatively short survival time following initial diagnosis.

The best responses are seen in patients with lymphoma and small cell lung cancer. Other types of lung cancer have fewer long-term responses. Only 10% to 20% of all patients are alive 2 years after therapy. This is probably due to the nature of the underlying malignancies.[108] Of patients with lymphoma, 45% have survived to 30 months, compared to 10% of patients with lung cancers.[115,117,118]

Although a diagnosis of SVCS may not offer long-term survival, with prompt diagnosis and treatment it can be managed and therefore allow improvement in the patient's quality of life. See pp. 430-431 for nursing management of SVCS.

SYNDROME OF INAPPROPRIATE ANTIDIURETIC HORMONE SECRETION

DEFINITION

The syndrome of inappropriate antidiuretic hormone secretion (SIADH) is a disorder of water balance. Antidiuretic hormone (ADH), also called arginine vasopressin, regulates the body's water balance.[87] SIADH is characterized by elevated serum blood levels of antidiuretic hormone (ADH), excessive water retention, and hyponatremia.[87,123,143,160]

ETIOLOGY AND RISK FACTORS

SIADH develops in 1% to 2% of patients with cancer.[55,143,164] Approximately two thirds of patients with documented SIADH have a neoplasm. The most common malignant disease associated with this syndrome is lung cancer, and 87% of these cases are small (oat)

Nursing Management

The nursing care of patients with SVCS begins with astute assessment skills. Identification should be made of those patients considered to be at risk, followed by close observation and baseline data collection. Documentation of vital signs, mental status, appearance, and level of activity are essential to facilitate detection of changes. Subtle changes in subjective complaints or objective parameters should be reported to the physician. Once a diagnosis of SVCS has been established, the role of the nurse continues to be important.[26,68,76,84,107]

NURSING DIAGNOSIS

- Ineffective breathing patterns related to venous congestion in the upper torso

INTERVENTIONS

- Determine current respiratory status:
    Observe for signs and symptoms of respiratory distress (dyspnea, shortness of breath, tachypnea, air hunger, stridor, orthopnea).
    Assess lungs. Observe ventilatory movements (rate and depth), patency of airway, use of accessory muscles, clubbing of fingernails, discoloration of nail bed or mucous membranes.
    Palpate chest for fremitus, crepitance, deviation of the trachea, or nonsymmetrical chest expansion.
    Percuss chest for density/consolidation and displacement of organs.
    Auscultate chest for breath sounds.
    Monitor laboratory and other respiratory function tests, CBC, electrolytes, arterial blood gases, chest x-ray, scans.
- Assist with breathing and pulmonary toilet:
    Positioning for comfort and enhanced chest expansion
    Deep breathing and coughing every 2 hours
    Pursed lip breathing
    Frequent mouth care
    Suctioning if necessary
- Provide oxygen and mechanical ventilation as indicated.
- Administer respiratory medications and steroids as prescribed.

NURSING DIAGNOSES

- Potential for decreased cardiac output related to decreased venous return related to vena cava obstruction
- Potential for impaired gas exchange related to venous congestion related to vena cava obstruction

INTERVENTIONS

- Assess patient for changes in cardiac function:
    Check blood pressure and pulse every 2 to 4 hours as indicated.
    Observe patient for signs of impedance of venous blood flow from the upper torso (plethora of the face; thoracic and neck vein distention; facial, trunk, and arm edema, especially in the morning; dyspnea, tachypnea, cough; cyanosis; mental status changes).
    Monitor laboratory values (CBC, arterial blood gases, chest x-ray, ECG, scans).
- Provide oxygen therapy as ordered.
- Position patient for comfort and enhancement of venous drainage from upper torso:
    Elevate and support upper extremities, especially if edematous.
    Avoid constrictive clothing.
    Maintain a cool room temperature.
    Avoid closed-in areas if possible.
- Prevent activities that increase intrathoracic or intracerebral pressure (Valsalva's maneuver, vomiting, bending over, stooping).
- Assist patient with physical activities as needed.
- Provide measures to decrease anxiety:
    Relaxation techniques
    Antianxiety medications

NURSING DIAGNOSES

- Potential for alteration in cerebral tissue perfusion related to upper torso venous stasis and decreased cardiac output
- Potential for alteration in thought process related to decreased cerebral tissue perfusion and impaired gas exchange

INTERVENTIONS

- Assess organ systems for malfunction related to ischemia.
- Note any changes in mental status.
- Monitor laboratory values closely.
- Administer vasoactive drugs as ordered.
- Provide oxygen as prescribed.
- Institute safety measures as indicated.

NURSING DIAGNOSIS

- Potential for impaired skin integrity in the chest/thorax area related to the effects of SVCS and/or radiation therapy

INTERVENTIONS

- Explain effects of SVCS and/or radiation on skin and prepare patient for temporary changes (edema, discoloration, pruritis).
- Outline proper skin hygiene:
  Use mild soap and tepid water and pat dry.
  Avoid use of lotions, creams, ointments, powders, and perfumes on skin in the treatment field.
- Wear loose cotton clothing on the chest.
- Protect chest from direct sunlight.
- Avoid application of heat to the area being treated.
- Report any discomfort to physician and nurse.

NURSING DIAGNOSIS

- Potential for impaired swallowing related to inflammation of the esophagus related to vena cava obstruction and/or effects of radiation therapy

INTERVENTIONS

- Assess patient's ability to swallow liquids and solids.
- Observe closely for aspiration.
- Provide analgesics as indicated.
- Change diet to avoid irritating foods (spicy or coarse).
- Avoid alcohol and tobacco use.
- Provide frequent mouth care.
- Alter medication schedule and form or rate (decrease pill size, liquids, etc.) as needed.
- Provide adequate hydration and nutrition.

As the acute phase of SVCS passes, the patient will be ready to become more involved in self-care, and anticipatory guidance can be given to facilitate continued therapy and detection of any changes in condition.

cell carcinoma. In fact, 50% of patients with small cell lung cancer have impaired water excretion.*

SIADH may be the presenting symptom in patients with small cell lung cancer.[38] Other cancers associated with SIADH include cancer of the duodenum and pancreas, lymphoma, thymoma, and mesothelioma. Several chemotherapeutic agents, cisplatin, cyclophosphamide, vinblastine, and vincristine have demonstrated the inappropriate release of ADH.[79,123,143]

The incidence of SIADH is rising because of the increased incidence of small cell lung cancer and other cancers associated with the ectopic production of ADH.[38]

Nonmalignant conditions that can account for SIADH are central nervous system disorders, pulmonary infections, asthma, the use of positive pressure respirators, the administration of certain medications, hypoadrenalcorticism, lupus erythematous, and acute intermittent porphyria.[87]

PATHOPHYSIOLOGY

All body fluids are solutions containing various concentrations of solute (salt) and solvent (fluid or water). The concentration of salt in body fluid creates an osmotic pressure. Measurement of osmotic pressure is referred to as osmolality or osmolarity. It is expressed in osmols (Osm) or milliosmols (mOsm) per kilogram of either water (osmolality) or solution (osmolarity). In a steady state, normal osmolality is maintained at a constant level of 280 to 300 mOsm/kg.[158,160] The osmolarity and volume of the extracellular fluid and the

urine are maintained by a balance of fluid intake and urinary excretion.

Fluid intake is maintained by the thirst mechanism located in the hypothalamus (Figure 19-16). Lack of water increases the osmolality of the extracellular fluid, which activates the sensation of thirst. Fluid intake is then increased to restore the fluid balance. If excess fluid is ingested, it is excreted to maintain the balance.[79]

The second portion of the osmolarity-regulating system is urinary excretion. The amount of urine excreted by the kidneys depends on how much fluid is reabsorbed and circulated throughout the body.[83,123] This regulation of fluid intake and output through the kidneys is controlled by the presence of ADH in the kidneys.

ADH is produced by the hypothalamus and transported to the posterior pituitary where it is stored. Changes in ADH production and secretion (increase or decrease) are controlled by receptors in the kidneys, heart, and brain, in response to extracellular or intravascular volume[55,83,123] (Figure 19-16). ADH secretion is extremely sensitive and responds to a 1% to 2% change in osmolality.

When plasma osmolarity is increased or plasma volume is decreased, ADH is secreted from the pituitary gland. Once in the kidneys, ADH increases the permeability of the distal tubule and the collection duct, which allows more water reabsorption. This enhanced amount of water enters the vascular system, diluting solutes, lowering plasma osmolarity, and resulting in concentrated urine excretion. Decreased plasma or blood volume also stimulates ADH secretion. A moderate increase in ADH occurs with a 10%

---

*References 33, 38, 55, 86, 107, 123, 124.

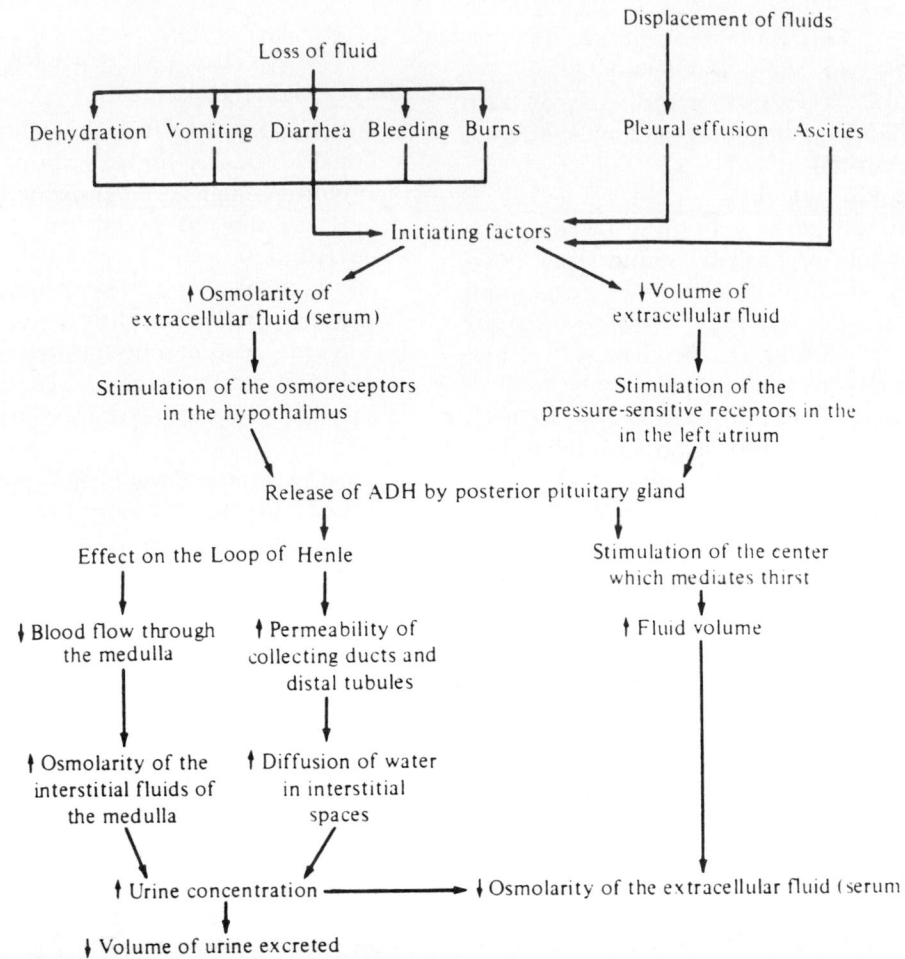

Figure 19-16 Feedback mechanism regulating the release of ADH. (From Yasko JM: Syndrome of inappropriate antidiuretic hormone secretion. In Yasko JM, editor: Guidelines for cancer care: symptom management, Reston, Va, 1983, Reston Publishing Co.)

blood loss, and a 25% blood loss can produce 20 to 50 times the normal rate of ADH secretion.[83] This response maintains arterial blood pressure.

If plasma osmolarity is decreased, as in the presence of excessive water intake, ADH secretion is halted. This decreases the permeability to water of the renal distal tubule and the collecting duct, allowing more water to be excreted as dilute urine. An increase in plasma or blood volume also stops the release of ADH. The drinking of alcohol also inhibits ADH secretion. In summary, the thirst mechanism and the ADH feedback mechanisms (Figure 19-16) regulate body fluids and maintain a constant osmolality.[79, 123]

A variety of conditions can disrupt the body fluid regulating system and cause the inappropriate secretion of ADH. Three pathophysiologic mechanisms are responsible for SIADH:

- Inappropriate secretion of ADH from the supraoptic-hypophyseal system. This mechanism results from CNS disorders such as head trauma, stroke, meningitis, brain abscess, CNS hemor-

rhage, CNS tumors (both primary and metastatic), encephalitis, and Guillain-Barré syndrome. Postoperative patients, patients in shock, patients experiencing status asthmaticus, pain, or high stress levels, and patients on positive pressure breathing may also experience SIADH through this mechanism. These conditions increase intrathoracic pressure and/or decrease venous return to the heart. Cardiac output decreases, leading to decreased plasma volume, stimulating ADH secretion.[83]

- ADH or an ADH-like substance is secreted by cells outside of the supraoptic-hypophyseal system, referred to as ectopic secretion. Infections within the pulmonary system such as those caused by bacteria or viruses may release ADH by this mechanism. This may also be one process leading to SIADH seen in patients with a malignancy.

- The action of ADH on the renal distal tubules is enhanced. Various drugs can stimulate or potentiate the release of ADH. These include narcotics such as morphine, nicotine, tranquilizers, barbiturates, general anesthetics, potassium supplements, thiazide diuretics, hypoglycemia agents such as chlorpropamide (Diabinese), clofibrate (Atromid-S), acetaminophen (paracetamol, Tylenol), isoproterenol, and four antineoplastic agents: cisplatin (Platinol), cyclophosphamide (Cytoxan), vinblastine (Velban), and vincristine (Oncovin).[83,123]

Patients with cancer may have SIADH resulting from any one of these three mechanisms. Intrathoracic or mediastinal tumors can increase intrathoracic pressure, resulting in a decreased venous return and decreased cardiac output, which stimulates the release of ADH. Patients with small (oat) cell lung cancer (50%), pancreatic cancer, lymphomas, and thymomas have demonstrated synthesis and secretion of ADH or an ADH-like substance from the neoplastic tissue.[143,160] Patients receiving chemotherapy that includes cisplatin (Platinol), cyclophosphamide (Cytoxan), vinblastine (Velban), or vincristine (Oncovin) have the potential to develop SIADH.

SIADH is associated with water excess and is due to the ectopic production of ADH. ADH increases the permeability of the kidney to water, promoting water reabsorption and decreasing urinary output. This may be associated with hyponatremia. Hyponatremia may be due to excessive loss of sodium or excessive gain of water. It is always due to a relatively greater water concentration than sodium concentration.[38]

However, hyponatremia is not solely diagnostic of SIADH. Some other disorders may also stimulate SIADH. In hypothyroidism and hypoadrenocorticism, the hormone deficiency is responsible, but the exact mechanism is unknown. Finally, SIADH can also be seen with hyponatremia secondary to sodium depletion (renal disease, vomiting, diarrhea, or diabetic acidosis) hypokalemia, glucocorticoid deficiency, third-spacing, and dilutional hyponatremia related to congestive heart failure, renal failure, or ascites related to liver disease.[38,55,87,124]

CLINICAL FEATURES

The clinical syndrome resulting from inappropriate secretion of ADH has the following features[38,55,123,143,160]:

- Hyponatremia (serum sodium less than normal level of 135 to 147 mEq/L)
- Decreased osmolality of serum and extracellular fluid (less than normal level of 280 to 300 mOsm/kg)
- Excessive water retention (water intoxication)
- Urine osmolarity greater than appropriate for plasma osmolarity, producing less than maximally dilute urine (abnormally high urine specific gravity)

- Continued urinary excretion of sodium (sodium in urine greater than 20 mEq/L) (washing of sodium in urine)
- Absence of fluid volume depletion (normal skin turgor and blood pressure)
- Suppression of plasma renin
- Normal renal, adrenal, and thyroid function

The symptomatology experienced by the patient with SIADH depends on the degree of duration of water retention and hyponatremia. Excessive water retention continues in spite of a decrease in the osmolality of serum and extracellular fluid. Urine is concentrated, the extracellular fluid expands, and this results in hyponatremia. Patients complain of thirst, anorexia, nausea, and vomiting. There is weight gain, lethargy, and muscle weakness. Irritability, personality changes, and mental confusion may occur and lead to seizures and coma.[38,55,123,124]

DIAGNOSIS

A differential diagnosis of SIADH is sometimes difficult since any one of the clinical features may be absent. Therefore, the presence of all of the features is not required for diagnosis. To support a clinical diagnosis of SIADH, a water loading test may be performed safely if the serum sodium is greater than 125 mEq/L and if the patient is asymptomatic.[15] Patient preparation for the test requires nothing by mouth and no nicotine for 12 hours. Serum osmolality levels and serum, BUN, creatinine, Na^+, K^+, and Cl^- levels are obtained. The patient is weighed.

The water loading test is performed in the following manner[160]:

- Instruct the patient to remain recumbent during the duration of the test, which is 5 to 6 hours.
- Administer 300 ml of water 1 hour before test begins to replace insensible fluid losses during the period of nothing by mouth.
- Administer water (20 ml/kg) within 30 minutes.
- Collect urine hourly for 5 hours.
- Monitor patient for nausea, abdominal pain, feeling of fullness, desire to defecate, fatigue, shortness of breath, and chest pain.
- Calculate urine volume, osmolality, and specific gravity as follows:

	NORMAL RESULTS	RESULTS SEEN WITH SIADH
Urine volume	80% excreted	<40% excreted
Urine osmolality	100 to 1,000 mOsm/kg	<100 mOsm/kg
Specific gravity	1.015 to 1.025	<1.003

Serum and urine levels of ADH, which would be elevated in the presence of SIADH, can also be measured.

TREATMENT MODALITIES

The primary treatment of choice for SIADH is to treat or eliminate the underlying cause. Other medical orders would include:

- Discontinue any medications that might cause SIADH.
- Restrict fluids to 500 to 1000 ml/24 hr depending on the severity until there is an increase in the plasma osmolality. This may take 4 to 10 days. The slowest response is seen in patients with ADH-secreting tumors.[160]
- Administer pharmacologic agents that interfere with the action of ADH on the renal tubules and induce polyuria, such as lithium carbonate (300 mg/day) or demeclocycline, a tetracycline derivative (600 mg to 1200 mg/day) (greater renal toxicity is seen with 1200 mg/day).[143] The total drug dose is divided and given 2 or 3 times a day.
- If symptoms of water intoxication are severe, administer hypertonic (5% NaCl) solution with or without furosemide (Lasix) via volumetric pump.

Currently no drugs are available that directly suppress the synthesis or release of ADH from malignant tissue, but effective tumor treatment and/or the use of lithium carbonate or demeclocycline have produced a resolution of the syndrome. Lithium carbonate disrupts the action of ADH on the kidneys, resulting in polyuria. Demeclocycline interferes with the action of ADH, producing an isotonic or hypotonic urine and an increase in serum sodium.[123]

Serum sodium levels should be monitored very closely during treatment for SIADH. Correction of the serum sodium should be limited to a rate of rise of 0.5 to 1 mEq/L/hr to minimize the risk of central pontine myelinolysis leading to long-lasting neurologic damage.[143]

PROGNOSIS

SIADH can be successfully treated as evidenced by a return to normal levels of serum and extracellular osmolality, serum sodium and urine osmolality, and specific gravity. The rapidity and duration of response is highly dependent on the underlying cause.

SIADH usually resolves with tumor regression, but it can persist despite control of the tumor. It may recur, suggesting tumor progression but recurrence is sometimes seen with stable disease during the maintenance phase of therapy. Neurologic impairment from water intoxication is usually reversible and does not require long-term rehabilitation.[38]

If the underlying cause is not eliminated, the SIADH may be a chronic problem and require ongoing intermittent management.[38,55,86]

Nursing Management

The primary nursing intervention for a patient diagnosed with SIADH is patient education and emotional support to facilitate patient compliance.[49,82,107,121]

NURSING DIAGNOSES

- Alteration in fluid volume: excess related to fluid retention (due to SIADH) and possible hyponatremia
- Potential for fluid volume deficit related to fluid restriction as treatment for SIADH

INTERVENTIONS

- Assess for signs or symptoms of alteration in fluid volume:
  Excess — rales, shortness of breath, neck vein distention, weight gain, edema of sacrum and/or lower extremities
  Deficit — dry mucous membranes, poor skin turgor, weight loss, rapid thready pulse, orthostatic hypotension, restlessness
- Auscultate lungs for breath sounds every 4 hours.
- Monitor cardiac function and tissue perfusion.
- Monitor intake and output closely:
  Restrict fluids as ordered (500 to 700 ml/24 hours).
  Allocate fluids per shift as per discussion with patient.
  Give pills and medications with meals to allow flexibility with fluid rations.
  Monitor intravenous infusions carefully using a flow regulator.
  Accurately measure urine output. Intake and output should be almost equal until serum sodium is within normal limits.

- Obtain a daily weight.
- Monitor laboratory values (serum electrolytes, BUN, creatinine, calcium, magnesium) with special attention to the following:

  Serum plasma osmolality. As SIADH progresses, plasma osmolality decreases, which causes the brain to swell and level of consciousness (LOC) to decrease. Therefore, serum osmolality can predict LOC.
  Serum sodium. Hypernatremia may result from overcorrection of low serum levels. Accompanying signs and symptoms of hypernatremia include thirst, dry mucous membranes, irritability, lethargy, and seizures.

- Obtain urine osmolality and specific gravity.
- Monitor skin integrity and provide skin care.

NURSING DIAGNOSIS
- Potential for alteration in oral mucous membranes related to fluid restriction

INTERVENTIONS
- Thoroughly assess the oral cavity daily.
- Provide oral care every 2 to 4 hours as needed:
  Use mouth washes with little to no alcohol.
  Discourage smoking and drinking alcohol.
  Avoid spicy and mechanically harsh foods.
  Use mouth moisturizers and artificial saliva as needed.

NURSING DIAGNOSIS
- Potential for alteration in thought processes related to low serum sodium

INTERVENTIONS
- Assess neurologic status:
  Determine level of consciousness, noting any changes in sensorium.
  Check muscles and tendon reflexes for twitching.
  Monitor for seizure activity if serum sodium < 120 mEq/L.
- Initiate safety precautions:
  Monitor patient activities.
  Assist patient with transfer and ambulation.
  Use bed rails at night.
- Increase safety measures if there is a change in LOC or a serum sodium < 120 mEq/L:
  Orient frequently to time and place.
  Pad bed rails.
  Use restraints as necessary.
  Implement seizure precautions: padded tongue blade and airway at bedside; no oral thermometers.

Many patients with extreme hyponatremia cannot recollect much of their experience during the SIADH event. This points out the need to provide measures to ensure safety and to reduce anxiety.

CONCLUSION
Successful management of patients with oncologic complications requires expertise from all members of the health care team. It requires in-depth knowledge in oncology, but also in many related areas such as immunology, pharmacology, cardiopulmonary and critical care. The nurse is in a pivotal role as coordinator of the care and as patient advocate to help the patient and family deal with the impact of the illness on their lives.

BIBLIOGRAPHY
1. Abraham J and Polomano R: Disseminated intravascular coagulation. In Polomano RC and Miller SE, editors: Understanding and managing oncologic emergencies, Monograph, Columbus, Ohio, 1987, Adria Laboratories.
2. Anderson RP and Li W: Segmental replacement of superior vena cava with spiral vein graft, Ann Thorac Surg 36(1):85, 1983.
3. Bailes BK: Disseminated intravascular coagulation principles, treatment, nursing management, AORN J 55(2):517, 1992.
4. Baird S, editor: Prevention and management of neutropenia in the cancer patient, Oncol Nurs Forum Suppl 17(1):3, 1990.
5. Bajorunas DR, editor: Advances in the hypercalcemia of malignancy, Semin Oncol 17(Suppl 5):1, 1990.
6. Baldwin PD: Epidural spinal cord compression secondary to metastatic disease: a review of the literature, Cancer Nurs 6(6):441, 1983.
7. Barbiere CC: Are you listening? Cardiac tamponade: diagnosis and emergency intervention, Crit Care Nurse 10(4):7, 1990.
8. Barbiere CC: Cardiac tamponade: diagnosis and emergency intervention, Crit Care Nurse 10(4):20, 1990.
9. Barry S: Septic shock: special needs of patients with cancer, Oncol Nurs Forum 16(1):31, 1989.
10. Bass J and others: Superior vena cava syndrome: report of a new operative technique, J Natl Med Assoc 72(11):1105, 1980.
11. Beattie S and Meinhardt SL: Transesophageal echocardiography: advanced technology for the cardiac patient, Crit Care Nurse 12(8):42, 1992.
12. Berger NA: Introduction: An overview of oncologic emergencies, Semin Oncol 16(6):461, 1989.
13. Bick R: Disseminated intravascular coagulation and related syndromes: etiology, pathophysiology, diagnosis and management, Am J Hematol 5(3):265, 1978.
14. Bockheim CM: What is the role of edtidronate

in the treatment of hypercalcemia? Highlights Antineoplast Drugs 7(3):59, 1989.

15. Boh D and VanSon A: The water load test, Am J Nurs 82(1):112, 1982.

16. Bradof J, Sands MJ, and Lakin PC: Symptomatic venous thrombosis of the upper extremity complicating permanent transvenous pacing: reversal with streptokinase infusion, Am Heart J 104(5):1112, 1982.

17. Brandt B: A nursing protocol for the client with neutropenia, Oncol Nurs Forum 11(2):24, 1984.

18. Braunwald E: Pericardial disease. In Braunwald E and others, editors: Harrison's principles of internal medicine, ed 11, New York, 1991, McGraw-Hill Book Co.

19. Briening EP: Septic shock: tough cases that teach the most, RN 51(9):36, 1988.

20. Britton D and Yasko JM: Hypercalcemia. In Yasko JM, editor: Guidelines for cancer care: symptom management, Reston, Va, 1983, Reston Publishing Co.

21. Bruckman JE and Bloomer WD: Management of spinal cord compression, Semin Oncol 5(2):135, 1978.

22. Buchsel PC: Managing infections in the neutropenic oncology patient. In Challenges in treatment and management, Proceedings of the Sixth National Conference on Cancer Nursing, Atlanta, 1992, American Cancer Society.

23. Byrne TN: Spinal cord compression from epidural metastases. N Engl J Med 327:614, 1992.

24. Calafato A and Jessys AL: Body fluid composition, alteration in: hypercalcemia. In McNally JC and others, editors: Guidelines for oncology nursing practice, ed 2, Philadelphia, 1991, WB Saunders Co.

25. Carlson A: Infection prophylaxis in the patient with cancer, Oncol Nurs Forum 12(3):56, 1985.

26. Cawley M: Alteration in cardiac output, decreased: related to superior vena cava syndrome. In McNally JC and others, editors: Guidelines for oncology nursing practice, ed 2, Philadelphia, 1991, WB Saunders Co.

27. Ciszewski M: Spinal cord compression. In Brown MH and others, editors: Standards of oncology nursing practice, New York, 1986, John Wiley & Sons.

28. Clark JC, McGee RF, and Preston R: Nursing management of responses to the cancer experience. In Clark JC and McGee RF, editors: Core curriculum for oncology nursing, ed 2, Philadelphia, 1992, WB Saunders Co.

29. Colman RW and Rubin RN: Disseminated intravascular coagulation due to malignancy, Semin Oncol 17(2):172, 1990.

30. Concilus EM and Bohachick PA: Cancer: peri-cardial effusion and tamponade, Cancer Nurs 7(5):391, 1984.

31. Coward D: Cancer-induced hypercalcemia, Cancer Nurs 9(3):125, 1986.

32. Cowcher K and Hanks GW: Long-term management of respiratory symptoms in advanced cancer, J Pain Symptom Mgt 5(5):320, 1990.

33. Culpepper RN, Porter GA, and Roddam RF: Why is the serum sodium low? Patient Care 20(7):94, 1986.

34. Dangel RN: Injury, potential for, related to disseminated intravascular coagulation (DIC). In McNally JC, and others, editors: Guidelines for oncology nursing practice, ed 2, Philadelphia, 1991, WB Saunders Co.

35. Deisseroth A and Wallenstein R: Use of hematopoietic growth factors. In DeVita VT, Hellman S, and Rosenberg AS, editors: Cancer: principle and practice in oncology, ed 3, Philadelphia, 1989, JB Lippincott Co.

36. Delaney TF and Oldfield EH: Spinal cord compression. In DeVita VT, Hellman S, and Rosenberg SA, editors: Cancer: principle and practice in oncology, ed 3, Philadelphia, 1989, JB Lippincott Co.

37. Desser RK, Brown CM, and Bitran JD: The management of malignant pleural effusions, Monograph, Evansville, Ind, 1984, Bristol-Myers Co.

38. Dietz K and Flaherty AM: Oncologic emergencies. In Groenwald SL and others, editors: Cancer nursing principles and practices, ed 2, Boston, 1990, Jones and Bartlett Publishers.

39. Donoghue M: Spinal cord compression. In Yasko JM, editor: Guidelines for cancer care: symptom management, Reston, Va, 1983, Reston Publishing Co.

40. Donoghue M: Superior vena cava syndrome. In Yasko JM, editor: Guidelines for cancer care: symptom management, Reston, Va, 1983, Reston Publishing Co.

41. Dutcher JP: Bleeding and coagulopathy. In Dutcher JP and Wiernik PH, editors: Handbook of hematologic and oncologic emergencies, New York, 1987, Plenum Medical Book Co.

42. Dyck S: Surgical instrumentation as a palliative treatment for spinal cord compression, Oncol Nurs Forum 18(3):515, 1991.

43. Einzig AI: Hypercalcemia in malignancy. In Dutcher JP and Wiernik PH, editors: Handbook of hematologic and oncologic emergencies, New York, 1987, Plenum Medical Book Co.

44. Ellerhorst-Ryan JM: Septic shock: understanding and managing a crisis. In Challenges in treatment and management, Proceedings of the Sixth National Conference on Cancer Nursing, Atlanta, 1992, American Cancer Society.

45. Epstein C and Bakanauskas A: Clinical management of DIC: Early nursing interventions, Crit Care Nurs 11(10):42, 1991.

46. Estes ME: Management of the cardiac tamponade patient: a nursing framework, Crit Care Nurse 5(5):17, 1985.

47. Fuen LG and Thurer R: Tube drainage and intrapleural therapy for malignant pleural effusions: a portfolio of case reports, Monograph, Evansville, Ind, 1990, Bristol-Myers Co.

48. Fingar BL: Sclerosing agents used to control malignant pleural effusions, Hospital Pharmacy 27:622-628, July, 1992.

49. Finley JP: Nursing care of patients with metabolic and physiological oncological emergencies. In Clark JC and McGee RF, editors: Core curriculum for oncology nursing, ed 2, Philadelphia, 1991, WB Saunders Co.

50. Frommel L, Mesa D, and Outlaw E: Septic shock. In Brown MH and others, editors: Standards of oncology nursing practice, New York, 1986, John Wiley & Sons.

51. Gentzch P: Mobility, impaired physical, related to spinal cord compression. In McNally JC and others, editors: Guidelines for oncology nursing practice, ed 2, Philadelphia, 1991, WB Saunders Co.

52. Gilbert MR and Grossman SA: Incidence and nature of neurologic problems in patients with solid tumors, Amer J Med 81:951, 1986.

53. Gilbert RW, Kim J, and Posner JB: Epidural spinal cord compression from metastatic tumor: diagnosis and treatment, Ann Neurol 3(1):40, 1978.

54. Glover DJ and Glick JH: Managing oncologic emergencies involving structural dysfunction, CA 35(4):238, 1985.

55. Glover DJ and Glick JH: Oncologic emergencies. In Holleb AI, Fink DJ, and Murphy GP, editors: American Cancer Society textbook of clinical oncology, Atlanta, 1991, American Cancer Society.

56. Gobel BH and Lawler PE: Malignant pleural effusions, Oncol Nurs Forum 12(4):49, 1985.

57. Gray BH and others: Safety and efficacy of thrombolytic therapy for superior vena cava syndrome. Chest 99:54, 1991.

58. Griffin J: Be prepared for the bleeding patient, Nursing 16(6):34, 1986.

59. Grossman SA and Lossignol D: Diagnosis and treatment of epidural metastases, Oncology 4(4):47, 1990.

60. Gulcap R and Dutcher JP: Fever and infection. In Dutcher JP and Wiernik PH, editors: Handbook of hematologic and oncologic emergencies, New York, 1987, Plenum Medical Book Co.

61. Gulcap R and others: Comparative study of pamidronate disodium and etidronate disodium in the treatment of cancer-related hypercalcemia, J Clin Oncol 10(1):134, 1992.

62. Harnett S: Septic shock in the oncology patient, Cancer Nurs 12(4):191, 1989.

63. Henry P, Seery R, and Outlaw EM: Hypercalcemia. In Brown MH and others, editors: Standards of oncology nursing practice, New York, 1986, John Wiley & Sons.

64. Hewitt JB and Janssen WR: A management strategy for malignancy-induced pleural effusion: long-term thoracostomy drainage, Oncol Nurs Forum 14(5):17, 1987.

65. Hilderley LJ: Spinal cord compression: the nurse's role in early detection and rehabilitation. In Challenges in treatment and management, Proceedings of the Sixth National Conference on Cancer Nursing, Atlanta, 1992, American Cancer Society.

66. Hilton G and Frei J: High-dose methylprednisolone in the treatment of spinal cord injuries, Heart Lung 20(6):675, 1991.

67. Hogan CM: Sexual dysfunction related to disease process and treatment. In McNally JC et al, editors: Guidelines for oncology nursing practice, ed 2, Philadelphia, 1991, WB Saunders Co.

68. Hunter JC: Nursing care of patients with structural oncological emergencies. In Clark JC and McGee RF, editors: Core curriculum for oncology nursing, ed 2, Philadelphia, 1992, WB Saunders Co.

69. Hydzik CA: Alteration in cardiac output, decreased: related to cardiac tamponade. In McNally JC and others, editors: Guidelines for oncology nursing practice, ed 2, Philadelphia, 1991, WB Saunders Co.

70. Joiner GA and Kolodychuk GR: Neoplastic cardiac tamponade, Crit Care Nurse 11(2):50, 1991.

71. Jenkins J: Pleural effusion. In Baird SB, editor: Decision making in oncology nursing, Philadelphia, 1988, BC Decker, Inc.

72. Jennings BM: Improving your management of DIC, Nursing 9(5):60, 1979.

73. Johndrow PD and Thornton S: Syndrome of inappropriate antidiuretic hormone: a growing concern, Focus Crit Care 12(5):29, 1985.

74. Joshi J: Epidemiology of infections in cancer patients, Mediguide Infec Dis 9(2):1, 1989.

75. Kanner R: Epidural spinal cord compression. In Dutcher JP and Wiernik PH, editors: Handbook of hematologic and oncologic emergencies, New York, 1987, Plenum Medical Book Co.

76. Kern L and Omery A: Decreased cardiac output in the critical care setting, Nurs Diagnosis 3(3):94, 1992.

77. Khandheria BK and Oh J: Transesophageal echo-

cardiography: state-of-the-art and future directions, Am J Cardiol 69, June: 61H, 1992.

78. Klein DM and Witek-Janusek L: Advances in immunotherapy of sepsis. Dimens Crit Care Nurs 11(2):75, 1992.

79. Kliger A and Lovett D: Electrolyte abnormalities in cancer patients. In Yarbro J and Bornstein R, editors: Oncologic emergencies, New York, 1981, Grune & Stratton, Inc.

80. Kraemer K: Superior vena cava syndrome. In Johnson BL and Gross J, editors: Handbook of oncology nursing, New York, 1985, John Wiley & Sons.

81. Kralstein J and Frishman W: Malignant pericardial disease: diagnosis and treatment. In Dutcher JP and Wiernik PH, editors: Handbook of hematologic and oncologic emergencies, New York, 1987, Plenum Medical Book Co.

82. Kratcha-Sveningson L: Body fluid composition, alteration in: syndrome of inappropriate antidiuretic hormone (SIADH). In McNally JC and others, editors: Guidelines for oncology nursing practice, ed 2, Philadelphia, 1991, WB Saunders Co.

83. Lane G and Peirce AG: When persistence pays off, Nursing 12(1):44, 1982.

84. Larkin M and Benson LM: Ineffective airway clearance. In Clark JC and McGee RF, editors: Core curriculum for oncology nursing, ed 2, Philadelphia, 1992, WB Saunders Co.

85. Lazarus HM, Creger RJ, and Gerson SL: Infectious emergencies in oncology patients, Semin Oncol 16(6):543, 1989.

86. Lind JM: Ectopic hormonal production: nursing implications, Semin Oncol Nurs 1(4):251, 1985.

87. Lindaman C: SIADH is your patient at risk? Nursing 22(6):60, 1992.

88. Littleton M: Pathophysiology and assessment of sepsis and septic shock, Crit Care Nurs Q 11(1):30, 1988.

89. Lokich J and Goodman R: Superior vena cava syndrome, JAMA 321(1):58, 1975.

90. Mahon SM: Signs and symptoms associated with malignancy-induced hypercalcemia, Cancer Nurs 12(3):153, 1989.

91. Mangan CM: Malignant pericardia effusions: pathophysiology and clinical correlates, Oncol Nurs Forum 19(8):215, 1991.

92. Marcus SL and Fuks JZ: Syndrome of inappropriate antidiuretic hormone secretion and hyponatremia. In Dutcher JP and Wirnik PH, editors: Handbook of hematologic and oncologic emergencies, New York, 1987, Plenum Medical Book Co.

93. Mayer DK: Cardiac tamponade. In Baird SB, editor: Decision making in oncology nursing, Philadelphia, 1988, BC Decker, Inc.

94. Mayer DK: Spinal cord compression. In Baird SB, editor: Decision making in oncology nursing, Philadelphia, 1988, BC Decker, Inc.

95. Mayer DK: Superior vena cava syndrome. In Baird SB, editor: Decision making in oncology nursing, Philadelphia, 1988, BC Decker, Inc.

96. Mayer DK: Disseminated intravascular coagulation. In Baird SB, editor: Decision making in oncology nursing, Philadelphia, 1988, BC Decker, Inc.

97. Mayer DK: Hypercalcemia. In Baird SB, editor: Decision making in oncology nursing, Philadelphia, 1988, BC Decker, Inc.

98. Mayer DK: Inappropriate antidiuretic hormone syndrome. In Baird SB, editor: Decision making in oncology nursing, Philadelphia, 1988, BC Decker, Inc.

99. Mayer DK: Septic shock. In Baird SB, editor: Decision making in oncology nursing, Philadelphia, 1988, BC Decker, Inc.

100. McFadden ME and Sartorius SE: Multiple systems organ failure in the patient with cancer. Part I: Pathophysiologic perspectives, Oncol Nurs Forum 19(5):719, 1992.

101. McFadden ME and Sartorius SE: Multiple system organ failure in the patient with cancer Part II: Nursing implications, Oncol Nurs Forum 19(5):727, 1992.

102. McGillick K: DIC: the deadly paradox, RN 45:41, 1982.

103. McMorrow ME and Cooney-Daniello M: When to suspect septic shock, RN, 54(10):32, 1991.

104. Meriney DK: Application of Orem's conceptual framework to patients with hypercalcemia related to breast cancer, Cancer Nurs 13(5):316, 1990.

105. Meriney DK: Diagnosis and management of acute promyelocytic leukemia with disseminated intravascular coagulopathy: A case study, Oncol Nurs Forum 17(3):379, 1990.

106. Mersky C: DIC: identification and management, Hosp Pract 17:83, 1982.

107. Miaskowski C: Oncologic emergencies. In Baird SB, McCorkle R, Grant M, editors: Cancer nursing a comprehensive textbook. Philadelphia, 1991, WB Saunders Co.

108. Miller SE: Superior vena cava syndrome. In Polomano RN and Miller SE, editors: Understanding and managing oncologic emergencies, Monograph, Columbus, Ohio, 1987, Adria Laboratories.

109. Miller SE and Campbell DB: Malignant pericardial effusions. In Polomano RC and Miller SE,

editors: Understanding and managing oncologic emergencies, Monograph, Columbus, Ohio, 1987, Adria Laboratories.

110. Miller SE and Campbell DB: Pleural effusions in malignant disease. In Polomano RC and Miller SE, editors: Understanding and managing oncologic emergencies, Monograph, Columbus, Ohio, 1987, Adria Laboratories.

111. Mizock B: Septic shock—a metabolic perspective, Arch Intern Med 144(3):579, 1984.

112. Moores DWO: Malignant pleural effusion, Semin Oncol 18(Suppl 2):59, 1991.

113. Morse LK, Heery ML, and Flynn KT: Early detection to avert the crisis of superior vena cava syndrome, Cancer Nurs 8(4):228, 1985.

114. Mundy G: Options for correcting hypercalcemia of malignancy, Hospital Therapy, Feb:52, 1988.

115. Nissenblatt M: Oncologic emergencies, Am Fam Phys 20(2):104, 1979.

116. Olopade OI and Ultmann JE: Malignant effusions, CA 41(3):167, 1991.

117. Parish J and others: Etiologic considerations in superior vena cava syndrome, Mayo Clin Proc 56(7):407, 1981.

118. Perez CA, Presant CA, and VanAmburg AL: Management of superior vena cava syndrome, Semin Oncol 5(2):123, 1978.

119. Perry A: Shock complications: recognition and management, Crit Care Nurs Q 11(1):1, 1988.

120. Pilapil F: Disseminated intravascular coagulation (DIC). In Brown MH and others, editors: Standards of oncology nursing practice, New York, 1986, John Wiley & Sons.

121. Pizzo PA and Myers J: Infections in the cancer patient. In DeVita VT, Hellman S and Rosenberg SA, editors: Cancer: principles and practice in oncology, ed 3, Philadelphia, 1989, JB Lippincott Co.

122. Poe CM and Radford AI: The challenge of hypercalcemia in cancer, Oncol Nurs Forum 12(6):29, 1985.

123. Poe CM and Taylor LM: Syndrome of inappropriate antidiuretic hormone: assessment and nursing implications, Oncol Nurs Forum 16(3):373, 1989.

124. Portlock C and Goffinet D: Manual of clinical problems in oncology, ed 2, Boston, 1986, Little, Brown & Co.

125. Rahko PS and Shaver JA: Superior vena cava syndrome, Hosp Med 21(7):83, 1985.

126. Ratnoff OD: Hemostatic emergencies in malignancy, Semin Oncol 16(6):561, 1989.

127. Reichel J and Menon L: Pulmonary emergencies in oncology. In Dutcher JP and Wiernik PH, editors: Handbook of hematologic and oncologic emergencies, New York, 1987, Plenum Medical Book Co.

128. Rice V: Shock, a clinical syndrome: an update, Part 1 an overview of shock, Crit Care Nurse 11(4):20, 1991.

129. Rice V: Shock, a clinical syndrome: an update, Part 2 the stages of shock, Crit Care Nurse 11(4):74, 1991.

130. Rice V: Shock, a clinical syndrome: an update, Part 3, therapeutic management, Crit Care Nurse 11(4):34, 1991.

131. Rice V: Shock, a clinical syndrome: an update, Part 4 nursing care of the shock patient, Crit Care Nurse 11(7):28, 1991.

132. Rodriquez M and Dinapoli RP: Spinal cord compression, Mayo Clin Proc 55(7):442, 1980.

133. Rooney A and Haviley C: Nursing management of disseminated intravascular coagulation, Oncol Nurs Forum 12(1):15, 1985.

134. Rosch J and others: Gianturco expandable wire stents in the treatment of superior vena cava syndrome recurring after maximum tolerance radiation, Cancer 60(6):1243, 1987.

135. Rosetti A: Nursing care of patients treated with intrapleural tetracycline for control of malignant pleural effusion, Cancer Nurs 8(2):103, 1985.

136. Ruckdeschel JC: Management of malignant pleural effusion: An overview. Semin Oncol 15(suppl. 3):24, 1988.

137. Ruckdeschel JC and others: Intrapleural therapy for malignant pleural effusions, a randomized comparison of bleomycin and tetracycline, Chest 10(6):1528, 1991.

138. Sahn SA: Diagnosis pleural effusion, Hosp Med, 28(9):66, 1992.

139. Schruber JA: Impaired gas exchange. In Clark JC and McGee RF, editors: Core curriculum for oncology nursing, ed 2, Philadelphia, 1992, WB Saunders Co.

140. Sculier JP and others: Superior vena cava obstruction syndrome in small cell lung cancer, Cancer 57(4):847, 1986.

141. Shoemaker WC: Early diagnosis and management of pericardial tamponade, Hosp Med 14(11):7, 1978.

142. Siegrist C and Jones J: Disseminated intravascular coagulopathy and nursing implications, Semin Oncol Nurs 1(4):237, 1985.

143. Silverman P and Distelhorst CW: Metabolic emergencies in clinical oncology, Semin Oncol 16(6):504, 1989.

144. Siskind MM: A standard of care for the nursing diagnosis of ineffective airway clearance, Heart Lung 18(5):477, 1989.

145. Smith EL: Dyspnea and quality of life, Quality of Life—A Nursing Challenge 1(1):31, 1992.

146. Smith LH and Van Gulick AJ: Management of neutropenic enterocolitis in the patient with cancer, Oncol Nurs Forum 19(9):1337, 1992.

147. Spain RC and Wittlesey D: Respiratory emergencies in patients with cancer, Semin Oncol 16(6):471, 989.

148. Spross J and Stern R: Nursing management of oncology patients with a superior vena cava obstruction syndrome, Oncol Nurs Forum 6(3):3, 1979.

149. Theologides A: Neoplastic cardiac tamponade, Semin Oncol 5(2):181, 1978.

150. Tripp A: Hyper and hypocalcemia, Am J Nurs 769(7):1143, 1976.

151. Trounson LW: Nursing diagnosis and the syndrome of inappropriate antidiuretic hormone, J Postanesth Nurs 1(4):244, 1986.

152. Truett L: The septic syndrome, Cancer Nurs 14(4):175, 1991.

153. Utley JR: Relief of superior vena cava syndrome with spiral vein bypass grafting, J S C Med Assoc 81:489, 1985.

154. Varricchio CG and Jassak PF: Acute pulmonary disorders associated with cancer, Semin Oncol Nurs 1(4):269, 1985.

155. Warrell RP and Bockman RS: Metabolic emergencies. In DeVita VT, Hellman S and Rosenberg SA, editors: Cancer: principles and practice in oncology, ed 3, Philadelphia, 1989, JB Lippincott Co.

156. Wilson JK and Masaryk TJ: Neurologic emergencies in cancer patients, Semin Oncol 16(6):490, 1989.

157. Wood HA and Ellerhorst-Ryan JM: Ineffective breathing pattern. In McNally JC and others, editors: Guidelines for oncology nursing practice, ed 2, Philadelphia, 1991, WB Saunders Co.

158. Yahalom J: Superior vena cava syndrome. In DeVita VT, Hellman S, and Rosenberg SA, editors: Cancer: principles and practice in oncology, ed 3, Philadelphia, 1989, JB Lippincott Co.

159. Yasko JM: Septic shock. In Yasko JM, editor: Guidelines for cancer care: symptom management, Reston, Va, 1983, Reston Publishing Co.

160. Yasko JM: Syndrome of inappropriate antidiuretic hormone secretion. In Yasko JM, editor: Guidelines for cancer care: symptom management, Reston, Va, 1983, Reston Publishing Co.

161. Yasko JM and Schafer SL: Disseminated intravascular coagulation. In Yasko JM, editor: Guidelines for cancer care: symptom management, Reston, Va, 1983, Reston Publishing Co.

162. Yasko JM and Schafer SL: Neoplastic pericardial tamponade. In Yasko JM, editor: Guidelines for cancer care: symptom management, Reston, Va, 1983, Reston Publishing Co.

163. Zehner LC and Hoogstraten B: Malignant effusions and their management, Semin Oncol Nurs 1(4):259, 1985.

164. Zimberg M and Mahon SM: Understanding delirium: an impediment of quality of life, Quality of Life—A Nursing Challenge 1(1):3, 1992.

UNIT III

CANCER TREATMENT MODALITIES

CHAPTER 20

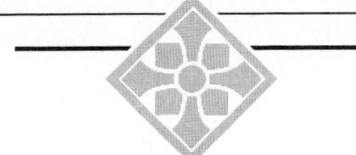

Surgery

Karen A. Pfeifer

The four primary modalities for the treatment of cancer are surgery, chemotherapy, radiation therapy, and biotherapy. Surgery can be the initial and preferred treatment of choice for many cancers. Advances in surgical techniques, a better understanding of the metastatic patterns of individual tumors, and intensive postoperative care have now made it possible for tumors to be removed from almost any part of the body.[15,16,33]

If cancer is diagnosed early enough and remains localized, surgery can effect a cure. Of the 40% of cancer patients treated by surgery alone, one third are cured. However, the key is to find the cancer while it is still localized. Surgical treatment failures are due primarily to the presence of metastasis at the time of initial diagnosis. Metastasis has occurred in 50% of cancer patients by the time their tumor is of sufficient size to be clinically detected.[7,16,24,27,42]

Approximately 90% of cancer patients experience some type of surgical intervention for diagnosis, initial treatment, or management of complications.[7] The nurse may encounter the cancer patient anywhere along this continuum. It is imperative that the nurse have a strong foundation of knowledge about surgical oncology upon which comprehensive plans of care can be designed and evaluated.

HISTORICAL PERSPECTIVE

Surgery is the oldest recorded form of curative treatment for cancer. At one time, surgery was the only effective method of cancer diagnosis and treatment. The first recorded surgical excision of a tumor is in the Edwin Smith Papyrus from the Egyptian Middle Kingdom (approximately 160 BC). However, Ephraim MacDowell is credited with describing modern surgical approaches to cancer in the United States. In 1809, he successfully excised a 22-lb ovarian tumor from Mrs. Jane Todd Crawford, who subsequently survived 30 years. This was the first of 13 ovarian resections performed by MacDowell, and it served as a great stimulus to the advancement of elective surgery. Other major individuals in the evolution of surgical oncology include Albert Theodore Billroth, who performed the first laryngectomy, gastrectomy, and esophagectomy during the period between 1860 and 1890. In the 1890s, William Stewart Halsted clarified the principles of en bloc tumor resections by his development of the radical mastectomy.[11,16,18,30,33]

However, in the early days of cancer surgery, surgical conditions were not optimal, and the operative procedures often resulted in severe postoperative disfigurement, rapid local recurrence of the cancer, or death. These outcomes were largely the results of undeveloped surgical techniques and intraoperative and postoperative problems (e.g., excessive blood loss and difficult anesthesia). Modern advances such as asepsis, improved anesthesia techniques, blood transfusions, the use of antibiotics, tracheostomy to alleviate airway obstruction, and nasogastric decompression of the stomach have increased the safety of surgical oncology.[11,33]

The preferred treatment for many years was to remove the cancer and as much of the surrounding tissue as possible. Therefore, the majority of the surgical procedures were radical in nature. In the mid-1950s, it was noted that despite the technical sophistication of these radical procedures, the mortality rates associated with certain cancer sites were not improving (e.g., breast cancer). Many cancers that were thought to be local processes were discovered to be systemic diseases with metastatic lesions. It then became evident that surgery alone, regardless of the magnitude of the procedure, was not effective for all cancers.[3]

APPLICATIONS FOR SURGICAL ONCOLOGY

Surgery has several applications in oncology as described below (see Figure 20-1).

Diagnosis of Disease

A histologic diagnosis is critical to planning treatment, because it is the only definitive diagnostic method and different types of cancer respond differently to treatment. The surgeon must obtain a tissue sample for histologic study when appropriate. Surgical techniques that are used to obtain tissue samples for examination include: *incisional biopsy* (where a wedge of tumor tissue is secured from tumors larger than 3 cm in diameter), *excisional biopsy* (where the entire tumor mass, usually less than 2 to 3 cm in diameter, and a margin of surrounding normal tissue are removed), *needle biopsy* (where core tissue samples are aspirated via a needle), or *endoscopy* (where small portions of tumors are removed with forceps following visual examination). The type of biopsy technique depends on a tumor's location, size, and growth characteristics (Table 20-1).[11,15,30,43]

The biopsy site should be in an area that will be removed at the time of surgery, or the biopsy should contain the total tumor. Incision lines should be made in cosmetically acceptable areas or folds of skin if possible. The specimen obtained for examination must contain normal tissue and tumor tissue for comparison by the pathologist. It must be intact and not crushed or contaminated. Only positive findings are definitive.[11,15,33]

The current trend is for a *two-step process*. The biopsy is performed first, followed by a period of time (usually within 2 weeks) before performing the surgical procedure. This accomplishes two things: (1) it allows the patient and/or significant others to begin adjusting to the diagnosis and (2) it allows the patient and/or significant others additional time to make decisions about treatment options.[15]

Staging of Disease

Diagnosis includes determining the type and extent of cancer at one point in time, or staging the disease. Tumor stage provides information relating to quantity and location of disease and prognosis.

Surgical staging is reserved for tumors that are inaccessible, difficult to evaluate, and incorrectly staged by any other means. A staging laparotomy (or diagnostic laparotomy) may be performed before radical surgery so that hidden intraperitoneal, lumboaortic, or liver metastasis can be ruled out. Staging laparotomy can also be done to obtain tissue samples and determine disease sites. In lymphoma, a staging laparotomy includes an exploratory laparotomy with splenectomy and biopsy of the liver and retroperitoneal lymph nodes. Metal clips are sometimes placed on organs to define the tumor and mark specific areas for future radiation therapy.[15,46]

Treatment of Disease

Surgical treatment of the cancer process focuses on five primary areas: primary treatment, adjuvant treatment, salvage treatment, palliative treatment, and combination treatment.

PRIMARY TREATMENT.　Primary treatment involves the removal of a malignant tumor and a margin of adjacent normal tissue. The goal is curative by the reduction of the patient's total body tumor burden. Cure can be accomplished through the following interventions. *Local excision* is the simple excision of a tumor and a small margin of normal tissue. This form is often used to treat skin cancer. *Wide excision* or *en bloc dissection* involves removal of the primary tumor, regional lymph nodes, intervening lymphatic channels, and involved neighboring structures. Examples include radical mastectomy, radical neck dissection, and abdominal-perineal resection. The second form of wide excision is *extended wide excision*, in which wide tumor infiltration in a particular region is removed. *Surgical treatment of cancer in situ* is accomplished by several special surgical techniques. These techniques cause little or no mutilation.[16,30,42,43]

ADJUVANT TREATMENT.　Adjuvant treatment involves the removal of tissues to decrease the risk of cancer incidence, progression, or recurrence. Adjuvant treatment includes *cytoreductive therapy*, also known as *debulking*, which is surgery to remove a large tumor burden. If the number of cancer cells can be reduced to a very small amount by surgical intervention, any remaining cancer cells are more likely to be destroyed by other systemic treatment. Cytoreductive therapy is commonly used in the treatment of ovarian cancer and neuroblastoma and other childhood tumors. Adjuvant therapy also includes *prophylactic surgery*, which is surgery performed on organs with underlying conditions that have a high incidence of subsequent cancer. For example, ulcerative colitis carries with it a high incidence of cancer of the colon. Approximately 40% of patients with total involvement of the colon will ultimately die with colon cancer. A colectomy may very well be warranted. The decision to do the surgery is based on (1) the statistical risk of cancer based on medical/family history, (2) the presence or absence of symptoms, (3) the degree of difficulty in diagnosing a cancer early should it develop, and (4) postoperative appearance and function.*

SALVAGE TREATMENT.　Salvage treatment involves the use of an extensive surgical approach to treat local recurrence after implementing a less extensive pri-

---

*References 7, 11, 16, 30, 33, 42, 43, 46, 48.

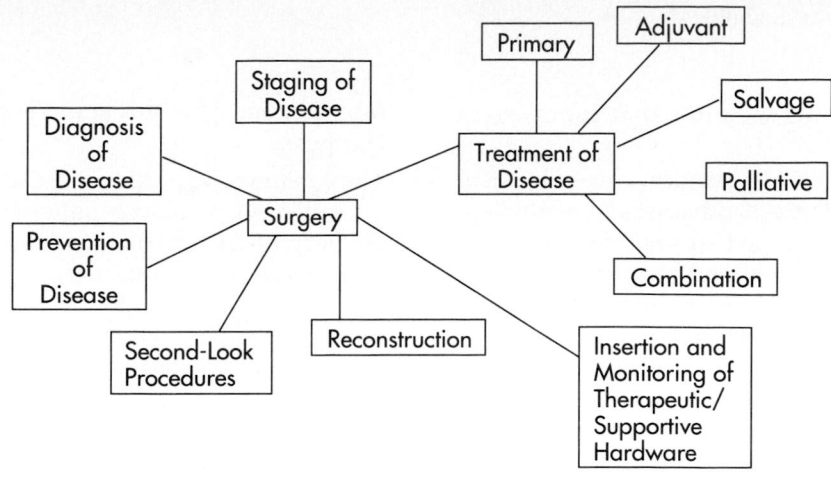

Figure 20–1 Applications for surgical oncology.

Table 20–1 Biopsy Techniques*

Type	Purpose	Technique	Advantages	Disadvantages
Incisional biopsy	Histologic study	Removal of a portion of tumor Secures a wedge of tumor tissue Usually performed at the tumor margin Performed on tumors larger than 3 cm in diameter	Usually done under local anesthesia Simple method to obtain diagnosis	Negative report does not eliminate possibility of cancer Specimen may not be large enough Tumor margins may not be defined Additional surgery required to remove tumor
Excisional biopsy	Histologic study Cure/control	Removal of the entire tumor mass with a margin of surrounding normal tissue Most common type of biopsy performed Performed on tumors that are small (2 to 3 cm) and accessible	Usually done under local anesthesia Can be definitive therapy—tumors of the lip, nose, ear, breast Quick, simple removal of tumor at time of biopsy Decreased cost	Cells may be implanted into tissue and incision, causing local recurrence
Needle biopsy	Histologic study	Aspiration of core tissue samples through a special needle inserted into the tumor Samples may be fluid or tissue Performed during surgery or via percutaneous route	Simple to perform Reliable Inexpensive Creates little disturbance in surrounding tissue Done under local anesthesia Does not require hospitalization	Specimen may not be large enough Needle may miss the tumor Improper handling may distort cells Risk of injury to adjacent structures Possible seeding of tumor cells along needle tract
Endoscopy (Bite biopsy)	Histologic study	Small portions of tumors are removed with forceps following visual examination Tumors of the gastrointestinal, genitourinary, and pulmonary tracts often diagnosed by this method	Allows access to tumors that might not otherwise be accessible except by laparotomy or thoracotomy Creates little disturbance in surrounding tissue Introduction of flexible instruments has made endoscopy more tolerable for the patient and easier for the surgeon	Risk of injury—perforation, hemorrhage

*References 11, 15, 30, 33, 38, 43.

mary approach (e.g., mastectomy after lumpectomy and radiation therapy).[43]

PALLIATIVE TREATMENT.   Surgical cures are not always possible. Nevertheless, advances in technology and research have lengthened survival for many cancer patients. However, prolonged survival brings with it the complications of disease or treatment. Surgery in these cases is then redirected from cure to palliation. Palliative surgery is used to decrease disease or treatment-related symptoms without trying to cure the cancer surgically. It is performed to prolong life and ensure a more comfortable quality of life for the patient and significant others. The benefit of palliative treatment depends on the biologic pace of the cancer, the patient's projected life expectancy, and expected treatment outcomes. Examples of palliative procedures include:

- Bone stabilization
- Relief of life-threatening obstruction or bleeding
- Removal of solitary metastasis (e.g., cerebral or hepatic)
- Treatment of oncologic emergencies (e.g., perforation, abscesses, spinal cord compression, hypersplenism)
- Treatment of complications from chemotherapy and radiation therapy (e.g., skin breakdown, fistulas, perforation, radiation proctitis)
- Ablative surgery, or removal of a hormone source, thereby altering the hormonal environment that encourages development and growth of a tumor (e.g., oophorectomy, orchiectomy, adrenalectomy)
- Management of cancer pain (e.g., nerve blocks, cordotomy, neurectomy, rhizotomy, sympathectomy, lobotomy, thalamotomy, tractotomy)

The goals of palliative surgery are to cure or relieve distressing symptoms, provide more comfort for the patient, and to prevent symptoms that will occur if the patient goes untreated.*

COMBINATION TREATMENT.   Combination treatment involves the use of surgery with other treatment modalities with the goals of improving tumor resectability, decreasing the extent of tumor removed, limiting the change in physical appearance and functional ability, and improving treatment outcomes. Examples include preoperative chemotherapy, radiation therapy, or biotherapy; intraoperative chemotherapy or radiation therapy; and postoperative chemotherapy, radiation therapy, or biotherapy. Current research in this area is aimed at timing of combination therapies, sequencing of combination therapies, and identifying those combination therapies that are most effective in controlling cancer with minimal effects.[2,43]

---

*References 1, 7, 11, 13, 16, 30, 42, 43, 46.

Insertion and Monitoring of Therapeutic/Supportive Hardware

Therapeutic/supportive hardware can be surgically implanted to promote patient comfort and/or ease delivery of treatment. (See Table 20-2 for additional information on this hardware.[43])

Second-Look Procedures

Second-look procedures involve follow-up surgery within a predetermined time frame after the original surgery and/or adjuvant treatment to check for the presence or absence of disease. Sites and volume of residual tumor are identified and resected when possible. Second-look procedures are usually done for those cancers that tend to recur locally (e.g., ovarian cancer). They may also be done to assess response to other treatment modalities or to evaluate residual disease following other treatment modalities. Second-look procedures are becoming more uncommon today because of the availability of other laboratory tests, diagnostic procedures, and tumor markers to assess treatment response.[43]

Reconstruction

The need to remove a sufficient margin of normal tissue around a tumor's border sometimes involves extensive surgical resection, bringing with it disfigurement and considerable impairment of function. Reconstructive surgery involves the reconstruction of anatomic defects caused by cancer surgery. Its purpose is to improve function and/or cosmetic appearance.[15,43,46]

Reconstructive surgery may be immediate and permanent, immediate and temporary, or postponed for safety reasons or until suitable graft tissue can be prepared and transferred. Those cancer surgeries requiring the largest number of subsequent reconstruction surgeries are surgery of the head and neck (facial reconstruction), breasts (breast reconstruction after mastectomy), and superficial tissues of all sites (skin graft after resection for melanoma). The *choice of method* depends on site, extent, loss of substance, chances of permanent cure, age, psychologic and general condition of the patient, availability of free skin grafts, and suitable internal prostheses.[46]

Teaching about options for reconstruction and counseling are usually begun before primary surgical therapy is initiated. Patients often fear that their desire for reconstructive surgery will be interpreted as vanity by family, friends, and health care personnel. They must be helped to see that reconstruction is desirable, positive, and sometimes necessary for achieving an optimal level of functioning.[15]

Prevention of Disease

Cancer prevention can entail *preventive surgery*. Surgery is the preferred treatment for precancerous and

Table 20–2 Therapeutic Hardware[21,34,35,43]

Type	Advantages	Disadvantages
Ventricular reservoirs	Increase patient comfort and decrease anxiety because of easy access Convenient use in the home setting Improved medication tolerance Duration of remission rates is often lengthened	Infection Catheter occlusion Catheter displacement
Central venous catheters (Short-term use)	Multiple lumen catheters permit simultaneous delivery of potentially incompatible medications and fluids Provide easy access to the vascular system for delivery of intravenous fluids, medications, parenteral hyperalimentation, and blood/blood products and for obtaining blood samples Increase patient comfort by reducing the number of venipunctures	Infection, especially the result of lack of cuff and subcutaneous tunnel Catheter displacement Severed catheter Possible restriction of patient activity Possible body image disturbance Requires sterile dressing changes, often prohibiting the patient from learning to care for catheter at home Frequent maintenance required
(Long-term use)	Multiple lumen catheters permit simultaneous delivery of potentially incompatible medications and fluids Provide easy access to the vascular system for delivery of chemotherapy, intravenous fluids, other medications, parenteral hyperalimentation, and blood/blood products and for obtaining blood samples Increase patient comfort by reducing the number of venipunctures Can be connected to internal or external pumps for continuous drug delivery Patient and/or significant other can learn to care for the catheter, permitting in-home use	Infection Catheter occlusion Catheter displacement Severed catheter Possible restriction of patient activity Possible body image disturbance Frequent maintenance required
Implantable vascular access devices	No external component—less disturbance in body image, lessened chance for infection, and increased comfort Provide easy access to the vascular system for delivery of chemotherapy, intravenous fluids, other medications, parenteral hyperalimentation, and blood/blood products and for obtaining blood samples Less interference with clothing Fewer restrictions on activities Minimal care required—infrequent need for irrigation No dressings, caps, or clamps Can be connected to external pumps for continuous drug delivery	Catheter occlusion Catheter displacement Port/catheter disconnection System may only be accessed through the skin—needle stick still required Improper surgical placement of the port (too deep; angled) can make access difficult Rotation of port

Adapted with permission from Szopa TJ: Surgery. In Ziegfeld CR, editor: Core curriculum for oncology nursing, ed 2, Philadelphia, 1992, WB Saunders Co.

in situ lesions of all epithelial surfaces (e.g., skin, oral cavity, and cervix). Benign polyps of the cervix, bladder, colon, and stomach are often removed surgically to reduce the risk of future cancer. Although rare, a second mastectomy is sometimes performed on those women with a high potential for developing a second breast cancer.[16]

PRINCIPLES OF SURGICAL ONCOLOGY

When considering surgery for the patient with cancer, the surgeon critically evaluates the following: tumor factors, tumor cell kinetics, and patient variables.

Tumor Factors

ANATOMIC LOCATION.   Tumor location can prevent or impede access for removal. The surgeon must decide whether the area of tumor can be encompassed by regional excision. Some tumors cannot be surgically treated because an adequate margin of normal tissue cannot be removed. Those tumors that involve or are attached to vital structures usually do not benefit from surgical resection. Superficial and well-encapsulated tumors are the most easily removed by surgery.[11,15,16]

HISTOLOGIC TYPE.   Certain histologic types of cancer are not treated by surgery because these cancers are disseminated at the outset of diagnosis. Examples include lymphomas, leukemias, and small cell cancer of the lung.[11]

TUMOR SIZE.   Smaller tumors are less likely to have spread and the patient is more likely to be cured by surgery. However, patients with larger tumors respond more favorably to surgery than to other treatment modalities. Whereas chemotherapy and radiation therapy require an excellent blood and oxygen supply in order to cause cell destruction, surgery does not. Therefore, surgical removal of large localized tumors that have necrotic centers and poor blood supplies is also an effective treatment procedure.[11,16]

Tumor Cell Kinetics

GROWTH RATE OR BIOLOGIC AGGRESSIVENESS. Well-differentiated, slow-growing tumors that consist of cells with long cell cycles lend themselves best to surgical resection. These tumors are more likely to be confined locally and have a smaller chance for invasion and dissemination. Poorly differentiated, rapid-growing tumors are less amenable to surgery.[15,16]

INVASION.   Any cell that remains after cancer therapy carries with it the potential for recurrence if that cell can reproduce. Therefore, any surgery that is intended to be curative must include resection of normal tissue around the tumor to ensure removal of all cancer cells. Some cancers (e.g., melanomas) invade deeply into tissues, requiring radical surgery or eliminating surgery as a treatment option.[15]

The first operation performed for removal of a cancer has a better chance for success than subsequent operations after recurrence. Therefore, the surgeon's knowledge of invasive tumor patterns is critical for planning the most effective treatment.[15]

METASTATIC POTENTIAL OR PATTERN AND EXTENT OF METASTATIC SPREAD.   Some tumors metastasize late or not at all. Even when advanced, these tumors may be cured by aggressive surgery. Other tumors are known to metastasize to certain regional lymph nodes, and cure may be achieved by removal of the tumor-bearing organ and its nearby lymph nodes. Other tumors predictably metastasize early. Surgery may not be warranted for these tumor types. Alternatively, it may be used to remove all visible tumor before the patient begins adjuvant treatment or to resect remaining disease after several courses of chemotherapy.[15,40]

Evidence of spread into blood or lymph vessels indicates a poorer prognosis, and less favorable results are achieved by surgery. If a patient has widespread metastatic disease, surgical resection alone will usually result in a 50% or greater probability of local recurrence. Such a patient may require more treatment than simple surgical resection of a tumor.[11,16]

Patient Variables

GENERAL STATE.   The patient's general health state plays a major role in determining the efficacy of surgery. As with any treatment, surgical risk must be compared to the probability of long-term recovery. Cancer patients are clearly at increased risk for developing complications postoperatively and/or succumbing to clinical problems.[16]

HOST RESISTANCE OR IMMUNE COMPETENCE. The patient's ability to initiate an immunologic response to the cancer cells that remain after surgery is critical. The person with cancer is less likely to be able to mount an effective immune response. However, the ability to resist infection has been shown to be closely related to total body tumor burden. Surgery can reduce the patient's tumor burden, thus improving immune status.[15,16]

DESIRE FOR TREATMENT.   The patient's desire for treatment must be carefully assessed by the surgeon. Even though surgery may be the most effective measure for tumor control, it is not appropriate for a patient who does not want an operation.[11,31]

QUALITY OF LIFE.   Research has shown that some radical surgeries are not justified. Either they do not improve the end result, or they interfere with the patient's welfare. Selection of surgery as a treatment choice must include consideration of the quality of the patient's life when treatment is complete.[15]

Evaluation of tumor factors, tumor cell kinetics, and patient variables permits the establishment of the following fundamental principles that guide the surgical oncologist[11,15,30,42,43]:

- Wide surgical incisions are usually made. Surgical excision of a tumor includes removal of the tumor and a wide margin of normal tissue surrounding it. The surgeon's goal is to ensure a tumor-free border.
- Removal of the tumor-bearing organ and adjacent lymph nodes is preferred if serious morbidity or disfigurement can be avoided. Surgery is done in a manner that will produce satisfactory appearance and function.
- The surgeon will do as much surgery as necessary to eliminate the tumor and as little surgery as possible to accomplish that purpose.
- Careful surgical techniques are employed to prevent the potential escape of tumor cells into the general circulation (seeding). These techniques include glove and instrument changes when a second area of the body requires surgery, early ligation of blood vessels and lymphatics that supply the tumor, and wound irrigation with tumoricidal solutions (0.5% formaldehyde or sterile water). Such measures reduce the risk of recurrence.
- Human tissue is friable, especially if the area has been irradiated previously. Minimal palpation and manipulation of the tumor (no-touch technique) minimize damage to tissue and seeding and local recurrence.
- The greatest chance for a surgical cure is at the time of the first surgical intervention.
- Slow-growing, localized tumors are more amenable to surgical intervention than are rapidly-growing ones that have metastasized early.
- A bloodless surgical field is important for gross observation of the tumor at all times.
- Surgical removal of a primary tumor can change the growth patterns of metastatic lesions, probably by changing residual tumor cell kinetics.
- Reconstruction and rehabilitation are essential components of comprehensive cancer therapy.
- Surgery is being used more frequently in conjunction with other treatment modalities (combination treatment).

SPECIAL SURGICAL TECHNIQUES

Several special surgical techniques are used in the treatment of cancer. These include electrosurgery, cryosurgery, chemosurgery, lasers, and photodynamic therapy.

Electrosurgery

Electrosurgery eliminates cancer cells by using the cutting and coagulating effects of high-frequency electrical current applied by needles, blades, or elec-

trodes. This technique may be an alternative treatment for certain cancers of the skin, oral cavity, and rectum.[16,42]

Cryosurgery

Cryosurgery involves application of liquid nitrogen probes to selectively destroy tumor tissue. Cryosurgery destroys cancerous or precancerous cells by deep-freezing them. The site thaws naturally and becomes gelatinous, healing spontaneously. Most healing is complete in 6 to 8 weeks. Carbon dioxide, Freon, and nitrous oxide are the three common gaseous freezing agents used. Cryosurgery is often used in skin cancer and precancerous and cancerous gynecologic lesions. It has also been found to be effective in some brain, prostate, and oral cavity cancers. Most patients require only one treatment.[16,30,42,43]

Chemosurgery

Chemosurgery, the combined use of layer-by-layer surgical resection of tissue and topical application of chemotherapeutic agents, was first described by Dr. Frederic Mohs in 1941 and is performed today in only a few centers in the United States. In chemosurgery (also known as Mohs' technique), excised tissue is mapped in location to the wound. This allows the surgeon to remove mostly malignant tissue and little or no normal tissue, minimizing disfigurement.[30,43]

Lasers

Laser (an acronym for light amplification by stimulated emission of radiation) therapy is used for local excision. A contact tip or "laser scalpel" provides a focused form of energy within a precise location and depth of tissue. Lasers destroy cancer cells by intensive thermal energy and can be used for cancers of the larynx, female reproductive tract, and skin.[9,22,30,43]

Photodynamic Therapy

Photodynamic therapy involves the intravenous injection of a light-sensitizing agent (hematoporphyrin derivative [HPD]) with uptake by cancer cells, followed by exposure to a laser light within 24 to 48 hours of injection. This results in fluorescence of cancer cells and cell death. Photodynamic therapy is used for determining extent of disease and response to treatment.[43,45]

TYPES OF EQUIPMENT IN SURGICAL ONCOLOGY

Several types of equipment and hardware are used in surgical oncology.

Ventricular Reservoir (Ommaya Reservoir)

A ventricular reservoir consists of a mushroom-shaped silicone dome that provides direct access to ventricular cerebrospinal fluid. The dome, approxi-

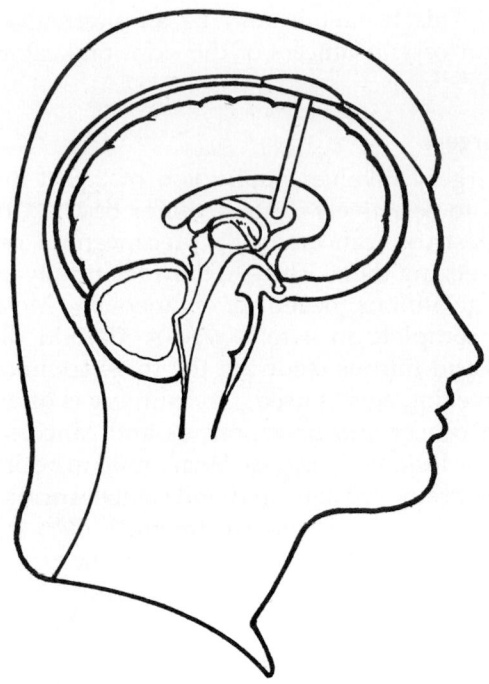

Figure 20–2 The Ommaya reservoir. (From Brager B and Yasko J: Care of the client receiving chemotherapy, Reston, VA, 1984, Reston Publishing Co, Inc.)

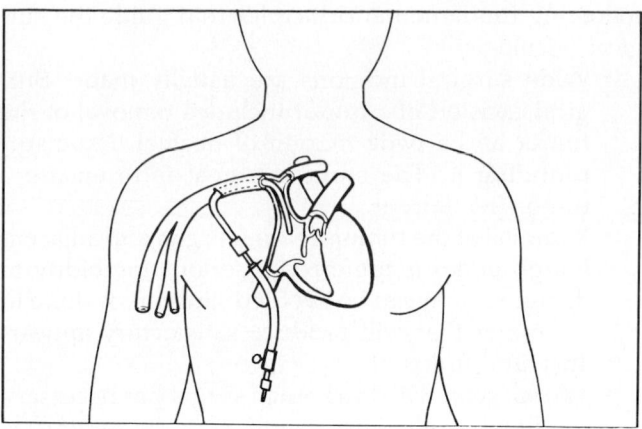

Figure 20–3 Anatomic location of long-term central venous catheter. (From LaRocca JC and Otto SE: Pocket guide to intravenous therapy, ed 2, St Louis, 1993, Mosby.)

mately 3.4 cm in diameter, is attached to a silicone catheter. Ventricular reservoirs have three primary uses: (1) they more predictably and consistently deliver medication (e.g., chemotherapy drugs and pain medication) directly into the subarachnoid space and cerebrospinal fluid *(intrathecal administration),* (2) they permit cerebrospinal fluid to be sampled for pathologic examination, and (3) they permit cerebrospinal fluid pressure to be measured (Figure 20-2 and Table 20-2).[21]

Central Venous Catheters

Central venous catheters are available for short- and long-term use. In short-term use, central venous catheters are used for brief intermittent or continuous administration of intravenous fluids, medications, parenteral hyperalimentation, or blood/blood products. They may also be used for obtaining blood samples. Most short-term central catheters are inserted via the subclavian or jugular vein and terminate in the superior vena cava near the right atrium. Most catheters have no cuff and do not pass through a subcutaneous tunnel (Table 20-2).[21,34]

Long-term central venous catheters are used when a prolonged course of parenteral therapy is expected. The silicone catheter is surgically placed percutaneously or by venous cutdown. The catheter is implanted via the subclavian or jugular vein, with the tip terminating in the superior vena cava near the

right atrium. The catheter is then threaded subcutaneously to an exit site in the chest, usually to the right or left of midline. The procedure is usually done under local anesthesia. A Dacron cuff forms a seal around the catheter. This cuff stabilizes the catheter and reduces infection by preventing retrograde migration of organisms. The catheter may also be sutured in place to secure catheter placement. Central venous pressure can be measured by connecting the catheter's lumen to a manometer. Examples include the Hickman, Broviac, and Groshong catheters.[21,34] (See Figure 20-3 and Table 20-2.)

Implantable Vascular Access Device (IVAD)

The IVAD system consists of a self-sealing silicone rubber septum enclosed in a metal or plastic port that is attached to a silicone catheter (Figure 20-4). The port is surgically implanted beneath the skin, generally in the chest region. The catheter is then threaded subcutaneously and terminates in a body cavity, organ, epidural space, or blood vessel (e.g., peritoneal cavity, heart, or hepatic artery) (Figure 20-5). The procedure may be done on an inpatient or outpatient basis. Chemotherapy, intravenous fluids, pain and other medications, and blood/blood products can be given intermittently or continuously via the port. The system is accessed by a needle puncture through the skin into the port's septum. Noncoring needles must be used when accessing the port to prevent damage to the silicone septum (Figure 20-6). Intravenous fluids are to be administered only through a venous port. Several commercially made ports are available in single or double lumens and lower profile ports for the smaller patient. Examples are the Infuse-A-Port, Port-A-Cath, and LifePort.[21,35] This technology also extends to the peripheral vasculature with the peripheral access port for those pa-

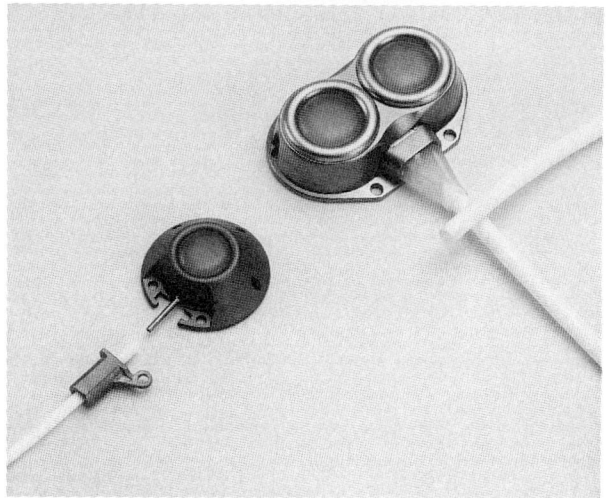

Figure 20–4   LifePort II dual lumen and Lo-Profile Ports. (Courtesy of Strato Medical Corporation, Beverly, Mass.)

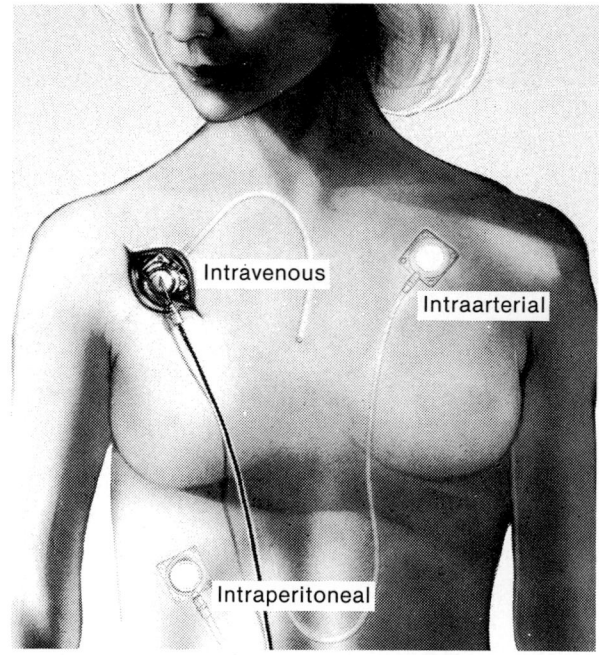

Figure 20–5   Location and termination sites for implanted infusion ports. (Courtesy of Pharmacia Deltec, Inc., St. Paul, Minn.)

tients whose disease prohibits the use of a traditional central venous access. (See Table 20-2.)

Brachytherapy

In brachytherapy, or internal radiation, sealed radioactive isotopes are temporarily or permanently inserted within body tissues (e.g., interstitial placement of iridium implants in breast cancer) or into hollow cavities (e.g., intracavitary placement of cesium implants in the vagina for cervical cancer). A specific

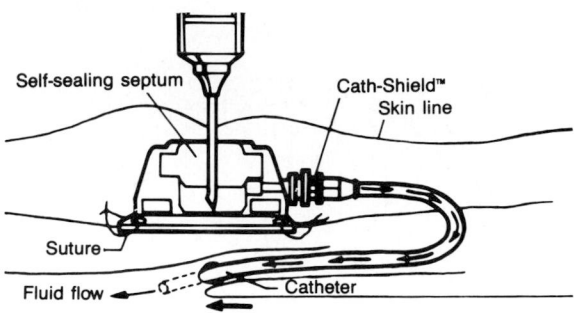

Figure 20–6   Cross-section of implantable port with needle. (Courtesy Pharmacia Deltec, Inc., St. Paul, Minn.)

dose of radiation is delivered continually over hours or days. This method allows delivery of high, concentrated doses of radiation to a specific part of the body, while minimizing the radiation dose to normal tissues. Sealed radioactive sources include seeds, threads, needles, and ribbons.[5,17]

Arterial Catheter

An arterial catheter can be surgically placed for the purpose of delivering higher concentrations of chemotherapy to a localized region *(regional chemotherapy)*. This alleviates some of chemotherapy's systemic side effects.

There are two types of regional chemotherapy. In the first type, a catheter is inserted percutaneously into the arterial system to perfuse an entire region, usually a limb. The vessel is isolated from the general circulation by a pump oxygenator that provides extracorporeal circulation. Ten times the amount of chemotherapy that can be given systemically is infused into the region. The drug is cleared from the isolated circulation by infusing dextran, followed by whole blood. An example is regional intra-arterial limb perfusion for melanoma or soft tissue sarcoma.

In the second type of regional chemotherapy, a catheter, e.g., an implantable vascular access device, is inserted into the tributary artery of the region where the tumor is located. An example is intra-arterial infusion of the liver by intrahepatic placement of a catheter, using an ambulatory infusion pump for continuous infusion chemotherapy.[25,30,46]

Tenckhoff Catheter

The Tenckhoff catheter may be surgically placed for the treatment of malignant ascites as often occurs with lymphomas and cancers of the ovary, colon, or stomach. In this instance, the Tenckhoff catheter is used for the administration of intraperitoneal chemotherapy. The catheter is inserted into the peritoneal cavity under local anesthesia and has an internal Dacron cuff (Figure 20-7).[25]

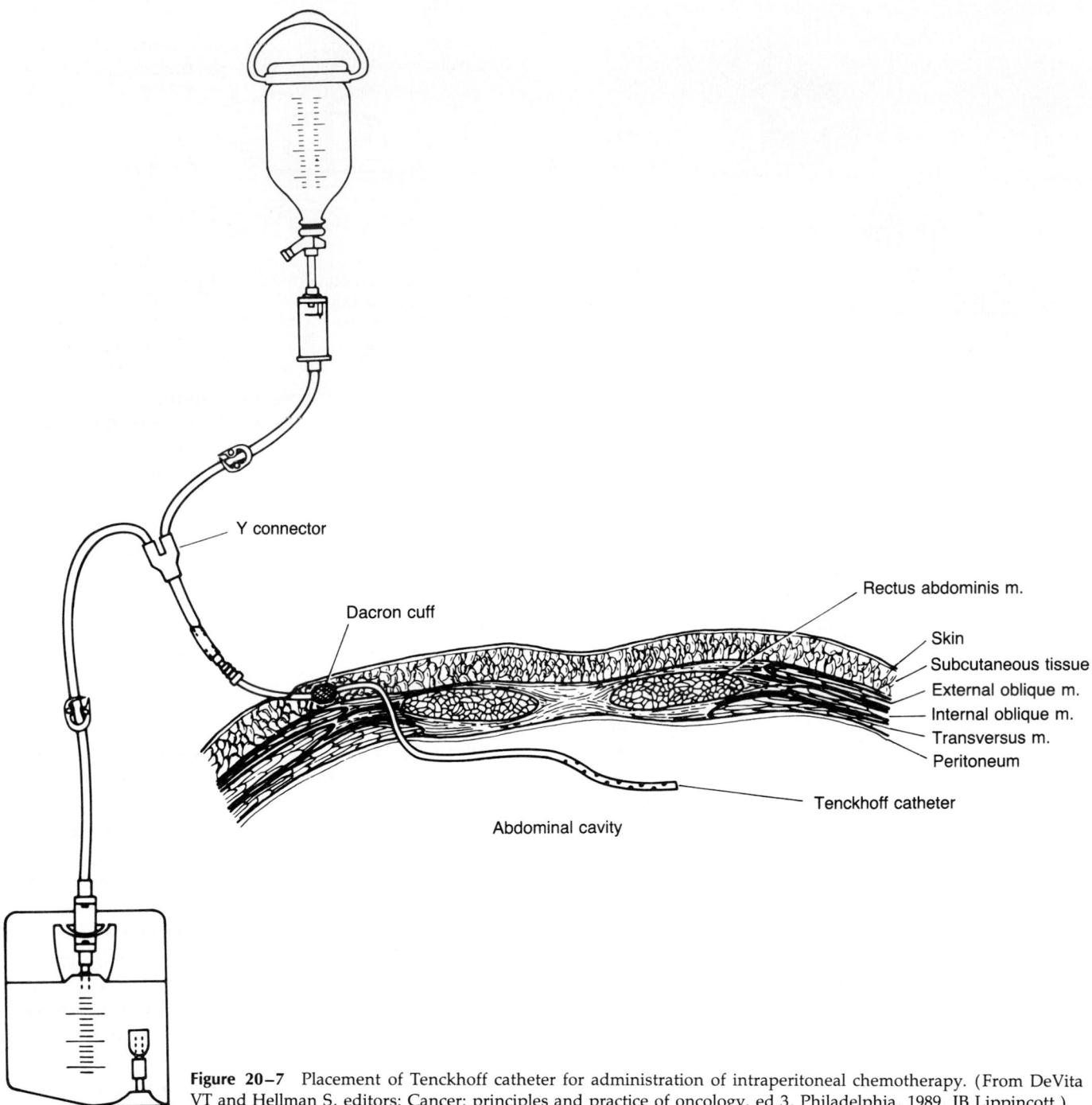

Y connector

Dacron cuff

Rectus abdominis m.

Skin
Subcutaneous tissue
External oblique m.
Internal oblique m.
Transversus m.
Peritoneum

Tenckhoff catheter

Abdominal cavity

Figure 20–7 Placement of Tenckhoff catheter for administration of intraperitoneal chemotherapy. (From DeVita VT and Hellman S, editors: Cancer: principles and practice of oncology, ed 3, Philadelphia, 1989, JB Lippincott.)

Implanted Infusion Pumps

Implanted infusion pumps are used for continuous regional infusion of chemotherapy or pain or other medications to specific body sites by way of an artery, vein, or the spinal fluid. Bolus injections may also be given by the pump's side port. Examples of ports include the Infusaid Model 400, SynchroMed® Infusion Pump, and Therex 3000 (Figure 20-8).

These pumps have no external components and are accessed percutaneously. The pump is placed in a subcutaneous pocket of tissue, usually in the left lower quadrant of the abdomen. The pump may also be placed in a pocket of tissue in the right or left subclavian fossa. The silicone catheter (outlet catheter) most commonly terminates in the hepatic artery, for treatment of liver cancer or liver metastasis; the superior vena cava, for systemic infusion of chemotherapy; or the spinal fluid, for pain management.[36]

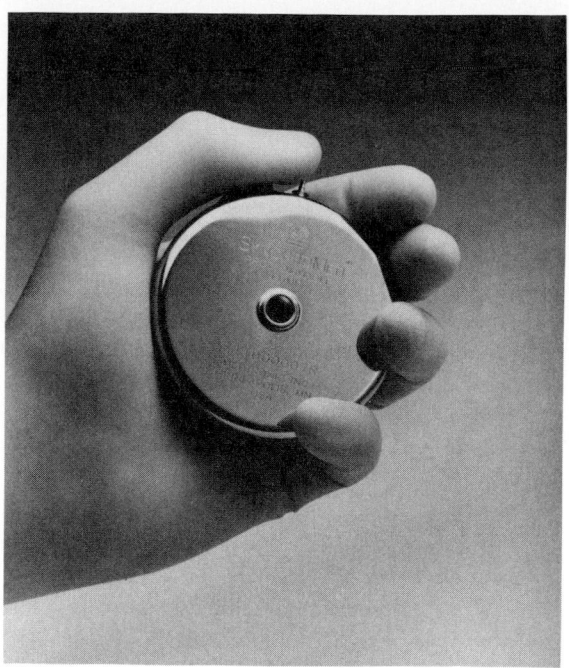

Figure 20–8 SynchroMed® infusion pump. (Courtesy of Medtronic, Inc., Minneapolis, Minn.)

SPECIAL CONSIDERATIONS IN SURGICAL ONCOLOGY
Nutrition

Protein-calorie malnutrition is a common problem in hospitalized cancer patients. Approximately 30% to 50% of hospitalized cancer patients experience moderate to severe degrees of malnutrition, resulting from their primary tumor and/or the diagnostic or treatment regimens used in the management of their disease. Protein-calorie malnutrition generally results from (1) decreased oral intake, (2) increased enteral losses as a result of malabsorption or intestinal fistulas, and/or (3) increased nutritional requirements due to hypermetabolism or the presence of a tumor.[6,7,23,47]

The nutritionally compromised cancer patient is a poor surgical risk. When subjected to the stress of surgery, the patient is unable to preserve lean body mass and enters into negative nitrogen balance. The results are (1) poor wound healing, (2) anemia, (3) infection, (4) sepsis, (5) pneumonia, (6) further malnutrition, and (7) increased morbidity. Nutritional management is aimed first at reversing protein-calorie malnutrition and preventing weight loss. Once this has been accomplished, the nutrition plan can be as aggressive as the cancer treatment plan. The optimal duration of nutrition support varies with each cancer patient.[7,15,28,39]

Blood Disorders

Preoperative nursing management of the cancer patient must include an accurate assessment of hemodynamic parameters and an understanding of abnormal clotting factors.[15]

Anemia is common among cancer patients and should be corrected preoperatively with packed red cell transfusions to a hematocrit equal to or greater than 35. In addition, some conditions (e.g., liver failure, uremia, and leukemia) are associated with platelet dysfunction. It is generally accepted that 50,000 functionally active platelets per cubic millimeter are sufficient for surgery. An insufficient preoperative platelet count can result in postoperative bleeding and fatal hemorrhage, especially if the patient receives large volumes of blood products.[2]

The cancer patient is highly susceptible to changes in the hemostatic system, particularly hypercoagulability and thrombosis. Shortened partial thromboplastin and prothrombin times and elevated clotting factors have been observed. Postoperative deep vein thrombosis is more likely to develop in cancer patients than in other surgery patients. Early postoperative ambulation is therefore critical. Cancers commonly associated with recurring deep vein thrombosis are cancers of the brain, pancreas, stomach, and lung.[15,20]

Complications of Multimodal Therapy

Radiation can cause fibrosis and obliteration of lymphatic and vascular channels, causing long-term damage to underlying tissues. Postoperative wound healing is thus affected in the patient who has been irradiated previously in the same area. Tissue that has been irradiated is not biologically normal, and once surgery disrupts tissue integrity, infection, wound dehiscence, and necrosis can occur.[15,37,49]

Certain chemotherapy drugs (methotrexate, cyclophosphamide, 5-fluorouracil, and doxorubicin) change the histology of healing surgical incisions and decrease tensile strength of wounds at specific times during the postoperative period. Wound strength is significantly impaired when chemotherapy is administered within the first 4 days of surgery. This highlights the need for nonabsorbable sutures and delay of chemotherapy when extensive surgical resection is required.[12,15,37,41]

Chemotherapy drugs often decrease the cancer patient's red blood cell, white blood cell, and platelet counts. The nadir may not occur for 10 to 14 days after initial drug administration. Monitoring of the patient's blood counts and knowledge of the drug's schedule and effects can alert the nurse to potential complications of wound infection and bleeding.[15]

Some chemotherapy drugs are toxic to specific organ systems, producing long-term side effects that can increase the cancer patient's risk of surgical complications. For example, preoperative administration of bleomycin can predispose the patient to postoperative acute adult respiratory distress syndrome. Interstitial fibrosis can occur with bleomycin and can increase surgical pulmonary complications. Diuretics, aggressive pulmonary hygiene, and fluid restriction can prevent interstitial pulmonary edema associated with preoperative bleomycin therapy. Preoperative administration of adriamycin or daunomycin (cumulative dose of 500 mg/m² or more) increases the risk of intraoperative and postoperative congestive heart failure and pulmonary edema. During surgery, the patient's fluid balance must be carefully monitored and controlled. Preoperative digitalis may be given to increase ventricular contractility. A Swan-Ganz catheter may be inserted to monitor physiologic parameters in the intraoperative and postoperative phases.[15]

Surgical Risks in Older Patients

All surgical procedures must be considered high-risk for the older cancer patient. Careful preoperative assessment of physiologic parameters and correction of nutritional deficits and fluid and electrolyte imbalances should begin as early as possible. If a careful baseline assessment is completed preoperatively and if the older patient is thoroughly instructed regarding postoperative management, then many complications can be avoided. Hypoxemia is the most common anesthesia-related problem in the older cancer patient. Age, obesity, and preexisting pulmonary disease all predispose the patient to hypoxemia, with the potential postoperative outcomes being pulmonary

Table 20–3 Physiologic Changes Related to the Aging Process

Physiologic Changes	Effects	Potential Postoperative Complications
CARDIOVASCULAR		
Decreased elasticity of blood vessels	Decreased circulation to vital organs	Shock (hypotension), thrombosis with pulmonary emboli, delayed wound healing, postoperative confusion, hypervolemia, decreased response to stress
Decreased cardiac output	Slower blood flow	
Decreased peripheral circulation		
RESPIRATORY		
Decreased elasticity of lungs and chest wall	Decreased vital capacity	Atelectasis, pneumonia, postoperative confusion
Increased residual lung volume	Decreased alveolar volume	
Decreased forced expiratory volume	Decreased gas exchange	
Decreased ciliary action	Decreased cough reflex	
Fewer alveolar capillaries		
URINARY		
Decreased glomerular filtration rate	Decreased kidney function	Prolonged response to anesthesia and drugs, overhydration with intravenous fluids, hyperkalemia, urinary tract infection, urinary incontinence
Decreased bladder muscle tone	Stasis of urine in bladder	
Weakened perineal muscles	Loss of urinary control	
MUSCULOSKELETAL		
Decreased muscle strength	Decreased activity	Atelectasis, pneumonia, thrombophlebitis, constipation, or fecal impaction
Limitation of motion		
GASTROINTESTINAL		
Decreased intestinal motility	Retention of feces	Constipation or fecal impaction
METABOLIC		
Decreased gamma globulin level	Decreased inflammatory response	Delayed wound healing, wound dehiscence, or evisceration
Decreased plasma proteins		
IMMUNE SYSTEM		
Fewer killer T cells	Decreased ability to protect against invasion by pathogenic microorganisms	Wound infection, wound dehiscence, pneumonia, urinary tract infection
Decreased response to foreign antigens		

From Phipps WJ, Long BC, Woods NF, and Cassmeyer VL, editors: Medical-surgical nursing: concepts and clinical practice, ed 4, St Louis, 1991, Mosby.

edema, myocardial infarction, decreased cardiac output, pulmonary thromboembolism, and aspiration pneumonia.[8]

Emergency surgery for cancer in the older patient carries greater risk than elective surgery. The older patient is at risk during emergency surgery because of declines in organ function and an increase in accompanying disease, e.g., cardiovascular disease. In addition, the increased morbidity after emergency surgery is associated with a decline in immune system competency in the older patient.[8,19]

One of the major problems facing the oncology nurse is the early detection of postoperative problems in the older patient due to a lack of recognition that a change in the patient's condition has occurred. Continuity of nursing care and thorough assessment from the preoperative to the postoperative phase avoid such problems.[32]

See Table 20-3 for additional information on the physiologic changes related to the aging process that can affect surgical outcome.

FUTURE DIRECTIONS AND ADVANCES IN SURGICAL ONCOLOGY

As the primary treatment measure, surgical oncology may have reached its potential. It is hard to envision how more complex surgical procedures could improve the results currently achievable, except in the area of reconstruction. The current research with radiotagged antibodies will hopefully lead to earlier detection of tumors that will facilitate surgical cures for certain cancers. Less extensive surgery may be even more prevalent in the future, such as the current tendency to do less extensive mastectomies for breast cancer. Both laser surgery and microsurgery will continue to bring even greater precision to surgical oncology.[26]

Text continued on p. 464.

Nursing Management

Nursing care of the surgical cancer patient is very similar to the nursing care required for any surgery patient. However, the nurse must be aware of the problems that are unique to the cancer disease process. Unlike other surgery patients, the cancer patient's comprehensive plan of care must include nursing management of the psychosocial and existential aspects of and complications specific to the cancer.[15]

PREOPERATIVE CARE

Preoperative nursing care of the cancer patient focuses on assessment and intervention. In order to accomplish these tasks effectively, the nurse must know the answers to the following questions[30]:

- *What is the purpose of the surgery?* Is it diagnosis, staging, cure, or palliation? Each purpose has a different meaning for the patient. By knowing the purpose of surgery, the nurse can better comprehend the patient's behavior. A patient in whom the diagnosis of cancer has been recently made will exhibit different behaviors than the patient with metastatic disease who undergoes palliative surgery for relief of intractable pain.
- *What kind of surgery will be performed?* The nurse must know what preoperative preparation or care is required (e.g., bowel preparation, nutritional supplementation); where incisions will be made and how long they will be; and what devices will be attached to the patient (e.g., catheters, drains, chest tubes).
- *What has the patient and/or family been told about the surgery, diagnosis, and possibilities for future treatment?* Patients often hear only the words "cancer" and "surgery." Everything else is a blur. Therefore, information needs to be repeated frequently.

Once answers to these questions have been obtained, preoperative nursing care of the cancer patient can then focus on reducing anxiety, enhancing physical well-being, and teaching.[42]

Reducing Anxiety

Cancer has a profound psychologic impact on patients and their significant others. Complex emotional responses are evoked, often resulting in hopelessness, powerlessness, and severe depression. Patients often react to the idea of surgery with apprehension and may be resentful, angry, anxious, and even panicked about the impending operation. The basis for these powerful reactions lies in the patient's fear of death from surgery or anesthesia and fear of pain and mutilation.[16,29]

Misconceptions and fears about surgery may be influenced by others close to the patient. Patients often expect outcomes similar to those of friends and relatives, especially if the outcome of their surgery was negative. The patient's prior experience with surgery also affects preoperative outlook and recovery; if previous operations were difficult, problems are often encountered in subsequent ones.[29]

Tumors that are visibly evident to the patient and, more importantly, to others, impact more on the patient's psychologic response to cancer. Tumors located away from vital organs are often viewed by cancer patients as less serious than those in vital structures. Tumors that involve the sex organs cause patients to question their sexuality and ability to function sexually and reproduce.[30]

Some preoperative fear is normal, even positive, because it encourages the patient to take the surgery seriously and make realistic plans for coping with it. For some patients, the question, "How do you think this surgery will change your life?" encourages the patient to explore fears, talk about related anxieties, and begin planning for change. This type of communication forms the basis for a supportive, trusting, and therapeutic relationship that will endure throughout subsequent readmissions to the hospital.[16,29,42]

Enhancing Physical Well-Being

The cancer patient may be debilitated as a result of advanced disease or the type of symptoms and/or length of time symptoms have been present. Enhancement of the patient's physical well-being in the preoperative period includes alleviation of physical symptoms such as pain, diarrhea, nausea and vomiting, fatigue, bowel obstruction, and malnutrition. Stress-related symptoms, such as insomnia and headaches, can also be minimized. Side effects of preoperative chemotherapy or radiation therapy increase

the patient's chances of developing postoperative physical and/or emotional problems. Proper preoperative treatment and management of these side effects will directly affect the patient's response postoperatively.[42] See Table 20-4 for information specific to preoperative assessment of physiologic parameters in the surgical oncology patient.

Teaching

Anxiety appears to be more severe in those patients who do not have accurate information about their impending surgery. During the preoperative period, concern about the disease or diagnosis is often replaced by concern about the impending surgery. Nurses are in a primary position to correct misconceptions and fill in the gaps about surgical procedures. Honestly and clearly answering questions about the site, type, and extent of surgery, as well as probable pain, discomfort, or any bodily changes, will often reduce and not increase the patient's level of anxiety. Information should be provided and repeated as needed.[42]

Preoperative patient teaching will be most successful if the nurse develops an individually tailored teaching plan based upon a thorough assessment of knowledge deficits. These deficits must be handled as any other nursing diagnosis, and the nursing pro-

Table 20—4 Preoperative Assessment of Physiologic Parameters[25,44]

Physiologic Parameters	Factors That Increase Surgical Risk	Assessment Factors	Laboratory Tests/Others
Nutritional status	Debilitation and malnourishment as a result of disease and/or previous therapy	Anorexia Eating habits Special diets Food restrictions Food preferences Availability of food Supplementation Nausea Vomiting Stomatitis Smell or taste changes Recent weight loss	Decreased serum albumin
Cardiovascular system	Congestive heart failure as a result of previous and prolonged chemotherapy	Dyspnea Fatigue Anorexia Nausea Vomiting Abdominal distention Right upper quadrant pain Tachycardia Weak, thready pulse Hypotension Rapid, labored respiration Frothy, blood-tinged sputum Moist rales Displaced apical pulse Weight gain Peripheral edema Dilation of peripheral veins	Increased pulmonary capillary pressure Decreased cardiac output Increased right atrial pressure

Table 20—4   Preoperative Assessment of Physiologic Parameters—cont'd

Physiologic Parameters	Factors That Increase Surgical Risk	Assessment Factors	Laboratory Tests/Others
Pulmonary system	Pulmonary edema and/or fibrosis as a result of previous and prolonged chemotherapy	Nasal flaring Retractions Tachypnea Labored, noisy breathing Diaphoresis Rales Wheezing Persistent cough Frothy, blood-tinged sputum Restlessness Confusion Hypotension Tachycardia Lethargy Intake and output Sudden weight gain Swollen feet or ankles Chest pain	Decreased vital capacity Decreased minute volume Decreased cardiac output $PaCO_2$ PaO_2 pH K^+ Na^+ Pulmonary capillary wedge pressure Pulmonary artery pressure Sputum specimens for culture and sensitivity Serial chest x-ray reports
Genitourinary system	Renal insufficiency as a result of previous and prolonged chemotherapy	Frequency of voiding Dysuria Anuria Infection Urine (color, clarity	Decreased creatinine clearance Increased BUN Increased uric acid levels Increased serum creatinine levels
Fluid and electrolyte status	Dehydration and electrolyte imbalance as a result of disease and/or previous therapy Hypovolemia as a result of disease	Intake and output Vomiting Diarrhea Bleeding	K^+ Mg^{++} Ca^{++} H^+
Liver function status	Metastatic liver disease	Jaundice Ascites Vague upper abdominal pain Anorexia Weight loss Splenomegaly Esophageal varices Fever of unknown origin Dependent edema	Total bilirubin
Hematologic factors	Platelet dysfunction as a result of disease and/or previous therapy Hypercoagulability as a result of disease Anemia as a result of disease	Easy bruising Excessive bleeding Dyspnea Fatigue Previous thrombophlebitis	Prothrombin time Partial thromboplastin Platelet count RBC count WBC count Hemoglobin Hematocrit
Potential for postoperative complications	Preoperative infection as a result of immunocompetence and/or previous therapy Previous radiation therapy	Sneezing Cough Sore throat Fever Skin lesions Rashes Radiation skin damage in relation to anticipated surgical incision	WBC count Throat culture Sputum culture

PREOPERATIVE PATIENT TEACHING PRIORITIES

Include information regarding:
- The surgery to be performed
- General preoperative activities and rationale
- General postoperative behaviors expected of the patient and rationale
- Techniques such as TCDB, incisional splinting, ROM exercises, incentive spirometry
- Types of apparatus to be used before and after surgery
- Plan of care and rationale for procedures
- Anticipated care settings, equipment and experiences related to surgery
- Self-care strategies to prevent and minimize complications of surgery

Outcomes of preoperative teaching:
The patient and/or significant other is able to:
- State that anxiety is decreased regarding surgery
- Demonstrate an understanding of preoperative procedures and routines by return demonstration, verbal feedback, etc.
- Demonstrate an understanding of postoperative procedures and routines by return demonstration, verbal feedback, etc.
- Participate in postoperative procedures and care

cess must serve as the basis for developing the teaching plan. Learning needs and goals or outcomes must be mutually identified and agreed upon by the patient and/or family and the nurse. See the box above for preoperative teaching priorities and desired outcomes.[4,42]

POSTOPERATIVE CARE

Postoperative nursing care of cancer patients depends on type of cancer, type of surgery performed, previous treatment, and preexisting physiologic deficits. Like preoperative care, postoperative care focuses on the physical and psychologic needs of patients.[30]

Physical Needs

All surgery patients' immediate postoperative needs are primarily physical. From the moment the patient arrives in the recovery room or special care unit, certain definitive goals act as guides throughout the remaining postoperative course. These goals are to prevent postoperative complications and to promote cardiovascular function, tissue perfusion, respiratory function, nutrition and elimination, fluid and electrolyte balance, renal function, rest and comfort, wound healing, and early movement and ambulation.[25,30] The reader is referred to any general surgical nursing text for a thorough discussion of these common postoperative goals.

Psychologic Needs

As patients are aroused from anesthesia, their first questions are often ones such as, "Do I have cancer? Did the doctor get all of it? Did the cancer spread? Did the doctor remove my (colon, leg, breast, etc.)?" The patient's questions should not be answered until recovery from the effects of anesthesia is complete, and the surgeon or referring physician has had time to see the patient and offer an adequate explanation. However, the nurse must ensure that a supportive environment is provided when test results are shared with the patient and family.[30]

All cancer patients must make psychologic changes. For some patients, the diagnosis of cancer may mean changes in lifestyle, occupation, or school or job attendance and performance. The threat of change can be so great that, occasionally, the cancer patient may become psychologically immobilized. Without incorporation of necessary psychologic changes, the cancer patient is at risk of not complying with the demands of therapy. The new sick role may also be incompatible with the patient's self-concept, making it difficult for the patient to temporarily rely on others for needed care.[30,42]

After surgery, patients slowly come to the realization that they have cancer. This realization may initiate feelings of helplessness, depression, and grief. Patients often grieve over real or imagined changes in body image and self-worth. Changes in body image may be difficult for the cancer patient to positively incorporate. When the patient is unable to fully accept the physical changes after surgery, conflict occurs between the way the body actually looks and the way the patient mentally pictures the body. This form of denial is usually followed by recognition of reality, grief, and depression. Patients who attach great psychological significance to the lost body part may believe the surgery has compromised the body's internal structure and complain of frailty. These patients frequently restrict their physical and sexual activities unnecessarily, feeling their bodies are vulnerable. Appropriate nursing measures will help the patient adapt to changes in body image. The nurse can assist patients by acknowledging the painfulness of the loss and by ensuring that they grieve in a safe, nonjudgmental environment.[29,30,42]

For most patients, cancer and death are synonymous words, and all cancers are considered one disease. This attitude reflects a lack of knowledge about different types of cancer. The diagnosis can initially isolate such patients from others. The patient's ability to make decisions may be changed by this same lack of knowledge. After the diagnosis is confirmed, most patients strive to regain their decision-making power. One way of doing this is by learning about the diagnosis, therapy, and hospital routines.[30]

It is important that the nurse assess the type and degree of support that significant others provide to the patient. The patient's postoperative anxiety level will often decrease when the nurse encourages family support and availability. However, the nurse must remember that cancer and surgery are crisis situations for the entire family. Initially the family may be emotionally and psychologically immobilized by the diagnosis, and family members may neglect themselves or not know where to turn for services. The nurse can share information on motel accommodations and restaurants and make other referrals as necessary. Sometimes, even simple decision making is overwhelming for the family in crisis. Often, family members want to support the patient but do not know what to say or do. The nurse can guide family members by helping them identify things to do.[29,30]

Nurses must be aware of the psychologic issues affecting cancer surgery patients in order to provide the most appropriate care and encourage their patients to adapt positively to the demands of disease and therapy.[29] See Chapters 26 and 30.

GERIATRIC CONSIDERATIONS

- Physiologic changes: cardiovascular, respiratory, renal, gastrointestinal, immune, metabolic, and musculoskeletal systems may be compromised (see Table 20-3)
- Anesthesia risk for hypoxemia
- Postoperative risk for pulmonary edema, myocardial infarction, decreased cardiac output, pulmonary thromboembolism, and aspiration pneumonia
- Discharge plan will require assessment for need of additional resources, such as home-care agency, American Cancer Society and/or social services

---

RECOMMENDED POSTOPERATIVE NURSING DIAGNOSES AND INTERVENTIONS FOR THE SURGICAL ONOCOLOGY PATIENT[14,25,42]

NURSING DIAGNOSES

- Body image disturbance:
  - Related to surgical removal of body part
  - Related to diagnosis of cancer

- Coping, ineffective family compromised
  - Related to diagnosis of cancer

- Coping, ineffective individual
  - Related to diagnosis of cancer
  - Related to potential life-style changes

- Fluid volume deficit: potential
  - Related to surgical procedure
  - Related to excessive fluid loss from abnormal routes (indwelling tubes)
  - Related to excessive fluid loss from postoperative nausea/vomiting
  - Related to inability to receive or absorb fluids

INTERVENTIONS

- Encourage patient to discuss feelings and concerns with health care providers and significant others.
- Help patient identify, label, and express feelings about the significance of the lost body part, treatment modalities, and anticipated prognosis.
- Promote acceptance of positive/realistic body image.

- Provide opportunities for expression of feelings.
- Provide information to assist patients and their families in working through their emotional reactions to the diagnosis, treatment, and prognosis.

- Provide opportunities for patient to express feelings about the diagnosis and prognosis.
- Assist patient in meeting adaptations or changes in activities and relationships.

- Monitor vital signs.
- Assess capillary refill time.
- Measure intake and output.
- Monitor electrolyte values.
- Measure urine specific gravity.
- Monitor hemoglobin and hematocrit.
- Assess oral mucous membranes.
- Assess skin turgor.
- Administer intravenous or oral fluids as ordered by the physician.
- Administer antiemetics as ordered by the physician.

Adapted with permission from Friel M: Concepts related to the nursing care of surgical oncology patients. In Vredevoe D, Derdiarian A, and Sarna L, editors: Concepts of oncology nursing, Englewood Cliffs, NJ, 1981, Prentice-Hall; and Thompson JM and others: Clinical nursing, ed 2, St Louis, 1989, Mosby.

NURSING DIAGNOSES — cont'd

- Fluid volume deficit

  Related to surgical procedure (loss of 15% to 20% of total blood volume during surgery)

- Gas exchange, impaired

  Related to embolization of thrombus

- Infection: potential for

  Related to preoperative immunocompromised status as a result of disease and/or previous therapy

  Related to break in skin integrity (surgical incision)

  Related to urinary retention due to surgical procedure

- Injury: potential for

  Related to peritonitis secondary to breakdown of anastomosis caused by decreased tissue healing resulting from chemotherapy, radiation therapy, poor nutritional status, and/or tumor

INTERVENTIONS — cont'd

- Maintain strict bedrest with patient supine and head of bed elevated slightly.
- Limit all activities.
- Monitor vital signs every 5 to 15 minutes.
- Administer drugs as ordered to maintain BP, increase cardiac output.
- Maintain patent IV for drug administration.
- Administer fluids and volume expanders as ordered.
- Monitor urine output.
- Assess skin for color, temperature, and elasticity.
- Maintain accurate intake and output.
- Monitor arterial blood gases.
- Administer oxygen as ordered.
- Monitor respiratory rate and pattern.
- Monitor hemodynamic parameters as ordered.

- Observe for signs/symptoms of pulmonary embolus:

    Chest pain
    Dyspnea
    Tachypnea

- Assess for presence of risk factors.
- Obtain cultures as ordered and report results.
- Monitor vital signs (increased pulse; low-grade, intermittent fever).
- Observe body secretions, excretions, and exudates for signs of infection; report abnormalities.
- Monitor hydration and electrolyte balance.
- Monitor changes in WBC count.
- Wash hands before and after contact with patient.
- Prevent patient's exposure to infected visitors or staff.
- Turn patient frequently; instruct in deep breathing.

- Monitor wound site (edema, redness, undue pain).
- Verify orders for wound care.

- Observe amount, color, specific gravity, and odor of urine output.
- Administer antibiotics as ordered.
- Assess for abdominal pain.
- Force fluids.

- Assess for signs/symptoms:

    Moderate to severe abdominal pain
    Burning ache aggravated by any motion, even respiration
    Anorexia
    Nausea
    Vomiting
    Fever within 48 hours after surgery
    Chills, thirst, scanty urine
    Inability to pass feces or flatus
    Abdominal distention

NURSING DIAGNOSES — cont'd	INTERVENTIONS — cont'd

Tachycardia with weak, thready pulses
Rapid, shallow respirations
Tachypnea

Related to postoperative intestinal obstruction secondary to adhesions from radiation therapy

- Assess for signs/symptoms:
  Vomiting
  Abdominal cramping
  Constipation

Related to hypercoagulability and postoperative inactivity

- Assess calves daily
- Observe for signs/symptoms of thrombophlebitis:
  Calf pain
  Calf tenderness
  Homan's sign
  Dilated superficial veins
  Edema of involved extremity

- Knowledge deficit
  Related to such areas as self-care, activities related to health care regimen, decision-making regarding health

- At every interaction, assess for knowledge deficits.
- Use patient's theories about illness as a starting point for teaching, and continually seek patient's perception.
- During interactions, assess frequently to see if patient understands, accepts diagnosis.
- Simplify information to conform to patient's terms, thought patterns, and daily routines.
- Give explicit directions.
- Be accessible to patient for questions.
- Demonstrate to patient and family how to use information.
- Reinforce correct use of information.
- Teach patient how to rehearse mentally a necessary health action.
- Make certain patient is actively involved in decisions about own care.
- Offer peer support network and opportunity for patient to watch others successfully mastering similar health care problems.
- Provide instruction in multiple modalities (visual, written, discussion), so that patient will remember it in various ways.
- Provide materials to take so that the patient can review and use the new knowledge. (See Geriatric Considerations box on p. 459.)

- Mobility, impaired physical
  Related to surgical removal of limb

- Assist patient with ambulation; control distance.
- Have patient use walker, cane, or wheelchair as needed as assistive devices.
- Minimize environmental barriers.
- Encourage use of involved limb.
- Change patient's position slowly.
- Encourage moderate physical exercise, adequate rest, and performance of range of motion exercises.
- Balance nutritional intake; supplement protein.
- Discuss "phantom" pain with patient and family.

NURSING DIAGNOSES — cont'd

- Nutrition, altered, less than body requirements
    Related to surgical procedure for cancer that interferes with mechanical process of eating
    Related to surgical procedure for cancer that interferes with absorption of essential salts and nutrients

- Pain
    Related to surgical procedure
    Related to complications at therapeutic hardware's insertion sites

INTERVENTIONS — cont'd

- Assess for signs/symptoms of protein-calorie malnutrition:
    Edema
    Dyspigmentation of the hair
    Easy pluckability of the hair
    Muscle wasting
    Dermatosis
- Review results of anthropometric test, dietary analysis, and clinical exam.
- Perform nutrition assessment:
    Assess problem area, food preferences, patterns and behaviors related to food intake, intake and output, and calorie count.
- Encourage good mouth care.
- Provide relaxed environment without pain.
- Observe presentation of food.
- Encourage family to bring in favorite foods when allowed.
- Consult with dietitian to provide diet and supplements that meet patient's needs.
- Care for and monitor intravenous total parenteral nutrition.
- Care for feeding tubes.
- Provide nutrition teaching for patient and family before discharge.

- Incorporate the following in assessing patient's pain status:
    Location/Characteristics
    Onset
        Frequency
        Intensity, using 0-5 scale
        Quality
        Effective pain control measures
        Ineffective pain control measures
        Pain expression style
        Movement
        Muscle tone
        Emotional distress
        Effect of pain on postoperative activities
        Effect on sleep/wake pattern
- Identify strategies that eliminate or control pain.
- Explore strategies that have been successful in the past.
- Identify strategies that patient values as essential for pain reduction.
- Administer medication per physician's orders and protocols using appropriate delivery system:
    Monitor effect at frequent intervals.
    Graphically record pain assessment data.
    Provide physician with evidence of need to change medication.
- Intervene at onset of pain
- Position for comfort
- Provide distraction

NURSING DIAGNOSES — cont'd

INTERVENTIONS — cont'd

- Suggest and instruct patient in relaxation techniques: short simple techniques with nurse directing for acute pain.
- Pace activities and plan activities ahead of time.
- Provide supportive environment.
- Use several pain reduction strategies.

- Skin integrity, impaired: potential
    Related to tissue damage and/or poor tissue healing as a result of chemotherapy, radiation therapy, and/or poor nutritional status.

- Observe incision site for hematomas (swelling, discoloration).
- Assess patency of any drains.
- Assess for signs/symptoms of dehiscence:
    Rapid onset of serosanguineous drainage
    Popping sensation
- Assess for signs of impending evisceration.
- Check use of abdominal binders for obese patients.

- Skin integrity, impaired
    Related to tissue damage and/or poor tissue healing as a result of chemotherapy, radiation therapy, and/or poor nutritional status.

- Assess for signs/symptoms of dehiscence:
    Monitor amount and color of drainage.
    Call physician immediately.
    Obtain vital signs.
    Prepare patient for surgery
- Assess for signs of evisceration:
    Apply sterile moist towels over extruded intestine or omentum.
- Prepare patient for surgery.

- Tissue perfusion, altered (peripheral)
    Related to lymphedema secondary to lymph node dissection

- Do not obtain BP measurements, venipunctures, withdraw blood, or inject medication into affected limb.
- Assess for signs/symptoms of lymphedema: affected limb becomes red, warm or unusually hard or swollen.
- Elevate affected limb above the level of the heart on pillows
- Observe for infection secondary to lymphedema.
- Teach importance of good hygiene.
- Encourage progressive exercise of affected limb.

    Related to hypercoagulability and postoperative inactivity

- Bedrest.
- Limit self-care activities.
- Raise affected limb above level of right atrium.
- Do not use knee gatch.
- Assess quality and location of pain.
- Administer analgesics as ordered.
- Measure calf or thigh or both daily and record.
- Assess circulation of affected extremity and check pulses in all extremities. Use Doppler sensor if pulses seem absent.
- Use elastic stockings as ordered.
- Obtain vital signs every 4 to 8 hours.
- Administer anticoagulant therapy as ordered.
- Monitor PT and PTT studies.
- Initiate a progressive exercise program.
- Instruct patient to apply support stockings before ambulating, avoid standing for long periods.

DISCHARGE PLANNING

The goal for the cancer patient is to develop or regain independence. This can be achieved by encouraging patients to participate in activities of daily living and learning new self-care measures early in their hospitalization in preparation for discharge. However, in their eagerness to help patients, family members often try to do everything for them. This response serves only to foster dependence in patients and contributes to their feelings of helplessness. The nurse must guide the patient and family in understanding the significance of the patient's early steps toward independence.[30]

Nurses sometimes mistakenly assume that, once the patient is discharged from the hospital, the patient will receive the care, attention, and support needed at home. However, some patients dread their discharge from the hospital almost as much as their admission to it. Some patients become very dependent on the hospital and their new sick role, particularly if their home life is unstable. A supportive home environment will probably remain so after the patient's discharge from the hospital. However, an unstable home environment (e.g., in which poor communication and strained relationships exist) is likely to worsen after surgery. Whether the patient is able to adjust to changes in physical appearance or function is largely determined by the family's reaction to these same issues. If the patient feels rejected at home, the patient may fear rejection from society at large.[29]

Discharge planning must therefore begin when a patient is admitted to the hospital and continue throughout the hospital stay. The nurse's assessment must include information about the family and family situation; the patient's knowledge about the disease, treatment, and available resources; the social setting; school and/or work; and diet. The health care team can then begin to make appropriate plans to ease the transition from hospital to home. Many times, preparing the home to receive the patient takes longer than the hospitalization. Members of the health care team must be consulted for their evaluations of the family's ability to care for the patient. Evaluation may reveal that home care by private or visiting nurses or admission to an extended care facility may be needed when the patient leaves the hospital. If the family is experiencing communication problems and emotional

---

> ### POSTOPERATIVE PATIENT TEACHING PRIORITIES
>
> *Include information regarding:*
> - Changes in self-care activities and other activities resulting from surgery
> - Progressive return to maximum activity level
> - Anticipated discharge medications
> - Wound management
> - Proper use of assistive or prosthetic devices
> - Symptoms to observe for: fever, pain, vomiting, diarrhea, bleeding, malnutrition
> - Who and when the patient should call if problems arise
> - Where to get additional information about cancer or treatment
> - Where support groups are located and how to contact: Reach to Recovery, Make Today Count
> - Resources or agencies that might be helpful to the patient: physical therapy, occupational therapy, speech therapy, ostomy outpatient clinics, prosthetic fitting devices, home care agencies
> - Where the patient can get medical supplies
> - Follow-up care that may be needed
> - When the patient can return to work
> - Any job retraining that may be necessary
> - When the patient can drive a car
> - When the patient can resume sexual activity

---

difficulties, the health care team might consider referral to family therapy or a family support group.[29,30]

Most cancer patients are not completely recovered from their surgery at the time of discharge from the hospital. Therefore, the information identified in the box above should be given to the patient in writing before discharge.

The astute nurse institutes and documents discharge planning based on a thorough admission assessment and history and makes every attempt to involve family members early in the process. If needed, referrals are made to appropriate members of the health care team so that all possible issues are addressed well before the patient's discharge from the hospital.

Discharge planning allows patients and their families to prepare for living with cancer outside the hospital. Postoperative needs and concerns are anticipated early by the nurse, allowing the cancer patient and family to face the challenges that lie ahead.[30]

CONCLUSION

Current trends in tumor biology and interdisciplinary cancer management have changed previous reliance on surgery as the only curative form of cancer therapy and precipitated changes in the extensiveness of surgical resections. By combining surgery, radiation therapy, chemotherapy, and biotherapy, disease-free intervals have been significantly expanded.[15]

In spite of known limitations, surgery continues to be an important treatment modality for cancer. The nurse may encounter the cancer surgery patient at the time of initial diagnosis or when the patient returns for reconstructive surgery after several years of disease-free existence. This demands flexibility on the part of the nurse and a strong understanding of the foundations and principles of surgical oncology nursing.

BIBLIOGRAPHY

1. Anseline PF and others: Radiation injury of the rectum, Ann Surg 194:716, 1981.
2. Baird RM and Rebbeck PA: Impact of preoperative chemotherapy for the surgeon, Recent Results Cancer Res 103:79, 1986.
3. Bender CM and Yasko JM: Nursing role in management: problems with abnormal cell growth. In Lewis SM and Collier IC, editors: Medical-surgical nursing: assessment and management of clinical problems, ed 3, St. Louis, 1992, Mosby.
4. Brown MH and others: Standards of oncology nursing practice, New York, 1986, John Wiley & Sons, Inc.
5. Bucholtz JD: Implications of radiation therapy for nursing. In Clark JC and McGee RF, editors: Core curriculum for oncology nursing, ed 2, Philadelphia, 1992, WB Saunders Co.
6. Butler J: Nutrition and cancer: a review of the literature, Cancer Nurs 3:131, April 1980.
7. Daly JM and DeCosse JJ: Principles of surgical oncology. In Calabresi P, Schein PS, and Rosenberg SA, editors: Medical oncology: basic principles and clinical management of cancer, New York, 1985, Macmillan Publishing Co.
8. Derby SA: Cancer in the older patient. In Ashwander P, Belcher AE, Mattson EAH, Moskowitz R, and Riese NE, editors: Oncology nursing: advances, treatments and trends into the 21st century, Rockville, MD, 1990, Aspen Publishers, Inc.
9. Dixon J: Current laser applications in general surgery, Ann Surg 207(4):355, 1988.
10. Duke JH and Miller TA: Salt and water: fluid and electrolyte problems. In Condon R and DeCosse J, editors: Surgical care, Philadelphia, 1980, Lea & Febiger.
11. Eilber FR: Principles of cancer surgery. In Haskel CM, editor: Cancer treatment, ed 2, Philadelphia, 1985, WB Saunders Co.
12. Falcone RE and Nappi JF: Chemotherapy and wound healing, Surg Clin North Am 64:779, 1984.
13. Forbes J: Principles and potential of palliative surgery in patients with advanced cancer, Recent Results Cancer Res 108:134, 1988.
14. Friel M: Concepts related to the nursing care of surgical oncology patients. In Vredevoe D, Derdiarian A, and Sarna L, editors: Concepts of oncology nursing, Englewood Cliffs, NJ, 1981, Prentice-Hall.
15. Frogge MH and Goodman M: Surgical therapy. In Groenwald SL, Frogge MH, Goodman M, and Yarbro CH, editors: Cancer nursing: principles and practice, ed 2, Boston, 1990, Jones and Bartlett Publishers.
16. Griffiths MJ, Murray KH, and Russo PC: Oncology nursing: pathophysiology, assessment, and intervention, New York, 1984, Macmillan Publishing Co.
17. Haibeck S: Intraoperative radiation therapy, Oncol Nurs Forum 15(2):143, 1988.
18. Hill G: Historic milestones in cancer surgery, Semin Oncol 6(4):409, 1979.
19. Howland WS: Preoperative evaluation of the cancer patient for emergency surgery. In Turnbull AD, editor: Surgical emergencies in the cancer patient, Chicago, 1987, Year Book Medical Publishers.
20. Kempin S, Gould-Rossbach P, and Howland WS: Disorders of hemostasis in the critically ill cancer patient. In Howland WS and Carlon GC, editors: Critical care of the cancer patient, Chicago, 1985, Year Book Medical Publishers.
21. LaRocca JC and Otto SE: Pocket guide to intravenous therapy, ed 2, St Louis, 1993, Mosby.
22. Lehr P: Surgical lasers: how they work, current applications, AORN J 50(5):972, 1989.
23. Lindsey A, Piper B, and Stotts N: The phenomenon of cancer cachexia: a review, Oncol Nurs Forum 9(2):38, 1982.
24. Liotta LA: Mechanisms of cancer invasion and metastasis. In DeVita VT Jr, Hellman S, and Rosenberg SA, editors: Important advances in oncology, Philadelphia, 1985, JB Lippincott Co.
25. Luckmann J and Sorensen KC: Medical-surgical nursing: a psychophysiologic approach, ed 4, Philadelphia, 1991, WB Saunders Co.
26. Maxwell M: General principles of therapy. In Groenwald SL, Frogge MH, Goodman M, and Yarbro CH, editors: Cancer nursing: principles and practice, ed 2, Boston, 1990, Jones and Bartlett Publishers.
27. Morton DL, Sparks FC, and Haskel CM: Oncology. In Swartz SI, editor: Principles of surgery, ed 4, New York, 1984, McGraw-Hill.
28. Mullen J: Consequences of malnutrition in the surgical patient, Surg Clin North Am 61(3):465, 1981.
29. Office of Cancer Communications: Coping with cancer: a resource for the health professional, Bethesda, 1982, US Department of Health and Human Services.
30. Pack R and Lynds BG: Surgical intervention. In McIntire SN and Cioppa AL, editors: Cancer

nursing: a developmental approach, New York, 1984, John Wiley & Sons, Inc.

31. Patterson WB: Principles of surgical oncology. In Rubin P, editor: Clinical oncology for medical students and physicians: a multidisciplinary approach, ed 6, New York, 1983, American Cancer Society.

32. Patterson WB: Surgical issues in geriatric oncology, Semin Oncol 16:57, 1989.

33. Rosenberg SA: Principles of surgical oncology. In DeVita VT Jr, Hellman S, and Rosenberg SA, editors: Cancer: principles and practice of oncology, ed 3, Philadelphia, 1989, JB Lippincott Co.

34. Scelsi DB and Tenenbaum L: Central venous catheters. In Tenenbaum L, editor: Cancer chemotherapy: a reference guide, Philadelphia, 1989, WB Saunders Co.

35. Scelsi DB and Tenenbaum L: Implanted infusion ports. In Tenenbaum L, editor: Cancer chemotherapy: a reference guide, Philadelphia, 1989, WB Saunders Co.

36. Scelsi DB and Tenenbaum L: Implanted infusion pumps. In Tenenbaum L, editor: Cancer chemotherapy: a reference guide, Philadelphia, 1989, WB Saunders Co.

37. Shamberger R: Effect of chemotherapy and radiotherapy on wound healing: experimental studies, Recent Results Cancer Res 98:17, 1985.

38. Sherman CD: Principles of surgical oncology. In Kahn SB and others, editors: Concepts in cancer medicine, New York, 1983, Grune & Stratton, Inc.

39. Shiplacoff TA: Concepts in surgical oncology. In Vredevoe D, Derdiarian A, and Sarna L, editors: Concepts of oncology nursing, Englewood Cliffs, NJ, 1981, Prentice-Hall.

40. Silberman AW: Surgical debulking of tumors, Surg Gynecol Obstet 155(3):577, 1982.

41. Smith RW, Sampson MK, and Lucas CE: Effects of vinblastine, etoposide, cisplatin and bleomycin in rodent wound healing, Surg Gynecol Obstet 161(4):323, 1985.

42. Snyder CC: Oncology nursing, Boston, 1986, Little, Brown and Co.

43. Szopa TJ: Implications of surgical treatment for nursing. In Clark JC and McGee RF, editors: Core curriculum for oncology nursing, ed 2, Philadelphia, 1992, WB Saunders Co.

44. Thompson JM and others: Clinical nursing, ed 2, St Louis, 1989, Mosby.

45. Tootla J and Easterling A: PDT: destroying malignant cells with laser beams . . . photodynamic therapy, Nurs 19(11):48, 1989.

46. Veronesi U: Principles of cancer surgery. In Holland JF and Frei E III, editors: Cancer medicine, Philadelphia, 1982, Lea & Febiger.

47. Willard MP, Gilsdorf RB, and Price RA: Protein-calorie malnutrition in a community hospital, JAMA 243:1720, 1980.

48. Wong RJ and DeCosse JJ: Cytoreductive surgery, Surg Gynecol Obstet 170(3):276, 1990.

49. Yasko J: Care of the client receiving external radiation, Reston, VA, 1982, Reston Publishing Co.

CHAPTER 21

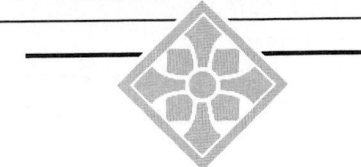

Radiation Therapy

Ryan Iwamoto

Radiation therapy is a localized treatment that is used alone or in conjunction with other treatments such as surgery, chemotherapy, or both. In certain situations, combining radiation therapy with other therapies maximizes cure rates because of the effect of the other therapies on radioresistant cells.[41] Radiation therapy may be administered prior to surgery to treat undisturbed tissues and to decrease the tumor size to make resection feasible. Radiation therapy may also be delivered after surgery to treat cancer cells that may be disseminated beyond the surgical margins. In other instances, radiation is used before and after surgical resection. Chemotherapy may be combined with radiation therapy to control subclinical disease and enhance the local effect of radiation.

Radiation therapy is used for several purposes:[11] to cure by eradicating disease, allowing the person to live a normal life span; to control the growth and spread of the disease, allowing the person to live for a time without symptoms; to prevent microscopic disease, as with cranial irradiation for certain types of lung cancers; and to improve a person's quality of life by relieving or reducing symptoms associated with advanced cancer. These symptoms include pain from bone metastasis; uncontrolled bleeding from the tumor; tumor obstruction around major blood vessels, gastrointestinal tract, kidneys, ureters and trachea; spinal cord compression; and symptoms related to brain metastasis.[11] The box at right summarizes the uses of radiation therapy.

DEFINITION

Radiation therapy is the use of high energy ionizing rays or particles to treat cancer. Approximately 60% of all persons with cancer will be treated with radiation therapy at some point during their illness.

USES OF RADIATION THERAPY

Radiocurable cancers

Skin
Hodgkin's disease—early stages
Breast—early stage following lumpectomy
Seminoma
Uterine cervix—stage II
Larynx—disease confined to vocal cords; with or without surgery
Prostate
Bladder
Anal canal

Adjuvant therapy

Bladder—preoperative radiation therapy
Breast—later stages; chest wall recurrence
Head and neck
Brain
Lung
Esophagus
Rectum
Soft-tissue sarcoma

Prophylactic therapy

Whole brain for lung cancer

Palliative therapy

Pain from bone metastasis
Bleeding—uncontrolled from tumor
Pressure—superior vena cava syndrome, spinal cord compression, brain metastasis

---

HISTORICAL PERSPECTIVE

Since the late nineteenth century when radium, radioactivity, and x-rays were discovered, radiation has been used to treat cancer. Radiation was one of the earliest ways cancer was treated. The first successful radiation treatment for cancer was reported in 1898.

At that time, large doses were delivered in a single treatment, which resulted in many complications. Between 1920 and 1940, studies were conducted to evaluate the effects of radiation on tissues, and fractionation of the dose (dividing the total dose into several small increments) was started.

With the invention of the vacuum tube, treatment with higher energies to deeper tissues was possible. In 1952, the first patient was treated with cobalt. Linear accelerators were developed in the mid-1950s and provided treatment rays with deeper penetration and less scatter to normal tissues. Over the past 100 years, the specialty of radiation oncology has advanced with the use of computer technology, the refinement of treatment machines and advancements in radiobiologic science.

PRINCIPLES OF RADIATION THERAPY

High-energy ionizing radiation destroys the cancer cell's ability to grow and multiply. Some cells are directly damaged by the ionizing rays or particles. However, more cells are indirectly affected when the ionizing rays or particles penetrate the cell's nucleus and interact with the water content of the nucleus to form oxygen radicals. These unstable radicals then cause damage to the cell's DNA with breakage of one or both chromosomal strands. Immediate cell death may occur if the chromosomal damage is irreparable. Some cells survive in spite of the chromosomal damage. However, these cells are unable to divide and die at the time of mitosis. As a result of radiation, some cells become giant cells, which continue to function but are unable to divide. These cells gradually degenerate and die.

The radiosensitivity of cancer cells is dependent upon several factors:
- Type of cell (see Table 21-1)
- Phase of cell life—cells in the resting stage are less sensitive to radiation than those in active cellular division
- Division rate of the cell—rapidly dividing cells are more sensitive to radiation than slowly dividing cells because more cells will be in the active cellular division stage
- Degree of differentiation—poorly differentiated cells are more sensitive to radiation therapy than well-differentiated cells
- Oxygenation—well-oxygenated tissues are more sensitive to radiation therapy because oxygen is needed to form the chemically active substances

Normal cells are also affected by the ionizing radiation. The sum total of the effects upon each cell in the tissue accounts for the side effects of radiation therapy. However, normal cells are generally better able to repair the chromosomal damage done by the radiation. The treatments are delivered to kill as

Table 21–1   Radiosensitivity of Various Tumors and Tissues

Tumors	Relative Radiosensitivity
Lymphoma, leukemia, seminoma, dysgerminoma	High
Squamous cell cancer of the oropharyngeal, glottis, bladder, skin, and cervical epithelia; adenocarcinomas of alimentary tract	Fairly high
Vascular and connective tissue elements of all tumors; secondary neurovascularization; astrocytomas	Medium
Salivary gland tumors, hepatomas, renal cancer, pancreatic cancer, chondrosarcoma, and osteogenic sarcoma	Fairly low
Rhabdomyosarcoma, leiomyosarcoma, and ganglioneurofibrosarcoma	Low

From Rubin P: Principles of radiation oncology and cancer radiotherapy. In Rubin P, editor: Clinical oncology for medical students and physicians, New York, 1983, American Cancer Society, p 60. Copyright 1983 by the American Cancer Society. Reprinted by permission.

many cancer cells as possible while minimizing the damage to normal cells. Body tissues have limits to the amount of radiation that can be tolerated. Exceeding those limits can result in serious complications[5] (Table 21-2).

Radiation dose is recorded as the absorbed energy per unit mass.[41] The Systeme Internationale Unit for radiation dosage, the Gray, has replaced the rad (radiation absorbed dose). One Gray (Gy) equals 100 rads; 1 cGy equals 1 rad.

ADMINISTRATION OF RADIATION THERAPY

Radiation therapy can be delivered in many ways. External beam radiation (teletherapy) uses a treatment machine placed at some distance from the body. Radiation can also be delivered by implanting a sealed radioactive source in or near the cancerous area to provide a localized treatment. This is called *brachytherapy*. The radioactive source may be placed within the body temporarily or permanently depending on the given situation. For brachytherapy patients receiving a temporary implant, isolation in a hospital room may be required while the implant is in place.

In other circumstances radioactive materials are injected intravenously or taken orally for a systemic effect (nonsealed sources). The radioactive substance travels to areas of the body requiring treatment. Thyroid cancer is frequently treated with radioactive iodine in this manner.

Tumor-specific antibodies that have been coupled with radioactive isotopes combines the science of immunology with radiation therapy to maximize tumor

Table 21–2 Minimal and Maximal Tolerance Dose of Various Organs

Organ	Injury	Minimal Tolerance Dose $TD_{5/5}$* (cGy)	Maximal Tolerance Dose $TD_{50/5}$† (cGy)	Whole or Partial Organ (Field Size or Length)
Bone marrow	Aplasia,	250	450	Whole
	pancytopenia	3,000	4,000	Segmental
Liver	Acute and chronic	2,500	4,000	Whole
	hepatitis	1,500	2,000	Whole (strip)
Stomach	Perforation, ulcer, hemorrhage	4,500	5,500	100 cm
Intestine	Ulcer, perforation,	4,500	5,500	400 cm
	hemorrhage	5,000	6,500	100 cm
Brain	Infarction, necrosis	5,000	6,000	Whole
Spinal cord	Infarction, necrosis	4,500	5,500	10 cm
Heart	Pericarditis,	4,500	5,500	60%
	pancarditis	7,000	8,000	25%
Lung	Acute and chronic	3,000	3,500	100 cm
	pneumonitis	1,500	2,500	Whole
Kidney	Acute and chronic	1,500	2,000	Whole (strip)
	nephrosclerosis	2,000	2,500	Whole
Fetus	Death	200	400	Whole

*$TD_{5/5}$ = Minimal tolerance dose. The dose, given to a population of patients under a standard set of treatment conditions, that will result in no more than a 5% rate of severe complications within 5 years after treatment.
†$TD_{50/5}$ = Maximal tolerance dose. The dose, given to a population of patients under a standard set of treatment conditions, that will result in a 50% rate of severe complications within 5 years after treatment.
From Rubin P, Cooper R, Phillips TL, editors: Radiation biology and radiation pathology syllabus, Set RT 1: Radiation oncology. Chicago, 1975, American College of Radiology. Reprinted by permission.

treatment while minimizing normal tissue toxicity.[12,83] These antibodies are designed to be attracted to specific antigens on certain tumor cells while sparing normal tissues. They are produced in animals and injected intravenously into the patient. When the radiolabeled antibodies are administered in the bloodstream, it seeks out the tumor and the radioactivity attached to the antibody directly treats the cancer cells. There are few acute side effects associated with antibody administration. Allergic reactions may be noted during or soon after the injection of the antibodies. Bone marrow suppression, particularly thrombocytopenia, may be noted 4 to 6 weeks after antibody administration.[12]

EXTERNAL RADIATION THERAPY
Treatment Planning

Before radiation treatments can begin, a plan is developed to determine the best way to deliver the treatments. A major part of the planning process is the localization procedure which uses a simulator (Figure 21-1). A *simulator* is a machine that simulates the treatment machine in its movement and positioning. Depending on the area being treated, a variety of radiographic studies such as CT scans, MRI studies, barium enemas, and intravenous pyelograms help define the exact area within the body that needs treatment (Fig-

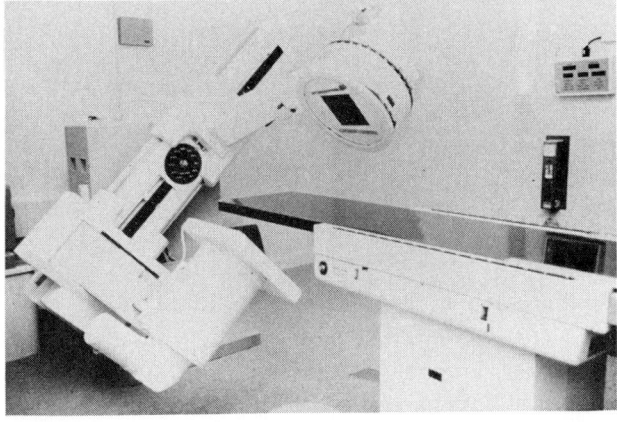

Figure 21–1 The simulator, which simulates the treatment machine, is used during the localization procedure. (Photo courtesy of Virginia Mason Clinic, Seattle, Wash.)

ure 21-2). Marks or small tattoos placed on the body are used to position the patient for treatment. These marks assure that treatment delivery will be consistent. Special plastic or plaster forms or molds may be constructed to help support and assist the patient to maintain a precise position during each treatment (Figure 21-3). The area of treatment is shaped with

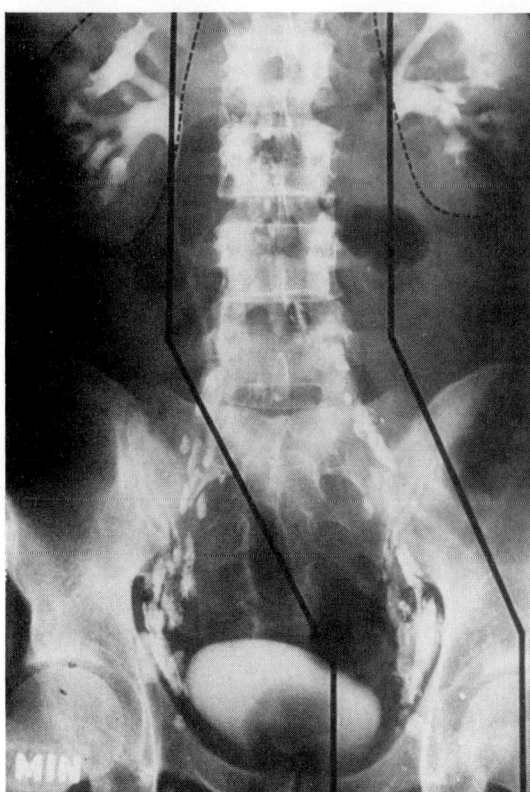

Figure 21–2 Simulation film. The radiation oncologist determines the treatment area using radiographic studies. The treatment area of this patient is the paraaortic and left inguinal lymph nodes. (Photo courtesy of Virginia Mason Clinic, Seattle, Wash.)

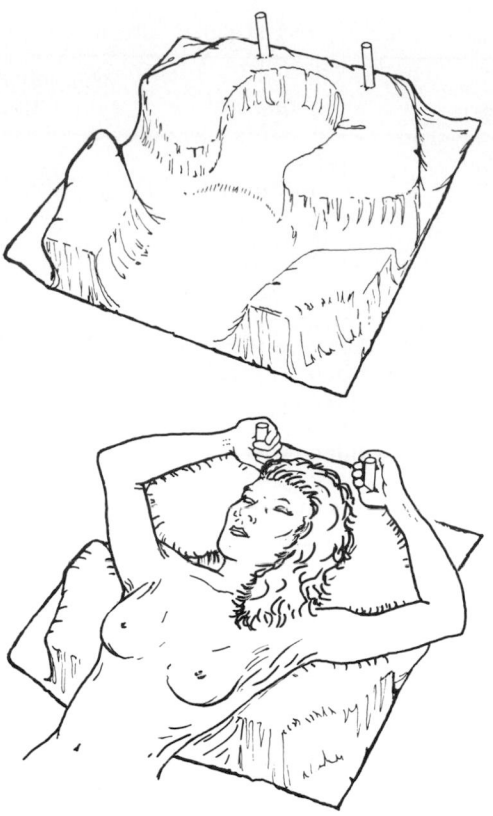

Figure 21–3 The Alpha-cradle is used to help women maintain their position for radiation therapy to the breast. The cradle is individually sized so that the woman is able to conform to the exact position necessary for treatment. (Photo courtesy of Virginia Mason Clinic, Seattle, Wash.)

special shielding devices called blocks. These blocks, made of lead or high-density alloys, help to minimize radiation exposure to normal tissues near the treatment area. A compensating filter may be used to differentially absorb the radiation beam to provide a uniform dose to the treatment volume. The treatment planning session usually lasts 1 to 2 hours.

Treatment Delivery

External radiation treatments are administered daily, Monday through Friday, for 2 to 8 weeks. Palliative treatments, such as for pain from bone metastasis, may be delivered at higher daily doses for fewer numbers of treatment. The actual treatment takes 2 to 5 minutes. More time is spent carefully positioning the patient on the treatment table.

A variety of machines are used in radiation therapy, depending on the type and extent of the tumor. These machines vary according to the energy produced as well as ionizing particles delivered (Table 21-3). Linear accelerators are commonly used in cancer therapy (Figure 21-4). The higher the energy produced by the machine, the greater the depth of penetration of the radiation beam. With higher energies the maximum effect of the radiation occurs below the skin surface and the dose to the skin is minimized;

thus the term skin-sparing effect. There is also less radiation scatter with higher energies of radiation (Figure 21-5).

The number of treatments delivered during a course of radiation therapy depends on the type and extent of cancer, the area treated, and dose. Because a single large dose of radiation is too toxic to normal tissues, the total radiation dose is divided into small daily doses or fractions to be given over time. This process is called *fractionation*. The dose is usually the same each day. With fractionation of the total dose more radiation can be delivered to the tumor while minimizing the damage to normal tissues because fractionation allows normal cells to repair the sublethal damage after each treatment.[41] Fractionation also increases damage to the tumor because of reassortment of cells into radiosensitive phases of the cell cycle and an increased oxygenation in the tumor.[36] Large tumors usually contain cells that are far from a capillary network and as a result are hypoxic. As the tumor shrinks over time, oxygenation increases within the tumor as more cells have access to the capillary blood flow. As a result, this improves the radiation's effectiveness.

Table 21–3 Treatment Machines

Machine	Treatment Beam	
KILOVOLTAGE Mechanical	X-rays	Low-level energy; superficial treatment; scatter of radiation beam; intracavitary therapy
MEGAVOLTAGE Cobalt-60 radioactive source is in head of machine; replaced every 5 to 10 years because of decay of the isotope	Gamma rays (1-4 MeV)	Deeper penetration than kilovoltage; below skin level; less scatter
SUPERVOLTAGE Linear accelerators Betatron Cyclotron	 X-rays and electrons (4-35 MeV) Electrons Protons, neutrons, or electrons	 Less scatter; deep tumors More DNA double-strand injury; less oxygen dependent; less cell cycle specific

MeV, million electron volts; the energy of an electron accelerated across 1 million volts.

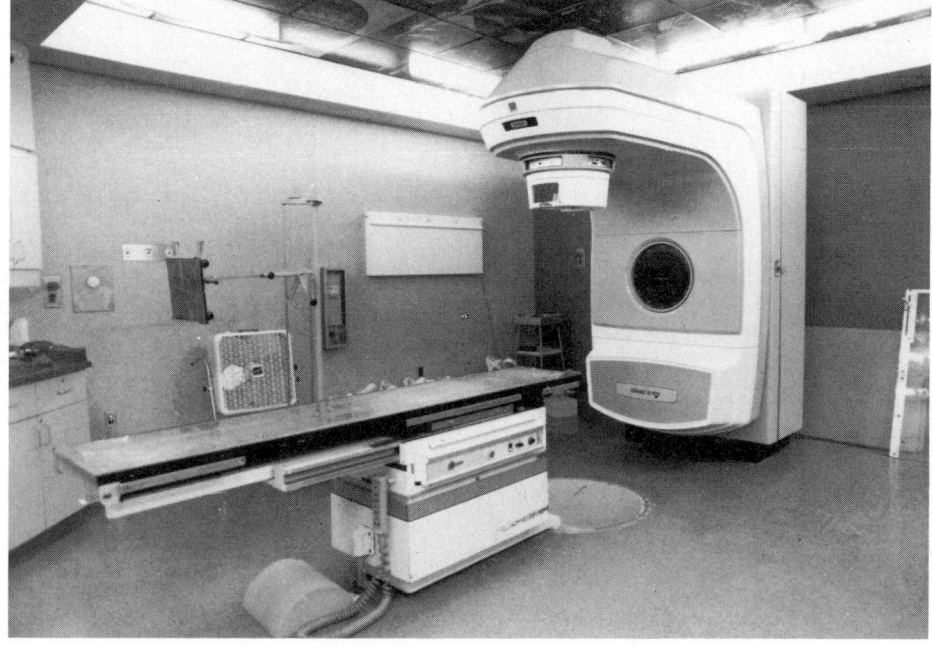

Figure 21–4 Linear accelerator provides supervoltage treatment. (From Belcher AE: Cancer nursing, St Louis, 1992, Mosby.)

Some treatment schemes deliver treatments two to three times a day with at least 5 to 6 hours between each fraction. This is called *hyperfractionation*. Hyperfractionation may improve the treatment of large tumors, tumors with excessive bleeding and brain tumors.[83] The increased fractionation theoretically affects more mitotically active cells each day.

FUTURE DIRECTIONS AND ADVANCES IN RADIATION THERAPY
Total Body Irradiation
Leukemic cells are radiosensitive. In conjunction with bone marrow transplantation, supralethal radiation in the form of total body irradiation and chemotherapy are administered to reduce the tumor volume and provide immunosuppression to prevent the rejection of the marrow graft.[30] A variety of techniques provide a homogeneous dose of radiation to the entire body (Figure 21-6). Doses range from 8 to 14 Gy, depending on fractionation. Acute side effects include nausea and vomiting, parotitis, anorexia, diarrhea, and fatigue.[27] Effects such as stomatitis, pancytopenia, and interstitial pneumonitis occur during the weeks following total body irradiation. Delayed effects of total body irradiation include gonadal insufficiency and cataracts.[4]

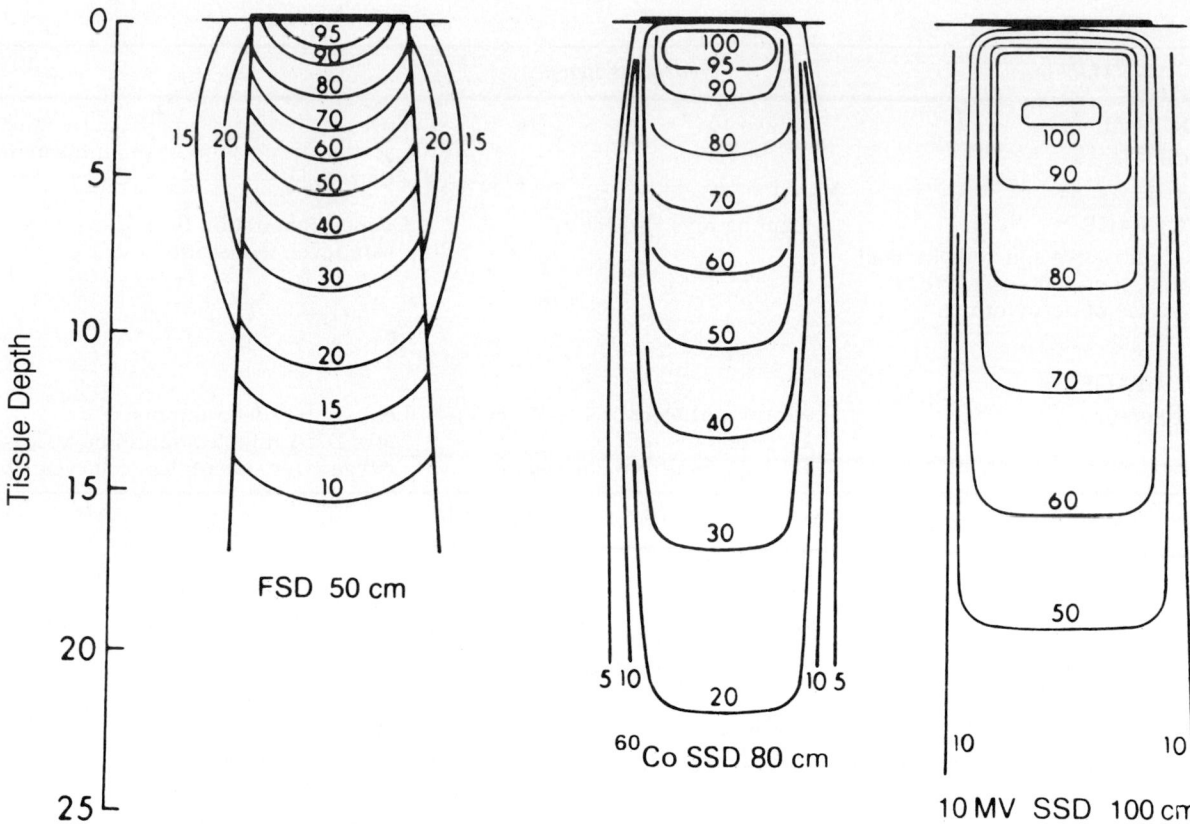

Figure 21–5 Isodose distributions (percent of dose delivered) comparing increasing energies: kilovoltage (250 kVp), megavoltage (cobalt), and supervoltage (10 mV). FSD is equal to focal skin distance, or the distance from the focal spot in the x-ray tube to the skin of the patient. SSD is equal to source-surface distance, or the distance from the front surface of the source of radiation to the surface of the patient. As the energy increases, the superficial tissues are spared, with the maximal radiation dose occurring below the skin surface. This results in less skin reactions and less side scatter. (From Keller BE and Rubin P: Basic concepts of radiation physics. In Rubin P, editor: Clinical oncology for medical students and physicians, New York, 1983, American Cancer Society.)

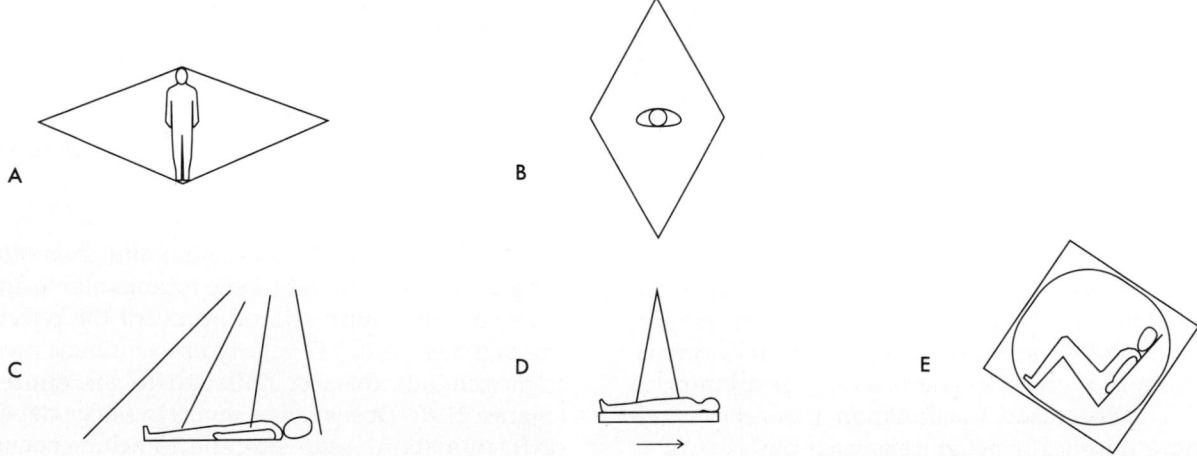

Figure 21–6 Methods of delivery of total body irradiation. **A,** Lateral opposed beams. **B,** Floor and ceiling parallel opposed beams. **C,** Supine and prone treatment using three matching fields. **D,** Supine and prone—patient moves horizontally through treatment beam field. **E,** Horizontal shrinking field technique—patient in sitting position. (From Quast U: Total body irradiation, Radiother Oncol 9:95, 1987, and Novack DH and Kiley JP: Total body irradiation, Front Radiat Ther Onc 21:69, 1987.)

Half-Body Irradiation

When patients have numerous painful areas from bone metastasis located in the upper or lower half of the body, half-body irradiation may be utilized to provide expedient pain relief. This procedure delivers a single treatment to the upper or lower half of the body and frequently results in dramatic pain relief.[83] When the upper body is treated, premedication with antiemetics is necessary. Hypotension, fever, and chills can occur and may require brief hospitalization following the treatment. With mid-body irradiation, bone marrow depression and diarrhea as well as nausea and vomiting can occur. Lower body irradiation can result in bone marrow depression and diarrhea.

Hyperthermia

The use of heat, or *hyperthermia*, with radiation therapy has shown some promise in the treatment of locally advanced solid tumors.[25,64,65,75] Heat is cytotoxic by affecting the cell membranes and causing damage of lysosomal vesicles within the cell, which in turn release digestive enzymes that cause cell death. Hyperthermia enhances the effects of radiation therapy on certain radioresistant and hypoxic tumor cells because heat affects more S-phase (synthesis) cells and poorly vascularized tumors are less able to dissipate the heat. The heat may also help to make permanent the radiation-induced chromosomal damage within the tumor cells, rendering them unable to repair the damage.

Hyperthermia is usually applied immediately after a radiation treatment. The number of treatments depends on the tumor site and its extent. Approximately 72 hours between treatments provide maximum benefits from hyperthermia.[64]

Hyperthermia is applied locally or regionally. Local hyperthermia may be accomplished with microwaves, ultrasound, deep heating with electromagnetic wave applicators, and interstitial hyperthermia with probes implanted in or near the tumor. Regional hyperthermia involves perfusing heated solutions through a part of the body. The optimal therapeutic temperature is 41° to 45° C for approximately 45 minutes.[64] Interstitial temperature probes are usually inserted within the body part as well as placed superficially to monitor the heat. Close monitoring of the heat is required to obtain optimal heating with minimal discomfort and side effects. Side effects associated with hyperthermia include local discomfort and skin reactions ranging from transient erythema to edema and blisters. Hyperthermia enhances the skin reactions associated with radiation therapy.[83] Careful assessments for signs of infections are necessary. Hyperthermia with ultrasound has occasionally been associated with substantial pain, requiring the procedure to be stopped.[80]

Hyperthermia is also being used with interstitial brachytherapy to treat tumors of the head and neck, breast, prostate, and rectum.[8] After catheters are placed within the tissues, hyperthermia is applied for approximately 1 hour. The catheters are then immediately loaded with the radioactive sources for a prescribed length of time. A second 1 hour treatment with hyperthermia is then administered following the removal of the radioactive sources.

The use of hyperthermia can compound the patient's anxiety associated with radiation therapy. The fears of "being heated" and "being burned" are frightening perceptions that nurses can help patients confront and understand.

Intraoperative Radiation Therapy

Intraoperative radiation therapy provides direct visualization and treatment of tumors to control local recurrence of cancer.[2,32] After surgical exposure, a targeting cone is placed directly on the tumor site. This cone helps to displace normal tissues and thus minimize toxicities. The treatment machine is carefully aligned with the cone. All persons leave the treatment room for the 15 to 25 minutes it takes to deliver the fairly large dose of electron irradiation (approximately 2000 cGy). Anesthesia personnel monitor the patient through a closed-circuit television. Intraoperative radiation is used to treat locally advanced abdominal cancers such as gastric, pancreatic, colorectal, bladder, cervical, and retroperitoneal sarcomas. Complications and side effects, no greater than with radiation therapy or surgery, may include nausea, vomiting, and anorexia.[32,35] No increased risk for poor wound healing or postoperative infection has been reported, and severe complications such as neuropathy have been few.[15] Coordination between departments and disciplines is required to provide this complex therapy.[2,3,35]

Radiosensitizers

Chemical radiosensitizing compounds are used to increase the lethal effects of radiation therapy.[21,36] Nonhypoxic sensitizers such as iododeoxyuridine (IUdR) incorporate into the DNA and increase the susceptibility of the cell to radiation damage. Hypoxic cell sensitizers such as metronidazole, misonidazole, SR2508, and Ro-03-8799 increase oxygen to hypoxic cells and promote damage of the DNA, preventing cell repair. Depending on the agent, side effects include peripheral neuropathy, nausea and vomiting, and skin rashes. Certain chemotherapeutic agents such as cyclophosphamide or cisplatin are also being used as radiosensitizers and are given in conjunction with radiation therapy.

Stereotactic External-Beam Irradiation

Stereotactic irradiation involves treatment of relatively small intracranial volumes with a three dimensional distribution of the treatment beam.[56] This technique decreases the radiation dose to normal tissues. Benign conditions such as arteriovenous malformations and malignancies such as astrocytomas and brain metastases are treated with stereotactic external-beam irradiation. Various methods such as gamma units using cobalt ("gamma knife") and modified cobalt or linear accelerator units are used. To perform this treatment, a stereotactic frame is fixed to the patient's skull and used to target the treatment beam. Treatment is usually given in a single fraction. Steroid medications are used to minimize cerebral edema.

Text continued on p. 489.

Nursing Management

NURSING CARE RELATED TO EXTERNAL RADIATION THERAPY

Understanding the principles of radiobiology is the key to understanding symptom management. The side effects associated with radiation therapy are localized and depend on area treated, volume of tissue irradiated, fractionation, total dose, type of radiation, and individual differences. Variations of side effects will be observed among people receiving similar courses of treatment. A delay between the time of radiation exposure and the time the effects are seen can vary from days to weeks to months depending on the cell's metabolic activity. Early reactions occur during or within weeks after treatment. Some symptoms do not subside until 2 or more weeks after treatment has ended. Delayed reactions occur months to years following therapy. Since radiation therapy has its greatest effect on rapidly dividing cells, the epithelial tissues such as mucous membranes and the skin are most susceptible to its effects. Selected nursing diagnoses related to radiation therapy are listed as follows:

NURSING DIAGNOSES

- Impaired skin integrity related to radiation therapy
- Infection related to skin breakdown
- Activity intolerance related to radiation therapy
- Altered nutrition, less than body requirements related to anorexia
- Altered oral mucous membrane related to head and neck irradiation
- Sensory-perceptual alterations: gustatory, related to head and neck irradiation
- Impaired swallowing related to esophagitis
- Alteration in comfort related to cough
- Altered nutrition, less than body requirements, related to nausea and vomiting
- Diarrhea related to pelvic irradiation
- Altered patterns of urinary elimination related to pelvic irradiation
- Ineffective individual coping related to alopecia
- Disturbance in self-esteem related to alopecia
- Anxiety about radiation therapy
- Knowledge deficit about radiation therapy and self-care measures

General Side Effects

SKIN

Certain skin reactions are normal and expected with radiation therapy.[39] The skin overlying the areas being treated may develop a reaction as soon as 2 weeks into the course of treatment.[20,43,44,77,82] Skin erythema may range from mild, light pink to deep and dusky.[43] Increased skin sensitivity and slight edema may also appear. As treatment continues, the skin reaction can progress, with the skin becoming slightly to moderately dry, itchy, and flaky (dry desquamation). In some cases the skin develops mild to severe moist desquamation, in which the epidermal layers of the skin slough, leaving a raw, painful area that may drain serous exudate.[20,39] Areas of moist desquamation generally heal within several weeks.[77]

Skin reactions vary but tend to be greater in those receiving large doses of radiation.[82] Also, treatments with electron beams usually produce more intense skin reactions because of the superficial concentration of the radiation dose. Some treatments involve the use of a bolus material placed on the skin to increase the skin dose. In addition, certain treatments are given from a tangential angle as opposed to perpendicular to the treatment site. These techniques can increase the skin reaction.[43,62,77] Certain areas of the skin such as areas covering bony prominences or surgical wounds tend to be more sensitive to the effects of radiation than others.[38] Areas having skin folds such as the axilla, under the breasts, perineum, groin, and gluteal fold are also at increased risk for developing a skin reaction because of increased warmth and moisture and lack of aeration.[43,77] The skin on the face is also particularly sensitive to the effects of radiation. Skin reactions may also occur where the radiations exit, that is, on the opposite side of the body from where the treatment is delivered. Evaluating the angle of the treatment beam will help determine where these reactions may occur. When chemotherapy is used in conjunction with radiation therapy, the patient is at higher risk of developing a skin reaction.[63]

Special consideration needs to be given to patients receiving pelvic irradiation following low anterior or anterior-posterior resection for rectal cancer. The surgical wound site is at increased risk for skin breakdown because the perineum is generally within the treatment field. The radiation oncologist may have the buttocks taped apart during the actual radiation treatment to minimize the skin reaction.[38] If a stoma such as colostomy or ileostomy is included in the treatment field, the stoma appliance and skin barrier can act as a bolus material and enhance the skin reaction. Daily assessments of the skin are necessary and removal of the skin barrier and appliance may be required during the actual treatment to minimize peristomal skin breakdown.[38]

Before beginning radiation therapy, instruct the patient to protect the skin and minimize sources of irritation and trauma. Nursing diagnoses related to skin care include "Actual or potential for impaired skin integrity" and "Potential for infection related to skin breakdown." Assess the patient's usual skin care. Unintentional enhancement of skin reactions may occur if patients use products contraindicated during radiation therapy. These include compresses, ointments, and other remedies prescribed before diagnosis and treatment.[43] Plan to educate the patient and family about skin care during radiation therapy. Cleanse the skin with lukewarm water as needed and pat rather than rub the skin with a towel to dry. Avoid using soaps. When soap is necessary, use only nondeodorant, unperfumed soaps. Powders, perfumes, and deodorants should not be applied to the irradiated skin, as they can dry and irritate the skin. Avoid the use of cornstarch in the axilla, groin, and gluteal folds.[44,78] Shaving with a razor blade within treatment areas should be avoided. An electric razor may be used if there is no skin irritation. Protect the treated skin from cold, heat, and sun. Only loose-fitting cotton clothing should be worn close to the skin.[20,44] Tight, restrictive clothing such as bras and belts over the treated area may chafe the skin and should not be worn.[39] In addition, avoid placing adhesive tape over the irradiated skin, as this will further irritate the skin.

If the skin becomes dry, the patient may complain of tenderness and pruritus. A nonperfumed hydrophilic moisturizing lotion that contains no heavy metal ions may be applied to the skin upon the recommendation of the radiation oncologist or radiation oncology nurse. Avoid having lotion on the skin during treatment, because the lotion may increase the skin reaction. Remove excess lotion with a soft washcloth before treatment. Although topical steroids can help decrease pruritus and tenderness because of vasoconstriction, they must be used with extreme caution. Steroid creams and ointments can cause thinning of the skin and delay skin healing.[38] Fluorinated preparations are not recommended because they cause more vasoconstriction and thinning of the skin.[38,43] Steroid preparations should not be used for moist skin reactions.[78]

For moist desquamation, normal saline irrigations or cool compresses may be applied to the affected area three to four times a day to soothe the skin. Cleansing with half-strength to third-strength hydrogen peroxide and saline followed by a rinse with saline may also be used.[11,39,82,90] Caution with use of ointments and salves is important to avoid increasing the skin reaction. A thin layer of A&D ointment, lanolin, or Aquaphor may be applied to the moist desquamation.[36,43,44] In some instances, treatment is stopped and zinc oxide or silver sulfadiazine cream is put either directly on the skin or on a nonadherent dressing (Telfa pad or combine dressings), which is then applied to the moist reaction.[43] Hydrocolloid dressings have been found effective to heal dermatitis and moist desquamation.[59,69] These dressings may be left on the skin reaction for up to 5 days to provide comfort. No increase in infection rates has been reported. Assess for signs of infection and culture suspicious lesions and drainage.[87] With painful skin reactions, systemic analgesics are sometimes necessary, especially at bedtime, to allow the patient to rest.

If moist desquamation occurs in the perineum, then sitz baths, perineal compresses, and protective emollients may all be used.[38] A hand-held blow dryer may be used on cool setting to dry the perineum. These reactions are painful, and treatment is frequently stopped for a time to allow the tissues to heal.

Once radiation therapy is completed, the skin usually heals within a few weeks. Although the acute tenderness and erythema diminish within 2 weeks, the patient may be left with a tanned skin within the treatment field, which will usually subside.[20] The irradiated skin may also remain more sensitive to heat or cold and develop a sunburn more readily than untreated parts of the body.[39,45,78] The patient should continue to protect the irradiated skin by avoiding direct sun exposure by using clothing such as scarves and hats. A sunblock with a high sun protection factor (SPF) should be used when sun exposure is unavoidable. Delayed effects of the skin from radiation include fibrosis and atrophy of the skin, telangiectasia, and lymphedema as a result of fibrosis of the lymph glands.[87] These delayed effects occur because of changes in the vascular component of the skin leading to tissue damage.[77] Recall phenomenon occurs months to years after a course of radiation therapy. In this phenomenon, skin, mucous membrane, or pul-

Table 21—4   Nursing Care of Irradiated Skin

When treatment begins:	• Assess skin integrity
	• Instruct patient to minimize trauma and protect the skin within the treatment field:
	  —Cleanse skin with lukewarm water as needed.
	  —Avoid use of soaps, powders, perfumes, deodorants.
	  —Avoid shaving.
	  —Protect skin from cold, heat, sun.
	  —Wear loose-fitting clothing over treatment site.
	  —Avoid adhesive tape on irradiated skin.

If dry desquamation occurs:	• Use a hydrophilic moisturizing lotion two to three times a day (e.g., Aquaphor®). • Remove excess lotion from skin before daily treatment.
If moist desquamation occurs:	• Saline irrigations or cool compresses may be used three to four times a day. • Apply hydrocolloid dressing for comfort (e.g., DuoDerm®). • If treatment is withheld, zinc oxide or silver sulfadiazine may be applied to skin reaction and covered with a nonadherent dressing. • Culture suspicious lesions and drainage. • Use analgesics as necessary.
When treatment is completed and skin is healed:	• Instruct the patient to protect the irradiated skin by avoiding exposure to sun, heat, or cold. • Use of sunblock when sun exposure is unavoidable.

monary reactions occur with the treated area when certain chemotherapeutic agents such as dactinomycin and doxorubicin are given systemically. These reactions are generally more severe than the skin reactions seen during radiation therapy and subside within 2 weeks.[39] Evaluate the patient and family's understanding of potential and actual skin reactions and appropriate care and protection of the skin. Table 21-4 summarizes guidelines for skin care.

FATIGUE

Fatigue, the subjective feeling of tiredness, is experienced by many people receiving radiation therapy.[40,52,66] The etiology of fatigue is not well understood.[90] Fatigue may result from tumor breakdown, which releases by-products into the blood stream. Another theory suggests an increased basal metabolic rate, which quickly uses the body's energy stores. Fatigue may occur after treatment each day and become chronic as treatment continues.[40,52,82] Variations, including less fatigue on Sundays because there is no treatment over the weekend, have been reported.[40] Fatigue is compounded by pain, depression, anorexia, infection, anemia, and dyspnea.[1] Although the level of fatigue varies among individuals, most people are able to continue their work and usual activities. Fatigue may persist weeks to months after the completion of radiation therapy and gradually disappear.[52]

A nursing diagnosis of "Actual or potential activity intolerance" can be made for the person receiving radiation therapy. Assess for the presence and pattern of fatigue. Evaluate factors that increase or decrease fatigue. Monitor blood counts for anemia, which can compound fatigue.

Assist patients and families to understand that fatigue can occur with radiation therapy. Help patients to evaluate their activities so they can pace themselves throughout the day and plan for rest periods or naps as needed. Determining the times of the day when extra energy is needed can help a person to plan rest periods through the day and evening. Taking a nap immediately after returning home from treatment helps some to have energy for the rest of the day.[44,45,90] Plan for assistance with transportation, purchase and preparation of food, child care, and other activities of daily living. Evaluate the need for assistive devices such as a cane or walker. These measures can help minimize exertion with certain activities and decrease fatigue.[1,44,90] If the patient is experiencing pain, assure adequate pain management with pharmacologic and nonpharmacologic measures. In addition, assure that the person is maintaining an adequate nutritional intake.[90] People with recent weight loss who are undergoing therapy will need additional nutritional supplementation. This supplementation will help the patient maintain or improve nutritional status and minimize fatigue. A dietitian is an excellent resource to help plan the patient's nutritional program. Evaluate the patient's and family's understanding of the causes of fatigue and their ability to modify activities to maintain or improve function.

ANOREXIA

Loss of appetite, or anorexia, sometimes is a result of cancer itself but also may come from cancer therapy. As with fatigue, the mechanisms causing anorexia are unclear. Contributing factors include inactivity, medications, and inability to ingest and digest foods.[45] The patient has a loss of appetite, which can result in weight loss and progressive fatigue.

Assess the loss of appetite in patients receiving radiation therapy. The nursing diagnosis "Altered nu-

Table 21-5 Guidelines for Frequency of Blood Counts—Joint Center for Radiation Therapy

Site	No Prior Chemotherapy	Previous Chemotherapy <1 Year	Previous Chemotherapy >1 Year	Concomitant Chemotherapy
Breast	Baseline, 3 weeks later if taking Tamoxifen	Weekly—every other week	Every 3 weeks	Bi-weekly—weekly
Head/Neck	Every 3 weeks	Every other week	Every 3 weeks	Bi-weekly—weekly
Whole Brain	Baseline only	Weekly	Every 3 weeks	Weekly
Hodgkins	Weekly	Weekly	Weekly	Bi-weekly
Lung/Esophagus*	Weekly—every other week	Weekly—every other week	Weekly	Bi-weekly—weekly
Spine†	Weekly—every other week	Weekly	Weekly	Bi-weekly—weekly
Pelvis* Prostate	Every other week	Every other week	Weekly—every other week	Weekly
Colon	Every other week	Weekly	Weekly	Bi-weekly—weekly
GYN	Every other week	Weekly	Weekly	Bi-weekly—weekly

*Depends upon field size, hx of previous irradiation.
†Depends upon the presence and extent of metastatic disease.
From Hirshfield-Bartek J et al: Monitoring the myelosuppression effects of radiation therapy, Oncol Nurs Forum 15:547, 1988.

trition, less than body requirements" is made for the person with anorexia. Discuss with the patient and family the fact that anorexia sometimes occurs in people undergoing radiation therapy and suggest ways to overcome this problem. Assist the patient and family to plan ways to improve appetite to help the patient eat adequately and maintain body weight.

Frequent small meals rather than three large ones can help make eating less overwhelming and allow more food to be consumed throughout the day. Instruct the patient and family to have high-calorie, high-protein foods readily available at all times. Specially prepared nutritional supplements and carefully selected convenience foods can provide additional calories and protein. Because radiation treatments are given daily and considerable time is spent commuting to and from treatments, suggest that the patient carry snacks to consume during the commute. Some patients have found that having a meal at a restaurant each day is a special treat to look forward to. Consult a dietitian to determine the nutritional needs of the patient and plan additional ways to meet those needs. Help the patient and family understand the importance of nutrition during therapy. Evaluate their ability to utilize suggestions to enhance appetite and maintain optimal nutrition (see Chapter 27).

BONE MARROW SUPPRESSION

When large volumes of active bone marrow are treated with radiation, a decrease in bone marrow function occurs.[90] These treatment areas include the pelvis, spine, sternum, ribs, metaphyses of long bones, and skull.[45] Blood counts must be monitored routinely. The fall in blood counts usually develops slowly.

However, if chemotherapy is combined with radiation therapy, the blood counts can fall precipitously and must be closely followed. Table 21-5 describes guidelines for frequency of blood counts. Factors affecting the frequency of obtaining blood counts include treatment site, use of other myelosuppressive therapies, stage of disease, and age of patient.

Assess for infections, bleeding, and fatigue. Plan and implement education for the patient and family about precautions for neutropenia, thrombocytopenia, and anemia.[19] Transfusions of blood products are sometimes used, and in some cases radiation therapy is withheld for a while to allow the blood counts to recover. Evaluate the patient's and family's understanding and use of self-care measures and precautions for bone marrow suppression.

Site-Specific Side Effects

HEAD AND NECK

Radiation therapy is given to the head and neck for cancers of the mouth, tongue, and larynx. Some problems are stomatitis, xerostomia, dental caries, taste changes, osteoradionecrosis, and hypopituitarism.[89]

Stomatitis

Stomatitis, or irritation of the mucosa in the mouth and oropharynx, can occur as the radiation affects the rapidly dividing cells of the oral mucosa. The patient may first note a tenderness in the mouth. This tenderness may be accompanied with mild to moderate erythema and edema of the mucosa. A whitish pseudomembrane may form on the surface of the mucosa. This membrane should be left undisturbed. Eventually this membrane pulls away from the underlying tissue, leaving a painful and friable ulcer.[6] Bleeding often results when stomatitis is severe. Superimposed bacterial, fungal, and/or viral infections can also occur. The mucosal reaction may be enhanced by metallic tooth restorations in adjacent areas, which cause electron back scatter of radiation. During treatments a material with a low atomic number such as a piece of gauze or an oral stent made of dental acrylic is sometimes placed between the tooth and mucosa to minimize this reaction.[49,53]

Mouth care is crucial for the person receiving radiation therapy for head and neck cancer. Tooth brushing and flossing, if tolerated, after meals and at bedtime will help remove debris from the teeth and gingiva. If tooth brushing becomes too painful, warm saline rinses and gentle swabbing with moistened gauze or a tooth sponge may be better tolerated. Instruct the patient and family on mouth care, including inspecting the oral cavity each day. Poorly fitting dental prostheses should not be worn until evaluated by a dentist; nor should the prosthesis be used when the mouth and gingiva become painful, because the prosthesis can cause more irritation and lead to mucosal breakdown. Oral pain is controlled with topical anesthetics or systemic analgesics. Viscous lidocaine, dyclonine hydrochloride, diphenhydramine, and Mylanta provide topical pain relief. Nonsteroidal antiinflammatory agents provide topical pain relief as well as antiinflammatory actions.[73]

Instruct the patient to use a soft, bland diet to make chewing and swallowing easier, allowing the patient to maintain nutrional intake. Topical thrombin can be applied to control minor areas of bleeding in the mouth and topical or systemic antibiotics are used to control oral infections.[67]

Xerostomia

Xerostomia, or dryness of the mouth, may occur 1 to 2 weeks into therapy. When the treatment field includes the salivary glands, the saliva changes from a thin to a thick, sticky, and acidic fluid that is unable to cleanse the mouth. As a result, debris adheres more readily to the teeth. The patient may note difficulty speaking, problems with retention of dentures, and difficulty eating certain foods such as crackers, breads, and peanut butter. With higher doses of radiation, xerostomia may remain a chronic problem.[23] Older patients are at higher risk for xerostomia because of normally decreased levels of oral secretions.

Instruct the patient to perform mouth care before meals to help relieve xerostomia. Assist the patient and family to assess food choices and preparation to appropriately modify the patient's diet. Sauces, gravies, and other liquids taken with meals can moisten dry and thick foods. Frequent sips of fluids and atomizer mists are helpful. Sucking on sugarless sour candies can help stimulate salivation. Commercially available saliva substitutes such as Moi-Stir, Oralbalance, and Mouth Kote provide temporary relief of xerostomia. Two to three milliliters of solution are placed in the mouth and swished to coat the mucosal surfaces. Products containing lemon or glycerin should be avoided, as these may cause further irritation and drying of the mucosa.[85,88] Lemon juice also decalcifies teeth.[88] Commercial mouthwashes should be avoided because many contain alcohol and/or flavoring agents that further irritate the mucosa. Patients may find a room humidifier used at bedtime helps decrease mucosal dryness and minimize the frequency with which they awaken to drink fluids.[54]

Tooth decay and caries

Tooth decay and caries become rampant as a result of xerostomia.[23] Cariogenic bacteria adhere to the teeth and flourish in the acidic environment. Before treatment a dentist evaluates the patient and provides prophylaxis, including extraction of teeth with extensive decay. A daily program of fluoride application on debris-free teeth is important to prevent caries.[23,45,90] The fluoride is applied once or twice a day using specially constructed trays. These trays are filled with fluoride gel and placed over the teeth for approximately 5 to 10 minutes. The patient may expectorate the excess gel, but should not rinse the mouth or drink fluids for at least 30 minutes. Since xerostomia often becomes a chronic problem, the use of fluoride must be continued even after radiation therapy is completed to prevent tooth decay.

NURSING DIAGNOSES FOR PERSONS RECEIVING HEAD AND NECK IRRADIATION (FLOOR OF MOUTH)

Pretreatment phase

- Anxiety regarding radiation therapy.
- Knowledge deficit related to radiation therapy and self care measures.

INTERVENTIONS

- Allow verbalization of fears, concerns, questions.
- Provide education:
    Use of radiation therapy for cancer of the floor of the mouth.
    Potential side effects (stomatitis, taste changes, xerostomia, fatigue, and skin changes) and appropriate self-care measures.

NURSING DIAGNOSES FOR PERSONS
RECEIVING HEAD AND NECK IRRADIATION
(FLOOR OF MOUTH) — cont'd

Pretreatment phase — cont'd

INTERVENTIONS — cont'd

- Consult dentist for evaluation and fluoride prophylaxis.
- Inspect mouth.

Treatment phase

- Altered oral mucous membrane related to head and neck irradiation.

- Inspect mouth daily: assess for stomatitis, infections
- Review mouth care:
  Brush and floss teeth if tolerated.
  As stomatitis progresses, use moistened gauze instead of toothbrushing and flossing.
  Rinse with normal saline at least four times a day.
- Provide soft, bland diet.
- Maintain hydration.
- Use saliva substitute and moisten foods for xerostomia.
- Offer topical anesthetics or analgesic medications prior to meals to relieve oral pain.
- Monitor weight.

- Sensory-perceptual alterations: gustatory, related to head and neck irradiation.

- Instruct patient to perform mouth care before and after meals.
- Experiment with different foods and tastes such as cold cooked chicken.

- Impaired skin integrity.

- Review skin care measures.
  Protect skin.
  Avoid using soap on the skin within the treatment field(s).
  Avoid constricting clothing or jewelry around the neck.
  Avoid shaving.
  Use moisturizing lotion if dryness occurs.
- If moist desquamation occurs:
  Burows compresses four times a day.
  Hydrocolloid dressings applied to desquamated areas.

- Activity intolerance.

- Evaluate activities.
- Plan rest periods during the day.
- Assist in securing community resources:
  Transportation to and from treatment center.
  Food purchasing and preparation.

Posttreatment phase

- Altered oral mucous membrane related to head and neck irradiation.

- Assess oral status (xerostomia, taste changes); inspect mouth.
- Review importance of oral hygiene and frequent visits to the dentist.
- To prevent osteoradionecrosis, continue prophylactic fluoride treatments.
- Review importance of minimizing alcohol and tobacco intake to reduce the risk of oral complications.

Taste change

Taste changes occur as the taste buds are affected by the radiation.[18] Occasionally patients report a bad or peculiar taste in the mouth. For instance, certain red meats may taste rancid or coffee may taste extremely bitter. In other cases there is a decrease in some or all taste sensations.[14] This can be very frustrating for patients who already have a loss of appetite and are trying to increase their nutritional intake. Although some recovery of taste may occur, alterations can persist 7 years or longer.[61] Therefore follow-up assessments of taste changes and their influence on nutrition should be ongoing.[81]

Mouth care should be performed before and after each meal. Experimenting with different foods and using additional seasonings, if tolerated, can help make food more palatable.[28] If red meats are a problem, use other sources of protein such as fish and poultry. Marinating meats in wine or sweet and sour sauce before and during cooking can mask unpleasant tastes. Serving foods cold or at room temperature also blunts peculiar tastes.

Osteoradionecrosis

Osteoradionecrosis, a late and chronic effect of radiation therapy, usually occurs in the mandible. Trauma to the bone such as tooth decay and infections heal poorly because of compromised bone structure and can lead to necrosis of the bone. Patients who continue to consume tobacco and/or alcohol are at a greater risk for developing this serious complication.[23] Another risk factor is poorly fitting dentures, which abrade the mucosa. The mucosal breakdown can eventually reach the mandible. Treatment of osteoradionecrosis may include antibiotic therapy, surgical removal of the necrotic bone, and hyperbaric oxygen therapy to promote healing of the bone.[3,4,16,60,87]

Nursing care includes teaching and reinforcing the need to maintain good oral hygiene with frequent visits to the dentist for evaluation. Minimizing mouth irritants such as tobacco and alcohol as well as evaluating fit and comfort of dentures will help decrease risk factors associated with osteoradionecrosis. See Chapter 12 for more detailed information.

The nursing diagnoses "Altered oral mucous membrane related to head and neck irradiation" and "Sensory-perceptual alterations: gustatory, related to head and neck irradiation" are used when patients have alterations in the oral cavity as a result of radiation therapy. Assess mouth care practices and inspect the oral cavity for mouth changes. Evaluate the patient's ability to perform appropriate mouth care, minimize irritation, and prevent infections.

Hypopituitarism

The symptoms of hypopituitarism are associated with decreased secretions of cortisol, thyroxine, and sex

Table 21–6 Signs and Symptoms of Hypopituitarism

Pituitary Deficiency	Target Organ Deficiency	Signs and Symptoms
ACTH	Cortisol	Fatigue, weakness, weight loss, anorexia, nausea, postural dizziness, muscle weakness, hypoglycemia
TSH	Thyroxine	Dry skin and hair, fatigue, edema, pallor, cold intolerance, hoarseness, weight gain, delayed deep tendon reflexes, alopecia, lethargy, mental and physical slowness, constipation
LH, FSH	Estrogen	Amenorrhea, decrease in sexual libido
	Testosterone	Decrease in sexual libido
GH		Short stature in children Asymptomatic in adults
PRL		Failure of lactation

From Schultz PN: Hypopituitarism in patients with a history of irradiation to the head and neck area: diagnoses and implication for nursing, Oncol Nurs Forum 16:823, 1989.

hormones[74] (see Table 21-6). The symptoms may develop slowly within the first year after radiation therapy or up to 24 years following treatment. During times of stress such as surgery or acute illness, the consequences of hypoadrenalism can be life threatening.[74] Adrenal insufficiency is treated with adrenocortical replacement, and sex hormone deficits are replaced with appropriate hormone therapy.

CHEST

Radiation therapy is given to the chest for lung cancer, lymphoma, cancers involving the mediastinum including the esophagus, and breast cancer. Common side effects of radiation therapy to the chest are esophagitis and cough. Late effects include pneumonitis and rarely, lung fibrosis. With current tissue-sparing techniques for treating breast cancer, the dose to the lung and esophagus is minimized, and these patients have little if any of the above-mentioned effects.

Esophagitis

Esophagitis occurs if part of the esophagus is within the treatment field. Approximately 2 to 3 weeks from the start of therapy the patient may note difficulty or pain with swallowing and complain of a "lump in the throat." Esophagitis can become so severe that radiation treatments must be withheld for a short time. The nursing diagnosis of "Impaired swallowing related to esophagitis" is made when the patient experiences esophagitis. Assist the patient and family to plan a soft, bland, or liquid diet that provides a high calorie and protein intake. Use of anesthetic and coating mouth rinses before meals can decrease the discomfort associated with eating and allow the patient to continue with therapy. Hilderley[42] described the beneficial use of a mouthwash containing viscous lidocaine, diphenhydramine elixir, and Mylanta taken 15 minutes before meals to relieve esophagitis. Other oral liquid pain medications may be used to numb the throat and relieve dysphagia.[24] Occasionally systemic analgesics taken half an hour to an hour before meals are needed to obtain an acceptable level of pain relief. Evaluate the patient's and family's understanding and use of measures to relieve esophagitis and maintain an optimal nutritional intake.

Cough

A cough may develop or increase if lung tissue is within the treatment field, as with treatment for lung cancer. Initially the cough may be productive as trapped material is released by the previously blocked alveoli.[82] However, as treatment continues, the mucosa dries out and the cough becomes nonproductive. Assess the character, intensity, and frequency of cough and monitor changes in lung sounds. The nursing diagnosis "Alteration in comfort related to cough," is made if the patient develops a cough. Assist the patient to plan measures to relieve the cough. Make sure the patient has an adequate fluid intake. Humidification of the air and avoiding irritants such as smoke can reduce the cough. Use of cough preparations that contain codeine may be indicated for severe dry, hacking coughing that results in fatigue or disrupts sleep. Monitor for signs and symptoms of respiratory infection and instruct the patient to avoid sources of infection. Evaluate the patient's use of measures to minimize cough and risk of respiratory infections.

Radiation pneumonitis

Radiation pneumonitis can occur approximately 1 to 3 months after radiation therapy to the lung.[45,82] At first there may be an unproductive cough that eventually becomes productive. The symptoms include fever and dyspnea. The effect is similar to the adult respiratory distress syndrome (ARDS). Radiation pneumonitis is treated with steroids, bed rest, and antibiotics for any superimposed infections.[82,90]

Radiation fibrosis

Radiation fibrosis may occur 6 to 12 months after treatment is completed. This consequence of radiation therapy is a restrictive disease of the lung. Lung fibrosis is seen primarily within the treated area of the lung and usually develops in areas of previous pneumonitis.[65] The primary symptom is shortness of breath. Treatment of radiation-induced lung fibrosis is limited to symptomatic control of dyspnea and supportive care.

ABDOMEN

Gastritis may occur if part of the stomach is within the treatment field. A soft and bland diet is tolerated best. Antacids may be used if needed.

"Altered nutrition, less than body requirements, related to nausea and vomiting" occurs if a large part of the abdomen, including the stomach, paraaortic area, and/or small bowel is within the treatment field. Nausea and vomiting usually occur within the first 6 hours following treatments and may last for 3 to 6 hours.[90] In rare instances nausea may persist for longer periods. Assess patients for occurrence and pattern of nausea and vomiting. Prophylactic use of antiemetics before treatment each day and as needed following treatment can minimize and relieve nausea and vomiting from radiation therapy. For severe nausea and vomiting, around-the-clock antiemetics are recommended.

Relaxation techniques and distraction such as listening to soothing music and engaging in an enjoyable activity can help control nausea.[11] Using relaxation techniques before and after treatments help minimize the anxiety that can exacerbate nausea.[90] Plan dietary modifications to minimize nausea and vomiting. A diet that is low in fat, low in sugar, and easily digested is best tolerated. Soups, broths, and other fluids should be consumed to maintain fluid intake and prevent dehydration (see Chapter 27). Evaluate the patient's and family's understanding of the potential and actual causes of nausea and vomiting. Also evaluate their ability to use appropriate measures to reduce or relieve nausea and vomiting and maintain the patient's nutritional status.

PELVIS

Diarrhea and cystitis commonly occur when the pelvis is being treated for gynecologic cancer, prostate cancer, testicular cancer, rectal cancer, or lymphomas. Diagnoses include "Diarrhea related to pelvic irradiation" and "Altered patterns of urinary elimination related to pelvic irradiation."

Diarrhea

Diarrhea occurs as the bowel lining atrophies and resorption of fluids from the colon is decreased.[90] Malabsorption of bile salt may also cause diarrhea.[62] Diarrhea can occur 2 to 3 weeks into treatment and last throughout the course of therapy. Some patients produce an increased number of stools; others produce loose, watery stools with cramping.[45] In certain instances treatment may be interrupted to allow the bowel to recover. Occasionally chronic enteritis develops.

Assess the patient's usual bowel pattern. If diarrhea occurs, help the patient and family plan measures to minimize diarrhea. Instruct the patient and family on the use of a low-residue diet. Decreasing the amount of fat in the diet can also be helpful because fats are difficult to digest. If milk products are not tolerated, they should be avoided. If the diarrhea persists while the patient is on a low-residue diet, antidiarrheal medication such as diphenoxylate atropine or loperamide HCl may be indicated. If diarrhea tends to occur after meals as a result of the gastrocolic reflex, the antidiarrheal medication should be taken before meals. Tenesmus of the anal sphincter is controlled with antispasmodic and anticholinergic medications.[45] Evaluate the patient's and family's understanding and use of measures to minimize diarrhea and tenesmus in order to maintain the patient's usual pattern of elimination.

Cystitis

Cystitis occurs if the bladder is within the treatment field. Symptoms include dysuria, small bladder capacity, urinary frequency and urgency, nocturia, and urinary hesitancy. Rarely, bleeding occurs. Hyperbaric oxygen therapy has shown therapeutic benefits in treating chronic radiation-induced cystitis that is refractory to conventional therapy.[72,86] Hyperbaric oxygen therapy increases tissue oxygenation and promotes vascularization and formation of granulation tissue. Patients sit in a hyperbaric oxygen chamber and receive 100% oxygen for approximately 2 hours. Up to 60 treatments are delivered once or twice a day.

Assess and monitor symptoms of cystitis, including signs of hematuria. Instruct the patient to maintain an adequate fluid intake.[45] As symptoms occur, bladder infections must be ruled out or treated. Obtain urine specimens for analysis and culture. Bladder analgesics such as phenazopyridine can relieve cystitis. Antispasmodic medications can provide some relief from bladder spasms. Evaluate the patient's understanding of the causes of cystitis and ways to relieve symptoms.

Erectile dysfunction

Erectile dysfunction following pelvic radiation may occur in men as a result of fibrosis of the pelvic vasculature and damage of pelvic nerves. A decrease in the ability to attain and maintain an erection occurs gradually and may be permanent. Allow the patient and his partner to discuss concerns and feelings regarding changes in sexual functioning and body image. Consultation with a urologist may include a discussion of pharmacologic interventions and prostheses that may be used.

Vaginal stenosis

When the vaginal vault is included in the treatment field, vaginal stenosis may develop and cause dyspareunia and difficulties with pelvic examinations. Vaginal stenosis can be minimized or prevented by use of a vaginal dilator. While lying supine with knees bent, the well-lubricated dilator is inserted into the vagina, withdrawn, and reinserted for 5 to 10 minutes.[37] Vaginal dilation needs to be performed three times a week for at least 1 year.

Ovarian failure

Ovarian failure occurs with small amounts of radiation and produces symptoms associated with menopause; hot flashes, amenorrhea, decreased libido, and osteoporosis.[26,90] Older women are at a higher risk of ovarian failure than younger women. Replacement hormonal therapy with midcyclic estrogens and progesterone reverses the clinical effects of early menopause. In certain circumstances the ovaries can be shielded from radiation.[90] In one technique, oophoropexy, the ovaries are surgically placed outside the treatment field.

Testicles

The testicles are usually shielded from radiation. However, if exposure is needed or unavoidable, spermatogenesis will stop and usually results in permanent sterility.

Issues related to sexuality need to be explored with sensitivity. As physical changes occur, the patient and his or her partner need to explore ways to satisfyingly express their sexuality and feelings (see Chapter 31).

BRAIN
Cerebral edema

When the brain is treated for primary brain tumor or brain metastasis, assessment for symptoms of cerebral edema is crucial. Cerebral edema occurs as tissues around the tumor become inflamed. These symptoms include headaches, nausea, vomiting, seizures, vision changes, motor function disabilities, slurred speech, and changes in mental status. Steroids are usually indicated during the course of treatment to minimize cerebral edema. If symptoms occur or increase, an evaluation is needed and may indicate a need to adjust the steroid dosage. Steroids may be needed on a continuing basis to control edema. Plan to assure patient safety in the home and workplace as well as during transportation to and from the treatment center. Evaluate the patient's and family's understanding of the cause of cerebral edema and the signs and symptoms they should monitor and report.

Alopecia

Alopecia, which occurs within the treatment area, depends upon the dose and extent of radiation to the scalp. The hair loss may be regional or patchy, depending on the treatment technique. Alopecia starts when the dose to the scalp reaches 2500 to 3000 cGy, and the hair gradually thins over 2 to 3 weeks.[45] With large doses of radiation (>4000 cGy) as in the treatment for primary brain tumors, the hair loss is per-

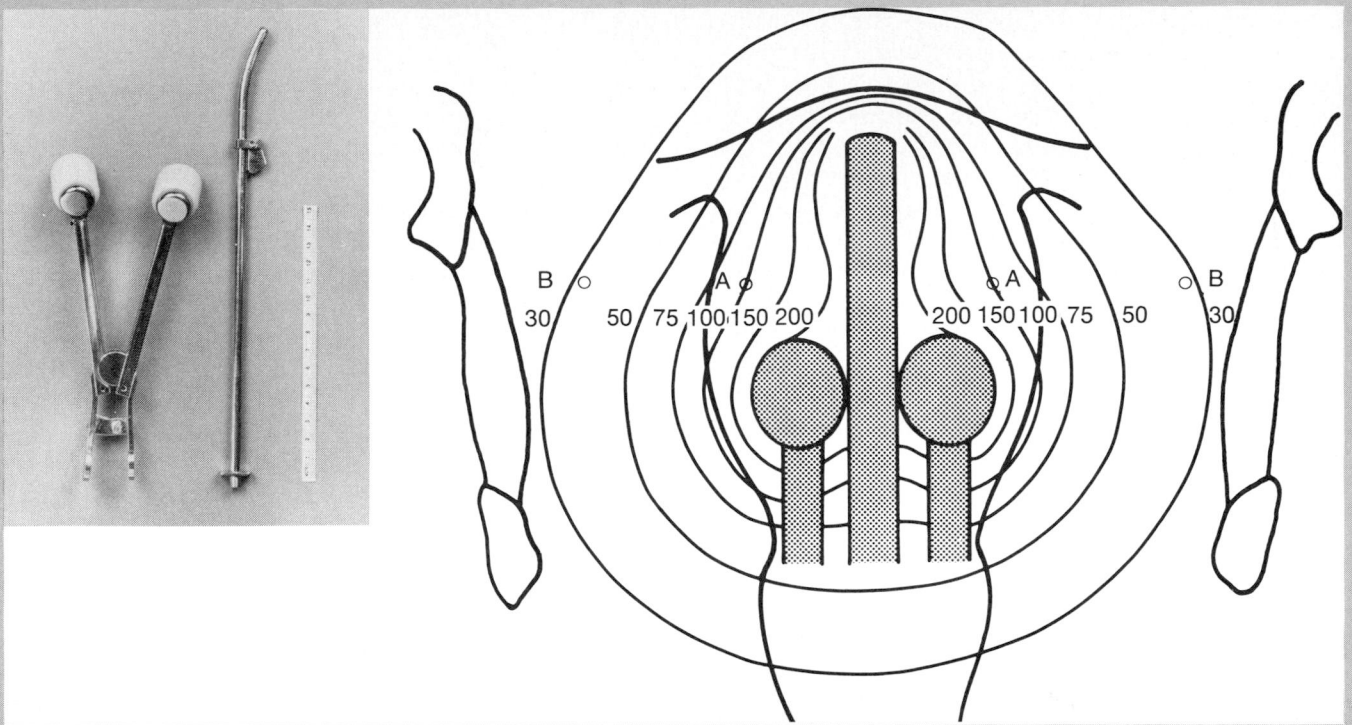

Figure 21–7   The Fletcher-Suit applicator is one of many kinds of applicators used to deliver intracavitary irradiation for carcinomas of the cervix and endometrium. The long central tamdem is placed in the uterine cavity. (To the right is a section of tubing used to hold the radioactive sources and place them in the hollow tamdem.) The movable sleeve on the tamdem marks the cervical os, permitting localization of the os on radiographs as a reference point for computerized dosimetry. The colpostats are placed in the lateral fornices. The entire apparatus is held in place with vaginal packing. After the applicator is in place, radiographs are taken to determine the accuracy of placement. Computerized dosimetry is then done to determine the best loading pattern and the length of time required for the treatment. Finally the radium or cesium sources are put in place. (Photo courtesy of Virginia Mason Clinic, Seattle, Wash.; drawing from DiSaia P and Creasman W: Clinical gynecological oncology, ed 4, St Louis, 1993, Mosby.)

manent.[90] With small doses such as those given for palliative purposes alopecia is more variable. Hair loss may occur directly opposite the treatment site, where the x-rays exit. Regrowth of hair may start 2 to 3 months after completion of therapy.[62,77]

Hair texture and color

Changes in hair texture and color may also occur. The scalp may develop pruritus and become very dry or peel. The scalp needs protection along guidelines for skin care outlined earlier in this chapter. Gentle brushing and combing of hair is recommended. Permanent waves and hair coloring are contraindicated because they can irritate the scalp.[45] Using a scarf, turban, hat, or cap to protect the scalp from the wind, cold, and sun is advisable. A wig may be worn. Assure that the wig lining is comfortable and does not further irritate the scalp. A mild shampoo may be used, but excessive shampooing should be avoided. The potential or actual loss of hair can be traumatic for the patient. Nursing diagnoses are "Ineffective individual coping related to alopecia" and "Disturbance in self-esteem related to alopecia." Help the patient cope with the psychologic effects by recognizing the importance of

alopecia, approaching the patient with gentleness, honesty and caring, and allowing verbalization of fears, grief, and anger. Prepare the patient and family in advance for alopecia. Assess its significance. Provide information on what can be done to cover and care for the scalp. These activities communicate understanding of the loss and offer support to the patient as she or he adapts to the change in body image.[90]

INTERNAL RADIATION THERAPY
Brachytherapy

Radioactive implants deliver relatively large amounts of radiation to a specific site over a short time.[37] Tumors may be treated with an implant alone, but more commonly, an implant is done following a course of radiation therapy to provide a boost of radiation to the tumor.[83] Cancers of the brain, tongue, lips, esophagus, lung, breast, vagina, cervix, endometrium, rectum, prostate, and bladder may be treated with brachytherapy. Implants are usually placed temporarily within the body cavity or structure with specifically designed applicators (Figure 21-7). The radioactive material, ribbons, wires, seeds, capsules, needles, or tubes are encapsulated (sealed), so there is no contamination of bodily fluids. The radioactive isotopes are usually placed in the body with an afterloading technique of placing the applicators (needles, plastic or metal tubes) in the body in the operating room or under fluoroscopy. The applicators are sutured in or near the tumor. After the patient returns to the hospital room, the radioactive isotopes are placed within the applicators. With this procedure, exposure of staff members to radiation is minimized. The implant remains in the body for the prescribed length of time.

Intracavitary placement of implants within the vagina or uterus is performed with general or spinal anesthesia.[37] The vagina is packed with gauze to stabilize the applicator and separate the bladder and rectum from the radioactive source. Patients usually have a bowel cleansing before the applicator placement and are placed on a low residue diet and diphenoxylate atropine to prevent a bowel movement during the time of the implant. Postoperative pain is managed with oral or parenteral medications.

With cervical and vaginal implants, the patient may experience fatigue and dysuria following the implant. Women may resume sexual intercourse within 2 to 3 weeks following the implant.[37] Since a decrease in normal vaginal secretions may occur, use of a water-based lubricant is recommended. Vaginal stenosis can also occur. Routine vaginal dilation is recommended to maintain the integrity of the vaginal walls.

Interstitial radioactive implants with needles, wires, seeds, or catheters are placed directly into the tissues. These implants may be temporary or permanent. Head and neck cancers are commonly treated with temporary interstitial implants. Goals of nursing care include minimizing airway obstruction and instructing the patient to perform oral care with saline irrigations every 3 to 4 hours. Nasogastric tube feedings are used to provide a high protein and calorie liquid diet. Since talking is difficult and should be avoided, the patient communicates with a writing pad or specially created flash cards. With head and neck implants, the patient is permitted to get out of bed but must remain in the hospital room. Elevating the head of bed to 30 to 45 degrees will help minimize tissue swelling and aspiration of oral secretions.

Temporary interstitial implants of the breast are performed approximately 2 weeks after a course of external beam radiation therapy to provide more radiation to the site of tumor excision. Catheters are placed under general anesthesia, and radioactive sources are placed within the catheters once the woman returns to her hospital room.

Interstitial brain implants for recurrent brain tumors allows treatment of a highly localized area within the brain. Catheters are placed using a sterotactic frame with CT guidance.[55]

In some instances permanent low-level radioactive implants may be placed percutaneously or intraoperatively in or near tumor masses. The level of radioactivity is low, so radiation precautions are usually not required. Permanent interstitial implants with radioactive iodine seeds are placed intraoperatively or with transrectal ultrasound guidance within the prostate gland to treat prostate cancer.[33] The radioactive source has a short half-life, and the patient's body tissues effectively shield any radiation. Patients are instructed to filter urine for seeds that may pass through the urine, use condoms when having sexual intercourse, and to avoid close contact with pregnant women and children while the radioactive source decays.

Radioactive isotopes that deliver a high dose rate of radition to a limited volume of tissue allows site specific treatments over a shorter period of time. Treatments can be delivered within a few hours and can be done in the outpatient setting. The use of a remote afterloading brachytherapy device decreases staff exposure to the high dose isotopes used during therapy.[51] If the patient requires direct care, the sources can be momentarily removed through the applicators by remote control before nurses enter the room.

Providing patients with education about the implant; the process, its effects and how to manage those effects is crucial. Brandt[7] studied the informational needs of 22 patients receiving brachytherapy and found that most patients desired the maximum information about their illness. Symptom management, activity restrictions during the implant, causes of their current symptoms and how the implant could affect those symptoms were items that the patients identified as important to know before the implant. After the implant, the patients identified information about when to call the doctor, the potential side effects of treatment, and how to manage those side effects as the most important items.

Nonsealed Radioactive Therapy

When radioactive isotopes are injected intravenously or taken orally (nonsealed sources), the patient and the body secretions may be radioactive, and nursing care must follow specific radiation safety precautions.[31] Depending on the isotope used, the patient usually must be isolated because of radioactivity for approximately 3 to 4 days. The amount of radioactivity emitted is carefully monitored during the patient's hospitalization. Table 21-7 describes the different radioactive isotopes used in cancer therapy.

Table 21–7 Radioactive Isotope Chart

Isotope	Emission	Half-Life*	Source	Use	Administration
^{131}I (iodine)	Gamma rays†	8.05 days	Unsealed	Thyroid cancer	Oral, intravenous
^{32}P (phosphorus)	Beta particles‡	14.3 days	Unsealed	Malignant pleural or peritoneal effusion	Intrapleural; intraperitoneal in colloid form
^{192}Ir (iridium)	Beta particles Gamma rays	74.4 days	Sealed	Cancers of head and neck, breast, bronchus, brain; sarcomas	Interstitial and intracavitary
^{125}I (iodine)	Gamma rays	60.2 days	Sealed	Cancers of prostate, bladder, brain, bronchus	Interstitial
^{137}Cs (cesium)	Beta particles Gamma rays	30.0 years	Sealed	Gynecologic cancers	Intracavitary in an applicator
^{226}Ra (radium)	Beta particles Gamma rays	1602 years	Sealed	Head and neck cancer	Intracavitary and interstitial

*Time required for isotope to lose 50% of its radioactivity.
†Gamma rays: highly ionizing electromagnetic radiation emitted from radioactive isotopes; patient's body does not effectively shield gamma rays.
‡Beta particles: ionizing particles with moderate penetrating ability; the patient's body effectively shields the radiation when the isotope is injected.
Adapted from Gillick M: Radiation therapy: internal radiation, Cancer Nurs 2(4):314, 1979.

MINIMIZING NURSE'S EXPOSURE TO RADIATION

Nurses play a major role in dispelling the patient's and family's fears and misconceptions about radiation therapy. When working with patients with internal radiation therapy, nurses need to be aware of their own concerns so that care can be provided thoroughly and effectively while minimizing radiation exposure.[76] Nursing inservices about radiobiology and radiation safety principles combined with discussions and practice laboratories can help clarify how nurses can protect themselves and still provide comprehensive nursing care. Fear is highly contagious, and nurses need to develop awareness of their behaviors and its impact on patients. National and state regulations keep individual exposure below levels that produce somatic or genetic damage.[31,76]

When the nurse works with patients with a radioactive implant or systemic radiation, he or she should anticipate the patient's needs and use the principles of time, distance, and shielding to minimize radiation exposure.[31,37]

• Time
  Minimize time spent in close proximity to the patient. Radiation exposure is directly related to the time spent within a specific distance of the source of radioactivity.
  Use time efficiently by organizing patient care activities and assembling necessary supplies before entering the patient's room. Before leaving the patient's room, place personal items within

---

INVERSE SQUARE LAW

Radioactive Source

Meters	0 1 2 3 4 5 6 7 8
Exposure rate	1/1 1/4 1/16 1/64

If the exposure at 1 m from the radioactive source is x, the exposure at 2 m is one fourth of x, and at 4 m, one sixteenth.

According to the inverse square law, exposure decreases as the distance from the radioactive source increases according to the formula.

$$\text{Exposure rate} = \frac{1}{(\text{distance})^2}$$

---

reach of the patient to avoid needing to reenter the room. Direct care is usually limited to one-half hour per person per shift. Encourage the patient to perform self care activities.

• Distance
  Maximize the distance from the radioactive material. The amount of radiation decreases according to the inverse square law. Visit frequently with the patient at the door to the patient's room. See box above.

• Shielding
  When appropriate, use shielding to decrease exposure to radiation. With radium or cesium implants, a lead bed shield 1 inch thick is needed to attenuate the radiation. These shields are

usually placed at the patient's bedside. Most nursing care is provided from behind the shields. The lead aprons used in diagnostic radiology are not sufficiently thick to stop gamma rays and therefore are not recommended.[45]

Table 21-8 describes some general guidelines for working with patients receiving internal radiation therapy.

Table 21—8   Guidelines for Internal Radiation Therapy

	Sealed Sources	*Unsealed Sources*
Preparation of the patient	Instruct patient and family on procedure and visitation restrictions. Isolation is a temporary requirement and the nursing staff is available for all needs, but, by necessity, the nurse will work quickly and remain in the room for essential activities only. Preoperatively, patients may require bowel cleansing or placement of Foley catheter, as with cervical/vaginal implants.	
Room assignment	Private room usually required.	Private room only.
Restrictions on staff and visitors	No one under 18 years of age and no one who is or may be pregnant. Time spent close to the patient must be limited as much as possible. Visits with the patient from the doorway are usually permitted for longer periods.	
Shielding	Stay behind lead shields. Lead aprons are not effective.	Lead aprons are not effective.
Level of patient's activity	Patient remains in room. Depending on location of implant, the patient's activities may be limited to bedrest. In some instances raising the head of the bed may also be limited. Diversional activities such as watching television or reading a book are recommended.	Patient remains in room. Bathroom privileges if tolerated. Patient should care for self.
Body fluid precautions	Body fluids and materials are not radioactive. No special precautions are necessary for handling these materials.	Secretions from the patient may be radioactive: a. Wear gloves when handling equipment or objects that may have come in contact with body fluids or materials, e.g., urinals, bedpans, and emesis basins. b. Wash gloves before removing and place in designated waste container. c. Wash hands thoroughly with soap and water after gloves are removed. d. Disposable shoe covers may be put on before entering the patient's room and removed before exiting, especially if patient is incontinent. e. Disposable items such as eating utensils, cups, and plates should be used. f. Nondisposable items such as equipment and linens should not be removed from the patient's room until checked for radioactivity. Soiled items should be placed in a plastic bag, sealed, and left in the patient's room until checked for radioactivity. g. Stool, urine, and emesis are usually discarded in the toilet in the patient's room. Instruct patient to flush toilet 2 to 3 times after each use. h. Vomiting, stool or urinary incontinence, and excessive sweating may produce radioactive contamination of the room and linen. Use gloves to dispose of the material in the toilet,

Continued.

Table 21–8 Guidelines for Internal Radiation Therapy—cont'd

	Sealed Sources	*Unsealed Sources*
		if appropriate, or in plastic bags, which are left in the patient's room for monitoring. i. If skin becomes contaminated, wash affected area immediately with soap and water. j. If clothing becomes contaminated, have level of radioactivity evaluated before leaving the immediate area. k. Take special room preparation and additional precautions according to specific institution's policies.
Special precautions	a. Check linens, clothing, and bedpans for signs of dislodged implant. If implant is dislodged, do not touch it, but notify the physician immediately. If forceps are available, the source may be picked up with them and placed in an available container such as an emesis basin. The container should be placed in a distant corner of the room from the door. Immediately notify the physician. b. Dressings and packings should not be changed unless ordered by the physician.	
Discharge of patient from the hospital	Patient is no longer radioactive once implant is removed and placed within a lead-lined container.	Patient is discharged when total body retention of the radioactive isotope is at a safe level. After patient is discharged, the patient's room and all items in it are surveyed for any residual radioactivity.

Nursing Management

HELPING PATIENTS AND FAMILIES COPE WITH RADIATION THERAPY

Radiation therapy can sound frightening, and many patients approach it with apprehension. The nurse is in a vital position to help the patient and family cope with this treatment and its sequelae.[46] Since most patients receive radiation therapy as an outpatient, self-care is supported by nurses through assessment, symptom management, and education.[84,89] Education can increase the patient's treatment-related knowledge while decreasing anxiety and general emotional distress during treatment.[68] The nursing diagnoses "Anxiety regarding radiation therapy" and "Knowledge deficit related to radiation therapy and self-care measures" may be used. Support and counsel the patient who may need help to sort through his or her feelings about radiation therapy. Specifically assess the patient's expectations and concerns about therapy.

Patients are very interested in learning about their disease and treatment and ways to minimize symptoms and care for themselves.[57] Dodd[22] studied the self-care behaviors of patients receiving radiation therapy and found that patients identified themselves and physicians as the most frequent source of information about self-care behaviors. Nurses were cited much less frequently.

Patient education is challenging when faced with decreased time to provide the education, and patient and family variables such as anxiety, symptom distress, and lack of resources.[17] Identifying the major teaching needs and tailoring the education for the patients so that it is provided over a period of time helps make the information less overwhelming. A weekly patient newsletter is one way that information can be given to patients and families throughout treatment.[34,79]

Concrete objective information describing the common physical sensations experienced, the environmental surroundings, and information about timing of events helps to decrease the amount of disruption to the patient's usual activities during and after radiation therapy.[48] Educate the patient and family about the therapy and its side effects: what occurs, when it may occur, how long it lasts, and what they can do to manage the problem. Describe to the patient what he or she may experience[82]:

- The patient may be in the treatment room for about 20 minutes, but the actual treatment lasts only 2 to 5 minutes.
- The patient must lie on a hard table.
- The patient must remain alone in the room for the actual treatment.
- The patient may hear a buzzing, clicking, or whirring sound from the treatment machine.
- The machine may rotate around the patient, depending on how the treatment is delivered.
- The treatment itself is painless.

Many myths, fears, and anxieties surround radiation therapy. Many patients have heard from others about someone else's experience with radiation; the burns, disfigurement, and pain. Explain to the patient and family that not all treatments cause the same problems and that as technology advances, some side effects have become less frequent and not as severe.

The treatment machines are large and can be intimidating as they closely hover over the patient. Some patients fear being crushed by the machine or parts of it. For some patients, being alone in the treatment room during the treatment reinforces the loneliness of having cancer.

A common misconception about external radiation therapy is the fear of radioactivity. Many people mistakenly believe that the patient is radioactive. Assure the patient and family that with external radiation the patient is *not* radioactive. There is no residue of radiation on the patient, and therefore the patient should not be isolated from family or friends.

Community resources are available and can be gathered to assist the patient and family. These resources include a variety of services through the American Cancer Society, visiting nurses, home parenteral nutritional services, Meals on Wheels, accommodations for out-of-town patients, and transportation assistance for daily treatment.

Patient-teaching priorities for external and internal beam radiation therapy and geriatric considerations are given in the following boxes.

PATIENT TEACHING PRIORITIES: EXTERNAL BEAM RADIATION THERAPY

Instruct the patient and family about:
  Use of radiation therapy to treat cancer.
  Events that occur before, during, and after a course of radiation therapy: consultation, simulation, daily treatment, routine evaluations during course of therapy, and follow-up.
  Time factors: length of simulation, length of daily treatment, length of course of radiation therapy.
  Environmental information: description of surroundings, treatment room, and machine.
  Effects and side effects of radiation therapy (general and site-specific):
    That radiation therapy is a localized treatment and expected side effects are general as well as site-specific.
    What happens, why it occurs.
    When these effects are experienced.
    How long these effects last and when they resolve.
    That patient is *not* radioactive; there is no need to isolate the patient from family and friends.
  Measures that patients and families can use to minimize or prevent side effects:
    General effects: skin care, nutrition, energy conservation.
    Site-specific effects.
  Delayed effects to monitor: skin care, fatigue, site-specific effects.
  Follow-up care: routine follow-up with health care providers and adherence to recommendations for healthy living.

PATIENT TEACHING PRIORITIES: INTERNAL RADIATION THERAPY—SEALED AND NONSEALED SOURCES

Instruct the patient and family about:
  Use of internal radiation therapy to treat cancer.
  Patient preparation before therapy.
  Procedures involved in the therapy.
  Visitation restrictions: no one under 18 years of age, no one who is or may be pregnant.
  Isolation requirements: temporary isolation, patient remains in room, nursing care for essential activities only, time spent in close proximity will be limited. If the patient with nonsealed radioactive source has bathroom privileges, the patient is instructed to flush the toilet 2 to 3 times after each use.
  Patient activity may be restricted depending on the procedure; diversional activities such as watching television or reading a book are recommended.
  Discharge from the hospital: monitor for delayed effects such as fatigue; pelvic implants: diarrhea, urinary symptoms such as bladder infections, women are instructed to perform vaginal dilation 3 times a week for up to 1 year after the implant.

GERIATRIC CONSIDERATIONS

Compromised body systems in the elderly place them at risk for developing side effects sooner and with greater severity:

Skin: monitor for excessive dryness and early skin reactions.

Energy stores may be depleted and increase fatigue.

Medications prescribed for symptom management may need dosage adjustments to minimize adverse reactions.

Head and neck irradiation: normally decreased oral secretions predispose the elderly for oral complications.

Check the fit and comfort of oral prostheses.

Taste acuity may be altered prior to start of irradiation.

Sexuality: assess changes experienced. Provide education about the effects of radiation therapy. Because of the importance of preventing vaginal stenosis so that vaginal intercourse and pelvic examinations are feasible, instruct women who have received radiation therapy involving the vaginal vault to perform vaginal dilation 3 times a week for up to 1 year. Radiation therapy further decreases vaginal secretions. Women are instructed to use water-based lubricants for comfort. Some men experience erectile dysfunction with aging as a result of vascular changes. Pelvic irradiation may further damage the pelvic vasculature and cause nerve damage. Provide counseling or referral to specialist.

Social concerns:

Radiation therapy is usually delivered Monday through Friday for up to 7 weeks. The elderly may need to rely on public transportation or family and friends for daily transportation. In many situations, the patient is caring for a spouse or child and being away from home is difficult without a caretaker. Many elderly are on fixed incomes, and the added expense of therapy, transportation, out-of-town housing, and additional medications needed during therapy is a hardship.

CONCLUSION

Nurses have always been involved in the development of radiation oncology as a specialty, whether being at the bedside of the patient receiving radiation therapy, delivering the treatment, or helping to calm the confused or frightened patient on the treatment table. The fears and concerns of patients have changed very little and the impact of the diagnosis of cancer remains profound.

In a collaborative role with the radiation oncology team, the nurse provides continuity and quality patient care.[9,10] The nurse is in a prime position to assess, plan for, and evaluate interventions to prevent, minimize, or relieve side effects associated with radiation therapy.[9,10] In working with nurses in the hospital, home care and ambulatory settings, and with patients and families, the nurse helps to improve the patient's quality of life throughout treatment and rehabilitation.

BIBLIOGRAPHY

1. Aistars J: Fatigue in the cancer patient: a conceptual approach to a clinical problem, Oncol Nurs Forum 14:25, 1987.
2. Bane C and Rich TA: Intraoperative radiation therapy, AORN J 37(5):835, 1983.
3. Bane CL and Shurkus LM: Caring for intraoperative radiation patients, AORN J 37(5):840, 1983.
4. Barrett A, Nicholls J, and Gibson B: Late effects of total body irradiation, Radiother Oncol 9:1131, 1987.
5. Bentel GC, Nelson CE, and Noell KT: Elements of clinical radiation oncology. In Bentel GC, Nelson CE, and Noell KT, editors: Treatment planning and dose calculation in radiation oncology, ed 4, New York, 1989, Pergamon Press.
6. Beumer J, Curtis T, and Harrison RE: Radiation therapy to the oral cavity: sequelae and management, part 1, Head Neck Surg 1:301, 1979.
7. Brandt B: Informational needs and selected variables in patients receiving brachytherapy, Oncol Nurs Forum 18:1221, 1991.
8. Brandt BB and Harney J: An overview of interstitial brachytherapy and hyperthermia, Oncol Nurs Forum 16:833, 1989.
9. Bruner DW: Report on the radiation oncology nursing subcommittee of the American College of Radiology task force on standards development, Oncology 4:80, 1990.
10. Bruner DW, Iwamoto R, Keane K, and Strohl R, editors: Manual for radiation oncology nursing practice and education, Pittsburgh, 1992, Oncology Nursing Society.
11. Bucholtz J: Radiation therapy. In Ziegfeld CR, editor: Core curriculum for oncology nursing, ed 2, Philadelphia, 1992, WB Saunders.
12. Bucholtz JD: Radiolabeled antibody therapy, Semin Oncol Nurs 3:67, 1987.
13. Campbell-Forsyth L: Patients' perceived knowledge and learning needs concerning radiation therapy, Cancer Nurs 13:81, 1990.
14. Conger A: Loss and recovery of taste acuity in

patients irradiated to the oral cavity, Radiat Res 53:338, 1973.

15. Cromack DT and others: Are complications in intraoperative radiation therapy more frequent than in conventional treatment? Arch Surg 124:229, 1989.

16. Davis JC, Dunn JM, Gates GA, and Heimbach RD: Hyperbaric oxygen, Arch Otolaryngol 105:58, 1979.

17. DeMuth JS: Patient teaching in the ambulatory setting, Nurs Clin North Am 24:645, 1989.

18. DeWys W and Walters K: Abnormalities of taste sensation in cancer patients, Cancer 36:1888, 1975.

19. Dietz KA: Radiation therapy: external radiation, Cancer Nurs 2(2):129, 1979.

20. Dietz KA: Radiation therapy: external radiation, Cancer Nurs 2(3):233, 1979.

21. Dische S: Chemical sensitizers for hypoxic cells: a decade of experience in clinical radiotherapy, Radiother Oncol 3:97, 1985.

22. Dodd MJ: Patterns of self care in cancer patients receiving radiation therapy, Oncol Nurs Forum 11:23, 1984.

23. Dreizen S and others: Prevention of xerostomia-related dental caries in irradiated cancer patients, J Dent Res 56:99, 1977.

24. Dunne CF: Oral analgesics to relieve radiation-induced esophagitis, Oncol Nurs Forum 18:785, 1991.

25. Emami B and Perez CA: Combination of surgery, irradiation, and hyperthermia in treatment of recurrences of malignant tumors, Int J Radiat Oncol Biol Phys 13:611, 1987.

26. Feldman JE: Ovarian failure and cancer treatment: incidence and interventions for the premenopausal woman, Oncol Nurs Forum 16:651, 1989.

27. Ford R and Ballard B: Acute complications after bone marrow transplantation, Semin Oncol Nurs 4:15, 1988.

28. Gallucci BB and Iwamoto RR: Taste alterations in patients with cancer: nursing care of the cancer patient with nutritional problems, Report of the Ross Oncology Nursing Roundtable 40, 1981.

29. Gillick K: Radiation therapy-internal radiation, Cancer Nurs 2:314, 1979.

30. Glasgow G: Total body irradiation for bone marrow transplantation. In Withers HR and Peters LJ, editors: Innovations in radiation oncology, Berlin, Heidelberg, New York, 1988, Springer-Verlag.

31. Godwin CL, Bucholtz JD, and Wall SC: Hidden hazards on the job, part 3, radiation, Nursing Life Nov/Dec:43, 1985.

32. Goldson AL: Past, present and prospects of intraoperative radiotherapy, Semin Oncol 8:59, 1981.

33. Greenburg S, Petersen J, Hansen-Peters I, and Baylinson W: Interstitially implanted I-125 for prostate cancer using transrectal ultrasound, Oncol Nurs Forum 17:849, 1990.

34. Hagopian GA: The effects of a weekly radiation therapy newsletter on patients, Oncol Nurs Forum 18:1199, 1991.

35. Haibeck SV: Intraoperative radiation therapy, Oncol Nurs Forum 15:143, 1988.

36. Hall EJ: Radiobiology for the radiologist, ed 3, Philadelphia, 1988, JB Lippincott Co.

37. Hassey K: Demystifying care of patients with radioactive implants, Am J Nurs 85:788, 1985.

38. Hassey KM: Skin care for patients receiving radiation therapy for rectal cancer, J Enterostom Ther 14:197, 1987.

39. Hassey KM and Rose CM: Altered skin integrity in patients receiving radiation therapy, Oncol Nurs Forum 9:44, 1982.

40. Haylock PJ and Hart LK: Fatigue in patients receiving localized radiation, Cancer Nurs 2:461, 1979.

41. Hendrickson FR and Withers HR: Principles of radiation oncology. In Holleb AI, Fink DJ, and Murphy GP, editors: American Cancer Society textbook of clinical oncology, Atlanta, 1991, American Cancer Society.

42. Hilderley L: Relieving radiation esophagitis, Oncol Nurs Forum 13:71, 1986.

43. Hilderley L: Skin care in radiation therapy: a review of the literature, Oncol Nurs Forum 10:51, 1983.

44. Hilderley LJ, Hassey KM, and Dudjak LA: Nursing management of the patient receiving radiation therapy, Pub No 3480.04-PE, Atlanta, 1988, American Cancer Society, Inc.

45. Hilderley LJ: Radiotherapy. In Groenwald SL, editor: Cancer nursing principles and practice, ed 2, Boston/Monterey, 1990, Jones and Bartlett Publishers, Inc.

46. Hilderley LJ: The role of the nurse in radiation oncology, Semin Oncol 7:39, 1980.

47. Hirshfield-Bartek J and others: Monitoring the myelosuppressive effects of radiation therapy, Oncol Nurs Forum 15:547, 1988.

48. Johnson JE and others: Reducing the negative impact of radiation therapy on functional status, Cancer 61:46, 1988.

49. Jones D and Hafermann MD: A radiolucent bite-block apparatus, Int J Radiat Oncol Biol Phys 13:129, 1986.

50. Jordan LN and Buck SS: A teaching booklet for patients receiving high dose rate brachytherapy, Oncol Nurs Forum 18:1235, 1991.

51. Jordan LN and Mantravadi RVP: Nursing care of the patient receiving high dose rate brachytherapy, Oncol Nurs Forum 18:1167, 1991.

52. King KB and others: Patients' descriptions of the experience of receiving radiation therapy, Oncol Nurs Forum 12(4):55, 1985.

53. Klevenhagen SC, Lambert GD, and Arbabi A: Backscattering in electron beam therapy for energies between 3 and 35 MeV, Phys Med Biol 27:363, 1982.

54. Ladd L: The dry mouth dilemma, Oncol Nurs Forum 18:785, 1991.

55. Lamb S and Gutin PH: Interstitial radiation for treatment of primary brain tumors using the Brown-Roberts-Wells stereotaxic system, J Neurosurg Nurs 17:22, 1985.

56. Larson DA, Wasserman TH, Drzymala RE, and Simpson JR: Stereotactic external-beam irradiation. In Perez CA and Brady LW, editors: Principles and practice of radiation oncology, ed 2, Philadelphia, 1992, JB Lippincott Co.

57. Lauer P, Murphy SP, and Powers MJ: Learning needs of cancer patients: a comparison of nurse and patient perceptions, Nurs Res 31:11, 1982.

58. Mansfield MJ and others: Hyperbaric oxygen as an adjunct in the treatment of osteoradionecrosis of the mandible, J Oral Surg 39:585, 1981.

59. Margolin SG and others: Management of radiation-induced moist skin desquamation using hydrocolloid dressing, Cancer Nurs 13:71, 1990.

60. Marx RE: A new concept in the treatment of osteoradionecrosis, J Oral Maxillofac Surg 41:351, 1983.

61. Mossman K, Shatzman A, and Chencharick J: Long term effects of radiotherapy on taste and salivary function in man, Int J Radiat Oncol Biol Phys 8:991, 1982.

62. Mulkerin LE: Practical points in radiation oncology, Garden City, NY, 1979, Medical Examination Publishing Co., Inc.

63. O'Rourke ME: Enhanced cutaneous effects in combined modality therapy, Oncol Nurs Forum 14:31, 1987.

64. Overgaard J: The current and potential role of hyperthermia in radiotherapy, Int J Radiat Oncol Biol Phys 16:535, 1989.

65. Perez CA and others: Hyperthermia. In Perez CA and Brady LW, editors: Principles and practice of radiation oncology, ed 2, Philadelphia, 1992, JB Lippincott Co.

66. Piper BF, Lindsey AM, and Dodd MJ: Fatigue mechanisms in cancer patients: developing nursing theory, Oncol Nurs Forum 14:17, 1987.

67. Preston FA: Management of oral bleeding caused by thrombocytopenia, Oncol Nurs Forum 10:59, 1983.

68. Rainey L: Effects of preparatory patient education for radiation oncology patients, Cancer 56:1056, 1985.

69. Roof LM: The use of Vigilon primary wound dressing in the treatment of radiation dermatitis, Oncol Nurs Forum 18:133, 1991.

70. Rubin P: Principles of radiation oncology and cancer radiotherapy. In Rubin P, editor: Clinical oncology for medical students and physicians, New York, 1983, American Cancer Society.

71. Rubin P, Cooper R, and Phillips T: Radiation biology and radiation pathology syllabus, 1975, American College of Radiology.

72. Schoenrock GJ and Ciani P: Treatment of radiation cystitis with hyperbaric oxygen, Urology 27:271, 1986.

73. Schubert MM and Newton RE: The use of benzydamine HCl for the management of cancer therapy-induced mucositis: preliminary report of a multicentre study, Int J Tissue React 9(2):99, 1987.

74. Schultz PN: Hypopituitarism in patients with a history of irradiation to the head and neck area: diagnoses and implications for nursing, Oncol Nurs Forum 16:823, 1989.

75. Scott R and others: Hyperthermia in combination with definitive radiation therapy: results of a phase I/II RTOG study, Int J Radiat Oncol Biol Phys 15:711, 1988.

76. Sedhom LN and Yanni MIY: Radiation therapy and nurses' fears of radiation exposure, Cancer Nurs 8:129, 1985.

77. Sitton E: Early and late radiation-induced skin alterations, part 1: mechanisms of skin changes, Oncol Nurs Forum 19:801, 1992.

78. Sitton E: Early and late radiation-induced skin alterations, part 2: nursing care of irradiated skin, Oncol Nurs Forum 19:907, 1992.

79. Sporkin E: A newsletter for radiation therapy patients (abstract), Oncol Nurs Forum 14(suppl): 149, 1987.

80. Storm FK, Morton DL, and Bull JMC: Hyperthermia, American Cancer Society, Inc, Pub No 3364-PE, 1984.

81. Strohl R: Taste sensations after radiation therapy, Oncol Nurs Forum 10:80, 1983.

82. Strohl RA: The nursing role in radiation oncology: symptom management of acute and chronic reactions, Oncol Nurs Forum 15:429, July/August, 1988.

83. Strohl RA: Radiation therapy: recent advances and nursing implications, Nurs Clin North Am 25:309, 1990.

84. Tighe MG, Fisher SG, Hastings C, and Heller B: A study of the oncology nurse role in ambulatory care, Oncol Nurs Forum 12:23, 1985.

85. Van Drimmelen J and Rollins HF: Evaluation of a commonly used oral hygiene agent, Nurs Res 18:327, 1969.

86. Weiss JP and others: Treatment of radiation-induced cystitis with hyperbaric oxygen, J Urol 134:352, 1985.

87. Wescott WB: Dental management of patients being treated for oral cancer, CDAJ 13:42, 1985.

88. Wiley SB: Why glycerol and lemon juice? Am J Nurs 69:342, 1969.

89. Woodtli MA and Van Ort S: Nursing diagnoses and functional health patterns in patients receiving external radiation therapy: cancer of the head and neck, Nurs Diagn 2:171, 1991.

90. Yasko JM: Care of the client receiving external radiation therapy, Reston, Va, 1982, Reston Publishing Co., Inc.

CHAPTER 22

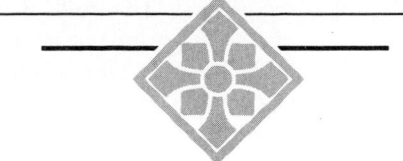

Chemotherapy

Shirley E. Otto

About 1,170,000 people were diagnosed as having cancer in 1993. More than one half of these people will receive systemic chemotherapy as a form of treatment due to disease recurrence, secondary therapy after a local treatment, and/or for treatment of hematologic disease. The primary focus of chemotherapy is to prevent cancer cells from multiplying, invading adjacent tissue, and/or developing metastasis.[9,18,34]

DEFINITION

Chemotherapy is the use of cytotoxic drugs in the treatment of cancer. It is one of the four modalities—surgery, radiation therapy, chemotherapy, and biotherapy—that provide cure, control, or palliation. Chemotherapy is systemic as opposed to localized therapy such as surgery and radiation therapy. There are four ways chemotherapy may be used[18]:

- *Adjuvant therapy*—a course of chemotherapy used in conjunction with another treatment modality (surgery, radiation therapy, and biotherapy) and aimed at treating micrometastases
- *Neoadjuvant chemotherapy*—administration of chemotherapy to shrink the tumor prior to surgical removal of the tumor
- *Primary therapy*—the treatment of patients with localized cancer for which there is an alternative but less than completely effective treatment
- *Induction chemotherapy*—the drug therapy given as the primary treatment for patients with cancer for which no alternative treatment exists
- *Combination chemotherapy*—administration of two or more chemotherapeutic agents in the treatment of cancer, allowing each medication to enhance the action of the other or to act synergistically with it (an example of combination che-

motherapy is the widely known MOPP regimen of nitrogen *m*ustard, vincristine [*O*ncovin], *pro*carbazine, and *p*rednisone, used to treat patients with Hodgkin's disease)[3,24,27]

HISTORICAL PERSPECTIVE

Systemic therapy in the form of metallic salts (arsenic, copper, lead) began with Egyptian and Greek civilization. This practice continued for centuries with limited success. Each generation of people had their own specific remedy for various illnesses. In the late 1880s some bacterial compounds were developed. None of these methods proved reliable and effective in the treatment of these varied illnesses.[18]

Research for chemotherapy began in the early 1900s with Paul Ehrlich's use of rodent models of infectious diseases to develop antibiotics. Further developments led to the use of rodents to test potential cancer chemotherapeutic agents. An additional discovery in drug development was the result of servicemen's exposure to mustard gas during World Wars I and II.[3,18,29] This exposure to mustard gas led to the observation that alkylating agents caused marrow and lymphoid suppression in humans. This experience resulted in the use of these agents in the treatment of Hodgkin's and other lymphomas, and was first attempted at Yale's New Haven Medical Center in 1940. Because of the secret nature of the gas warfare program, this work was not published until 1946. Chemotherapy as a treatment modality was introduced in the late 1950s and became established in medical practice in the 1970s.

Since the onset of cytotoxic drug research, thousands of chemical agents have been tested for their ability to destroy cancer cells. There are now more than 100 cytotoxic agents available for commercial and/or experimental use with approval by the Federal Drug Administration.[18]

PRINCIPLES OF CHEMOTHERAPY
Cell Generation Cycle
The cell cycle is the sequence of events resulting in the replication of DNA and equal distribution into daughter cells called *mitosis*. Normal cells and cancer cells go through the same division cycle, characterized by the following phases: G_0—resting or dormant phase; G_1—phase in which protein synthesis takes place in preparation for the S phase-DNA synthesis; and G_2—phase for further protein synthesis in preparation for the M phase—mitosis and cell division. The generation time, or length of time it takes for a cell to complete the phase or cycle, varies from hours to days. Chemotherapeutic drugs are most active against frequently dividing cells, or in all the phases of the cell cycle except G_0. Normal cells with rapid growth changes most commonly affected by chemotherapeutic agents include bone marrow (platelets and red and white blood cells), hair follicles, mucosal lining of the gastrointestinal tract, skin and germinal cells (sperm and ova). Chemotherapy is given according to schedules that are most effective for tumor kill and are planned to allow recovery of the normal cells.[9,18,23]

Tumor Growth
The regulatory mechanism controlling the growth of cancer cells differs from that of normal cells. Unlike normal cells, cancer cells grow via a pyramid effect; however, they grow at the same rate as the tissue from which they originated (e.g., breast cancer develops at the same rate of growth as normal breast tissue development). The time required for a tumor mass to reach a certain size is called doubling time. Tumors probably have undergone approximately 30 doublings from a single cell before they are clinically detected. Between the seventh and tenth doubling time there is the possibility for the tumor to shed cells, a process called *micrometastasis*. During the early stages of tumor growth, doubling time is more rapid than at later stages. This pattern of growth is called *Gompertzian function*. Tumor cells are more sensitive than normal cells to chemotherapy agents that are toxic to rapidly dividing cells.[39]

Curative treatment for cancer is targeted at killing the stem cells responsible for the neoplastic disease clone. In an attempt to understand the growth of the tumor cells, investigators are trying to identify tumor-specific stem cells and then determine which cytotoxic drug is most effective against the tumor. Many investigators have tried to increase the efficiency of chemotherapy through the use of assays to assess the response of the tumor clone to specific chemotherapy agents.[40,46]

The role of tumor growth and cell kinetics is important in understanding the action of cytotoxic therapy. Hematologic diseases such as leukemia and lymphoma have many rapidly dividing cells. When chemotherapy is initiated there is the potential for rapid and extensive cellular destruction due to the nature of the bone marrow stem cells and the rapidly dividing cancer cells. The treatment implications for these diseases and others are discussed later in the chapter.[34,35]

Refer to Chapter 1, Pathophysiology, for a detailed discussion of the cell generation cycle and properties of tumor growth.

Drug Classification
Chemotherapeutic agents are classified according to their pharmacologic action and their interference with cellular reproduction. The basic groups and their potential action are as follows:

- *Cell-cycle phase specific* drugs are active on cells undergoing division in the cell cycle; examples include antimetabolites, vinca plant alkaloids, and miscellaneous agents such as asparaginase and dacarbazine. These drugs are most effective against actively growing tumors that have a greater proportion of cells cycling through the phase in which the drug attacks the cancer cell. Cell cycle phase specific drugs are given in minimal concentration, via continuous dosing methods.[9,24]

- *Cell-cycle phase nonspecific drugs* are active on cells in either a dividing or resting state; examples include alkylating agents, antitumor antibiotics, nitrosureas, hormone and steroid drugs, and miscellaneous agents such as procarbazine. These agents are active in all phases of the cell cycle and may be effective in large tumors with few active cells dividing at the time of administration. Drugs of this nature are often given as single bolus injections.

The mechanisms of most chemotherapeutic drugs is targeting of the DNA of the cell in some manner. This action may result in direct interference with the DNA, inhibition of enzymes related to RNA or DNA synthesis or both, and/or destruction of the cells' necessary proteins.[9,18,24]

A general description of each drug classification follows, and detailed information regarding the specific drugs in each class can be found in Appendix 22-1 at the end of this chapter.

- Alkylating agents are cell cycle phase nonspecific. They act primarily to form a molecular bond with the nucleic acids, which interferes with nucleic

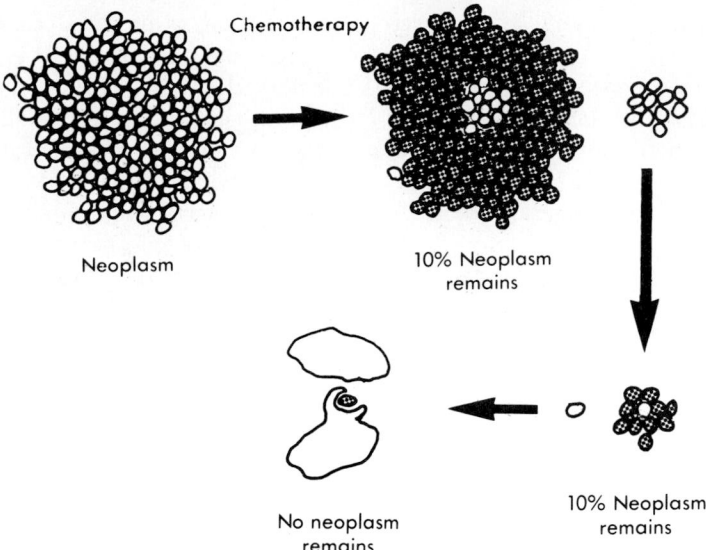

Figure 22–1 Cell kill hypothesis. (From Goodman MS: Cancer: chemotherapy and care. Bristol Laboratories, Division of Bristol-Myers Co, Evansville, Indiana.)

acid duplication, preventing mitosis. This category of drugs has similar phase activity to that observed in radiation therapy, with two peaks of maximum lethal activity, one in G_2 to M phase, and one near the G_1 S phase boundary.

- Antibiotics (antitumor agents) are cell cycle phase non-specific. These drugs disrupt DNA transcription and inhibit DNA and RNA synthesis.
- Antimetabolites are cell-cycle phase specific. They exhibit their action by blocking essential enzymes necessary for DNA synthesis or become incorporated into the DNA and RNA so that a false message is transmitted.
- Hormones are cell cycle phase non-specific. These chemicals, secreted by the endocrine glands, alter the environment of the cell by affecting the cell membrane's permeability. By manipulating hormone levels, tumor growth can be suppressed. Hormone therapies are not cytotoxic and therefore not curative. Their purpose is prevention of cell division and further growth of hormone-dependent tumors.
- Antihormonal agents derive their antineoplastic effect from their ability to neutralize the effect of or inhibit the production of natural hormones used by hormone-dependent tumors.
- Nitrosureas are cell-cycle phase nonspecific. They have the ability to cross the blood-brain barrier. Their action is similar to that of the alkylating agents; DNA and RNA synthesis are both inhibited.
- Corticosteroids provide an antiinflammatory effect on body tissues (e.g., they reduce intracranial or spinal cord compression and suppress lymphocytes). They may also promote a feeling of well-being as well as increased appetite.
- Vinca plant alkaloids are cell-cycle phase specific. They exert a cytotoxic effect by binding to microtubular proteins during metaphase, causing mitotic arrest. The cell loses its ability to divide and so dies.
- Miscellaneous agents may be cell-cycle phase specific or nonspecific or both. These drugs act by a variety of mechanisms. For example, *L*-asparaginase is unique; it is an enzyme product that acts primarily by inhibiting protein synthesis.[25,26,34,36]

Cell Kill Hypothesis

A single cancer cell is capable of multiplying and eventually killing the host. Every tumor cell must be killed to cure cancer. With each course of the drug therapy a given dose of chemotherapeutic drug kills only a *fraction, not all*, of the cancer cells present (Figure 22-1). Repeated courses of chemotherapy must be used to reduce the total number of cancer cells. This cardinal rule of chemotherapy, that is, the inverse relationship between cell number and curability, was established by Skipper and colleagues[9,19] in the early 1960s.

Factors Considered in Drug Selection[9,19]

- Patient's eligibility for chemotherapy (confirmed diagnosis; bone marrow, nutritional, hepatic, and renal status; expectation of longevity; history of chemotherapy and radiation therapy)

- Cancer cell type (e.g., squamous cell, adenocarcinoma)
- Rate of drug absorption (e.g., treatment interval and routes—oral, intravenous, intraperitoneal)[8]
- Tumor location (many drugs do not cross the blood-brain barrier)
- Tumor load (larger tumors are generally less responsive to chemotherapy)
- Tumor resistance to chemotherapy (tumor cells can mutate and produce variant cells distinct from the tumor stem cell of origin)[18,39-41]

Combination Chemotherapy

Chemotherapeutic drugs are most frequently given in combination. This enhances the effect of the drugs on the tumor cell kill. Considerations for drugs used in combination include verified effectiveness as a single agent, results in increased tumor cell kill, increased patient survival, presence of a synergistic action, varied toxicities, different mechanisms of action, and administration in repeated courses to minimize the immunosuppressive effects that might otherwise occur.[27,34,36] Combination chemotherapy provides additional benefits not possible with single drug treatment, such as maximal cell kill within the range of toxicity tolerated by the host for each drug, a broader range of coverage of resistant cell lines in a heterogeneous tumor population, and prevention or slowing of the development of new resistant lines.[38,40,42,60]

COMBINATION CHEMOTHERAPY REGIMENS

Breast
CMF—Cyclophosphamide, Methotrexate, 5-Fluorouracil
FUVAC—5-Fluorouracil, Vinblastine, Adriamycin, Cyclophosphamide

Lung
CAV—Cisplatin, Adriamycin, Vinblastine
CAMP—Cyclophosphamide, Adriamycin, Methotrexate, Procarbazine

Hodgkin's
ABVD—Adriamycin, Bleomycin, Vinblastine, Dacabazine
MOPP—Nitrogen Mustard, Oncovin, Prednisone, Procarbazine

Lymphoma
CHOP-BLEO—Cyclophosphamide, Adriamycin, Oncovin, Prednisone, Bleomycin
PROMACE-CytaBOM—Prednisone, Oncovin, Methotrexate, Adriamycin, Cyclophosphamide, Etoposide-Cytarabine, Bleomycin, Leucovorin, Dexamethasone, Trimethoprim Sulfa

Testicular
VBP—Vinblastine, Bleomycin, CisPlatin
VPV—VP-16 (etoposide), CisPlatin, Vinblastine

Because numerous cellular variants exist within a metastasis by the time it is detected, therapy for metastatic disease is often directed toward characteristics of the secondary tumor rather than the primary tumor. Combination chemotherapy rather than single sequential therapy maximizes therapeutic response by addressing the diversity of cellular response.[27] See examples of commonly used combination therapies in the box on this page.

CHEMOTHERAPY ADMINISTRATION
Calculation of Drug Dosage

Drug dosage for cancer chemotherapy is based on body surface area (BSA) in both adults and children. Drug calculations should be verified by a second person to ensure accuracy of the dose. The dosage range of a drug may vary with different drug regimens.[10,19,45]

The dosages of some drugs are calculated proportionally to the BSA of the patient. BSA is calculated in square meters (m^2). A nomogram is used to correlate height with weight to determine BSA (Figure 22-2). The drug dose is ordered in milligrams per square meter. For example[10,53,59]:

> Height = 68 inches
> Weight = 150 pounds
> m^2 = 1.80 BSA
> Dose = 75 mg/m^2
> $1.80 \times 75 = x$ dose
> x = 135 mg dose

Drug Reconstitution

Pharmacy staff should reconstitute all drugs and pre-prime the intravenous tubings under a class II biologic safety cabinet. In certain conditions (short-term stability of drug after mixing with unknown required administration time, e.g., intrathecal injection of methotrexate using preservative free diluent) nurses may be required to reconstitute medications. When preparing and reconstituting the drugs use aseptic technique in accordance with current manufacturer's recommendations. Immediately label all the syringes of reconstituted drugs with the name of the drug.[19,45] Many chemotherapeutic agents are colorless and cannot be distinguished from one another after reconstitution.[25] (See safe handling recommendations for drug preparation guidelines later in this chapter.)

Guidelines for Administration
ROUTES
Oral Route. Emphasize importance of compliance by the patient with prescribed schedule. Plan and assess for drugs with emetic potential to be taken with meals; drugs requiring hydration (cytoxan) need to be taken early in the day.
Subcutaneous and Intramuscular Route. Demonstration with a return demonstration may be needed if the

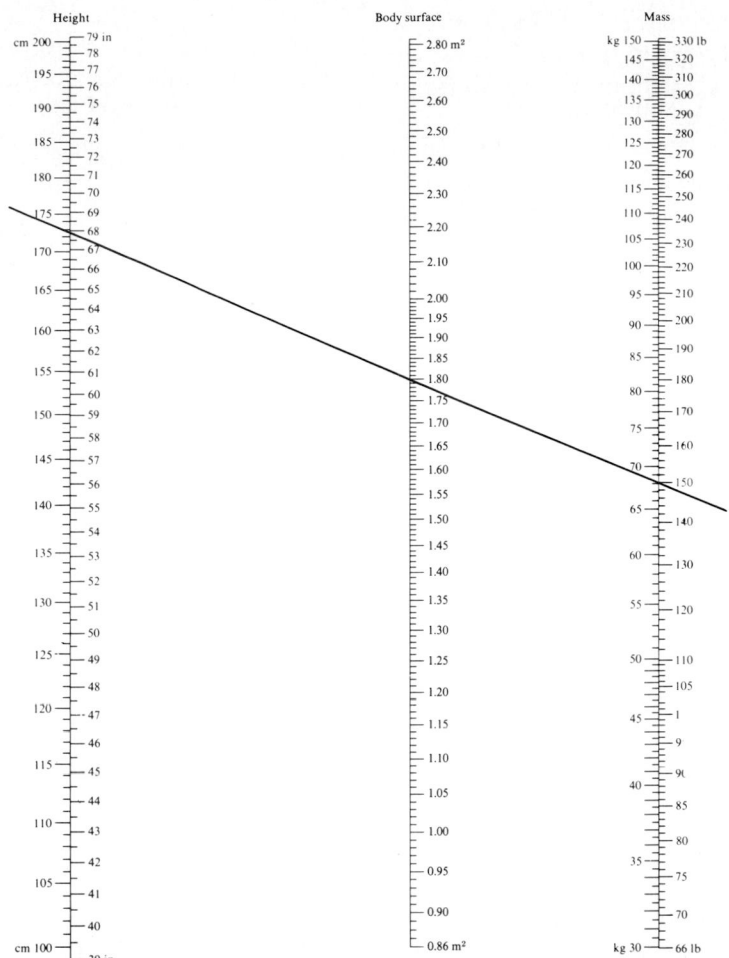

Figure 22–2 Body surface area of adults: nomogram for determination of body surface from height and mass, based on the formula of Dubois and Dubois, Arch Intern Med 17:863, 1916: $S = M^{0.425} \times H^{0.725} \times 71.84$, or $\log S = \log M \times 0.425 + \log H \times 0.725 + 1.8564$ (S, body surface in cm^2; M, mass in kg; H, height in cm). (Courtesy CIBA-GEIGY, Ltd, Basel, Switzerland.)

patient is giving self-injections. Be sure to rotate injection sites for each dose.[49]

Topical Administration. Cover surface area with a thin film of medication; instruct the patient to wear loose-fitting cotton clothing. Wear gloves and be sure to wash hands thoroughly after procedure. Caution the patient not to touch ointment.[52]

Intra-arterial Route. This requires catheter placement in an artery near the tumor; because of arterial pressure, administer the drug in a heparinized solution through an infusion pump. Throughout the infusion, monitor vital signs, color and temperature of extremity, and potential for bleeding at site. Instruct the patient and family about care of catheter and infusion pumps (e.g., routine filling and maintenance of the infusion pump) if chemotherapy is given at home.[25]

Intracavity Route. Instill the drug into the bladder through a catheter and/or through a chest tube into the pleural cavity. Follow prescribed premedication dosage to minimize local irritation.

Intraperitoneal Route. Deliver the drug into the abdominal cavity through the implantable port and/or external suprapubic catheter (for example Tenckhoff). Warm the infusate solution with dry heat to body temperature before administration. Monitor the patient for abdominal pressure, pain, fever, and electrolyte imbalance after infusion; measure abdominal girth.[20]

Intrathecal Route. Reconstitute all intrathecal medications with *preservative-free* sterile normal saline or sterile water. Infusion of medication may be given through an Ommaya reservoir, implantable pump, if available, and/or through lumbar puncture. Usually the volume of medication via an Ommaya reservoir or lumbar puncture is 15 ml or less. Maintain sterile technique throughout the procedure. The medication should be injected *slowly*. If chemotherapy drugs (Cytarabine and/or Methotrexate) are given in high doses, monitor patient closely for potential neurotoxicity. Only a physician may administer intrathecal

drugs via an Ommaya reservoir or lumbar puncture.[36]
Intravenous Route.   May be given through central venous catheters or peripheral venous access. Methods of administration include the following[50,51]:

- Push (bolus)—medication administered through syringe directly into the vein
- Piggyback (secondary setup)—drug administered using a secondary bag (bottle) and tubing; primary infusion concurrently maintained throughout drug administration[50,51]
- Side arm—drug administered through syringe and needle into the side port of a running (free-flowing) intravenous infusion
- Infusion—drug added to the prescribed volume of fluid IV bag or bottle.

Check for blood return before, during, and after infusion of chemotherapeutic drugs.[50,51] Follow the agency guidelines for frequency of monitoring continuous chemotherapeutic infusions. For continuous infusion of a vesicant drug, suggestions include validating blood return every 2 hours; for continuous infusion of a non-vesicant drug, validate blood return every 4 hours.[40,44]

Vein Selection and Venipuncture

Many chemotherapeutic agents irritate veins and surrounding tissues. Venipuncture sites must be changed on a planned basis every 48 hours to reduce the possibility of phlebitis and infiltration. Peripheral sites should be changed daily before administration of vesicants. Veins suitable for venipuncture feel smooth and pliable, not hard or sclerotic. Select a vein that is large enough to allow adequate blood flow around the IV device.

Selection of the appropriate site and equipment is determined by the patient's age, vein status, drugs to be infused, and expected period of infusion. The extremity should be observed and palpated. Use distal veins first, and choose a vein above areas of flexion. The distal veins of the hands and arms should be used first and subsequent venipuncture should be proximal to previous sites. Select the shortest catheter with the smallest gauge appropriate for the type and duration of the infusion. Veins commonly used include the basilic, cephalic, and metacarpal (Figure 22-3).

Large veins on the forearm are the preferred site. If a drug does extravasate in this area, there is maximum soft-tissue coverage to prevent functional impairment. Avoid the antecubital fossa and the wrist because an extravasation in these areas can destroy nerves and tendons, resulting in loss of function.[50,51]

Procedure for Chemotherapeutic Drug Administration

- Verify the patient's identification, drug, dose, route, and time of administration with the physician's order.

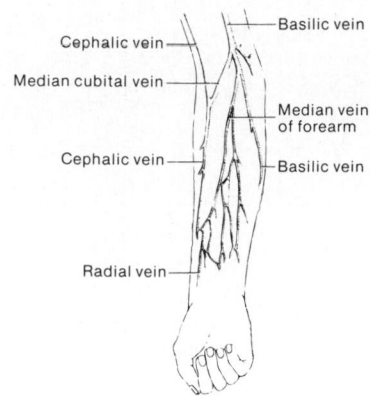

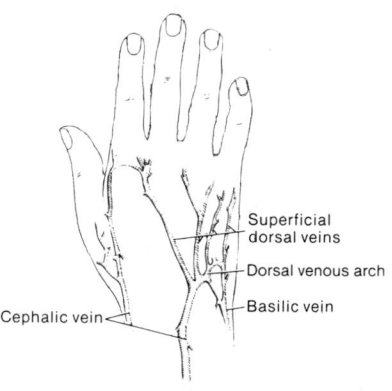

Figure 22–3   Venous anatomy. (From Perry A and Potter P: Clinical nursing skills and techniques, St. Louis, 1986, Mosby.)

- Review drug allergy history with the patient.
- Anticipate and plan for possible side effects or major system toxicity (Tables 22-1 and 22-2)
- Review appropriate laboratory data and other tests.
- Verify informed consent for treatment.
- Select appropriate equipment and supplies.
- Calculate the dose and reconstitute the drug using aseptic technique; follow safe handling guidelines.
- Explain the procedure to the patient and the patient's family.
- Administer antiemetics or other prescribed medications.
- Initiate peripheral IV site and/or prepare central venous access site.
- Administer chemotherapeutic agents.
- Monitor the patient at scheduled intervals throughout the course of drug administration.
- Dispose of all used supplies and unused drugs in approved puncture-proof, leakproof containers outside of patient area.
- Document procedure according to agency policy and procedure.

Documentation Recommendations

- Site assessment before and after infusion or injection of chemotherapeutic drug

Table 22–1 Teaching the Patient to Manage Most Common Side Effects of Chemotherapeutic Drugs

Side Effects	Points to Cover
ACHES AND PAINS **Nursing action:** Assess location, quality, and duration of pain.	Pain medication should be taken on a regular schedule. Side effects of pain medicine are constipation, dry mouth, and drowsiness. Strategies for rest and relaxation include music, progressive relaxation exercise, distraction, and positive imaging.
ALOPECIA *Hair loss:* Adriamycin, cyclophosphamide, daunorubicin, dacarbazine, vinblastine, mitoxantrone, taxol. *Hair thinning:* 5-Fluorouracil, methotrexate, bleomycin, vincristine, etoposide, Edatrexate.[5,7] **Nursing action:** Discourage use of scalp tourniquets for patients with diseases that originate with or metastasize to the scalp.	Hair loss occurs 10 to 21 days after drug treatment. Hair loss is temporary, and hair will regrow when drug is stopped. Hair loss may occur suddenly and in large amounts. Select wig, cap, scarf, or turban before hair loss occurs. Avoid use of hair dryers, curling irons, and harsh or frequent shampoos. Keep head covered in summer to prevent sunburn and in winter to prevent heat loss.
ANOREXIA **Nursing action:** Assess dietary history and monitor serum albumin and transferrin levels.[11,15,38]	Eating is a social event; eat with others in a pleasant area with soft music and attractive settings. Freshen up before meals. For example, use mouth care, take exercise. Eat small, frequent meals (five to six meals daily). Avoid drinking fluids with meals to prevent feeling of fullness. Concentrate on eating foods high in protein, for example, eggs, milk products, peanut butter, tuna, beans, peas. Breakfast may be the moset tolerable meal of the day; try to include one third of daily calories at this time. Monitor and record weight weekly; report weight loss.
CONSTIPATION Drugs associated with potential: vincristine, vinblastine, and narcotics. **Nursing action:** Determine normal bowel habits; advise the patient not to strain with bowel evacuation. Respond immediately to the urge to defecate.[5,7]	Increase intake of high-fiber foods, for example whole grain products, bran, fresh fruit, raw vegetables, popcorn. Increase fluid intake to 2 to 3 quarts of liquids daily; take fresh fruit juices, prunes, and/or hot liquids on waking. Follow prescribed use of stool softener. Follow prescribed physician orders if no bowel movement for 3 days or more.
CYSTITIS Drug associated with potential: cyclophosphamide and ifosfamide. **Nursing action:** Observe urine for color and amount, and assess frequency of voiding; advise patient to take oral cyclophosphamide early in the day.[5,45]	Increase fluid intake to 3 quarts daily. Empty bladder at least every 4 hours, especially at bedtime and at least once during the night. Report increasing symptoms of frequency, bleeding, burning on urination, pain, fever, and chills promptly to the physician.
DIARRHEA **Nursing action:** Monitor serum fluid and electrolytes, and monitor number, frequency and consistency of diarrhea stools.	Avoid eating high-roughage, greasy, and spicy foods, alcoholic beverages, tobacco, and caffeine products; avoid using milk products or use boiled skim milk. Eat a bland diet. Increase fluid intake to 3 quarts of liquids daily (weak, tepid tea, bouillon, grape juice). Record number and consistency of daily bowel movements; report information to the physician. Follow prescribed medication schedule if problem persists beyond 1 day. Cleanse rectal area after each bowel movement.
DEPRESSION **Nursing action:** Assess for changes in mood and affect.	Set small goals that are achievable daily. Participate in enjoyable and diversionary activities, for example music, reading, outings. Share feelings and concerns with someone.

Continued.

Table 22–1 Teaching the Patient to Manage Most Common Side Effects of Chemotherapeutic Drugs—cont'd

Side Effects	Points to Cover
FATIGUE **Nursing action:** Assess for possible causes (anemia, chronic pain, stress, depression, and insufficient rest or nutritional intake).	Conserve energy and rest when tired; plan rest periods. Plan for gradual accommodation of activities into lifestyle. Monitor dietary and fluid intake daily.
HEMATOPOIETIC CHANGES *Leukopenia:* most myelosuppressive agents produce WBC nadir 7 to 14 days after drug administration. Myelosuppression will be severe and prolonged with increased dosage of: Busulfan 2-6 Grams Carboplatin 2-4 Grams Cyclophosphamide 5-10 Grams Cytarabine 3-6 Grams Etoposide 2-4 Grams Methotrexate 2-6 Grams **Nursing action:** Monitor white blood count and differential; change equipment as indicated, for example, O_2 setup, IV supplies; teach sexual hygiene.	Avoid sources of infection, for example people with bacterial infections, colds, sore throats, flu, chicken pox, measles, and cold sores, people recently vaccinated with live attenuated viruses (MMR, DPT). Avoid having fresh fruit, plants, and flowers at or near bedside. Avoid cleaning animal litter boxes. Maintain good personal hygiene, for example bathe daily, wash hands before eating and preparing food, clean carefully after bowel movements, keep nails clean and clipped short and straight across. Maintain adequate fluid intake. Conserve energy; get adequate rest and exercise. Prevent trauma to skin and mucous membranes. Avoid elective dental work or surgery. Avoid enemas, rectal suppositories and temperatures, and catheterizations. Use toothettes or nonabrasive dental cleaning devices. Report signs and symptoms of infection immediately to the physician; for example, fever of 38° C or greater, cough, sore throat, a shaking chill, and painful or frequent urination, and vaginal discharge.
Thrombocytopenia: drugs associated with a delayed cumulative effect: mitomycin, and nitrosureas[36,42,60] **Nursing action:** Monitor platelet counts; observe bleeding precautions; apply firm pressure to venipuncture site for 3 to 5 minutes; monitor pad count on menstruating women; monitor environment for sharp objects.	Avoid use of straight-edge razor, power tools, physical activity causing injury. Avoid use of drugs containing aspirin. Humidify the air; use lotion and lubricants on skin and lips. Avoid invasive procedures; no intramuscular injections. Discourage bare feet when ambulatory. Use sanitary pads instead of tampons. Report the following signs and symptoms immediately to the physician: bleeding gums, increasing bruising, petechiae, purpura, hypermenorrhea, tarry-colored stools, blood in urine, or coffee-ground emesis.
Anemia **Nursing action:** Monitor hematocrit and hemoglobin, especially during drug nadir.	Adjust physical activity to accommodate periods of rest. Report the following signs and symptoms promptly to the physician: fatigue, dizziness, shortness of breath, and palpitations.
NAUSEA AND VOMITING **Nursing action:** Premedicate with antiemetic before nausea begins, for example, one-half hour before meals; patient may require routine antiemetics for 3 to 5 days following some chemotherapy protocols; monitor fluid and electrolyte status.[11,15,33,42]	Eat frequent, small meals. Avoid greasy and fatty foods and very sweet foods and candies. Avoid unpleasant sights, odors and tastes. Cold foods, salty foods, dry crackers, and dry toast may be more tolerable. If vomiting is severe, restrict diet to clear liquids and notify the physician. Consider diversionary activities, for example music therapy and relaxation techniques, recall strategies that were successful during pregnancy or other times of stress. Report weight loss to physician.
MUCOSITIS, RECTAL **Nursing action:** Monitor for electrolyte imbalance and granulocyte count; monitor number, consistency, and amount of bowel movements and urine output; assess for rectal bleeding.	Eat low-residue and easily digestible foods. Increase intake of liquids to replace fluid loss. Follow prescribed medication schedule, for example antidiarrheal and pain-control drugs. Wash rectal area with soap and water following each bowel movement; pat or air dry skin.

Table 22–1 Teaching the Patient to Manage Most Common Side Effects of Chemotherapeutic Drugs—cont'd

Side Effects	Points to Cover
MUCOSITIS, VAGINAL Symptoms occur 3 to 5 days after chemotherapy and subside 7 to 10 days after therapy.	Report pain, ulceration, or bleeding of mucous membranes lining the perineum and vagina to physician. Sitz bath with warm salt water may provide relief of vaginal itching and odor. Use hydrogen peroxide (one-quarter strength) with warm water after voiding to rinse perineal area.[55] Avoid commercial douches, tampons, and deodorant-containing vaginal pads or liners.
PHARYNGITIS AND ESOPHAGITIS Symptoms are often first noted by difficulty or pain in swallowing; may progress to ulceration and infection. **Nursing action:** Monitor for inability to swallow.	Eat a soft pureed or liquid diet. Follow prescribed medication schedule to relieve discomfort. Report to the physician symptoms that persist more than 3 days.
SKIN CHANGES **Nursing action:** Perform ongoing skin assessment.	Maintain good personal hygiene, wash underclothes/clothing in contact with skin with a mild detergent. Use topical preparations to minimize itching. Avoid use of perfume and perfumed lotion. Avoid scratching to prevent infection. Avoid wearing rough fabrics, tight fitting clothes (panty hose/jeans).
STOMATITIS (ORAL) Symptoms occur 5 to 7 days after chemotherapy and persist up to 10 days.[37]	Continue brushing regularly; use soft toothbrush. Use nonirritant mouthwash, for example, salt, soda and water solution, for at least four times daily. (¼ tsp. salt, 8 oz. H_2O, pinch of soda) Avoid irritants to the mouth, for example, tobacco, alcoholic beverages, spices, and commercial mouthwashes.[13] Avoid wearing dentures until mouth soreness heals. Maintain good nutritional intake; eat soft or liquid foods high in protein; add sauces or gravies in food to make food soupier. Follow prescribed medication schedule, for example drugs for oral candidiasis. Report promptly to physician persistent symptoms, and if white patches occur on tongue, back of throat, or gums.

From Otto SE: Chemotherapy administration. In LaRocca JC and Otto SE, editors: Pocket guide to intravenous therapy, ed 2, St. Louis, 1993, Mosby.

- Establishment of blood return before, during, and after IV and intraarterial infusion of chemotherapy
- Establishment of catheter or device patency before, during, and after infusion of chemotherapy (e.g., intraperitoneal, intrathecal)
- Patient and family education about chemotherapy protocol—potential side effects and toxicities, self-management of side effects, and schedule of follow-up blood counts, tests, and procedures
- Chemotherapeutic drug, dose, route, and time
- Premedications, postmedications, other infusions, and supplies used for chemotherapy regimen
- Any complaints by the patient of discomfort and

symptoms experienced before, during, and after chemotherapeutic infusion[50,51]

SAFE HANDLING OF CHEMOTHERAPEUTIC AGENTS

The number and usage of chemotherapeutic agents have increased considerably in recent years. A concern among health care workers has emerged regarding the potential occupational hazard associated with the handling of these drugs. Clinical studies have indicated that many agents are carcinogenic, mutagenic, and teratogenic or any combination of the three. Exposure to these chemotherapeutic agents can

Table 22–2 Major System Toxicity or Dysfunction and Nursing Management

Toxicity/Dysfunction	Nursing Management
CARDIAC TOXICITY Drugs associated with potential: doxorubicin, cyclophosamide, mitoxantrone, and daunorubicin.	Verify baseline cardiac studies, for example, ECG, ejection fracture; cardiac enzymes, before drug administration. Monitor cardiac status and report symptoms of tachycardia, shortness of breath, distended neck veins, galloping heart rhythm, and ankle edema. Monitor and record total cumulative dose of drug in the patient's medical record; adriamycin approximate maximum lifetime dose is 550 mg/m².
HEMATOPOIETIC TOXICITY (see Table 16-1)	
HEPATIC TOXICITY Drugs associated with potential: adriamycin, asparaginase, carmustine, lomustine, methotrexate, mercaptopurine, mithramycin, streptozocin, cytarabine, busulfan, and cyclophosamide.	Monitor liver function studies, for example lactic dehydrogenase (LDH), bilirubin, prothrombin time, and liver function tests—serum glutamic-oxaloacetic transaminase (SGOT) and serum glutamic-pyruvic transaminase (SGPT). Report to the physician signs of jaundice, tenderness over the liver, and urine and stool color changes.
HYPERSENSITIVITY REACTION Drugs associated with potential: asparaginase, doxorubicin (local erythema), bleomycin, etoposide, taxol, and teniposide.[5,36,40,60]	Review the patient's allergy history. Monitor for symptoms of hypersensitivity and anaphylaxis, for example agitation, urticaria, rash, chills, cyanosis, bronchospasm, abdominal cramping, and hypotension; onset may be rapid or delayed; advise the patient to report subjective symptoms promptly. Ensure proper medical equipment is nearby and in good working condition. Emergency drugs for intervention should be readily available. When administering a drug with potential for a reaction, give a test dose,[45] monitor vital signs, and observe for allergic response. If allergic response occurs, stop drug administration and notify the physician immediately.
METABOLIC ALTERATIONS Hypocalcemia	Monitor serum level; observe for muscle cramping, tingling of extremities, depression, and tetany.
Hypercalcemia	Monitor serum level; observe for anorexia, constipation, nausea, vomiting, polyuria, and mental status change.[53]
Hypoglycemia	Monitor serum and urine levels; observe for weakness, diaphoresis, hunger, headache, and tachycardia.
Hyperglycemia	Monitor serum and urine levels; observe for thirst, hunger, glucosuria, and weight loss.
Hyperuricemia (potential with treatment of highly proliferative tumors, for example leukemia and lymphoma).[36]	Monitor serum and urine levels, daily intake and output. Initiate prescribed drug therapy (for example allopurinol) to inhibit the formation of uric acid before administration of chemotherapy drug. Provide vigorous hydration, for example oral and IV fluid intake (2000 to 3000 ml), beginning 12 to 24 hours before initiation of chemotherapy.[42] Alkalinize urine to pH ≥ 7.0 by administration of IV NaHCO₃. Report pain, chills, fever, and diminished urinary output.[31]
Hypokalemia	Monitor serum level; observe for muscle weakness, twitches, paralytic ileus, and polyuria.
Hyperkalemia	Monitor serum level; observe for confusion, complaints of numbness or tingling, weakness, and cardiac arrhythmias.
Hypomagnesemia	Monitor serum level; observe for personality changes, anorexia, nausea, vomiting, lethargy, weakness, and tetany.

Table 22–2 Major System Toxicity or Dysfunction and Nursing Management—cont'd

Toxicity/Dysfunction	*Nursing Management*
METABOLIC ALTERATIONS—cont'd	
Hypernatremia	Monitor serum level. Observe for symptoms of thirst: dry mucous membrane, poor skin turgor, rapid thready pulse, restlessness, lethargy, and weight loss.
Hyponatremia	Monitor serum level. Observe for symptoms of rales, shortness of breath, distended neck veins, weight gain, edema of sacrum and/or lower extremities, increasing mental status changes, and seizures.
NEUROTOXICITY Drugs associated with potential: vincristine, vinblastine, intrathecal cytarabine, methotrexate infusions, high-peak plasma levels of 5-fluorouracil, and high doses of cytarabine and cisplatin.[24,26,27,28]	Monitor and report weakness, numbness, and tingling sensation of hands, arms, and feet; also monitor and report hoarseness, jaw pain, hallucinations, mental depression, decreased or absent deep tendon reflexes, slapping gait or foot drop, severe constipation, and paralytic ileus.
OTOTOXICITY Drug associated with potential: cisplatin.	Verify baseline audiogram. Monitor and report tinnitus, hearing loss, and vertigo.
PULMONARY TOXICITY Drugs associated with potential: bleomycin, busulfan, carmustine.	Verify baseline respiratory function. Individuals older than age 70 have increased risk. Monitor respiratory status and report dyspnea, dry cough, rales, tachypnea, and fever.
REPRODUCTIVE SYSTEM DYSFUNCTION Drugs associated with potential: chlorambucil, cyclophosphamide, mechlorethamine, vincristine; hormonal agents (IM, Sub-Q), flutamide, leuprolide, and zoladex; oral/tamoxifen.[4,24,26,27]	Assess for nature and frequency of sexual dysfunction. Counsel the patients regarding avoidance of pregnancy during and sperm banking before chemotherapy; provide information on contraceptives.[55] Inform the patient of potential for temporary or permanent infertility and loss of libido. Women may have symptoms including amenorrhea, hot flashes, insomnia, dyspareunia, and vaginal dryness; estrogen therapy may help manage these symptoms.[9,15,55] Birth control practices are recommended by most practitioners for 2 years following chemotherapy, as this provides for evaluation of disease responses, avoidance of possible teratogenic drug effects, and in male patients recovery of spermatogenesis. See Chapter 31 for further information.
RENAL SYSTEM TOXICITY Drugs associated with potential: cisplatin, cyclophosphamide, methotrexate, mithramycin, streptozotocin, and ifosfamide.	Verify baseline renal function. Assess 12 to 24 hour urine creatinine level before treatment. Encourage adequate fluid intake. Monitor intake and output, weigh changes. Report diminished output to physician, for example, less than 500 ml in 24 hours.[31,42]

From Otto SE: Chemotherapy administration. In LaRocca JC and Otto SE: Pocket guide to intravenous therapy, ed 2, St Louis, 1993, Mosby.

come by inhalation, absorption, and digestion.[2,57,61] Safe handling guidelines should be used when implementing policy and procedure within each agency that prepares, administers, stores, or disposes of supplies or unused chemotherapeutic agents.*[2,57]

---

*Recommendations for safe handling of chemotherapeutic drugs are available from the Occupational Safety and Health Administration (OSHA), National Cytotoxic Study Commission, and American Society of Hospital Pharmacists.

Safe handling practice guidelines cover the following:

- Drug preparation
- Drug administration
- Disposal of supplies and unused drugs
- Management of spills
- Care of patients receiving chemotherapy (e.g. linen contamination, patient excreta)
- Staff education
- Employment practice regarding reproductive issue

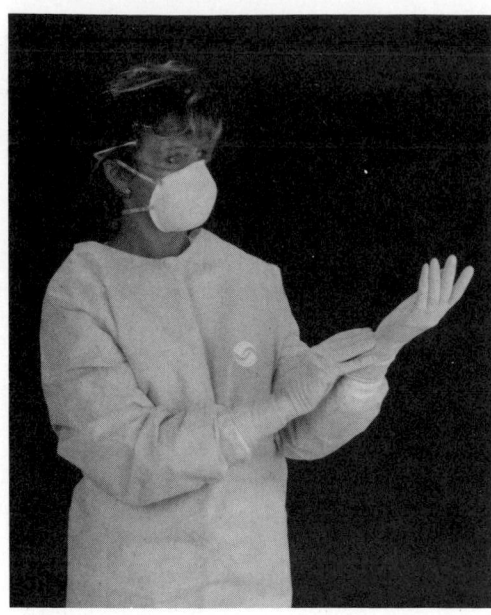

Figure 22–4 Female wearing gloves, gown, eyewear, and mask. (Courtesy Biosafety Systems, Inc., San Diego, Calif.)

Drug Preparation

To ensure safe handling, all chemotherapeutic drugs should be prepared according to the package insert in a class II biologic safety cabinet (BSC). Venting to the outside is desirable where feasible. Personal protective equipment includes disposable surgical latex gloves and a gown made of lint-free low-permeability fabric with a closed front, long sleeves, and elastic or knit cuffs. Wear eye-protective splash goggles or a face shield when preparing drugs if not using a biologic safety cabinet.[2,57]

Change gloves between preparation and administration of the drug and at least every 30 minutes during preparation and administration.

Suggestions to minimize exposure include the following:

- Wash hands before and after drug handling.
- Limit access to drug preparation area.
- Keep labeled drug spill kit near preparation area.
- Apply gloves before drug handling.
- Prepare drugs using aseptic technique.
- Avoid eating, drinking, smoking, chewing gum, applying cosmetics, and storing food in or near drug preparation area.
- Place absorbent pad on work surface.
- Use Luer-Lok equipment.
- Open drug vials and ampules away from body.
- Vent vials with a hydrophobic filter needle or pin to prevent spray of drug.
- Wrap alcohol wipe around neck of ampule before opening.
- Prime lines containing drugs inside BSC using original drug vial or a zip-close plastic bag.
- Cover tip of needle with sterile gauze or alcohol wipe when expelling air from syringe.
- Label all chemotherapeutic drugs.
- Clean up any spills immediately.
- Transport drugs to delivery area in a leakproof container.

Drug Administration

- Wear protective equipment (gloves, gown, and eyewear; Figure 22-4).[2,14,50,57]
- Inform the patient that chemotherapeutic drugs are harmful to normal cells and that protective measures used by personnel minimize their exposure to these drugs.
- Administer drugs in a safe and unhurried environment.
- Place a plastic-backed absorbent pad under the tubing during administration to catch any leakage.
- Do not dispose of any supplies or unused drugs in patient care areas. (See the section on disposal of supplies below.)

Disposal of Supplies and Unused Drugs

- Do not clip or recap needles or break syringes.
- Place all supplies used *intact* in a leakproof, puncture-proof, appropriately labeled container.
- Place all unused drugs in containers in a leakproof, puncture-proof, appropriately labeled container; keep these containers in every area where drugs are prepared or administered so that waste materials need not be moved from one area to another.[50,57]
- Dispose of containers filled with chemotherapeutic supplies and unused drugs in accordance with regulations of hazardous wastes, for example, licensed sanitary landfill or incineration at 1000° C.

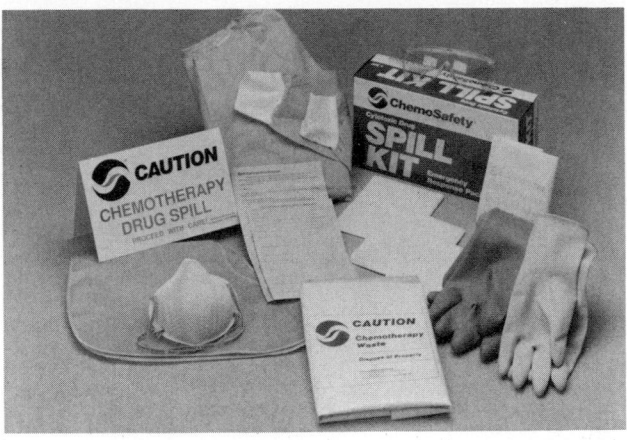

Figure 22–5 Chemotherapy spill kit. (Courtesy Biosafety Systems, Inc., San Diego, Calif.)

Management of Chemotherapy Spills

Chemotherapy spills should be cleaned up immediately by properly protected personnel trained in the appropriate procedures. A spill should be identified with a warning sign so that other persons will not be contaminated. The following are recommended supplies and procedures to manage a chemotherapy spill on hard surfaces, linens, personnel, and patients[3,50,57]:

SUPPLIES
- Chemotherapy spill kit (Figure 22-5):
    Respirator mask for airborne powder spills
    Plastic safety glasses or goggles
    Heavy-duty rubber gloves
    Absorbent pads to contain liquid spills
    Absorbent towels for cleanup after spill
    Small scoop to collect glass fragments
    Two large waste disposal bags
- Protective disposable gown
- Containers of detergent solution and clear tap water for postspill cleanup
- Puncture-proof and leak-proof container approved for chemotherapy waste disposal
- Approved, specially labeled, impervious laundry bag
- Eyewash faucet adapters or fountain in or near work area[57]

PROCEDURE FOR SPILL ON HARD SURFACE
- Restrict area of spill.
- Obtain drug spill kit.
- Put on protective gown, gloves, goggles and if powder spill respirator mask.
- Open waste disposal bags (double bag).
- Place absorbent pads gently on the spill; be careful not to touch spill.
- Place saturated absorbent pad in waste bag.
- Cleanse surface with absorbent towels using detergent solution and wipe clean with clean tap water.

- Place all contaminated materials—for example gown, gloves, saturated absorbent pads, and towels—in double-bagged waste disposal bags.
- Discard waste bag and contents in approved container.
- Wash hands thoroughly with soap and water.[57]

PROCEDURE FOR SPILL ON LINEN
- Restrict area of spill.
- Obtain drug spill kit.
- Obtain specially marked, approved laundry bag and a labeled impervious bag.
- Put on protective gown, gloves, goggles.
- Remove soiled, contaminated linen from the patient's bedside.
- Place linen in approved, specially marked impervious laundry bag.
- Contaminated linen should be washed two times in laundry; laundry personnel should wear surgical latex gloves and gown when handling this material.
- Clean contaminated area with absorbent towels and detergent solution.
- Place all contaminated supplies used for management of spill in waste disposal bag and discard in approved waste disposal container.
- Wash hands thoroughly with soap and water.[57]

PROCEDURE FOR SPILL ON PERSONNEL OR PATIENT
- Restrict area of spill.
- Obtain drug spill kit.
- Immediately remove contaminated protective garments or linen.
- Wash affected skin area with soap and water.
- Eye exposure: immediately flood the affected eye with water for at least 5 minutes; obtain medical attention promptly.
- Follow procedures for contaminated linen.
- Notify the physician if drug spills on patient.

DOCUMENTATION
- Document in the patient's medical record management of drug spill and notification of the patient's physician.
- Document on the agency's approved forms management of spill occurring on hard surface, linen, or personnel.[57]

Caring for Patients Receiving Chemotherapeutic Drugs

Personnel handling blood, vomitus, or excreta from patients who have received chemotherapy within the previous 48 hours should wear disposable surgical latex gloves and gowns to be appropriately discarded after use. Linen contaminated with chemotherapeutic drugs, blood, vomitus, or excreta from a patient who has received these drugs within 48 hours before should be placed in a specially marked impervious laundry bag according to procedures for drug spills on linen.[14,57,61]

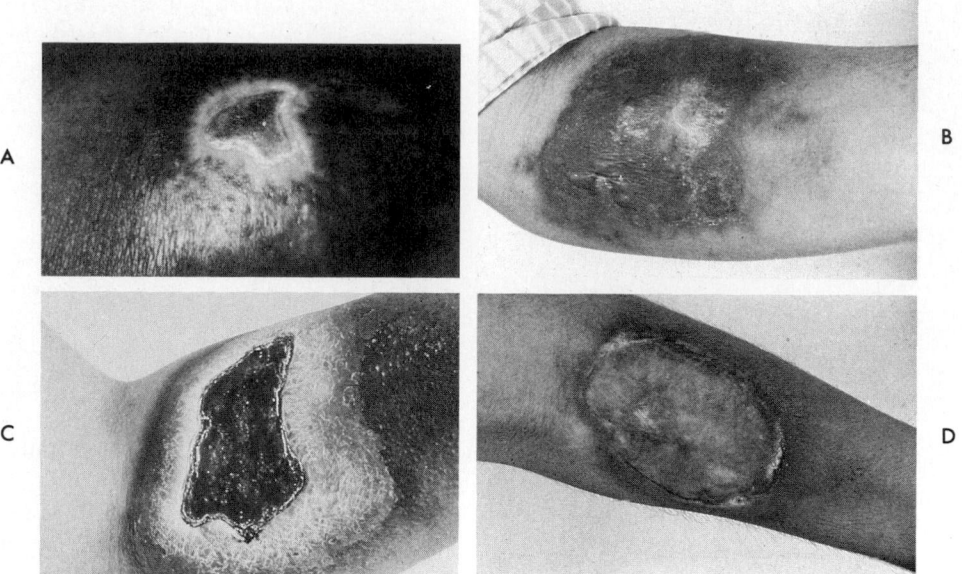

Figure 22–6   *A,* Resulting cutaneous effects of vesicant extravasation; note central necrosis surrounded by erythema and induration. *B,* Lateral progression of initial cutaneous effects occurring over a period of weeks. *C,* Eschar requiring surgical debridement eventually develops. *D,* Wide surgical excision of involved area on forearm. (Courtesy of Robert Dorr, University of Arizona, Progressions 2(4)4; 1990, Mosby.)

Staff Education

All personnel involved in any aspect of the handling of chemotherapeutic agents should receive an orientation to chemotherapy drugs, including their known risks, relevant techniques and procedures for handling, the proper use of protective equipment and materials, spill procedures, and medical policies covering personnel handling chemotherapeutic agents who are pregnant or actively trying to conceive children (per OSHA requirements). Evaluation of staff compliance may be achieved by regular quality monitoring.[7,14,16,57]

Employment Practices Regarding Reproductive Issues

The handling of chemotherapeutic agents by women who are either pregnant or actively trying to conceive and by those who are breast-feeding remains a sensitive and unsettled issue. Some suggest offering these personnel the opportunity to transfer to areas that do not involve chemotherapeutic agents. All safe handling guidelines should be practiced with utmost care by all pregnant personnel.[4,9,14]

Extravasation Management

Extravasation is the accidental infiltration of vesicant or irritant chemotherapeutic drugs from the vein into the surrounding tissues at the IV site. A vesicant is an agent that can produce a blister and/or tissue destruction. An irritant is an agent that is capable of producing venous pain at the site of and along the vein with or without an inflammatory reaction. Injuries that may occur as the result of extravasation include sloughing of tissue, infection, pain, and loss of mobility of an extremity. The degree of tissue damage is related to several factors such as: drug vesicant potential, drug concentration, the quantity of drug extravasated, duration of tissue exposure,[1,6,31,44] veinpuncture site/device, and needle insertion technique and individual tissue responses (Figure 22-6).

Because of the harmful effect of vesicants on tissues, studies using human subjects are limited, so controlled clinical trials demonstrating effectiveness of treatment have been difficult to attain. Most extravasation interventions have been based on preclinical studies using animal model systems including mice, pigs, rabbits, and dogs. Treatment strategies for extravasation management include the use of specific antidotes and guidelines for immediate intervention to minimize the tissue damage. Prevention of the extravasation and prompt intervention are the key elements for successful extravasation management. Tissue destruction resulting from drug extravasation may be subtle and progressive. Initial symptoms include pain or burning at the IV site, progressing to erythema, edema, and superficial skin loss (Figures 22-7 and 22-8). Tissue necrosis may not develop for 1 to 4 weeks after the drug extravasation.*

---

*References 1, 6, 17, 21, 22, 31, 44.

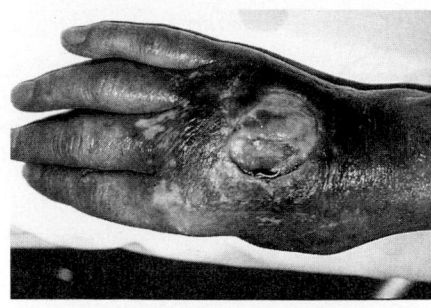

Figure 22–7 Doxorubicin extravasation in dorsum of right hand; note depth of wound. (From Progressions 2(4)4; 1990, Mosby.)

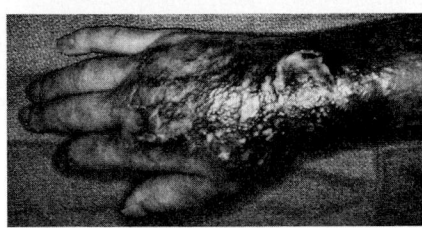

Figure 22–8 One month after doxorubicin extravasation in dorsum of right hand. (Courtesy of Robert Dorr, University of Arizona, Progressions 2(4)4; 1990. Mosby.)

GENERIC NAME	TRADE NAME
Nonvesicant Chemotherapeutic Drugs	
Asparaginase	Elspar
Bleomycin	Blenoxane
Carboplatin	CBDCA
Cisplatinum	Cisplatin
Cyclophosphamide	Cytoxan
Cytarabine	Ara-C, Cytosar
Floxuridine	FUDR
Fludarabine	Fludara
Fluorouracil	5-FU
Ifosfamide	Naxamide
Methotrexate	Mexate
Taxol	
Thiophosphoramide	Thiotepa
Topotecan	

Chemotherapeutic Drugs with Vesicant Potential	
Amasacrine	AMSA
Bisantrene	ADAH
Dacarbazine	DTIC-Dome
Dactinomycin	Actinomycin D, Cosmegen
Daunorubicin	Cerubidine, Daunomycin
Doxorubicin	Adriamycin
Epirubicin	Epi-Epidoxrubicin
Esorubicin	Eso-Deoxydoxorubicin
Idarubicin	Ida-Idamycin
Mechlorethamine	Nitrogen Mustard, Mustargen
Mitomycin	Mutamycin
Mitoxantrone	Novantrone
Vinblastine	Velban
Vincristine	Oncovin

GENERIC NAME	TRADE NAME
Chemotherapeutic Drugs with Irritant Potential	
Carmustine	BCNU
Etoposide	VP-16, VePesid
Mitoguazone	Methyl-GAG, MGBG
Plicamycin	Mithracin
Streptozocin	Zanosar
Teniposide	VM-26
Vindesine	Eldisine

Controversial Topics*[,50,51]

The management of extravasation of chemotherapeutic drugs involves some controversial issues.

USE OF ANTECUBITAL FOSSA FOR DRUG ADMINISTRATION

Favor
- Larger veins permit more rapid infusion of drug.
- Larger veins permit potentially irritating drugs to reach the general circulation sooner with less irritation.

Oppose Antecubital Fossa Access
- Arm mobility is restricted.
- Infiltration may cause extensive reconstructive efforts.
- Early infiltration may be difficult to assess.
- Potential for venous fibrosis; blood drawing from antecubital fossa may be more difficult.

METHODS OF DRUG SEQUENCING

Favor Administering Vesicants First
- Vascular integrity decreases over time.
- Initial assessment of vein patency is most accurate.
- Possibility of diminishing patient awareness of symptoms related to drug infiltration.

Favor Administering Vesicants Last
- Vesicants are irritating and may increase fragility of veins.
- Venous spasm may occur at onset of drug administration and alter assessment of venous access.

NEEDLE OR CATHETER SIZE

Favor Large (18- or 19-) Gauge
- Irritating chemotherapeutic agents can reach circulation sooner with less irritating effect on the peripheral veins.

Favor Small (20- to 23-) Gauge
- Smaller-gauge devices are less likely to puncture the wall of a small vein.
- Increased blood flow around a smaller-gauge device increases dilution of chemotherapeutic agents.
- Phlebitis may be minimized with a smaller-gauge device.

---

*Adapted from Oncology Nursing Society Task Force: Cancer chemotherapy guidelines and recommendations for nursing education and practice, 1992 guidelines, Pittsburgh, 1992, The Oncology Nursing Society.

Prevention of Extravasation[31,44,50,51]

Nursing staff responsibilities for the prevention of extravasation include the following:

- Knowledge of drugs with vesicant potential (see list on p. 507)
- Skill in drug administration
- Identification of risk factors, for example multiple venipunctures, previous treatment
- Anticipation of extravasation and knowledge of approved management protocol
- Obtaining a new venipuncture site daily if peripheral access used
- Consideration of central venous access for difficult peripheral access
- Most sources recommend 24 hour vesicant infusion via central venous access *only*
- Administration of drug in a quiet, unhurried environment
- Testing vein patency without using chemotherapeutic agents
- Providing adequate drug dilution, for example side port infusion via free-flowing intravenous infusion
- Careful observation of access site and extremity throughout the procedure
- Validation of blood return from intravenous site before, during, and after vesicant drug infusion
- Educating patients regarding symptoms of drug infiltration, for example pain, burning, and stinging sensations at intravenous site

Protocol for Extravasation Management at a Peripheral Site

Agency policy and procedure for management of extravasation with the responsible physician's prescription should be easily accessible to the staff. The approved antidotes should be readily available, and the following procedure should be initiated with a physician's prescription as soon as extravasation of a vesicant or irritant agent is suspected or occurs.[31,44,50,51]

- Stop the chemotherapeutic drug.
- Leave the needle or catheter in place.

Table 22–3 Chemotherapeutic Vesicant Drugs with Recommended Antidotes

Drug	Antidote
ALKYLATING AGENT Mechlorethamine (nitrogen mustard)	Isotonic Sodium thiosulfate Dilute 1.6 ml sodium thiosulfate 25% with 8.4 ml of sterile water; inject 1 to 4 ml through existing IV access; inject subq if IV access is removed Apply ice pack and/or cold compresses

Table 22–3 Chemotherapeutic Vesicant Drugs with Recommended Antidotes—cont'd

Drug	Antidote
ANTIBIOTICS Actinomycin D Dacarbazine Daunorubicin Doxorubicin Epirubicin* Esorubicin* Idarubincin* Mithramycin Mitomycin C Piroxanthrone*	Hydrocortisone 100 mg/ml Inject 0.5 ml IV through existing IV line and 0.5 ml subcutaneously into extravasated site; apply cold compresses Dexamethasone 4 mg/ml Inject 0.5 ml IV through existing IV line and 0.5 ml subcutaneously into extravasated site; apply cold compresses/ice packs immediately, *do not* apply pressure *Alternative protocol* Topical DMSO 1 to 2 ml of 1 mmol DMSO 50% to 100% Apply topically one time at the site; apply cold compresses
BISANTRENE	Sodium bicarbonate 1 mEq/ml Mix equal parts of sodium bicarbonate with sterile normal saline (1:1 solution); resulting solution is 0.5 mEq/ml Inject 2 to 6 ml (1 to 3.0 mEq) IV through existing IV line and subcutaneously into the extravasated site; apply cold compresses
VINCA ALKALOIDS Vinblastine Vincristine	Hyaluronidase (Wydase) 150 U/ml Add 1 ml sterile sodium chloride Inject 1 to 6 ml (150 to 900 U) subcutaneously into the extravasated site with multiple injections; apply warm compresses
LOCAL ANTIDOTE[21] (may be used for daunorubicin, doxorubicin, and mitomycin)	Topical cooling may be achieved using: Ice packs Cooling pad with ice water circulating Cryogel packs changed frequently Cooling of site to patient tolerance for 24 hr. Elevate and rest extremity 24-48 hr.†

*Limited information available.
†References 6,17,31,44,50,51.

- Aspirate any residual drug and blood in the IV tubing, needle or catheter, and suspected infiltration site.
- Instill the IV antidote (Table 22-3).
- Remove the needle
- If unable to aspirate the residual drug from the IV tubing, remove needle or catheter.
- Inject the antidote subcutaneously clockwise into the infiltrated site using 25-gauge needle; change the needle with each new injection.
- Avoid applying pressure to the suspected infiltration site.
- Photograph the suspected area of extravasation according to agency's policy and procedure for documentation and follow-up.
- Apply topical ointment if ordered.
- Cover lightly with an occlusive sterile dressing.
- Apply cold or warm compresses as indicated (see Table 22-3).
- Elevate the extremity.
- Observe regularly for pain, erythema, induration, and necrosis.
- Documentation of extravasation management:
  Date
  Time
  Needle or catheter size and type
  Insertion site
  Drug sequence
  Approximate amount of drug extravasated
  Nursing management of extravasation
  Photo documentation
  Patient complaints and statements
  Appearance of site
  Physician notification
  Follow-up measures
  Nurse's signature

Anaphylaxis

Nursing personnel administering chemotherapy in all settings are recommended to follow the listed guidelines for drug preparation, administration and disposal, vein selection, documentation of drug infusion, venous access device and possible side effects, teaching the patient about self-management of most common side effects, and management of chemotherapy spills and drug extravasation.[16,44] In addition to these guidelines, all nursing personnel should be alert and prepared for the possible complications of anaphylaxis. The drugs and supplies necessary to manage these complications must be readily available.[5,25]

The nurse must be informed and prepared for the specific drugs known to be at risk for anaphylaxis. Test dosing prior to infusion of the drug and following the infusion precautions will decrease the anaphylaxis occurrence (see Table 22-4).[34,36]

Emergency medications and supplies for management of anaphylaxis include the following:
- Injectable aminophylline, diphenhydramine hydrochloride (Benadryl), dopamine, epinephrine, heparin, hydrocortisone
- Oxygen setup, tubing cannula, or mask and airway device
- Suction equipment
- IV fluids (isotonic solutions)
- IV tubings and supplies for venous access

Prompt and effective nursing intervention for anaphylaxis decreases complications. The nurse must be alert to the signs and symptoms of an anaphylactic response to a chemotherapeutic drug. All or some of these symptoms may be present: anxiety, hypotension, uticaria, cyanosis, respiratory distress, abdominal cramping, flushed appearance, chills. The calm and reassuring presence of the nurse will facilitate in the management of these symptoms, which proceeds as follows[50]:
- Immediately stop the drug infusion.
- Maintain an intravenous line with isotonic saline.
- Position the patient for comfort and to promote perfusion of the vital organs.
- Notify the physician, nursing agency and/or emergency medical services.
- Maintain the airway and anticipate the need for cardiopulmonary resuscitation.
- Monitor the vital signs according to agency policy.
- Administer the appropriate medications with an approved physician's order.
- Follow the nursing agency's protocol for follow-up care (e.g., evaluation of the patient by a physician).
- Document the incident in the patient's medical record.

An anaphylaxis occurrence will be very upsetting to the patient and family. Follow up care is required to diminish their anxiety and to monitor delayed side effects. Instruct the patient and family on the pertinent drug side effects, when and where to call for assistance, and what symptoms (shortness of breath, rash on body increasing in size and intensity, flushed appearance, fever, chills, abdominal cramping, and a feeling of anxiousness) require immediate health care intervention.[52,54]

ALTERNATIVE CARE SETTINGS

Improved drug delivery, cost containment, and considerations of the quality of life have affected trends in chemotherapy administration. Management of symptoms such as control of nausea and vomiting and innovative pain management have reduced the need for hospitalization. Options to give chemotherapy in outpatient settings include ambulatory care

Table 22–4   Chemotherapeutic Drugs with Anaphylactic Potential

Drugs	Signs and Symptoms	Precautions
Asparginase (Elspar)	Respiratory distress, increased pulse, respirations, hypotension, facial edema, anxiety, flushed appearance, hives, itching. Risk for anaphylaxis increases with each dose	Test dose prior to initial IV/IM dosing. Monitor 30 min/IM; 60 min/IV post drug administration. Keep vein open IV normal saline prior, during, and 30/60 post IV administration of Asparginase. Initiate drug infusion slowly (mg/m²/titrate infusion). Code cart, O_2, suction equipment, drugs for anaphylaxis at or near patient's bedside.
	Test Dose Procedure: Prepare 10,000 IU Asparginase with 5 ml NS. Inject 0.1 ml of this solution (200 IU) into 9.9 ml NS. Inject intradermally 0.1 ml of this concentration (20 IU) to make a wheal in inner aspect of arm. Observe wheal for 60 min for erythema, swelling, and itching prior to infusion.	
Bleomycin	Dyspnea, hypotension, increased pulse and respiration, rash	Test dose prior to initial IV dosing. Initiate drug infusion slowly (10-20 ml/15 min). Monitor vital signs and auscultate breath sounds Q4hr during and for 24 hours postinfusion and/or on scheduled basis in outpatient setting.
	Test Dose Procedure: Inject 2 U Bleomycin intradermal to make a wheal in inner aspect of arm. Observe for erythema, edema, and itching prior to first 2 doses of Bleomycin infusion.	
Etoposide (VP-16)	Hypotension, bronchospasm, chest pain, increased pulse, respirations, facial flush, fever, chills, diaphoresis	Initiate drug infusion slowly (10-20 ml/15 min). Infuse total volume over at least 60 minutes. Monitor vital signs Q15 min × 4; Q30 min × 2 and Q4hr, during and 24 hours post infusion.
Taxol	Hypotension, dyspnea with bronchospasm, urticaria, abdominal and extremity pain, angioedema and diaphoresis. Incidence is increased with shorter infusions.	Ensure recommended premedications are given prior to taxol infusion. Dexamethasone 20 mg PO 12 and 6 hr; diphenhydramine 50 mg IV bolus 30 to 60 min; cimetidine 300 mg IV infusion 30 to 60 min; antiemetic (e.g., Zofran) 10 mg in 50 ml IV infusion over 15 min. Obtain baseline vital signs; then monitor q15 min × 4; Q1 hr × 4; then Q4 hr during the infusion. Code cart, O_2, suction equipment, and drugs for anaphylaxis at or near bedside.
Teniposide (VM-26)	Severe hypotension, anxiety, increased pulse, respirations, fever	Initiate drug infusion *slowly* (10-20 ml/30 min). Total infusion time 60-120 min. Monitor vital signs Q15 min. × 4; Q30 min × 2, during and post infusion; then monitor Q4hr × 24 hr.

Data from American Hospital Formulary Service, American Society of Hospital Pharmacists, Inc., Bethesda 1992, Physicians Desk Reference, Medical Economics Data, New Jersey 1993.

centers, physicians' offices, extended care facilities, and home health agencies. Certain principles of chemotherapy administration and standards of care for patients must be maintained by the staff regardless of the setting.[50,51,55,61]

Home health care will expand in the next decade. The oncology patient is now and will continue to be a major segment of this population of patients. Criteria specific to home administration of chemotherapy include: care giver(s) able and willing to assist; pa-

tient's physical condition stable and within the range of home care capabilities; stable and suitable living conditions, including cleanliness, plumbing, refrigeration, telephone; and access to emergency assistance.[6,12,55]

Patients and family members involved in chemotherapy drug infusion and/or management of side effects require verbal, written, demonstration, and/or return demonstration procedural information. Following are suggested nursing interventions to facilitate teaching the patient and family about drug administration in the home.[52,54]

Interventions

- Assess the patient's ability and willingness to learn, the availability of care giver, environment at home, ability to assume self-care, and compliance with treatment regimen.
- Describe the purpose, schedule, and procedure of the chemotherapeutic regimen.
- Explain to the patient the possible side effects of chemotherapeutic drugs (nausea and vomiting, anorexia, stomatitis, constipation, diarrhea, alopecia, and skin and hematopoietic changes).[24]
- Instruct the patient or the care giver about dealing with specific side effects.[15]
- Review symptoms such as temperature elevation over 38° C, severe constipation or diarrhea, persistent bleeding from any site, sudden weight gain or loss, shortness of breath, pain not relieved by prescribed medications, and severe nausea and vomiting more than 24 hours after treatment. Emphasize the importance of promptly reporting these symptoms to the physician.[25]
- Instruct the patient or the care giver regarding management of infusion devices.[52]
- Validate aseptic technique and skills of the patient or the care giver for prescribed self-administration and discontinuation of chemotherapeutic drugs.
- Explain safe handling precautions for administration and disposal of chemotherapy.[12,16]
- Provide information and a list of resources for obtaining, storing, and disposing of drugs and supplies. Also provide a schedule of follow-up tests and care.[30,48]
- Record the drug, dose, route, and time given in home and provide this information to the agency responsible for care management.[48,49]
- Discard all unused drugs and used supplies into a recommended puncture-proof, leakproof container. Return this container to the appropriate agency for disposal (Fig. 22-9).[50,51]
- Use plastic sheeting to protect bedding or furniture if incontinence is possible.
- Carefully handle linen contaminated by chemotherapeutic drugs and excreta, and wash twice, separately from all other linen.[55,57]
- It is recommended that the patient receive the first chemotherapy dose in an acute care or outpatient setting.

FUTURE DIRECTIONS AND ADVANCES IN CHEMOTHERAPY

Future directions in chemotherapy offer many exciting opportunities. The use of effective adjuvant, neoadjuvant, combination chemotherapies, and che-

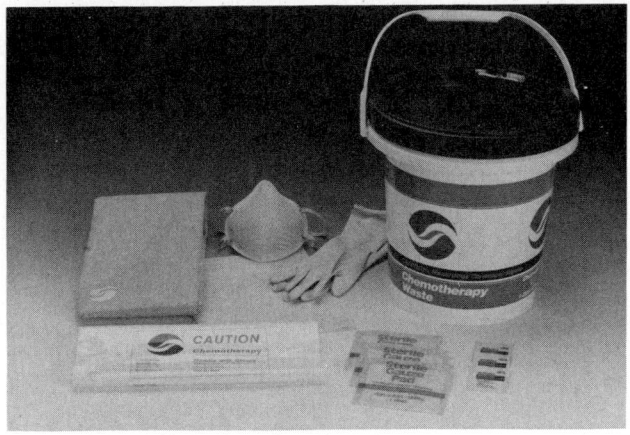

Figure 22–9 Home health care kit. (Courtesy Biosafety-systems, Inc., San Diego.)

motherapy in combination with other treatment modalities will increase. Ongoing drug research will focus on new drug development and dose intensity schedules for most of the major cancer diseases. Drugs currently demonstrating clinical efficacy include: topotecan/breast cancer; piroxantrone/breast, melanoma; edatrexate/non-small cell lung and head and neck cancers; and taxol/used in many solid tumors.[60,62]

Other ways that will increase effectiveness of chemotherapy drugs is to protect the body from serious side effects. The development of the colony-stimulating factors, granulocyte colony-stimulating factor (G-CSF), and granulocyte-macrophage colony-stimulating factor (GM-CSF) has allowed for the delivery of chemotherapy with a lessened degree and incidence of leukopenia/infection and allows for the potential for aggressive dose intensification of chemotherapeutic regimens. ICRF-187, also known as ADR-529, has been studied as an antineoplastic agent and, more significantly, as a protective agent against the cardiotoxic effects of doxorubicin and related anthracyclines.[24,36,40,42]

Another major problem limiting the efficacy of chemotherapy drugs is the presence of drug resistance at the onset of therapy or the development of resistance during the course of therapy. Multidrug resistance phenomenon is being explored in depth, and the clinical implications of the potential role of topoisomerase II in resistance are beginning to be delineated. Finally, the use of chemotherapy agents 13-cisretinoic acid plus interferon for mycosis fungoides, 4-HPR for transitional cell cancer of the bladder, beta-carotene for head and neck stage I, II, and melanoma, and tamoxifen for breast cancer in all the chemoprevention trials will present many exciting challenges for all oncology nurses.[26,28,30,35,41]

Text continued on p. 516.

Nursing Management

Nursing management of the patient receiving chemotherapy requires multiple assessment and intervention strategies. Nursing care begins with a thorough understanding of the patient's condition; goal of therapy; drug dose, route, schedule; administration principles; and potential side effects. Additional nursing management includes monitoring responses to therapy, reassessing and documenting signs and symptoms, and communicating pertinent information to other members of the health care team. Ongoing psychosocial evaluation and patient teaching components require astute nursing interventions. Multiple resources are available at the local and national level. The Oncology Nursing Society, American Cancer Society, National Cancer Institute, and Leukemia Society all provide lay and professional educational materials.[12,47,51,57]

NURSING ASSESSMENT AND INTERVENTION

Chemotherapeutic drugs may cause adverse side effects and major system toxicity and dysfunction. Side effects and toxicity vary in severity according to the patient's individual response to the drug therapy. The most frequent side effects are myelosuppression, nausea, and vomiting. Myelosuppression can be a dose-limiting toxicity.[8] Myelosuppression, stomatitis, mucositis, and skin integrity are discussed extensively in Chapter 29. The chemotherapeutic drugs work by destruction and/or suppression of new leukocytes, platelets, and erythrocytes. Monitor these effects through an evaluation of the blood count at scheduled periodic intervals. The time or level at which a blood count reaches its lowest point is the nadir. The nadir varies with individual drugs but usually occurs between 7 and 21 days after the administration of chemotherapeutic drugs.

Nausea and vomiting are often the most distressing side effects of chemotherapy.[54] Nausea and vomiting may be acute, anticipatory, delayed, or persistent. *Acute* nausea and vomiting occur within 1 to 2 hours of treatment and last for approximately 24 hours. *Anticipatory* nausea and vomiting occur before the treatment. Nausea and vomiting after the initial 24 hours of treatment may be referred to as delayed or persistent. Cisplatin in particular is associated with this symptom. An estimated 60% of patients experience delayed emesis after cisplatin even if emesis is adequately controlled during the first 24 hours.[33]

Assessing and reporting their frequency, severity, patterns, and duration aid in prevention and management of symptoms. Prevention is best for nausea and vomiting. Behavioral interventions such as relaxation, distraction, and guided imagery may help with anticipatory nausea and vomiting. Allowing the patient to sleep through the peak hours of nausea and vomiting and/or chemotherapy may diminish these symptoms. Administration of antiemetics 30 to 60 minutes before chemotherapy also alleviates the symptoms. Antiemetics should be continued at scheduled intervals throughout the expected duration of nausea and vomiting.[15,42]

In the past 10 to 15 years antiemetic research has had a profound effect on the treatment of chemotherapy-induced nausea and vomiting. The incidence of these side effects is related to the emetic potential of the chemotherapy drug, the dose, route, schedule, duration, and combinations of administration (Table 22-5).[33,42] The combination of antiemetic drugs with

Table 22-5 Emetic Potential of Common Chemotherapy Drugs

Mild Potential	Moderate Potential	Severe Potential
Bleomycin	Carboplatin	Cisplatin
Busulfan	Carmustine	Cyclophosphamide
Chlorambucil	Cytarabine	Dacarbazine
Etoposide	Daunorubicin	Dactinomycin
5-Fluorouracil	Doxorubicin	Mechlorethamine
Hydroxyurea	Ifosfamide	Streptozotocin
Mercaptopurine	Lomustine	
Methotrexate	Mitomycin C	
(low dose)	Mitoxantrone	
Tamoxifen	Procarbazine	
Vinblastine	Taxol	

Table 22-6 Selected Parenteral Antimetic Regimens

Drug	Dosage	Schedule
Metoclopramide (Reglan)	1-3 mg/kg IV	30 min before and 90 min after chemotherapy, then Q4hr PRN
Dexamethasone (Decadron)	20 mg IV	30-40 min before chemotherapy
Lorazepam (Ativan) *or*	1.5 mg/m² IV	30 min before chemotherapy
Diphenhydramine (Benadryl)	50 mg IV	30 min before chemotherapy
(The above drugs are used in varying doses and schedules depending upon severity of emetic episode.)		
Ondansetron (Zofran)	0.15 mg/kg in 30-50 ml; infuse over 15-30 min	30 min before chemotherapy, then in 4 and 8 hr after the initial dose

From American Society of Hospital Pharmacists, Inc., 1993, Bethesda, MD.

different mechanisms, round-the-clock administration, and higher dosages have been shown to be more effective than single-agent dosing and PRN schedules.[11] Several agents now used as single agents or in combination are metoclopramide, haloperidol, dexamethasone, lorazepam and prochlorperazine (Tables 22-6 and 22-7). Many of these drugs act on the chemoreceptor trigger zone in the brain by blocking dopamine receptors.[11,15,43]

Although these antiemetics have demonstrated effectiveness, they are associated with undesirable side effects: sedation, extra-pyramidal reactions, anxiety, mood changes, and diarrhea. Another major drawback is that most of these drugs are administered IV and are usually not feasible for outpatient use and children.[33,48]

The development and use of the 5-HT3 antagonists (Odansetron/Zofran) has made new strides in effective antiemetic therapy. Although more costly than previous antiemetic drugs, the dosing schedule is less frequent (0.15 mg/kg 30 minutes before chemotherapy, then in 4 and 8 hr after the initial dose). Side effects thus far are mild: headache, constipation, and transient elevated liver enzymes. Ondansetron has demonstrated effectiveness as an oral agent and may be suitable for outpatient therapy and children.[11,15,43]

The remaining side effects listed in Table 22-1 such as aches and pains, alopecia, anorexia, constipation, cystitis, diarrhea, depression, fatigue, mucositis, pharyngitis, and stomatitis have listed nursing actions and points to cover for patient/family teaching. The nurse's responsibilities include evaluating patient's response to drugs, teaching the patient or care giver self-management interventions, and monitoring various laboratory data, signs, and symptoms reported by the patient. The information will be useful in developing the plan of care for the patient receiving chemotherapy.*

Pertinent information related to the major system toxicities: cardiac, hematopoietic, hepatic, hypersensitivity, neurologic, ototoxicity, pulmonary, reproductive, and renal; and metabolic alterations (Table 22-2) has *dose limiting restrictions* for many of the drugs. If symptoms occur and the chemotherapy drug dose and/or schedule is *not altered/evaluated* the potential for *irreversible side effects* are increased. All of the toxicities listed in Table 22-2 require astute observations and interventions by all the health care team members.[5,8,27,30]

Selected nursing diagnoses and interventions appropriate for the patient receiving chemotherapy are listed below. Additional nursing diagnoses may be ascertained by assessing the patient's health, psychosocial issues, and/or specific side effects of the chemotherapy drugs. Further circumstances that may affect patient responses include the setting in which the drug is administered (acute care/home care), activities of daily living needs, and life-style changes.[5,7,9]

NURSING DIAGNOSIS

Knowledge deficit related to chemotherapeutic side effects

- Assess educational level, ability, desire to learn, and barriers to learning.
- Assess knowledge level relative to cancer, pre-

*References 24, 26, 28, 30, 32, 34.

Table 22–7 Selected Oral Antiemetic Regimens

Drugs	Dosage	Schedule
Chlorpromazine hydrochloride (Thorazine)	10, 25, 50, 100, 200 mg tablets; 75, 150, 200, 300 mg SR capsules	Give 30–75 mg in 2-4 hr in divided doses; 1 hr before chemotherapy administration; then every 4-6 hr PRN.
Dronabinol	2.5, 5, 10 mg SR capsules	Give 1-3 hr before chemotherapy administration; then 4-6 doses per day every 2-4 hr. Maximum 15 mg/m² per dose.
Ondansetron	8 mg (12 yrs of age and older)	Give initial dose 8 mg tablet 30 min prior to chemotherapy. Maximum dose 3 times a day for 2 to 3 days.
	4 mg (4-11 yrs old)	Give initial dose 4 mg tablet 30 min prior to chemotherapy. Maximum dose 3 times a day for 2 to 3 days.
Prochlorperazone (Compazine)	5, 10, 25 mg tablets; 10, 15, 30 mg SR capsules	Give 10–25 mg 1 hr before chemotherapy administration; 15–30 mg SR capsules every 12 hr. Then repeat *one* of above doses every 3-4½ hr.
Promethazine (Phenergan)	12.5, 25, 50 mg tablets	Give 25–50 mg 1 hr before chemotherapy administration; then 12.5–25 mg 4 times per day.
Trimethobenzamide hydrocloride (Tigan)	100, 250 mg capsule	Give 250 mg 1 hr before chemotherapy administration; then 250 mg 4 times per day.

From Physician Drug Reference, Medical Economics Data, Medical Economic Co, Inc., N.J., 1993, and American Hospital Formulary Service, 1993.

vious experience with the diagnosis, and treatment of cancer.

- Evaluate understanding relative to the specific diagnosis, disease process, and potential treatment planned.
- Assess previous experience with chemotherapy.
- Determine availability of caregiver to participate in patient's care and treatment process.
- Assess patient/family needs for consultation with varied resources (e.g., I can Cope Support Group, Reach to Recovery, Look Good-Feel Better, Ostomy, and Laryngectomy Support Groups[16,32,34]).

Oral mucous membrane, alteration in, related to side effects of drugs[8,25,37]

- Assess history of alcohol use, tobacco use, or other risk factors.
- Obtain current history of current treatment; radiation therapy, chemotherapy, surgery, and biotherapy.
- Query the patient about his usual regimen for oral hygiene and the date of last dental exam.
- Assess the oral mucosa; palate, tongue, gums, teeth, lips, floor of mouth, and inner aspects of cheeks. Note redness, ulcerations, bleeding, white patches, and color, amount, and consistency of saliva.

Injury, potential for, related to alteration in immune system; clotting factors[24-26]

- Monitor CBC, hemoglobin, PT, PTT, and platelet count.
- Assess type of therapy (chemotherapy, radiation therapy) and current drugs (aspirin, anticoagulants), which may alter bleeding and clotting time.
- Assess factors (fever, sepsis, altered hepatic function, and bone marrow function) that may alter clotting process.
- Identify potential date of nadir for platelets.
- Observe and report symptoms: bruising, bleeding from venous access sites, nose, gums, vagina, rectum; hemoptysis, hematemesis; black, tarry, and/or gross blood in stools; increase in usual menstrual flow, change in vital signs, and spontaneous petechiae or hematomas.

Nutrition, alteration in: less than body, requirement related to nausea and vomiting[33,38,40]

- Assess the amount, color, consistency and frequency of emesis, and nauseous episodes.
- Determine what factors facilitate and/or prevent nausea and vomiting.
- Query the patient about strategies in the past that were helpful in management of nausea and vomiting.

- Assess baseline weight prior to illness, onset of illness, changes since onset of treatment, weight 1 month ago, and note weight gains/losses.
- Monitor laboratory values: serum albumin, serum transferrin level, CBC, and electrolytes.
- Assess dietary history: food habits, food likes/dislikes, and amount and type of food eaten at breakfast, lunch, supper, and snacks.
- Note altered bowel habits and presence of other related GI distress (heartburn, feeling of fullness, cramping).
- Consult with dietary services and/or plan with patient recommendations for nutritional intake (cold foods, salads, cheeses, fruits, salty foods, colas) that will stimulate appetite and facilitate calorie intake.

Sensory-perceptual alteration: visual related to photosensitivity, auditory related to ototoxicity[40,42,52]

- Determine chemotherapy and/or other treatment-related protocol that may affect sensory alterations.
- Assess severity of symptoms regarding compromises in patient's activities in daily living.
- Assess environmental conditions (light, noise, room temperature).
- Determine onset of sensory alteration; severity, changes in duration, and/or other discomforting symptoms.
- Instruct patient regarding precautions to follow: photosensitivity (wear sun glasses when outside, dim room lights, driving and/or work-related restrictions), ototoxicity (limit/restrict environmental noise), inform health care team regarding presence of symptoms and restrictions for work-related, driving, and/or activities of daily living.

Disturbance in self-concept related to alopecia[5,7]

- Inform patient that hair loss is temporary and hair will regrow when the treatment is stopped; usual hair growth returns 2-6 months.
- Provide resources for purchase/loan of wigs, scarves, and caps.
- Inform patient about health care measures for scalp protection: use of gentle shampoos, avoidance of hair dryers and curling irons, permanents, and hair dying; protect scalp in winter and summer (cold/heat loss) and wear protective covering when outdoors.
- Encourage sharing of feelings regarding body image changes. Inform patient about American Cancer Society support groups (e.g., I Can Cope, Look Good-Feel Better).

Alteration in comfort: pain related to bone metastasis, pruritus, and mucositis[8,24,25]

- Determine onset, location, duration, severity, intensity, and radiation of symptoms.
- Assess symptoms with patient/family suggestions: What makes the symptoms/discomfort better? What makes the symptoms/discomfort worse? For example: types and frequency of interventions; treatments related interventions related to hygiene, nutritional, and pain; time of intervention regarding food intake and mobility.
- Provide physician prescribed medications and/or treatment interventions.
- Encourage relaxation/meditation/distraction strategies to facilitate coping with discomfort and enhanced effects of medications/treatment interventions.
- Monitor electrolyte imbalance and granulocyte count.
- Assess the skin, especially hidden areas (between toes, skin folds of breasts, buttocks, perineal area) on a scheduled basis; report changes and findings promptly.

Infection, potential for, immunosuppression, break in skin, or contamination of supplies[8,30,32,47]

- Monitor CBC and acute granulocyte count.
- Monitor expectation of nadir related to chemotherapy.

- Instruct and monitor prudent handwashing technique: prior to any nursing intervention, before/after meals, after bathroom use, and prior to any treatment-related activity for self-care.
- Restrict visitors with potential infections or recently immunized with attenuated live vaccines (DPT, MMR).
- Monitor food intake: instruct regarding restrictions (no fresh vegetables/fruits) and consult with nurse prior to eating food brought in to hospital.
- Ensure cleanliness of room and supplies used in routine care; change all supplies on a scheduled basis.
- Examine all sterile supplies prior to use; note expiration date for sterility, observe for any defect or interruption of integrity of the product, and use sterile technique when opening and using the product.

Patient teaching priorities and geriatric considerations are given in the boxes on this page.

PATIENT TEACHING PRIORITIES FOR CHEMOTHERAPY[32,34,47,48,52]

Assess willingness, readiness to learn, and barriers to learning (acuity of illness, sensory deficits, pain, and/or fear and anxiety regarding diagnosis/treatment).

Inform patient/family about schedule of activities for chemotherapy administration and monitoring of laboratory and diagnostic tests.

Encourage practice and repetition of newly learned skill to enhance the learner's performance for at risk procedures.

Validate aseptic technique and skills of the patient or the caregiver for prescribed self-administration and discontinuation of chemotherapy drugs.

Provide written materials such as those from the National Cancer Institute "Chemotherapy and You." "What Are Clinical Trials All About," 1-800-4-CANCER telephone number, and other materials as needed.

Teach and review specific drugs and related side effects the patient may experience, and when, where, how, and who to call if problems.

Provide information and list of resources for obtaining, storing, and disposing drugs and supplies.[45,49]

GERIATRIC CONSIDERATIONS[52,54]

Potential for cardiac, renal, respiratory, and hepatic systems compromise: medication dosage and/or schedule of administration may be altered.

High-dose drug regimens have been associated with increased toxicity (e.g., neurotoxicity with high-dose cytarabine—patients over 50 years old are particularly susceptible to this toxicity).

Consider neuromuscular and sensory deficits that may be present, such as visual and hearing losses and arthritic joints; plan individualized teaching sessions; use printed materials with large print for reading ease; return demonstration techniques may require more simplistic steps to facilitate patient/family ease in learning the required technique.

Consider age-related changes in body function accommodations; bowel and bladder tonicity (unable to hold large volume hydration, unable to retain large volume bowel cleansing preparations); provide prompt and frequent elimination needs.

Premedications may cause drowsiness; encourage patient/family to utilize transportation resources (family, public, American Cancer Society) if receiving chemotherapy and/or required laboratory tests monitoring.

Query the patient/caregiver regarding over-the-counter and/or previous physician prescribed medications; some of these medications may alter bleeding and clotting times and/or interfere with prescribed chemotherapy medications.

Assess ability of patient and caregiver and determine if additional resources, such home-care agency, Meals on Wheels, and social services for financial assistance, are needed.[7,30,36]

CONCLUSION

Nurses have major responsibilities in caring for patients who receive chemotherapeutic agents. It is important that nurses know treatment goals, drug classifications with modes of action, principles of tumor growth and cell kill, and administration protocols. Chemotherapeutic agents should be administered only by nurses who have been educated and are skilled in the various procedures. Patient and family education on the many aspects of chemotherapy (e.g., procedure, potential side effects and toxicities, and follow-up care) requires competent nursing assessment and intervention. The nurse should encourage the patient and family to be an integral part of planning and implementing care. Keeping abreast of all the new drugs and their implication along with the above responsibilities offers many challenges for the nurse in the varied settings of oncology practice.

BIBLIOGRAPHY

1. Alberts DS and Dorr RT: Case report: topical DMSO for mitomycin-c-induced skin ulceration, Oncol Nurs Forum 18(4):693, 1991.
2. American Society of Hospital Pharmacists: ASHP technical assistance bulletin on handling cytotoxic and hazardous drugs, Am J Hosp Pharm 47(5):1033, 1990.
3. Baird and others: Cancer Nursing: a comprehensive textbook, Philadelphia, 1991, WB Saunders Co.
4. Barnicle MM: Chemotherapy and pregnancy, Semin Oncol Nurs 8(2):124, 1992.
5. Barton-Burke MS and others: Potential toxicities and nursing management. In Cancer chemotherapy: A nursing process approach, Boston, 1991, Jones and Bartlett Publishers Inc.
6. Beason R: Antineoplastic vesicant extravasation, INS 13(2):111, 1990.
7. Bender C: Implications of antineoplastic therapy for nursing, In Clark JC and McGee RF editors, Core curriculum for oncology nursing, ed 2, 1992, Philadelphia, WB Saunders Co.
8. Bjergaard J and others: Increased risk of myelodysplasia and leukaemia after etoposide, cisplatin, and bleomycin for germ-cell tumours, Lancet 338(8):359, 1991.
9. Brown JK and Hogan CM: Chemotherapy, In Groenwald SL, Frogge MH, Goodman M, and Yarbro CH: Cancer nursing principles and practice, Boston, 1992, Jones and Bartlett Publishers Inc.
10. Brown M and Mulholland JL: Drug calculations: Process and problems for clinical practice, ed 4, St. Louis, 1992, Mosby.
11. Button D: Recent developments in the management of emesis with the 5-HT3 antagonist granisetron, Semin Oncol Nurs 6(suppl 1):14, 1990.
12. Carey PJ and others: Appraisal and caregiving burdens in family members caring for patients receiving chemotherapy, Oncol Nurs Forum 18(8):1341, 1991.
13. Caruso CC and others: Cooling effects and comfort of four cooling blanket temperatures in humans with fever, Nursing Research 41(2):68, 1992.
14. Caudell KA and others: Quantification of urinary mutagens in nurses during potential antineoplastic agent exposure: A pilot study with concurrent environmental and dietary control, Cancer Nurs 11(1):41, 1988.
15. Clark RA and others: Antiemetic therapy: management of chemotherapy-induced nausea and vomiting, Semin Oncol 5(2):53, 1989.
16. Creaton EM and others: A hospital-based chemotherapy education and training program, Cancer Nurs 14(2):79, 1991.
17. Dahlstrim KK and others: Fluorescence microscopic demonstration and demarcation of doxorubicin extravasation. Experimental and clinical studies, Cancer 65(4):1722, 1990.
18. DeVita VT Jr.: Principles of chemotherapy, In DeVita VT Jr., Hellman S, and Rosenberg SA, editors: Cancer: Principles and practice of oncology, ed 3, Philadelphia, 1989, JB Lippincott Co.
19. Dison N: Simplified drugs and solutions for nurses, ed 10, St. Louis, 1992, Mosby.
20. Doane LS, Fisher LM, and McDonald TW: How to give intraperitoneal chemotherapy, AJN 90(4):58, 1990.
21. Dorr RT: Antidote vesicant chemotherapy extravasation, Blood Review 4:41, 1990.
22. Dorr RT and others: High levels of doxorubicin in the tissues of a patient experiencing extravasation during a 4-day infusion. Cancer 64(12):2462, 1989.
23. Dudjak LA: Cancer metastasis. Semin Oncol Nurs 8(1):40, 1992.
24. Fields SM and Von Hoff DD: New anticancer agents, Highlights on Antineoplastic Drugs, 10(2):16, 1992.
25. Finley RS: Drug interactions in the oncology patient, Semin Oncol Nurs 8(2):95, 1992.
26. Galassi A: The next generation: New chemotherapy agents for the 1990s, Semin Oncol Nurs 8(2):83, 1992.
27. Gatzemeier U and others: Combination chemotherapy with carboplatin, etoposide, and vincristine as first-line treatment in small-cell lung cancer, J Clin Oncol 10(5):818, 1992.
28. Gosland MP and Lum BL: The 1991 ASCO and AACR meetings: a focus on drug resistance and

dose intensification. Highlights on Antineoplastic Drugs, 9(3):56, 1991.

29. Groenwald SL and others: Cancer nursing: Principles and practice, ed 2, Boston, 1990, Jones and Bartlett.

30. Gullatte MM and Graves T: Advances in antineoplastic therapy, Oncol Nurs Forum 17(6):867, 1990.

31. Hessen JA: Protocol for treatment of vesicant antineoplastic extravasation, Hosp Pharm 24(9):705, 1989.

32. Hiromoto BM and Dungan B: Contract learning for self-care activities, a protocol study among chemotherapy out-patients, Cancer Nurs 14(3):148, 1991.

33. Hogan CM: Advances in the management of nausea and vomiting, Nurs Clin North Am 25(2):475, 1990.

34. Irani MA: Improving chemotherapy patient outcomes. Highlights on Antineoplastic Drugs, 10(1):5, 1992.

35. Jenkins J: Biology of cancer: current issues and future prospects, Semin Oncol Nurs 8(1):63, 1992.

36. Kane B and Kuhn JG: Therapeutic drug monitoring in antineoplastic drug development. Highlights on Antineoplastic Drugs 10(2):21, 1992.

37. Kenny SA: Effect of two oral care protocols on the incidence of stomatitis in hematology patients, Cancer Nurs 13(6):345, 1990.

38. Lin EM: Nutrition support making the difficult decisions, Cancer Nurs 14(3):261, 1991.

39. Lind J: Tumor cell growth and cell kinetics, Semin Oncol Nurs 8(1):3, 1992.

40. Lobert S and Correia JJ: Antimiotics in cancer chemotherapy, Cancer Nursing 15(1):22, 1992.

41. Madeya ML and Pfab-Tokarsky JM: Flow cytometry: an overview, Oncol Nurs Forum 19(3):459, 1992.

42. Maher M: The conduct of clinical trials in the area of emesis control, Semin Oncol Nurs 6(suppl 1):10, 1990.

43. Marty M and others: Comparison of 5-hydroxtryptamine 3 (serotonin) antagonist ondansetron (GR38032F) with high-dose metoclopromide in the control of cisplatin-induced emesis, N Engl J Med 322(12):816, 1990.

44. McCaffrey D and Engelking C: Ten fallacies associated with the nature and management of chemotherapy extravasation, Progressions 2(4):3, 1990.

45. McGovern K: 10 Golden rules for administering drugs safely, Nursing 22(3):49, 1992.

46. McMillan SC: Carcinogenesis, Semin Oncol Nurs 8(1):10, 1992.

47. McNally JC and others: Guidelines for oncology nursing practice, ed 2. Philadelphia 1991, WB Saunders Co.

48. Meade CD and others: Readability of American Cancer Society patient education literature, Oncol Nurs Forum 19(1):51, 1992.

49. Newton M and others: Reviewing the "big three" injection routes, Nursing 22(2):34, 1992.

50. Oncology Nursing Society Cancer Chemotherapy: Guidelines and recommendations for nursing education and practice, 1992, Pittsburgh, Pa.

51. Oncology Nursing Society Clinical Practice Committee Module V of the Cancer Chemotherapy guidelines revised, Oncol Nurs Forum 16(2):275, 1989.

52. Padberg RM and Padberg LF: Strengthening the effectiveness of patient education: applying principles of adult education, Oncol Nurs Forum 17(1):65, 1990.

53. Richardson JK and Richardson LI: The mathematics of drugs and solutions with clinical application, St. Louis, 1990, Mosby.

54. Schulmeister L: Establishing a cancer patient education system for ambulatory patients, Semin Oncol Nurs 7(2):118, 1991.

55. Stevens KR: Safe handling of cytoxic drugs in home chemotherapy, Semin Oncol Nurs 5(2):15, 1989.

56. Tsavaris NB and others: Conservative approach to the treatment of chemotherapy-induced extravasation, J Derm Surg Oncol 16(6):519, 1990.

57. US Department of Labor, Office of Occupational Medicine, Occupational Safety and Health Administration: Work practice guidelines for personnel dealing with cytotoxic (antineoplastic) drugs, No 8-1.1, Washington, DC, 1993, US Government Printing Office.

58. Viner CV and others: Ondansetron: a new safe and effective antiemetic in patients receiving high-dose melphalan, Cancer Chemother Pharmacol 25(6):449, 1990.

59. Weinstein SM: Math calculations for intravenous nurses, INS 13(4):231, 1990.

60. Wujcik D: Current research in side effects of high-dose chemotherapy, Semin Oncol Nurs 8(2):102, 1992.

61. Xistris D and Schulmeister L: Complying with the new OSHA regulations. Problem solving in Office Oncology Nursing, 6(4):1, 1992.

62. Yarbro JW: Oncogenes and cancer suppressor genes, Semin Oncol Nurs 8(1):30, 1992.

Appendix 22–1 Most Commonly Used Chemotherapeutic Drugs

Class	Route	Dose (mg/m²)	Infusion Solution	Infusion Duration	Nadir	Major Side Effects/Toxicities	Nursing Action
ALKYLATING AGENTS							
Busulfan (Myleran)	PO	2-6	NA	NA	Delayed	Myelosuppression, nausea, vomiting, pulmonary fibrosis	Promote compliance; Increased toxicity with high dosage
Carboplatin (CBDCA)	IV / IP	250-500	0.5-2 mg/ml D₅W	>30 min	21 days	Myelosuppression, nausea, vomiting, mild nephrotoxicity and neurotoxicity	Hydration; premedicate with antiemetics; Drug decomposes if mixed in NS
Chlorambucil (Leukeran)	PO	0.1-0.3 mg/kg	NA	NA	7-14 days	Myelosuppression, sterility, stomatitis	Promote compliance
Cisplatin	IV / IV / IP, IA	50-120 / 15-20	1,000 ml/NS / 150 ml/NS	>6 hr / 1 hr	3 wk	Nausea, vomiting, renal neurotoxic damage, ototoxicity, electrolyte imbalance	Hydration, I&O; obtain 12-24 hr creatinine clearance
Cyclophosphamide (Cytoxan)	IV / High-dose IV / PO	400 / 1-1.5 g / 50-200	20 mg/ml/SW / 100 ml SW / NA	Bolus / 60 min / NA	7-14 days	Nausea, vomiting, alopecia, myelosuppression, hemorrhagic cystitis, cardiotoxic pneumoniitis	Hydration, I&O; obtain 12-24 hr creatinine clearance, force fluids, void frequently
Estramustine	PO	600	NA	NA	None	Toxicity, nausea, vomiting, gynecomastia; cardiac toxicity	Educate patient about side effects; drug may be given in divided doses
Hexamethylmelamine (HMM, HXM)	PO	150	NA	NA	21-28 days	Myelosuppression, neurotoxicity, anorexia, nausea, vomiting	Premedicate with antiemetics
Ifosfamide (Isophosphamide Naxamide)	IV	700-2,000	50-100 mg/ml DW	Bolus or continuous infusion	7-14 days	Myelosuppression, nephrotoxicity, nausea, vomiting, phlebitis, neurotoxicity, alopecia, hemorrhagic cystitis	Provide hydration, monitor I&O; administer MESNA concomitantly
Mechlorethamine (Nitrogen mustard)	IV / Topical	1-6 / 10 mg dissolve in 50 ml H₂O; apply daily to weekly	10 mg/10 ml NS/SW	1 ml/min	7-21 days	Severe nausea, vomiting, extravasation, myelosuppression	Vesicant; use in <60 min after reconstitution
Melphalan (Alkeran)	PO	Dose will vary according to protocol			7-14 days	Nausea, vomiting may occur with high-dose, myelosuppression	Promote compliance
Thiotepa	PO / IV / Instill bladder	6-10 / 8.0	NA / NS/SW 60 mg/60 ml D/W	NA / Bolus >30 min; weekly	7-28 days	Myelosuppression, headache, fever, occasional nausea	Observe for reactions

Drug	Route	Dose	Dilution	Administration	Nadir	Toxicities/Side effects	Nursing considerations
ANTIBIOTICS							
Bleomycin	IV IM SC	10-20 u/m² 10 10	5 u/ml/NS 15 u/ml/NS 15 u/ml/NS	IM test dose; then 1 u/min q wk q wk	7 days	Fever, chills, pulmonary toxicity, hyperpigmentation, alopecia, stomatitis, hypotension	Auscultate breath sounds at least bid Test dose prior to initial dosing
Dactinomycin (Actinomycin D)	IV	1-2	Dilute to concentration; 0.5 mg/ml SW	1-5 min	7-14 days	Potentiates effects of radiation therapy, myelosuppression, alopecia	Vesicant; administer free-flowing IV
Daunorubicin (Cerubidine, Daunomycin)	IV	30-60	1 mg/ml/SW	1 ml/min	7-14 days	Myelosuppression, alopecia, nausea, vomiting, stomatitis, red urine, cardiotoxic	Vesicant; cumulative dose 500-600 mg/m²
Doxorubicin (Adriamycin)	IV	50-75	5 mg/ml/SW	1 ml/min	7-14 days	Myelosuppression, alopecia, nausea, vomiting, diarrhea, red urine	Vesicant; cumulative dose 550 mg/m²; incompatible with many drugs (e.g., Heparin)
Idarubicin (Idamycin)	IV	18-25 mg	1 mg/1 ml/NS	Bolus 1 ml/min	7-14 days	Myelosuppression, alopecia, nausea, vomiting, mucositis	Vesicant; administer free-flowing IV
Mitomycin C (Mutamycin)	IV	10-20	Dilute to concentration; 0.5 mg/ml D₅W/NS	1 ml/min	Delayed	Myelosuppression, alopecia, nausea, vomiting, fever, stomatitis, urine color change	Vesicant
Mithramycin (Plicamycin, Mithracin)	IV	25-50 µg/kg	150 ml/D₅W	>30 min	Rapid	Thrombocytopenia, hepatotoxicity, nausea, vomiting, phlebitis	Vesicant; monitor liver and kidney function tests
ANTIMETABOLITES							
Cytarabine (Ara-C, Cytosar)	IV	100-200	Dilute 1 ml/20 mg	Bolus >60-min or 24-hr continuous infusion; infuse over 60 min; <60 min increases toxicity	5-7 days	Potent myelosuppressant, anorexia, alopecia, nausea, vomiting, hepatotoxicity, neurotoxicity with increased dosage and intrathecal administration; conjunctivitis	Monitor for neurotoxicity with high dose; force fluids; administer antiemetics; use decadron eye drops as prophylactic measure
	High dose IV	3 g Variable	1 ml/50 mg 50 mg/ml (>300 mg/m²)				
	IT	20/30 mg	Use preservative-free solution	Slowly			
	SC	10 mg	20 mg/ml 20 mg/ml	NA			

Continued.

Appendix 22–1   Most Commonly Used Chemotherapeutic Drugs — cont'd

Class	Route	Dose (mg/m²)	Infusion Solution	Infusion Duration	Nadir	Major Side Effects/Toxicities	Nursing Action
ANTIMETABOLITES — cont'd							
Floxuridine (FUDR)	IA	0.1–0.6 mg/kg	Convenient volume	24-hr continuous infusion	7–14 days	Myelosuppression, oral and gastrointestinal ulceration, nausea, vomiting	Observe and patient teaching for arterial catheterization
Fluorouracil (5-FU)	IV	400–600	1,000 ml/NS	24-hr continuous infusion	7–14 days	Myelosuppression, alopecia, skin rash, nausea, vomiting, ataxia, diarrhea, stomatitis	Observe; incompatible with anthracyclines; observe and patient teaching for arterial catheterization
	IV	500	ml/NS	Bolus			
	IA	20–30 mg/kg	ml/NS	24-hr continuous infusion			
Fludarabine (Fludara)	IV	30 mg/m² × 5 days	30 ml D$_5$W/NS	15–30 min	7–14 days	Myelosuppression, flu-like syndrome, nausea and vomiting, dyspnea	Decreases Cd-4 lymphocytes
Hydroxyurea	IV	500–3,000	100 ml D$_5$W/NS	Over 30 min	7–14 days	Myelosuppression, stomatitis, alopecia, dysuria, nausea, vomiting, allergic reactions	Observe; oral daily dose may be given in divided doses with meals
	PO	1,000 mg/qd					
Methotrexate (Mexate)	IV	25–40	10–25 ml DW/NS	Bolus	7–14 days	Oral and gastrointestinal ulceration, myelosuppression, stomatitis, renal toxicity, nausea, vomiting, diarrhea	Dosage 1 g/m² or > require hydration, alkylinization of urine and folinic acid rescue
	IV	7,500 with rescue	100 ml DW/NS	>10 min			
	IM	25	2 ml/NS	NA			
	IT	12	10 ml preservative-free DW	1–5 min			
6-Mercaptopurine (6-MP)	PO	100	NA	NA	7–14 days	Myelosuppression, hepatotoxicity, stomatitis, anorexia	Promote compliance
6-Thioguanine (6-TG)	PO	100	NA	NA	Delayed	Myelosuppression, nausea, vomiting	Promote compliance
HORMONES							
Androgens							
Fluoxymesterone (Halotestin)	PO	10–30 mg qd	NA	NA	None	Nausea, vomiting, edema, liver function abnormalities, virilization in the female	Educate the patient about virilization

Drug	Route	Dosage				Side effects	Patient education
Testosterone	PO IM	Variable 100 mg 3×/wk breast	NA	NA	None	Mild fluid retention, monitor FBS with diabetes mellitus	Educate the patient: female—masculinization and menstrual irregularity; male—gynecomastis, impotence
Progestins							
Megestrol acetate (Megace)	PO	40-80 mg qd	NA	NA	None	Mild fluid retention, hypercalcemia with breast cancer	Teach patient to recognize and report side effects
Medroxyprogesterone acetate (Provera)	PO	400-800 mg/ 2×/wk	NA	NA	None	Mild fluid retention, hypercalcemia with breast cancer	Teach patient to recognize and report side effects
Medroxyprogesterone acetate (Depo-Provera)	IM	400-800 mg/ 2×/wk	NA	NA	None	Acute local hypersensitivity, possible IM injections	Teach patient to recognize and report side effects
Estrogens							
Diethylstilbestrol (DES)	PO	10/breast 0.5-1.5/prostate	NA	NA	None	Breakthrough bleeding, spotting, premenstrual-like syndrome, feminization in males	Instruct patient about changes
Conjugated estrogen (Premarin)	PO	10 mg tid breast 1.25-2.5 mg tid prostate	NA	NA	None	Breakthrough bleeding, premenstrual-like syndrome	Educate patient about changes
Chlorotrianisene (TACE)	PO	12-25 mg qd prostate	NA	NA	None	Increase or decrease in weight, breakthrough bleeding	Educate patient about changes
ANTIHORMONAL AGENTS		Dosage not administered by m^2 and may be given in divided dosages					
Aminoglutethimide (Cytadren)	PO	500/1000 mg qid	NA	NA	Unknown	Myelosuppression, dermatitis, masculinization, drowsiness, lethargy, weakness	Monitor for neurotoxicity
Flutamide (Eulexin)	PO	250-750 mg tid	NA	NA	Unknown	Gynecomastia, hepatotoxicity, libido effect	Educate patient about changes
Leuprolide (Leupron)	SC/IM	Variable	NA	NA	None	Impotence, amenorrhea, hot flashes	Educate patient about changes
Mitotane	PO	2-16 g/day	NA	NA	Unknown	Nausea, vomiting	Administer in divided doses
Tamoxifen (Nolvadex)	PO	10-20 mg bid	NA	NA	None	Hot flashes, nausea, vomiting, transient bone or tumor pain	Educate patient regarding changes
Zoladex (Goserelin)	IM	3.6 mg monthly	NA	NA	None	May increase bone pain, hot flashes, decreased libido, impotence, gynecomastia	Educate patient regarding changes

Continued.

Appendix 22–1 Most Commonly Used Chemotherapeutic Drugs — cont'd

Class	Route	Dose (mg/m²)	Infusion Solution	Infusion Duration	Nadir	Major Side Effects/Toxicities	Nursing Action
NITROSUREAS							
Carmustine (BCNU)	IV	25-125	100 mg/ml D₅W	>30 min	3-6 wk	Myelosuppression, stomatitis, nausea, vomiting, hepatotoxic pneumonitis, pulmonary fibrosis	Administer slowly: vein irritant; Contains alcohol; patient may feel inebriated
Lomustine (CCNU)	PO	70-150	NA	NA	4-5 wk	Nausea, vomiting, thrombocytopenia, myelosuppression	Administer at bedtime with antiemetics
Semustine (MeCCNU)	PO	150-200	NA	NA	Delayed 4-8 wk	Myelosuppression, nausea, vomiting, renal and hepatic toxicities	Administer on empty stomach with antiemetics
Streptozocin (Zanosar)	IV	0.5-1.5 g	100 mg/ml DW	>15 min	Variable	Mild myelosuppression, diarrhea, nausea, vomiting, chills, acute hypoglycemia	Administer slowly: vein irritant
CORTICOSTEROIDS							
Dexamethasone (Decadron)	IV IM PO	Dose varies with reason for drug	NA NA	Bolus NA	None	Gastrointestinal fluid and electrolyte disturbances, possible neuromusculoskeletal imbalances	Teach patient about side effects; IV rapid bolus may cause rectal itching
Hydrocortisone (Solu-Cortef)	IV	Dose varies with reason for drug	NA	Bolus	None	Fluid and electrolyte disturbance	Teach patient about side effects
Prednisone (Deltasone)	PO	40-100 mg/day	NA	NA	None	Fluid and electrolyte disturbance, manifestations of latent diabetes mellitus	Instruct patient to take medications after meals with gradual tapering after long-term use; teach side effects of drug
Prednisolone	PO	40 mg	NA	NA	None	Similar in action to prednisone	Same as prednisone
VINCA PLANT ALKALOIDS							
Vinblastine (Velban)	IV	4-20	mg/ml/NS	1 ml/min	5-9 days	Myelosuppression, stomatitis, neurotoxicity, alopecia	Vesicant; monitor for neurotoxicity
Vincristine (Oncovin)	IV	0.5-2	mg/ml/NS	1 ml/min	5-7 days	Neurotoxicity, constipation, alopecia, stomatitis	Vesicant; monitor bowel function and neurotoxicity

Drug	Route	Dose	Dilution	Rate	Nadir	Side effects	Comments
Vindesine (Eldisine)	IV	2-4	mg/ml/NS	1 ml/min	7-10 days	Myelosuppression, constipation, alopecia, neuropathy	Vesicant; monitor bowel function and neurotoxicity
Podophyllin alkaloids							
Etoposide (VP-16)	IV	50-100	50 ml/NS	Over 30-60 min	7-10 days	Nausea, vomiting, leukopenia, anemia, alopecia, hypotension	Administer drug slowly; may test dose before infusion
	PO	400 mg	NA	NA			
Teniposide (VM-26)	IV	50-130	100-250 ml/NS	Never give IV push; slow IV infusion only	7-10 days	Anaphylaxis, myelosuppression, severe hypotension, alopecia	Vesicant; slow infusion only; may test dose before infusion. High dose VP-16: use glass container for solution (solution will melt tubing) and give in nonfiltered tubing (e.g., albumin tubing)
MISCELLANEOUS AGENTS							
Asparaginase (Elspar)	IV	1,000 IU kg/day 2-20 days	2,000 U/ml NS	1 ml/min	None	Anaphylactic shock, nausea, vomiting, hyperglycemia, hepatotoxic	Monitor closely. Follow anaphylaxis protocol; test dose prior to initial dosing
	IM, Subq	6,000 IU kg 3×/wk	5,000 U/ml NS	NA			
Dacarbazine (DTIC-Dome)	IV	75-1,450	10 mg/ml DW	10-15 min or 24-hr continuous infusion	Delayed 7-21 days	Myelosuppression, venous spasm, flu-like syndrome, paresthesia, pruritus	Vesicant; premedicate with antiemetics
Levamisole	PO	1-5 mg/kg	NA	NA	None	Mild gastrointestinal complaints	Observe
Leucovorin	PO IV	200-500 mg/m² × 3 days/1 week	500 mg/m²; 250 ml/NS		7-14 days	Allergic reaction, irritant, myelosuppression, diarrhea, stomatitis, dehydration	Increased toxicity with increased dosage
Leustatin (cladribine, 2-CdA)	IV	0.09 mg/kg/day	10 mg vial/1 mg/ml; prepare 24 hr continuous 7 day infusion in 100 ml NS	100 ml via continuous infusion × 7 days	7-14 days	Myelosuppression, fever, nausea, rash, injection site reaction	Incompatible with D5W; calculate dose by multiplying patient's weight in kg by 0.09 mg (120 lb ÷ 2.2 lb/kg = 54.5 kg; 54.5 kg × 0.09 mg = 4.9 mg/day); prepare central venous access ambulatory pump
Mitoxantrone (DHAD)	IV	15	10 ml/NS or D_5W	>30 min	9-21 days	Myelosuppression, diarrhea, nausea, vomiting, phlebitis, bluish discoloration of urine, alopecia	Vesicant; monitor lab values, teach side effects

Continued.

Appendix 22–1 Most Commonly Used Chemotherapeutic Drugs — cont'd

Class	Route	Dose (mg/m²)	Infusion Solution	Infusion Duration	Nadir	Major Side Effects/ Toxicities	Nursing Action
MISCELLANEOUS AGENTS — cont'd							
Pentostatin (2'-deoxyco-formycin)	IV	4 mg/m² Q14 days	1 mg/ml	5 min or more	None	Myelosuppressive, rash, nausea, vomiting, diarrhea, stomititis, elevated liver enzymes, *neurotoxic*, cough, shortness of breath	Monitor laboratory values; assess neurologic toxicities and other side effects
Procarbazine (Matulane)	PO	100-150	NA	NA	Delayed 4-6 wk	Myelosuppression; avoid use of narcotics, epinephrine, antihistamines	Incompatible with ethanol, antidepressants, food rich in tyramine will get hypertensive crisis
Taxol	IV	200	500 ml/NS	4-24 hr	7-14 days	Alopecia, nausea and vomiting, neutropenia, skin rash, *allergic reaction*, cardiac arrhythmias	Ensure recommended premedications are given prior to taxol infusion; follow anaphylaxis protocol; monitor vital signs and cardiac dysrhythmias; prepare Taxol solution in a glass bottle and infuse via non-PVC tubing

NA, not applicable; *SW*, sterile water; *D₅W*, dextrose water 5%; *NS*, normal saline; *PO*, by mouth; *SC*, subcutaneous; *IM*, intramuscular; *IV*, intravenous; *IP*, intraperitoneal; *IT*, intrathecal; qd, daily, qid, four times a day; bid, twice a day; tid, three times a day.
Adapted from Chabner BA and Myers CE: Clinical pharmacology of cancer chemotherapy. In DeVita VT, Hellman S, Rosenberg SA, editors: Cancer: principles and practice of oncology, ed 4, Philadelphia, 1993, JB Lippincott Co.

Appendix 22–2 Investigational Drugs: Phase II Drugs[21,22,29]

Drug	Disease Evaluation	Toxicities
Amonafide	Acute myelocytic leukemia, esophagus, ovarian, sarcoma	Myelosuppression, alopecia, diarrhea, nausea and vomiting, seizure, dyspnea, rash, temporary orange tint in urine
Didemnin B	Brain, prostate, melanoma, non-small cell lung	Anaphylaxis, myalgia, myopathy Anorexia, nausea and vomiting, diarrhea, transient hepatotoxicity; may induce insulin-dependent diabetes
Diaziquone (AZQ)	Brain	Myelosuppression, alopecia, gastrointestinal distress
Dihydroxyazacytidine (DHAC)	Mesothelioma	Myelosuppression, chest pain, nausea and vomiting, diarrhea, stomatitis, pleural effusion
Edatrexate (10-EdAM)	Head and neck, mets. bladder, non-small cell lung	Leukopenia, nausea and vomiting, diarrhea, mucositis, stomatitis, respiratory infection, pulmonary fibrosis, fatigue, alopecia
Fazarabine	Brain, lung	Myelosuppression, pulmonary emboli, nausea and vomiting
Merberone	Gastrointestinal, hepatic, melanoma, renal	Myelosuppression, myalgia, nausea and vomiting, hypouricemia, diarrhea, stomatitis, alopecia, phlebitis
Pala	Colon (synergestic with 5-FU)	Nausea and vomiting, diarrhea, stomatitis, skin rash
Piroxantrone (Oxantrazale)	Breast, gastric, head and neck, melanoma, pancreas, renal, sarcoma	Myelosuppression, alopecia, nausea and vomiting, hyponatremia, stomatitis, fatigue, diarrhea, vesicant, cardiotoxic
Taxol	Breast, colon, gastric, head and neck, non-small cell lung, melanoma, renal	Myelosuppression, mucositis, alopecia, hypersensitivity, allergic reaction, neuropathy, cardiac arrhythmias
Topotecan	Lung, ovary, hepatic, gastric, ovary, renal, skin	Neutropenia, thrombocytopenia, alopecia, nausea and vomiting, rash, fever, microscopic hematuria, myelosuppression, nephrotoxicity, dermatitis
Trimetrexate (TMXT, TMQ)	*Pneumocystitis carinii*	Myelosuppression etc.

From Southwest Oncology Group Research Protocols, Southwest Oncology Group; National Cancer Institute, 1993.

Appendix 22–3 Investigational Drugs: Phase I Drugs[21,22,29]

Drug	Disease Evaluation	Toxicities
Adozelesin	Preclinical: leukemia, lung, melanoma, colon, pancreas, ovary	Undetermined
Biantrazole	Breast	Myelosuppression, alopecia, nausea and vomiting, phlebitis
Crisnatol mesylate	Glioma	Somnolence, dizziness, blurred vision, unsteady gait, confusion, vertigo, nystagmus
Camptothecan (CPT-11)	Colon, lung, cervix, ovary	Myelosuppression, gastrointestinal toxicities, alopecia, anorexia
Gemcitabine	Breast, colon, lung, head and neck, pancreas	Myelosuppression, dermatitis, fever, flu-like syndrome, hypotension, alopecia, mucositis, elevated liver enzymes
Ilmofosine	Renal, colon, breast, lung	Intravascular hemolysis, nausea and vomiting, diarrhea, phlebitis, fever
Suramin	HIV, Kaposi sarcoma, ovary, hormone resistant prostate, refractory lymphoma	Adrenocortical insufficiency, transient parathesia, muscle weakness, rash, coagulopathy, myelosuppression, liver function test abnormality
Taxotere	Breast, lung, ovary, pancreas	Neutropenia, alopecia, dermatitis, mucositis, phlebitis, mild anaphylactic reaction
Terephthalamidine	Hodgkin's seminoma	Anorexia, nausea and vomiting, weight loss, weakness
Tetraplatin (Ormaplatin)	Esophagus, gastric	Myelosuppression, nausa and vomiting, mild parathesia
Toremifene	Breast	Vaginal discharge, hot flashes, mild sweating
Vinorelbine (Navelbine)	Hodgkin's, ovary, breast	Leukopenia, nausea and vomiting, alopecia, constipation, decreased deep tendon reflexes, phlebitis

From Fields SM and Von Hoff DD: New anticancer agents, Highlights on Antineoplastic Drugs 10(2):16, 1992.

CHAPTER 23

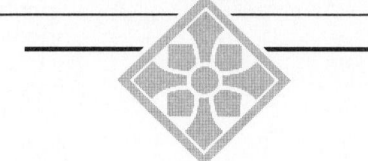

Biotherapy

Paula Trahan Rieger

The rapid introduction of novel agents and approaches has opened an exciting era in cancer therapy. Traditionally, surgery, radiation therapy, and chemotherapy, either singly or in combination, have been the mainstays of cancer therapy. Recently, however, biotherapy, or biologic therapy, has emerged as an important fourth modality for treating cancer.[45,144]

Oncology nurses whose patients receive biotherapy need a basic understanding of the immune system, the rationale for this therapy, and its primary clinical agents. (See Chapter 29 for a review of the immune system.) This chapter reviews the history of immunotherapy and other biotherapy approaches, scientific advances that led to clinical trials with biologic agents, the rationale for the use of these agents, their clinical indications, and the associated nursing care for patients receiving them.

THEORY OF IMMUNE SURVEILLANCE

Host defense mechanisms protect the body by detecting and eliminating substances that are recognized as "foreign" or "non-self." The theory of immune surveillance, refined and expanded by McFarlane Burnet,[29,86,110] states that certain cells undergo neoplastic transformation but are recognized by the immune system as foreign and subsequently destroyed. At first T cells were thought to be primarily responsible for this reaction, but it is now known that other immune cells such as natural killer (NK) cells and macrophages are also involved.[110] If an atypical cell somehow escapes detection or destruction, a clinically detectable tumor eventually develops.

Although this theory remains controversial, many clinical phenomena and laboratory observations support it. Spontaneous tumor regression has been observed in patients with solid tumors such as melanoma and renal cancer and with acute leukemia[186]; that is, tumors shrank or patients entered remission without treatment. Some of these regressions have been associated with infectious complications, which may suggest an immunologic mechanism.[86,186,140]

Immunologic defense mechanisms are relatively weak in the young and the aged, and the incidence of malignancy in humans peaks correspondingly during early childhood and old age. In these periods impaired or immature defense mechanisms may allow abnormal cells to escape immune surveillance and proliferate.

An increased incidence of cancer is also seen in patients with immune deficiencies resulting from immunosuppressive therapy or other causes, including individuals undergoing chronic immunosuppressive therapy for the maintenance of organ allografts. Patients with immunodeficiences exhibit a higher incidence of malignancies, especially lymphoid malignancies, than does the general population.[110,155]

The fact that immune cells infiltrate tumors also supports this theory. Pathologic examination of surgical specimens shows infiltration by lymphocytes, macrophages, and plasma cells, and it has been suggested that immune mechanisms may be responsible for decreasing the growth rate of tumors.[144]

A variety of experiments lend further support to the theory of immune surveillance. Neonatal thymectomy causes mice to accept tumor transplants, whereas mice possessing normal thymic function reject the transplants.[4] The use of antilymphocyte serum and immunosuppressive therapy in animals can increase the incidence and development of both spontaneous tumors and those induced by viruses and chemical carcinogens. Lymphocytes appear essential in the recognition and destruction of aberrant cells.[86]

If, as this evidence suggests, immune surveillance is an important part of antitumor host defense, how do transformed cells escape detection by the immune system? Krueger[110] proposes four basic mechanisms: (1) a basic defect in function of effector cells responsible for immune surveillance; (2) an imbalance of the immune response to the tumor; (3) malignant cells not sufficiently immunogenic to elicit an immune response; and (4) production of blocking factors that interfere with the immune response to tumors.

Although skepticism remains regarding the theory of immune surveillance, it remains an attractive explanation for the occurrence of cancer. Further experimentation will continue to clarify the relationship between the immune system and malignant cells.

HISTORICAL PERSPECTIVE

The observation of interactions between the immune system and malignant cells led to the development of therapies that could manipulate this natural process. Traditionally, this field has been known as immunotherapy.[146]

The immunotherapy of cancer can be divided into two approaches, active and passive. *Active immunotherapy* consists of giving a tumor-bearing host agents that are designed to elicit an immune response capable of retarding or eliminating tumor growth. The two types of active immunotherapy are specific and nonspecific. *Active specific* immunotherapy is immunization with tumor cells or tumor-cell extracts, either alone or in vaccines. *Active nonspecific* immunotherapy is an attempt to boost overall immunity through the use of adjuvants such as bacterial extracts. The latter approach was based on the observation that adjuvants administered in animal systems could cause tumor regression. It was also based on the idea that those with tumors have diminished defense mechanisms.[86,186]

Passive immunotherapy is the administration or transfer of previously sensitized immunologic reagents such as antisera (which contain sensitized antibodies) or immune-reactive cells to a tumor-bearing host. These reagents directly or indirectly mediate antitumor responses. The term *adoptive immunotherapy* is still used to refer to the passive transfer of sensitized cells such as lymphocytes or macrophages.[86,185,186]

Principles for immunotherapy of human cancer are based mainly on knowledge gained from animal experiments. First, immunotherapeutic approaches appeared most successful for small tumor burdens. Therefore, tumor burden was to be reduced by conventional treatment, followed by immunotherapy. Second, the host had to be immunocompetent, or immunocompetence had to be restored, for immunotherapy to be maximally effective. Third, the timing of immunotherapy was crucial. How long after conventional treatment should immunotherapy be started to allow for restoration of immunosuppressive effects was a concern. Fourth, the site of immunization for active immunotherapy, especially specific active immunotherapy, was extremely important. Active specific immunotherapy was often given in tumor-free lymphatic drainage areas.[86]

Initial attempts at boosting the immune systems of cancer patients to destroy tumors used a variety of microorganisms, fractions of microbial products, or other immunomodulators. Since the 1960s many clinical studies have attempted nonspecific stimulation of the immune system by using such products as bacille Calmette-Guerin (BCG) or its methanol extraction residue (MER), *Corynebacterium parvum (C. parvum)*, and levamisole. Although initial trials seemed positive, well-controlled prospective randomized trials did not show significant overall survival gains in the arm utilizing immunotherapy.[144]

The failure of these early trials to establish immunotherapy as a major modality most likely occurred for a variety of reasons such as the lack of purity and definition of immunotherapeutic agents, lack of analogy between animal model systems and humans, variability of experimental procedures, and inadequate administration of immunotherapeutic agents.[144,186]

TECHNOLOGIC ADVANCES

During the 1970s and 1980s several scientific and technologic developments led biologic therapy to emerge as a major modality in the treatment of cancer. Our overall understanding of the relationship between host defense mechanisms and cancer and of the basic biology of cancer has improved. Recombinant DNA technology has allowed the production of large quantities of highly purified products from the human genome, as hybridoma technology has done for highly purified, highly specific immunoglobulin reagents. Methods of growing large volumes of effector cells in culture have been developed, and advances in computer hardware and software have led to the isolation and purification of biologic molecules.[71,144]

These discoveries have led to the modern era of biotherapy. The use of this term is more appropriate than heretofore because this field encompasses a much broader basis than only the immune system. Although the use of agents affecting the immune system remains a subcategory, biotherapy includes treatments affecting other biologic responses such as growth and differentiation factors, chimeric molecules (genetically engineered molecules that may have some parts added or removed to tailor them for a particular use, as when a chimeric monoclonal antibody has part human and part murine fragments), and agents that may affect the ability of tumor cells to metastasize.

BIOTHERAPY DEFINED

Biotherapy may be defined as treatment with agents derived from biologic sources and/or affecting biologic responses. The majority of its agents are derived from the mammalian genome.[144] The subcommittee on biologic response modifiers (BRMs) to the National Cancer Institute Division of Cancer Treatment defines BRMs as "agents or approaches that modify the re-

lationship between tumor and host by modifying the host's biologic response to tumor cells with a resultant therapeutic effect."[129]

The explosion of biotherapy research, coupled with the aforementioned technologic advances, has led to the use of numerous agents both commercially and in clinical trials. Although nonspecific immunomodulating agents such as BCG and *C. parvum* are still used, a variety of newer agents such as interferons, interleukins, monoclonal antibodies, and hematopoietic growth factors are now undergoing clinical investigation (Tables 23-1 and 23-2). Many of these

Table 23-1 Biologic Activities of Cytokines

Cytokine	Abbreviation	Biologic Activity
Interferon-α or β	IFN-α or β	Exerts antiviral activity; induces MHC Class I antigen expression; augments NK cell activity; has fever-inducing and antiproliferative properties.
Interferon-γ	IFN-γ	Induces MHC Class I and Class II antigens; activates macrophages and endothelial cells; augments NK cell activity; exerts antiviral activity; augments or inhibits other cytokine activities.
Interleukin-1 α or β	IL-1 α or β	Activates resting T cells; makes early hematopoietic progenitors more sensitive to later acting factors (hemopoietin 1 activity); induces CSF production by accessory cells; induces fever, sleep, ACTH release, neutrophilia, and other acute-phase responses; activates endothelial cells and macrophages; mediates inflammation, catabolic processes, and nonspecific resistance to infection; stimulates synthesis of other cytokines.
Interleukin-2	IL-2	Is a cofactor for growth and differentiation of T and B cells; augments lymphocyte killer activity; induces production of other cytokines.
Interleukin-3	IL-3	Stimulates early growth of granulocyte, monocyte, erythrocyte, and megakaryocyte progenitor cells; supports mast-cell growth; induces acute nonlymphocytic leukemia blasts to proliferate.
Interleukin-4	IL-4	Is growth factor for activated B cells; induces MHC Class II antigens on B cells; promotes IgG secretion; is growth factor for resting T cells; enhances cytolytic activity of cytotoxic T cells; supports mast-cell growth; synergizes with other growth factors to promote colony growth.
Interleukin-5	IL-5	Induces proliferation and differentiation of eosinophil progenitors.
Interleukin-6	IL-6	Induces B-cell differentiation; enhances Ig secretion by B cells; synergizes with other growth factors to promote colony growth; synergizes with IL-1 in stimulating T-cell proliferation.
Interleukin-7	IL-7	Supports the growth of B-cell precursors.
Tumor necrosis factor α or β	TNF α or β	Is cytotoxic for some tumor cells; induces fever, sleep, and other systemic acute-phase responses; activates endothelial cells and macrophages; mediates inflammation, catabolic processes, and septic shock; stimulates synthesis of other cytokines.
Granulocyte colony-stimulating factor	G-CSF	Stimulates growth of granulocyte colonies and activates mature granulocytes; increases antibody-dependent, neutrophil-mediated cytotoxicity; induces in vitro differentiation of leukemia cell lines; stimulates proliferation of leukemic progenitors.
Granulocyte-macrophage colony-stimulating factor	GM-CSF	Stimulates growth of granulocyte, monocyte, and early erythrocyte progenitors, and less, megakaryocyte progenitors; activates mature granulocytes and monocytes; enhances antibody-dependent, cell-mediated cytotoxicity; may stimulate proliferation of leukemic progenitors.
Macrophage colony-stimulating factor	M-CSF	Stimulates growth of monocyte colonies; supports in vitro survival of monocytes; activates mature monocytes; enhances antibody-dependent, monocyte-mediated cytotoxicity.

From Oettgen HF and Old LJ: The history of cancer immunotherapy. In DeVita VT, Hellman S, and Rosenberg SA, editors: The biologic therapy of cancer, Philadelphia, 1991, JB Lippincott Co, p. 111.

Table 23–2 Clinical Status of Major Biologic Response Modifiers

Agent	Status/Indication
INTERFERONS	
Interferon-α	
Interferon-α 2a (Roferon-A,® Roche Lab.)	FDA-approved for hairy-cell leukemia, AIDS-related Kaposi's sarcoma
Interferon-α 2b (Intron-A,® Schering Corp.)	FDA-approved for hairy-cell leukemia, AIDS-related Kaposi's sarcoma, condyloma acuminata, chronic hepatitis non-A, non-B/C, and chronic hepatitis B
Interferon-α leukocyte (Aiferon,® Purdue Fredrick)	*Condyloma acuminata*
Interferon-β	In clinical trials
Interferon-γ	
Interferon γ 1b (Actimmune,® Genentech)	FDA-approved for chronic granulomatous disease
INTERLEUKINS	
IL-1-α	In clinical trials
IL-1-β	In clinical trials
IL-2 (Proleukin,® Cetus)	FDA-approved for the treatment of renal cell cancer
IL-4	In clinical trials
IL-5	Preclinical study
IL-6	In clinical trials
HEMATOPOIETIC GROWTH FACTORS	
GM-CSF (Prokine,® Hoechst-Roussel) (Leukine,® Immunex)	FDA-approved for the acceleration of myeloid recovery in patients with non-Hodgkin's lymphoma, acute lymphoblastic leukemia, and Hodgkin's disease undergoing autologous BMT
G-CSF (Neupogen,® Amgen)	FDA-approved to decrease incidence of infection in patients with nonmyeloid malignancies receiving myelosuppressive anticancer drugs
M-CSF	In clinical trials
IL-3	In clinical trials
Erythropoietin	
Epogen® (Amgen)	Indicated for the treatment of anemia in patients with chronic renal failure
Procrit® (Ortho-Biotech)	Indicated for the treatment of anemia in patients with chronic renal failure, the treatment of anemia related to therapy with Zidovudine (AZT) in HIV-infected patients, and the treatment of anemia in cancer patients on chemotherapy

Table 23–2 Clinical Status of Major Biologic Response Modifiers—cont'd

Agent	Status/Indication
MONOKINES	
Tumor Necrosis Factor (TNF)	In clinical trials
MONOCLONAL ANTIBODIES (MoAbs)	
OncoScint®, Cytogen	FDA-approved for diagnostic imaging of colon and ovarian cancer
EFFECTOR CELLS	
Lymphokine Activated Killer Cells (LAK)	In clinical trials
Tumor Infiltrating Lymphocytes (TILS)	In clinical trials
Gene-altered TILS	In clinical trials

are naturally occurring body substances that act as messengers between cells. A generic term for these messengers is *cytokine*, which refers to protein products from cells that serve as cell regulators. More specifically, lymphokines are products of lymphocytes, and monokines are products of monocytes. The name *interleukin* refers to proteins that act as messengers between cells.[58,186]

A system of classification is often useful for looking at the agents' mechanisms of action. However, the way many BRMs work against tumors is not fully understood. Many agents may have more than one antitumor mode of action, and with certain agents it is often difficult to determine which mode of action is most important to the antitumor effect. It may be one action or the combination of several. In addition, many agents have both immunologic actions and other biologic effects.

In general, BRMs can be classified into three major divisions: agents that augment, modulate, or restore the host's immunologic mechanisms; agents that have direct antitumor activity (cytotoxic or antiproliferative mechanisms); and agents that possess other biologic effects (those that affect differentiation or maturation of cells, that interfere with the ability of a tumor cell to metastasize, or that affect initiation or maintenance of neoplastic transformation).[37,109]

MAJOR AGENTS IN USE

INTERFERONS

Interferon (IFN) was first characterized in 1957 by virologists Isaacs and Lindemann.[95] They found that this newly discovered protein was produced by virally infected cells and was capable of protecting other cells from viral infection. A great deal has been learned since about the IFN system and its biologic effects. Interferon has proved effective in the treatment of several malignancies and viral diseases.

There are three major classes, according to antigenic type: alpha, beta, and gamma. While alpha- and beta-IFNs are primarily produced by leukocytes and fibroblasts respectively, gamma-IFN is made primarily by T-lymphocytes. The interferons may be termed a family of glycoprotein hormones possessing pleiotropic biologic effects.[16,63]

Biologic Effects

All IFNs mediate their cellular effect after binding to a specific receptor. Alpha-and beta-IFN share a receptor, while gamma-IFN use a different one. The interferons possess a wide range of biologic effects: antiviral, antiproliferative, and immunomodulatory. Exactly how they exert their antitumor effects is unknown. It is unclear which of their many biologic effects may be most important in obtaining tumor responses, for example direct effects versus immune stimulation. This is further complicated by the likely diversity of patients' responses to the agents and the differing effects of IFN on different diseases. In addition, there are differences in biologic effects between different classes of interferon.[16,76]

The antiviral activity of IFN renders uninfected cells resistant to attack by the offending virus as well as by a variety of other viruses. Internalization of the IFN-receptor complex causes a sequence of events that results in the production of antiviral proteins and enzymes. Both in vitro and in vivo experimentation have demonstrated the antiproliferative effects of IFN. Although the exact mechanism is unknown, IFN causes extension of all phases of the cell cycle and lengthens overall cell generation time. The proteins also may inhibit DNA and protein synthesis to block the growth of tumor cells. Cellular proto-oncogenes play an important role in the regulation of cell growth, and IFNs are known to inhibit expression of proto-oncogenes.

A variety of immunomodulatory effects have been described for the IFNs; these differ for the different classes of IFN. In vitro, IFN increases the killing potential of NK cells by recruiting pre-NK cells and enhancing the cytotoxic activity of activated cells. Low doses of IFN appear to stimulate antibody production, but higher doses have a suppressive effect. Gamma-IFN appears to be a more potent activator of macrophage function than alpha- or beta-IFN; however, all three are capable of inducing tumoricidal activity and increasing phagocytosis. Interferons are capable of affecting the production of other lymphokines that regulate immune responses. Little is known about the positive and negative feedback regulation between IFNs and other lymphokines. Current investigations will continue to define the immunomodulatory effects on IFNs and their interactions with other cytokines.[16]

Phenotypic Effects

Interferon is also capable of affecting the phenotypic properties of neoplastic cells. In vitro studies have shown that IFN can enhance differentiation of certain cell lines. IFN can also induce or enhance expression of HLA antigens and increases tumor-associated antigens in melanoma and other cell lines. This may improve endogenous host antitumor activity.[16,76]

Clinical Indications

Initial clinical trials with IFN were carried out in the early 1970s using the Cantell preparation of leukocyte IFN (alpha-IFN), which was manufactured by Kari Cantell and coworkers at the Finnish blood bank.[31] Although supplies of leukocyte IFN were scarce, expensive, and very impure, a few important pharmacologic studies were done. The National Cancer Institute (NCI) in 1975 and the American Cancer Society in 1978 expanded this work. Although initial trials showed responses in patients with breast cancer and lymphoma, large-scale clinical trials have not supported widespread efficacy in these two diseases. Large-scale clinical trials with IFN became possible during the 1980s with the advent of recombinant DNA technology. Large quantities of very pure IFNs of all types are now available because of these industrial-scale production methods.[156]

The Food and Drug Administration (FDA) approved two recombinant alpha-IFN products for the treatment of hairy-cell leukemia (HCL) in 1986: IFN-α 2b (Intron® A) and IFN-α 2a (Roferon® A). The use of these IFNs in high doses is also approved for the treatment of AIDS-related Kaposi's sarcoma.[171,190] Since then, Intron® A has received additional approvals for the treatment of condyloma acuminata, chronic hepatitis non-A, non-B/C, and chronic hepatitis B.[190]

The treatment of HCL with alpha-IFN has shown dramatic antitumor effects. Doses as low as 3 million units per day have been shown to be of benefit in as many as 95% of patients.[162,164] The median time to response is 4 to 6 months, and most patients must remain on maintenance doses indefinitely to maintain clinical benefits. Other diseases against which alpha-IFN has shown efficacy include chronic myelogenous leukemia,[212,213] low-grade lymphomas,[76,130] multiple myeloma,[76,130] melanoma,[76] renal cell cancer,[76] ovarian carcinoma (intraperitoneal route), and superficial bladder carcinoma (Tables 23-3 and 23-4). (For a comprehensive review see Figlin,[60] Foon,[63] Goldstein and colleagues,[76] Kirkwood and Ernstoff,[103] Rosenberg and associates,[186] and Yarbro et al.[228]) Beta-interferon remains under clinical investigation. Although

Table 23–3 Response of Various Hematological Malignancies to IFN-α

Tumor Type	Response Rate*
Hairy-cell leukemia	80–90%
Chronic myelogenous leukemia	
Newly diagnosed	70–80%
Advanced	10–25%
Philadelphia-negative myeloproliferative disorders	
Essential thrombocythemia and polycythemia vera	75%
Cutaneous T-cell lymphomas	
No prior therapy	80%
Previously treated	55%
Non-Hodgkin's lymphomas (relapsed)	
Low grade	40–50%
Intermediate and high grade	15%
Hodgkin's disease (relapsed)	20%
Multiple myeloma	
No prior therapy	50%
Previously treated	15–25%
Chronic lymphocytic leukemia	10–15%
Acute leukemia	10–20%

*Responses signify a partial or complete regression of tumor.
From Kurzrock R, Talpaz M, and Gutterman JU: Other tumors. In DeVita VT, Hellman S, and Rosenberg SA, editors: The biologic therapy of cancer, Philadelphia, 1991, JB Lippincott Co.

Table 23–4 Response of Various Solid Tumor IFN-α

Tumor Type	Response Rate*
Cervical intraepithelial neoplasia	80–90%
Basal cell cancer	90%
Superficial bladder cancer	60–70%
Malignant neuroendocrine tumors	30–80%
Kaposi's sarcoma (AIDS-related)	35%
Ovarian cancer	
Parenteral	10–15%
Intraperitoneal	40%
Gliomas	30%
Renal cell cancer	15–20%
Nasopharyngeal cancer	20%
Melanoma	10–15%
Colorectal cancer	<10%
Osteogenic sarcoma	<10%
Lung (small and non-small cell)	<10%
Breast cancer	<10%

*Responses signify partial or complete tumor regression.
From Kurzrock R, Talpaz M, and Gutterman JU: Other tumors. In DeVita VT, Hellman S, and Rosenberg SA, editors: The biologic therapy of cancer, Philadelphia, 1991, JB Lippincott Co.

gamma-interferon remains under investigation for the treatment of cancer,[21,119] it is commercially available for the treatment of chronic granulomatous disease.[73]

Interferon continues to be explored as a single agent and in combination with other BRMs and chemotherapeutic agents.[138] One exciting development is the combination of IFN and fluorouracil (5-FU) for the treatment of colon cancer. A pilot study conducted by Wadler and co-workers[222] in 1989 reported a response rate of 81% with 13 of 16 previously untreated patients with advanced colon carcinoma. These results led to other investigators attempting to duplicate Wadler's regimen and to evaluate this combination in other cancers. In subsequent trials, the combination of 5-FU and alpha-IFN has shown promise; however, the ultimate role of this combination will be clarified only upon completion of randomized trials comparing it to single-agent therapy with 5-FU or to 5-FU with folinic acid.[154]

An occasional problem in patients receiving chronic treatment with alpha-IFN is development of neutralizing antibodies. Although the clinical significance of this phenomenon is uncertain, in a number of clinical trials the development of neutralizing antibodies has been associated with resistance to therapy. Factors that may contribute to formation of antibodies are immunogenicity, underlying disease, routes of administration, dosing regimens, and duration of treatment. It has been difficult to determine the true incidence of antibody formation. Additional factors that may be important are blood sampling time and assay methodology. Until comparative studies are well controlled for these variables, the formation of antibodies and their effect will remain controversial.[61]

Administration

In spite of numerous clinical trials the optimal dose, route, and frequency of administration for interferon are yet to be determined. The most common routes of administration are intramuscular and subcutaneous, although IFN is also given intravenously, intralesionally, intraperitoneally, intravesically, intra-arterially and intrathecally.[104,186]

Pharmacokinetics differ by types of IFN and route of administration. Intravenous administration results in rapid clearance with a half-life of 4 to 8 hours. With subcutaneous or intramuscular administration, peak serum levels occur at about 6 to 8 hours, and complete clearance occurs by 16 to 24 hours.[79] IFN is metabolized in the kidneys, and most metabolites are completely reabsorbed. Although at first IFN was given by a predetermined standard dosage, it is now more commonly prescribed by body surface area (million units/m²). Dosage requirements for alpha-IFN vary among patients and diseases. A rough classification for dosage is given in Table 23-5. In general, the higher the dose, the more severe the side effects and inhibition of the patient's performance status.

Alpha-interferon is supplied commercially as a sterile lyophilized powder with accompanying diluent or as a sterile solution. It must be stored in a refrigerator at 2° to 8° C. The vial should not be shaken when the powder is reconstituted, as this will make the medication foam. For further information, such

Table 23-5 Interferon Dosage

Interferon Protocol	Dose (million units/m²)
Low dose	0-3
Intermediate dose	3-10
High dose	>10

as the availability of differing vial strengths, and shelf-life stability, see the manufacturer's product literature.[171,190]

Handling issues are a concern to all oncology nurses. To date there has been no formal research on the safest way to handle IFNs or other BRMs. Many institutions place BRMs in the same classification as chemotherapy, instructing staff to follow institutional policy on the handling and disposal of cytotoxic drugs. Patients taught to self-administer interferon are advised to dispose of vials, needles, and syringes in a puncture-resistant container. Guidelines for disposal of used equipment in the home setting are available from the U.S. Environmental Protection Agency. In some clinical trials, patients are requested to return unused vials to the dispensing institution.[82]

Side Effects

The toxicity of interferon has been well established. In general, side effects are similar for all classes of interferon, with slight variations according to dosage, schedule, and type. Although at higher doses the effects of IFN can be quite debilitating, side effects are generally reversible upon cessation of therapy. Because interferon is generally given as long-term therapy, side effects can be divided into those occurring early (acute) and those occurring as therapy progresses (late or chronic). Some side effects occur only occasionally or rarely.

Nearly all patients beginning therapy with IFN have flulike symptoms. Although symptoms may be severe at first, tachyphylaxis (adjustment to symptoms over time) prevents them from becoming dose limiting. Symptoms include chills 2 to 4 hours after injection followed by fever spikes up to 40° C. Patients may have headaches, myalagias, arthralgias, and malaise. High-risk patients (e.g., those with a history of cardiac problems and debilitated patients) should be premedicated, monitored closely, and kept well hydrated.

Chronic side effects tend to increase in intensity after patients have been on therapy for several weeks and to maintain their level of intensity. Of prime concern are fatigue and anorexia with resultant weight loss; these can become dose limiting. The patient's interferon therapy may have to be halted or the dosage reduced if these side effects become too severe. Patients also experience lethargy, lack of concentration,[1] neutropenia, mild thrombocytopenia, elevated

transaminase levels, proteinuria, and asymptomatic hypotension.

A number of side effects are less widespread; they vary in frequency between individual patients and in intensity depending on dose. These include gastrointestinal effects such as nausea, vomiting, diarrhea, and altered taste (patients complain of foods tasting metallic or bitter). Patients may exhibit central nervous system or neurologic changes such as depression, mood alterations, decreased libido, memory problems,[1] EEG abnormalities, and peripheral neuropathies. Inflammation at the injection site, reactivation of herpes simplex, rash, exacerbation of psoriasis, and mild alopecia (thinning of hair as opposed to full-scale hair loss) have all been reported. Lab values should be watched for changes indicating anemia, hypercalcemia, hyperkalemia, elevated BUN, and elevated lactate dehydrogenase.[163,186]

In general, patients receiving low doses tolerate side effects well. Although not proved by research, a frequent recommendation is that IFN be given at bedtime so that patients will sleep through the worst of the side effects. The most common life-threatening toxicity is acute cardiac failure, which is extremely rare. It is generally recommended that patients with a strong history of cardiovascular disease not be placed on IFN therapy.

INTERLEUKINS

The term *interleukin* literally means "between leukocytes." Traditionally, when biologic proteins were characterized, they were given acronyms based on their functional properties (e.g., T-cell growth factor [TCGF]). When genes for these cytokines were ultimately cloned, it was found that a number of these substances were in fact the same molecule. At international symposia the terminology interleukins was agreed upon to name these biologic proteins. Hence, as more of these cytokines are discovered and their amino acid sequences established, they are named numerically, for example IL-5 and IL-6[42,53,70] (see Table 23-1).

Research has progressed through the discovery of IL-12.[161] This section will concentrate on interleukin-2 (IL-2), which received FDA approval in 1992 and will briefly cover other interleukins that are making their way into clinical trials. Interleukin-3 will be covered under the discussion of hematopoietic growth factors.

Interleukin-1

Interleukin-1 (IL-1) was originally described as an endogenous pyrogen and lymphocyte activating factor.[52] It is a complex and heterogeneous molecule now known to be produced by a variety of cells. Its biologic activities include serving as an endogenous pyrogen, inducing the release of lymphokines from activated

T cells and fibroblasts, enhancing antibody responsiveness through synergism with other lymphokines that affect B cell function, inducing the proliferation of fibroblasts, serving as a chemotactic factor for neutrophils, macrophages, and lymphocytes, and serving as a mediator of the inflammatory response.[52,210] Two genes coding for proteins with IL-1 properties have been discovered. These have been termed *interleukin-1-alpha (IL-1-a)* and *interleukin-1-beta (IL-2-β)*. Both share the same cell surface receptor and various biologic activities.

Several phase I trials have evaluated IL-1 in patients.[40,44] In general, these studies demonstrated a delayed increase in leukocytes and platelets. In patients receiving IL-1-β post-treatment with 5-FU, it appeared to exert a myeloprotective effect.[40] Further studies evaluating IL-1 in this capacity are in progress. A study by Vadhan-Raj and co-workers[217] demonstrated that IL-1-α increased circulating platelet counts and enhanced platelet recovery following treatment with carboplatin (CBDCA) in patients with ovarian cancer. Common toxicities experienced in these phase I trials were chills and fever, constitutional symptoms (headache, myalgias, arthralgias, fatigue, and nausea), hypotension at higher doses, tachycardia, and inflammation at injection sites. Occasional toxicities, especially at doses of greater than 300 ng/kg, were cardiac arrhythmias, reversible renal insufficiency, abdominal pain and transient CNS changes. Future trials will continue to evaluate the myeloprotective effect of IL-1, as well as its role in the pathology of septic shock, inflammatory bowel disease, and autoimmune diseases such as rheumatoid arthritis.[210]

Interleukin-2

Interleukin-2 is a glycoprotein mainly produced by activated T-helper cells. First discovered in 1976 by Morgan and co-workers,[134] it was originally named T-cell growth factor. Since then, intensive research has proved IL-2 to be a potent modulator of immune responses. The release of IL-2 in vivo occurs in response to two signals presented to T lymphocytes. The first is activation of T cells by antigen or mitogen, and the second is through interactions with IL-1. Like many polypeptide hormones, IL-2 exerts its biologic effects by binding to membrane-bound receptors on certain immune cells. It is now known that the IL-2 receptor has low-affinity and high-affinity forms. Hence, a resting cell may display very few IL-2 receptors. Once activated, it may display thousands of receptors and respond to activation by IL-2.[16,42]

BIOLOGIC EFFECTS.   The biologic effects of IL-2 are numerous and have been well documented.* IL-2 supports the growth and maturation of subpopulations of T cells both in vitro and in vivo, stimulates cytotoxic T cells, stimulates the proliferation and activity of NK cells, and develops the capacity in lymphoid cells incubated with IL-2 to lyse fresh tumor cells. These cells, known as lymphokine-activated killer (LAK) cells, have served as the basis for adoptive immunotherapy regimens. IL-2 also enchances antibody responses by activating other lymphocytes to produce lymphokines important to B cell function (IL-4 and IL-6), stimulates the expression of its own cell surface receptor, and induces the release of other lymphokines such as gamma-IFN and granulocyte-macrophage colony-stimulating factor (GM-CSF) that can mediate physiologic effects. Both in vitro and in vivo studies have demonstrated that IL-2 can reverse immune deficiencies in mice and humans. It appears that there are no differences in activity between naturally occurring IL-2 and the recombinant forms available.

CLINICAL INDICATIONS.   In 1992, IL-2 was approved by the FDA for the treatment of renal cell cancer.[34] (For a complete chronology on the clinical investigation of IL-2, see Parkinson,[152] Rosenberg,[184,185] and Rosenberg and co-workers.[186]) The first phase I clinical evaluations of IL-2 began in 1983 with IL-2 obtained from a human lymphoma tumor cell line. Although production methods limited supplies, a few clinical trials were conducted for patients with malignant tumors or acquired immune deficiency syndrome (AIDS). Therapy was given intravenously and produced minimal side effects. However, no therapeutic responses were seen.[115,116]

When the DNA sequence coding for IL-2 was elucidated, recombinant DNA technology made possible the production of large quantities of purified IL-2. As a result, phase I trials using recombinant IL-2 (rIL-2) were initiated in 1984.[116] Concurrently, studies conducted by Rosenberg[185] showed that adoptive immunotherapy with LAK cells was well tolerated by patients. These LAK cells were generated from fresh peripheral blood lymphocytes obtained through lymphocytapheresis and then incubated with IL-2.

In 1984 studies of the combination of IL-2 and LAK cells began. Results reported by Rosenberg and associates[185] in December 1985 showed that of 25 patients, 11 exhibited tumor responses. These responses were seen in patients with melanoma, renal cancer, and colorectal and pulmonary adenocarcinoma.

The excitement over these results generated an explosion of clinical trials with IL-2. Numerous clinical trials have evaluated a variety of doses, routes of administration, and schedules for IL-2. Trials have been conducted using IL-2 alone and in combination with LAK cells. Although patients with a variety of cancers have been treated, the majority of trials have focused on patients with renal cell cancer and melanoma because of the successes seen in these solid tumors.

---

*References 16, 42, 70, 109, 185, 206.

Rosenberg and colleagues have conducted prospective randomized studies to determine whether LAK cell administration with IL-2 is more effective than IL-2 alone. Early results showed no significant difference between the two arms; however, with longer follow-up (median of 50.2 months) treatment with LAK cells and IL-2 appears to yield improved survival in patients with melanoma as compared to IL-2 alone.[182]

Research efforts continued to find cells with more potent antitumor activity. A new subpopulation of lymphocytes, denoted *tumor-infiltrating lymphocytes (TILs)*, appeared to have greater efficacy in the treatment of experimental tumors than did LAK cells. TILs are obtained by removing tumor specimens from the host. Human TILs are T cells and can be isolated by growth in single-cell suspensions. They appear to be less dependent on adjunctive systemically administered IL-2 than are LAK cells. Early clinical trials using IL-2 plus TILs by Rosenberg and co-workers reported remissions in 11 of 20 patients with metastatic melanoma treated with this combination. Work continues on how to achieve the optimal therapeutic benefit and to find predictors of response.[182,214]

The combination of IL-2 with other cytokines, monoclonal antibodies, and chemotherapy is another active area of focus. Preclinical studies in animal models have shown antitumor activity to be enhanced by use of the above combinations.[62,138,139,152,208] Phase I and II trials evaluating the efficacy of these combinations continue. Other studies have evaluated a long-acting IL-2 (PEG IL-2) that could be administered once a day. Evaluation of chimeric molecules is an active area of pursuit. One such example is the use of an IL-2 molecule with diptheria toxin attached that is administered to patients whose malignancies express the IL-2 receptor. Phase I and II trials with this molecule,[160] as well as its evaluation for the treatment of rheumatoid arthritis continue. Over the next several years we will see increased use of IL-2 in the clinical setting as research defines optimal dosing and schedules and its concomitant use with effector cells and other biologic or chemotherapeutic agents.[72,85,106,208]

ADMINISTRATION.   As with other BRMs the optimal therapeutic dosage, route, and schedule for IL-2 have yet to be determined. The most common route of administration is intravenous, using either bolus or continuous infusion.[34] Investigations continue to evaluate other routes such as subcutaneous, intraperitoneal, and intra-arterial. The trend in dosing is towards expression of the dose in common international units. The recommended dose for Proleukin® is 600,000 IU/kg every 8 hours by a 15-minute IV infusion for a total of 14 doses.[34]

Pharmacokinetic studies show rapid initial plasma clearance (6 to 7 minutes) after bolus administration. With longer infusions, however, a more prolonged clearance is seen (half-life of approximately 30 minutes). These observations suggest a multicompartmental model of pharmacokinetics.[13,115,116] Inactivation appears to occur in the kidneys, with inactive metabolites excreted in the urine.

Other concerns about drug administration that are important to nurses include the following: handling procedures, which are determined by hospital policy; manufacturer's instructions for administration, how long the drug is stable in solution, and whether the drug can pass through a micropore filter; and evaluation of compatibility with concomitant medications such as antiemetics and vasopressors.[166]

SIDE EFFECTS.   Although responses to therapy with IL-2 are seen, severe systemic toxicities associated with high-dose IL-2 therapy make it difficult to tolerate. The range and severity of toxicity seen with IL-2 are related to and influenced by dose, schedule, and concomitant use of adoptive immunotherapy, other BRMs, and chemotherapy.[203]

How many side effects arise from IL-2 remains a mystery. While IL-2 may directly cause some side effects, the induction of other cytokines by IL-2 may also play a role. One encouraging note is that the majority of IL-2-related side effects disappear once therapy is completed. IL-2 is often administered on a cyclic basis similar to that of chemotherapy. This gives patients an opportunity to recuperate between cycles or courses, although cumulative toxicity does occur with repeated cycles. Patients have exhibited a marked decline in performance status over time, and more severe toxicity and impairment have been observed as the dose increases. Because the toxicity of existing IL-2 regimens can be severe enough to require hospitalization, future trials will continue to search for dosage schedules that can maximize therapeutic responses with a more acceptable level of toxicity.[152] See box on page 535 for an overall summary of IL-2 side effects by system.

As with other BRMs, patients receiving IL-2 have constitutional or flulike symptoms. These include chills followed by fever up to 40° C, headache, myalgias, arthralgias, and general malaise. Pretreatment with acetaminophen and indomethacin or another nonsteroidal antiinflammatory drug (NSAID) helps control these side effects. With continuous infusions of IL-2, the above medications are often necessary around the clock to control fevers.

The major cardiovascular and pulmonary toxicity associated with IL-2 administration stems from cumulative, dose-related fluid imbalances caused by a capillary leak syndrome. Shortly after administration a rapid decrease in systemic vascular resistance occurs, and fluids shift from the vascular bed to the interstitium. This causes a drop in mean arterial blood pressure, increased cardiac output, and an increase in heart rate.[186]

INTERLEUKIN-2 TOXICITIES

Constitutional symptoms
Chills, fever
Headaches
Malaise
Myalgias, arthralgias
Fatigue
Nasal congestion

Cardiovascular system
Hypotension
Decreased systemic vascular resistance
Tachycardia
Atrial arrhythmias
Edema
Weight gain
Ascites

Pulmonary system
Pulmonary edema
Dyspnea
Decreased PO_2

Renal function
Oliguria
Increased BUN, creatinine
Proteinuria
Azotemia

Gastrointestinal system
Nausea and vomiting
Diarrhea
Decreased appetite
Mucositis
Glossitis
Xerostomia

Endocrine system
Hypothyroidism

Integumentary system
Erythema
Erythematous rash
Dry skin
Pruritus
Dry desquamation

Central nervous system
Confusion, disorientation
Somnolence
Lethargy
Combativeness
Psychoses
Anxiety
Depression

Hematologic function
Anemia
Thrombocytopenia
Eosinophilia
Lymphopenia

Hepatic function
Increased bilirubin
Elevated SGOT, SGPT, LDH

Related laboratory values
Hypophosphatemia
Hypocalcemia
Hypomagnesemia
Decreased serum albumin

Other
Potential for catheter-related sepsis

From Rieger PT and Weatherly B: Can your nursing skills meet the challenge of a patient receiving IL-2? Dimen Onco Nur 3(3):9, 1989.

Weight gains as much as 10% of baseline weight have been observed in high-dose trials.[186] Fluid retention is usually manifested as peripheral edema and abdominal ascites. These effects may progress to interstitial pulmonary edema with subsequent dyspnea and decreased PO_2 levels in some patients. In extreme cases of respiratory distress, patients require intubation.[57,113]

Although clinically patients appear fluid overloaded, in reality they are hypovolemic. This hypovolemia leads to hypotension, decreased central venous pressure (CVP), and renal hypoperfusion. These physiologic changes place an increased demand on the heart, and transient arrhythmias may be observed. Because of this, patients usually undergo rigorous pretherapy screening for underlying cardiac problems before beginning therapy with IL-2. Medical treatment includes administration of colloid solutions (5% albumin), judicious use of fluids to avoid pulmonary edema, and the use of vasopressors.[152,186,205]

The multiple hemodynamic abnormalities associated with IL-2 therapy often lead to the development of renal hypoperfusion and prerenal azotemia. Renal toxicity is evidenced by oliguria, proteinuria, azotemia, and increases in BUN and creatinine levels.[108] These effects, seen at various doses, usually return to baseline after therapy. Medical treatment includes fluids, diuretics (if blood pressure and CVP are within normal limits), and pressors such as low-dose dopamine to stimulate renal blood flow.

Acute gastrointestinal effects are common with IL-2. Nausea and vomiting closely parallel chemotherapy-associated nausea and vomiting. Patients often complain that food odors increase nausea. Unfortunately, for some patients, IL-2-associated nausea and vomiting have proved resistant to pharmacologic treatment. Often the aggressive use of multiple antiemetics around the clock is required. In addition, patients lose their appetite; therefore weight loss over time becomes a major concern. Diarrhea may be acute or chronic and is often watery and profuse. Mucositis, glossitis, and xerostomia can further damage nutritional status.

Baseline assessment of mental status is important in patients receiving IL-2. CNS toxicity may be manifested as confusion, lethargy, decreased concentration, extreme somnolence, depression, hallucination, paranoia, combativeness, agitation, and nightmares.[43] Occasionally, these toxicities are severe enough to cause the delay or discontinuation of therapy.

Skin changes occurring with IL-2 therapy are profound and cumulative; they are a major source of discomfort for patients. Varying degrees of erythema, erythematous rash, pruritus, dryness, and occasionally dry desquamation may all be seen either alone or in combination (Figures 23-1 and 23-2). Skin biopsies have not elucidated the etiology of these skin changes. Aggravation of underlying dermatologic conditions as well as recall phenomena may also be seen.

Patients may develop neutropenia, thrombocytopenia, or anemia. In programs using lymphocytapheresis, anemia is often exacerbated. With prolonged IL-2 administration, marked eosinophilia often occurs. The clinical significance of this is uncertain, although it may be responsible for the fluid shifts observed.[107]

Significant lymphopenia occurs within minutes of IL-2 administration. However, rebound lymphocytosis occurs within 24 hours after discontinuation of a treatment. As with other IL-2 side effects, these changes are usually reversible upon cessation of therapy.

Patients receiving IL-2 often have several abnormal lab values. Patients should be monitored for increased bilirubin, elevated hepatic enzymes (aminotransferases, lactate dehydrogenase), hypomagnesemia, hypophosphatemia, hypocalcemia, decreased serum albumin, and respiratory alkalosis. Replacement therapy should be instituted as appropriate.

The incidence of catheter-related sepsis appears higher in patients receiving high doses of IL-2. Currently, trials are in progress evaluating the use of prophylactic antibiotics in this patient population. It is often difficult to differentiate signs of infection from those associated with IL-2; therefore, patients must be monitored closely.[152]

In patients receiving adoptive immunotherapy with either LAK or TILs, the majority of side effects are attributable to IL-2. Chills and fever are the major side effects noted with cell infusions. These are readily treatable with meperidine. A further risk is that of infection, because lymphocytes incubated in culture medium for 3 to 4 days may be contaminated with viruses or bacteria.[186] (See Table 23-6 for medications frequently used during IL-2 therapy.)

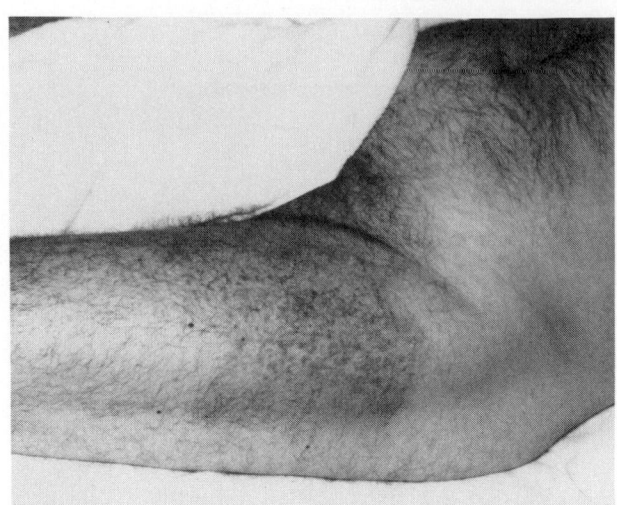

Figure 23–1 Skin rash and erythema (on thigh) shortly after starting therapy with IL-2. (From Rieger P and Weatherly B: Can your nursing skills meet the challenge of a patient receiving IL-2? Dimens Oncol Nurs 3(3), Fall 1989.)

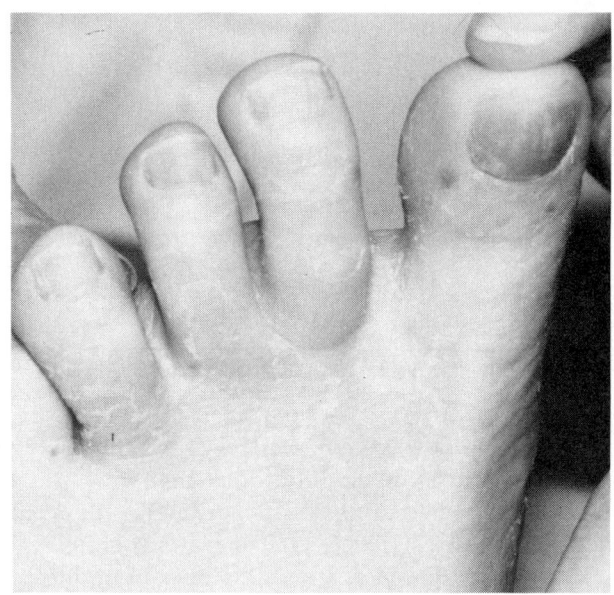

Figure 23–2 Skin desquamation in patient who receives IL-2. (From Rieger P and Weatherly B: Can your nursing skills meet the challenge of a patient receiving IL-2? Dimens Oncol Nurs 3(3), Fall 1989.)

Interleukin-4

Primarily produced by activated T cells, IL-4 has a number of biologic effects. It stimulates the growth of resting B cells in vitro; it increases production of immunoglobulin in vitro; it may stimulate certain T-cell lines in vitro; it produces CSF-like activity in vitro; and it may stimulate growth and maturation of mast

Table 23–6   Frequent Concomitant Medications Used During IL-2 Therapy

Medication	Dose/Frequency/Route	Side Effect Treated
Acetaminophen	650 mg q4h PO/PR	Fever, myalgia
Indomethacin	50-75 mg q8h PO/PR	Fever, myalgia
Meperidine	25-50 mg IV prn	Chills
Ranitidine HCl*	50 mg q8h IV	Gastritis
Albumin 5% (12.5 g/250 ml)	250 ml prn IV	Oliguria, hypotension
Droperidol	1 mg IV q4-6h, IV prn	Nausea
Prochlorperazine	25 mg q3-4h, PR prn	Nausea
Promethazine	50 mg q3-4h, PR prn	Nausea
Aluminum hydroxide 200 mg	30 mL q3-4h, PO prn	Gastric upset
Magnesium hydroxide 200 mg		
Simethicone 20 mg		
Thiethylperazine maleate	10 mg q3-4h, PO prn	Nausea
Loperamide	2 mg q3h, PO prn	Diarrhea
Diphenoxylate HCl (2.5 mg)	q3-4h, PO prn	Diarrhea
Atropine sulfate (25 µg)		
Codeine sulfate	30-60 mg q3-4h, PO prn	Diarrhea
Opium tincture (deodorized)	2-4 gtt q3-4h, PO prn	Diarrhea
Hydroxyzine HCl	10-20 mg q6h, PO prn	Itching
Sodium bicarbonate 6 tsp/1,500 ml	swish and spit	Dry, sore mouth
Diphenhydramine HCl	25-50 mg q3-4h, PO prn	Itching
Oatmeal powder	Apply locally prn	Itching
Lubriderm 8 oz with 0.25% camphor, 0.25% menthol, and 0.25% phenol	Apply locally prn	Itching
Lidobenalox oral	5 ml q3-4h, PO prn	Pharyngitis
Triazolam	0.25 mg qhs, PO prn	Insomnia
Lorazepam	0.5 mg q3-4 PO prn	Anxiety
Flurazepam HCl	15-30 mg qhs PO prn	Insomnia
Dopamine HCl	400 mg/250 ml; (2 µg/kg/min)	Oliguria, hypotension
Phenylephrine	100 mg/250 ml, titrate IV to maintain blood pressure (0.1-2.5 µg/kg/min)	Hypotension
Magnesium sulfate	1 g IV prn (over 1 hr)	Hypomagnesemia
Oxacillin	150 mg/kg/1d IV	Prevent catheter sepsis

Abbreviations: PO = orally; PR = rectally; q = every; IV = intravenously; prn = as needed; tsp = teaspoon.
From Lotze MT and Rosenberg SA: Interleukin-2: clinical applications. In DeVita VT, Hellman S, and Rosenberg SA, editors: The biologic therapy of cancer, Philadelphia, 1991, JB Lippincott Co.

cells in vitro. The full range of biologic effects and clinical potential remains to be determined.[42,98]

Several phase I trials have evaluated tolerance of IL-4 in patients, utilizing several routes of administration: IV bolus, short-term IV infusion, and subcutaneous injection.[67,97] Toxicities experienced were low-grade delayed fevers, nausea, reversible elevation in liver enzymes, and nasal congestion. Occasional toxicities, especially at higher doses were chills, hypotension, and edema with weight gain. Rare instances of therapy complicated by gastroduodenal erosion or ulceration have been reported.[187] A phase II outpatient dose and schedule have been established at 5 mcg/kg/day by the subcutaneous route. Phase II trials are in progress with greatest interest in hematologic malignancies (multiple myeloma, indolent lymphoma, B-CLL, intermediate grade lymphoma, Hodgkin's disease, and CML).

HEMATOPOIETIC GROWTH FACTORS

Colony-stimulating factors (CSFs) are a family of glycoprotein hormones responsible for the proliferation, differentiation, and maturation of hematopoietic cells in vitro. They also stimulate functions of certain mature leukocytes.[38] The four classic CSFs are granulocyte-macrophage colony-stimulating factor (GM-CSF), granulocyte colony-stimulating factor (G-CSF), macrophage colony-stimulating factor (M-CSF), and IL-3 (multi-CSF). All are produced in recombinant form. GM-CSF and G-CSF have both received regulatory approval whereas clinical trials with IL-3 and M-CSF are in progress. The characterization of other hematopoietic CSFs is also being pursued. After in-vitro studies elucidate their biology, the next step will be assessment of their clinical efficacy in vivo.[68] For the four classic CSFs, current investigations attempt to further define appropriate dosages, schedules, and routes of administration as well as the diseases and conditions for which these agents are best used.[11,125,126]

The CSFs were discovered through research into the process and regulation of hematopoiesis. These glycoproteins were detected because of their mandatory and unique role in stimulating hematopoietic

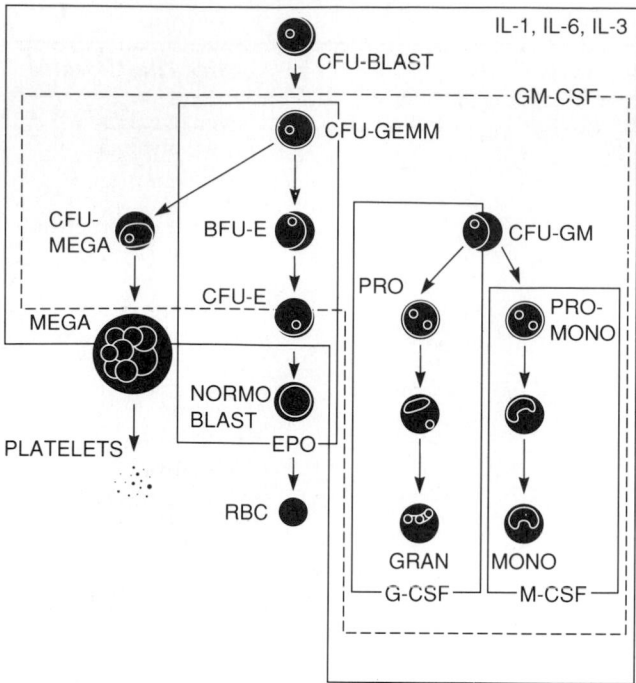

Figure 23–3 Regulation of hematopoietic cell development. CFU, Colony-forming unit. CFU-GEMM, CFU-granulocyte erythroid macrophage-megakaryocyte. Mega, megakaryocytes. CFU-GM, DFU-granulocyte macrophage. Pro, promyelocyte. Mono, monocyte. Gran, granulocyte. (From Gabrilove J: Overview of CSFs, Semin Hematol 26(2) Suppl 2, April 1989.)

cells to proliferate[54] (Figure 23-3). The use of semisolid colonal assay systems to culture hematopoietic cells revealed that specific regulatory molecules (CSFs) were necessary to sustain progenitor cells and to form colonies. The ability to clone these agents greatly enhanced the ability to study them. There appear to be overlapping functions as well as synergism between different CSFs. As these are all receptor-mediated molecules, differences in effects on different hematopoietic lineages may be related to the distribution of receptors.[126,127]

To understand the CSFs, one needs a basic understanding of hematopoiesis, or the production and development of blood cells. This process normally occurs in the bone marrow, where cells of various lineages proliferate, differentiate, and mature. Most blood cells possess a relatively short life span. Therefore they must be constantly produced to offset continual turnover. For example, baseline levels of granulocytes and macrophages are maintained within a narrow range. However, the body has a remarkable ability to increase production in response to stresses such as infection and inflammation. Factors thought to be important in the control of hematopoiesis are the bone marrow microenvironment, cell-to-cell interaction, and humoral substances.[230]

The process starts with a multipotent or pluripotent stem cell. These cells have the capacity for self-re-

newal and the ability to form multilineage colonies, although they are relatively quiescent under normal circumstances. Cells become successively more proliferative during differentiation, and their capacities to renew themselves and to form multilineage colonies become more restricted. The factors controlling hematopoiesis have not been entirely delineated. Constitutive substances that may affect the lineage commitment status of a cell are being investigated. CSFs appear more important in the stress response, and they seem to help control the number of effector cells in the immune response.[30,81]

BIOLOGY AND CLINICAL APPLICATIONS. Biologic activity of the CSFs is summarized in Table 23-7. In vitro studies suggested that the CSFs may have clinical value in a variety of settings. CSF clinical trials continue to evaluate (1) reducing cancer treatment morbidity by decreasing myelosuppression (both intensity and duration) and the incidence of febrile neutropenia; (2) improvement in survival by allowing patients to receive chemotherapy treatments on schedule; (3) speeding marrow recovery after bone marrow transplant; (4) restoring bone marrow function in aplastic anemia, myelodysplastic syndrome, myelomas, leukemias, and acquired and congenital neutropenias; (5) combining CSFs with other BRMs to enhance effector cell functions further; (6) treating leukemia by promoting terminal cell maturation; and (7) treating burns, overwhelming sepsis-related infections, and parasitic infections.[68,75,125,132]

GM-CSF

Of all the CSFs, GM-CSF has received the most extensive clinical evaluation. Early clinical trials evaluated its application in patients with AIDS,[77] myelodysplastic syndromes and aplastic anemia,[218,219] and in cancer patients after chemotherapy[12] and autologous bone marrow transplant.[22] All studies showed dose-dependent increases in leukocytes, especially neutrophils, eosinophils, and monocytes. The duration of neutropenia appeared shorter after chemotherapy, and leukocyte recovery was enhanced after transplant, compared with controls. Overall, no significant effects on platelet recovery were seen. Counts rose during therapy in a dose-dependent manner but fell rapidly once therapy was discontinued. In general, courses were well tolerated, and side effects were dose dependent. Recombinant human GM-CSF Prokine® (Sargramostim) and Leukine® (Sargramostim) received regulatory approval in 1991 for the acceleration of myeloid recovery in patients with non-Hodgkin's lymphoma (NHL), acute lymphoblastic leukemia (ALL), and Hodgkin's disease undergoing autologus bone marrow transplantations (BMT).[87,92] Issues to be addressed in future trials include evaluation of GM-CSF's effects on the incidence and seriousness of neutropenic infections after chemother-

Table 23–7 Biologic Activity of CSFs

GSF	Colonies Stimulated	Known Cellular Sources	Cell Functions Enhanced in Vitro
GM	Neutrophil, monocyte/macrophage, eosinophil	T-cells, endothelial cells, and fibroblasts	Inhibits neutrophil migration Increases neutrophil chemotactic response Augments ADCC Activates monocytes/macrophages Appears to synergize with IL-3
G	Neutrophils	Monocytes, endothelial cells, fibroblasts	Enhances chemotactic response and phagocytosis of neutrophils Augments ADCC Enhances neutrophil migration
M	Monocytes/macrophages	Monocytes, endothelial cells, fibroblasts	Monocyte cytotoxicity Stimulates monocyte ADCC
Interleukin-3	Mixed, myeloid, erythroid, megakaryocytic, basophilic	T-cells	Appears to synergize with other CSFs Enhances ADCC and phagocytosis in mature eosinophils Enhances monocyte function (complete range of activities needs further delineation)

ADCC, antibody-dependent cellular cytotoxicity.

apy or transplant, the timing of therapy in relationship to chemotherapy administration,[132,216] long-term toxicity, and the antitumor effect in both solid tumors and leukemias.

ADMINISTRATION.   GM-CSF is manufactured by several pharmaceutical companies, so there may be variations in the different products that affect administration. Nurses should consult pharmacy resource personnel about filterability and stability issues. Pharmacology studies show GM-CSF has a relatively short half-life, with the second phase lasting 1 to 3 hours.[33] In early trials, GM-CSF was given by IV infusion (continuous infusion, bolus); however, subcutaneous administration is also used.

It is difficult to define a standard dose for GM-CSF, not only because it is a relatively new agent, but also because different sources of GM-CSF are manufactured in different systems (bacterial versus yeast versus mammalian cells) and different bioassays are used to evaluate its strength.

In general, doses of 125 to 250 $\mu g/m^2$ (3 to 5 $\mu g/kg$) are fairly well tolerated. The recommended dose for Prokine® and Leukine® is 250 $\mu g/m^2/day$ for 21 days as a 2 hour IV infusion beginning 2 to 4 hours after the autologous bone marrow infusion.[87,92] Toxicity is dose related, and the dose-limiting side effects are myalgias, arthralgias, capillary leak syndrome with edema, and pericardial and pleural effusions occurring at doses greater than 16 to 32 $\mu g/kg$.[12]

SIDE EFFECTS.   Side effects are affected by the dosage, route of administration, patient population, and setting used (postchemotherapy, post–bone marrow transplantation). Common side effects are constitutional symptoms (chills and fever), bone pain, fatigue, and anorexia. Other reported side effects are rashes, flushing, phlebitis,[77] gastrointestinal disturbances, erythema at the injection site, hypotension, fluid retention, pericarditis, pleural and pericardial effusions, thrombocytopenia, and thrombus formation at the catheter tip.[12] These effects are generally reversible with cessation of therapy.*

G-CSF

The majority of clinical trials investigating G-CSF focused on its use after chemotherapy.[137] Trials with combination chemotherapy for urothelial carcinoma[69] and high-dose chemotherapy for small-cell lung cancer[23] demonstrated a decreased duration of severe neutropenia after G-CSF therapy. Gabrilove's study showed that patients who received G-CSF had fewer days of antibiotic therapy and a decreased incidence and severity of mucositis and were more likely to be able to stay on their chemotherapy schedules than other patients. Patients exhibited a dose-dependent increase in leukocyte counts, mainly because of an increase in absolute number of neutrophils. Counts fell rapidly once therapy was stopped. G-CSF has also been investigated in neutropenia from other causes.[58] In patients with hairy-cell leukemia, for example, G-CSF dramatically increased the absolute neutrophil count.[74]

---

*References 12, 22, 81, 118, 218, 219.

Table 23–8 Clinical Potential of GM-CSF and G-CSF

Adjunct to standard chemotherapy
• Reduce morbidity
• Allow full doses to be delivered on time
Permit dose intensification of chemotherapy
• Reduce the morbidity of autologous or allogeneic marrow or peripheral stem-cell transplantation
• Allow larger doses of drugs to be administered
• Increase the frequency of chemotherapy cycles
Reversal of marrow failure
• Malignancies with marrow infiltration, chronic lymphatic leukemia, hairy-cell leukemia, lymphoma
Differentiation-inducing agents
• Myelodysplastic syndromes
• Myeloid leukemia
Recruitment of malignant cells prior to chemotherapy
• Myeloid leukemia
Direct anticancer effects

From Metcalf D and Morstyn G: Colony-stimulating factors: general biology. In DeVita VT, Hellman S, and Rosenberg SA, editors: Biologic therapy of cancer, Philadelphia, 1991, JB Lippincott Co.

Table 23–9 Adverse Observations Associated with CSF Administration

GM-CSF	G-CSF
Bone pain	Bone pain
Lethargy	
Rash	
First-dose effect	
Fever	
Thrombophlebitis	
Elevated AP, γGT, LDH*	Elevated AP and LDH
Hypoalbuminaemia	Elevated urate level
Pericarditis	Sweet syndrome (acute febrile neutrophilic dermatosis)
Fluid retention	
Progression of myelodysplastic syndromes with 15% or more marrow blast cells	? Progression of myelodysplastic syndromes with more than 15% blasts
? Transient fall in platelets at high dose	? Transient fall in platelets at high dose
Reactivation of autoimmune thrombocytopenia	

*AP = alkaline phosphatase; LDH = lactic dehydrogenase; γGT = gamma glutamyl transpeptidase.
From Metcalf D and Morstyn G: Colony-stimulating factors: general biology. In DeVita VT, Hellman S, and Rosenberg SA, editors: Biologic therapy of cancer, Philadelphia, 1991, JB Lippincott Co.

Recombinant human G-CSF Neupogen® (Filgrastim) received FDA approval in 1991. It is indicated to decrease the incidence of infection in patients with non-myeloid malignancies receiving myelosuppressive anti-cancer drugs associated with a significant incidence of severe neutropenia with fever. The recommended starting dose of Neupogen® is 5 µg/kg/day, administered subcutaneously or intravenously as a single daily injection.[7] Therapy is generally well tolerated, with medullary bone pain as the only consistent toxicity reported. This pain is usually mild to moderate in severity and is generally well controlled with non-narcotic analgesics. Erythema is occasionally seen at the site of subcutaneous injections. (See Tables 23-8 and 23-9 for a review of GM-CSF/G-CSF clinical uses and toxicity.)

M-CSF

Due to its inherent biologic activity, considerable interest exists for the use of M-CSF, alone or in combination with other biologic agents, for the treatment of malignancy.[15] Early phase I trials are in the process of evaluating dosage and toxicity for both the subcutaneous and intravenous route. In trials evaluating subcutaneous administration doses up to 12,800 µg/m^2 have been administered. In general, toxicity has been mild consisting of local reaction, arthralgia, and fatigue. At the highest dose levels thrombocytopenia and monocytosis have been observed.[28] Future trials will further define dosage and evaluate the efficacy of M-CSF in treating cancer.

Interleukin-3

The ability of IL-3 to target multipotential committed progenitor cells provides a strong rationale for its eval-

uation in the treatment of bone marrow failure states.[199] Phase I/II clinical trials are now in progress evaluating the use of IL-3 alone and in combination with other CSFs for patients with bone marrow failure, normal hematopoiesis but advanced malignancy, or prolonged cytopenia post radiotherapy and/or chemotherapy.[89,111] In trials with IL-3 alone, all studies showed a delayed increase in leukocytes (granulocytes, eosinophils, and basophils), and occasional increases in platelets and reticulocytes. Both subcutaneous and intravenous routes were used, with doses up to 1000 µg/m^2/day being fairly well tolerated.

The most common toxicities experienced were low-grade fever and headaches with occasional flushing, erythema at injection sites, bone pain, lethargy, and nausea and vomiting. Future trials will continue to further refine dosage and the application of IL-3 in bone marrow failure states, and its ability to provide a myeloprotective effect post chemotherapy or radiotherapy. In vivo simian studies with IL-3 have shown marked stimulation when it is given in combination with GM-CSF.[54] Preliminary clinical results suggest that this combination may have a synergistic effect on hematopoietic progenitor cells and be of value in reducing chemotherapy induced neutropenia.

ERYTHROPOIETIN

Epogen®[10] (recombinant human erythropoietin) and Procrit are FDA approved as treatment for chronic anemia in end-stage renal disease after phase I and II trials demonstrated clinical efficacy.[56] Physiologically, erythropoietin is produced in response to decreased oxygen levels. The recombinant form is produced in cultured mammalian cells. When receiving it intravenously three times a week, virtually all patients achieved normalization of hematocrit (Hct) and were transfusion independent. Therapy is well tolerated in general, and the majority of side effects (hypertension, seizures, increased clotting of venous access grafts) appear to be related to increased Hct. Patients are generally started at a dosage of 50 to 100 U/kg three times a week intravenously or subcutaneously. Maintenance doses are generally titrated in 25-unit increments to keep the Hct in a chosen target range, for example 36% to 38%. In 1993, Procrit® received regulatory approval for the treatment of anemia in cancer patients on chemotherapy.[149,227]

TUMOR NECROSIS FACTOR

Discovered in 1975 in the serum of animals treated with injections of BCG or *C. parvum* followed by endotoxins, tumor necrosis factor (TNF) is a protein that selectively targets transformed cells.[16] Normal human fibroblasts appeared insensitive to TNF. These findings generated considerable interest in the use of TNF in the treatment of cancer. The gene for TNF has been isolated, identified, and cloned to produce recombinant TNF (rTNF). Further investigations have analyzed TNF's relationships with other cytotoxic factors produced by immune effector cells. Cachectin was isolated by Beutler and colleagues,[19] who believed it to be important in the pathogenesis of cachexia. Amino acid sequencing and cloning techniques proved human cachetin and TNF to be the same molecule.[19,215] This TNF, primarily produced by activated macrophages, is termed *TNF-alpha*. Another cytokine, lymphotoxin, which shares biologic activity with TNF-alpha, has been termed *TNF-beta*. It is produced primarily by lymphocytes. This section will focus on TNF-alpha.

Biologic Effects

Although primarily synthesized in vivo by activated macrophages, TNF is also produced by lymphocytes, NK cells, astrocytes, and microglial cells of the brain. This polypeptide hormone, pivotal in the pathogenesis of infection, inflammation, and injury, participates in the beneficial processes of host defense and tissue homeostasis. TNF interacts with high-affinity receptors on normal tissue cells, with resultant internalization of the receptor-ligand complex. Details of this process remain unclear.

Biologic activities of TNF that may be responsible for its antitumor effects: it is cytotoxic or cytostatic to some human tumor cells; it promotes the induction of other mediators (IL-2 and GM-CSF)[66,215]; it enhances chemotactic, phagocytic, and cytotoxic activity of macrophages and neutrophils; and it causes the induction of several cell-surface antigens. It also serves as the primary mediator of endotoxic shock[128] and as a growth factor by stimulating fibroblasts and mesenchymal cell proliferation.[16,215]

Clinical Indications

Both preclinical studies in animal models and human clinical trials have evaluated the effectiveness of TNF as an antitumor agent. An overview of phase I experience with TNF in the United States indicates that more than 200 patients with a variety of malignancies have received therapy with TNF. However, to date therapeutic responses are unimpressive.*

An editorial by Frei[66] concludes that until the cellular mechanisms of TNF cytotoxicity and tumor cell resistance are understood, clinical trials will not be able to exploit the full potential of this agent. Current efforts are focused on phase II investigations and on evaluating combination therapy of TNF with other cytokines,[138,139] and chemotherapy (actinomycin).

Administration

TNF has been administered by intramuscular, subcutaneous, intravenous[20,202] (via both bolus and continuous infusion), and intraperitoneal routes. The maximum tolerated dose as defined in phase I trials varies with route and schedule. TNF has not received FDA approval and is therefore administered only in investigational settings.

Pharmacy resource personnel should be consulted about stability, filterability, and other administration concerns (e.g., intravenous lines are often preprimed with albumin and normal saline before TNF administration). Handling procedures should follow hospital policy.

Side Effects

Toxicity associated with TNF has been well documented in early clinical trials.[131] Side effects are similar to those seen with other biologic agents, are dose dependent, and in general resolve upon discontinuation of therapy. Dose-limiting toxicities with IV administration have been constitutional symptoms and shocklike manifestations, including fever and hypotension.[59] As with interferon, patients may exhibit tachyphylaxis to many of the side effects.

Common side effects include fever, severe chills or rigors, fatigue, myalgias, headache, soreness at the injection site (erythema and tenderness), nausea and/or vomiting, and loss of appetite with resultant weight loss. Pretreatment with meperidine is often

---

*References 20, 35, 59, 66, 131, 204.

helpful in controlling chills and rigors. Depending on dose and schedule, these side effects may lessen or disappear with subsequent doses.

Occasional side effects include hematologic changes (leukopenia, thrombocytopenia), cardiovascular changes (hypotension, dizziness), hepatic changes (elevated transaminases, hyperbilirubinemia), elevated triglycerides, and decreased serum cholesterol. These changes are usually reversible with cessation of therapy. Hypotension can generally be managed with fluid administration. For higher IV doses of TNF (≥ 100 $\mu g/m^2$), patients are often prehydrated.

Although rare, more severe toxicity associated with changes in the central nervous or respiratory systems has occurred.[135] Neurologic deficits observed include transient ischemic attacks and strokelike symptoms. Patients who develop these symptoms should be removed from the study and evaluated to determine the etiology of the symptoms. Respiratory insufficiency, evidenced primarily by dyspnea, has also been observed. Morice and associates[135] monitored 19 patients receiving subcutaneous or intravenous TNF. All but 2 demonstrated impairment of gas exchange as measured by DLCO, a measurement of alveolar gas exchange. This toxicity appeared to be dose related but resolved in the majority of patients with the cessation of therapy.

MONOCLONAL ANTIBODIES

Monoclonal antibodies (MoAbs), produced by the fusion of antibody-producing cells and myeloma tumor cells (hybridomas) have been shown to be highly specific for a single target antigen. With the development of hybridoma technology in 1975,[105] large amounts of pure antibodies with a predetermined specificity could be produced. This rekindled interest in the use of antibodies for the diagnosis and treatment of cancer. Their potential was implicated in the early 1900s, when Paul Ehrlich observed that antiserum from tumor-bearing mice when injected into tumor-bearing animals of the same strain was capable of causing tumor rejection. He termed these antibodies magic bullets and proposed using them as carriers to deliver drugs and toxins to tumor cells.[55]

An antigen is any substance that the body recognizes as foreign and attacks with an immune response. The humoral immune response produces immunoglobulins against the invading antigen from B-cell derived plasma cells. These immunoglobulins, or antibodies, react specifically with the antigenic determinants or epitopes of the inducing antigen. The antigenic determinants are parts of the antigen recognized by the antibodies. Each antigen has any number of epitopes, depending on the complexity of its structure. Individual B cells produce an antibody spe-

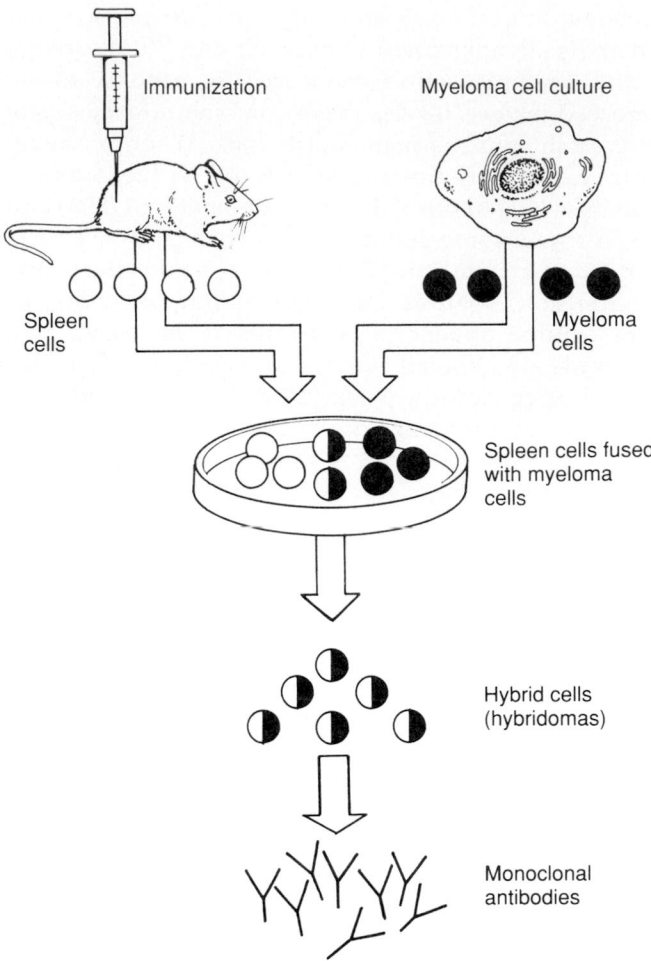

Figure 23–4 Monoclonal antibody production.

cific for a single antigenic determinant. Therefore, when an antigen invades the body, a variety of antibodies against it are produced.

Hybridoma technology begins with immunizing a mouse with a chosen antigen (Figure 23-4). After the mouse mounts an immune response, its spleen is removed to obtain B lymphocytes producing antibodies. Because lymphocytes cannot grow indefinitely in culture, they are fused with mouse myeloma cells (plasma cells) to immortalize the antibody-producing B lymphocytes. These new cells, *hybridomas,* can grow indefinitely in culture and produce antibodies with predetermined specificity—MoAbs. The next step is to select and clone for the desired antibody. Once the desired hybridoma is obtained, it can be frozen for future use, grown in culture to produce continuous quantities of MoAbs, or reinjected into mice and grown as tumors to produce MoAbs in ascites fluid.

As previously discussed, when the body encounters a foreign substance, an immune response is mounted. It has long been hypothesized that tumor cells express cell-surface molecules (antigens) different from those expressed on normal cells. Antigens found only on malignant cells are termed *tumor-specific antigens* (TSA), whereas antigens also found on normal tissues but to a greater degree in malignant cells are termed *tumor-associated antigens* (TAA).[17,49,50] The majority of malignant cells express TAA. One example is oncofetal antigens, which are normally expressed on embryonic cells and later reexpressed on malignant cells. Whereas most current therapies are toxic for both malignant and normal cells, MoAbs can be used to attack the tumor cell directly. Theoretically, antibody therapy is the most tumor-specific approach to cancer treatment.[49,50]

Biology and Clinical Applications

UNCONJUGATED ANTIBODY. Numerous clinical trials have been conducted with native MoAbs—those not bound to drugs, toxins, or isotopes—for a large number of malignancies. An unconjugated antibody may demonstrate an anticancer effect in several ways. One is to mediate an antitumor cytotoxic effect through complement-dependent cytotoxicity or antibody-dependent cellular cytotoxicity. The constant region (F_c) of the immunoglobulin reacts with either the first component of the complement system or with immune effector cells; the end result is tumor cell lysis.[84] Tumor cells express a variety of receptors important for growth and proliferation advantages. A second approach employs MoAbs directed against cell surface receptors involved in proliferation such as the epidermal growth factor (EGF) receptor. The intent is to block or downgrade the number of available receptors, thereby inducing an antiproliferative effect.[124] An extensively studied approach is the use of anti-idiotype antibodies. Idiotypes are the variable regions of the immunoglobulin molecule that contain the antigen-combining region. A malignant B cell clone produces cells that express and occasionally secrete a specific antibody. Infusions of antibodies directed against a B-cell lymphoma idiotype may suppress that clone back to its baseline.[27,46,50] Another approach, actually a method of passive immunization, uses antibodies as surrogate tumor antigens to stimulate an immune response against the tumor. For example, suppose a murine antibody (AB1) is selected to recognize a certain TAA. A second antibody (AB2) is raised against the idiotype of AB1. This second antibody, AB2, is an antiidiotype antibody. The patient is immunized with this antibody. An antiidiotype response to AB2 produces a third antibody, AB3. This third antibody has the same capacity to react with the desired TAA as AB1 because its idiotype is the mirror image of this antigen. In essence, by receiving AB2, the patient becomes self-immunized, developing his or her own human antibodies against the tumor. This technique is also used to immunize

against invading organisms such as viruses because it avoids vaccination with whole virus or viral antigens. Whether this method can produce sufficient antibodies for an antitumor effect is unknown.[49,50,84]

The first MoAb clinical trials were conducted in patients with hematologic malignancies—leukemias and lymphomas. There soon followed trials evaluating MoAbs in solid tumors such as melanoma, colorectal cancer, prostate cancer, breast cancer, and lung cancer.[49,50,63,64,186] To date this approach has led only to transient clinical responses.

Several problems can impact on the therapeutic efficacy and/or toxicity of MoAbs. A major concern is the development of human antimouse antibodies (HAMA) after murine MoAbs are administered.[200] HAMA may trigger immune complex formation, which mediates tissue damage, neutralization of MoAbs (preventing their binding to tumor cells), and alteration of MoAb clearance and organ distribution. Strategies being evaluated to abrogate the development of HAMA include the infusion of antibody fragments, infusion of large doses of MoAb to induce tolerance, immunosuppressive therapy, and the use of human[50] or chimeric (part murine/part human)[26,141] antibodies.

Another concern is antigenic modulation. Surface antigens decrease during this process, being either internalized and later reexpressed or shed from the cell surface. Antigenic modulation is especially problematic in hematologic malignancies. Within minutes of exposure to MoAbs, modulation can occur. Once circulating levels of MoAb decrease, antigen is reexpressed. Obviously, once modulation occurs, MoAbs cannot effectively bind to malignant cells. Strategies for circumventing this problem include administration of mixed MoAbs (a cocktail) to recognize different antigens and choosing MoAbs specific for nonmodulating antigens.[50,186]

Other problems include poor tumor vascularity (poor circulation inhibits delivery of MoAbs to the tumor site); cross-reactivity of MoAbs with normal tissues; tumor heterogeneity (expression of more than one TAA); lack of sufficient antigen expression on the tumor cell surface; and lack of in vivo cytotoxicity of the antibody alone. Clinical trials are evaluating strategies to overcome these obstacles so that the full therapeutic benefit of MoAbs can be realized.[50] For example, one area of focus is the combination of native MoAbs and other BRMs.

IMMUNOCONJUGATES. An active area of investigation is the conjugation of MoAbs to toxins (immunotoxins),[153,221] chemotherapy (chemoimmunotoxins), radioisotopes (radioimmunotherapy), and biologic response modifiers (immunobiologics).[78,84] The ricin A chain, a toxin, has been conjugated to several antitumor murine MoAbs, and clinical trials are progressing.[148,209] Clinical trials are investigating immunoconjugates of chemotherapeutic agents such as methotrexate, doxorubicin, and cisplatin to MoAbs. By selectively delivering these drugs to the tumor, investigators hope to increase tumor cell kill while avoiding systemic toxicity. Problems include acquired drug resistance and the need to deliver large amounts of drug (as opposed to small amounts with toxins) to the tumor.

Another exciting area is conjugation of radioisotopes to MoAbs. Two important advantages to this approach include the ability to kill antigen-negative bystander cells, and the lack of a need for internalization by the tumor cell to exhibit their cytotoxic effect. Clinical trials are in progress in this area.[84,102] Major problems with all types of conjugates include damage to normal tissue due to cross-reactivity and systemic toxicity should the MoAb and the conjugate dissociate.

DIAGNOSTIC IMAGING WITH RADIOLABELED ANTIBODIES. The use of radiolabeled MoAbs in diagnostic imaging has received intense study.[186] When low doses of radioisotopes such as indium-111 and iodine-131 are conjugated with MoAbs that react to specific tumor antigens, MoAbs can be used to locate both primary and metastatic tumors. The ability of radiolabeled MoAbs to detect tumors is being compared to conventional x-rays and isotope scans. In some instances, antibodies are more sensitive than conventional scans. Problems that are associated with radioimmunoimaging include tumor size (lesions <1 cm in size do not image well), tumor heterogeneity, nonspecific uptake of MoAbs by other organs (especially the liver and spleen), tumor vascularity, toxicities, and the HAMA response.

OTHER CLINICAL APPLICATIONS. For diagnosis, MoAbs may be used in the serologic detection of clinically unapparent tumors or to aid in the differential diagnosis of tumors that look alike on routinely processed light microscope specimens. The latter field, *immunohistochemistry*, has been used increasingly over the past several years. MoAbs have been used extensively to classify leukemias and lymphomas.[64]

MoAbs have also been used in bone marrow transplantation. One of the more severe complications of allogeneic transplantation is the development of graft-versus-host disease (GVHD). In an attempt to prevent the development of GVHD, MoAbs reactive with immunocompetent T cells are incubated in vitro with donor marrow before the marrow is infused into the recipient. An attractive therapeutic option in this area is the use of MoAbs to purge autologous marrow of lingering malignant cells prior to transplantation. (For a concise review, see Foon.[63,64]

The use of monoclonal antibodies and antibody conjugates continues to progress (Table 23-10). The

Table 23–10 Antibodies in Cancer Therapy

1. Antibodies
   Cytotoxic
   Regulatory
   Immunization
2. Immunoconjugates
   Radiolabeled antibodies
   Chemoimmunoconjugates
   Immunotoxins
   Immunobiologicals
3. Bone marrow transplantation
   Allogeneic
   Autologous

From Dillman RO: Antibody therapy. In Oldham RK, editor: Principles of cancer biotherapy, ed 2, New York, 1991, Marcel Dekker.

future holds further exploration and refinement of this area and investigation into the use of human monoclonal antibodies and chimeric monoclonal antibodies.[24,49,141]

ADMINISTRATION. At present most MoAbs remain investigational. Routes of administration for MoAbs include intravenous, intraarterial, intraperitoneal, and intralymphatic.[186] Dosage depends on investigational protocols and whether the MoAb is being used for diagnostic or therapeutic purposes.

Antibodies are generally diluted in normal saline and administered over several hours via an infusion pump to prevent accidental bolus infusion.[47,48] Handling procedures may vary among institutions; however, appropriate cytotoxic handling procedures should be used with chemoimmunoconjugates and immunotoxins. Radiation safety procedures should be employed whenever radiolabeled MoAbs are used. Pharmacy resource personnel should be consulted regarding filterability, solution compatibility, stability, and other pertinent issues.[188]

SIDE EFFECTS. Allergic reaction to mouse protein is a major concern for patients receiving murine MoAbs. The major acute toxicity is anaphylaxis, manifested as generalized flushing and/or urticaria, followed by pallor and/or cyanosis. Respiratory distress may also occur. If untreated, anaphylaxis can progress to systemic vascular collapse, unconsciousness, and death. Fortunately, its occurrence is rare. Treatment involves immediately stopping the antibody infusion and administering fluids and emergency drugs such as epinephrine, diphenhydramine, and hydrocortisone sodium succinate.

Subacute toxicity includes fever, chills and rigors, diaphoresis, malaise, urticaria, pruritus, nausea, vomiting, dyspnea, and hypotension. Fevers, chills, diaphoresis, and shaking rigors are often seen when MoAbs bind to circulating leukemic cells.[51] These toxicities can occur in the first 24 hours to 1 week after the infusion. They are usually easily treated before or during the infusion with acetaminophen, antihistamines, meperidine, or antiemetics.[47,48,188]

Serum sickness, the major delayed toxicity seen with MoAb therapy, can occur 2 to 4 weeks after infusion. It results from circulating immune complexes deposited in the tissues and presents symptoms such as urticaria, pruritus, arthralgias, generalized adenopathy, and flulike symptoms. Treatment includes aspirin, acetaminophen, and occasionally corticosteroids. Symptoms usually resolve as the complexes are cleared from the body.[48,51]

RETINOIDS

The retinoids are a class of agents consisting of vitamin A (retinol) and related derivatives (all-trans retinoic acid [RA] and 13-cis-retinoic acid [cRA]) that are involved in growth, reproduction, epithelial cell differentiation, and immune function. Specific effects of the retinoids on the immune system include enhancement of humoral antibody responses and certain cell-mediated immune responses, and improved phagocytosis by macrophages. The biologic effects of retinoids appear to occur from changes in gene expression that occur via specific nuclear receptors. Retinol and retinoic acid (RA) are known to bind to cellular retinol or RA binding proteins. These proteins facilitate the transfer of RA and retinol from the cytoplasm to the nucleus, where they bind to one of several nuclear RA receptors. This ultimately leads to the transcription of appropriate target genes through binding to specific DNA sequences.[207]

Preclinical studies with RA have demonstrated several potentially beneficial effects: induction of cell differentiation in both normal epithelial cells and certain tumor cell lines, and direct growth inhibition with/ without differentiation. Due to the unique biology of the retinoids, a number of clinical trials are evaluating their use in the treatment of cancer patients. Toxicity in these trials can be classified according to mucocutaneous, visual, skeletal, lipid, liver and teratogenic side-effects. Mucocutaneous toxicities are generally the most troublesome and include dryness of the mucosal tissues, erythema and desquamation of the skin, and chelitis. Due to the strong teratogenic effect of the retinoids, extreme caution should be exercised to avoid their use during pregnancy.[114,207]

A series of clinical studies with oral RA have demonstrated high complete remission rates (CR) in patients with acute promyelocytic leukemia (APL). Although many responses are not lasting despite continued therapy, the role of RA alone and in combination with conventional therapy for APL continues to be evaluated. Additional clinical trials, both phase I and II, are evaluating the use of RA in myelodysplastic syndrome, other hematologic malignancies (multiple myeloma, mycosis fungoides) and solid tumors (cervical, squamous cell cancer of the head and neck, breast, and prostate carcinoma).[207]

Another exciting area is the use of retinoids in the chemoprevention of upper aerodigestive tract carcinomas.[18] Clinical trials have evaluated the effectiveness of both natural agents and synthetic retinoids in reversing oral premalignant lesions. A randomized, placebo-controlled trial of 13-cRA has been reported by Hong and associates. Reversal of dysplasia occurred in 54% of the retinoid group and in only 10% of the placebo group. Two significant problems were encountered in this study: toxicity from 13-cRA and a relapse rate of over 50% within 3 months of stopping therapy. A second trial evaluated an induction phase with higher doses (1.5 mg/kg/day) followed by a 9-month maintenance program with either low-dose 13-cRA (0.5 mg/kg/day) or beta-carotene (30 mg/d). Preliminary data demonstrate that the relapse rate after 9 months is 8% in the low-dose 13-cRA group and 55% in the beta-carotene group. Other trials include evaluation of high-dose 13-cRA to prevent second primary tumors (SPT) in patients with squamous cell cancer of the head and neck. With a median followup of 42 months, only 6% of the 13-cRA group developed SPT as compared to 28% of the placebo group. An important direction for future chemoprevention trials will be establishing effective doses that decrease toxicity and evaluation of other retinoids such as RA.[114]

OTHER IMMUNOMODULATING AGENTS

This section briefly reviews agents that either boost immunologic responses (specifically or nonspecifically) or cause the induction of cytokines. Although many of these agents were more actively investigated in the 1960s and 1970s, they may still be encountered today. For example, they may now be used alone via different routes (intraperitoneal, intrapleural), or smaller subunits may be used in an attempt to elicit an immune response. Further possible uses include the combination of these agents with newer BRMs.

Bacillus Calmette-Guerin

Bacillus Calmette-Guerin (BCG) was used in first-generation immunotherapy trials.[86] Developed in the early 1900s, it is an attenuated form of the living bovine tubercle bacillus. It is believed to have a nonspecific immunostimulating effect. The initial work with BCG in animal models was done by Old and coworkers,[143] who demonstrated that BCG could stimulate the reticuloendothelial system and the immune response. Clinical trials reported by Mathé[120] in 1969 demonstrated positive therapeutic results of BCG therapy for children with acute lymphocytic leukemia (ALL). Although early trials with BCG in a multitude of settings appeared promising, further investigations did not support these results.[86,186] Trials with BCG continue. When one is comparing results of clinical trials with BCG, it is of prime importance to note variability in the strains of BCG used (Pasteur, Glaxo, Phipps, and so on), route of administration, dosage, and schedule. BCG is approved for the treatment of bladder cancer by intravesical instillation.[189]

BCG can be administered intralesionally; intradermally by scarification, the tine technique, or the Heafgun; or intracavitarily (to the pleura, peritoneum, or bladder). Side effects can include local inflammatory reactions, flulike symptoms, hypersensitivity, and the serious complication of disseminate BCG infection.

Levamisole

Levamisole is an orally active synthetic agent that is an isomer of tetramisole, a broad-spectrum antihelminthic agent.

Ergamisol® (Levamisole)[99] is now approved by the FDA for use with 5-FU as an adjuvant treatment for colon cancer (Duke's stage C). A randomized study showed Duke's C patients treated with levamisole and fluorouracil to have a higher 5-year survival rate than untreated patients.[112] Toxicity has been minimal with levamisole alone, and no more severe than expected for flourouracil alone, when the two drugs were combined.

Tumor Antigens

This form of therapy rests on the premise that tumor cells express immunogenic determinants that are not associated or that are associated to a lesser degree with normal cells. The immune system will theoretically recognize these cells as foreign and mount an immunologic response. Tumor vaccines employ tumor cells or purified components of tumor cell membrane. To increase the immunogenicity of the cells, the surface is often treated with viruses, irradiation, or neuramidase. Tumor vaccines are also given in combination with other immunostimulants such as BCG or *C. parvum*. Vaccines are usually administered by multiple intradermal injections, with patients receiving vaccines prepared from their own tumor cells. Although historically this approach has been unsuccessful, recent randomized phase II trials to evaluate active specific immunotherapy in colorectal cancer have proved efficacy. One hindrance has been the technical limitations of such individualized vaccines. The process is technologically complex, labor intensive, and expensive. Research with monoclonal antibodies may lead to the characterization and purification of reactive antigenic molecules that could be mass produced as a generic vaccine.[83]

Text continued on p. 553.

Nursing Management

Caring for patients receiving biotherapy can be challenging and exciting. For both the experienced and the novice oncology nurse, it represents a new focus. Many BRMs are now available for commercial use. With continuing research, biotherapy advances over the next few years will be exponential. Nurses working in this area have an opportunity to be on the cutting edge in developing standards of care for patients receiving biotherapy. Although for biotherapy the mode of action and pattern of toxicity differ from those for chemotherapy, nurses can draw on their expertise in management of chemotherapy-related side effects to meet the challenge of dealing with side effects unique to biotherapy.

POSSIBLE NURSING DIAGNOSES FOR PATIENTS RECEIVING BIOTHERAPY

Neurologic function
- Sensory/perceptual alterations (specify)
- Sleep pattern disturbance
- Social interaction, impaired
- Thought processes, altered

Renal function
- Urinary elimination, altered patterns

Hematologic function
- Potential for injury re: weakness or bleeding
- Potential for infection re: decreased WBC
- Activity intolerance re: anemia

Skin
- Skin integrity, impaired

Gastrointestinal system
- Nutrition altered less than body requirements
- Diarrhea
- Oral mucous membranes, altered
- Skin integrity, impaired, potential re: diarrhea

Cardiovascular system
- Tissue perfusion, altered re: hypotension
- Fluid volume deficit

Pulmonary system
- Impaired gas exchange, potential
- Anxiety re: respiratory distress

Miscellaneous
- Fatigue
- Activity intolerance

- Body temperature, altered, potential
- Pain
- Self-care deficit
- Knowledge deficit (specify)

Psychosocial adjustment
- Coping, ineffective, individual or family
- Decisional conflict (specify)
- Hopelessness
- Sexuality patterns, altered

ASSESSMENT AND PLANNING

From the first encounter, nurses play a key role in managing patients on biotherapy. (For the purposes of this chapter, the word *patient* will be assumed to include patient and family when applicable.) The physician will generally obtain a detailed history and physical examination before placing a patient on therapy. The physician explains the purpose of therapy, the treatment schedule, associated side effects, and financial concerns as appropriate. The physician also obtains informed consent when applicable. It is important that nurses understand the ethical and legal foundations of informed consent, for they serve as both educator and advocate for the patient.[100,118,169,188,220] The nurse may have to answer many questions the patient is either afraid or embarrassed to ask the physician. Within the scope of independent nursing practice, the nurse can do much to reinforce information and clarify misconceptions. Assessing whether patients understand their therapeutic plan is crucial, and this information should be relayed to other members of the health care team as appropriate.

The nurse should perform a baseline assessment using a body systems approach, including psychosocial concerns, before the patient starts therapy. This should include current symptoms related to disease or previous treatment, level of functional status, and hopes, fears, and expectations related to therapy. A medication profile should also be obtained, as many medications are contraindicated with certain biologic agents or can contribute to side effects. Initial assessment should also include evaluation of the patient's support systems. When biotherapy trials are investigational, the patient often receives therapy away from home and usual support systems. Patients may be concerned about finances; appropriate housing; family, friends, and job while they are away; loneliness; and fear of the unknown. It is especially helpful to allow patients to voice their concerns and resolve problems through appropriate referrals.

The nurse plays a crucial role in assessment of and tolerance to side effects while patients are on therapy. A basic understanding of the biology, mode of action, and side effects (acute and chronic) of the agent being administered are a must. This knowledge can be applied through regular, systematic assessment of the patient. It is necessary to evaluate symptoms for duration, frequency, and severity in order to plan appropriate care. Information and care plans should be documented in the patient's medical record.

The nurse must also assess the therapeutic plan in order to develop a plan of care and intervene appropriately. Such questions include the following:
- Will the therapy be given in the hospital, in an ambulatory care setting, or both? In the ambulatory care setting, assessment of the patient's compliance with the therapeutic plan is especially important.
- What types of laboratory tests (routine lab work, special lab work, and pharmacology) and diagnostic procedures will be required?
  What agent or agents will the patient receive, and what are the associated side effects?
- Is the agent under investigation or FDA approved?
- If under investigation, has informed consent been secured?
- What is the nature of the agent? Are there special handling precautions or storage requirements? Are any special equipment or emergency supplies needed?
- What type of teaching will the patient need (self-administration techniques, side effects and management, and so on)?
- What type of monitoring will be required? Are special vital signs necessary, such as orthostatic blood pressures?

With thorough assessment both before and during therapy the nurse can better formulate and update the patient's plan of care.*

HANDLING ISSUES

As previously mentioned, handling issues are of concern to all oncology nurses. Policies and procedures governing safe handling of cytotoxic agents during preparation, administration, and disposal are well established nationwide. However, there has been no formal research to date regarding the safest way to handle biologic agents. The nurse is advised to check institutional policy regarding handling of BRMs at the place of employment. The majority of BRMs do not directly affect DNA and are therefore not considered genotoxic substances. However, many institutions place them in the category of cytotoxic products requiring special handling. In the future, new generation BRMs may require special handling. The addition of chemotherapeutic agents or toxins to BRMs would necessitate special handling, and the addition of ra-

*References 24, 47, 91, 94, 100, 101, 122, 147, 188.

dioisotopes would require appropriate radiation safety procedures.

MANAGEMENT OF SIDE EFFECTS
Neurologic Side Effects

To ensure prompt recognition of CNS toxicity, patients should be assessed before therapy for baseline data and regularly during therapy for changes in level of consciousness, orientation, and mental status. Changes should be reported to the physician. The nurse should also evaluate the patient's medication profile for other drugs that can contribute to CNS toxicity. The patient should be taught which signs and symptoms to report. Family members are often the first to recognize subtle changes and should be encouraged to report them to the health care team. Often the nurse and the patient together can creatively deal with minor CNS changes, such as slowed thinking, decreased concentration, and memory problems.*

For more serious problems such as confusion, disorientation, and somnolence, safety concerns arise. Patients should be protected from injury when appropriate with fall precautions or bed sensors. Patients should be reoriented as needed. Especially in the intensive care unit, the nurse should allow normal periods of sleep and rest.

Patients on BRMs may suffer from depression. Allowing patients to verbalize their feelings is often helpful. However, a psychiatric consultation should take place when appropriate.

For a review of BRM related side effects and their frequency of occurrence see Table 23-11.

Renal Side Effects

In all treatment settings, patients should be evaluated for renal toxicity through assessment of BUN and creatinine levels, and changes should be reported to the physician. With IL-2 therapy, renal toxicity is more problematic. Patients should be placed on strict intake and output and be weighed regularly. Urine output is often decreased; therefore, intake and output will not usually balance. The physician usually sets a minimum output per shift that can be used as a guideline for reporting changes. Nursing also includes administration of fluids, diuretics, and pressors as ordered.[151,169,188,205]

Hematologic Side Effects

Patients are monitored for changes in complete blood count, including differential and platelet counts. When ordered, the coagulation profile should also be assessed. Signs and symptoms to report should be taught to the patient along with appropriate precautions (bleeding precautions for thrombocytopenia,

measures to guard against infection should white counts decrease, and conservation of energy for anemia) if a problem develops. Replacement therapy with blood and platelets should be administered as ordered.

Hepatic Side Effects

Nursing includes assessing the patient for changes in serum transaminases and bilirubin and for jaundice or hepatomegaly. Nursing diagnoses should be formulated as appropriate.

Skin Changes

Skin changes are most commonly seen with IL-2 and retinoid therapy, although rashes have been reported with IFN and GM-CSF. The baseline assessment of skin condition should include history of underlying skin conditions such as psoriasis. Patients should be taught signs and symptoms to be expected as well as an appropriate skin care routine. Skin should be observed daily for signs of infection and breakdown. Therapeutic measures for dry skin include gentle cleansing (avoid scrubbing the skin), tepid versus hot baths, frequent use of water-based lotions and creams, soft cotton clothing, and bath oils.[39,151,169,188,205] Patients should be taught to avoid the use of perfumed lotion, as it can further irritate already sensitive skin. Pruritus can also be a major problem. Helpful measures include antipruritic medications (often with around the clock administration), soft clothing, and the use of colloidal oatmeal baths.[41] In some cases a room humidifier has been helpful.[169] It is important to caution patients against the use of topical steroids, as this is contraindicated in many IL-2 protocols.

Irritation with resultant erythema and swelling may occur at subcutaneous injection sites. Patients should be reassured that this inflammatory reaction usually resolves in several days. Generally no treatment is necessary; however, if applications of cold or heat are considered, they should be verified with the physician.

Gastrointestinal Side Effects

Teaching the patient to maintain nutritional status is of prime importance, because anorexia and weight loss over time are common side effects of many biologics.[94,121] Baseline nutritional status and dietary intake should be assessed and documented. Measures commonly used with other oncology patients such as small, frequent meals and calorie supplements are appropriate here. A dietary consultant should be used as necessary. If weight loss becomes significant, tube feedings or hyperalimentation may have to be considered. Antiemetics usually abate nausea and vomiting; however, with IL-2 more aggressive around-the-clock therapy is usually necessary. Prophylactic an-

---

*References 82, 91, 100, 151, 169, 188, 205.

Table 23–11   Side Effects of Biological Response Modifiers

Agent	Alteration in Hematologic Lab Values	Alteration in Mental Status	Anaphylaxis	Anorexia	Bone Pain	Bronchospasm	Capillary Leak Syndrome	Chills	Desquamation	Diarrhea	Edema, Peripheral	Edema, Pulmonary	Fever	Fluid Retention	Flushing	Headache	Hives	Hypotension	Liver Enzymes	Mucositis	Myalgias	Nausea	Pruritis	Rash	Tachycardia	Weight Loss	Weight Gain	Other Side Effects
Interferon alpha and beta	+	O	R	+	O	R	R	+	R	O	R	R	+	R	O	+	R	O	+	R	+	O	O	O	O	+	R	Fever dissipates after first week
Interferon gamma	+	O	R	+	O	R	R	+	R	O	R	R	+	R	O	+	R	+	+	R	+	O	O	O	O	+	R	Fever higher and more persistent
GM-CSF‡	+	O	R	O	O	R	O	O*	R	O	R	R	+	R	O	O	R	O†	R	R		O	O	O	O	O	O	Erythema at injection site
G-CSF‡	+‡	R	R	R	O	R	R	R	R	R	R	R	R	R	O	R	R	R	O	R	R	R	R	R	R	R	R	
Monoclonal antibodies	O	R	O	O	R	O	O	O	R	R	R	R	O	R	O	O	O	O	R	R		R	O	O	O	R	R	Side effects depend on what is attached
Tumor necrosis factor	+	O	R	+	R	R	R	+	R	O	R	R	+	R	R	+	R	O	O	R	+	O	R	R	O	+	R	Severe rigors
Interleukin-2	+	O	R	+	R	R	+	+	O	+	+	O	+	+	+	+	R	+	+	O	+	+	+	+	+	+	+	Weight gain during treatment and weight loss (occurs over time due to decrease in appetite)

*Dose-dependent; as dose increases, chills are more regularly seen preceding fever.
†Patients may exhibit 10–20 mm decreases in systolic blood pressure; however, symptomatic hypotension is generally seen at higher doses given intravenously.
‡GM-CSF = Granulocyte-macrophage colony-stimulating factor; G-CSF = granulocyte colony-stimulating factor
+ = Common
O = Occasional
R = Rare

From Rumsey KA, Rieger PT, and Harle M: Nursing management of the patient receiving biological response modifiers. In Rumsey KA and Rieger PT, editors. Biological Response Modifiers: A Self Instructional Manual for Health Care Professionals. Chicago, 1992, Precept Press, p. 65.

tiemetic administration and an odor-free environment are often necessary with IL-2. Diarrhea is controlled through the use of antidiarrheal medications. Special consideration should also be given to the skin integrity in the perianal area through assessment, hygienic measures, and the use of barrier creams as indicated.

Mucositis may also occur, especially with IL-2 therapy. The oral cavity should be assessed and its condition documented. A pretreatment oral assessment by the dental oncologist to identify and treat preexisting oral disease may be recommended. Patients should be taught meticulous oral hygiene using saline and baking soda mouth rinses, soft toothbrushes, alterations in diet for comfort, and avoidance of solutions such as commercial mouthwashes that can exacerbate oral dryness. If dryness of oral mucous membranes is extreme, artificial saliva may be helpful.[169]

Cardiovascular/Pulmonary Side Effects

A thorough assessment of cardiopulmonary parameters is important with all biologic agents, but of extreme importance with IL-2 therapy because of the capillary-leak syndrome. Nursing specific for this syndrome includes evaluation of cardiovascular status by monitoring heart rate, blood pressure (including orthostatic checks), central venous pressure as indicated, and other cardiac indices. Accurate daily weight and strict intake and output measures are a must to evaluate fluid imbalances.[39,151,169,188,205] Patients should be assessed for edema and abdominal ascites. They should be taught reportable signs and symptoms and to rise from a lying to a sitting position slowly so as to avoid dizziness that may result from sudden drops in blood pressure. Bed rest may be indicated if systolic blood pressure consistently runs below 80 mm Hg and the patient is symptomatic. Nursing assessment of pulmonary status includes monitoring respiratory rate, ausculation of breath sounds, monitoring lab values of oxygenation, and heeding complaints of shortness of breath or altered breathing patterns. Patients should be taught which signs and symptoms to report and reassured that toxicity is dose related and reversible. Nurses should position patients for maximum respiratory effort.

Constitutional Symptoms

Chills followed by fever are seen with almost all biologic agents.[80] Patients should be told to expect this reaction and that tachyphylaxis will occur. As chills are usually transient and self-limiting, nursing primarily focuses on comfort measures. Patients are often premedicated with acetaminophen or other NSAIDs. They should be kept warm with blankets and warm clothing during chills and be instructed to avoid cold beverages. For severe chills, intravenous meperidine

may be necessary. Fevers are usually controlled with regular administration of acetaminophen. However, for prolonged or extreme temperature elevations, cool sponging or hypothermia blankets may be necessary. When therapy is initiated, vital signs including temperature are usually monitored for the first day or so. Many patients should monitor their temperature several times a day so that fever patterns can be established. One should never assume that all fevers in a patient receiving a BRM are related to it. Variables such as length of time the patient has been receiving the agent, comparison of the fever with the patient's usual fever patterns, spiking fevers in spite of administration of antipyretics, and other signs and symptoms of infection should all be considered. Appropriate interventions can then be instituted. Adequate fluid intake should be encouraged during high fevers to avoid dehydration. Acetaminophen, massage, and heating pads can be used as appropriate to control headache, myalgias, arthralgias, and bone pain.

Fatigue

Fatigue is common with many biologic agents, is usually chronic, and in some instances can be the dose-limiting side effect.[94,167] Its etiology is unknown, so nursing interventions are aimed at helping patients cope with this often distressing side effect. Although few tools can objectively measure fatigue, nurses can document the patient's fatigue by gathering data on the following: contributing factors such as anemia, stressors, depression, and other treatment regimens; diagnosis, disease stage, and prognosis; degree of immobility; manifestations of fatigue; and patterns of fatigue. What factors alleviate versus exacerbate fatigue? When is fatigue the greatest? How long does it persist?

Interventions focus on four areas: conservation of energy, nutritional management, stress management, and management of contributing factors (see Aistars,[2] Irwin,[94] Piper,[157-159] and Rieger[167]). When teaching patients about this side effect and its management, nurses should stress that this fatigue is chronic, not acute, and that more sleep often exacerbates the problem instead of alleviating it. Many patients fear that increased fatigue signals progression of disease. The nurse should reassure such patients that fatigue is an expected side effect of the medication. If fatigue becomes so severe that the patient's functional status is acutely impaired, therapy may have to be stopped or the dosage reduced.[2,157-159,223]

Allergic Reactions

Allergic reactions are most commonly associated with MoAb infusions.[46-48,188] Patients should be monitored regularly for vital signs, many as frequently as every

15 minutes, and observed closely. Emergency drugs must be kept at the bedside and a crash cart on hand. Nursing may include medication of the patient before or during therapy to prevent chills, fever, and urticaria. With certain MoAbs, fever is common, and should be evaluated for its relationship to the course of therapy (early versus late.)[48]

Psychosocial Difficulties

When investigational biotherapy is used, patients often have extreme optimism that therapy is going to help them, especially if there is no effective therapy for their particular disease or if they have failed several courses of therapy. Although hope is important, expectations should be realistic. The nurse can be instrumental in helping patients voice their hopes and fears, answering questions, and discussing patient expectations. Depression is often common, either as a side effect of biologics, related to fatigue, or as a result of failing therapy. The failure of therapy can be extremely difficult for patients, and the nurse's most effective tool is often her presence. Even when a cure is not possible, the nurse can foster hope that something can be done for the patient and reassure the patient that he or she will not be abandoned.

As previously mentioned, patients are often away from their usual support systems. Family dynamics are often disrupted, and therapy may be more difficult to tolerate than anticipated. Support groups, individual counseling, and simply ventilating their feelings to the nurse can all be helpful. Serving as an advocate for the patient, the nurse can make appropriate referrals to help resolve problems.[90]

Patient Instruction

The nurse is responsible for teaching patients about the particular biologic agent or agents they are to receive, for preparing them for participation in experimental trials, for describing side effects and how to cope with them, and for teaching self-administration of the medication.[136,168] Early assessment of the patient for learning needs and barriers (physical, psychological, and verbal deficiencies and dysfunctions), and use of appropriate written and audiovisual materials that will reinforce teaching (Figure 23-5) are key.* A teaching plan specific for the patient can then be formulated and documented in the medical record.

Sufficient time should be allotted to teach patients to administer their medication. This should always be anticipated with interferon therapy and CSFs. Patients need to learn how to reconstitute the medications (if applicable), how to draw up the proper dose, the proper technique for intramuscular or subcutaneous

---

*References 5, 6, 8, 172-180, 191-198.

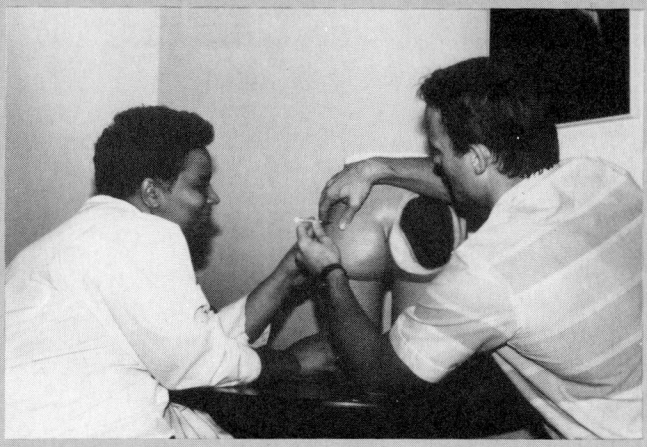

Figure 23–5 Nurse teaching patient self-administration of interferon.

injection, the proper technique for site selection and rotation, storage requirements for the medication, and proper disposal of needles and syringes at home. A variety of vital strengths are available for IFN. The nurse can exercise considerable latitude in selecting a strength that is easy for the patient to use and cost-effective. The nurse also should accommodate dose escalations if applicable without the need to reteach the patient continually. Many biologic agents require refrigeration or freezing, and therefore special arrangements for transport must be made. Patients are also instructed in reportable signs and symptoms. With CNS side effects, changes are often subtle. Family members are usually the first to recognize changes and can report them to the health care team. Many patients are asked to keep a daily log or diary of associated side effects, time and location of injections, and other medications used. If the patient is not self-sufficient, appropriate referrals should be made before discharge. Priorities for patient teaching in biotherapy and geriatric considerations are given in the boxes on p. 552.

Nursing Research

Biotherapy follows a pattern different from that of standard chemotherapy, often lasting months to years. The associated toxicities are complex, chronic, usually subjective, and prone to have a major effect on the quality of life.[25] The etiology of many side effects is unknown; this makes treatment difficult or empirical. A clearer understanding of the nature of these side effects is essential to the development of effective strategies for dealing with them. Biologic therapy is ripe with opportunities for research, including the conduct of nursing research in conjunction with clinical trials.[133]

One difficulty with research in this area is accu-

BIOTHERAPY PATIENT TEACHING PRIORITIES

Assessment

Time available
Learning needs
People available to teach
Barriers to learning
Resources needed

Teaching content

Treatment plan
   Goals of therapy
   Commercial versus investigational agent
   Treatment regimen
   Associated laboratory and diagnostic tests
   Special requirements
Side effects
   Expected side effects
   Management of symptoms experienced
   Reportable signs and symptoms
Self-Administration of BRMs
   Aseptic technique
   Reconstitution of powdered medications
   Drawing up the proper dose
   Proper site selection and rotation
   Administration of the injection
   Storage of the drug
   Proper disposal of equipment at home
Psychosocial/economic concerns
   Coping skills/resources
   Reimbursement resources

Documentation

Time frame for teaching
Patient/significant others taught
Tasks/information disseminated
Resources utilized
Evaluation/need for referrals

GERIATRIC CONSIDERATIONS

Factors affecting medication dosage and administration

- Alterations in hepatic and renal function may necessitate adjustment of dosage and or schedule.

- Decreases in cardiovascular function may require lower doses of biologic response modifiers (BRMs) such as interferon and interleukin-2 whose side effects may stress the cardiovascular system.
- Alterations in neurosensory/perceptual protective mechanisms may place elderly patients at higher risk for problems with CNS associated side effects of BRMs such as confusion, depression, memory loss, or slowed thinking.
- Decreased functional status may place patients at a higher risk for intolerance of fatigue associated with many BRMs.
- Altered nutritional intake (less than body requirements) may be increased due to anorexia associated with some BRMs.
- Decreased tissue, skin and mucous membrane integrity may place patients at higher risk for IL-2-related skin toxicity.
- Evaluation of the patients current medication profile should occur to determine drugs that may be contraindicated with BRMs and/or cause additive toxicity.

Factors affecting patient teaching

- Assess for neuromuscular and sensory deficits (e.g., vision problems, hearing losses, arthritic joints) that may inhibit teaching/learning. Utilize appropriate teaching tools for deficits present (e.g., large print, minimal illustrations for patient with vision problems).
- Assess for reading level and comprehension, as many people 65 and older have completed eight or fewer years of formal schooling. Utilize reading materials targeted for the appropriate reading level and/or audiovisual aids. Reinforce information presented often.

Factors affecting social support systems

- Approximately 30% of patients 65 or older live alone, the majority being women. The difficulties of living alone are often intensified by poverty, having few relatives or other social supports, and decreased functional status.
- Many BRMs are given on an outpatient basis; hence patients are required to learn self-care. Evaluation of formal and informal support networks, functional capacity and economic status should be incorporated into the nursing assessment, and referrals made to community resources as needed.
- Spouses should be evaluated for early indicators of caregiver role strain and appropriate interventions initiated.

Reference Boyle DM, and others: ONS position paper on cancer and aging, *Oncol Nurs Forum*, 19(6):913-933, 1992.

rately measuring symptoms.[65,123] Although observer-rated toxicity scales used in clinical trials have been adapted to accommodate symptoms associated with BRMs, often they are not sensitive enough for research purposes.[142] The subjective nature of most BRM-associated symptoms makes their measurement a challenge. Nursing research efforts need means to quantify side effects before interventions to prevent and control them can be studied.[211]

These research efforts might be focused on the development of tools to measure side effects, determination of the most effective time of drug administration to alleviate side effects, interventions to control or prevent toxicity, evaluation of teaching methods, evaluation of quality of life and symptom distress, and drug handling issues. Such studies have begun; however, a great deal of work remains to be completed.[96,170]

FUTURE DIRECTIONS AND ADVANCES IN BIOTHERAPY

Treatment with biologic agents is becoming more and more widespread, and we will continue to see new agents and novel combinations of agents make their way into the clinical setting.[145,226] It is imperative that oncology nurses be knowledgeable about biotherapy in order to care for patients receiving it. In their roles as educator, advocate, and care giver, nurses are key in facilitating management of patients receiving biologic agents. Over the next few years we will continue to see BRMs receiving FDA approval, which will increase their availability. Clinical trials will continue to define appropriate dosage, route, and clinical indications for many agents and combinations.[138,139] In addition, research efforts are now focusing on delineating the pathophysiology of BRM-associated side effects. It is hoped that these efforts will lead to improved tolerance of the more severe side effects.[165,201]

For years determination of the maximum tolerated dose has been the standard in chemotherapy trials. However, this approach may not be appropriate for biotherapy. Recent attention has focused on determining the optimal immunomodulatory dose. Lower doses may be more effective than the maximum tolerated dose in boosting an immune respone. In addition, determining the full range of biologic effects in vivo will assist in determining dosage. Investigators are also faced with the challenge of developing therapeutic regimens that maximize response yet are tolerable to patients, cost-effective, and realistically managed.[186]

Clinical investigations evaluating combinations of cytokines and of cytokines and chemotherapy continues to be an area of active focus. The availability of recombinant cytokines has led to evaluation of their efficacy in vivo as single-modality cancer therapy. Although clinical benefits have been achieved, few patients have been cured. An additional problem is the toxicity of cytokines when given at high doses. Is there a way to maximize response while achieving acceptable toxicity? Studies in animal models using combinations of cytokines have demonstrated synergism and a resultant increase in antitumor effect. Combining agents may make it possible to use smaller doses while maintaining therapeutic benefit. This has provided a rationale for the use of combinations of cytokines. Examples of combinations being investigated are alpha-IFN and IL-2, TNF and IL-2, and monoclonal antibodies and IL-2. It is hoped that effective combinations of BRMs with or without chemotherapy will result in improved therapeutic benefits and decreased toxicity.[138,139]

An exciting area of focus for the future is gene therapy, defined as the insertion of a functioning gene into the cells of a patient to correct an inborn genetic error or to provide a new function to the cell. Work in this area has been pioneered by Rosenberg and associates at the National Cancer Institute. Trials are in progress evaluating the insertion of the gene for TNF into TIL cells. Theoretically, TILs would secrete large amounts of TNF locally at the tumor site.[182,183]

Another area of promise is evaluation of new hematopoietic growth factors. Stem cell factor (SCF), or kit ligand, is a newly cloned growth factor that has growth promoting activities on a variety of hematopoietic cell lineages.[229] Preclinical studies indicate that SCF targets hematopoietic cells at or near the level of the pluripotent stem cell. SCF has also been shown to synergize with erythropoietin to increase both the number and size of erythrocyte precursors.[117] Clinical trials will soon begin to evaluate its potential therapeutic benefit in patients with cancer. Another factor soon to begin clinical trials is interleukin-6 (IL-6), a pleitropic cytokine involved in defense mechanisms and hematopoiesis. IL-6 was first recognized as acting on B cells to induce immunoglobulin secretion. In vitro work has shown IL-6 to synergize with IL-3 to support the proliferation of multipotent hematopoietic progenitor cells, and to induce the maturation of megakaryocytes. Work is also in progress evaluating the role of IL-6 in human myelomas.[3] Multicenter phase I trials with IL-6 are in progress. Additionally, phase I clinical trials are in progress evaluating a new fusion protein of GM-CSF/IL-3 termed PIXY321. These trials are evaluating its myeloprotective effect postchemotherapy. The future looks very promising for further clinical successes with hematopoietic growth factors.

A final area of concern is reimbursement. Because of recent economic trends in health care, funding agencies and third-party payors are often unwilling to underwrite the cost of phase I and II investigations for drugs not approved by the FDA. In the case of approved agents, they may be unwilling to pay for indications not included in the original FDA approval. Treatment with many BRMs can be costly in both the inpatient and ambulatory care setting; therefore this problem is of major importance to both patients and health care professionals.[224,225] Patients who receive investigational drugs as part of an approved clinical trial receive the drug at no cost; however, they are responsible for all other associated costs. In the case of an FDA-approved drug, patients must pay for the drug. Because extended therapy can be quite expensive, some pharmaceutical companies have programs to assist patients in receiving drugs if they are no longer able to pay or have reached a yearly maximum (cost assistance programs).* In addition, most pharmaceutical companies sponsor reimbursement hotlines that will assist patients and health care professionals with reimbursement concerns.

---

*References 9, 36, 88, 93, 150, 178, 181, 198.

CONCLUSION

Oncology nurses who care for patients receiving biotherapy are on the cutting edge of cancer therapy. They must stay abreast of continual changes, be knowledgeable about therapeutic agents and modalities, and develop standards of care and nursing interventions to manage toxicity. The possibilities for nurses to participate in this exciting new therapeutic modality are limitless.

BIBLIOGRAPHY

1. Adams F, Quesada JR, and Gutterman JU: Neuropsychiatric manifestations of human leukocyte interferon therapy in patients with cancer, JAMA 252:938, 1984.
2. Aistars J: Fatigue in cancer patients: a conceptual approach to a clinical problem, Oncol Nurs Forum 14(6):25, 1987.
3. Akira S and Kishimoto T: The evidence for interleukin-6 as an autocrine growth factor in malignancy, Semin Can Bio 3:17, 1992.
4. Allison AC and Taylor RB: Observations on thymectomy and carcinogenesis, Cancer Res 27:703, 1967.
5. Amgen, Inc. Getting ready for Epogen—Information for our dialysis patients (flip chart). Thousand Oaks, CA: Amgen, 1991.
6. Amgen, Inc. How to give yourself a subcutaneous injection (videotape). Thousand Oaks, CA: Amgen, 1991.
7. Amgen: Neupogen (Filgrastim), package insert, Thousand Oaks, CA, 1991, Amgen, Inc.
8. Amgen, Inc. Self-injection chart: step-by-step guide to subcutaneous self-injection (available English and Spanish). Thousand Oaks, CA: Amgen, 1991.
9. Amgen, Inc. Neupogen reimbursement hotline. (1-800-272-9376). Thousand Oaks, CA: Amgen, 1990.
10. Amgen, Inc., Epogen (Epoetin alfa), package insert, Thousand Oaks, CA, 1989, Amgen, Inc.
11. Andreef M and Welte K: Hematopoietic colony-stimulating factors, Semin Oncol 16(3):211, 1989.
12. Antman KS and others: Effect of recombinant human granulocyte-macrophage colony-stimulating factor on chemotherapy-induced myelosuppression, N Engl J Med 319(10):593, 1988.
13. Atkins MB and others: Phase I evaluation of recombinant interleukin-2 in patients with advanced malignant disease, J Clin Oncol 4(9):1380, 1986.
14. Baird SB (Ed): New perspectives on the management of myelosuppression, Oncol Nurs Forum 18(2) Suppl, 2, 1991.
15. Bajorin DF, Cheung NV, and Houghton AN: Macrophage colony-stimulating factor: Biological effects and potential applications for cancer therapy, Semin Hematol 28(2) Suppl 2:42, 1991.
16. Balkwill FR: Cytokines in cancer therapy, Oxford, 1989, Oxford University Press.
17. Bates SE and Longo DL: Use of serum tumor markers in cancer diagnosis and management, Semin Oncol 14(2):102, 1987.
18. Benner SE, Lippman SM, and Hong WK: Chemoprevention strategies for a lung and upper aerodigestive tract cancer, Cancer Res 52(9) suppl: 2758, 1992.
19. Beutler B and Cerami A: Cachectin: more than a tumor necrosis factor, N Engl J Med 316(7):379, 1987.
20. Blick M and others: Phase I study of recombinant tumor necrosis factor in cancer patients, Cancer Res 47:2986, 1987.
21. Bonnem EM and Oldham RK: Gamma interferon: physiology and speculation on its role in medicine, J Biol Response Mod 6:275, 1987.
22. Brandt SJ and others: Effects of recombinant human granulocyte-macrophage colony-stimulating factor on hematopoietic reconstitution after high-dose chemotherapy and autologous bone marrow transplantation, N Engl J Med 318 (14):869, 1988.
23. Bronchud MH and others: Phase I/II study of recombinant human granulocyte colony-stimulating factor in patients receiving intensive chemotherapy for small cell lung cancer, Br J Cancer 56:809, 1987.
24. Brophy LR and Rieger PT: Biotherapy. In Clark JC and McGee RF, editors: Core curriculum for oncology nursing, ed 2, Philadelphia, 1992, WB Saunders Co.
25. Brophy LR and Sharp EJ: Physical symptoms of combination biotherapy: A quality-of-life issue, Oncol Nurs Forum 18(1) suppl:25, 1991.
26. Brown BA and others: Tumor-specific genetically engineered murine/human chimeric monoclonal antibody, Cancer Res 47:3577, 1987.
27. Brown SL, Miller RA, and Levy R: Antiidiotype antibody therapy of B-cell lymphoma, Semin Oncol 16(3):199, 1989.
28. Budd GT and others: Phase I trial of subcutaneous (SQ) recombinant monocyte/macrophage-colony stimulating factor (rM-CSF) in patients with refractory malignancies, Blood 78(10) Suppl 1:8, 1991.
29. Burnet FM: The concept of immunological surveillance, Prog Exp Tumor Res 13:1, 1970.
30. Cannistra SA and Griffin JD: Regulation of the production and function of granulocytes and monocytes, Semin Hematol 25(3):173, 1988.
31. Cantell K and Hirvonen S: Preparation of human leukocyte interferon for clinical use, Tex Rep Biol Med 35:138, 1977.

32. Carroll-Johnson RM (Ed): A case management approach to patients receiving G-CSF. Oncology Nursing Society Monograph, 1992, Oncology Nursing Press, Inc.

33. Cebon J and others: Pharmacokinetics of human granulocyte-macrophage colony-stimulating factor using a sensitive immunoassay, Blood 72:1093, 1988.

34. Cetus Oncology Corp: Proleukin® (Aldesleukin) for injection, package insert, Emeryville, CA, 1992, Cetus Oncology Corp.

35. Chapman P and others: Clinical pharmacology of recombinant human tumor necrosis factor in patients with advanced cancer, J Clin Oncol 5:1942, 1987.

36. Chiron Corporation. Proleukin reimbursement line (1-800-775-7533). San Francisco, CA: Chiron, 1992.

37. Clark J and Longo D: Biological response modifiers, Mediguide Oncol 6(2):1, 1986.

38. Clark SC and Kamen R: The human hematopoietic colony-stimulating factors, Science 236:1229, 1987.

39. Corey BS and Collins JL: Implementation on an rIL-2/LAK cell clinical trial: a nursing perspective, Oncol Nurs Forum 13(6):31, 1986.

40. Crown J and others: A phase I trial of recombinant human interleukin-1 alone and in combination with myelosuppressive doses of 5-fluorouracil in patients with gastrointestinal cancer, Blood 78(6), 1420, 1991.

41. Dangel RB: Pruritus and cancer, Oncol Nurs Forum 13(1):17, 1986.

42. Dawson MM: Lymphokines and interleukins, Boca Raton, 1991, CRC Press.

43. Denicoff KD and others: The neuropsychiatric effects of interleukin-2/Lymphokine activated killer cell therapy, Ann Intern Med 107:293, 1987.

44. Dennis D and others: Biologic activity of interleukin 1 (IL-1) alpha in patients with refractory malignancies: Proc ASCO 11: #830, 1992.

45. DeVita VJ, Hellman S, and Rosenberg SA, editors: Biologic therapy of cancer, Philadelphia, 1991, JB Lippincott Co.

46. DiJulio JE: Treatment of B-cell and T-cell lymphomas with monoclonal antibodies, Semin Oncol Nurs 4(2):102, 1988.

47. Dillman JB: New antineoplastic therapies and inherent risks: monoclonal antibodies, biologic response modifiers, and interleukin-2, J Intravenous Nurs 12(2):103, 1989.

48. Dillman JB: Toxicity of monoclonal antibodies in the treatment of cancer, Semin Oncol Nurs 4(2):107, 1988.

49. Dillman RO: Antibody therapy. In RK Oldham, editor: Principles of cancer biotherapy, New York, 1991, Marcel Dekker.

50. Dillman RO: Monoclonal antibodies for treating cancer, Ann Intern Med 111:592, 1989.

51. Dillman RO and others: Toxicities and side effects associated with intravenous infusions of monoclonal antibodies, J Biol Response Mod 5:73, 1986.

52. Dinarello CA: Interleukin-1 and interleukin-1 antagonism, Blood 77(8):1627, 1991.

53. Dinarello CA and Mier JW: Lymphokines, N Engl J Med 317(15):940, 1987.

54. Donahue RE and others: Stimulation of hematopoiesis in primates by continuous infusion of recombinant human GM-CSF, Nature 321:872, 1986.

55. Ehrlich P: Studies in immunity, ed 2, New York, 1910, Wiley & Sons.

56. Eschbach JW and others: Correction of the anemia of end-stage renal disease with recombinant human erythropoietin, N Engl J Med 316(2):73, 1987.

57. Farrell MM: The challenge of adult respiratory distress syndrome during interleukin-2 therapy, Oncol Nurs Forum 19(3):475, 1992.

58. Fazio MT and Glaspy JA: The impact of granulocyte colony-stimulating factor on quality of life in patients with severe chronic neutropenia, Oncol Nurs Forum 18(8):1411, 1991.

59. Feinberg B and others: A phase I trial of intravenously administered recombinant tumor necrosis factor alpha in cancer patients, J Clin Oncol 6(8):1328, 1988.

60. Figlin RA: Biotherapy with interferon-1988, Semin Oncol 15(6) suppl 6:3, 1988.

61. Figlin RA and Itri LM: Anti-interferon antibodies: a perspective, Semin Hematol 25(suppl 3):9, 1988.

62. Figlin RA and others: Concomitant administration of recombinant human interleukin-2 and recombinant interferon alfa-2a: an active outpatient regimen in metastatic renal cell carcinoma, J Clin Oncol 10(3):414, 1992.

63. Foon KA: Biological response modifiers: the new immunotherapy, Cancer Res 49:1621, 1989.

64. Foon KA: Laboratory and clinical applications of monoclonal antibodies for leukemias and non-Hodgkins lymphomas, Curr Probl Cancer 13(2):63, 1989.

65. Frank-Stromborg M, editor: Instruments for clinical nursing research, Boston, MA, 1992, Jones & Bartlett.

66. Frei E and Spriggs D: Tumor necrosis factor: still a promising agent, J Clin Oncol 7(3):291, 1989.

67. Freimann J and others: Phase I studies of recombinant human interleukin-4 (IL-4), Proc ASCO 10, #725, 1991.

68. Gabrilove JL: Colony-stimulating factors: clinical status. In DeVita VT Jr, Hellman S, and Rosen-

berg SA, editors: Important advances in oncology, Philadelphia, 1991, JB Lippincott Co.

69. Gabrilove JL and others: Effect of granulocyte colony-stimulating factor on neutropenia and associated morbidity due to chemotherapy for transitional-cell carcinoma of the urothelium, N Engl J Med 318(22):1414, 1988.

70. Galazka AR and others: Lymphokines and cytokines. In RK Oldham, editor: Principles of cancer biotherapy, New York, 1991, Marcel Dekker.

71. Gallucci B: The immune system and cancer, Oncol Nurs Forum 14(suppl 6):3, 1987.

72. Gambacorti-Passerini C and Sondell PM: Problems, controversies, and perspectives on the clinical use of interleukin-2, Curr Opinion Oncol 2:1139, 1990.

73. Genentech: Actimmune (Interferon gamma 1b), package insert, San Francisco, CA, 1991, Genentech, Inc.

74. Glaspy JA and others: Therapy for neutropenia in hairy cell leukemia with recombinant granulocyte colony-stimulating factor, Ann Intern Med 109(10):789, 1988.

75. Glaspy JA and Golde DW: Clinical applications of the myeloid growth factors, Semin Hematol 26(2) suppl 2:14, 1989.

76. Goldstein D and others: Interferon therapy in cancer. In RK Oldham, editor: Principles of cancer biotherapy, New York, 1991, Marcel Dekker.

77. Groopman JE and others: Effect of recombinant human granulocyte-macrophage colony-stimulating factor on myelopoiesis in the acquired immunodeficiency syndrome, N Engl J Med 317(10):593, 1987.

78. Grossbard ML and Nadler LM: Immunotoxin therapy of malignancy. In DeVita VT Jr, Hellman S, and Rosenberg SA, editors: Important advances in oncology, Philadelphia, 1991, JB Lippincott Co.

79. Gutterman JU and others: Recombinant leukocyte A IFN: pharmacokinetics, single dose tolerance, and biologic effects in cancer patients, Ann Intern Med 96(5):549, 1982.

80. Haeuber D: Recent advances in the management of biotherapy-related side effects: flu-like syndrome, Oncol Nurs Forum 16(suppl 6):35, 1989.

81. Haeuber D and DiJulio JE: Hemopoietic colony stimulating factors: An overview, Oncol Nurs Forum 16(2):247, 1989.

82. Hahn MB and Jassak PF: Nursing management of patients receiving interferon, Semin Oncol Nurs 4(2):95, 1988.

83. Hanna MG and others: Fundamental and applied aspects of successful active specific immunotherapy of cancer. In RK Oldham, editor: Principles of cancer biotherapy, New York, 1991, Marcel Dekker.

84. Harris DT and Mastrangelo MJ: Serotherapy of cancer, Semin Oncol 16(3):180, 1989.

85. Heberman RB: Interleukin-2 therapy of human cancer: potential benefits versus toxicity, J Clin Oncol 7(1):1, 1989.

86. Hersh EM, Gutterman JU, and Mavligit G, editors: Immunotherapy of cancer in man: scientific basis and current status, Springfield, IL, 1973, Charles C Thomas.

87. Hoechst-Roussel Pharmaceuticals, Inc.: Prokine, package insert, Sommerville, NJ, Hoechst-Roussel, 1991.

88. Hoechst-Roussel Pharmaceuticals, Inc.: The Hoechst reimbursement information service (1-800-PROKINE). Sommerville, NJ: Hoechst-Roussel, 1991.

89. Hoelzer D, Seipelt G, and Ganser A: Interleukin 3 alone and in combination with GM-CSF in the treatment of patients with neoplastic disease, Semin Hematol 28(2) Suppl 2:17, 1991.

90. Hogan CM: Coping with biotherapy: physiological and psychosocial concerns, Oncol Nurs Forum 18(1) Suppl 1:19, 1991.

91. Hood LE and Abernathy E: Biological response modifiers. In Baird SB, McCorckle R, and Grant M, editors: Cancer nursing: comprehensive textbook, Philadelphia, 1991, WB Saunders Co.

92. Immunex Corporation: Leukine (Sargramostim), package insert, Seattle, WA, 1991, Immunex Corp.

93. Immunex Corporation: A reimbursement support program for Leukine (1-800-321-4669). Seattle, WA: Immunex, 1990.

94. Irwin MM: Patients receiving biologic response modifiers: overview of nursing care, Oncol Nurs Forum 14(6) (suppl 6):32, 1987.

95. Isaacs A and Lindemann J: Virus interference, Proc Soc Biol 147:257, 1957.

96. Jackson BS and others: Long-term biopsychosocial effects of interleukin-2 therapy, Oncol Nurs Forum 18(4):683, 1991.

97. Jakubowski A and others: A phase I trial of recombinant human IL-4 (rhIL-4) in patients with advanced cancer, Blood 78(10) Suppl 1: 427a (#1698), 1991.

98. Jansen JH and others: Interleukin-4: A regulatory protein, Blut 60:269, 1990.

99. Janssen Pharmaceutica: Ergamisol (levamisole hydrochloride), package insert, Piscataway, NJ, 1990, Janssen Pharmaceutica, Inc.

100. Jassak PF: Biotherapy. In Groenwald SL, Hansen Frogge M, Goodman M, and Yarbro CH, editors: Cancer nursing: principles and practice, ed 3, Boston, 1993, Jones and Bartlett.

101. Jassak PF and Ryan MP: Ethical issues in clinical research, Semin Oncol Nurs 5(2):102, 1989.

102. Kalnicki S and Bloomer WD: Antibody radiotherapy: current status. In Zalutsky MR, editor: Antibodies in radiodiagnosis and therapy, Boca Raton, CRC Press.

103. Kirkwood JM and Ernstoff MS: Interferons in the treatment of human cancer, J Clin Oncol 2(4):336, 1984.

104. Kirkwood JM and others: Comparison of intramuscular and intravenous recombinant-alpha 2 interferon in melanoma and other cancers, Ann Intern Med 103(1):32, 1985.

105. Kohler G and Milstein C: Continuous cultures of fused cells secreting antibody of predefined specificity, Nature 256:495, 1975.

106. Kolitz JE and Mertelsmann R: The immunotherapy of human cancer with interleukin-2: present status and future directions, Cancer Investig 9(5):529, 1991.

107. Kovach JS and Gleich GJ: Eosinophilia and fluid retention in systemic administration of interleukin-2, J Clin Oncol 4(5):815, 1986.

108. Kozeny GA and others: Effects of interleukin-2 immunotherapy on renal function, J Clin Oncol 6(7):1170, 1988.

109. Krown SE, Jacubowski A, and Houghton A: Biologic response modifiers. In Wittes RE, editor: Manual of oncologic therapeutics 1991/1992, Philadelphia, 1991, JB Lippincott Co.

110. Krueger GRF: Abnormal variation of the immune system as related to cancer. In Herberman RB, editor: Influence of the host on tumor development, Dordrecht, 1989, Kluwer Academic Publishers.

111. Kurzrock R and others: Phase I study of recombinant human interleukin-3 in patients with bone marrow failure, J Clin Oncol 9(7):1241, 1991.

112. Laurie JA and others: Surgical adjuvant therapy of large-bowel carcinoma: an evaluation of levamisole and the combination of levamisole and fluorouracil, J Clin Oncol 7(10):1447, 1989.

113. Lee RE and others: Cardiorespiratory effects of immunotherapy with IL-2, J Clin Oncol 7(1):7, 1989.

114. Lippman SM and Hong WK: Retinoid chemoprevention of upper aerodigestive tract carcinogenesis. In DeVita VT Jr, Hellman S, and Rosenberg SA, editors: Important advances in oncology, Philadelphia, 1991, JB Lippincott Co.

115. Lotze MT and others: In vivo administration of purified human interleukin-2: I. Half-life and immunologic effects of the Jurkat cell line derived IL-2, J Immunol 134:157, 1985.

116. Lotze MT and others: In vivo administration of purified human interleukin-2: II. Half life, immunologic effects and expansion of peripheral lymphoid cells in vivo with recombinant IL-2, J Immunol 135:2865, 1985.

117. Lyman AD and Williams DE: Biological activities and potential therapeutic uses of steel factor, Am J Ped Hem/Oncol 14(1):1, 1992.

118. Lynch M, Yanes L, and Todd R: Nursing care of AIDS patients participating in a phase I/II trial of recombinant human granulocyte-macrophage colony-stimulating factor, Oncol Nurs Forum 15(4):463, 1988.

119. Maluish AE and others: The determination of an immunobiologically active dose of interferon gamma in patients with melanoma, J Clin Oncol 6(3):434, 1988.

120. Mathé G and others: Active immunotherapy for acute lymphoblastic leukemia, Lancet 1:697, 1969.

121. Mayer D and others: Weight loss in patients receiving recombinant leukocyte-A interferon (IFNrA): a brief report, Cancer Nurs 7:53, 1984.

122. Mayer DK: Biotherapy: recent advances and nursing implications, Nurs Clin N Am 25(2):291, 1990.

123. McCorkle R and Young K: Development of a symptom distress scale, Cancer Nurs 1(3):373, 1978.

124. Mendelsohn J: Antibodies to growth factors and receptors. In DeVita VT Jr, Hellman S, and Rosenberg SA, editors: Biologic therapy of cancer, Philadelphia, 1991, JB Lippincott Co.

125. Mertelsmann R and Herrmann F, editors: Hematopoietic growth factors in clinical applications, New York, 1990, Marcel Dekker.

126. Metcalf D: The colony-stimulating factors: discovery, development and clinical applications, Cancer 65(10):2185, 1990.

127. Metcalf D: The granulocyte-macrophage colony-stimulating factors, Science 229:16, 1985.

128. Michie HR and others: Detection of circulating tumor necrosis factor after endotoxin administration, N Engl J Med 318(23):1481, 1988.

129. Mihich E and Fefer A, editors: Biological response modifiers: subcommittee report, Natl Cancer Inst Monogr, p. 63, 1983.

130. Mitsuyasu RT: The role of alpha interferon in the biotherapy of hematologic malignancies and AIDS-related Kaposi's sarcoma, Oncol Nurse Forum 15(6) Suppl 6:7, 1988.

131. Moldawer N and Figlin R: Tumor necrosis factor: Current clinical status and implications for nursing management, Semin Oncol Nurs 4(2):120, 1988.

132. Moore MAS: Does stem cell exhaustion result from combining hematopoietic growth factors with chemotherapy? If so, how do we prevent it? Blood 80(1):3, 1992.

133. Mooney KH and others: 1991 Oncology Nursing Society research priorities survey, Oncol Nurs Forum 18(8):1381, 1991.

134. Morgan DA, Ruscetti FW, and Gallo RC: Selective in vitro growth of T lymphocytes from normal human bone marrows, Science 193:1007, 1976.

135. Morice RC and others: Pulmonary toxicity of recombinant tumor necrosis factor (rTNF), Proc Am Soc Clin Oncol 6:29, 1987 (abstract).

136. Morra ME and Grant M (Eds.): Cancer patient education, Semin Oncol Nurs 7(2):79, 1991.

137. Morstyn G and others: Treatment of chemotherapy-induced neutropenia by subcutaneously administered granulocyte colon-stimulating factor with optimization of dose and duration of therapy, J Clin Oncol 1(10):1554, 1989.

138. Mulé JJ and Rosenberg SA: Combination cytokine therapy: Experimental and clinical trials. In DeVita VT Jr, Hellman S, and Rosenberg SA, editors: Biologic Therapy of Cancer, Philadelphia, 1991, JB Lippincott Co.

139. Mulé JJ and Rosenberg SA: Immunotherapy with lymphokine combinations. In DeVita VT, Hellman S, and Rosenberg SA, editors: Important advances in oncology, Philadelphia, 1991, JB Lippincott Co.

140. Oettgen HF and Old LJ: The history of cancer immunotherapy. In DeVita VT Jr, Hellman S, and Rosenberg SA, editors: Biologic therapy of cancer, Philadelphia, 1991, JB Lippincott Co.

141. Oi V and Morrison SL: Chimeric antibodies, Biotechniques 4:214, 1987.

142. Oken MM and others: Toxicity and response criteria of the Eastern Cooperative Oncology Group, Am J Clin Oncol 5(6):649, 1982.

143. Old LJ and others: The role of the reticuloendothelial system in the host reaction to neoplasia, Cancer Res 21:1281, 1961.

144. Oldham RK: Biotherapy: general principles. In Oldham RK, editor: Principles of cancer biotherapy, ed 2, New York, 1991, Marcel Dekker.

145. Oldham RK: Speculations for the 1990s. In RK Oldham, editor: Principles of cancer biotherapy, New York, 1991, Marcel Dekker.

146. Oldham RK and Smalley RV: Immunotherapy: the old and the new, J Biol Response Mod 2:1, 1983.

147. Oncology Nursing Society: Biological response modifiers: guidelines and recommendations for nursing practice, Pittsburgh, 1989, The Oncology Nursing Society.

148. Oratz R and others: Antimelanoma monoclonal antibody—ricin A chain immunoconjugate (XMMME-001-RTA) plus cyclophosphamide in the treatment of metastatic malignant melanoma: results of a phase II trial, J Biol Response Mod 9(4):345, 1990.

149. Ortho Biotech: Procrit (epoetin alfa), package insert, Raritan, NJ, 1993, Ortho Pharmaceutical Corp.

150. Ortho Biotech: PROCRIT line—(reimbursement hotline 1-800-553-3851). Raritan, NJ: Ortho-Pharmaceutical Co., 1991.

151. Padavic-Shaller K: IL-2: Nursing applications in a developing science, Semin Oncol Nurs 4(2):142, 1988.

152. Parkinson DR: Interleukin-2 in cancer therapy, Semin Oncol 15(6) Suppl 6:10, 1988.

153. Pastan I, Willingham MC, and Fitzgerald DJP: Immunotoxins, Cell 47:641, 1986.

154. Pazdur R and others: 5-fluorouracil and recombinant interferon alfa-2a: review of activity and toxicity in advanced colorectal carcinomas, Oncol Nurs Forum 18(1):11, 1991.

155. Penn I: Principles of tumor immunity: Immunocompetence and cancer. In DeVita VT Jr, Hellman S, and Rosenberg SA, editors: Biologic therapy of cancer, Phildelphia, 1991, JB Lippincott Co.

156. Pestka S: The purification and manufacture of human interferons, Scientific American 249:37, 1983.

157. Piper BF: Alteration in comfort: Fatigue. In McNally JC, Somerville ET, Miaskowski C, and Rostad M, editors: Guidelines for oncology nursing practice, ed 2, Philadelphia, 1991, WB Saunders.

158. Piper BF, Lindsey AM, and Dodd MJ: Fatigue mechanisms in cancer patients: developing a nursing theory, Oncol Nurs Forum 14(6):17, 1987.

159. Piper BF and others: Recent advances in the management of biotherapy-related side effects: fatigue, Oncol Nurs Forum 16(6) Suppl 6:27, 1989.

160. Platanias LC and others: Phase I study of genetically engineered DAB IL-2 in patients with hematologic malignancies, Blood 78(10) Suppl 1: 439a (#1748), 1991.

161. Podlaski FJ and others: Molecular characterization of interleukin-12, Arch Biochem Biophys 294(1):230, 1992.

162. Quesada JR, Gutterman JU, and Hersh EV: Treatment of hairy-cell leukemia with alpha interferons, Cancer 57:1678, 1986.

163. Quesada JR and others: Clinical toxicity of interferons in cancer patients: a review, J Clin Oncol 4:234, 1986.

164. Quesada JR and others: Interferon for induction of remission in hairy cell leukemia, N Engl J Med 310(1):15, 1984.

165. Rieger PT: The pathophysiology of selected symptoms associated with BRM therapy. Monograph, 1992, Cetus Corporation.

166. Rieger PT: Infusing interleukin-2 and dopamine, Oncol Nurs Forum 16(2):276, 1989.

167. Rieger PT: Management of cancer related fatigue, Dimens Oncol Nurs 2(3):5, 1988.

168. Rieger PT and Rumsey KA: Responding to the educational needs of patients receiving biotherapy. In Carroll-Johnson RM, editor: The biotherapy of cancer V—Monograph, Pittsburgh, 1992, Oncology Nursing Press, p. 10.

169. Rieger PT and Weatherly B: Can your nursing skills meet the challenge of a patient receiving IL-2? Dimens Oncol Nurs 3(3):9, 1989.

170. Rieker PP, Clark EJ, and Fogelberg PR: Perceptions of quality of life and quality of care for patients with cancer receiving biological therapy, Oncol Nurs Forum 19(3):433, 1992.

171. Roche Laboratories: Roferon-A package insert, Nutley, NJ, 1990, Hoffman-LaRoche, Inc.

172. Roche Laboratories. Roferon-A subcutaneous self-administration instruction review (flipchart). Nutley, NJ: Hoffmann-LaRoche, 1990.

173. Roche Laboratories. The right combination to increase survival and improve quality of life. Nutley, NJ: Hoffmann-LaRoche, 1990.

174. Roche Laboratories. Managing your patients on Roferon-A: Guidelines for the health professional, Nutley, NJ, 1990, Hoffmann-LaRoche, Inc. (Hotline 1-800-7-Roferon).

175. Roche Laboratories. At home with your Roferon-A therapy: Patient Guide (available English and Spanish), Nutley, NJ, 1990, Hoffmann-LaRoche, Inc.

176. Roche Laboratories. At home with Roferon-A therapy (videotape and audiotape cassette). Nutley, NJ: Hoffmann-LaRoche, 1990.

177. Roche Laboratories. The right start with Roferon-A managing side effects (videotape). Nutley, NJ: Hoffmann-LaRoche, 1990.

178. Roche Laboratories. Roferon-A cost assistance program (videotape). Nutley, NJ: Hoffmann-LaRoche, 1990.

179. Roche Laboratories. Roferon-A subcutaneous self-administration instruction review (flipchart). Nutley, NJ: Hoffmann-LaRoche, 1990.

180. Roche Laboratories. The right combination to increase survival and improve quality of life. Nutley, NJ: Hoffmann-LaRoche, 1990.

181. Roche Laboratories. Roferon-A cost assistance program: program guide (reimbursement hotline 1-800-443-6676). Nutley, NJ: Hoffmann-LaRoche, 1989.

182. Rosenberg SA: The immunotherapy and gene therapy of cancer, J Clin Oncol 10(2):180, 1992.

183. Rosenberg SA: Gene therapy of cancer. In: DeVita VT Jr, Hellman S, and Rosenberg SA, editors: Important advances in oncology, Philadelphia, 1991, JB Lippincott Co.

184. Rosenberg SA: Adoptive immunotherapy for cancer, Sci Am 262(5):62, 1990.

185. Rosenberg SA: Immunotherapy of patients with advanced cancer using interleukin-2 alone or in combination with lymphokine activated killer cells. In DeVita VT Jr, Hellman S, and Rosenberg S, editors: Important advances in oncology, Philadelphia, 1988, JB Lippincott Co.

186. Rosenberg SA, Longo DL, and Lotze MT: Principles and applications of biologic therapy. In Devita VT Jr, Hellman S, and Rosenberg S, editors: Cancer: Principles & practice of oncology, ed 3, vol 1, Philadelphia, 1989, JB Lippincott Co.

187. Rubin JT and Lotze MT: Acute gastric mucosal injury associated with the systemic administration of interleukin-4, Surgery 111(3):274, 1992.

188. Rumsey KA and Rieger PT, editors: Biological response modifiers: a self-instructional manual for health professionals, Chicago, IL, 1992, Precept Press.

189. Schellhammer PF, Ladaga LE, and Fillion MB: Bacillus Calmette-Guerin for superficial transitional cell carcinoma of the bladder, J Urol 135:261, 1986.

190. Schering Corp: Intron A: Interferon alpha-2b recombinant for injection, Kenilworth, NJ, 1992, Schering Corp.

191. Schering Corp: Living with Intron A (kit). Kenilworth, NJ: Schering, 1991.

192. Schering Corp: Self-administration of Intron A: step-by-step subcutaneous technique, Kenilworth, NJ, 1991, Schering Corp.

193. Schering Corp: Taking control of your therapy, Kenilworth, NJ, 1991, Schering Corp.

194. Schering Corp: Flexible dosing chart: Intron A. Kenilworth, NJ: Schering, 1990.

195. Schering Corp: Intron A: A practical guide for oncology nurses, Kenilworth, NJ, 1990, Schering Corp.

196. Schering Corp: Self injection of Intron A, Kenilworth, NJ, 1990, Schering Corp. (videotape).

197. Schering Corp: Intron-A: a day-by-day guide, Kenilworth, NJ, 1989, Schering Corp.

198. Schering Corp: Schering patient assistance program: IRIS, an innovative approach to reimbursement (1-800-521-7157). Kenilworth, NJ: Schering, 1989.

199. Schrader JW: Interleukin-3: the pan-specific hemopoietin. In Schrader JW, editor: Lymphokines, vol 15, San Diego, 1988, Academic Press, Inc.

200. Schroff RW and others: Human anti-murine immunoglobulin responses in patients receiving monoclonal antibody therapy. Cancer Res 45:879, 1985.

201. Sergi JS: The physiology of the flu-like syndrome and the cardiopulmonary and renal symptoms associated with BRM therapy, Cetus Corp (1991) (monograph).

202. Sherman M and others: Phase I study of recombinant human tumor necrosis factor administered as a five-day continuous infusion, J Clin Oncol 6(2):344, 1988.

203. Siegel JP and Puri RK: Interleukin-2 toxicity, J Clin Oncol 9(4):694, 1991.

204. Silverman P and Berger NA: Recent clinical experience with tumor necrosis factor and advances in understanding its physiologic function and cellular activities, Curr Opinion Oncol 2:1133, 1990.

205. Simpson C, Seipp CA, and Rosenberg SA: The current status and future applications of interleukin-2 and adoptive immunotherapy in cancer treatment, Semin Oncol Nurs 4(2):132, 1988.

206. Smith KA: Interleukin-2, Sci Am 262(3):50, 1990.

207. Smith MA and others: Retinoids in cancer therapy, J Clin Oncol 10(5):839, 1992.

208. Sondel PM and others: The cellular immunotherapy of cancer: current and potential uses of interleukin-2, Crit Rev Oncol Hematol 9(2):125, 1989.

209. Spitler L and others: Therapy of patients with malignant melanoma with a monoclonal antimelanoma antibody ricin A chain immunotoxin, Cancer Res 47:1717, 1987.

210. Starnes HF: Biological effects and possible clinical applications of interleukin 1, Semin Hematol 28(2) Suppl 2:34, 1991.

211. Strauman JJ: The nurse's role in the biotherapy of cancer: nursing research of side effects, Oncol Nurs Forum 15(6) Suppl 6:35, 1988.

212. Talpaz M and others: Hematologic remissions and cytogenic improvement induced by recombinant human interferon A in chronic myelogenous leukemia, N Engl J Med 314:(17)1065, 1986.

213. Talpaz M and others: Interferon alpha in the therapy of CML, Br J Haematol 79 Suppl 1:38, 1991.

214. Topalian SL and others: Immunotherapy of patients with advanced cancer using tumor infiltrating lymphocytes and recombinant interferon-2: a pilot study, J Clin Oncol 6(5):839, 1988.

215. Tracey KJ, Vlassara H, and Cerami A: Cachectin tumor necrosis factor, Lancet 1:1122, 1989.

216. Vadhan-Raj S and others: Abrogating chemotherapy-induced myelosuppression by recombinant granulocyte-macrophage colony-stimulating factor in patients with sarcoma: protection at the progenitor cell level, J Clin Oncol 10(8):1266, 1992.

217. Vadhan-Raj S and others: Interleukin-1 (IL-1) increases circulating platelet (plt) counts and reduces carboplatin (CBCDA) induced thrombocytopenia, Proc ASCO 11: #710, 1992.

218. Vadhan-Raj S and others: Stimulation of myelopoiesis in patients with aplastic anemia by recombinant human granulocyte-macrophage colony-stimulating factor, N Engl J Med 319 (25):1628, 1988.

219. Vadhan-Raj S and others: Effects of recombinant human granulocyte-macrophage colony-stimulating factor in patients with myelodysplastic syndromes, N Engl J Med 317(25):1545, 1987.

220. Varrichio CG and Jassak PF: Informed consent: an overview, Semin Oncol Nurs 5(2):95, 1989.

221. Vitetta ES and Thorpe PE: Immunotoxins. In DeVita VT Jr, Hellman S, and Rosenberg SA, editors: Biologic therapy of cancer, Philadelphia, 1991, JB Lippincott Co.

222. Wadler S and others: Fluorouracil and recombinant alfa-2a-interferon: an active regimen against advanced colorectal carcinoma, J Clin Oncol 7(12):1769, 1989.

223. Winningham ML: How exercise mitigates fatigue: Implications for patients receiving cancer therapy. In Carroll-Johnson RM, editor: The biotherapy of cancer V—Monograph. Pittsburgh, 1992, Oncology Nursing Press, Inc.

224. Wittes RE: Paying for patient care in treatment research—who is responsible? Cancer Treat Rep 71(2):107, 1987.

225. Yasko JM and Ver Furth M: Closing comments: economic trends, Semin Oncol Nurs 8(2):156, 1992.

226. Yarbro JW: The new biology of cancer: future clinical applications, Semin Oncol 16(3):254, 1989.

227. Yarbro JW, Bornstein RS, and Mastrangelo MJ: Management of anemia in oncology, Semin Oncol 19(3) Suppl 8:1, 1992.

228. Yarbro JW, Bornstein RS, and Mastrangelo MJ: Interferon: advances in biotherapy, Semin Oncol 18(5) Suppl 7:1, 1991.

229. Zsebo KM and others: Effect of recombinant rat stem cell factor on hematopoietic recovery after otherwise lethal total body irradiation, Blood 78(10) Suppl 1:374 (#1485), 1991.

230. Zucker-Franklin D and others: Atlas of blood cells: function and pathology, vol 1, Philadelphia, 1988, Lea & Febiger.

CHAPTER 24

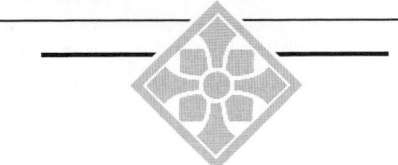

Bone Marrow Transplantation

Jill Grodecki Moore
Sandra Szekley

Bone marrow is a spongy tissue found in the inner cavities of bone. Normal functioning marrow is rich in progenitor or stem cells, which eventually proliferate into mature erythrocytes, leukocytes, and platelets (see Chapters 14 and 29 for further information). Bone marrow transplantation (BMT) is the process of replacing diseased or damaged bone marrow with normal functioning bone marrow. Bone marrow transplants (BMT) are used in the treatment of a variety of diseases and offers a chance for long-term survival.

HISTORICAL PERSPECTIVE

The first known documented cases of human bone marrow transplantation occurred as early as the 19th century. These early transplants were quite unscientific. Medical practitioners experimented with bone marrow as a treatment modality for poorly understood diseases for which there was no existing treatment. Bone marrow was injected into or sometimes even fed to patients. Some positive results occurred; however, these benefits were sporadic and the reasons for improvement were poorly understood. These primitive attempts were for the most part abandoned.

Later in the 20th century an interest in bone marrow transplantation again arose as an experimental approach for the treatment for some hematologic diseases. A variety of approaches were used and many important discoveries were made. Developments in antibacterial, fungal and viral therapies, blood banking techniques, chemotherapeutic regimens, growth factors, graft-versus-host disease (GVHD) prophylaxis and control, and tissue typing have made BMT a more effective, viable treatment option. The high-lights of these significant developments are summarized in Table 24-1.

TYPES OF BONE MARROW TRANSPLANTATION

There are two major types of BMT: autologous and allogeneic. The type of transplant is identified by the relationship of the recipient to the donor. An autologous BMT is a transplant in which the patient's own bone marrow is collected (harvested), placed in frozen storage (cryopreserved), and reinfused to the patient following the conditioning regimen. Therefore, the patient is their own donor. An allogeneic BMT is a transplant in which the patient receives someone else's bone marrow. There are several types of allogeneic BMT, each type named according to donor. They are: *syngeneic*—occurs when the donor is the patient's identical twin; *related*—the donor is related to the recipient and is usually a sibling; *unrelated*—the donor is no relation to the recipient.

For an autologous BMT to be successful, the following criteria have been suggested:
- The malignancy is responsive to chemotherapy and/or radiation therapy
- Marrow failure is the only dose-limiting toxicity of the effective treatment
- Tumor burden and drug resistance are minimal
- The bone marrow is free of tumor cells or clones.[36]

Autologous BMT is primarily used for the treatment of diseases in which the patient's own bone marrow contains adequate stem cells that can eventually generate functioning erythrocytes, leukocytes, and platelets. For example, autologous BMT is not a viable option for the treatment of aplastic anemia since the patient's bone marrow is lacking stem cells. It can,

Table 24-1   Significant Historical Events in Marrow Transplantation

Year	Researcher	Significant Finding
1896	Quine	Attempted BMT by injecting or feeding bone marrow to patients. Poor results.
1939	Osgood et al.	Attempted to cure aplastic anemia by massive IV injections of marrow cells.
1950	Relders et al.	Attempted BMT in dogs. Adequate doses of bone marrow, but inadequate radiation exposure did not allow for sufficient immunosuppression for engraftment.
1951	Lorenzo et al.	Demonstrated that guinea pigs and mice exposed to lethal radiation could be protected by infusion of bone marrow.
1955	Lindsley et al.	Radiation protection described earlier was result of growth of donor bone marrow.
1956	Ford et al.	Cytogenetic techniques used to show that radiation protection was due to transfer and survival of donor marrow cells.
1957	Thomas et al.	Large quantities of bone marrow could be safely infused IV; one patient showed transient engraftment. Estimated necessary dose of marrow cells and warned against GVHD reactions.
1959	Thomas et al.	Demonstrated that IV infusion of marrow from identical twin could protect against lethal radiation doses in patients with refractory leukemia.
1964	Mathe	First to achieve enduring bone marrow graft in patient with leukemia.
1968	Epstein et al.	Detected DL-A antigen in dogs and showed that marrow grafts between litter mates were almost always successful.
1968	Gatti et al.	Performed first marrow transplant from a matched sibling for an infant with immunodeficiency.
1975	Thomas et al.	Performed series of successful transplants using HLA-A identical siblings.

however, be a treatment option for patients with limited disease in their bone marrow.

The major criterion for an allogeneic BMT is finding a suitable donor. Tissue typing of the patient and potential donors is the first step in identifying whether a patient has a compatible donor. To determine a person's tissue type, a small amount of peripheral blood is drawn and antigens on the surface of the leukocytes are analyzed. These antigens make up the human leukocyte antigen (HLA) system, which plays a role in immune surveillance by constantly identifying "self" from "non-self."[46]

There are a pair of antigens at several sites on the white blood cells, called *loci*. Three of these loci, the HLA-A, HLA-B, and HLA-DR, are important in determining whether a patient and potential donor are compatible. The best match is one in which the antigens of the patient and potential donor match at all three loci. Matching at the A, B, and DR loci minimizes the risk of graft-versus-host disease (GVHD) and graft rejection.

The antigens that make up the HLA system are inherited from one's parents. Each offspring receives a set of antigens, referred to as a *haplotype*, from each parent (Figure 24-1). Thus, the best chance of finding a matched donor occurs among full siblings. Statistically, each sibling has a one in four (25%) chance of receiving the same haplotypes from the same parents (Figure 24-1). It is possible, but unlikely, that parents and/or children of a patient will match, since they are usually only a one haplotype (half) match. In general,

	Mother		Father	
	M-1	M-2	F-1	F-2
A	1	2	3	9
B	5	7	12	13
DR	1	2	4	5

	Child #1		Child #2		Child #3		Child #4	
	M-1	F-1	M-1	F-2	M-2	F-1	M-2	F-2
A	1	3	1	9	2	3	2	9
B	5	12	5	13	7	12	7	13
DR	1	4	1	5	2	4	2	5

Figure 24-1   HLA inheritance.

relatives outside the immediate family have approximately the same chance of matching as someone from the general population. Overall, the chances of matching someone in the general population are approximately one in 20,000 depending on how common the individual's haplotypes are.

When possible donors are identified from HLA typing, a mixed lymphocyte culture (MLC) is performed. The MLC is done to further ensure compatibility between donor and patient. A small amount of peripheral blood is drawn from each person, and the patient and donor lymphocytes are grown in a culture for 4 to 5 days to assess their reaction to one another. A very stimulating culture indicates an increased chance of their marrow interacting adversely, whereas a nonstimulating culture indicates patient and donor have a better chance of interacting compatibly.

A third test being done is DNA typing, which has made the HLA typing process even more accurate. This "fingerprinting" technique uses DNA to identify antigens by amplifying and examining their various protein chains. This procedure has shown that previously identified antigens that were thought to be identical are actually different; this will no doubt have tremendous impact on the accuracy and importance of identically matched HLA antigens in the future.

Mismatched donors are utilized in allogeneic transplants for which there is no true match. Mismatches currently considered for transplant are either one or two antigen mismatches. The mismatch can occur at either the A, B, or D loci. The higher the number of mismatches, the higher the incidence of GVHD or graft rejection and the poorer the chances of the patient's survival.[2]

Mismatching does not refer to ABO incompatibility. Corrections can be made to overcome ABO incompatibility so that, for example, a patient with blood type "O" can receive a BMT from a donor with blood type "A." When ABO incompatibility occurs, the donor's erythrocytes can be removed from the transfusable bone marrow prior to transplant. Therefore, the donor's erythrocytes are not infused and side effects from the ABO incompatibility are minimized. The recipient will eventually sero-convert to the donor's blood type.

The last option for donor availability is the attainment of an unrelated donor. The National Marrow Donor Registry Program (NBMDR) was established in 1987 for this purpose. The registry contains over 600,000 available bone marrow donors, all of whom have had tissue typing completed and have expressed a desire to donate bone marrow. The registry search determines which listed donors have compatible typing with the recipient patient. There are also several other donor registries containing approximately 500,000 donors located throughout the world that are available for searches. It is not inconceivable that a patient in the United States could receive bone marrow from a donor located somewhere in Europe, Asia, Africa, or anywhere else in the world. The system is an anonymous one. When chosen, the donor does not know who is receiving the marrow and the recipient does not know from which donor the marrow came or where that donor is located. Hundreds of BMTs have been made possible as a result of efforts of the NBMDR.

Peripheral Blood Stem Cell

Although stem cells have been traditionally harvested from bone marrow cavities, functional hematopoietic stem cells can be found circulating in peripheral blood as well. These peripheral stem cells can be effectively transplanted as evidenced in 1986 when reports re-

vealed that six medical facilities from around the world had transplanted autologous PBSC into various patients with a variety of diseases.* PBSC transplants continue to be used today for the treatment of several types of malignant diseases.

PBSC are collected through the process of aspheresis, which extracts the various blood cells, separates them, retains the peripheral stem cells, and returns the remaining cells back to the patient. This is accomplished by an apheresis machine to which the patient is connected via IV lines, usually for 2 to 6 hours. Typically, 6 to 8 apheresis sessions are required to collect a sufficient number of peripheral stem cells for transplantation. The concentration of stem cells in bone marrow can be 100 times greater than in the peripheral system.[10] After collection, the peripheral stem cells are cryopreserved to be transplanted at a later time.

There are several advantages to this type of collection process—it can be done on an outpatient basis, the patient does not undergo general anesthesia, no operating room suite expenses are incurred, and the patient does not experience the pain associated with multiple bone marrow aspirations.[25] The possible side effects of this harvesting method include light-headedness, coldness, numbness around the lips, or cramping in the hands.[10] Disadvantages of PBSC include: placement of central venous catheter to accommodate the process of apheresis, potential for labor intensity (PBSC can require 5 to 10 collections), and additional resources that may be required for storage of the PBSC product. The patient receiving the PBSC may also experience increased toxicities related to the preservative DMSO.[10]

Transplantation of PBSC is performed in the same way as an autologous BMT. The side effects noted include hemoglobinuria, red urine, hypertension, fever, chills, vomiting, tachypnea, elevated serum bilirubin, cough, diarrhea, elevated serum creatinine, flushing, and headache.[24] Studies have suggested that these side effects may be more frequent in patients who received a large volume of PBSC or in patients whose dose of stem cells contain a large volume of red blood cells.[24]

There are a number of significant reasons why PBSC transplants are advantageous. PBSC may be of value when bone marrow is invaded with tumor and is unsuitable for harvesting. It is thought that tumor cells in the peripheral blood circulate in few numbers compared to bone marrow and that peripheral blood tumor cells have decreased ability to proliferate.[8] Thus, transplantation becomes an option for patients with tumor invaded marrow.

Due to prior radiation or chemotherapy, some pa-

---

*References 7, 11, 23, 27, 35, 40.

Table 24–2 Diseases Treated with Bone Marrow Transplantation

Type	Disease
Malignant	Acute myelogenous leukemia
	Acute lymphocytic leukemia
	Chronic myelogenous leukemia
	Myelodysplastic syndrome
	Hodgkin's disease
	Non-Hodgkin's lymphoma
	Multiple myeloma*
	Breast cancer*
	Neuroblastoma
	Testicular cancer*
	Ewing's sarcoma*
	Rhabdomyosarcoma*
	Wilm's tumor*
	Malignant melanoma*
	Lung cancer*
Non-malignant	Aplastic anemia
	Myelofibrosis
	Wiskott-Aldrich syndrome
	Severe combined immunodeficiency syndrome
	Mucopolysacharoidosis
	Osteopetrosis
	Lipid storage diseases*
	Thalassemia*
	Paroxysmal nocturnal hemoglobinuria*

DISEASES TREATED WITH PBSC TRANSPLANTATION[10]

Acute leukemia
Brain tumors
Breast cancer
Hodgkin's disease
Multiple myeloma
Neuroblastoma
Non-Hodgkin's lymphoma
Ovarian cancer
Small cell lung cancer
Testicular cancer

*Role of BMT is still under investigation.

Table 24–3 Survival Rates (Approximate 5-year Disease-Free Survival [DFS] of Patients Receiving Autologous or Matched Sibling BMTs)

AUTOLOGOUS TRANSPLANTS	
Disease	DFS
AML (1st CR)	40-50%
AML (2nd CR)	20%
ALL (1st CR)	40-50%
ALL (2nd CR)	20%
CML (chronic)*	10%
Hodgkin's disease	35-55%
Non-Hodgkin's	20-75%
Breast cancer*	16-30%

ALLOGENEIC TRANSPLANTS	
Disease	DFS
AML (1st CR)	25-60%
ALL (1st CR)	40-60%
ALL (2nd CR)	30-60%
CML (chronic)	65%
CML (accelerated)	30%
CML (blastic)	15%
Hodgkin's disease	25-55%
Non-Hodgkin's	20-65%
Multiple myeloma*	30%

*Limited number of patients and follow-up.

tients have a minimal number of available stem cells in their bone marrow. Since these patients have an inadequate number of bone marrow stem cells, bone marrow transplantation is not an option. There may be a sufficient number of peripheral stem cells that can be harvested, however, making transplantation a viable option for these patients.

To increase the number of circulating PBSC, colony stimulating factors (CSF) such as GM-CSF can be administered.[21] This can decrease the apheresis collection time and can result in a more rapid neutrophil recovery after transplant, thereby possibly shortening the hospitalization of the patient.[25] Some institutions are currently using PBSC in combination with traditional autologous BMT to achieve this rapid immune reconstitution.[19]

INDICATIONS FOR BONE MARROW TRANSPLANTATION

Bone marrow transplantation is a treatment modality for a variety of malignant and nonmalignant diseases (Table 24-2). Most BMTs are performed for malignancies, particularly those of hematologic origin. The type and stage of the disease, the patient's age and performance status, and donor availability determine the type of transplant that can be done and the chances of survival. Table 24-3 identifies approximate 5-year disease-free survival for autologous and allogeneic transplants. Allogeneic transplants are more frequently done for leukemia and nonmalignant diseases. Autologous transplants are more common in the treatment of malignant lymphoma and solid tumors.

Hematologic Malignancies
LEUKEMIA
For acute lymphocytic leukemia (ALL) and acute myelogenous leukemia (AML), allogeneic BMT is the primary type of transplant done. The best results are achieved when the transplant is done in first complete remission (CR), the patient is less than 45 years old, and the donor is a matched sibling.[9] Autologous or unrelated donor transplants may be used for patients without a matched sibling.[9,17] Currently, the success

of these BMTs is comparable to patients receiving intensive postremission chemotherapy.[9]

For chronic myelogenous leukemia, allogeneic BMT is the only treatment option that is curative.[29,30] The disease phase at the time of transplantation is the factor most strongly associated with treatment success.[30] Patients who have a BMT in the chronic phase have higher rates of success. The best results are seen in young patients, transplanted in chronic phase within a year of the diagnosis.[12]

LYMPHOMA

BMT in the malignant lymphomas, Hodgkin's and non-Hodgkin's, is very widely used as a salvage treatment. Due to the high chemotherapy and radiation sensitivity of these tumors, patients with lymphoma are optimal candidates for BMT.[45]

Autologous, allogeneic, and recently PBSC transplants are used, although autologous transplants are most frequent due to better donor availability and decreased complications. Autologous BMT also allows for treatment of older patients, which is especially important in non-Hodgkin's lymphoma.[45]

Patients with lymphoma who have good performance status, have had less than two prior chemotherapy regimens, and have a low tumor burden at the time of transplant have the best survival rates.[45] In Hodgkin's disease, BMT is usually indicated for patients who fail to achieve a complete response to three or four courses of chemotherapy or who are in early relapse after initial complete response.[20,22,31] In non-Hodgkin's lymphoma, BMT is usually indicated for patients who have relapsed after an initial complete response or who remain responsive to chemotherapy but have residual disease.[20,22,45] For patients with residual disease or highly aggressive non-Hodgkin's lymphoma, BMT should be carried out as a consolidation.[20]

OTHER HEMATOLOGIC MALIGNANCIES

Myelodysplastic syndrome and multiple myeloma are also being treated with bone marrow transplantation. Myelodysplastic syndrome is generally treated similarly to patients with leukemia. They do not, however, have as favorable a success rate. This population of patients has a more difficult tumor burden to overcome since it is frequently a secondary malignancy.

Currently, multiple myeloma is receiving increased attention as a disease in which BMT may be a useful treatment option. Clinical trials of allogeneic and autologous BMTs are being done. It is too early to tell if allogeneic transplantation is curative since patients' bone lesions post transplant have remained unchanged and a longer follow up is necessary to determine the antitumor efficacy of BMT. Autologous BMT for multiple myeloma has shown a reduction in tumor mass with significant improvement in bone pain.[5,20] Since the tumor grows slowly, the goal of autologous transplantation is to extend the active life of patients with multiple myeloma.[5]

Solid Tumors

BMT for solid tumors is based on the rationale of rescuing patients from the bone marrow suppressant effects of higher than standard dose chemotherapy and/or radiation. For BMT to be effective, the disease must be responsive to treatment that cannot be given in higher doses due to bone marrow suppression.[46] Although BMTs are currently being performed on a variety of solid tumors, most are still considered investigational. The diseases currently receiving the most attention and study are breast cancer and neuroblastoma. Other tumors for which BMT has shown some positive responses are: Ewing's sarcoma, malignant melanoma, rhabdomyosarcoma, testicular cancer, and Wilm's tumor.

BREAST CANCER

Autologous BMT and PBSC transplants as a treatment modality for breast cancer has generated increased interest and investigation. Studies of BMTs in patients with advanced metastatic disease have shown favorable response and have further increased interest in performing transplants earlier in the disease process. Transplants are now beginning to focus on women relapsing after conventional therapy and those at high risk for relapsing.[17] Although 20% of patients with advanced disease achieved a complete response, the low number of subjects and the brief period of follow-up make these results inconclusive.[17] Further clinical trials are necessary to address issues regarding the efficacy of autologous and PBSC transplants in breast cancer.

NEUROBLASTOMA

Neuroblastoma is the most frequent pediatric solid tumor treated with BMT. Approximately 60% of patients have advanced disease and only a 10% chance of cure with conventional therapy.[32,37] Recent studies of autologous BMT in these patients suggests an overall 5-year disease-free survival of 20% to 40%.[17,37] Again the small number of patients and the brief follow-up makes these results encouraging but inconclusive. Further clinical trials are needed to determine if autologous BMT provides optimal treatment.[17,37]

Non-Malignant Diseases

Aplastic anemia and severe combined immunodeficiency syndrome (SCIDS) are the most common non-malignant diseases for which BMT is a treatment modality. Both diseases are related to a failure or absence of proliferative cells resulting in life-threatening immunosuppression. Allogeneic BMT is used primarily to reconstitute the proliferative cell population.[1,46]

APLASTIC ANEMIA

Allogeneic BMT is responsible for approximately 80% overall survival in aplastic anemia.[1] Patients who have had blood product transfusions prior to BMT have a higher rate of graft rejection. Therefore, at the time of diagnosis HLA typing is done on the entire family. All patients younger than age 45 should be considered for BMT. Although patients are immunosuppressed due to the disease, a conditioning regimen is usually administered.[46] This is especially true of patients who have received transfusions.

SCIDS

The earliest successful BMTs were in patients with SCIDS.[1] Most patients with SCIDS will die within 1 year of diagnosis and, since this disease occurs so early in life, a matched sibling donor may be unavailable.[1,46] For these reasons, the use of a haplo-identical parent and in some instances matched unrelated donors is considered.[1] Approximately 70% of patients receiving a matched BMT will be cured.[1,46] The survival rate is slightly lower for patients receiving a haplo-identical parent match due to the increased incidence of graft rejection and GVHD.[1] Since the disease has already immunosuppressed the patient, there is usually no conditioning regimen given.

BONE MARROW TRANSPLANTATION PROCEDURE
Pretreatment Work Up

An extensive evaluation is performed on the bone marrow transplant recipient prior to transplant. This is done to establish the recipient's physical and psychosocial status. For allogeneic transplants, the donor is also thoroughly assessed. The assessment is done on an outpatient basis and includes a variety of tests, procedures, and consults (see box at right). A team approach is usually used and typically includes psychology, social work, surgery, chaplaincy, and radiology in addition to nursing and medicine.

The patient's family and/or significant other are also included in this process. These evaluations alert the BMT team to potential problems that can occur, such as physical hindrances, negative coping mechanisms, or financial difficulties. This assessment also ensures that the patient has adequate support systems to aide him or her throughout the rigorous process of bone marrow transplant.

Marrow Harvest

Harvesting is the process of obtaining bone marrow for transplantation. This procedure occurs in the operating room, typically under general anesthesia. Bone marrow is obtained by performing multiple punctures with a large bore needle into the patient's posterior and occasionally the anterior iliac crests. Usually two physicians work simultaneously, one on

---

PRETRANSPLANTATION EVALUATION

Bone marrow recipient
History and physical examination
Bone marrow biopsy and aspiration with cytogenetics
Chemistry profile
Complete blood count, platelets, reticulocyte count
ABO and Rh typing
Coagulation profile
Serum immunoelectrophoresis
Quantitative immunoglobulins
Hepatitis screen
Cytomegalovirus, HIV, and herpes simplex virus titers
Urinalysis, creatinine clearance, and protein quantification
Chest x-ray
Electrocardiogram, echocardiogram, or radionucleotide ventriculogram
Pulmonary function testing
Sinus x-ray
Allergy testing
Audiology consult
Physical therapy consult
Dental consult
Dietary consult
Social work consult
Psychology/Psychiatry consult
Opthamology consult
Surgery consult—insertion of multiple lumen catheter

Bone marrow donor
History and physical examination
Chemistry profile
Complete blood count, platelet count
ABO and Rh typing
Hepatitis screen
Cytomegalovirus, HIV, and herpes simplex virus titers
Chest x-ray
Electrocardiogram
Urinalysis

---

either side of the patient. Multiple punctures are necessary since each aspiration obtains only 2 to 5 ml of bone marrow.

The amount of bone marrow collected depends on the size of the recipient and donor as well as the type of bone marrow transplant (autologous vs. allogeneic). Usually 10 cc per kilogram of body weight will yield the amount of needed stem cells. Therefore, a 50 Kg patient would contribute approximately 500 cc of bone marrow, and, if obtaining about 5 cc per aspiration, then approximately 100 aspirations are required to obtain the desired 500 cc of marrow.

Once collected, the marrow is mixed with a heparinized solution, filtered to remove bone fragments and fat, and placed in a blood bag. It is at this point that the marrow can be treated or purged. Purging is the process of removing residual malignant cells from the marrow for autologous transplant. It is performed using monoclonal antibodies or chemotherapeutic agents. Marrow collected for allogeneic BMT may also be treated. One such treatment is that of T-cell depletion, which is the process of removing T lymphocytes from the marrow in order to prevent acute GVHD. If an ABO incompatibility exists, the red cells may also be removed from the allogeneic marrow.

When an allogeneic bone marrow transplant is to occur, then the marrow is immediately transfused into the recipient. The marrow will usually be brought directly to the recipient's room from the operating room. For an autologous transplant, the collected marrow is mixed with the preservative dimethylsulfoxide (DMSO), placed in a blood bag, and cryopreserved. It will be thawed and transplanted at a later date.

Following bone marrow harvest, the postoperative recovery time is minimal. A large pressure dressing will have been applied to the iliac crests. Nursing responsibilities following bone marrow harvest include routine postoperative care such as maintaining comfort and mobility, care of the dressing, and monitoring vital signs and blood counts. Postoperatively patients can expect discomfort at the sites for approximately 1 week. This discomfort can typically be relieved with acetaminophen. In an allogeneic BMT, the donor's psychological and emotional needs must not be overlooked. Many donors experience anxiety over whether or not the bone marrow transplant will be a success or a failure. Nursing must allow for the ventilation of donor feelings and offer support.

Conditioning Regimens

The conditioning regimen is the process of preparing the patient to receive bone marrow. It accomplishes three vital functions: obliterate the malignant disease; destroy the patient's preexisting immunologic state; and create space in the marrow cavity for the proliferation of the transplanted stem cells.[43] In effect, conditioning regimens destroy the patient's own bone marrow. The proliferation of new erythrocytes, leukocytes, and platelets cannot occur unless new functioning bone marrow is given to the patient. Upon completion of the conditioning regimen, the patient must receive a bone marrow transplant or die.

The conditioning regimen consists of high-dose chemotherapy with or without total body irradiation. There are several regimens using various combinations of chemotherapy and/or radiation that last 4 to 10 days (Table 24-4). Cyclophosphamide, carmustine, etoposide, busulfan, cytarabine, and methotrexate are all common chemotherapeutic agents used in conditioning regimens. The regimen chosen depends on the type of disease and the amount and response to previous radiation or chemotherapy.[28]

In addition to the occurrence of severe myelosuppression, the patient may experience many other side effects (Table 24-5). Most of these are immediate responses to the chemotherapy and/or radiation and can continue for several weeks following BMT. Management of these side effects focuses on control of the symptoms, prevention of further complications, and maintenance of patient comfort (Table 24-5). Long-term effects, such as cataracts and gonadal dysfunction, also can occur and are discussed in the section on complications.

Transplantation of Marrow

Following completion of the conditioning regimen, the bone marrow must be infused. If the regimen was one in which chemotherapy was the last treatment given, there is a rest period of 24 to 72 hours prior to transplant. This rest period is necessary because of the drug's half-life. When compared to the donor search, extensive pretransplant work-up, and toxic conditioning regimen, most patients describe the actual transplantation of marrow as quite anticlimactic.

For autologous transplants, the frozen marrow is brought to the recipient's room for transplant. The bag of marrow is thawed in a normal saline bath, drawn up in large syringes, and given rapid IV push via central venous catheter. The entire process takes approximately 20 to 30 minutes depending on the volume of bone marrow being transplanted. Patients often experience minimal shortness of breath due to the rapid infusion of bone marrow as well as nausea and vomiting due to the preservative dimethylsulfoxide (DMSO). DMSO also gives off a strange garlic-like odor as it is excreted via the patient's respiratory system for 24 to 48 hours following autologous BMT.

For allogeneic transplants, the marrow is infused on the same day as it is collected. This procedure resembles a red blood cell transfusion in that the bag of marrow is hung and transfused via the patient's central venous catheter. Unfiltered tubing must be used in order to prevent precious stem cells from becoming trapped and not getting infused. The total time of infusion depends on the amount of marrow, but usually lasts between 1 and 5 hours. Possible side effects in an allogeneic transplant are similar to those that can occur with a blood transfusion; shortness of breath, chills, fever, rash, chest pain, and hypotension. These reactions are more likely to occur if the marrow is ABO incompatible. If reactions do occur, they are treated with additional diphenhydramine, hydrocortisone, epinephrine, and/or oxygen therapy as the situation requires.

Table 24-4   Common Conditioning Regimens

Busulfan/Cyclophosphamide

Day	−7	−6	−5	−4	−3	−2	−1	0
Busulfan 1 mg/kg every 6 hrs	X	X	X	X				
Cyclophosphamide 60 mg/kg/day					X	X		
Rest day							X	
Transplant day								X

Busulfan/Cytarabine/Cyclophosphamide

Day	−9	−8	−7	−6	−5	−4	−3	−2	−1	0
Busulfan 1 mg/kg every 6 hrs	X	X	X	X						
Cytarabine 2 gm/m² every 12 hrs					X	X				
Cyclophosphamide 60 mg/kg/day							X	X		
Rest day									X	
Transplant day										X

Cyclophosphamide/Total Body Irradiation (TBI)

Day	−6	−5	−4	−3	−2	−1	0
Cyclophosphamide 60 mg/kg/day	X	X					
Rest day			X				
TBI 200 Gy BID				X	X	X	
Transplant day							X

Cyclophosphamide/Etoposide/Carmustine

Day	−7	−6	−5	−4	−3	−2	−1	0
Cyclophosphamide 1.8 gm/m²/day	X	X	X	X				
Etoposide 200 mg/m² every 12 hrs	X	X	X	X				
Carmustine 600 mg/m²/day					X			
Rest day						X	X	
Transplant day								X

Cyclophosphamide/Total Body Irradiation (TBI)

Day	−8	−7	−6	−5	−4	−3	−2	−1	0
Cyclophosphamide 50 mg/kg/day	X	X	X	X					
TBI 300 Gy every day					X	X	X*	X	
Transplant day									X

Cyclophosphamide

Day	−5	−4	−3	−2	−1	0
Cyclophosphamide 50 mg/kg/day	X	X	X	X		
Rest day					X	
Transplant day						X

*Lungs shielded for this dose

Patients may be premedicated with diphenhydramine and/or hydrocortisone in order to prevent or minimize these reactions. In both transplant procedures emergency equipment is always available at the patients bedside. The physician is also available throughout the entire transplant. The nursing staff is responsible for closely monitoring vital signs as well as for signs and symptoms of reaction. Teaching is also an important aspect of nursing care. The patient and family/significant other will have been exposed to much information about this procedure prior to its occurrence; however, several questions always arise along with patient and family anxiety on this eventful day. Some patients view their transplant day as a "birthday" of sorts as in their eyes they are given a new chance at life.

Engraftment Period

The engraftment period is the time immediately post transplant when the transfused stem cells migrate, by some unknown phenomenon, to the recipient's bone marrow space and begin to regenerate. This usually takes 2 to 3 weeks and is evidenced by increasing blood counts. During this period the patient experiences severe pancytopenia and immunosuppression. Immediate complications that can occur include infection and bleeding. The patient's care during this time focuses on prevention of and early treatment of infection and bleeding. Patients typically receive numerous antibiotics and blood components during this time (Tables 24-6 & 24-7).

Since infections and bleeding can be major complications immediately after BMT, one goal is to

Table 24-5 Side Effects of Conditioning Regimens

	Major Side Effects	*Management*
Busulfan	Nausea, vomiting, diarrhea, seizures (possible during administration and up to 48 hours after last dose)	Administer antiemetic at scheduled intervals. Check emesis for busulfan tablets and replace 1 for 1. Establish seizure precautions and monitor for seizure activity. Administer anticonvulsant at scheduled intervals as ordered. See Chapter 22.
Carmustine (BCNU)	Nausea, vomiting, diarrhea Hypotension Alcohol intoxication (drug is reconstituted in an alcohol base) Stomatitis Veno-occlusive disease (hepatic failure occurs in first 4 weeks)	Administer antiemetic at scheduled intervals. Monitor BP throughout administration. Maintain adequate hydration. Monitor for possible intoxication, maintain safe environment, and keep patient in bed during administration and several hours afterward. Monitor for ascites, edema, and elevated liver function. Administration diuretics, lactulose, albumin, and fluid restriction as ordered. See Chapter 22.
Cyclophosphamide (Cytoxan)	Nausea, vomiting, diarrhea Hemorrhagic cystitis Alopecia Cardiac toxicity	Administer antiemetic at scheduled intervals. Maintain adequate hydration. Monitor for blood in urine. Maintain continuous bladder irrigation as ordered and provide foley catheter care. Administer MESNA and pain medications as ordered. Ensure that EKG is done and checked prior to administration of each dose. See Chapter 22.
Cytarabine (Ara-C)	Nausea, vomiting, diarrhea Erythema Neurotoxicity Hemorrhagic conjunctivitis Alopecia	Administer antiemetics at scheduled intervals. Monitor palms and soles for erythema, provide creams and assistance with ADLs as needed. Monitor for cerebellar toxicity—ataxia. Administer steroid eye drops at scheduled intervals up to 48 hours after last dose. See Chapter 22.
Etoposide (VP-16)	Nausea, vomiting, diarrhea Hypotension Alopecia	Administer antiemetics at scheduled intervals. Monitor BP throughout administration. Maintain adequate hydration. See Chapter 22.
Total body irradiation (TBI)	Nausea, vomiting, diarrhea Stomatitis Alopecia Veno-occlusive disease Fever Parotitis Erythema	Administer antiemetics 30 minutes before treatment and immediately following. Monitor for ascites, edema, and elevated liver function. Administer diuretics, lactulose, albumin, and fluid restriction as ordered. Monitor temperature every 2 to 4 hours and observe fever pattern. Assess for signs and symptoms of infection. Administer antipyretics as ordered. Apply hot/cold packs to affected areas. Administer pain medications as ordered. Monitor skin integrity and keep skin clean and dry. Avoid harsh soaps and irritants. If desquamation occurs, use dressings, ointments only as ordered. See Chapter 21.

shorten the length of the pancytopenic period. A relatively new and exciting development that aides in this process are the hematopoietic growth factors (see Chapter 23 for further information). These include, but are not limited to, granulocyte-macrophage colony stimulating factors (GM-CSF), granulocyte colony stimulating factors (G-CSF), and interleukin 3 (IL-3).

These factors affect the function of mature myeloid cells as well as the ability to stimulate the proliferation of myeloid precursor cells at various stages of differentiation.[33]

GM-CSF and G-CSF are both myeloid stimulating factors. GM-CSF (Sargramostin) activates mature granulocytes and macrophages and has a multi li-

Table 24-6 Common Antibiotics, Antifungals and Antivirals

Medication	Route/Dose	Indications/Precautions
ANTIBIOTICS		
Cefoperazone	IV 2 gms every 8 hours	Suspected gram negative sepsis. Infuse over 30 minutes. Not approved for pediatric patients. Monitor prothrombin time and for diarrhea. Administer vitamin K as ordered.
Ceftazidine	IV 150 mg/kg/day every 8 hours	Suspected gram negative sepsis. Infuse over 30 minutes. Maximum dose 2 gms every 8 hours. Monotherapy for pediatric patients, second line therapy for adults. Monitor for diarrhea and development of drug resistance.
Norfloxicin	PO 400 mg BID	Reduction of bowel flora, anaerobes. Administer on empty stomach. Do not administer with antacids or carafate. Monitor for rash, nausea, vomiting, and diarrhea. Discontinue when granulocyte recovery is maintained.
Penicillin VK	PO 250 mg BID	Prophylaxis of gram positive infections post BMT. Check for allergy to penicillin. Monitor for rash.
Tobramycin	IV 5 mg/kg/day	Suspected gram negative sepsis. Infuse over 20 to 30 minutes. Do not administer at same time as ceftazidine, cefoperozone. Monitor peak and trough blood levels. Monitor for nephrotoxicity (elevated BUN and creatinine) and ototoxicity (ataxia, diminished hearing).
Trimethoprim-sulfamethoxazole	PO 1 DS tablet BID IV 15-20 mg/kg/day	Prophylaxis of *Pneumocystis carinii* pneumonia post BMT. Avoid with sulfa allergy. Administer per transplant center protocol. Monitor for rash, decreasing WBC and increasing BUN and creatinine.
Vancomycin	IV 1 gm every 12 hours (adult) IV 40 mg/kg/day (pediatrics) PO 125 mg every 6 hours	Suspected or proven gram positive infections. Infuse over 60 minutes. PO is used for *C. difficile* enterocolitis only (not absorbed orally). Monitor peak and trough blood levels. Monitor for nephrotoxicity (elevated BUN and creatinine) and ototoxicity (ataxia, diminished hearing).
ANTIFUNGALS		
Amphotericin B	IV 0.5-1 mg/kg/day	Treatment of fungal infections resistant to fluconazole. Infuse through D_5W only over 3 to 6 hours. Administer test dose at initiation of therapy (1 mg in 100 ml D_5W). Monitor for increased temperature and chilling rigor during infusion. Premedicate with diphenhydramine, acetominophen, or hydrocortisone as ordered. Monitor electrolytes and for nephrotoxicity.
Fluconazole	PO 500 mg BID IV 100-200 mg/day	PO for reduction of bowel flora (used with norfloxacin). IV for treatment of fungemia. Monitor for overgrowth of resistant strains of fungus—surveillance cultures. Monitor for elevated liver function tests and nephrotoxicity. Discontinue PO when granulocyte recovery is maintained.

Table 24-6   Common Antibiotics, Antifungals and Antivirals—cont'd

Medication	Route/Dose	Indications/Precautions
ANTIVIRALS		
Acyclovir	PO or IV 250-500 mg/M² every 8 hours	Prophylaxis and treatment of herpes simplex or cytomegalovirus. Infuse over 2 hours (doses >500 mg must be diluted in 500 ml of fluid). Monitor for increased BUN and creatinine.
Ganciclovir	IV 2.5 mg/kg every 8 hours IV 5 mg/kg every 12 hours	Prophylaxis and treatment of cytomegalovirus (CMV). Infuse over 1 hour, handle administration and disposal using chemotherapy precautions. Administer with immunoglobulin for cases of CMV pneumonitis. Monitor for decreased WBC and increased BUN and creatinine. Colony stimulating factors may be given to maintain WBC.
Foscarnet	IV 40-60 mg/kg every 8 hours	Second line therapy for herpes simplex or cytomegalovirus infections. Monitor for electrolyte disturbances, nephrotoxicity and decreased WBC. Monitor for seizure activity.
Immunoglobulin	IV 0.4 gm/kg every week × 6 PO 50 mg/kg/day every 6 hours	IV prophylaxis for herpes simplex and cytomegalovirus. IV treatment for CMV pneumonitis in conjuction with ganciclovir. PO treatment of rotovirus. Administer IV slowly 20 to 30 ml/hr. Monitor for chills, hypotension, and increased temperature during infusion.

neage factor. GM-CSF is indicated for the acceleration of myeloid recovery in patients with NHL, ALL, and Hodgkin's disease undergoing autologous BMT. G-CSF (Filgrastin) is lineage specific and regulates the production of neutrophils within the bone marrow. It reduces the incidence of infection as manifested by febrile neutropenia in patients with non-myeloid malignancies who are receiving myelosuppressive anti-cancer drugs associated with severe neutropenia and fever.

IL-3 has the additional potential of assisting even earlier multilineage progenitor cells to maturation and therefore may also have an impact on hastening platelet and red cell recovery after BMT.[34] This could lead to decreased bleeding problems for the patient and therefore require less blood transfusion therapy. The administration of IL-3 with or without GM-CSF or G-CSF may have an even greater impact on granulocyte recovery than the use of single agents.[15,42]

COMPLICATIONS OF MARROW TRANSPLANTATION

BMT recipients experience toxic complications associated with the immunosuppressive therapy necessary to allow the graft to occur. The major complications characteristic of BMT are: graft rejection, infections, pneumonitis, graft-versus-host disease

(GVHD), and recurrence of original disease (Table 24-8).

Graft Rejection

Rejection in marrow transplantation is not as frequent and does not have the same impact as in solid organ transplants. In BMT the diagnosis of rejection or graft failure is not well defined and with better pretransplant conditioning and blood product administration the occurrence of rejection has decreased.[1] Failure is infrequent in patients who have received unmanipulated marrow from an HLA-identical donor.[14]

Infection

Alterations in the integrity of physical barriers and severe granulocytopenia from the pretransplant regimen sets up an environment for serious bacterial and fungal infections during the first 6 weeks post-BMT.[41] Most of the time the causative agents are from the patient's own microflora, particularly from the GI tract and integumentary system. Common agents are gram-positive and gram-negative bacteria, such as *Staphylococci, E. coli,* and *Pseudomonas.*[1] Fungal infections are less common than bacterial infections, accounting for only 10% to 15% of systemic infections.[41]

Viral infections occur at varying times post-BMT. Herpes simplex and CMV are causative agents gen-

Table 24-7   Blood Component Therapy

Component	Indications	Special Considerations
PACKED RED BLOOD CELLS (PRBC)	Hemoglobin <8.0 gm Patient is symptomatic Active bleeding	Type and crossmatch is necessary Infuse over 2 to 4 hours Monitor for transfusion reaction (fever, chills, urticaria)
• Leukocyte poor PRBC Leukocytes are removed during transfusion	Patient has experienced febrile transfusion reactions Patient is at risk for alloimmunization	Infuse through a special filter (Pall)
• Washed PRBC Blood is washed with 1000 ml normal saline and repacked prior to transfusion	Patient has known severe allergic reaction to plasma and leukocytes	Infuse at 20-30 gtts/min until completion of unit Unit expires within 24 hours of washing
PLATELET CONCENTRATES	Platelet count <20,000 Active bleeding Prior to minor procedures or surgery	ABO compatibility preferred but not necessary One hour or 24 hour post-transfusion increments are monitored to determine effectiveness Splenomegaly, DIC, fever, sepsis may increase demand Monitor for transfusion reactions Prophylaxis with diphenhydramine, acetominophen, hydrocortisone
• Random donor (RDP) Several units (6-10) harvested from whole blood are pooled into one bag	Patient has had no prior transfusions Patient has had no reactions or alloimmunization	Units expires about 4 hours after pooling
• Leukocyte poor RDP Leukocytes are removed prior to or during transfusion	Patient is at risk for alloimmunization Patient has experienced febrile transfusion reactions	Unit is either centrifuged and leukocytes mechanically trapped (Leukotrap) or a special filter (Pall) is used for infusion)
• Single donor (SDP) Platelets are collected by pheresis from one donor	Patient is refractory to RDP Patient is at risk for alloimmunization	Try to match ABO/Rh of patient Usually transfuse with special filter (Pall) Unit expires within 24 hours of collection
• HLA matched Platelets are collected by pheresis from a donor whose HLA typing closely matches patient	Patient is refractory to RDP and SDP Patient is at risk for alloimmunization	Patient must have been HLA typed Unit expires within 24 hours of collection
• Resuspended platelets Plasma is removed from pooled units and an equivalent amount of normal saline is added	Patient has experienced severe reaction to platelet concentrates despite prophylaxis	Prophylaxis is usually needed
FRESH FROZEN PLASMA	Patient has had multiple PRBC transfusions Abnormal coagulation factors	Provide ABO compatible component Transfuse immediately after thawing
IRRADIATED COMPONENTS Gamma radiation delivered to blood components inactivates lymphocytes within the product	Severely immunocompromised patients at risk for GVHD	Component is not radioactive Component should be labeled as being irradiated Red blood cells and platelets are not affected

Table 24-8   Major Complications Following BMT

Complication	Appearance	Signs/Symptoms	Management
GRAFT REJECTION	1-4 weeks	Absent/prolonged neutropenia Partial marrow recovery Hypoplasia Hemolysis	Blood component therapy Retransplantation
INFECTION			
Bacterial	1-5 weeks	Fever	Maintain protective environment
Fungal	1-5 weeks	Dry, nonproductive cough	
Viral		Change in breath sounds	Provide good hygiene
Herpes	1-3 months	Erythema—oropharynx/catheter site	Monitor vital signs frequently
Cytomegalovirus	3 months	Diarrhea	Frequent head-to-toe systems assessments
Varicella zoster	1st year	Lesions—skin or mucous membranes	Administer colony stimulating factors
		Hypotension	CMV negative blood products
			Administer broad spectrum antibiotics
			Administer acyclovir and/or ganciclovir
			Intravenous immunoglobulins
PNEUMONITIS			
Interstitial	1-4 months	Fever	CMV negative blood products
Toxic	1-6 months	Dry nonproductive cough	Leukocyte poor blood products
		Shortness of breath	Colony stimulating factors
		Tachypnea	Ganciclovir
		Interstitial changes on x-ray	Intravenous immunoglobulins
ACUTE GVHD	3-14 weeks	Maculopapular skin rash Nausea, vomiting, uncontrollable diarrhea Jaundice Elevated liver function tests Hepatomegaly	Immunosuppression with cyclosporine-A, steroids, and/or methotrexate Symptomatic treatment of skin, GI tract, and/or liver
CHRONIC GVHD			
Skin	months-years	Hyper- or hypo-pigmentation; patchy erythematous scaling; thickening, hardening resembling scleroderma; hair loss in involved areas	Immunosuppresion with cyclosporine-A, steroids, azathioprine (Imuran), and/or thalidomide (investigational)
Mouth		White striae and erythema on mucosa; decreased salivary flow with dryness of mouth	Symptom management of affected organ or system
Eyes		Dryness, redness, itching/burning; corneal thickening	
Sinuses		Chronic sinusitis; predisposition to gram positive infections	
GI tract		Difficulty swallowing; retrosternal pain; abdominal discomfort; diarrhea	

Continued.

Table 24–8   Major Complications Following BMT—cont'd

Complication	Appearance	Signs/Symptoms	Management
CHRONIC GVHD—cont'd			
Pulmonary		Productive cough; progressive dyspnea, wheezing, pneumothorax	
Vagina		Inflammation; dryness; stenosis	
Muscle		Occasional polymyositis; proximal weakness	
GU tract		Cystitis; mild nephrotic syndrome	
Hematopoietic		Eosinophilia; thrombocytopenia; hypoplastic marrow; marrow fibrosis	
Lymphoid		Hypocellularity and atrophy of lymph tissues; functional asplenia	
Endocrine		Decreased growth rates; delayed pubertal development; autoimmune hyperthyroidism	
Nervous system		Entrapment neuropathy; peripheral neuropathy; myasthenia gravis	
LATE EFFECTS			
Cataracts	1-6 years	Loss of vision Dryness	Surgical intervention
Gonad dysfunction	variable	Infertility Menopause	Replacement sex hormones Psychosexual counseling
Growth failure	variable	Impaired growth of facial skeleton and dentition (<6 y/o) Absent growth spurts No height changes	Supplemental growth hormone Replacement sex hormones
Hypothyroidism	1-15 years	Dry skin Hoarse speech Lethargy/apathy Weight gain with appetite loss Increased susceptibility to cold	Replacement hormones
Secondary malignancy	months-years	Specific to disease	Determined by type and extent of disease as well as by patient's physical and psychological status
RECURRENCE	months-years	Signs/symptoms of original disease	Determined by extent of disease and patient's physical and psychological status

erally in the first 3 to 6 months post-BMT. Varicella zoster is usually not seen until later in the first year post-transplant.[1] Viral infections are also commonly associated with the incidence of chronic GVHD and can occur at any time during the course of chronic GVHD.[1,3]

During the first 6 weeks post-transplant, prevention of infections is the most important step in counteracting infections. Maintaining protective environments, good hygiene, frequent monitoring of vital signs, and head-to-toe assessments are very important. The greater the speed of marrow recovery, the less the incidence of bacterial and fungal complications.[41] For this reason there is a strong interest in the benefits of growth factors to stimulate engraftment.

Pneumonitis

The most significant viral infection is that caused by CMV and is closely related to the incidence of interstitial pneumonitis. Greater than 50% of interstitial pneumonitis is caused by CMV.[1] Interstitial pneumonitis peaks in incidence around 2 to 3 months post-BMT and has a 60% mortality rate.[1,41,44] The risk factors for interstitial pneumonitis are: total body irradiation, presence of GVHD, advanced age of patient (>45 years), prior lung injury, and CMV serologic status of recipient and/or donor.[1,41]

Since CMV infection is a significant complication, screening for CMV during the pretransplant work up is routine. This screening is valuable to identify patients at risk, evaluate the need for prophylaxis, and to guide clinical steps if an infection is suspected.[47] Screening consists of serologic testing of the recipient and donor for CMV. The incidence of recipient seropositivity pretransplant is 40% to 70%.[47] In an allogeneic transplant a sero-positive donor may transmit CMV to a sero-negative recipient. In autologous transplants a sero-negative patient may convert to sero-positive due to blood product transfusion.

Prevention, early detection, prompt treatment, and immune restoration is important to a successful outcome.[44] One means of preventing CMV transmission is to provide sero-negative blood products to BMT recipients who are sero-negative and have a sero-negative marrow source. Since this can put a great strain on the blood bank an alternative is to provide leukocyte depleted blood components.[47] This is commonly accomplished by the use of special filters during the transfusion of the blood product. Prophylaxis with acyclovir or ganciclovir in CMV sero-positive recipients has also been used to decrease the chance of CMV infections. However, their use in this manner must be weighed against the risk of bone marrow toxicity as a side effect.[47] The most successful treatment of CMV is ganciclovir and intravenous immunoglobulins (IVIG).

Graft Vs. Host Disease

Graft vs. host disease (GVHD) is a complication that can occur following allogeneic BMT. It is an immune mediated reaction of the newly grafted marrow to the body of the recipient. Two types of GVHD have been identified: acute and chronic. They are distinguished from each other by the target organs, pathology, and timing post-transplant. Chronic GVHD may occur following acute GVHD but not necessarily. A patient may also develop chronic GVHD without ever having had acute GVHD.

ACUTE GVHD

Acute GVHD is typically defined as occurring before 100 days following BMT. There is a 45% incidence in HLA matched sibling donor transplants and greater than 75% incidence in HLA mismatch related donor transplants.[12] The risk factors related to the incidence of acute GVHD are: advanced patient age (>45 years); HLA mismatch; and donor-recipient sex mismatch.[41] The skin, GI tract, and liver are the primary target organs of acute GVHD. The occurrence of acute GVHD also prolongs immune deficiency.

Skin involvement is characterized by a maculopapular rash that can proceed to a desquamating dermatitis.[1] A biopsy of the skin is necessary to confirm the diagnosis and rule out other causes for the rash. In the first 20 days post-BMT this can be difficult due to changes in the skin related to the conditioning regimen.[1] The GI involvement is typically characterized by nausea, vomiting, and diarrhea. Again, a biopsy of the GI mucosa is the only definitive way to make a diagnosis. The pathologic changes seen in the GI tract are similar to those seen in the skin. In both the skin and the GI mucosa secondary infections can occur because the acute GVHD has altered their integrity. Liver involvement is characterized by jaundice, elevated liver function studies, and hepatomegaly.

Acute GVHD can range from mild to life threatening and is graded to distinguish its severity (Table 24-9). In its mildest form acute GVHD typically can be controlled and actually benefits those patients transplanted for malignancies. Patients with acute GVHD have a decreased incidence of disease recurrence.[12]

Since acute GVHD can be a life-threatening complication, means of preventing its occurrence are routinely administered. One of the most common means of preventing GVHD is the use of Cyclosporine-A (CsA), steroids, and/or methotrexate (MTX). All of these agents provide immunosuppression following BMT and are given according to a scheduled regimen (Table 24-10). Since GVHD is immune mediated, suppressing immune reactions following BMT should prevent its occurrence. The T cells have been identified as the primary culprit in GVHD. Depleting the marrow of T cells prior to infusion into the recipient has greatly reduced the incidence and severity of acute GVHD.[12] However, the incidence of graft rejection and/or relapse is also significantly increased.[12]

Treatment for acute GVHD centers around increasing immune suppression. This is primarily achieved through increasing dosages of CsA and steroids. Typically these are increased or initiated only for the acute GVHD to be controlled, then are tapered back to the scheduled dosage pattern. If there is limited or no response to the increase then further increases are made.

CHRONIC GVHD

The onset of chronic GVHD is typically post 100 days post-transplant; however, it can occur at 70 days or up to years post-transplant. It affects as many as 50%

Table 24-9 Acute GVHD Severity Grading

Stage	Skin	Liver	GI Tract
+	Maculopapular rash <25% of body surface	Bilirubin 2-3 mg/100 ml	Diarrhea >500 ml/day
+ +	Maculopapular rash 25%-30% of body surface	Bilirubin 3-6 mg/100 ml	Diarrhea >1000 ml/day
+ + +	Generalized erythroderma	Bilirubin 6-15 mg/100 ml	Diarrhea >1500 ml/day
+ + + +	Generalized erythroderma with bullous formation (>2 cm vesicle) and desquamation	Bilirubin >15 mg/100 ml	Severe abdominal pain with or without ileus

Table 24-10 Example Immunosuppression Schedule

Day of BMT	Cyclosporine-A	Methylprednisolone
−2	IV 5 mg/kg/day continuous infusion	
+4	IV 3 mg/kg/day continuous infusion	
+8		IVP 0.5 mg/kg BID
+15	IV 3.75 mg/kg/day continuous infusion	IVP 0.375 mg/kg BID
+23		IVP 0.25 mg/kg BID
+29	PO 7.5 mg/kg BID	
+31		PO 0.125 mg/kg BID
+36	PO 5 mg/kg BID	
+38		PO 0.25 mg/kg × 1
+40		PO 0.25 mg/kg × 1
+42		PO 0.25 mg/kg × 1
+84	PO 4 mg/kg BID	
+98	PO 3 mg/kg BID	
+120	PO 2 mg/kg BID	
+181	Discontinue	

of matched sibling transplants and is life threatening in about 5% of cases.[1,3] It is characterized by scleroderma-like features and persistent immunodeficiency.[1] It is a systemic multi-organ syndrome that resembles collagen-vascular diseases.[3] Chronic GVHD can be a continuation of acute GVHD, can occur after acute GVHD has resolved, or can occur without any acute GVHD preceding it. The risk factors related to incidence are: advanced age of recipient (>45 years), occurrence of preceding acute GVHD, T cell replete marrow, and female donor to male recipient.[3]

Almost every organ in the body can be affected by chronic GVHD (Table 24-8). The basic affect is that of dermal thickening, fibrosis, and dryness. Bacterial, fungal, and viral infections are common in patients with chronic GVHD and are the most frequent cause of death.[3] Late interstitial pneumonitis occurs fre-

quently. Mortality is highest in patients with progressive acute to chronic GVHD and those with multi-organ involvement.[39]

Recurrence

Disease or recurrence remains the most significant problem post-BMT. It is the major factor related to patient mortality greater than 3 months after BMT.[1,34,41] Relapse is more frequent following autologous BMT due to hidden malignant cells in the transplanted marrow.[1,41] In allogeneic BMT the presence of GVHD is associated with decreased incidence of recurrence.[12] In a few patients recurrent leukemia has been identified as being of donor origin, leading to the possibility that the leukemic environment of the recipient stimulated the susceptible donor cells.[1]

Late Effects

Long-term effects of BMT can occur several months to several years post-transplant. Late effects are a common concern as more patients survive disease-free for upward of 20 years post-BMT.[14,26] The more common effects are: cataracts, hypothyroidism, growth failure, gonadal dysfunction, and secondary malignancies. The late effects of BMT are of particular concern in the pediatric population and for patients with the possibility of cure with less intensive treatment.[26]

CATARACTS

Cataracts are of concern primarily in patients who receive TBI. Since radiation is more commonly being given in fractionated doses, the incidence of cataracts has decreased. Patients receiving TBI in a single dose have an 80% incidence of cataracts versus a 20% incidence when TBI is given in fractionated doses.[14,26] Patients receiving conditioning regimens of chemotherapy only do not have significant risk of developing cataracts.

GONADAL DYSFUNCTION

Sexual development is impaired in both males and females. Older patients (>40 years) are less likely to recover their reproductive functioning.[14] Following

TBI most females (90%) experience ovarian failure and require hormone replacement.[14,26] Males, following TBI, will recover production of testosterone but have absent or abnormal spermatogenesis.[14,26] If TBI is not used as part of the conditioning regimen, both males and females have a better chance of recovering gonadal functioning. There are several reports of patients having children post-transplant.[14]

GROWTH FAILURE

Impairment of growth is a common problem in children after BMT. Again, the incidence is high in those children who received TBI.[26] Of children who received TBI, 40% to 55% have decreased growth hormone, causing a retardation of spinal growth and the pubertal growth spurt.[14,26] Administration of growth hormone has shown some effect on growth velocity and some catch up in growth can occur.

HYPOTHYROIDISM

The incidence of hypothyroidism is also related to preparation with TBI. Thyroid function is affected in up to 60% of patients receiving single dose TBI and up to 25% in those receiving fractionated TBI.[14] Patients who have received conditioning regimens of chemotherapy only usually have normal thyroid function.[14]

SECONDARY MALIGNANCY

New malignancies may develop 6 months to years following BMT. TBI, immunosuppression, immunodeficiency, viral infection, chronic immune stimulation, and genetic predisposition are factors that have been identified with increased risk of second malignancy post-BMT.[14] Radiation appears to be the most important risk factor. Non-Hodgkin's lymphoma is the most frequently reported new malignancy and develops more often in donor cells.[26] The incidence of leukemia and solid tumors as secondary malignancies is rare. Most often the appearance of leukemia is a recurrence of the original disease.[26] Overall, BMT recipients have a sixfold to sevenfold higher tumor incidence than nontransplanted individuals.[14]

FUTURE DIRECTIONS AND ADVANCES IN BONE MARROW TRANSPLANTATION

According to data from the International Bone Marrow Transplant Registry, the number of patients undergoing BMT continues to increase annually. Future advances will include increasing numbers of autologous transplants, upper age limit for allogeneic transplants by a decade, transplants from mismatched or unrelated donors, and expansion of the donor pool. Alternative stem cell sources (e.g., autologous blood stem cell and cord blood stem cell transplantation) and transplantation of CD34 stem cells will provide more BMT options.

Important advances in conditioning regimens and the prevention and treatment of post-transplant complications will occur by extended uses of newer and more potent drugs. Biotherapy drugs such as biologic response modifiers, cytokines, and colony stimulating factors used to reduce relapse and enhance hematologic function will have continued exploration.

Immunotoxins (Orthozyne-H65-RTA used in corticosteriod-resistant AGVHD) and varied dosing schedules for cyclosporin, immunoglobulin, and ganiclovir are in Phase I and Phase II clinical trials.

Outpatient resources and transplantation via the outpatient mode will continue to expand. Third-party reimbursement, length of hospital stay, and financial resources for medications used in transplant recovery will have ongoing scrutiny. Advances in all of these areas require continued basic research in transplant biology and the efforts of the International Bone Marrow Transplant Registry, which provides invaluable analysis of worldwide bone marrow transplant data.[10,14,17,29,39]

Text continued on p. 582.

Nursing Management

Bone marrow transplantation is a strenuous medical treatment that in and of itself can be life threatening. As with any major medical treatment and life threatening situation faced by our patients and families, the general stresses that affect the patient and family must be addressed. These stresses are not necessarily unique to transplant; however, throughout the transplant process there are periods of transition when these general stresses increase in occurrence and/or intensity.

Prior experiences affect a patient/family examination of the risks and benefits of transplant. For some patients, the decision to have a transplant comes on the heels of being informed that they have a life-threatening illness and transplant must be done as soon as possible and is the only chance of cure. For other patients, the decision for transplant comes after a course or more of chemotherapy and living with their disease for a period of time pretransplant. Still other patients are informed at the time of diagnosis that a transplant is the only curative option and needs to be done within a certain time frame. Also affecting the patient's reaction to transplant is the ability to locate a donor if they cannot be their own donor and do not have a match within their family.

The idea of transplantation as a treatment option

generally creates a wide spectrum of emotional reactions. Patients may experience anxiety, fear, depression, denial, grieving, and hopefulness all at different times. Coping styles that the patient and family have relied on in the past will be those they most likely fall back on at this time. Dysfunctional or disruptive coping behaviors, such as substance abuse, may resurface. Past or current psychiatric problems may also become intensified.

Everyday life for these patients and their families will be disrupted by transplantation. There will be changes in patients' roles within the family. When the transplant center is a distance from home, the family may be separated for several months. The relocation of the patient and a family member may be necessary. Child care as well as elder care can be affected by changes in the roles of family members. New routines also have to be incorporated into family life. Lifestyle changes following transplant may be permanent or temporary and can be a major disruption on family life.

The financial impacts of transplant can be devastating to families. Transplantation is a costly treatment. This is due to the numerous resources necessary to care for the patient. The cost of housing, food, dependent care, and transportation can seriously affect the financial status of any family. Reimbursement continues to vary based on the third-party payor and the disease being treated. Third-party payors may detail which diseases they accept as being treatable by transplantation and which are experimental. Very rarely are the costs of searching for an unrelated donor covered by third parties. They may cover the cost of the patient's care throughout the transplant, but the cost of searching for an unrelated donor is not covered.

Donors for allogeneic transplants also have special considerations that need to be addressed. The most important is the one of choice. Potential donors need to be adequately educated as to their role in a transplant if they are a match. It is the donor's choice to donate. In families with less then ideal relationships, this can be a challenge. Donors also need to be aware that agreeing to donate carries some amount of responsibility for the recipient's health. However, they must also understand that once they have donated, they have no control over what happens to the recipient. This is especially important in cases where patients develop GVHD.

Caring for patients undergoing BMT requires comprehensive and consistent nursing management. Patient/family teaching is key to providing assistance to patients and family members throughout the transplant process. Table 24-11 outlines the teaching priorities by stage of transplantation. Examples of nursing diagnosis and interventions for patients undergoing BMT follow.

Nursing Management

NURSING DIAGNOSES	INTERVENTIONS
Body image disturbance, potential Related to treatment process	Encourage patient to verbalize feelings about appearance and perceptions of life style changes. Validate perceptions and assure that responses are appropriate. Promote acceptance of positive, realistic body image. Suggest ways that the patient can cope with body image changes
Comfort, alteration, potential Related to side effects of treatment regimens	Assess patient's pain: Location Onset Frequency Intensity Quality Identify effective pain control measures. Administer medications as ordered and needed. Assess for effectiveness of pain control measures. Intervene at onset of pain. Instruct patient in relaxation techniques (see Chapter 28).

Table 24-11 Patient/Family Teaching Priorities

Topic	Pretransplant	During Transplant	Post-transplant
Transplant Process			
Donor identification	X		
Tissue typing	X		
Recipient workup	X		
Donor workup	X		
Goal of transplant	X	X	
Duration of process	X	X	
Conditioning regimen	X	X	
Bone marrow harvest	X	X	
Immunosuppression	X	X	X
Unit environment	X	X	
Central Venous Catheter			
Insertion	X	X	
Catheter care		X	X
Routine Care			
Hygiene/skin care	X	X	
Oral care	X	X	
Nutrition	X	X	
Infection precaution	X	X	
Bleeding precautions	X	X	
Side Effects			
Nausea/vomiting	X	X	
Diarrhea	X	X	
Alopecia	X	X	
Stomatitis	X	X	
Seizures	X	X	
Hypotension	X	X	
Cystitis	X	X	
Acral erythema	X	X	
Conjunctivitis	X	X	
Fever	X	X	
Parotitis	X	X	
Complications			
Graft rejection	X	X	X
Infections	X	X	X
Pneumonitis	X	X	X
GVHD	X	X	X
Late effects	X	X	X
Recurrence	X	X	X
Supportive Care			
Blood components	X	X	X
Antibiotics	X	X	X
Antifungals	X	X	X
Antivirals	X	X	X
Parenteral nutrition	X	X	X
Psychosocial			
Coping strategies	X	X	X
Sexuality	X	X	X
Socialization	X	X	X
Resources	X	X	X
Discharge			
Follow-up schedule		X	X
Medications		X	X
Diet		X	X
Activity	X	X	X
Precautions	X	X	X
Work/school	X	X	X
Emergency contact	X	X	X

NURSING DIAGNOSES — cont'd

Coping, ineffective, individual
Related to transplant process
Related to potential life style changes

Coping, compromised, family
Related to transplant process
Related to role changes

Fluid and electrolyte imbalance, potential for
Related to treatment process

Growth and development, altered
Related to late effects of treatment

Infection, potential for
Related to myelosuppression
Related to immunosuppression

INTERVENTIONS — cont'd

Assess patient's level of distress and anxiety related to:
Uncertainty of future
Bothersome symptoms
Changes in self-concept
Assess for signs of maladaptive or risky behaviors that interfere with responsible health practices.
Identify patient's support system, resources and communication patterns.
Assess patient's ability to problem solve.
Listen attentively and provide support.
Encourage verbalization of fears.
Assist patient with problem solving as needed.
Provide reassurance that anxiety or distress are common feelings among transplant patients.
Initiate referrals to social work, psychology, or community resources as appropriate (see Chapter 30).

Assess past family relationships and coping patterns.
Provide opportunities for family to express feelings.
Assist family members in adapting to changes in roles and activities as appropriate.
Listen attentively and provide support.
Encourage communication and positive interaction between patient and family.
Initiate referrals to social work, psychology, or community resources as appropriate.

Monitor patient's
Intake and output
Weight
Abdominal girth
Edema
Serum electrolytes
Blood urea nitrogen
Hemoglobin and hematocrit
Assess patient for signs of fluid overload or dehydration.
Administer diuretics as ordered.
Maintain fluid restrictions as needed.

Monitor patient's growth according to standard growth charts.
Assess for accomplishments of normal growth and developmental tasks.
Monitor for learning disabilities.
Provide referrals for educational and emotional support as needed.
Administer growth hormone as ordered and assess for response.

Assess for signs and symptoms of infection:
Fever
Cough
Erythema

NURSING DIAGNOSES — cont'd	INTERVENTIONS — cont'd
	Institute measures to prevent exposure to potential sources of infection:
	Meticulous handwashing
	Meticulous hygiene
	Good oral hygiene after meals
	Monitor white blood count and differential.
	Monitor vital signs and head-to-toe systems assessments frequently.
	Obtain cultures of blood, urine, stool, sputum as ordered and appropriate.
	Administer antibiotics, antifungals, antivirals, and antipyretics as ordered.
	Instruct patient and family in prevention of infections.
	Monitor culture results and serum antibiotic levels as needed.
	Implement protective isolation precautions per hospital policy.
	Minimize invasive procedures.
Injury, potential for	Monitor platelet count and anticipate nadir.
Related to thrombocytopenia	Assess for signs and symptoms of bleeding:
	Petechiae
	Ecchymosis
	Epistaxis
	Vaginal or rectal bleeding
	Administer platelet transfusions as ordered.
	Observe patient for signs of transfusion reaction and response to transfusions.
	Teach patient to avoid:
	Shaving with razor
	Flossing teeth
	Picking nose or scabs
	Forceful nose-blowing
Knowledge deficit	Evaluate patient and family readiness to learn.
Related to transplant process	Identify barriers to learning such as language, physical deficiencies, psychological deficiencies, intellectual development.
	Determine patient and family knowledge of the transplant process.
	Review information patient and family have already been given.
	Provide written or audiovisual education materials and review with patient and family.
	Allow adequate time for verbalization of questions, concerns and fears.
	Reinforce and clairfy information as needed.
Nutrition, altered: less than body requirements	Assess nutritional intake and monitor calorie counts.
Related to effects of treatment process	Assess for causes of decreased nutritional intake:
	Nausea and vomiting
	Xerostomia
	Taste changes

NURSING DIAGNOSES — cont'd

Sexuality patterns, altered
  Related to treatment process
  Related to late effects

Skin integrity, impaired, potential
  Related to treatment process
  Related to GVHD

INTERVENTIONS — cont'd

Provide small frequent meals.

Initiate referral to dietician for assessment of food preferences and appropriateness of diet (see Chapter 27).

Assess for physical symptoms that may affect libido.

Assess for fear, anxiety, depression, and diminished self-concept.

Promote open communication about sexual issues by bringing up the subject.

Instruct patient on appropriate hygiene and contraceptive measures (see Chapter 31).

Assess impaired area every shift for:
  Color
  Scaling
  Bleeding
  Drainage
  Tenderness

Avoid use of harsh soaps, hot water, perfume, deodorant, and based creams.

Maintain meticulous hygiene with antibacterial soap.

Instruct patient to avoid activities and clothing that irritate affected areas.

Instruct patient to avoid exposure to the sun and use sun screen when outdorrs.

Use therapeutic beds and pain medications as needed for severe skin GVHD (see Chapter 29).

CONCLUSION

Bone marrow transplantation via autologous and allogeneic methods and/or the peripheral blood stem cell process offers many patients with life-threatening diseases cure and new hope for the future. Since the availability of the National Marrow Donor Registry Program, DNA typing, and multiple blood component therapy resources, options have increased for the patient requiring this treatment. Continued clinical research exploring treatment regimens, multi-recovery agents (hematopoietic growth factors), and antibiotic/antifungal/antiviral drugs will be ongoing challenges. Financial reimbursement continues to vary based on the third-party payor and out-of-pocket expenses for the recipient/donor/family are currently the most unsettled issues facing the patient/family. Many opportunities exist for nurses in this challenging practice environment.

The following is a list of resources and support services for patients and families undergoing bone marrow transplantation.

1. Aplastic Anemia Foundation of America
   Baltimore, Maryland
2. American Cancer Society
   Atlanta, Georgia
3. BMT Newsletter
   Highland Park, Illinois
4. Cancer Information Service
5. Candlelighters Childhood Cancer Foundation
   Washington DC
6. Corporate Angel Network
   White Plains, New York
7. Immune Deficiency Foundation
8. Leukemia Society of America
   New York, New York
9. LIFE-SAVERS Foundation of America
   Covina, California
10. National Bone Marrow Donor Program
    St. Paul, Minnesota
11. National Cancer Institute
    Washington DC
12. National Coalition of Cancer Survivorship
    Albuquerque, New Mexico
13. Oncology Nursing Society Bone Marrow Transplant Special Interest Group
    Pittsburgh, Pennsylvania

14. Ronald McDonald Houses and Children's Charities
Chicago, Illinois

BIBLIOGRAPHY

1. Abramowsky CR and Coccia PF: Bone marrow transplantation in pediatrics. In Abramowsky CR and Colvin RB, editors: Organ transplantation in children, Basel, 1989, Karger.
2. Applebaum FR: Bone marrow transplantation. In Wittes RE, editor: Manual of oncologic therapeutics, Philadelphia, 1988, JB Lippincott Co.
3. Atkinson K: Chronic graft-versus-host disease following marrow transplantation, Marrow Transplantation Reviews 2:1, 1992.
4. Ayash LJ and others: Hepatic venoocclusive disease in autologous bone marrow transplantation of solid tumors and lymphomas, J Clin Oncol, 8:1699, 1990.
5. Barlogie B and Gahrton G: Bone marrow transplantation in multiple myeloma, Bone Marrow Transplant 7:71, 1991.
6. Belec RH: Quality of life: Perceptions of long-term survivors of bone marrow transplantation, Oncol Nurs Forum 19:31, 1992.
7. Bell AJ and others: Peripheral blood stem cell autografting, Lancet 1:1027, 1986.
8. Benisinger WI and Berenson RJ: Peripheral blood and positive selection of marrow as a source of stem cells for transplantation, Prog Clin Biol Res 337:93, 1990.
9. Bernasconi C and others: Allogeneic versus autologous bone marrow transplantation versus intensive post remission chemotherapy in acute leukaemias, Bone Marrow Transplant 4(Suppl 4):65, 1989.
10. BMT Newsletter, Peripheral stem cell transplants, BMT Newsletter, 11:1, 1992.
11. Castaigne S and others: Successful haematopoietic reconstitution using autologous peripheral blood mononucleated cells in a patient with acute promyelocytic leukemia, Br J Haematol 62:209, 1986.
12. Champlin RE: T-cell depletion for bone marrow transplantation: Effects on graft rejection, graft-versus-host disease, graft-versus-leukemia, and survival, Cancer Treat Res 50:99, 1990.
13. Chielens D and Herrick E: Recipients of bone marrow transplants: Making a smooth transition to an ambulatory care setting, Oncol Nurs Forum 17:857, 1990.
14. Deeg HJ: Delayed complications of marrow transplantation, Marrow Transplant Rev 2:10, 1992.
15. Donahue RE and others: Human IL-3 and GM-CSF act synergistically in stimulating hematopoiesis in primates, Science 241:1820, 1988.
16. Ersek M: The process of maintaining hope in adults undergoing bone marrow transplantation for leukemia, Oncol Nurs Forum 19:883, 1992.
17. Gale RP, Armitage JO, and Dicke KA: Autotransplants: Now and in the future, Bone Marrow Transplant 7:153, 1991.
18. Gaston-Johansson F, Franco T, and Zimmerman L: Pain and psychological distress in patients undergoing autologous bone marrow transplantation, Oncol Nurs Forum, 19:41, 1992.
19. Gianni AM and others: Rapid and complete hematopoietic reconstitution following combined transplantation of autologous blood and bone marrow cells. A changing role for high dose chemo-radiotherapy?, Hematol Oncol 7:139, 1989.
20. Gorin NC: Autologous bone marrow transplantation in hematological malignancies, Am J Clin Oncol 14(Suppl 1):S5, 1991.
21. Haas R and others: Successful autologous transplantation of blood stem cells mobilized with recombinant human granulocyte/macrophage colony-stimulating factor, Exp Hematol 18:94, 1990.
22. Jones RJ: Autologous bone marrow transplantation in hematologic malignancies, Curr Opin Oncol 3:234, 1991.
23. Kessinger A and others: Reconstitution of human hematopoietic function with autologous cryopreserved circulating stem cells, Exp Hematol 14:192, 1986.
24. Kessinger A and others: Cryopreservation and infusion of autologous peripheral stem cells, Bone Marrow Transplant 5:25, 1990.
25. Kessinger A: Autologous peripheral stem cell transplantation, Marrow Transplant Rev 25, 1992.
26. Klob HJ and Bender-Gotze CH: Late complications after allogeneic bone marrow transplantation for leukaemia, Bone Marrow Transplant 6:61, 1990.
27. Korbling M and others: Autologous transplantation of blood-derived hematopoietic stem cells after myeloablative therapy in a patient with Burkitt's lymphoma, Blood 67:529, 1986.
28. Lum LG and Storb R: Bone marrow transplantation. In Flye MW, editor: Principles of organ transplantation, Philadelphia, 1989, WB Saunders Co.
29. Marks DI and Goldman JM: Bone marrow transplantation in chronic myelogenous leukemia, Marrow Transplant Rev 2:17, 1992.
30. McGlave P: Bone marrow transplants in chronic myelogenous leukemia: An overview of determinants of survival, Semin Hematol 27:23, 1990.
31. McMillan A and Goldstone A: What is the value of autologous bone marrow transplantation in the treatment of relapsed or resistant Hodgkin's disease?, Leuk Res 15:237, 1991.

32. Moss TJ: Bone marrow transplantation for solid tumors in pediatrics, Cancer Treat Res 50:279, 1990.

33. Peters WP: The myeloid colony stimulating factors: Introduction and overview, Semin Hematol 28(Suppl 2):1, 1991.

34. Rabinowe SN and others: The impact of myeloid growth factors on engraftment following autologous bone marrow transplantation for malignant lymphoma, Semin Hematol 28(Suppl 2):6, 1991.

35. Reiffers J and others: Successful autologous transplantation with peripheral blood hematopoietic cells in a patient with acute leukemia, Exp Hematol 14:312, 1986.

36. Santos GW: Overview of autologous bone marrow transplantation (ABMT), Int J Cell Cloning 3:215, 1985.

37. Seeger RC and Reynolds CP: Treatment of high-risk solid tumors of childhood with intensive therapy and autologous bone marrow transplantation, Ped Clin North Am 38:393, 1991.

38. Steeves RH: Patients who have undergone bone marrow transplantation: Their quest for meaning, Oncol Nurs Forum 19:899, 1992.

39. Sullivan KM: Prevention and treatment of chronic graft-versus-host disease, Marrow Transplant Rev 2:8, 1992.

40. Tilly H and others: Haemopoietic reconstitution after autologous peripheral blood stem cell transplantation in acute leukemia, Lancet 11:154, 1986.

41. Tutschka PJ: Early complications of bone marrow transplantation in children and adults, Bone Marrow Transplant 4(Suppl 4):22, 1989.

42. Ulich TR and others: Acute and subacute hematologic effects of multi-colony stimulating factor in combination with granulocyte colony stimulating factor in vivo, Blood 75:48, 1990.

43. Vitale V, Barra S and Frazone P: Total body irradiation in the conditioning regimen for hematological malignancies, Bone Marrow Transplant 8(Suppl 1):28, 1991.

44. Volker DL: Clinical characteristics of cytomegalovirus infection, Nursing Acumen 3:1, 1992.

45. Vose JM, Armitage JO, and Bierman PJ: Bone marrow transplantation for Hodgkin's disease, non-Hodgkin's lymphoma, and multiple myeloma, Cancer Treat Res 50:259, 1990.

46. Whedon MB, editor: Bone marrow transplantation principles, practice and nursing insights, Boston, 1991, Jones and Bartlett Publishers.

47. Whedon MB: Cytomegalovirus-seronegative autologous bone marrow transplant patient, Nursing Acumen 3:4, 1992.

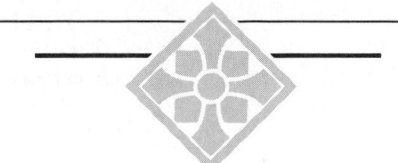

CHAPTER 25

Cancer Clinical Trials

Linda Meili

Oncology as a medical and nursing specialty has grown rapidly over the past 20 years. The efforts of a nation-wide network of physicians and nurses performing clinical trials resulted in improved surgical outcomes, new chemotherapy agents, less toxic radiation therapy, and the testing of numerous biologic agents and growth hormones. Many cancers once fatal are now curable, and many other cancers are considered chronic diseases with many long-term survivors.

Nurses are at the forefront of this battle against cancer. Oncology nurses now administer first-time treatments given to patients. In clinical trials, nurses ensure that treatments are given safely and that patients are monitored closely for known and unknown side effects. Nurses perform numerous expanded roles in all phases of clinical trials. Nurses are much more than participants in medical trials, however. Nurses are independent clinical researchers who study the human response to disease and treatments. Clinical trial patients present nurses with the opportunity to identify and study the effects, responses, and sequelae of new medical therapies and to define appropriate nursing interventions.

This chapter provides the framework for understanding the history, purpose, and implementation of clinical trials. The roles of the oncology nurse as direct caregiver, educator, advocate, coordinator, administrator, and researcher are discussed.

HISTORICAL PERSPECTIVE OF CLINICAL TRIALS

The United States federal government founded the National Institutes of Health (NIH) in 1887. The purpose of the NIH is to support research in the causes, diagnosis, prevention, and cure of human disease.[46] As one of the largest biomedical research facilities in the world, the NIH is part of the U.S. Department of Health and Human Services.

Many of the early clinical trials in this country focused on the prophylaxis and treatment of infectious diseases.[45] By the 1930s, cancer was identified as a major health problem requiring a large-scale, national plan of action. In 1937, Congress unanimously passed the National Cancer Institute Act, which appropriated $700,000 to establish the National Cancer Institute (NCI), now the largest of the 12 NIH institutes. The NCI expected to break new theoretical ground by conducting its own research, promoting research in other institutions, and coordinating cancer-related activities throughout the country.[12] The NCI underwent numerous reorganizations and expansions over the next decades.

The Warren Grant Magnuson Clinical Center was established in 1953 on the NIH campus. The Clinical Center is shared by the NIH institutes that are conducting combined laboratory and clinical studies. Both inpatients and ambulatory care patients from all over the world participate in cancer clinical trials at this facility. Travel, nursing care, and medical care are provided to these patients at no cost.[46]

The trials performed within the NIH Clinical Center are called *intramural* research studies. *Extramural* trials are those NCI-sponsored studies conducted at universities, medical schools, and hospitals across the country. Extramural research programs are supported by grants, contracts, or cooperative agreements and utilize about 80% of the funds appropriated to the NIH by Congress.[46]

The post-World War II years brought successes in cancer treatment with the development of new chemotherapy agents. The National Chemotherapy Program, funded through congressional appropriations in 1955, was devoted to testing new chemicals that might prove to be effective antineoplastic agents. The Cancer Chemotherapy National Service Center at the NCI functioned as a pharmaceutical house to move new drugs into both the intramural and extramural trials. In 1965, the program expanded to include international drugs.

The motivated efforts of a public and private campaign ultimately resulted in the signing of the National Cancer Act in 1971. This created a national cancer program administered by the NCI with its director appointed by and reporting to the president of the United States. This legislation was a landmark in the history of cancer treatment and research. Increased power and funding created new opportunities for physicians, improving the quality and increasing the accessibility of cancer care for patients across the country.

In 1991 on the twentieth anniversary of the National Cancer Act, Harold Freeman, chairman of the President's Cancer Panel, testified before a house panel and listed the following accomplishments in cancer treatment[8]:

- Fewer amputations in osteosarcoma patients
- 50% survival in acute lymphocytic leukemia, improved from 28%
- Improvement in 5-year survival of women with breast cancer from 85% to 91%
- Prostate cancer 5-year survival 71%, up from 50%

The following programs, initiated by the NCI since 1971, increased the number of cancer specialists and organized a structure to coordinate national research and to translate research advances into clinical practice.

Oncology Training Programs

The NCI funded fellowship programs in medical oncology and radiotherapy. There were 100 medical oncologists in the 1960s; now there are more than 4000.[12] The first certifying examinations for medical oncologists were in 1974. The increased numbers of radiation therapists and medical oncologists allowed movement of this specialty from predominantly university settings into community hospitals and into many less urban settings.

Comprehensive Cancer Centers

The National Cancer Act of 1971 formally authorized the Cancer Centers Program.[12] The NCI was challenged to develop a network of specialized and comprehensive cancer centers to serve as a national resource for research and a multidisciplinary treatment approach, as well as a community resource through outreach programs and cancer control.[11] Designation as a comprehensive cancer center requires meeting eight criteria established by the NCI. These include basic research, mechanisms for technology transfer, clinical research, program of high priority clinical trials, cancer prevention and control research, research training and continuing education programs, cancer information services, and community service and outreach activities.[11] In 1993, there were 28 comprehensive cancer centers, a tremendous increase since the year of the National Cancer Act when there were only three.

Cooperative Research Groups

Cooperative research groups consist of researchers who jointly develop and conduct cancer treatment clinical trials in a multi-institutional setting.[11] These groups are funded by the National Cancer Institute through cooperative agreements. The cooperative group program started wth the National Chemotherapy Service Center funding in 1955. The original purpose of the groups was to test the new chemotherapy agents developed at the NCI. The scope of the program has broadened through the years and current areas of research include evaluation of multimodality therapies, basic science, supportive care, quality of life, and chemoprevention trials.[11] The results of cooperative group research are reported through group-wide meetings and published in scientific journals.

The goals of cooperative group research are:
- To improve survival and quality of life for cancer patients
- Conduct basic scientific research on cancer biology, pathology, epidemiology, supportive care
- To serve as a research base for the conduct of cancer control research
- To conduct oncology nursing research[11]

Cooperative groups share common goals, but may differ in their clinical focus. The focus may be the multimodality treatment of all adult cancers or all pediatric cancers. Other groups focus on a specific type of cancer or specific type of treatment. There are currently 13 cooperative groups funded by the NCI. These groups are listed in the box on p. 587. The names of certain groups imply a geographic focus (Southwest Oncology Group), however they include members from across the country and some international locations as well.

Cooperative groups are generally similar in structure. They are composed of an operations office, statistical center, and various standing committees. The operations office manages the administrative affairs of the group and houses the group chairman. The statistical center, which may be in a different location, houses the group biostatistician and protocol data coordinators. This office handles protocol registration,

NCI-FUNDED COOPERATIVE RESEARCH GROUPS

Brain Tumor Cooperative Group (BTCG)
Cancer and Leukemia Group B (CALGB)
Children's Cancer Study Group (CCSG)
Eastern Cooperative Oncology Group (ECOG)
European Organization for Research and Treatment of Cancer (EORTC)
Gynecological Oncology Group (GOG)
Intergroup Rhabdomyosarcoma Study (IRS)
National Surgical Adjuvant Project for Breast and Bowel Cancers (NSABP)
National Wilms' Tumor Study (NWTS)
North Central Cancer Treatment Group (NCCTG)
Pediatric Oncology Group (POG)
Radiation Therapy Oncology Group (RTOG)
Southwest Oncology Group (SWOG)

quality control of date, and ongoing statistical analysis of protocols. Each cooperative group has standing disease and discipline committees that represent the group's focus.

The role of oncology nurses in cooperative research groups has strengthened over the past decade. Most cooperative groups have a standing nurse oncologist committee with the chairperson being a member of the Board of Governors. Nurses review protocols prior to activation to assess the impact of the proposed treatment on the nursing unit. Nurses also are principal investigators or coinvestigators on companion studies and cancer control studies. The issue of nursing research in clinical trials is addressed later in this chapter.

Community-Based Research Programs

COOPERATIVE GROUP OUTREACH PROGRAM. The Cooperative Group Outreach Program (CGOP), implemented in 1976, was the NCI's first comprehensive effort to extend participation in clinical trials to community physicians. The objectives of the program are to make state-of-the-art cancer treatment available to patients in the community setting, adding to the pool of patients on clinical trials. The program consists of individual community oncologists, surgeons, or radiation therapists contracting with a member institution of a cooperative group to register patients on research protocols. The amount of funding the CGOPs receive is based on the number of eligible patients they enter on studies.[11]

COMMUNITY CLINICAL ONCOLOGY PROGRAM. The Community Clinical Oncology Program (CCOP) was initiated by the NCI in 1983 to disseminate state-of-the-art cancer research to patients in community settings. CCOP institutions are groups of community-based physicians who are linked to cooperative groups and cancer centers that serve as their research bases.[11]

This mechanism is beneficial to the patients, the community, and the NCI. Patients now have access to investigational therapies without traveling to a geographically distant treatment center. The local medical community benefits through opportunities for education and exchange of information. The National Cancer Institute benefits by having available more patients potentially eligible for registration on clinical trials.

All studies available for CCOP participation through the 17 research bases are assigned a "credit" value by the NCI. Generally, treatment studies are assigned one to two credits per patient depending on the complexity of the study. CCOPs are required to accrue at least 50 treatment credits each year.

CANCER CONTROL. Cancer control is the reduction of cancer incidence, morbidity, and mortality through an orderly sequence from research or interventions (including their impact on populations) to the broad, systematic appreciation of the research results.[29] With the National Cancer Act in 1971, cancer control activities were formalized as part of the National Cancer Program and recognized as a distinct program entity. With the creation of the Division of Cancer Control and Rehabilitation (DCPC) at the NCI in 1974, a national effort for effective intervention was made possible for the first time.[32] DCPC research priorities include tobacco-use control; diet, nutrition, and cancer prevention; chemoprevention; early detection; and access to state-of-the-art diagnosis and treatment.

Cancer control research is implemented through the cooperative group mechanism. Each cooperative group has a standing cancer control committee composed of interested oncology nurses, physicians, epidemiologists, and statisticians. Cancer control concepts are developed and submitted to the DCPC for review. Once the concept is approved, a protocol is developed and resubmitted to the NCI for final review, approval, and eventual activation by the research group. In 1986, the NCI mandated CCOP participation in cancer control research. CCOPs are required to accrue 50 cancer control credits per year. Cancer control studies are usually assigned a portion of credit (0.1, 0.3, 0.5) per patient registered.[11]

Oncology nurses, well-versed in the clinical trials mechanisms, are primarily responsible for the implementation, data collection, and conduct of the study.[34] Oncology nurses may evolve into independent prevention investigators in trials that treat well populations with essentially toxic agents.[75] Examples of current NCI-approved cancer control trials are listed in Table 25-1.

MINORITY-BASED CCOPS.   The CCOP model was

Table 25-1   Current Cooperative Group Cancer Control Research Studies

Name	Description
NSABP/P-1	A clinical trial to determine the worth of tamoxifen for preventing breast cancer
URCC/1990M	Control of vasomotor symptoms associated with tamoxifen therapy in postmenopausal women with breast cancer
MDACC/DM 89-089	Utility of a panel of intermediate markers in predicting colonic adenomatous polyp recurrence
SWOG-9041	Chemoprevention of recurrent adenomas and second primary colorectal carcinoma
POG 9284/85	Barriers to enrollment onto frontline therapeutic clinical trials

expanded in 1993 when the NCI funded 13 minority-based CCOPs. These are located in areas that serve ethnic minorities and poor populations. Minority-based CCOPs accrue patients on both treatment and cancer control studies.

Non-NCI Supported Research

Although the NCI supports a large network of cancer centers, cooperative research groups, and community programs, the majority of cancer clinical trials are not NCI sponsored. While comprehensive cancer centers and university hospitals contribute patients to NCI studies, they also conduct their own cancer research activities. These research studies are developed by physician investigators in their own institution. Studies include early trials with new chemotherapy or biologic agents, as well as comparative randomized trials to identify new or more effective drug combinations. Cancer clinical trials are also conducted by radiation therapists in these institutions.

The pharmaceutical industry sponsors many clinical trials to evaluate new agents. The pharmaceutical company contracts with institutions or individual investigators to register patients in their studies. In recent years, there has been a striking increase in clinical trials conducted by private pharmaceutical firms, largely related to a marked expansion in the field of biotherapeutics.[11]

DRUG DEVELOPMENT

The NCI is the largest, single sponsor of studies using antineoplastic agents. More than 100 such agents are currently in clinical testing and even a larger number are in preclinical testing.[11] New drugs are also developed by pharmaceutical companies. Agents at the NCI are developed through the Investigational Drug Branch (IDB), a division of the Cancer Therapy and Evaluation Program (CTEP). The development of new agents, whether through IDB or industry, is extremely costly in terms of labor, time, and financial resources.

Identification

The first and most obvious step is the discovery of the new agent. There are two basic approaches for the selection of chemicals to be tested: the empirical

and the rational. The empirical approach is a systematic screening of chemicals from a wide variety of plant, animal, and mineral sources. For example, didemnin B, an agent currently under study, was derived from the sea squirt; vincristine, an effective commercially available drug, was extracted from the vinca alkaloid plant. The emphasis on natural products is due to the observation that many human diseases are successfully treated by these substances.[15]

Drawbacks of the traditional discovery process are that thousands of substances must be screened to find one that has activity in human cancer. After investing large amounts of time and money, it is still unknown why the response is produced or how it may be improved. Rational drug design addresses these shortcomings by trying to identify the cell receptor site responsible for a given effect and, through a systematic process, specifically design compounds to stimulate or inhibit the receptor. Techniques of molecular biology refined in the biotechnology industry and computer technology aid in this process. The Division of Cancer Treatment at the NCI has established a grant program, the National Cooperative Drug Discovery Groups. These groups promote collaboration among scientists from academia, government, and industry in developing new cancer agents.[25,44,45]

Drug Screening

Identified compounds are entered into the NCI's Division of Cancer Treatment's drug testing program. Computer analysis and application of specific criteria for selection reduce the chance of duplicating drugs already under evaluation. The NCI selects approximately 10,000 of the 40,000 available substances for further testing.[33] These 10,000 compounds then undergo a screening process that utilizes both animal and human tumor systems. The tumor system most commonly used from 1955 to 1975 was the murine L1210 leukemia system. Tumors of uniform and predictable behavior were transplanted into mice, and the new drugs were given to the mice to evaluate tumor shrinkage and prolonged survival. This screening system was eventually found to be effective in selecting drugs active against leukemias and lymphomas, but ineffective against solid tumors.[15] Now the initial screening is performed in a system called the P388 mouse leukemia. Approximately 250 agents will demonstrate antitumor effect in this system and advance to a tumor panel consisting of human tumors transplanted into immunodeprived ("nude") mice. The current panel includes L1210 leukemia, B16 melanoma, M5076 mouse tumor, and MX-1, a human mammary xenograft.[33] The agent must show efficacy in at least one of the tumors to advance to further testing. The human tumor cloning system developed in 1980 can grow human cancer cells in culture for the purpose of anticancer drug screening. This system has identified effective drugs that showed no activity in the P388 screening system.[15]

Formulation and Production

Ten of the compounds that successfully pass through the screening system will be selected for identification, purification, and definition of chemical structure. Large amounts of the drug must be produced so there is sufficient quantity for further testing. The agent Taxol is a recent example of a drug production problem. This agent, known to be effective against ovarian cancer and possibly lung and breast cancer, is found in the bark of the Pacific yew tree. A hugh volume of yew bark must be harvested to produce even small quantities of Taxol. The fact that a particular type of owl, an endangered species, inhabits these trees set the stage for debate among the scientific community, conservationists, and the government. Currently, private companies are conducting research to synthetically manufacture this agent.

Toxicity Testing

Preclinical testing for drug toxicity is required once formulation and production problems are solved. Usually seven to nine compounds are tested per year. The goals of toxicology studies are to predict the safest starting dose for clinical trials and the prediction of organ system toxicity.[25] Toxicity testing is done in mice. Testing used to be done in a number of larger animals, but this was expensive and did not increase the safety of the drugs.[15] The mice are used to develop a dose-response curve. The lethal dose in 10%, 50%, and 90% of the animals is determined. The dose that is lethal in 10% of the mice, called the LD10, is used to establish an initial dose for human trials. To maximize safety, if an unknown compound is being given in humans, only 10% of the LD10 is used at first.

Investigational New Drug Application

Before a drug can be studied in humans, its sponsor, either the NCI or a pharmaceutical company, submits an Investigational New Drug Application (IND) to the Food and Drug Administration (FDA) to request permission to evaluate the agent in human cancer.[79] The sponsor may begin to investigate the drug 30 days after the FDA has received the application.[49] The development process for a new drug is lengthy and costly, taking approximately 12 years and 50 to 70 million dollars from screening to commercial availability.[33]

Physician Approval

Physicians participating in the human clinical trials of investigational drugs must first be approved by the FDA. The FDA requires that these physicians, by medical training and experience, can assume responsibility for compliance with the protocol requirements for drug administration, data monitoring, and toxicity reporting. The physicians sign an agreement that outlines their responsibilities in clinical research, Form FDA 1573.[41]

Clinical trials are carefully controlled experiments aimed at utilizing the smallest number of subjects to determine with statistical confidence the effectiveness of treatments and, at the same time, maintain patient safety.[44] The primary goal of clinical cancer research is to identify treatments that ultimately translate into improved quality of life and improved survival.[56]

Several steps must occur before a clinical trial is implemented. The first is the design and writing of the cancer treatment protocol and second, the approval of regulatory boards.

CANCER PROTOCOLS

A protocol is a formal document written to clearly describe the proposed experiment.[56] Both cancer treatment and cancer control experiments are written as protocol documents. Protocols provide the rationale for the proposed study, the study objectives or questions to be answered, and a concise description of the treatment involved. Protocols are written in a similar format and contain the same basic elements regardless of whether the study originates in a cancer center, cooperative group, or pharmaceutical company. The protocol is written by the principal investigator and must be approved by the study sponsor prior to distribution to participating investigators. The protocol is then followed by everyone involved in the study— physicians, nurses, data managers, pharmacists, study sponsor, and statisticians. The protocol document may be revised or amended as needed by the study sponsor throughout the course of the clinical trial. It is helpful to have a set of protocol notebooks with all the active studies near the area (hospital oncology unit or clinic setting) where protocol patients are evaluated and treated.

Table 25-2 lists the basic elements of a protocol, describes the purpose of each element, and presents nursing actions to be taken in evaluating and treating protocol patients.

Table 25—2 Protocol Elements, Purpose, and Nursing Interventions

Protocol Element	Purpose	Nursing Interventions
Objectives Background	Defines intent of study Describes previous studies and justification for current study	Objectives and background of study should be well understood and incorporated in patient/family teaching plan to ensure adequacy of informed consent process and enhance the patient's understanding and compliance.
Drug information	Describes animal toxicology studies, human toxicity previously observed, mechanisms of drug action, drug storage, preparation, administration, supplier	Adequate knowledge of drugs, especially investigational drugs, required before drug administration. Demonstrate knowledge of safe dose range, expected side effects, correct preparation, administration, and organs of drug excretion and metabolism.

Patient eligibility	Defines parameters of patient participation
	   Disease confirmation
	   Major organ function
	   Performance status
	   Medical history
		Accurate assessment of cancer history and previous treatments applicable to eligibility. Evaluate performance status. Evaluate required hematologic and chemistry results. Assess radiologic tests for bidimensionally measurable disease. Ensure all prestudy tests are performed within required time frame.

Treatment plan	Details initial and subsequent doses, administration guidelines and schedule, duration of treatment	Verify BSA for all doses. Verify initial and subsequent dose calculations. Validate method of drug administration. Ensure correct dose modifications for subsequent courses based on criteria defined by protocol. Patient/Family teaching regarding side effects, self-care, and administration schedule for drugs Additional medications include antiemetics, laxatives, and antidiarrheal agents
Study parameters	Schedule of required evaluations and treatment	Patient/family teaching about follow-up blood counts, office visits, hospitalizations, appointments for scans and x-rays Ensure required tests and labs are performed with results available before ordering the next treatment Provide patient/family with phone numbers of appropriate contacts for questions.

Criteria for response	Defines response:
	   Complete remission
	   Partial remission
	   Stable disease
	   Increasing disease
		Demonstrate knowledge of current disease status
		Assess response at required intervals per protocol incorporating physical exam findings and radiologic and biochemical results
		Emotional support of patients during response evaluation and change in response requiring change in treatment plan

Discipline review	Verification of correct pathologic diagnosis and/or radiation therapy treatment by a designated review panel	Ensure required slides, blood samples, films, etc., are submitted to correct address within the required time. Coordinate these activities with other departments (lab, pathology, radiation therapy).
Data submission	Defines required data forms and submission intervals	Complete data forms ensuring all submitted information is found in the patient's medical record. Verify accurate documentation of treatment, required lab and radiology parameters, toxicity and response evaluations. Submit within time constraints of research group.

Table 25–2 Protocol Elements, Purpose, and Nursing Interventions—cont'd

Protocol Element	Purpose	Nursing Interventions
Statistical considerations	Defines accrual goals, study design, and statistical analysis	Know expected number of patients to be accrued, expected length of study.
Toxicity criteria	Grading of treatment-related toxicities according to standardized scale	Ensure use of correct scale. Accurately assess and document toxicities in patient chart. Record toxicity grade on flow sheets at required intervals. Delineate between side effects of disease and treatment. Patient/family teaching regarding symptom management. Appropriate medical and nursing interventions to lessen morbidity of disease process or treatment or both.
Informed consent	Sample form that must be modified to meet institutional guidelines	Verify IRB approval date before patient registration. All protocols must be initially approved, followed by annual full board review. Verify patient has given informed consent before telephone registration. Provide patient with copy of consent.
Adverse drug reaction (ADR) reporting	Defines ADR and reporting responsibilities	Demonstrate knowledge of previously reported drug toxicities. Inform physician of possible observed ADR. Do thorough clinical investigation to determine whether adverse effect is due to the study drug. Notification of appropriate authorities and submission of required reporting forms according to time frame.

ETHICAL ISSUES/REGULATIONS

Before a clinical trial can be initiated in an institution certain ethical and regulatory conditions must be met. First, the study must be approved for human use by the institutional review board and the patient must voluntarily give his or her consent to participate.

History

These conditions, aimed at the protection of human subjects, developed over the last 50 years. The Nuremberg trials of 1947 exposed the horrors of human experimentation performed on Nazi concentration camp prisoners during World War II. In 1949, the Nuremberg code set forth standards for physicians and scientists conducting biomedical experiments on human subjects.[73] These codes set forth the absolute requirement of "voluntary consent of the human subject."[63] Unfortunately, several examples of subject abuse in medical research occurred in the United States. There was no regulation on clinical research in the United States before 1960. The Tuskegee Study, begun in Macon County, Alabama in 1932 under the auspices of the United States Public Health Service, left hundreds of black men with syphilis untreated so that long range effects of the disease could be studied. This study, intended to last 6 months, continued until 1973, when the Department of Health, Education, and Welfare halted it only after the national media reported the story the year before.[28,43,65] Another example of failure to disclose research information was the Willowbrook experiment conducted between 1956 and 1970 on between 700 and 800 retarded children. Consent was given by parents to enroll their children in this study to better understand hepatitis and to possibly develop more effective vaccines. Incentives were used to gain parental consent including earlier admission of their child to the hospital and better hospitalization conditions for children on the study.[43,74]

The Helsinki declaration, passed by the World Health Organization in 1964 and revised in 1975, provided recommendations to guide physicians in biomedical research.[45] In the United States in 1966, the first research regulations were issued by the Surgeon General's Office requiring internal review for all research protocols.[28,50] The Congress strengthened this regulation in 1974 by passing the National Research Act (PL98-348), which required review of all human subjects research by an institutional review board before any grants or contracts could be funded.[28,50] The National Commission for the Protection of Human Subjects of Biomedical and Behavioral Research ("the commission") was created by the 1974 National Research Act. The commission published a series of reports and recommendations on human research. This information, known as the "Belmont Report," was published in 1979.[4]

The three ethical principles stated in the Belmont report are:

- Respect for persons (autonomy)
- Minimization of risk and maximization of benefits to the subjects (beneficence)
- Fairness in the distribution of research burdens and benefits (justice)

These three principles are the foundation of institutional review board (IRB) and informed consent.

Institutional Review Boards

To protect human subjects from research abuses, the Department of Health and Human Services (DHHS) requires all federally funded institutions to have institutional review boards. The Office for Protection from Research Risks (OPRR) is the administrative subdivision of DHHS that negotiates assurances of compliance with individual institutions.

The assurance program requires that all cooperative group clinical protocols are subjected to full board review before human research subjects can be recruited and at least annually thereafter. Each institution must send IRB certification information to the cooperative group's operations office.

The institutional review board is composed of at least five members with professional competence, experience, and qualifications. The board should include both men and women and should represent a variety of backgrounds, races, and cultural considerations. At least one member should be a nonmedical professional and one person must have no direct affiliation with the institution performing the research.

The protocol review process provides the investigator, the institution, and the patient with the assurance that the research is medically and ethically sound.[45]

Informed Consent

Before a research subject can be registered on an IRB-approved research study, the DHHS requires that informed consent must be given by the subject. Informed consent is defined as "the knowing consent of an individual or his legally authorized representative so situated as to be able to exercise free power of choice without inducement or any element of force, fraud, deceit, distress, or any other form of constraint or coercion."[14]

Information must be provided in a language understandable to the subject. It is not complete unless the patient understands what he or she has been told and is able to use the information to decide whether to participate in the study. The physician must verify that the patient understood what was read and heard.

Patients must be allowed to ask questions, and the physician should question the patient to determine the patient's level of understanding.

Required Elements[46]

- Statement of research, purpose of the research, expected duration of participation, description of procedures including identification of any experimental procedures
- Description of risks and benefits of the study treatment
- Disclosure of alternative procedures or treatments that may be advantageous to the subject
- Description of confidentiality; disclosure of possibility of FDA inspection
- Explanation as to whether compensation and medical treatments are available if injury occurs
- Whom to contact about research, patient's rights, and research-related injury
- Instruction that participation is voluntary and results in no penalty or loss of benefits to which the subject is otherwise entitled

PHASES OF CLINICAL RESEARCH

There are three phases of clinical trials in humans: phase I, II, and III.

Phase I

The purpose of a phase I trial is to determine the maximum tolerated dose (MTD) in humans, to determine the most effective schedule of administration, and to identify and quantify toxic effects in normal organ systems. Studying the pharmacokinetics of the agent including drug absorption, distribution, metabolism, and excretion is a primary aim of these trials. The previous animal testing helps predict human toxicities, but careful and frequent monitoring of all human organ systems is required to define the dose-limiting toxicities.

Patients eligible for phase I trials have often been heavily pretreated with available standard therapies before having entered the study. Major organ function must meet the study eligibility criteria, life expectancy is required to be at least 1 to 2 months, and toxicity from previous treatments must be resolved. Objectively measurable disease is usually not a requirement in these trials since therapeutic response is not an endpoint of the study.

The initial drug dose in a phase I trial is one tenth of the dose that was lethal to 10% of the mice in toxicity testing. Three patients are entered at this dose, each about a week apart. Patients are then observed for toxicity for a specified period of time. When no irreversible, life threatening, or fatal toxicities have occurred, three more patients are entered at the next higher dose level. The MTD is usually defined within five dose escalations, thus a phase I trial requires 15 to 20 subjects.[33] The escalation of doses in tiers of patients is called the Fibonacci search method.[15] Efforts are underway to try to expedite dose escalation by using pharmacologic data to determine the starting dose to guide dose escalation, and to define the MTD using fewer subjects.[44]

Antitumor response or lack of response does not contribute directly to move the agent into phase II trials. Drugs are selected based on suggestion of therapeutic benefit. An effective agent may not produce responses in phase I trials because the optimal dose and schedule is unknown at the initiation of phase I studies.[45]

Phase I trails are usually performed in single institutions so the data can be monitored very closely by the study sponsor. Data is submitted biweekly and study summaries are required every 6 months to comply with FDA regulations. The first occurrence of any toxic reaction is reported by telephone to the Cancer Therapy and Evaluation Program for NCI sponsored drugs, for rapid information dissemination to other investigators using the agent.[15]

Not all cancer trials involve the use of chemotherapeutic agents. Trials may also investigate biologics, radiation therapy, surgical intervention, mechanical devices, or psychometric tools.[9] Cancer control studies all progress through the three phases of clinical trials.

Phase II

Phase II evaluation of a new anticancer drug is designed to determine whether or not the compound has objective antitumor activity in a variety of cancers. Attention is focused on the types of tumors that respond and the dose-response relationship. Unlike phase I studies, these trials are disease oriented. It is impossible to test the new drug in all types of cancer to see which ones respond, so the Drug Development Program of the NCI's Division of Cancer Treatment evolved the concept of *signal tumors*. These signal tumors include breast cancer, colorectal cancer, lung cancer, melanoma, acute leukemia, and lymphoma. These are the minimum numbers of cancers against which the new drug must be evaluated. This panel includes tumors that are at opposite extremes in sensitivity to chemotherapy and those that are leading causes of cancer deaths.[33] If a drug is inactive in these patients, it is likely to be inactive in other tumors.

Eligibility for a phase II study does require measurable or evaluable lesions since these areas are followed for tumor response. Depending on the drug and disease under study, previous treatment with chemotherapy and/or other treatment modalities may or may not be allowed. Adequate hematologic, he-

patic, renal, and cardiac parameters are specified by the protocol. Life expectancy of at least 8 weeks is required and patients must be capable of partial self-care to be eligible for most phase II trials.

The phase II study is a plan to ensure that adequate numbers of patients with the greatest probability of benefit are treated with the optimal dose and schedule of the drug. The recommended dose and schedule from phase I are tested in a variety of tumor types. The main problem in phase II trials is maintaining uniformity in treatment and study population. A phase II study will require 15 to 30 patients; each phase II drug is assigned by the NCI to two different cooperative groups.

The endpoints of a phase II trial may vary with the type of disease under study. For example, an endpoint of complete remission would not be realistic for a typically treatment-resistant disease such as metastatic melanoma. Because there is little effective treatment in this disease, the sole endpoints may be identifying the response rate and toxicity of the new agent.[56]

Phase III

A phase III trial establishes the value of the new treatment relative to standard treatments by a randomized or comparative study. The best role for the new drug must be defined. Different study methods that may be used to define this role are comparing the new drug to the best standard drug; using the new agent in a current, effective drug combination; and combined modality treatment versus the previous best single modality. There must be reasonable evidence to suggest that the new drug or combination of drugs is equivalent to or more effective than the currently accepted standard therapy.

Eligibility for a phase III trial is similar to phase II in that patients must have histologically confirmed disease that is bidimensionally measurable, have adequate major organ function, and be capable of performing at least partial self-care. Patients on phase III trials have received little or no previous therapy.

Phase III trials are large studies that involve hundreds of patients and multiple institutions. More phase III trials are being performed through the intergroup mechanism of the NCI, whereby several cooperative groups co-sponsor the study. This allows patients to be accrued from a wider geographic segment, thus allowing a more rapid completion and analysis of the study. Community-based programs contribute significant numbers of patients to phase III trials.

These trials are often randomized, meaning that the patient is arbitrarily assigned to one of two or more possible treatments. Neither the physician nor patient knows which treatment will be assigned until after informed consent is given and the registration is completed. The purpose of randomization is to remove potential biases in allocating patients to each treatment so that similar numbers of "like" patients receive each treatment.[56] Another advantage of randomized trials is that treatment groups can be "balanced" according to prognostic factors.[53] This stratification process may involve such variables as age, performance status, extent of disease, or prior therapy. This method assures that good and poor prognosis patients are distributed equally among all treatment arms so valid conclusions may be drawn when the study is completed.

The primary endpoint of a phase III trial is to improve upon existing treatment. Investigators will measure for higher complete response rates, increased disease-free survival, and longer overall survival. As treatment results improve, long-term toxicities become an important endpoint. Recently, more attention has focused on quality of life as a study endpoint.[61]

Nursing Management

Historically, nurses only provided physical care to the patients in clinical trials. Chemotherapy research was one of the first areas that emphasized active collaboration of nurses in research. The need for skilled chemotherapy nurses stimulated the development of role expansion. Nurses provided patient education regarding the various aspects of clinical trials. More recently, the role of nurses in clinical trials has expanded from the nurse as a participant in medical research to the nurse as principal investigator for independent research.

The roles of nursing in clinical trials include the areas of direct patient care, education, advocate coordination, administration, and independent research. These roles are accomplished by a variety of individuals who may include hospital staff nurse, ambulatory care nurse, research nurse, data manager, clinical nurse specialist, and unit manager. Maintaining coordinated efforts among these individuals requires skill in both organization and communication. Successful implementation and conduct of clinical trials results in safe patient care and generalizable research results.

Greater numbers of nurses than ever are actively involved in clinical trials because of the extension of these trials into the community. Nurses practicing in institutions that do not perform clinical trials still need a working knowledge of these studies because they may refer patients to centers for possible entry on a trial. The education and support an informed nurse can lend in this stressful situation are invaluable.

Nursing diagnoses and interventions for patients on Phase I, II, and III clinical trials are listed in the boxes on p. 595.

PATIENT CARE

The area of patient care includes the informed consent process, treatment administration, toxicity assessment, and documentation.

Informed Consent

In the past the nursing responsibility in the informed consent process consisted mainly of verifying that the signature on the consent document was that of the patient. Responsibility for disclosure was laid entirely upon the physician. Nurses answered questions to reinforce the physician's explanation.[13]

The changing role of the nurse and the autonomy of expanded roles, especially in ambulatory and clinical trials, brings new professional and legal responsibilities for informed consent to the nurse. Establishing the diagnosis and choosing a treatment plan are independent functions of the physician, but administering medical and nursing treatments and diagnosing and managing human responses to health problems are independent functions of the nurse. Clinical trials are an area of collaboration. The physician may introduce the idea of participation in a clinical trial and give an overview of the treatment, but often the protocol nurse must explain the details of the consent form and obtain the signature. In doing so, the protocol nurse accepts the delegated responsibility of providing information to aid the decision.[10,48]

The following factors assist in the process of informing the patient:

- Allow the patient to take the consent form home to read before making a decision.
- Write down treatment information.
- Draw a diagram of randomization and treatment schedule.
- Provide "What Are Clinical Trials All About" pamphlet from the NCI.
- Encourage the patient to call the NCI hotline (1-800-4-CANCER) for information regarding disease and treatment.
- Show audiovisual information about chemotherapy and side effects.

NURSING DIAGNOSES

- Knowledge deficit related to disease pathology and new diagnosis
- Knowledge deficit related to clinical trials process, randomization process, informed consent process
- Knowledge deficit related to experimental chemotherapy and side effects
- Conflict, decisional related to involvement in clinical trial vs. standard therapy
- Anxiety related to new diagnosis or disease progression
- Anxiety related to treatment with experimental agent or procedure
- Coping, ineffective; potential for related to new diagnosis or change in prognosis and new treatment
- Powerlessness related to involvement in a large clinical trial

- Assess the patient's anxiety level and integration of new information.
- Question the patient to determine whether he or she understands the treatment.
- Continue to review and reinforce information throughout treatment.

See Patient Teaching Priorities and Geriatric Considerations in the boxes on p. 596.

Treatment Administration

Protocol guidelines must be strictly followed so that results from a group of patients treated in precisely the same manner can be analyzed and the study repeated and validated.[9] The treatment nurse should always verify the body surface area calculation, protocol dose calculations and modifications, pretreatment lab values, and method of administration. Treatment nurses should be provided with protocol abstracts in the patient chart or a set of protocols in the treatment area to facilitate these activities. Experi-

---

NURSING INTERVENTIONS IN PHASE I, II, AND III CLINICAL TRIALS

Phase I

- Assess the adequacy of informed consent and notify the physician if the patient doesn't fully understand the risk-benefit relationship
- Know the mechanism of drug action, route of administration, absorption, metabolism, and excretion of drug
- Know results of animal toxicology studies to anticipate human toxicities
- Assess for, evaluate, and document unexpected adverse drug reactions
- Provide nursing care to minimize disease and treatment-related morbidity
- Understand disease process to distinguish between disease-related and treatment-related effects
- Carefully document objective and subjective response to treatment
- Document acute, chronic, delayed, and cumulative side effects
- Perform and document results of pharmacokinetic studies
- Participate in decisions concerning dose escalation, schedule manipulation, and determination of optimal dose

Phase II

- Know results of phase I drug studies:
    Side effects
    Dose-limiting toxicities
    Method of administration
    Drug metabolism and excretion
- Provide patient education and support:
    Treatment plan
    Expected side effects
    Symptom management
    Disease process

Phase III

- Ensure drug doses are calculated correctly
- Document toxicities and grade correctly
- Modify doses correctly and consistently
- Evaluate tumor measurements appropriately for response determination
- Ensure the patient's understanding of randomization process
- Assess for new and unexpected side effects of the drug
- Assess performance status
- Administer "Quality of Life" assessment tools
    Follow-Up After Treatment Completion:
- Teach the patient the importance of follow-up visits even years after treatment is completed
- Report data on survival and late effects until the patient dies
- Develop systems to maintain contact with patients who have moved or changed physicians
- Encourage patients to return to a healthful lifestyle in light of knowing cancer may recur
- Teach recommendations for screening and early detection appropriate to age
- Counsel other family members of patients at high risk for developing cancer

---

**PATIENT TEACHING PRIORITIES
CANCER CLINICAL TRIALS**

Cancer Control:
- Review American Cancer Society Guidelines on prevention strategies for diet, smoking cessation, and sun protection measures.
- Teach early detection measures (breast, skin, and testicular self-exam).
- Review Cancer Control Study Guidelines (purpose, treatment/drug schedule, and side effects of drugs); diagnostic exams preparation and schedule and follow-up plan.

Clinical Trials:
- Assess and clarify issues related to the informed consent, clinical trial, and randomization process.
- Review the purpose and treatment schedule; drugs and their related side effects; symptom management (e.g., fever, pain); appointments for diagnostic tests/x-rays; monitoring blood counts; return office/clinic visits and/or hospitalization; resources to contact for emergent care; and/or questions about clinical trials.

Ineffective Therapies:
- Use nonjudgmental approach in providing and/or clarifying information on ineffective therapies; offer reliable information from NCI, NIH, FDA, and AMA (e.g., pamphlets, resources to contact, and referrals for second opinions).

GERIATRIC CONSIDERATIONS

- Cancer Clinical Trials and Cancer Control Research have established eligibility criteria for patient accrual; refer to age-related guidelines.
- Consider sensory and neuromuscular deficits (e.g., visual, hearing, mobility) in selection of educational materials.
- Review current prescription and over-the-counter medication guidelines that may interact with scheduled drugs/treatments.
- Additional limitations such as fixed-income transportation, caregiver resources, and age-related functional status will require assessment and intervention strategies.

---

mental drugs may be administered by a staff nurse, clinic nurse, research nurse, or chemotherapy nurse.

Toxicity Assessment

The observation skills of oncology nurses are crucial to assess treatment-related toxicities in clinical trials. It is the nurse's observation of the patient after treatment that identifies the side effect profile and will ultimately be the basis for the care plan of patients on experimental treatment in the future.[55] It is the nurse that may be the first to recognize a side effect, perhaps even before the patient is aware of the experience.

Documentation

Accurate nursing documentation is the foundation of good clinical research. All data that are reported on flowsheets or case report forms must be verifiable in the patient's medical record. Nurses must take care to document treatments and assessments accurately. Study investigators can extrapolate hematologic toxicity from lab work, but cannot document other more subjective toxicities unless nursing documentation is objective. Areas requiring precise nursing assessment and documentation include: patient's level of activity, oral assessment, nausea, vomiting, anorexia, diarrhea, constipation, skin condition, and psychological changes. Inaccurate assessment or documentation of toxicities may result in patients receiving ineffective low dosages or toxicity-producing high doses in the subsequent course of therapy. The large box on p. 595 lists specific nursing responsibilities for phase I, II, and III clinical trials. Miaskowski has published excellent documentation forms that could be used to document nursing care for clinical trial patients.[57]

EDUCATOR
Patient Education

One of the vital roles in clinical trials is that of patient educator. The beginning of a clinical trial is a time of unique stress for the patient. The patient feels hopeful that the experimental therapy will work. There are also fears that it will not be successful and fear of unknown side effects. A list of nursing diagnoses for the clinical trial patient appears in the box on page 595.

The nurse can help the patient cope by describing the concept of clinical trials to the patient and family. Written information about the treatment schedule, side effects, and follow-up plan lend some structure for the patient. Provide a telephone number for the protocol nurse or assigned clinic nurse and instruct the patient to call with any questions. A telephone call from the protocol or clinic nurse the day following an outpatient treatment allows assessment of immediate side effects as well as assurance to the patient.

Nursing Education

Staff nurses are an integral component of the research team and must be knowledgeable about research protocols in which they are participating. Areas of education include the purpose and history of the protocol treatment, design of the study, previously observed toxicity, treatment administration, and management of side effects.

A clinical nurse specialist (CNS), when available in an institution, educates the staff about cancer treatment protocols and patient care. More frequently, however, the role of educator is found in a variety of other expanded nursing roles.[74] When available, research nurses are expert resources for information about the research process and details of particular protocols. Both the CNS and research nurse provide education and consultation about the research study. The primary focus of the CNS is nursing management of the patient and nursing skill development, whereas the priority of the research nurse is the successful implementation of the study.[74]

ADVOCATE

The nurse is an important advocate for the patient. Since the nurse is more accessible than the physician, the patient may feel more comfortable expressing fears or concerns to the nurse. The nurse advocates for the patient by ensuring that adequate information is given and that the patient has a clear understanding of the risk-to-benefit relationship as well as by ensuring adequate time for questions. The nurse must support the patient who refuses treatment or who wishes to withdraw from the study.

The nurse largely determines the quality of the informed consent. Oncology nurses have the competence, the rapport with clients, and the tradition of collaboration with colleagues to safeguard the right to informed consent.[16]

COORDINATOR

Cancer treatment protocols require the coordination of numerous hospital-based and outpatient services. These include hematology, chemistry, blood bank, pathology, pharmacy, hospital patient units, radiation therapy, and outpatient clinics. The research nurse is responsible for organizing and coordinating such activities as specimen collection for phase I pharmacokinetic studies, mailing blood, marrow, or tissue specimens to reference labs, and ensuring radiation ther-

apy materials are submitted for review. Good communication and interpersonal skills are required to accomplish these tasks. Without clear communication between departments, the patient may receive confusing or contradictory information and health care can become fragmented.[55]

ADMINISTRATOR

McEvoy and colleagues state that the role of the administrative nurse includes both coordinating the patients' care as well as coordination of the research project. The administrator is responsible for analyzing the impact of the research study to the resources available and the existing organizational structure within which the trial will take place.[21] Administrators work with study sponsors to coordinate the implementation and to negotiate funding for new studies. They may serve as liaison between hospital administration, physician investigators, the research staff, and the institutional review board. Information must be disseminated to many individuals within the research program. Characteristics of the nurse performing the administrative role of a clinical trial includes the ability to interact comfortably with a variety of professionals and to organize and implement group meetings.[55]

RESEARCHER

The role of nurses as merely data collectors for medical research has changed and expanded over the past decades of clinical trials. Nurses are independent investigators for nursing research studies. One purpose of nursing research in clinical trials is to evaluate patients' responses to treatment or disease.[55]

One method of implementing nursing research through the clinical trials mechanism is by "companion studies." Companion studies include nurse-sponsored studies "piggy-backed" on an existing medical study or a parallel study. The latter study is initiated in response to a nursing concern that may have been generated by observation of patients in an ongoing study. Some nursing studies are implemented through the cooperative group mechanism after being developed within the group's nursing committee. Funding for these studies is available through the cooperative group mechanism, the Division of Cancer Prevention and Control, and the NIH's Center for Nursing Research.[11]

Nurses may be involved with the generation of knowledge through identifying trends in patient experiences, dissemination of knowledge through presentation of research results, and utilization of knowledge by incorporating research results into their daily nursing practice.[22,55]

BARRIERS TO ACCRUAL ON CLINICAL TRIALS
Accrual

More than one million people will be diagnosed with cancer in 1993. Only 0.5% to 2.5% of these patients will be entered on a cancer clinical trial. Some patients are not eligible for studies, but less than 10% of patients eligible for NCI-sponsored studies will be registered.[79] In 1987, Friedman reported that in NCI-sponsored cooperative group trials, only 1% to 1.5% of potentially eligible breast cancer patients, 0.5% of rectal patients, and 1% of colon cancer patients were actually registered on study by their physicians.[24] This slow accession of patients is a contributing factor to three major cooperative group studies taking 32%, 113%, and 119% longer to complete than projected.[79] In studies where the endpoint is reduction in mortality, 18 to 24 months should be sufficient to accrue the needed number of patients. Given the present accrual rates, however, a duration of 3 to 8 years or more may be necessary to provide sample sizes of acceptable magnitude.[79]

In addition to the expense of keeping a trial open for an extended period, slow accrual also delays analysis of the study and, therefore, dissemination of new information into standard practice.

Strategies to Increase Accrual

CCOP.   The Community Clinical Oncology Program, as discussed previously in this chapter, was implemented by the NCI in 1983. A primary goal was to increase the available numbers of potentially eligible patients for clinical trials, thus improving accrual rates. Southwest Oncology Group (SWOG) figures attest to the community contribution: in 1983, the year CCOP accrual began, 209 CCOP patients were registered on SWOG studies. The following year the CCOP contribution jumped to 1230 patients.[19]

In 1988, over 50% of the 19,590 patients in NCI-approved clinical trials were entered in the community setting.[6] Even in the community setting, however, only approximately 30% of patients are eligible for participation and only 10% of these are registered.[39]

HIGH-PRIORITY TRIALS.   In 1988, the National Cancer Institute implemented the High-Priority Clinical Trials Program to enhance accrual to important cooperative group phase III trials. These studies are selected from existing cooperative group protocols because they require large numbers of patients, involve common malignancies, and answer important questions, the results of which will likely lead to improved patient survival.[11] Physicians who are not participating in clinical trials through the other available mechanisms may affiliate with a group as High Priority investigator. These physicians are reimbursed for the number of eligible patients they register on study. The most recent set of studies, Series IV High Priority Trials, are listed in Table 25-3. The High Priority Trials program has been successful in increasing patient accrual. These trials account for only 6% of currently active phase II studies, but accrue 27% of current phase III patients.[72]

Obstacles to Accrual

Various reasons and explanations are cited for poor patient accrual on clinical trials. Johansen and coworkers[47] group these obstacles into patient-related, nurse-related, and physician-related obstacles.

PATIENT-RELATED.   These authors identify potential patient-related barriers as financial costs (transportation, lodging, meals, loss of income); concerns of privacy and confidentiality; lack of interest in, disapproval of, or low opinions of clinical research; fear; anxiety; denial; and family influences.[47]

NURSE-RELATED.   Numerous nursing barriers to accruing patients on clinical trials also exist. Treating research patients increases the job responsibilities of nurses and conflicts in responsibility may arise. Many nurses do not have the opportunity for education regarding clinical research and feel ill prepared to assume these responsibilities. Lack of rewards and recognition for members of the research team and a lack of investigator/nurse and nurse/nurse collaboration may produce frustration.[47]

PHYSICIAN-RELATED.   Numerous authors discuss physician obstacles to registering patients on research

Table 25-3   National Cancer Institute-Sponsored Series IV High-Priority Trials

Name	Description
NSABP/B-24	Tamoxifen with lumpectomy and radiation for noninvasive breast cancer
INT-0115	Postoperative adjuvant therapy for non-small cell lung cancer
INT-0116	Adjuvant chemotherapy for gastric adenocarcinoma
CALGB-9082	High-dose chemotherapy with autologous bone marrow transplantation for stage II or III breast cancer
INT-0121	Evaluation of high-dose consolidation chemotherapy with autologous bone marrow transplantation for stage II or stage IV breast cancer
EST-1690	Postoperative adjuvant interferon alpha-2 for metastatic melanoma
EST-3886	Postoperative hormonal therapy for prostate cancer

studies.* An early study conducted by the National Surgical Adjuvant Breast and Bowel Project (NSABP) studies reasons surgical principal investigators chose not to enter patients in a large, multicenter, cooperative group trial. The clinical trial compared segmental mastectomy with postoperative radiation therapy, segmental mastectomy alone, and total mastectomy. Patient accrual was so far below expected accrual that it threatened the successful completion of the trial.[70] Ninety-seven percent of the 94 surveyed principal investigators responded to the survey. These physicians identified the following reasons for not entering eligible patients:

- Concern that the physician/patient relationship would be affected by a randomized clinical trial
- Difficulty with informed consent
- Dislike of open discussion involving uncertainty
- Perceived conflict between the role of scientist and clinician
- Practical difficulties in following procedures
- Feelings of personal responsibilities
- Feelings of personal responsibility if the treatments were found to be unequal

Additional factors that inhibit participation in clinical trials were identified in a 1989 American Medical Association survey. These factors include lack of time, bureaucratic administration of research, professional liability concerns, ethics of patient care, lack of interest, and reimbursement.[1] Three fourths of these physicians had a positive view of clinical trials, however.

FINANCIAL BARRIERS.   Financial barriers have become increasingly problematic over the past decade. There are two major areas of expense in cancer clinical trials.[78] The first area of expense is for the actual implementation and conduct of the trial and includes research personnel, data collection and analysis, and study monitoring. The other major area of expense is direct patient care, including the cost of drugs, tests, and hospitalization. Historically, these costs were shared by the treating institution, the NCI, the pharmaceutical companies, insurance companies, and the patient.[2] With a recessionary economy, spiraling health care costs, and increased competition for fewer government dollars, the burden of covering costs is shifting. The result of these changing economic conditions are that institutions and health professionals may be less able to participate in clinical trials without adequate reimbursement. For patients, decisions about participation in a clinical trial may be affected by the insurer's willingness to reimburse expenses.[47] One specific problem in reimbursement is the third-

party coverage for off-label use of chemotherapy agents. When the FDA approves the commercial use of an agent, it is for the specific condition listed on the package insert. Clinical trials and years of experience, however, often indicate that these agents are effective in conditions other than those listed on the label. These drugs become "standard care" and are prescribed for many patients. The General Accounting Office conducted a 1991 survey to determine the extent of off-label drug use in the practice of medical oncology.[26] Six hundred eighty respondents reported the recommendations they made to their last three patients and also designated agents they commonly use to treat specific malignancies. The survey found that one third of all prescribed drugs were for off-label indications and 44% of all combination drug treatments were off-label. Half of the respondents reported insurance reimbusement problems. The problem is that some insurers have considered off-label use of the drug to be "investigational" and, therefore, a nonreimbursable expense. This interpretation of off-label use has not been supported by the FDA, HCFA, or current state legislation and is actively being addressed in the cancer care arena.[2]

Strategies to Overcome Obstacles

Presently, clinical research in cancer is being threatened by inadequacies in the accrual of patients for clinical trials. A concerted effort by physicians, nurses, their respective professional organizations, and the National Cancer Institute can identify solutions to this accrual crises.

Education is an effective tool in overcoming many barriers. The National Cancer Institute through its "Patient to Patient" campaign is attempting to increase public knowledge about and acceptance of clinical trials. Products of this campaign include press releases, the brochures "What are Clinical Trials All About?" and "Cancer Treatments: Consider the Possibilities," and a videotape, "Patient to Patient: Cancer Clinical Trials and You." Patients can also be encouraged to call the NCI Hotline (1-800-4-CANCER) to get information about the disease, treatment centers, and available clinical trials. The Physicians Data Query (PDQ) data base now has treatment related information available by FAX. This program is called CancerFax and is accessed by dialing 301-402-5874 from the telephone on the FAX machine.

Anecdotal experience even at this early stage suggests that enhancing public awareness of and demand for access to clinical trials may be one of the most effective means of increasing accrual rates.[79]

Nurses are at the core of this patient education task. Patient education about clinical trials focuses on defining the purpose and relevance of cancer research,

*References 1, 2, 24, 26, 47, 70, 79.

including the significance of control groups and randomization.[47] Teaching is accomplished either in an individual setting with the patient and significant others or in a group setting. Participating in an American Cancer Society speakers' bureau provides opportunities to educate the public about the benefits of clinical trials. To overcome the obstacle of increased job responsibilities for nurses in clinical trials, Johansen and co-workers propose two strategies: adjusting the nurse/patient ratio when additional duties are required for clinical trial patients and demonstration of support of clinical research nurses by primary nurses and administrators.[47] The authors also suggest the following as forms of recognition for the nurses research involvement: coauthorships, attending educational conferences, and education material for the nursing unit. Physicians may reciprocate support by cooperating with associated nursing research. It is also suggested that recognition is influenced by the type and amount of research involvement and should be negotiated before trial implementation.[47]

Nurses can help increase patient accrual in several ways. Physicians can be better informed of available studies and eligibility requirements through improved verbal or written communications. Tumor registries and medical records departments can provide information on newly diagnosed patients whose charts are then evaluated by the research nurse for protocol eligibility. Nurses can coordinate prestudy testing and evaluation of results, as well as planning and troubleshooting potential barriers. These mechanisms decrease the amount of physician time required to prepare patients for registration. Since one of the main physician obstacles to registration is lack of time, these measures may increase physician enthusiasm regarding participation in clinical research.

In an effort to both reduce time involvement and costs of clinical trials most trial sponsors have review mechanisms to assure that studies are cost-conscious, yet maintain the scientific integrity necessary to fulfill clinical objectives.[34] This action results in decreasing the interval of expensive tests such as computed tomography (CT) scans and eliminating interesting but nonessential testing. Chemotherapy is often administered in the outpatient setting. Study sponsors are simplifying and standardizing data collection forms to decrease the amount of time required for record keeping. The Pediatric Oncology Group implemented electronic data transmission of protocol information from the participating institution to their statistical center. This started as a pilot project in 1991 and is being expanded to other institutions.

The NCI set an accrual goal of 50,000 new patients per year registered on clinical trials by 1992.[72] In May, 1991, at the semiannual meeting of the Clinical Trials Cooperative Group Chairmen, a general improvement in accrual rates was reported. Approximately 3700 more patients were registered on studies in 1990 than 1989. In 1992, a total of 22,709 patients were entered on phase I, II, and III trials.[72]

INEFFECTIVE CANCER THERAPIES

The American Cancer Society defines unproven cancer therapies as "those diagnostic tests or therapeutic modalities which are promoted for cancer prevention, diagnosis, or treatment and which are on the basis of careful review by scientists and/or clinicians not deemed proven or recommended for current use."[36] Furthermore, the American Society of Clinical Oncology's Subcommittee on Unorthodox Therapies states that the term *quackery* implies a knowing intent to misrepresent, whereas belief based on inadequate knowledge may be the underlying promotional incentive rather than the deliberate intent to defraud.[35] The important common feature to all these treatments is ineffectiveness.

The impact of ineffective therapies in today's society is tremendous. The numbers of patients subjected to ineffective therapies may never be known, but it is known that more than $2 billion is spent annually by people with cancer and those desiring an easy method to prevent cancer. Promoters of ineffective therapies accumulate millions every year, and the cancer patient, who may indeed be curable through conventional treatment, bears the financial burden of the promoter's financial gain.

The medical professional may perceive the cancer patient who seeks unproven therapy as naive. In fact, however, while patients discuss the latest "cure" through the extensive and accessible "underground" of patients sitting in our clinic waiting rooms, it may indeed be the health care professionals who are naive. Fear of discontinuation of medical treatment often precludes the verbalization of these ideas to physicians and nurses.

Historical Perspectives

Ineffective cancer treatments are nearly as old as our country. In 1748 George Washington and James Madison in the Virginia General Assembly appointed a committee to evaluate Mary Johnson's recipe for curing cancer. The cure, containing sorrel, black celandine, and spring water, was so well defended by testimonials from the "cured" that Mary Johnson was indeed awarded 100 pounds by the Assembly.[30] Numerous unproven treatments flourished, and advertisements by promoters abounded.

In 1906 Congress passed the Food and Drug Act. In 1910, the first time it was challenged, the Supreme Court ruled that it applied only to truthful labeling of ingredients in a product.[42] The court concluded that individuals could not be prosecuted for what was termed "mistaken praise" for their treatments.[54]

In 1912 President Taft urged Congress to pass tougher legislation. This produced the Sherley Amendment, which made it a crime to make false or fraudulent claims of therapeutic efficacy. However, it was the prosecution's responsibility to prove intent to defraud. An important piece of legislation, passed by Congress in 1938, finally required scientific proof of drug safety before marketing. A Supreme Court ruling in 1943 determined that the responsibility for establishing safety lies with the drug manufacturer.

In 1962 Congress further clarified the Food and Drug Act and added the essential element of proof of drug efficacy. This represents research in its current form: data are collected from animal studies evaluating safety and efficacy, an investigational new drug application is filed with the FDA, and upon approval of that application the drug enters human clinical trials. When all phases of clinical trials are complete, the company can market the drug if it is indeed safe and effective. The problem is that patients can still choose to use an ineffective and unproven therapy. The FDA is responsible for enforcement of the Food and Drug Act, which is difficult at best. The FDA's legal base is interstate commerce, so promoters operating entirely within a state can totally avoid FDA laws. The government has no control over ineffective therapies outside the country.

It is apparent that the health care profession cannot rely solely on governmental legislation and enforcement to protect patients from unproven and possibly dangerous treatments. The health care provider must help patients recognize these methods for what they are and make informed decisions regarding their cancer treatment.

Recognizing Ineffective Cancer Therapy

The American Society of Clinical Oncologists' Subcommittee on Unorthodox Therapies published its paper "Ineffective Cancer Therapy: A Guide for the Layperson" in 1983.[69] The committee identified 10 ways to recognize ineffective therapy:

1. *Is the treatment based on an unproven theory?* Promoters of ineffective cancer therapy are experts at using confusing scientific language in brochures. However, these claims are not backed with peer-reviewed publication in scientific journals. Encourage patients to use the National Library of Medicine Medlars Computer through their local reference library to determine whether the claims are published in scientific literature.

2. *Is there a need for special nutritional support when*

the remedy is used? People have believed in the medicinal power of certain foods for centuries, and we know proper nutrition is essential for good health. However, promoters may capitalize on the notion that certain natural foods can cure or prevent cancer. Many ineffective therapies claim that special food preparation or nutritional supplements are required to achieve the treatment's full effect.

3. *Is there a claim made for harmless, painless, nontoxic treatment?* These claims may be especially hard to resist, particularly when the promoter reinforces this with such phrases as "burning radiation," "poisonous chemotherapy," and "mutilating surgery."

4. *Are claims published frequently in the mass media?* Although promoters' claims are not published in scientific literature, they have an attentive audience in the media, often quick to publicize a "new cure" without full investigation. Since the FDA can enforce misleading drug labels but not media claims, the belief that "they couldn't say it if it weren't true" simply is not the case.

5. *Are claims of benefit the results of the power of suggestion?* Promoters rely heavily on testimonials of their "cured" clients. This can overwhelm the cancer patient, who doesn't know that some of these people never had cancer and that others who gave testimonials succumbed to cancer a short time later. Predictably, the placebo effect of any treatment when backed with faith and expectation can result in subjective improvements for short periods. The only scientifically valid evidence, however, is objective tumor response.

6. *Are the major promoters recognized experts in cancer treatment?* Many ineffective therapy promoters look like experts; they wear white coats and have framed degrees hanging in the office. Some are physicians but lack expertise in cancer research and care. The patient should check the Directory of Medical Specialists, which lists individuals who have recognition, special training, and experience in cancer research and treatment.

7. *Do promoters back up their claims with controlled studies?* Promoters claim excellent results from their treatment. However, the demonstration may be from patients' testimonials rather than controlled trials. Promoters may claim they don't have the staff or money to conduct such investigations. This claim is difficult to believe when they collect millions of dollars in profits every year.

8. *Is there a claim that only specially trained physicians*

can produce results with their drug, or is the formula a secret? Formulations of reputable cancer drugs are published in scientific journals, and the information is available to all physicians.

9. *Do the promoters attack the medical and scientific establishment?* Claims of a conspiracy of the medical community to prevent a cancer cure, thus securing the incomes of its members, are often voiced by promoters. However, members of the establishment also die of cancer, as do their loved ones. Ineffective promoters segregate themselves from the medical community, often performing their cures in hotel rooms and discouraging consultation with medical experts.

10. *Is there a demand for "freedom of choice" regarding drugs?* Americans revere the word "freedom," and so promoters claim the patient's freedom of choice would be limited if promoters weren't allowed to sell their products. The freedom to misrepresent facts in drug labeling and selling is no freedom at all, but simply a license to steal from the public.

A pamphlet discussing these 10 points, available from Adria Laboratories, is helpful for patients who want to evaluate an option for treatment.

Types of Ineffective Therapy

More than 100 types of ineffective therapy have been or are available. Table 25-4 lists some of the more common treatments and their rationale. The American Cancer Society and Food and Drug Administration have files on unproven treatments accessible to both professionals and lay persons.

PATIENT MOTIVATIONS FOR THE USE OF INEFFECTIVE THERAPY
Fear

The psychologic factors that influence a patient to seek ineffective therapies are multiple and complex, but the strongest motivator may be fear.[40] A Gallup poll in 1976 surveyed 1548 men and women about their fear of disease. Fifty-eight percent of the persons interviewed stated cancer was the disease they feared most.[62] Many people see cancer as a frightening, painful process ending in death. In addition to fear of death, the fear of an uncertain future, pain, mutilation, loss of family, dependence, costly medical care, and alienation dominate.[68]

Family Pressure

Add to these psychologic fears pressures from family and friends. In a sincere and well-meaning attempt to help, they look for a cure, determined to leave no stone unturned in their search. When cancer is diagnosed, people immediately relate success stories of others they know who may have been cured by conventional means, but they also tell stories of those cured by mystical and "innovative" means. Fear and pressure may lessen objectivity and increase vulnerability to the claims of ineffective therapy promoters. The family, as the patient's strongest support system, feels a responsibility to help decide on treatment and the patient, fearing alienation from family, may succumb to their wishes.

Recurrence and Progression

Many people resort to unproven therapies when the initial diagnosis is made; others who start with conventional therapy make that same decision when they find their disease has recurred or metastasized. A period of searching for a second opinion or reason for error in diagnosis is followed by anxiety, sometimes bordering on panic, and depression. Depression changes sleeping and eating patterns and impairs the ability to work and concentrate. The patient may reach a point of hopelessness and helplessness, knowing a cure may now be out of reach. At this time of emotional turmoil, thoughts may turn to pursuing unproven methods as a last resort.[37]

Mistrust of Medical System

Medical professionals would like to believe they are held in high regard by lay people, but this is not always true. Today's society has a medical sophistication unknown to previous generations. Health maintenance and prevention and treatment of disease are common topics in the national and local news. News from the latest *New England Journal of Medicine* may be heard on the nightly news before the issue arrives in the mail. While people are assuming more responsibility for their own health, they are actively assimilating new information. Some of this information includes knowledge of the side effects of conventional cancer treatments. They see alopecia, nausea, vomiting, lack of energy, and loss of appetite with chemotherapy. They see surgery that may cure but may result in disfigurement. The concept of radiation therapy is particularly frightening, since it cannot be seen or felt. The disillusionment some people feel with science and technology may carry over into the doctor's office, where this authority figure speaks in a medical language not easily understood and can easily rebuff patients who are already understandably apprehensive.

Promoters of ineffective therapies understand well the anxieties of patients in the conventional medical system. They deal with the apprehension, loss of control, and feelings of isolation very effectively by making the patient an active part of the treatment program. Coupled with a promise for cure without discomfort, a close camaraderie soon develops between

Table 25–4 Common Ineffective Treatments

Treatment	Rationale/Mechanism of Action	Comments
MACHINES/DEVICES		
Oscilloclast (Hubbard E meter, Drown radio therapeutic instrument, Orgon energy devices, Dotto electronic reactor)	Detect disharmonious disease-causing oscillations of body's electrons and adjust back to harmonious state.[60] Normalize bad vibrations or counteract harmful currents that cause cancer.[58]	Devices more commonly used at turn of century. FDA proved oscilloclast worthless and made it illegal.
DRUGS		
Koch antitoxin therapy	Developed reagent useful as oxidation catalyst and body stimulant antagonist to cancer cells. Process built upon normal cell metabolism and retarded functioning of anaerobic cancer cell.[17]	Developed in 1919 by W.F. Koch, MD, PhD. Popular in 1940s and 1950s. Treatment was extremely pure distilled water with one part per trillion of "reagent" glyoxylide.[54] Koch indicted in 1943 after FDA hearings; ended in mistrial after defense produced 104 witnesses offering testimonials. Koch moved to Brazil in 1948. Treatment is illegal in U.S. but can be obtained through underground medical community or in Mexico.[54]
Hoxsey method	"Restore body to physiologic normalcy."[38] Proposed that as a result of chemical imbalance, body cells matured and became cancerous.	Internal and external therapy—"pink medicine" and "black medicine." External treatment was paste applied to tumor. Federal court injunction stopped sales in 1960 after 10 years of litigation. FDA estimates patients spent more than $50 million on treatment. Available at Biomedical Center in Tijuana, Mexico.
Krebiozen (carcalon)	Stimulates body's inherent anticancer substances, hence slows or arrests growth of cancer.[36]	Endorsed by Andrew Ivy, MD, PhD, vice president of University of Illinois in 1951. Tested by NCI in 1961; substance identified as an amino acid found in all animal tissue. Later investigations showed samples contained mineral oil alone or with small amount of amyl alcohol and methylhydantoin.[30] Prescribed by thousands of doctors across the country. Many unsuccessful legal battles; FDA unable to outlaw because of intense pressure by supporters.[36] Continued to be dispensed until Ivy's death in 1977.
Laetrile	Cyanogenic glucoside, derived from variety of fruit and plant sources, was found too toxic in cancer treatment in 1920s. Purified in 1950s—beta-glucoronic analogue of amygdalin.[18] Theory: Cancer cells contain enzyme beta-glucosidase, which releases cyanide after drug administration. Normal cells low in enzyme so they are spared toxic effect while cancer cells are killed.[52] In 1970, transformed cyanogenic glycosides into substance dubbed B_{17}—labeled as vitamin ("vitamin theory").	Biggest success among unproven treatments in 1970s in spite of opposition by FDA and cancer research groups. NCI-sponsored clinical trial proved laetrile ineffective (1957-1977). Toxicity: fever, rash, headache, hypotension, vomiting, diarrhea, motor disturbances, agranulocytosis.
DMSO (Dimethylsulfoxide)	Combination therapy with DMSO allegedly yields decreased side effects of chemotherapy while potentiating its therapeutic effects. Theoretic basis suggests that the immune system of cancer patients forms a shell around cancer cells, and DMSO can penetrate the shell and enter the cell carrying with it any other drugs the patient is receiving.	ACS review of literature found no data supporting DMSO's antineoplastic activity.[71] FDA in 1978 approved use of 50% aqueous solution of DMSO (RIMSO-50) for relief of interstitial cystitis by bladder instillation. In 1983 ACS published statement that DMSO lacks scientific evidence of efficacy and declared it an unproven method.[71]

Continued.

Table 25–4 Common Ineffective Treatments—cont'd

Treatment	Rationale/Mechanism of Action	Comments
BIOLOGIC PRODUCTS		
Rand vaccine	Made from animal blood injected with material from human cancer collected from operating rooms.[3]	IND application failed. Production halted in 1967.[29]
Lewis method	Injections of coupled tumor protein antigen (CPTA).	
Helt cancer serum	Contains *E. coli* and *S. fecalis.*[29]	
METABOLIC THERAPIES		
Gerson diet	Cancer causes generalized tissue damage, especially in the liver. With tumor lysis, toxic degradation products appear in bloodstream, which leads to coma and death as a result of liver failure.[27] Theory: Cancer is caused by constipation or inadequate elimination of waste. Cure can be achieved through dietary manipulation. Basis for dietary recommendations: • Detoxifying of whole body • Providing essential contents of potassium • Adding oxidizing enzymes continuously (green leaf juice and fresh calf's liver juice)	Developed in 1920s by German physician. Currently more than 20 modifications of original program. Diet demands no foodstuffs other than fresh fruits and vegetables (chopped by Gerson-sold chopper) and oatmeal. No escape of steam during food preparation. No tobacco, alcohol, sodium, spices. Protein allowed only after sixth week of diet. Multiple additional iodine and niacin supplements used as well as coffee enemas.
Macrobiotic diet	Origins of cancer "rooted in the quality of the external factors that we are selecting and consuming."[51] Factors crucial to cancer prevention and control: overall blood quality, mental orientation, way of life. Specific causes of cancer result from excess of yin and/or yang foods. Health and happiness only result with proper balance of yin and yang, the two major world forces.[59]	Ten macrobiotic diets exist: diet no. −3 to diet no. 7, which is 100% brown rice. Foods eliminated gradually in progressing from diet no. −3 to no. 7. No scientific basis for this diet in cancer therapy. Nutritional value inadequate in vitamins, minerals, protein, calories.[51]
SPIRITUAL/MYSTICAL TECHNIQUES		
Psychic Surgery	Cancer can be removed from any part of the body without incisions by uses of prayers, "psychic surgeries," and massage. "Operation" done in hotel room. Body area covered with salve, then cotton-soaked square. Blood is splattered over site and a bloody piece of tissue held up. "Operative site" is wiped clean and diseased area is "whole" again.[65]	Patient's faith in method is major promotional factor. Arguments of simple faith used to counter scientific arguments. Psychic surgery done mostly in Philippines. Opposition believes done by sleight of hand using animal tissues and blood-filled capsules hidden by "psychic surgeon."
Spiritualists	Claim to have special healing abilities given by God. Rely on laying on of hands on the cancer site.	Patient must admit sinfulness and guilt to be cured.
Seances/Trances/Incantations	Invoke "mystical universal powers" to cure cancer. "Miracle injections" may be administered after trance is over.[64]	

the provider and patient, who are both on the outside of the medical system.

Nursing Role

Patients may perceive their physicians as too busy to answer questions about unproven methods, and so they frequently direct these queries to the nurse. Angry memories of curable patients who opted for laetrile may make the nurse's first emotional reaction to lecture the patient and tell him or her that these people have nothing to offer and only want money. This approach may quickly confirm the distrust for the medical community and encourage the patient to seek other treatment options. Patients need factual infor-

Table 25–4 Common Ineffective Treatments—cont'd

Treatment	Rationale/Mechanism of Action	Comments
PSYCHOLOGIC METHODS		
Simonton method	Attitude and stress may be crucial factors in the causation and cure of cancer. Uses relaxation and mental imagery to visualize cancer cells as weak and body as strong army attacking cancer cells.[67] Advocate that patients continue to receive conventional treatment in conjunction with their counseling sessions.	Founded by Carl and Stephanie Simonton. Established cancer counseling and research center in Ft. Worth, Texas. Entire program is described in their book *Getting Well Again.* While medical/scientific community supports notion that positive attitude promotes an optimal therapeutic response, there are no controlled studies to demonstrate objective response with this method. Individuals may feel guilty, believe their personality type caused cancer. Also may be encouraged to forgo standard treatment if they become overdependent on this method. Positive aspects of treatment include increased feelings of well being, promotion of relaxation, decreased feelings of helplessness, and adaptation to situation.
IMMUNOLOGIC THERAPY		
Immuno-augmentative therapy (IAT)	Immune stimulation enables body's normal defenses to destroy cancer cells. Treatment program consists of daily immunocompetence tests and immuno-augmentative therapy. Length of treatment ranges from 4 weeks to several months.[20]	Therapeutic approach based on reasonable scientific theory; scientific documentation of treatment results are lacking.[20] Lawrence Burton, PhD, a zoologist, founded treatment and uses it at the Immunology Researching Center in the Bahamas. He has publicized therapy widely but has not reported findings in scientific literature. Withdrew IND application after FDA requested further information. Some states have passed law protecting doctors who prescribe IAT from malpractice suits.[31]

mation delivered in a calm, objective, and nonjudgmental fashion. This is the appropriate time to evaluate what the patient has read or heard about the alternative therapy and what the perceived benefits are. What is the level of interest in the unproven method? What is the level of understanding about current therapy and treatment goals?

This is an important opportunity to provide accurate information about unproven methods. All currently accepted treatments were unproven at one time. The FDA and NCI protect patients by requiring proof of safety and efficacy before generalized use of a drug. The following interventions may help the patient evaluate unproven methods and improve nurse/patient relationships.

1. Explain how to access the Medlars system to determine scientific testing of treatment.
2. Check resources to verify promoter's cancer expertise:
   • Directory of Medical Specialists

   • American Federation of Clinical Oncologic Societies
   • American Association for Cancer Research
   • American Society of Clinical Oncology
   • National Cancer Institute Hotline (1-800-4-CANCER)
3. Offer reliable information:
   • "Ineffective Cancer Therapies" (Adria Laboratories)
   • "What Are Clinical Trials All About" (NCI)
4. Examine patient's expectation of current treatment plan.
5. Offer quality-versus-quantity of life information.
6. Help reestablish hope.
7. Identify ways to make patient and family more involved in treatment.
8. Referrals for a second opinion may increase confidence in current treatment or identify additional therapeutic alternatives.

If unproven methods or promotional techniques seem to the nurse or physician to warrant further legal investigation, the following organizations should be notified:

- The local health department
- Consumer protection office
- Medical society

The federal agencies and national organizations involved in the investigation, regulation, or reporting of such practices:

- Food and Drug Administration
- Federal Trade Commission
- U.S. Postal Service
- Consumer Product Safety Commission
- American Medical Association[28]

FUTURE DIRECTIONS AND ADVANCES IN CANCER CLINICAL TRIALS

Through clinical research and the clinical trials network, progress has been made in cancer treatment over the past 20 years. Combinations of surgery, radiation therapy, and chemotherapy have made a number of cancers curable. Even more cancers may become curable in the next two decades with the addition of biologic response modifiers to the therapeutic armamentarium.

Curable cancers include acute lymphoblastic leukemia in both children and adults, acute myeloblastic leukemia, Hodgkin's lymphoma, diffuse histiocytic and Burkitt's lymphoma, testicular tumors, Wilms' tumor, osteogenic sarcoma, and rhabdomyosarcoma.

Clinical trials also supply blood and tissue specimens for clinical research. This has greatly increased the knowledge of disease biology. Childhood acute lymphoblastic leukemia can now be subclassified into a variety of prognostic groups and the treatment tailor-made to yield the best outcome. Human tumor tissue can be cloned for testing with a variety of drugs to determine the most effective treatment. Polyglycoprotein, identified on the cell surfaces of some patients with multiple myeloma, ovarian cancer, and acute multiple myeloma, indicates a high risk for drug resistance. New tumor markers are being studied for prognostic significance. The study of oncogenes sheds further light on the biology of cancer. Advances in cytogenetic studies may identify high-risk subsets of patients requiring more aggressive therapy. Finally, the identification and mapping of the human genome will direct cancer research in this century and the next.

In 1986 the NCI presented its highly publicized Year 2000 goal: to reduce the mortality of cancer 50% by the year 2000. Since the National Cancer Program was established in 1971, much has been learned about the causes and cures of many forms of cancer. The source of the progress in understanding cancer has been a vigorous basic, clinical, and cancer research program. The knowledge gained about cancer can be used now to control a significant portion of the disease.[25,72]

One of the main emphases of the cancer control objectives is the prevention of cancer. The NCI identified the priority areas of research as chemoprevention, diet and nutrition, occupational cancer control, and screening and early detection.

These studies present new challenges and opportunities for oncology nurses. Rather than treatment of the patient with cancer, the healthy population will be the focus. Cancer control studies will take us into the community for many of the studies. New physician networks will be identified. From the NCI perspective of funding, cancer control trials will be as important as clinical trials.

CONCLUSION

No doubt these are exciting times for nurses involved in cancer research. New chemotherapy agents are being identified, the role of the biologic response modifier is being determined, technology is rapidly changing the world of diagnostics, and cancer control requires a new flexibility in systems. The challenges of cancer clinical trials are many, but the rewards justify our efforts.

BIBLIOGRAPHY

1. AMA Council on Scientific Affairs: Viability of cancer clinical research: patient accrual, coverage, and reimbursement, J Natl Cancer Inst 83(4):254, 1991.
2. Antman KH, Aldort LM, Yarbro JW, and others: Cost-effectiveness and reimbursement in patients' care, Semin Hematol 26(suppl):32, 1989.
3. Arje SL and Smith LV: The cruelest killers. In Barrett S and Knight G, editors: The health robbers, Philadelphia, 1976, George F Stickley Co.
4. Belmont Report: Ethical principles and guidelines for the protection of human subjects of research, DHEW Publication No. (05)-78-0012, Washington DC, 1978, US Government Printing Office.
5. Berlin NI: Unorthodox therapy. In Moosa AR, Robson C, and Schimpff SC, editors: Comprehensive textbook of oncology, Baltimore, 1986, Williams & Wilkins.
6. Bohigian G: Reliability of cancer research patient accrual, Presented at the American Medical Association Home of Delegates, Chicago, 1989.
7. Bujorian GA: Clinical trials: patient issues in the decision-making process, Oncol Nurs Forum 15(6):779, 1988.
8. The Cancer Letter, 17(40):6, October 18, 1991.
9. Cassidy J and Macfarlane DK: The role of the

research nurse in clinical cancer research, Cancer Nurs 14(3):124, 1991.

10. Chamorro T and Applebaum J: Informed consent: nursing issues and ethical dilemmas, Oncol Nurs Form 15(6):803, 1988.

11. Cheson BD: Clinical trials programs, Semin Oncol Nurs 7(4):235, 1991.

12. Closing in on a cure: solving a 5000 year old mystery, US Department of Health and Human Services, 1987.

13. Creighton H: Informed consent, Nurs Management 17(10):11, 1986.

14. Department of Health and Human Services: Protection of human subjects: informed consent. Washington DC, Federal Register, January 27, 1981, Part IX.

15. DeVita VT: Principles of chemotherapy. In DeVita VT, Hellman S, and Rosenberg SA, editors: Cancer principles and practice of oncology, ed 3, Philadelphia, 1989, JB Lippincott.

16. Donovan CT: Ethics in cancer nursing practice. In Groenwald S and others, editors: Cancer nursing: practice and principles, ed 2, Boston, 1991, Jones and Bartlett, Publishers.

17. Donsbach KW and Walker M: Metabolic cancer therapies, Huntington Beach, California, 1981, The International Institute of National Health Sciences, Inc.

18. Dorr R and Pazxinos J: The current status of laetrile, Ann Intern Med 89(3):389, 1978.

19. Durant J: Current status of clinical trials, Cancer 65(suppl):2371, 1990.

20. Easy cures for cancer still find support, JAMA 246(7):714.

21. Engelking C: Clinical trials: impact evaluation and implementation considerations. Semin Oncol Nurs 8(2):148, 1992.

22. Fawcett J: A typology of nursing research activities according to educational preparation, J Prof Nurs 1:75, 1985.

23. Freireich EJ: The design and planning of clinical trials. In Moosa AR, Robson MC, and Schimpff SC, editors: Comprehensive textbook of oncology, Baltimore, 1986, Williams & Wilkins.

24. Friedman MA: Patient accrual to clinical trials, Cancer Treat Rep 71:557, 1987.

25. Galassi A: New antineoplastic agents. In Hubbard SM, Greene PE, and Knobf MT, editors: Current issues in cancer nursing practice. Philadelphia, 1991, JB Lippincott Co.

26. General Accounting Office: Off label drugs: initial results of a national survey. Washington, DC, US General Accounting Office, (GAO/PEDM-91-12BR), 1991.

27. Gerson M: The cure of advanced cancer by diet therapy: a summary of 30 years clinical experimentation, Physiol Chem Physics 10:449, 1978.

28. Grady C: Ethical issues in clinical trials, Semin Oncol Nurs 7(4):288, 1991.

29. Grant guidelines for cancer control: areas of programmatic interest, US Department of Health and Human Services.

30. Grant RN and Bartlett I: Unproven cancer remedies—a primer. In Unproven methods of cancer management, New York, 1971, American Cancer Society.

31. Green S: Let's stop driving cancer patients to unproven treatments, Medical Work News 23(12):188, 1982.

32. Greenwald P, Cullen JW, and Weed D: Cancer prevention and control, Semin Oncol 17(4):383-390, 1990.

33. Gross J: Clinical research in cancer chemotherapy, Oncol Nurs Forum 13(1):59, 1986.

34. Guy JL: New challenges for nurses in clinical trials, Semin Oncol Nurs 7(4):297-303, 1991.

35. Henney JE: Unproven methods of cancer treatment. In DeVita VT, Hellman S, and Rosenberg SA, editors: Cancer principles and practice of oncology, ed 2, Philadelphia, 1985, JB Lippincott Co.

36. Holland J: The krebiozen story, JAMA 200:125, 1967.

37. Holland J: Why patients seek unproven cancer remedies: a psychological perspective, CA 32(1):10, 1982.

38. Hoxsey HM: You don't have to die, New York, 1956, Milestone Books.

39. Hunter CP, Frelick RW, Feldman AR, and others: Selection factors in clinical trials: results from the community clinical oncology physicians' patient log. Cancer Treat Rep 71:559, 1987.

40. Ingelfinger FJ: Cancer! Alarm! Cancer! N Engl J Med 293:1329, 1975.

41. Investigators' Handbook, Cancer Therapy Evaluation Program, Division of Cancer Treatment, National Cancer Institute, Bethesda, MD, 1986.

42. Jannsen WF: Cancer quackery: the past in the present, Semin Oncol 6:526, 1979.

43. Jassak PF and Ryan MP: Ethical issues in clinical research, Semin Oncol Nurs 5(2):102, 1989.

44. Jenkins J and Curt G: Implementation of clinical trials. In Baird SB, McCorkle R, and Grant M: Cancer nursing: a comprehensive textbook, Philadelphia, 1991, WB Saunders Co.

45. Jenkins J and Hubbard S: History of clinical trials, Semin Oncol Nurs 7(4):228, 1991.

46. Jenkins JF and Lake PC: Celebration of an era of public service at the National Institutes of Health and the National Cancer Institute, Cancer Nurs 11(1):58, 1988.

47. Johansen MA, Mayer DK, and Hoover HC: Ob-

stacles to implementing cancer clinical trials, Semin Oncol Nurs 7(4):260, 1991.

48. Kelly ME: Informed consent. In Northrup CE and Kelly ME, editors: Legal issues in nursing, St Louis, 1987, Mosby.

49. Kessler DA: The regulation of investigational agents, N Engl J Med 320(5):281, 1989.

50. Kreuger J: Safeguarding the rights of human subjects. In Davis A and Kreuger J, editors: Patients, nurses, and ethics. New York, 1980, AJN Company.

51. Kushi M: Macrobiotic approach to cancer, Wayne, NJ, 1982, Avery Publishing Group, Inc.

52. Laetrile: the political success of a scientific failure, Consumer Reports, Aug. 1977.

53. Leventhal BG: An overview of clinical trials in oncology, Semin Oncol 15(5):414, 1988.

54. Luursk J: Unproven methods of treatment. In Groenwald S, editor: Cancer nursing: practice and principles, Boston, 1987, Jones & Bartlett, Publishers.

55. McEvoy MD, Cannon L, and MacDermot ML: The professional role for nurses in clinical trials, Semin Oncol Nurs 7(4):268, 1991.

56. Melink TJ and Whitacre MY: Planning and implementing clinical trials, Semin Oncol Nurse 7(4):243, 1991.

57. Miaskowski C and Nielsen B: Documentation of the nursing process in cancer nursing. In Baird SB, McCorkle R, and Grant M, editors: Cancer nursing: a comprehensive textbook, Philadelphia, 1991, WB Saunders Co.

58. Miller NJ and Ruben JH: Unproven methods of cancer management, part I: background and historical perspectives, Oncol Nurs Forum 10(4):46, 1983.

59. Miller NJ and Ruben JH: Unproven methods of cancer management, part II: current trends and implications for patient care, Oncol Nurs Forum 10(4):46, 1983.

60. Milstead JC, Davis JB, and Dobelle M: Quackery in the medical device field, Proceedings from the Second National Congress on Medical Quackery, 1963.

61. Monipour CM and others: Quality of life endpoints in cancer clinical trials: review and recommendations, J Natl Cancer Inst 81:485, 1989.

62. Most feared diseases, Parade, February 6, 1977.

63. The Nuremburg Code, 1949. In Beauchamp T and Childress J, editors: Principles of Biomedical Ethics, ed 2, St Louis, 1981, Mosby.

64. Patrick PKS: Cancer quackery: information, issues, responsibility, action. In Marino LB, editor: Cancer nursing, St Louis, 1981, CV Mosby.

65. Psychic surgery can mean fiscal excision with tumor retention, JAMA 228:278, 1974.

66. Reiser J, Dyck AJ, and Curran WJ, editors: Ethics in medicine: Historical perspectives and contemporary concerns. Cambridge, MA, 1977, MIT.

67. Simonton OC: Unproven methods of cancer management, CA 32(1):58, 1982.

68. Spike J and Holland JC: The care of the patient with potentially fatal disease. In Strain J and Grossman S, editors: Principles of liaison psychiatry, New York, 1975, Appleton-Century-Crofts.

69. Subcommittee on unorthodox therapies, American Society of Clinical Oncology: Ineffective cancer therapy—a guide, J Clin Oncol 1:154, 1983.

70. Taylor KM, Margolese RG, and Soskolne CL: Physicians' reasons for not entering eligible patients in a randomized clinical trial of surgery for breast cancer, N Engl J Med 310(21):1363, 1984.

71. Unproven methods: DMSO, CA 33(2):122, 1983.

72. Update, National Cancer Institute, October 1993, Bethesda, MD.

73. Varricchio CG and Jassak PF: Informed consent: an overview, Semin Oncol Nurs 5(2):95, 1989.

74. Veatch RM: Case studies in medical ethics. Cambridge, MA, 1977, Harvard University Press.

75. Wheeler V: Preparing nurses for clinical trials: the cancer center approach, Semin Oncol Nurs 7(4):275, 1991.

76. Winn R: From opera to chemoprevention. Oncol Issues 7(2):13, 1992.

77. Wittes RE: Cancer emphasis in the clinical drug development program of the NCI. In DeVita T, Rosenberg SA, and Hellman S, editors: Cancer principles and practice of oncology, Update 1(12):1, 1987.

78. Wittes RE: Paying for patient care in treatment research—who is responsible? Cancer Treat Rep 71:107, 1987.

79. Wittes RE and Friedman MA: Accrual to clinical trials, J Natl Cancer Inst 80:884, 1988.

80. Young F and others: The FDA's new procedures for use of investigational drug in treatment, JAMA 259(15):2267, 1988.

UNIT IV

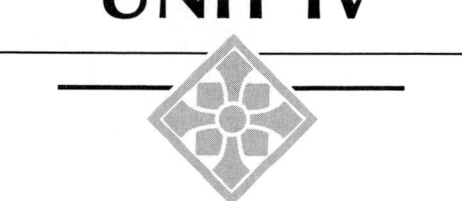

CANCER CARE SUPPORTIVE THERAPIES

CHAPTER 26

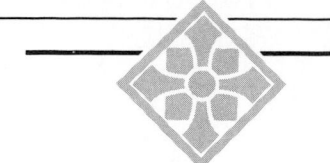

Home Care and Alternative Care Settings and Cancer Resources

Frances Cornelius

"Staff nurses increasingly are expected to assist hospitalized patients to make the transition between the acute care and community or convalescent setting. This transition is a complex and challenging task which requires data-gathering and decision-making skills."[1] The health care professional must be able to collect and analyze pertinent information in order to facilitate the development of an appropriate discharge plan.

The advent of rising health care costs and efforts to contain these costs have resulted in the increased emphasis upon home care and alternative care settings. Frequently, patients are discharged after only a short hospital stay when, in the past, they would have remained hospitalized for ongoing assessment and evaluation of their status and response to treatment. In addition, many cancer therapies that were previously only administered in acute care settings are now given routinely on an outpatient basis. The advances in cancer treatments as well as the availability of improved technology has made outpatient and home cancer treatment both safe and effective.

It is important to note that accompanying the decreased hospital stay there has been an increase in Emergency Department use and subsequent rehospitalization. "Patients who are frequent Emergency Room visitors or who have frequent readmissions to the hospital due to exacerbations of chronic illnesses are often patients who could or should have received home health care at an earlier time."[30] Leiby and Shupe[14] in their study identify the ill elderly as more at risk for hospitalization and recurrent hospitalizations and note that home health care does reduce the number of hospital readmissions. The authors further state that early discharge:

. . . results in less time during hospitalization for health professionals to instruct the patient in the self-care practices necessary to further their recovery within the home. This health teaching, therefore, needs to be continued after hospital discharge to lessen the chance of illness exacerbation and rehospitalization. And of course early discharge may mean that the patient remains acutely ill. Thus, nursing care is needed for the facilitation of the patient's self-care practices, health teaching, continuation of skilled assessments, and communication of changes in condition to the physician.[14]

Although the trend for more economical, home-based, family supported, cancer care and treatment is on the increase, it is important to note that demographic changes in our society and the decline of traditional extended family support systems necessitate utilization of alternative care settings such as extended care facilities. It is essential that the health care professional accurately assess and identify the specific needs of the client and, if available, the family's ability to take on the caregiving role. Identification of the presence or absence of adequate caregiving supports is central to determining if home care or alternative care settings are appropriate.

It is also imperative that health care providers, in particular the oncology nurse, be cognizant of all the variables that will affect the patient's response to treatment when he or she is at home or in alternative care settings. The goal is to ensure the patient's safety and facilitate the transition from the health care system. To accomplish this the oncology nurse must thoroughly assess and accurately identify the patient's/family's abilities, learning needs, as well as the en-

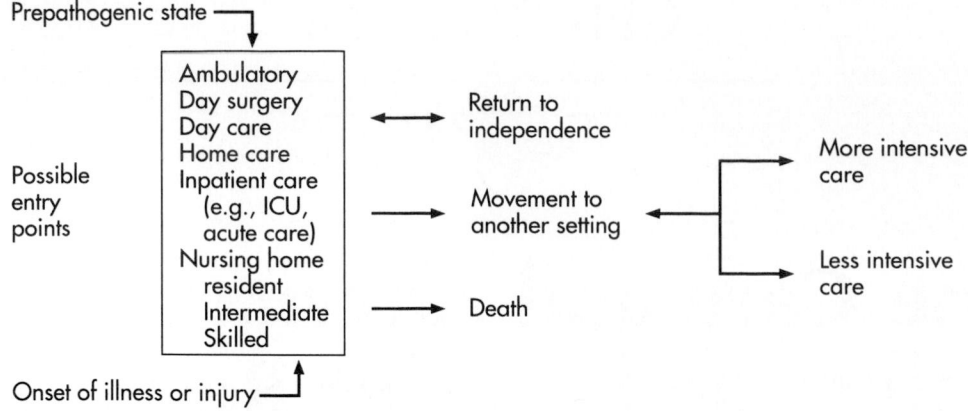

Prepathogenic state

Possible
entry
points

Ambulatory
Day surgery
Day care
Home care
Inpatient care
(e.g., ICU,
acute care)
Nursing home
resident
Intermediate
Skilled

Return to
independence

Movement to
another setting

Death

More intensive
care

Less intensive
care

Onset of illness or injury

Figure 26–1 Illness-Wellness continuum through discharge planning. (From Kelly K and McClelland E: Discharge planning: home care considerations. In Martinson IM and Widmer A, editors: Home health nursing, 1989, Philadelphia, WB Saunders Co.)

vironmental factors in the home that may interfere with the patient's safety and well-being.

Researchers have determined that supporting the caregiver in the caregiving role, particularly with the day to day management of care, is of paramount importance.[9,19,24] It has been determined "that the intervention most needed is the provision of assistance to family members caring for cancer patients. This intervention should be tailored to meet individual needs but must include information and skills relative to physical care, emotional support, and respite when possible."[24]

The discharge planning process is an organized systematic approach commonly utilized in the acute care setting to facilitate the transition from the hospital to home. It is important for the oncology nurse to be aware that the assessment and planning characteristic of discharge planning process should not be limited to the acute care setting. Patients seen in the outpatient oncology clinic have discharge planning needs also! In fact, this process is ongoing and should continue as the patient moves through a variety of health care settings during the course of their illness. A client-centered approach to provide continuity of care facilitates the delivery of holistic health services that serve the best interests of the client while assisting providers to plan services that are needs-based.[13]

In the literature, discussions regarding discharge planning focus primarily on the transition from the acute care setting. Upon examination, the process utilized in the hospital setting can be directly applied to the outpatient setting or any other health care setting in which a health care professional identifies discharge planning needs.

A model developed by Kelly and McClelland[13] achieves the balance between the realities of health care delivery today and the ideals of continuity of care

(Figure 26-1). Within this model, several key points are addressed:

1. Discharge planning can begin at any entry point in the health care system, not just as the client prepares to leave a 24-hour acute care setting.
2. Any point on the health continuum can serve as a basis for entry into the health care system. This may range from enrollment in a fitness clinic to a hospice program.
3. Movement through the care continuum may be multidirectional.
4. The intensity of care may be increased or decreased as the setting changes.[13]

THE DISCHARGE PLANNING PROCESS

THE ASSESSMENT

The oncology nurse in the acute care setting has a unique opportunity to perform a comprehensive assessment of the patient's strengths and limitations, over a period of days and sometimes weeks. This allows for the establishment of rapport between the nurse and patient. Frequently, when care is given over a period of days, the nurse's keen eye may note a patient care need that may not have been previously assessed. Granted, the in-patient setting is extremely hectic and frequently nurses do not have the luxury of spending extended periods of time with patients exploring their discharge needs when they, as well as the other patients in the nurse's care, have many needs that must immediately be addressed. Often, it becomes a matter of prioritization—What needs to be done now and what can wait? It is important to understand that discharge planning *cannot* wait until the day the patient is going home.

Similarly, the oncology nurse in the outpatient clinic setting also has the opportunity to assess for and identify the specific health care needs of the patient. Obviously, the time available to the clinic nurse is limited; however, a skilled practitioner can perform this task. It is expected that the experienced oncology nurse can very quickly and effectively assess, identify, and respond to new patient posthospitalization/post-clinic visit needs as these needs surface, if the nurse is continuously cognizant of the importance of discharge planning and has a workable discharge planning tool to facilitate the process.

The tool presented in this chapter was developed by Slevin and Roberts at St. Francis Medical Center, Peoria, Illinois, in 1987. It is a good example for discussion although there are many other tools currently available in the literature that are equally useful.[29]

Many factors must be considered prior to discharge and advance planning is imperative. Slevin and Roberts provide a helpful detailed approach to effective discharge planning transition from the acute care setting to the home setting. This process necessitates not only thorough assessment and evaluation but also extensive planning and coordination. The authors identify the patient admission data form and the chart as the initial sources of data for the discharge planner to screen and identify patients that may have discharge planning needs.

However, the experienced oncology nurse, while certainly utilizing secondary sources of data such as the patient's record, will, quite understandably, be relying upon his/her first-hand observations and assessment of the patient. No matter how the patient with posthospitalization or postclinic visit needs is identified, this screening process should be followed by (1) the client interview, (2) identification of the specific posthospitalization or postclinic problems or needs, and (3) development of a plan for solving client problems or needs. These three major components of the discharge planning process have specific subcomponents that, when addressed, both clarify and simplify the discharge planning process. These are discussed below.

The Client Interview

1. Introduction (if necessary)
2. Establish the relationship of the client to: *(a)* spouse, *(b)* family, including children, *(c)* neighbors, *(d)* church, and *(e)* senior citizen support activities.
3. Establish how the client's illness has affected his or her role and function in the family with special attention to: *(a)* financial support, *(b)* shopping, *(c)* meal preparation, *(d)* transportation, and *(e)* living arrangements.
4. Determine the client's prehospital daily routine.
5. Assess the client's learning and comprehension ability.
6. Assess the client's interest in discharge planning services.[29]

In addition to Slevin and Robert's six steps in the client interview, it is important to also determine the client's goals and expectations of treatment and rehabilitation. This very important factor is frequently overlooked by health care providers and is critical to the planning process.

Identification of Post-Hospital Problems and Needs

After the client interview has been completed and it is determined that some needs or potential problem areas exist and the client is interested in having discharge planning services, the next step is to clearly identify the specific needs. Slevin and Roberts identify the following factors warranting consideration at this stage of the planning process[29]:

1. Inadequate or no support system.
2. Inadequate financial resources.
3. Poor environmental conditions.
4. Inability to carry out treatment and medication regimen.
5. Inability to carry out activities of daily living.
6. Poor socialization.
7. Potential problems (i.e., related to disease progression or treatment.

These seven cues help clarify the specific and individual needs or problems of the client and give direction to the development of an individualized plan of care to address these concerns.

PLANNING
Development of a Plan for Solving Client Problem Needs

After the client's problems or needs have been identified, a collaborative process, involving the client, family or significant others, and health care professionals, should occur. At this time the oncology nurse should assist the client, family, and/or significant others to realistically look at their goals and expectations and subsequently develop a plan for care. This may entail placement in an extended care facility or linkage with community based agencies providing service in the home setting. With the diverse services available it is necessary to address the following items when assisting the client and family in this decision making process[29]:

1. Assist client or family to identify the specific problem(s).
2. Assist client or family to set priorities among the problems.
3. Assist the client or family to identify the services or resources needed.
4. Interpret services of the available resources of the client or family.
5. Establish financial status.
6. Work out details of selected plan with client or family.

7. Obtain client or family consent to contact the resources in their behalf.
8. Establish criteria for evaluation of the effectiveness of the plan. (Usually a follow-up telephone call. This will be discussed later in the chapter.)

At this point, it should be very apparent that the transition to home or alternative settings for care is highly complex and that it is necessary to consider many factors. It is important to keep in mind that health care is provided on a continuum and is a multidisciplinary effort. Utilize the resources available to you in your practice setting. If there is a discharge planner or social worker available in your institution, establish a collaborative relationship to facilitate the process for the benefit of your client. If such services are not available, network with your colleagues and professionals in the community.

Often, due to early discharge, there is not sufficient time to initiate all the appropriate referrals to community support services. In such cases the referrals may be made after the client is home. As it has been well documented that the caregiving role is very stressful, it is preferred that the professional doing the discharge planning make the initial contacts with the support services. A responsible family member may be willing to follow-up on a referral made by the professional. Be sure to give this individual the name of the referred agency, the phone number, and the agency contact person.

If the client needs skilled nursing care in the home setting make a referral to a skilled home care agency. Most hospitals have continuing patient care forms that must be completed when a referral is initiated. Include information about other identified needs and request that the home care agency's personnel assist client with the referral process. A list of national community resources is given in the Appendix. These organizations will help you identify available local community resources.

In addition to information about identified support needs, the referral for continuing patient care in the home care setting should also include information about significant factors related to this hospitalization, relevant past medical history, current medications and treatment orders, identified nursing problems, and results of recent diagnostic tests or bloodwork. Concise and comprehensive referrals are essential to facilitate the transition from the acute/ambulatory setting to home care. Keep in mind that while nurses in the hospital or ambulatory setting have ready access to the patient's extensive medical record, the home care nurse frequently has only the continuing patient care referral form. The information on the referral form is often not comprehensive, consequently making the home care nurse's job even more difficult.

"In summary, the transfer of information about a patient is essential to initiating prompt, effective care tailored to the specific needs of the patient. When accurate, timely information is available, the nurse who opens the case can accomplish the initial assessment more efficiently to facilitate continuity of care and assist the patient and family with the transition into home care."[16]

Assessing the Caregiver

In most institutions, assessment of supports of family, friends, and available organized institutions is routinely done if it has been determined that the client needs assistance in the home setting. Frequently, a primary caregiver, usually the spouse, has been identified and some in-hospital teaching has been initiated by the nurses prior to discharge. However, this is not enough. A caregiver assessment must also be done. As the trend for early discharge continues, "the family support system must assume greater responsibility for maintaining what is often a very aggressive post-hospitalization treatment plan."[6] The stress and anxieties associated with the caregiving responsibilities can be overwhelming. Often, unasked questions as well as feelings of inadequacy in their ability to properly and safely care for their loved one add to the caregiving burden. "Probably their greatest challenge is developing the confidence to do what is right for the patient. 'Have I changed the dressing correctly?' 'Have I suctioned the patient in the proper manner?' One question often leads to a hundred more! Teaching them not only the 'what to do's' but also the 'what to expect' is one of the best stress reducers."[6]

Feuer recommends that an extensive assessment of the caregiver also be conducted as part of the discharge planning process. He identifies 24 key issues and questions that should be addressed as part of this process[6]:

1. Has the caregiver's age been considered as well as the patient's?
2. Does the caregiver's mental and physical condition allow that person to assume this responsibility?
3. Will the caregiver live in the patient's home?
4. If the caregiver is not in the home, how accessible will that person be?
5. Who can provide some relief or free time for the caregiver?
6. Is the caregiver aware of the patient's medical condition?
7. Has the caregiver received instructions on administering medications, observing for possible side-effects and managing them?
8. Is the caregiver aware of the expected course of treatment?
9. If there is to be a change in the patient's condition,

does the caregiver know what problems to watch for?

10. If the patient's condition changes, does the caregiver know whom to call?

11. Does the caregiver know the name of the physician directing the home care plan?

12. If a home care agency will provide care at home, has the caregiver received the name and phone number of the company?

13. If the patient will be using medical equipment in the home, has the caregiver been given the name of the company which supplies it?

14. Has the caregiver been helped to develop a list of emergency phone numbers: a) community emergency numbers, b) rescue emergency numbers, c) physician, d) home care agency, e) equipment supplier, f) other family members, etc.?

15. Does the caregiver know about any follow-up medical appointments scheduled for the patient?

16. Has the caregiver been instructed in what not to do for the patient, as well as what to allow the patient to do for him/herself?

17. If prescriptions must be filled, are there immediate funds available to do this? Also, if a prescription is difficult to get at local pharmacies, advise caregiver where it is available.

18. Have questions regarding financial matters related to the patient's home care needs been arranged before discharge? Is the caregiver attending to financial matters?

19. If the caregiver can no longer assume responsibility, whom should he or she notify?

20. Does the caregiver have medications for the patient's first 24 hours home? If not, is there a plan developed to obtain these medications?

21. Has the caregiver been made aware of any appropriate support groups available in the community?

22. Have you supplied the caregiver with suitable educational materials regarding the patient's diagnosis?

23. Does the caregiver have the name and phone number of the person who arranged for home care services and who can be called to clarify issues or further explain services to be expected?

24. Has the discharge planner asked the caregiver if he or she has any questions or problems concerning the discharge, date, time, transportation home, or the services they will be receiving?

SETTINGS FOR CARE

In addition to the hospital, other settings for care include the home and extended care facilities.

Extended Care

Usually in the out-patient setting, extended care placement is not an identified need; however, it is wise to have a working knowledge about these resources. At times, family members may find the caregiving burden too overwhelming and request information on and assistance with extended care placement.

If it is determined that the client's care needs necessitate placement in an extended care facility, the extended care facility must then be identified that will most effectively meet the client's needs. There are four basic types of extended care facilities, which vary according to the amount and type of care needed by the client. These facilities include:

1. Skilled care facilities
2. Intermediate care facilities
3. Adult foster or sheltered care facilities
4. Residential care facilities

Skilled care facilities provide around-the-clock skilled nursing care and observation. In addition, there is frequent medical supervision. Intermediate care facilities provide around-the-clock basic nursing care for clients that are medically stable but unable to care for themselves. Adult foster or sheltered care facilities are for individuals that require a protective living arrangement that provides general supervision and assistance with bathing, dressing, meals, and other personal needs.[29]

Adult foster care is a viable option for adults needing care regardless of income or age. On the average, adult foster care tends to be less expensive than nursing home care. While there is some overlap between the populations served by nursing homes and foster care homes, residents in foster care tend to be less functionally impaired and less cognitively impaired than those in nursing homes.[23]

Residential care facilities are for individuals that no longer wish to live alone or have no place to live. In general, these facilities also provide similar services as a sheltered care facility and may occasionally, in times of illness, provide intermediate care for their residents.[29]

As there are many extended care facilities available it becomes an overwhelming task to select the best one. The State Long-Term Care Ombudsman office in your state will provide lists of certified extended care facilities that provide the various levels of care. This State Office will also provide information regarding reimbursement of these facilities by medicare or medicaid. This is a very helpful starting point for patients and their family members. It is recommended that the patient or significant other tour the facilities prior to making a selection.

Home Care

Home care has seen an increase in utilization in the last 10 years due to the implementation of DRGs and subsequent earlier discharges. The increase of consumerism and desire to exercise more control over personal health care has also been an influencing factor.

Home care is on the cutting edge of change in nursing and health care. In a time of increasing concern over federal health care expenditures, home care represents a humane, sensible, alternative to institutionalized care for an increasing number of Americans. It also offers other benefits, including eliminating the risk of nosocomial infection, maintaining patients' and families' social and cultural patterns, and promoting patients' self-esteem, independence, and personal involvement in care.[4]

Quite understandably, the option of home care services is very attractive to cancer patients and their families who face an illness that often strips away much of their sense of personal control.

There are two types of home care services available to health care consumers: traditional home care and high-technology home care. Traditional home care services generally provide skilled nursing care including patient assessment and intervention, patient and family education; rehabilitative services such as physical, occupational, and speech and language therapies; social work intervention and home health aide support.

Recent improvements in and the increasing availability of high technology in the home setting has made home care a viable option for cancer patients at all stages of treatment and illness. High-technology home care for patients with cancer generally refers to the home management of infusional therapies such as:

1. Antifungal therapy
2. Antibiotic therapy
3. Chemotherapy
4. Hemotherapy
5. Hydration therapy
6. Venous access device maintenance
7. Pain management
8. Total parenteral and enteral nutrition[17]

Home intravenous therapy is one of the most rapidly growing trends in the home care industry. Cost containment and the growing threat of communicable disease transmission in hospitals are the two major factors contributing to this trend.[20]

Not all patients with cancer are good candidates for home infusion therapy. These patients and their families must be properly screened prior to initiating such therapies in the home setting to ensure that the treatment is both safe and efficacious (Figure 26-2).

Patients that receive infusional therapy in the home must have a venous access device to ensure a reliable, safe, and patent access site. A variety of infusion pumps that are compact, reliable, and easy to manage are now available in the home setting and ensure that the prescribed medication is administered as ordered. Useful guides for management and care of central venous catheters and a general overview of infusion pumps are given in Tables 26-1 and 26-2.

1. The patient must want to receive therapy at home.
2. The patient must be medically stable for home treatment.
3. The patient should have a venous access device in place or adequate venous access via the peripheral route (or a plan must exist should peripheral access become exhausted).
4. The patient or caregiver must be able to care for the central line and demonstrate proficiency and competency in maintaining the access device.
5. The patient or caregiver must be knowledgeable of the therapy; this knowledge includes:
   a. Name of drug(s)—both infusional and adjunct medications
   b. Dosage(s)
   c. Potential side effects
   d. Actions to take to prevent or minimize side effects
   e. Potential adverse reactions to medication
   f. Storage of drug(s)
6. The patient or caregiver must be knowledgeable and proficient in the functioning of the infusion pump as follows:
   a. Operation of the pump
   b. Using the alarm system
   c. How to check if the pump is working
   d. Troubleshooting the pump
7. The patient's home environment must be conducive to home care (e.g., physical layout, telephone access, support person[s], running water, electricity).
8. The patient must have the financial means to pay for home treatment (e.g, insurance, private pay).
9. The patient or caregiver must have an emergency 24-hour number to call for problems (e.g., clinic RN, doctor's office, homecare agency).

Figure 26–2 Criteria for patient screening, home infusion therapy. (From Maloney CH and Preston F: Oncol Nurs Forum 19(1):77, 1992)

Total parenteral therapy and enteral therapy for cancer patients have been controversial issues from medical, ethical, and financial perspectives. Nevertheless, this form of treatment is quite commonly provided in the home setting. It is generally believed that improved nutritional status improves the quality of life, though not necessarily prolongs life. However, it is important to note that during the end-stage of illness, when vital organs begin to shut down, infusional therapies are not advised. This is particularly difficult for families to accept and understand as they frequently believe that since the patient is not eating or drinking, IVs are necessary. If the rationale for withholding, discontinuing, or decreasing fluids to keep vein open (KVO) is not clearly explained to families at this time, they may be concerned that the patient is being denied vital treatment. More information regarding home care for the terminally ill and symptom management can be obtained from several very helpful handbooks listed in the Cancer Resources Appendix (see Appendix).

Up to 70% of patients with cancer will experience pain during their illness and at least 90% of this cancer-related pain can be effectively relieved with existing pain management techniques. While the oral route of pain medication is the preferred method by pain experts, high-technology pain management is a reasonable option to patients whose pain can not be effectively controlled otherwise. The American Pain Society, a national chapter of the International Association for the Study of Pain, publishes a helpful booklet, *Principles of Analgesic Use in the Treatment of Acute Pain and Chronic Cancer Pain,* which can be obtained for a small fee. In addition, the American Pain Society may be contacted to obtain additional information regarding pain management and consult with another health care professional experienced in pain management techniques (see Appendix). See Chapter 28 for more in-depth information regarding pain management.

Given the advances in anti-cancer therapies as well as the availability of portable infusion pumps, chemotherapy administration in the home setting has become both safe and effective. Lokich[15] cites many advantages of continuous infusional chemotherapy: "(1) increased exposure to chemotherapeutic agents with continuous infusion, thereby increasing the tumorcidal effect, (2) an increased cumulative dose delivered to the tumor, and (3) a decrease in occurrence and severity of toxicities."[15] As a result this has become a more and more common practice in the home setting. It is important that patients receive their first dose of chemotherapy in an inpatient or outpatient setting to facilitate expedient and proper treatment if any untoward reactions occur. In addition, a plan for properly disposing of all biohazardous waste should be in place. See Chapter 22 for more detail.

As with chemotherapy, it is important that antibiotic and antifungal therapies be initiated in the inpatient or outpatient setting as untoward reactions commonly occur with these medications. Once the patient's tolerance to the medication has been established, this treatment modality in the home setting is preferable to extended hospitalization if the patient is medically stable.

It is obvious that the patient is generally more comfortable at home and the health care cost savings are considerable when such high-technology services are provided in the home setting. In addition, patient hospitalizations are reduced, there is increased quality of life for patients and their families, and patients have a sense of control and active participation in their treatment plan.

Geriatric Considerations

Ill elderly people generally want to be home among family and familiar surroundings. Family members feel inadequate in their abilities to properly care for their parent/spouse and may be reluctant to bring them home. This in turn may result in feelings of guilt and fears that they may be judged as uncaring. In addition, family members have feelings of guilt and helplessness associated with their parent's/spouse's illness. It is important that the nurse provide an opportunity for family members to discuss their fears, feelings, and concerns. Consideration should be also given to how this illness is affecting the family's ability to meet their continuing needs.[16]

McAnear[21] developed the following set of questions that enable the nurse to gain a more thorough awareness of the family's needs and coping abilities:

Needs
1. What difficulties is the family experiencing with the medical treatment? (This would include management and changes in course of illness.)
2. What are the sources of financial strain from direct and indirect costs related to the illness?
3. What changes are required in day-to-day living activities for the family?
4. In what manner has the illness fostered social isolation?
5. How have relationships within the family been affected?
6. What impact has the illness or its management had on the ability to meet their continuing needs?

Coping Strategies:
1. What is the level of knowledge and technical skill the family has gained concerning the illness and its treatment?
2. What strategies does the family employ to help maintain a sense of normalcy in family life?
3. Who are identified supportive people or groups and what do they provide for the family?
4. What activities do the family members use to enhance positive coping strategies?
5. Does this illness have any positive aspects or results as perceived by this family?

These questions are a good starting point for gathering assessment data. It is expected that, following the establishment of rapport with the family, each of these areas can be explored in more depth. Then the nurse and the family can work together to identify and implement mutually acceptable interventions that will promote optimal family functioning.[16]

It is important to provide the family with education to enable them to adequately care for their parent/spouse and to provide the necessary resources to support their primary caregiving role and to foster optimal family functioning.

There are many community resources available to aid and support families experiencing difficulties associated wtih caring for an elderly person who has cancer. These resources are listed in the Appendix.

Text continued on p. 623.

Table 26–1 Adult Central Venous Catheters: Recommended Nursing Management

Type	Heparinization	Dressing	Blood Sampling
CENTRAL VENOUS CATHETERS *Short-Term Use (2-8 weeks)* Subclavian Single Lumen Dual Lumen Triple Lumen	After each use, flash *each* lumen with 5 ml Normal Saline (N/S), then heparinized saline 2 ml (100 µ/ml). For catheter *not* in use, flush *each* lumen with heparinized saline 2 ml (100 µ/ml) *every 12 hours*	Daily sterile dressing change at the site for duration of catheter placement. Gauze dressing change every 24 hours; bio-occlusive change every 72 hrs. Change Luer-Lok injection caps *every 72 hours.*	Shut off all IVs for *one (1) full minute.* Withdraw 5 ml blood. Discard. Withdraw blood sample. Flush lumen with 5 ml N/S, then heparinize or resume IV. TPN-SHUT OFF IV 10 MINUTES.
PERIPHERAL INSERTED CATHETER Longline PICCs (Use gentle pressure on syringe plunger for PIC catheters)	After each use, flush lumen with 2 ml N/S, then heparinized saline 1 ml (100 µ/ml). For catheter *not* in use, flush lumen with heparinized saline 1 ml (100 µ/ml) every 12 hours.	Sterile dressing change after first 24 hours, then every 72 hours. Change Luer-Lok injection caps every 72 hours.	Shut off all IVs for *one (1) full minute.* Withdraw 1.5 ml blood. Discard. Withdraw blood sample. Flush lumen with 2.5 ml N/S then heparinize or resume IV. TPN-SHUT OFF IV 10 MIN ONLY blood sample from PIC catheter 3.8 Fr (18 gauge) or larger.
TUNNELED CATHETERS *Long-Term Use (1-3 years)* Broviac Hickman Quinton Raaf (single, dual and triple lumens)	After each use, flush *each* lumen with 5 ml N/S, then heparinized saline 2 ml (100 µ/ml). For catheter *not* in use, flush *each* lumen with heparinized saline 2 to 5 ml (100 µ/ml) daily/biweekly	Daily sterile dressing change at the exit site for at least 7 days. Gauze dressing change every 24 hrs; bio-occlusive change every 72 hrs. Thereafter, cleanse exit site daily (Betadine/alcohol). Optional daily clean dressing. Change Luer-Lok injection caps *weekly.*	Shut off all IVs for *one (1) full minute.* Withdraw 5 ml blood. Discard. Withdraw blood sample. Flush lumen with 5 ml N/S, then heparinize or resume IV. TPN-SHUT OFF IV 10 MINUTES.

GROSHONG

Single lumen Dual lumen Triple lumen	Does not require heparin to maintain catheter patency. *Use force when flushing.* Flush *each* lumen with 5 ml N/S after each use, except for TPN, then flush with 30 ml N/S. For catheter *not* in use, flush with 5 ml N/S weekly.*	Daily sterile dressing change at the exit site for at least 7 days. Gauze dressing change every 24 hrs; bio-occlusive change every 72 hrs. Thereafter, cleanse exit site daily (Betadine/alcohol). Optional daily clean dressing. Change Luer-Lok injection caps *weekly.*	Shut off all IVs for *one (1) full minute.* Withdraw 5 ml blood. Discard. Withdraw blood sample. Flush lumen with 30 ml N/S *vigorously,* then resume IV or apply injection cap.* TPN-SHUT OFF IV 10 MINUTES.

IMPLANTABLE VASCULAR ACCESS DEVICES

- Davol Port - Infuse-A-Port - Life Port - Omega Port - Port-A-Cath	After each use, flush *each* port with huber needle—10 ml N/S, followed by heparinized saline (100 µ/ml).† For port *not* in use, flush each port with 3 to 10 ml heparinized saline (100 µ/ml) *every 30 days* (venous placement). Intermittent flush >1/day use N/S and/or low dose/volume heparin.‡	Sterile bio-occlusive dressing when port accessed. Steri-strips at new incision site for 3 days. When incision site healed and port not accessed, no dressing required. When port is accessed for continuous infusion, change needle and extension tubing every 5-7 days.	Shut off all IVs for *one (1) full minute.* Withdraw 5 ml blood. Discard. Withdraw blood sample. Flush with 20 ml N/S followed by 3 to 10 ml heparinized saline (100 µ/ml)* or resume IV. TPN-SHUT OFF IV 10 MINUTES.
Tunneled catheters heparinization varies process	10-1000 µ/ml concentration; frequency daily, biweekly, weekly and amount 2-5 mL		

*Selected oncologists use 2 to 5 ml heparinized saline (100 µ/ml).
†Check manufacturer's specific recommendations regarding volume. Oncologists use heparin 10 ml (100 µ/ml).
‡Assess patient, disease, platelet count with frequency/volume/concentration of heparinization schedule.
§Use 5 ml or larger syringes when flushing and/or blood sampling from PIC catheter.

Table 26–2   General Overview of Ambulatory Infusion Pumps

CHARACTERISTICS OF PORTABLE SYRINGE INFUSION PUMPS*

Pump	Cost ($)	Wt	Dimensions†	Power Source(s)	Reservoir Type and Capacity	Accuracy	Flow Rate
AutoSyringe AS2F, Baxter Healthcare	1345	19.3 oz	7.2 inches × 2.9 inches × 2.5 inches	Rechargeable nickel cadmium battery (life = 5 days)	Syringe 1-44 mL; most brands	±4%	0.02-88 mL/hr
CADD-LD, Pharmacia Deltec	2995	9 oz	4.65 inches × 2.95 inches × 0.9 inches	9-V disposable alkaline battery	Syringe 10 mL	±3%	0-2.25 mL/hr
Infusaid MS26, Graseby Medical (Infusaid)	1435	175 g	165 mm × 53 mm × 23 mm	9-V disposable alkaline battery (life = 1.5 months or 500 full syringes)	Syringe 5-35 mL; most brands	±5%	1-99 mm/24 hr

CHARACTERISTICS OF PORTABLE PERISTALTIC CONTINUOUS-INFUSION PUMPS‡

Pump	Cost ($)	Wt (oz)	Dimensions (Inches)†	Power Source(s)	Reservoir Type and Capacity	Accuracy	Flow Rate
AutoSyringe AS30C, Baxter Healthcare	1295	9.7	4.5 × 4.0 × 1.5	9-V disposable battery (life = 2 wk at 0.5 mL/hr)	Proprietary bag 80 mL; any size external bag	±10% at low rate; ±5% at ≥5 mL/hr	0.5-9.9 mL/hr
Infumed 300, MedFusion Systems	1860	12	4.4 × 4.1 × 1.8	9-V disposable alkaline battery (life = 165 hr at 5 mL/hr)	Proprietary bags, 65, 150, and 250 mL; any size external bag	±5%	0.1-9.9 mL/hr
Cormed III, Bard	1895	11	4.7 × 3.4 × 0.96	9-V alkaline battery (life = 5.7 days); 3-V lithium backup (life = 3 yr)	Proprietary reservoirs 100 and 250 mL; external bag channel	±10%	0.1-9.99 mL/hr
CADD-1, Pharmacia Deltec	2595	15	6.3 × 3.5 × 1.1	9-V disposable alkaline battery (life = 5 days)	Proprietary cassettes 50 and 100 mL; remote reservoir adapter	±10%	1-90 mL/hr

*Pumping mechanism for all pumps is lead screw action.
†Dimensions in height × width × depth.
‡Pumping mechanism is rotary peristaltic action for AutoSyringe AS30C and linear peristaltic action for other pumps.

CHARACTERISTICS OF ELASTOMERIC RESERVOIR INFUSION PUMPS

Pump	Cost ($)	Wt	Dimensions (Inches)	Reservoir Capacity (mL)	Accuracy	Flow Rate
Singleday Infusor, Baxter Healthcare	35	30 g	6.5 long × 1.5 deep	65	± 10%	2 mL/hr
Multiday Infusor, Baxter Healthcare	70	30 g	6.5 long × 1.5 deep	65	± 10%	0.5 mL/hr
Daymate, Infusion Systems Corporation (Baxter)	40	2 oz	5 long × 2.5 deep	105	± 15%	2 mL/hr

CHARACTERISTICS OF PORTABLE PATIENT-CONTROLLED ANALGESIA (PCA) PUMPS

Pump	Cost ($)	Wt (oz)	Dimensions (Inches)	Power Source(s)	Reservoir Type and Capacity	Flow Rate	Special Features
CADD PCA 5800, Pharmacia Deltec*	3495	15	1.1 deep × 3.5 wide × 6.3 high	9-V alkaline battery (life = 5 days)	Proprietary cassettes 50 and 100 mL; remote reservoir adapter	0.05-20 mL/hr	Dose volume 0-3.95 mL; lockout 5-100 min; three lock levels for programming or operation; lockable pole clamp; programmable in mass (mg) using concentration or mL
Baxter PCA Infusion System†	37c	1	6.5 long	Elastomeric pressure	Balloon 60 mL	2 or 5 mL/hr (using two different Infusor models)	Dose volume 0.5 mL; maximum lockout 6 or 15 min; dose delivered dependent on drug concentration
Baxter PCA Basal/Bolus System§	62,‡# 77‡‖	1	6.5 long	Elastomeric pressure	Balloon 60 mL	0.5 mL/hr	Dose volume 0.5 mL; maximum lockout 15 or 60 min; dose delivered dependent on drug concentration
Bard Ambulatory PCA*	3195	11	4.7 wide × 3.4 high × 0.96 deep	9-V primary (typical life = 5-7 days); 3-V lithium, memory only (life = 3 years)	Bags 100 and 250 mL; external bag channel	0-20 mL/hr continuous	Dose volume 0-9.9 mL; lockout 3-240 min; programmable in volume (mL)

* Linear peristaltic pumping mechanism; basal, bolus, or basal/bolus infusion mode.
† Elastomeric pressure pumping mechanism; bolus infusion mode.
‡ Cost of infuser and control module.
§ Elastomeric pressure pumping mechanism; basal/bolus infusion mode.
# Has 15-minute lockout.
‖ Has 60-minute lockout.

Table 26–2   General Overview of Ambulatory Infusion Pumps — cont'd
CHARACTERISTICS OF IMPLANTABLE INFUSION PUMPS

Pump	Cost ($)	Wt (g)	Dimensions (mm)*	Power Source(s)	Usable Volume (mL) Reservoir	Flow Rate
Infusaid 100† 400†	3654 4656	187 208	87 × 28 87 × 28	Two-phase charging fluid	47 47	Preset generally at 1-6 mL/day
Infusaid 1000†	Not yet marketed	272	90.2 × 22.5	Two-phase charging fluid; lithium battery (typical life = 3.5-5 yrs)	22	0.001-0.5 mL/hr
Medtronics Synchro Med 8610/8610H infusion system‡	5850 pump; 6300 programmer	175	70.4 × 27.5	Lithium battery	18	0.009-0.9 mL/hr

Adapted from Kwan JW: Am J Hosp Pharm, 47(8) (Suppl 1); 1990.
*Dimensions in diameter × depth.
†Pumping mechanism is metal bellows with charging fluid.
‡Rotary peristaltic pumping mechanism.

Hospice

Any discussion of home care for clients with cancer would not be complete without considering Hospice and the vital care provided by health care professionals within this domain of practice. The advent of consumerism and the desire for increased control over the delivery and quality of care, particularly when all other treatment options have been exhausted or judged to be ineffective, has contributed to the increased public awareness of and interest in the hospice concept. Even though the term *hospice* is familiar to most, many do not understand the type of services provided under hospice.

A common misconception by both the public and health care professionals is that hospice is a specific type of extended care facility. *It is not.* Hospice is a philosophy of care that provides high quality, comprehensive care to persons with a terminal disease and their families. The setting for this care is usually in the home, however, hospitalization is available during acute medical crisis, impending death, or to give the family a short (2 to 5 days) respite. Medical crisis may include uncontrolled pain, nausea and vomiting, or other situations that may warrant a brief hospitalization until the client's symptoms are controlled.

In the early 1980s, formal acknowledgement of hospice treatment through reimbursement by Medicare and private insurance companies came about. This official recognition has made it easier for people to die at home by providing them with some financial and professional support, by setting standards to regulate the professional care they receive, and by educating physicians, nurses and the public about the home death alternative.[26]

The goal of hospice is to enhance the quality of life for the patient who is dying and for the surviving family members. Hospice care makes it possible for dying patients to live their last days in their own homes.[25] Hospice programs enable the terminally ill to remain comfortable in their own homes by providing the necessary support services. The hospice team is truly a multidisciplinary team of professionals, consisting of physicians, nurses, social workers, spiritual care advisors, pharmacists, nutritionists, and volunteers. Often, attorneys are available to provide legal aid to clients and their families. Most hospice programs provide ongoing bereavement services to families after the death of the client. For additional information about hospice and other support resources, see the Appendix.

Private Duty

There are many home care organizations that provide supplemental home care services on a fee for service basis. These additional services, such as nursing, nursing aides, companions, and housekeepers, can supplement available caregiving resources or provide care when there is no available caregiver, thereby preventing or delaying institutionalization. Private duty home care is often not included in most health insurances as a benefit, therefore it falls upon the patient or family to pay for this service. This can be a significant financial burden, however, when one considers the alternative of institutionalization, it can be well worth the expense. Agencies that provide these services are required by law to be licensed and can be found in your local yellow pages.

If the cost of such services through an agency is prohibitive for your client and family, you may suggest that they make arrangements with a friend or neighbor for light housekeeping, meal preparation, or sitter/companion services for nominal compensation.

Reimbursement Issues

Most health care insurances cover home care services. All require that the service is ordered by a physician and a medical plan of care is signed by the physician. Patients must also be *homebound*, unable to leave home without assistance of others and assistive devices. In addition, patients must also need skilled nursing care and have a medical condition that warrants ongoing assessment and evaluation. If the patient is medically stable for more than 2 weeks, he or she is no longer considered needy of ongoing skilled nursing service unless there are specific treatments ordered such as monthly foley catheter changes, vitamin B_{12} injections, etc.

The type of home care services vary from health insurance policy to health insurance policy. In many cases, prior approval is necessary. The medical plan of care must be reviewed and updated periodically and again signed by the physician. The certification periods, the specified time frame the plan of care is valid, is usually 30 or 60 days depending upon the payor (Table 26-3).

PATIENT AND FAMILY TEACHING

Nurses play a major role in educating individuals about cancer-detection methods, lifestyle risks, and treatment options.[22] Given the importance of this role, it is imperative that the oncology nurse be proficient in patient and family education.

The trend of consumerism in addition to the complex nature of cancer and current, often aggressive, treatment modalities necessitate improved, comprehensive patient and family education. "The goal of patient education is more than information giving; the intent is to provide individuals and their families support, with control, and knowledge to empower them to manage self-care deficits more effectively."[10] It has

Table 26–3 Payor Source Guidelines

Medical Insurance	Medicare	Medicaid	Blue Cross	HMO (HAP, GHP)	Commercial (Aetna, Prudential, etc.)
Prior authorization	No	No (restrictions vary state to state)	No (only Blue Care Network & FEP)	Yes	Varies
Medical plan of treatment signed by physician	Yes	Yes	Yes	Yes	Yes
Disciplines: Primary (may open case)	Nursing Physical therapy Speech therapy	Varies state to state: usual services: Nursing Physical therapy Speech therapy	Nursing P.T. O.T. S.T. MSS HHA	Varies with prior approval	Varies with benefit plan
Covered with primary discipline	MSS HHA O.T.	HHA	Nutrition (if agency certified for this service) ACCORDING TO BENEFIT PLAN		
Certification period	2 months 60-62 days	2 months 60-62 days (recent, must be done at 30 days)	30 days	60 days	60 days

Specifics related to illness
Specifics related to treatment and effects
Exercise/activity and rest
Safety
Financial issues
Insurance issues
Social interactions
Emotional concerns
Support groups/resources
Family concerns
Rehabilitation
Adaptive techniques
Returning to work
Long-term planning
Others: _____

_____

_____

_____

Figure 26-3 Sample topics for patients and families. (From Hileman JW: Identifying the needs of home care givers of patients with cancer, Oncol Nurs Forum 19(5):771, 1992)

1. Information about the underlying reasons for symptoms
2. Information about what symptoms to expect
3. Information about what to expect in the future
4. Information about treatment of side effects
5. Information about community resources
6. Honest and updated information
7. Ways to reassure my patient
8. Ways to deal with my patient's decreased energy
9. Ways to deal with the unpredictability of the future
10. Information about medications (side effects and scheduling)
11. Ways to encourage my patient
12. Information about my patient's psychological needs
13. Methods to decrease my stress
14. Ways of coping with my patient's diagnosis of cancer
15. Information about the type and extent of my patient's illness
16. Ways to cope with role changes
17. Information about the physical needs of my patient
18. Activities that will make my patient feel purposeful
19. Ways to be more patient and tolerant
20. Ways to deal with my depression
21. Ways to maintain a normal family life
22. Ways to discuss death with my patient
23. Ways to deal with my fears
24. Ways to combat fatigue
25. Ways to provide my patient with adequate nutrition

Figure 26-4 Top 25 Unmet needs of home caregivers. (From Hileman JW: Identifying the needs of home care givers of patients with cancer, Oncol Nurs Forum 19(5):775, 1992)

been well documented that patients and families with increased knowledge of their illness and treatment plan experience significantly less anxiety and stress.[24] Researchers have also noted that different patients have individual learning and informational needs. It is important that the oncology nurse consider individual differences when beginning patient or family teaching. As in the nursing process, a thorough assessment must take place. Determining what the patient or family member already knows is imperative to avoid boredom and "tuning out." Simply asking the individual if he or she is interested in obtaining additional information is a good first step. It is important to keep in mind that often the individual may not know what specific learning opportunities are available. It is helpful to have a list from which the individual may select appropriate topics (Figure 26-3). Hileman and colleagues[8] researched and identified the unmet needs of home caregivers of patients with cancer (Figure 26-4) and concluded that

most caregiver's unmet needs were psychological and informational. Oncology nurses in acute, community, clinic and outpatient settings appear to need to place an increased emphasis on the psychosocial and informational needs of family home caregivers. Because of shorter hospitalizations, nurses must begin this educational process early and continue the availability of counselling, especially on psychological and informational needs, after discharge. This could be done directly or by linking families to volunteer and professional community agencies with appropriate services.[8]

Mathis[18] in a study of educational wants of family caregivers determined that adults perceive that they need information about how to deal with real-life situations, and if given such information they will be motivated to learn. If such educational opportunities are not afforded, caregivers might reject the caregiving role.[18]

The oncology nurse must also assess for the appropriate instructional method for the individual. Literacy is a problem in the United States today with more than 20% of the general population functionally illiterate.[3] Illiteracy is more endemic among the elderly and the poor. Keeping this in mind, the oncology nurse should determine the reading capabilities of the client. This is not easily done. Many adults are embarrassed about the inability to read and over the years have become very skillful in covering up this deficit. Excuses such as "I don't have my glasses with me now. Can you read it to me?" or "I'll read it later" may serve as cues on which the nurse should follow-up. Other indicators identified by Meade and co-workers[22] include lack of interest in the material, expressions of frustration, lack of reading speed, and inability to answer questions about the content of the text. In addition to these informal methods of assessing reading ability the Wide-Range Achievement Test (WRAT) II developed by Janstak and Wilkinson is a helpful tool.[11] To assess the readability of written material or when developing your own written material, the Cloze procedure developed by Taylor may be utilized to make certain that the material is not written at too high a level.[31] Other readability formulas such as the Flesch Formula and the Forcast may also be utilized.[22]

Educational reading material is usually written at a sixth to eighth grade reading level. But even this may be too high! Glaser-Waldman, Hall, and Weiner[7] determined that 60% of their research sample of 101 hospital inpatients and outpatients could not read and understand material written at a sixth grade level.[7]

Meade and colleagues conducted an analysis of the readability of American Cancer Society (ACS) Patient Education Literature in 1991 and determined that ACS publications written prior to 1985 had a mean reading level of grade 12.7 while those written during and after 1985 had a mean reading level of grade 10.9. Of the 51 booklets analyzed in this study only six booklets were written at an 8.9 grade level or below, while 45 were written at ninth grade level or above.[22] In view of these results, it is important that the oncology nurse be cognizant of the importance of a multifaceted, creative approach to patient and family education. The findings of Meade and co-workers by no means negates the value of the written material available currently from ACS as well as other institutions. It is imperative that the oncology nurse be aware of the limitations of these materials, individualizing the teaching plan to meet the unique needs of each client. Utilize *all* available educational resources and modalities such as audiovisual, pictorial, didactic, as well as written material. These can only enhance and facilitate the learning process. It has been well documented that the use of multiple instructive modalities greatly improves the amount of learning that takes place. So, it is advisable to use a variety of teaching techniques. An extensive list of written educational materials is available in the Appendix.

Hiromoto and Dungan[10] recommend a contract learning protocol to provide a systematic and comprehensive approach to the individual's learning needs. The researchers have found that contract learning has had good results when utilized with adult learners as it includes concepts of independent, individualized, and self-directed learning.

Hiromoto and Dungan developed a useful learning needs assessment tool designed specifically for chemotherapy learning needs (Figure 26-5) and a form documenting the instructional material provided based upon the assessment (Figure 26-6). Ths example can assist development of an appropriate tool for one's own particular practice setting.[10]

The education process, like the nursing process, includes the steps of assessing, planning, implementing, and evaluating. The primary learner(s) in the family must be identified and his or her learning needs assessed. Following this assessment, a mutually acceptable plan to meet the identified educa-

Name _____ Date _____ Age _____

Diagnosis _____ Sex [   ] F [   ] M

Highest level of education [   ] Elementary

[   ] Intermediate   [   ] High School   [   ] College/University

[   ] Other _____

Patient's interest in learning is:

1	2	3	4
Total disinterest or defers to significant other	Minimal information desired	Moderate information desired	Desires all there is to know

Preferred learning method: [   ] Books [   ] Pictorial

[   ] Audiovisual   [   ] Other _____

Any reading or visual problems? [   ] no   [   ] yes _____

Any neurosensory impairments? [   ] no   [   ] yes _____

Questions related to:

Universal self-care requisites
[   ] Nutrition   [   ] Safety
[   ] Elimination   [   ] Financial
[   ] Activity & Rest   [   ] Social Interactions

[   ] Others _____

Developmental self-care requisites
[   ] Emotional Concerns   [   ] Family Concerns

[   ] Support Groups/Resources   [   ] Others _____

Health deviation self-care requisites
[   ] Illness   [   ] Treatment and Effects

[   ] Others _____

Are there any other questions? _____

I hereby acknowledge the above information to be an assessment of my current learning needs. I understand I am encouraged to participate in my health care utilizing self-care measures. I will have opportunities during my outpatient visits to seek further knowledge as questions or problems develop.

Client's signature _____ Date _____

Figure 26–5 Learning needs assessment tool. (From Hiromoto BM: Contract learning for self care activities, Cancer Nursing 14(3):148, 1991.)

Learning Interest #1

Chemotherapy: A Guide for patients with cancer (Adria pamphlet) (given to significant other)

Taking time (NIH booklet) (given to significant other)

Living with cancer (American Cancer Society—support group)

Other resources: _____

_____

Learning Interest #2

We care (American Cancer Society brochure)

Chemotherapy: A guide for patients with cancer (Adria pamphlet)

Living with cancer (American Cancer Society—support group)

Other resources: _____

_____

Learning Interest #3

Chemotherapy & you: A guide to self-help during treatment (NIH booklet)

Taking time (NIH booklet)

Nausea/vomiting (hospital's handout)

Symptom alert sheet for chemotherapy (hospital's handout)

Living with cancer (American Cancer Society—support group)

Chemotherapy slide show (OPTIONAL)   OR

Chemotherapy & you (Adria Laboratories picture book) (OPTIONAL)

Other resources: _____

_____

Learning Interest #4

Chemotherapy & you: A guide to self-help during treatment (NIH booklet)

Taking time (NIH booklet)

Nausea/vomiting (hospital's handout)

Symptom alert sheet for chemotherapy (hospital's handout)

Cancer terms: A guide for patients with cancer (Adria pamphlet)

Eating hints: Recipes and tips for better nutrition during cancer treatment

Living with cancer (American Cancer Society—support group)

Chemotherapy slide show (OPTIONAL)   OR

Chemotherapy & you—(Adria Laboratories picture book) (OPTIONAL)

Other resources: _____

_____

_____

Figure 26-6 Teaching material provided according to level of learning interests. (From Hiromoto BM: Contract learning for self care activities, Cancer Nursing 14(3):148, 1991)

tional needs is developed by nurse/teacher and client/learner. Appropriate teaching strategies are used to implement the plan, and it is mutually evaluated with the evaluation serving as a basis for further decision.[27] Addressing the educational wants and needs of the family caregiver is of top priority if the patient is to receive proper care and be able to remain in the comforts of his home.[19]

DISCHARGE INSTRUCTIONS

To help facilitate the transition to the home setting and ensure continuity of care and medical follow-up,

it is very important to clearly convey specific discharge instructions to the patient and/or family members at the time of discharge. Understandably, the time of discharge is particularly hectic and often instructions given at this time may not be remembered accurately or at all. Consequently it is advisable to have specific written instructions to review with and give the patient and family at the time of discharge.

Accessing the Health Care System

Many institutions have discharge instruction sheets that are completed by the nurse and include instructions regarding follow-up appointments and medications. But this is not enough. Patients and their families need to know how to access the health care system after discharge. They need to know the answers to such questions as:

Who should I call when questions arise that can't wait until the next appointment?

What should I expect?

When do I worry?

When should I call?

How can I reach these professionals?

What about after hours? Who is the contact person then?

As you can see, the list of questions can be endless. However they can be anticipated by the experienced professional. An individualized discharge instruction sheet (Figure 26-7) can be very helpful in reducing stress and anxiety.

In addition, the experienced oncology nurse, in either the inpatient or outpatient setting can anticipate any potential problems that may arise as a result of treatment or disease progression. In this case, it is appropriate for the nurse to provide the patient or responsible caregiver with information regarding anticipated problems (e.g., stomatitis associated with chemotherapy) and measures to manage these problems. If your institution does not have patient instruction sheets/pamphlets about common side effects or problems, there is a considerable amount of literature, for both professionals and patients, available from the American Cancer Society, The U.S. Department of Health and Human Services, and other organizations. Often, pharmaceutical companies provide informational pamphlets for patients as well as professionals (see Appendix).

Again, it is important to consider the client's reading ability and assess the readability of the written material you provide to the client. If the reading skills of the client or family member are limited, it may be more appropriate and indeed more effective for you to write out very simple instructions or information specifically tailored for the individual. Alternative teaching modalities such as audio or video tapes may also be effective teaching tools to augment any teach-

NAME: _____

MEDICATIONS: _____

        (name, dose, route, frequency, and common
        side effects)
_____
_____

TREATMENTS: _____

        (specify tx, procedure, frequency)
        or refer to attached handout of hospital
        treatment protocol
_____

WHEN TO CALL NURSE/DOCTOR:
IF TEMPERATURE IS 100° OR HIGHER
IF YOU HAVE PAIN THAT WON'T GO AWAY
IF YOU CAN'T KEEP FOOD OR LIQUIDS DOWN FOR 24 HOURS
    OR MORE
IF YOU HAVE NO BOWEL MOVEMENT FOR 3 OR MORE DAYS
IF YOU HAVE DIARRHEA FOR 24 HOURS OR MORE
IF YOU HAVE URINARY DIFFICULTIES
    PAIN OR BURNING
    BLEEDING
OTHER: _____
_____
_____

IMPORTANT PHONE NUMBERS:
DR. _____   _____ (phone)
NURSES' STATION   _____ (phone)
DISCHARGE PLANNER   _____ (phone)
HOME CARE AGENCY   _____ (name)

    _____ (contact person)   _____ (phone)
DURABLE MEDICAL EQUIP. SUPPLIER _____ (name)

    _____ (contact person)   _____ (phone)
    Items to be delivered: w/c, commode, cane, walker, shower
    chair, hospital bed,_____ (other) on ____ (date)

    _____ (please list)

YOUR NEXT APPOINTMENT WITH _____
IS ON _____ AT _____ AM/PM AT
THE ONCOLOGY OUT PATIENT CLINIC (include specific location).
    PLEASE CALL (clinic phone #) IF YOU ARE UNABLE TO KEEP
    THIS APPOINTMENT TO RESCHEDULE.

Figure 26–7 Discharge instruction. (From Slevin JB and Roberts AS: Discharge planning: a tool for decision making, Nursing Management 18(12):47, 1987)

ing plan (see Appendix for resources). You may even consider making your own audio tape for your patient, giving step by step instructions that your client and family would be able to follow more easily.

Follow-up Appointments

Central to an effective treatment of any cancer is consistent medical follow-up. Ongoing assessment and evaluation and subsequent modification of the treatment plan is critical as the trend for more aggressive posthospital treatment continues. Follow-up appointments are very important, yet, often difficult endeavors for patients and their families. There are several things that the nurse can do to help facilitate keeping follow-up appointments.

First and foremost is the almost universal concern about transportation. Often, patients do not have any transportation resources available to them. Frequently, this issue is not addressed at the time that the patient is given the follow-up appointment. It is important to ask the patient or family member if transportation is a problem. If so, they may be referred to local agencies that provide such services. The American Cancer Society and the American Red Cross are national organizations that have local offices that provide transportation to and from medical facilities at no charge or minimal cost. Many private companies provide transportation services for the disabled for a fee.

In addition to information about transportation resources, patients need to know what assistance is available when they arrive for their follow-up appointment. If a wheelchair is needed, how do they arrange to have one available? Most hospitals and clinics have wheelchairs available for such purposes. It is wise to check this out before the appointment. If a wheelchair is not available, the patient should be advised to arrange to bring his own.

At busy oncology clinics, follow-up appointments can become an all-day endeavor. Patients frequently are scheduled for blood work prior to their appointment with the physician and afterwards they may receive chemotherapy or be scheduled for other tests. It is wise to advise patients and their families to bring with them the medications that they may need to take while still at the clinic. In particular, be sure to tell patients to bring any p.r.n. medications, especially pain medications, with them also.

Tell patients and their families what to expect at the follow-up appointment, especially if the patient is going to receive a treatment or particular diagnostic test for the first time. Knowing what to expect greatly reduces fears and anxieties associated with the unknown.

In many health care settings, there is very little interaction between the various departments that provide cancer treatment. This often results in a breakdown in continuity of care as well as greatly diminishes interdepartmental, interdisciplinary collaboration, and collegiality.

Some institutions make interdepartmental experiences available as part of the orientation process. Such opportunities have direct benefits for both the patient and the health care professional. Drummand and Hagenstad[5] developed a program to provide inpatient oncology nursing staff with the opportunity to spend one half or full day in a full service oncology office. The authors found that this not only improved morale but also "improved communication between the oncology unit nurses and the oncology office staff and physicians."[5] In addition, this program fostered greater cohesiveness and collaboration between members of the oncology team.[5]

An added benefit of this program was the increased awareness of the outpatient diagnostic procedures, the prehospital admission process, and postdischarge care,[5] all of which is important information that the nurse can, in turn, share with his or her patient.[5]

Follow-up Phone Call

A follow-up phone call to patients and/or their families should be made within 24 to 48 hours after discharge. It is helpful to have a copy of the continuing patient care form and/or discharge instruction sheets to enable you to ask appropriate questions to facilitate obtaining accurate information about the patient's status. A helpful starting point is to ask the patient or family the following questions:

1. How are things going since you came home?
2. Have any problems occurred?
3. Do you have any questions that I can answer for you?

These questions can get things started, however, the nurse must ask specific questions related to the patient's illness and treatment plan to ensure accurate assessment of home situation. If during the conversation, it becomes apparent that things are not going well in the home, you may recommend that the patient be brought in to see the doctor.

Often, home care needs are not easily identified prior to discharge but once the patient is at home this need becomes apparent. If a home care referral has not been made, you may determine that, at this time, a referral is warranted and initiate this process.

Durable Medical and Adaptive Equipment

Durable medical equipment (DME) includes hospital beds, wheelchairs, and much more. There are many assistive devices currently available to patients and their families that can simplify home care management and also promote home safety. Essential equipment such as hospital beds, wheelchairs, and bedside commodes should be in the home at the time of discharge, however, some equipment and adaptive devices should not be ordered until a home evaluation can be done. While an experienced nurse can assess and evaluate home equipment needs, it is advisable that a physical or occupational therapist be consulted. These therapists have an extensive knowledge of available equipment and may be able to more effectively meet the patient's equipment needs.

Most insurances provide coverage for some DME; however, a physician's order is usually required. Some insurance companies require prior approval before the equipment can be delivered to the patient. DME companies can help with this process. See Table 26-3 for a general overview of insurance coverage and the Appendix for national durable medical and adaptive equipment resources. Also, DME companies in your community can be found in your local yellow pages.

COMMUNITY RESOURCES

There are many national and local community resources available to cancer patients and their families. The types of resources available range from personal services, informational services, social services, and support services. A phone call to the Cancer Information Service (1-800-4-CANCER) and the local American Cancer Society chapter is a good starting point when first attempting to identify resources available in your community.

Local community services often include agencies that provide and/or assist with:

1. Chore or housekeeping services
2. Adult day care
3. Socialization services (e.g., Friendly Visitor, In-Home Companion)
4. Nutritional services (e.g., Meals-on-Wheels, Nutrition sites, food supplements)
5. Financial savings and grant program
6. Transportation services

A list of national organizations that provide assistance to cancer patients and their families is included in the Appendix. These organizations will help you identify local community support services.

CONCLUSION

People with cancer move through a number of health care settings during the course of their illnesses. Inherent within this movement are encounters with many health care professionals. A successful transition through these settings is dependent upon the collaborative efforts of the health care providers. Ongoing communication is the key to the effectiveness of these efforts.[15]

In addition to collaboration, a thorough assessment and evaluation of the unique and specific care requirements of the patient must be performed in order to identify the appropriate community support services to facilitate the transition along the continuum. It is a challenge to meet the increasingly complex, multidimensional needs of patients with cancer and their families. We must be prepared and knowledgeable to successfully meet these needs.

Nursing Management

As previously discussed there are many essential steps necessary to facilitate transition to the home setting and ensure continuity of care. Assessment with planned interventions and an evaluation of the outcomes will enhance a smooth transition for the patient and family members. Following is an example of a nursing diagnosis: Impaired Home Maintenance Management with multiple assessment and intervention strategies that can be adapted to meet the varied individual client needs.

NURSING DIAGNOSIS

Impaired Home Maintenance Management related to: (specify)

- Inability to perform household activities secondary to side effects of chemotherapy
- Inability to perform household activities secondary to disease progression.

INTERVENTIONS

The following interventions apply to many individuals with impaired home management, regardless of etiology.

A. Assess for causative or contributing factors
  1. Lack of knowledge
  2. Insufficient funds
  3. Lack of necessary equipment or aids
  4. Inability to perform household activities (illness, sensory deficits, motor deficits)
  5. Impaired cognitive functioning
  6. Impaired emotional functioning
B. Reduce or eliminate causative or contributing factors if possible
  1. Lack of knowledge for home care
    a. Determine with the patient and family the information needed to be taught and learned.
      • Monitoring skills needed (pulse, circulation, urine)
      • Medication administration (procedure, side-effects, precautions)
      • Treatment procedures
      • Equipment use/maintenance
      • Safety issues (e.g., environmental)
      • Community resources
      • Follow-up care
      • Anticipatory guidance (e.g., emotional and social needs of family, alternatives to home care)
    b. Initiate the teaching and give detailed written instruction.
    c. Refer to a community nursing (home care) agency for follow-up.

2. Lack of necessary equipment or aids
  a. Determine the type of equipment needed, considering availability, cost, and durability.
  b. Seek assistance from agencies that rent or loan supplies.
    • Teach the care and maintenance of supplies that increase length of use.
    • Consider adapting equipment to reduce cost.
3. Insufficient funds
  a. Consult with social service department for assistance.
  b. Consult with service organizations for assistance
    • American Heart Association
    • The Lung Association
    • American Cancer Society
4. Inability to perform household activities
  a. Determine the type of assistance needed (e.g., meals, housework, transportation) and assist the individual to obtain them.
    • Meals
      Discuss with relatives the possibility of freezing complete meals that require only heating (e.g., small containers of soup, stew, casseroles).
      Determine the availability of meal services for ill persons (Meals on Wheels, church groups).
      Teach persons about foods that are easily prepared and nutritious (e.g., hardboiled eggs).
    • Housework
      Contract with an adolescent for light housekeeping.
      Refer to community agency for assistance.
    • Transportation
      Determine the availability of transportation for shopping and health care.
      Request rides with neighbors to places they drive routinely.
5. Impaired mental processes
  a. Assess the ability of the individual to safely maintain a household.
  b. Initiate appropriate referrals
6. Impaired emotional functioning
  a. Assess the severity of the dysfunction
  b. Initiate appropriate referrals.

C. Provide anticipatory guidance
   1. Discuss the implications of caring for a chronically ill family member.
      a. Amount of time involved
      b. Effects on other role responsibilities (spouse, children, job)
      c. Physical requirements (lifting)
   2. Share alternatives to reduce strain and fatigue of caretaking responsibilities.
      a. Acquire relief from responsibilities at least twice a week for at least 3 hours (sitter, neighbors, relatives)
      b. Enlist the aid of others to meet some of the needs of the ill person (hairdresser, transporting to physician's office)
      c. Plan to utilize at least 1 hour a day as leisure time (after ill person is asleep).

      d. Maintain contacts with friends and relatives even if only by phone; let friends know that you do use sitters so they can include you in some social activities.
      e. Allow the caretaker opportunities to share problems and feelings.
   3. Commend caregivers for their concern, diligence, and perseverance in caring for the loved one at home.
D. Initiate health teaching and referrals as indicated
   1. Refer to support groups (American Cancer Society, Encore, Y-Me).
   2. Refer to community nursing agency
   3. Refer to community agencies (volunteer visitors, meal programs, homemakers, adult day care)

BIBLIOGRAPHY

1. Aitken MJ: Matching models to environments: a planning guide to the selection of pediatric home care models, Home Health Care Nurse 7(2):13, 1989.
2. Cohen MH and Pinnick NP: Home care of children. In Martinson IM and Widmer A, editors: Home health care nursing, Philadelphia, 1989, WB Saunders Co.
3. Dixon E and Park R: Do patients understand written health information? Nursing Outlook 38(6):278, 1990.
4. Dolan MB: Community and home health care plans. Springhouse, PA: Springhouse, 1990.
5. Drummand PA and Hagenstad RR: Oncology outpatient experience: a unique approach to staff development, Nursing Management 18(9):88, 1987.
6. Feuer LC. Discharge planning: home caregivers need your support, too. Nursing Management 18(4):58, 1987.
7. Glazer-Waldman H, Hall K, and Weiner MF: Patient education in a public hospital, Nurs Research 34:184, 1985.
8. Hileman JW, Lackey NR, and Hassanein RS: Identifying the needs of home caregivers of patients with cancer, Oncol Nurs Forum 19(5):771, 1992.
9. Hinds C: The needs of families who care for patients at home: are we meeting them? Adv Nurs Pract 10:575, 1985.
10. Hiromoto BM and Dungan J: Contract learning for self-care activities, Cancer Nurs 14(3):148, 1991.
11. Jastak S and Wilkinson GS: Wide-range achievement test: revised administration manual, Washington, DC: Janstak Associates.

12. Johnston J and Clark B: Orientation to home care: maximizing Medicare reimbursement, Home Health Care Nurse 8:45, 1990.
13. Kelly K and McClelland E: Discharge planning: home care considerations. In Martinson IM and Widmer A, editors: Home health care nursing, Philadelphia, 1989, WB Saunders Co.
14. Leiby SA and Shupe DR: Does home care lessen hospital readmissions for the elderly? Home Health Care Nurse 10(1):37, 1992.
15. Lokich J: The delivery of cancer chemotherapy by continuous venous infusion, Cancer 50:2731, 1982.
16. Magilvy JK and Lakomy JM: Transitions of older adults to home care, Home Health Care Serv Quart 12(4):59, 1991.
17. Maloney CH and Preston F: An overview of home care for patients with cancer, Oncol Nurs Forum 19(1):75, 1992.
18. Mathis EJ: Top 20 educational wants of current family caregivers of disabled adults, Home Health Care Nurse 9(3):23, 1992.
19. Mathis EJ: Family caregivers want education for their caregiving roles, Home Health Care Nurse, 10(4):19, 1992.
20. McAbee RR, Grupp K, and Horn B: Home intravenous therapy: part I—issues. Home Health Care Serv Quart 12(3):59, 1991.
21. McAnear S: Parental reaction to a chronically ill child, Home Health Care Nurse 8(3):35, 1990.
22. Meade CD, Diekmann J, and Thornhill DG: Readability of American Cancer Society patient education literature, Oncol Nurs Forum 19(1):51, 1992.
23. Mehrotra CMN and Kosloski K: Foster care for

older adults: issues and evaluations, Home Health Care Serv Quart 12(1):115, 1991.

24. Perry G and Rhoades de Meneses M: Cancer patients at home: needs and coping styles of primary caregivers, Home Health Care Nurse 7(6):27, 1989.

25. Phillips K: Pediatric hospice: home care for the terminally ill child, J Home Health Care Pract 1(3):37, 1989.

26. Sankar A: Dying at Home: a family guide for caregiving, Baltimore: The Johns Hopkins University Press, 1992.

27. Shannon M: Skills in family teaching. In Martinson IM and Widmer A, editors: Home health care nursing, Philadelphia, WB Saunders Co.

28. Sherry D: Cost effectiveness and home care: myth or reality? Home Health Care Nurse 10(1):27, 1992.

29. Slevin AP and Roberts AS: Discharge planning: a tool for decision making, Nurs Manage 18(12):47, 1987.

30. Smith JB: Competition and continuity of care in home health nursing, Home Health Care Nurse 9(1):9, 1992.

31. Taylor WI: Cloze procedure: a new tool for measuring readability, Read J Quart 30:415, 1953.

APPENDIX
Cancer Resources

NATIONAL RESOURCES

About Face
Suite 1405
123 Elm Street
Toronto, Ontario Canada M5G-1E2
1-416-593-1448

A support organization for patients who are facially disfigured, their families and friends. Membership is $10.00 annually and benefits include a variety of publications, a video library, a reference library, and linkage through a computer network

Airport Owners and Pilots Association
Medical Department
412 Aviation Way
Frederick, MD 21701-4798
1-301-695-2139

This organization maintains a directory of medical transportation firms in the U.S. Contact the Airport Owners and Pilots Association to get a free copy of the directory.

American Cancer Society
1599 Clifton Road, N.E.
Atlanta, GA 30329
1-404-320-3333 (General Information)
1-404-329-7616 (Department of Nursing)
1-800-ACS-2345 (For Cancer Information)

Local facilities are listed in the telephone directory. The American Cancer Society provides a wide range of services encompassing the following:

- Information to the public on all sites of cancer, community resources, and rehabilitation programs
- Home care items for use by patients
- Transportation to assist cancer patients in getting to and from medical appointments
- Patient and family education programs to provide a better understanding of the disease and its management.
- Cancer Nursing News—a newsletter is mailed to nurses free upon request.

The following programs are offered by the American Cancer Society:

- *CanSurmount:* A short-term visitor program for patients with many types of cancer and families of patients. The one-to-one visit by a person who has experienced the same type of cancer offers functional, emotional, and social support.
- *I Can Cope:* A structured educational program that provides information and supportive materials to persons with cancer and their families.
- *International Association of Laryngectomees:* A program that provides information and supportive materials to laryngectomy patients. Laryngectomy visitors provide preoperative and postoperative support to patients who have recently undergone laryngectomy surgery.
- *Look Good, Feel Better:* A joint venture of American Cancer Society and the Cosmetic, Toiletry and Fragrance Association assists those recovering from cancer with the improvement of their quality of life through personal appearance and body image
- *Reach to Recovery:* A program that provides emotional support and practical information to women with breast cancer, especially those who have had a mastectomy. Postoperative visits are provided by women who have had a mastectomy, and literature and a temporary prosthesis are provided.
- *Ostomy Rehabilitation program*
- *Cancer Prevention and Early Detection programs* for the public.
- Resource, Information and Guidance for the general public and health care professionals

American Liver Foundation
1425 Tompton Avenue
Cedar Grove, NJ 07009
1-800-223-0179

The American Liver Foundation is a nonprofit organization that distributes educational materials, assists with transplant availability information, offers grants for research and, on the local level, conducts support groups and other activities.

American Lung Association
1740 Broadway
New York, NY 10019
1-212-315-8700

The American Lung Association is a nonprofit organization dedicated to eliminating lung disease and promoting lung health. The Association conducts programs to inform the public of air conservation, occupational health, smoking and health hazards, lung disease, and community health. It also provides professional educational programs, publications, films, fellowships, and research grants.

American Red Cross
P.O. Box 37243
Washington, D.C. 20013
1-202-639-3250

This nonprofit organization provides a wide range of support services to the community. Contact the American Red Cross branch in your area for specific information.

Appearance Concepts Consulting Group
Appearance Concepts Foundation
12543 Totem Lake, Suite 142
Kirkland, WA 98033
1-800-227-7730

The Appearance Concepts Consulting Group specializes in needs of women with cancer by providing professional beauty consultation and information about hair alternatives, makeup, skin care, and clothing. This organization offers training seminars for health care professionals, beauty and fashion professionals, and people with cancer or other cosmetic disabilities. The Appearance Concepts Foundation provides direct assistance to women who have limited financial resources utilizing goods and services that have been donated by product manufacturers and professionals and cosmetologists. The founder of this organization has written a book, *Beauty and Cancer,* and conducts a series of seminars and workshops on the topic.

Association for Applied Psychophysiology and Biofeedback
BF Training and Treatment Center
Suite 158, Southdale Medical Building
6545 France Avenue South
Edina, MN 55435
1-612-920-5700

This organization provides information on biofeedback as technique to help patients cope with pain. For more information and/or a referral to a trained specialist in your area write to AAPB, 10200 W. 44th Avenue, Suite 304, Wheatridge, CO 80033; include a stamped, self-addressed envelope

Association for the Care of Children's Health
3415 Wisconsin Avenue NW
Washington, DC 20016
1-202-244-1801

This is an international organization for healthcare professionals and parents coping with children living with illnesses which distributes booklets including *Chronic Illness and Handicapped Conditions* and *Preparing Your Child for Repeated Hospitalization,* as well as other resource materials.

Association for Research of Childhood Cancer
P.O. Box 251
Buffalo, NY 14225-0251
1-716-689-8922

This organization is made-up of parents who have lost children to cancer and people who support cancer research. This organization funds expansion and continuation of research in pediatric centers and provides money for pilot programs in cancer research. This group meets six times a year to support parents of children with cancer and also publishes a newsletter quarterly as well as the Parent/Child Handbook.

Better Together Club
c/o ConvaTec
P.O. Box 4291
Syosset, NY 11791-9706
1-800-422-8811

This is a nationwide club for ostomates created and funded by ConvaTec, an ostomy supply company. This club provides members with benefits including discounts on food, travel, entertainment, and a quarterly newsletter containing information on the latest medical and product news, travel hints, athletic tips, contests, and personal accounts of the emotional and practical aspects of living with an ostomy.

Cancer Care, Inc.
1180 Avenue of the Americas
New York, NY 10036
1-212-221-3300

A nonprofit social service agency founded to help cancer patients and their families cope with the impact of cancer. Psychological and financial support is provided. Counseling is available on both a group and individual basis.

Cancer Information Service
1-800-4-CANCER

The Cancer Information Service is available to answer questions by telephone from the general public, patients and their families, and health professionals. Printed materials on many topics related to cancer are available to callers without charge.

Candlelighters Childhood Cancer Foundation
1901 Pennsylvania Avenue, N.W.
Suite 1001
Washington, DC 20006
1-202-659-5136

A national organization of parents and families whose children have or have had cancer. Services include self-help and support groups, literature information, and referral to local and regional resources. (Many local chapters exist, and services may vary by locality.

Concern for Dying
250 W. 57th Street
New York, NY 10107
1-212-246-6962

A nonprofit educational organization that provides information regarding the living will, durable power of attorney, death and dying, and euthanasia. Psychological and legal counseling regarding terminal-care decision making are provided.

Encore
National Board, YWCA
726 Broadway
New York, NY 10003
1-212-614-2700

Encore is the national YWCA discussion and exercise program for women who have had breast cancer surgery. The program consists of floor and pool exercises and group discussion sessions that provide opportunities for sharing common concerns.

Ever Forward Foundation, Inc.
1101 S.W. Washington
Suite 101
Portland, OR 97205-9694
1-800-869-2995
1-503-224-9207 (fax)

Children that have cancer are eligible to become members of the Kangaroo Klub and will receive a membership packet containing various items (e.g., T-shirt, pen, etc.). Membership also includes the *One Year Program*, which includes a full year of age-appropriate communication and encouragement for the child (e.g., newsletters, cards, etc.) as well as gifts of encouragement, especially on holidays, birthdays, and other special occasions. The Kangaroo is chosen as the organization's mascot as Kangaroos cannot move backward, *only ever forward*.

Federation for Children with Special Needs
95 Berkley Street
Boston, MA 02116
1-800-331-0688 (voice or telecommunications device for the deaf)
1-617-482-2915

This organization is the headquarters of the "National Parent Resource Center Project" with regional offices throughout the United States. The Project works to assist and ensure collaboration between healthcare professionals and parents. Health and education counseling is available as well as a free newsletter.

International Association of Cancer Victors and Friends, Inc.
7740 W. Manchester Avenue, No. 110
Playa Del Rey, CA 90293
1-213-822-5032

This organization supports independent research for cancer treatments, disseminates information on chemotherapies, and provides education on nutrition and cancer as well as on carcinogens in air, food, and water. A quarterly publication, *Cancer Victors Journal*, is available through this organization as well as books, pamphlets, reprints of speeches, tapes, and referral lists.

Johanna's On Call to Mend Esteem
Cancer Rehabilitation Nurse Consultants
199 New Scotland Ave
Albany, NY 12208
1-518-482-4178

This non-profit cancer rehabilitation nursing service provides a wide range of preventative, restorative, supportive, and palliative nursing interventions for individuals with cancer. Educational services for the general public are available. This organization also publishes audiovisual and written material for public and professional education.

Leukemia Society of America
733 Third Avenue
New York, NY 10017
1-212-573-8484

A national and local organization for support of patients and families with leukemia and related disorders. Services include financial counseling, assistance with payment for outpatient drugs, laboratory costs, transportation, radiation therapy, and patient/family support groups.

Make A Wish Foundation of America
2600 North Central Avenue
Suite 936
Phoenix, AZ 85004
1-602-722-9474

This foundation is a non-profit organization that strives to fulfill the favorite wish of a child with a life-threatening or terminal illness. The organization will consider the wish of any child under the age of 18 anywhere in the world and covers all expenses related to granting that wish.

Make Today Count
101½ South Union Street
Alexandra, VA 22314-3323
1-703-548-9674

An international organization for persons with cancer or other life-threatening illnesses. Support groups and educational programs are provided. Brochures and handouts are available.

Medical Insurance Claims, Inc.
Kinnelon Professional Complex
170 Kennelon Road, Suite 10
Kinnelon, NJ 07405

This organization was established in response to the perceived need by the public for assistance in handling insurance claims. These services can be used by senior citizens, family members too involved with the illness of a loved one to deal with paper work. This organization has a full range of services for a fee, which includes filing claims and pursuing any missing information from health care providers to complete a claim.

National Association of Meal Programs
204 E. Street, N.E.
Washington, D.C. 20002
1-202-547-6157

This organization will provide referrals to the public regarding the nearest available meal preparation and delivery service in your area.

National Brain Tumor Foundation
323 Geary Street, Suite 510
San Francisco, CA 94102
1-415-296-0404

This organization supports research into causes and

treatments of brain tumors and offers information and support group referrals for patients and their families. An informational publication for brain tumor patients, *The Resource Guide*, and a newsletter, *Search*, are available through the foundation. A telephone consultation with a brain tumor survivor, nurse, or family member of a brain tumor patient can be arranged by calling this organization.

National Coalition for Cancer Survivorship
323 Eighth Street, S.W.
Albuquerque, NM 87102
1-505-764-9956

A network of independent organizations and individuals working in the area of cancer support and survivorship. The primary goal is to generate a nationwide awareness of cancer survivorship, NCCS facilitates communication between persons involved with cancer survivorship, promotes the development of cancer support activities, serves as a clearing house for information and materials on survivorship, advocates the interest of cancer survivors, and encourages the study of survivorship.

National Hospice Organization
1910 North Fort Meyer Drive, Suite 307
Arlington, VA 22209
1-703-243-5900

A nonprofit organization that provides literature and information about hospice to patients and their families and makes referrals to local, regional, and national resources.

National Lymphedema Network
2211 Post Street, Suite 404
San Francisco, CA 94115
1-800-541-3259

This organization provides educational information and a list of lymphedema support groups around the country.

National Neurofibromatosis Foundation, Inc.
141 Fifth Avenue, Suite 7-S
New York, NY 10010
1-800-323-7938
1-212-460-8980

This organization sponsors research, publishes educational materials, assists in the development of clinical centers and diagnostic protocols. Information packets about neurofibromatosis and support groups are available through this organization

Oley Foundation
214 Hun Memorial
Albany Medical Center
Albany, NY 12208
1-518-445-5079

This Foundation offers support to individuals receiving home parenteral and/or enteral nutrition therapy and their families. This organization has patient/family support groups and publishes a quarterly newsletter, *Lifeline Letter*. Services are provided free of charge to patients and their families.

Options Unlimited
76 East Main Street
Huntington, NY 11743
1-516-673-1150

Options Unlimited provides case management services for the coordination of care and services of patients with illnesses or injuries requiring long-term and/or critical medical care. This organization has a nationwide network of case management consultants, available on a fee basis, that will coordinate a variety of services, including working with insurance companies on billings and settlements, preparing the home for at-home patient care, and helping to find alternative financial assistance.

SKIP
(Sick Kids Need Involved People)
990 Second Avenue, 2nd Floor
New York, NY 10022
1-212-421-9160

SKIP is a national organization with the goal of providing case management and advocacy services to families of children with complex health care needs. These services are free and include identifying the services needed, helping families access those services to bring a child home from a medical facility, and locating financial aid resources. SKIP has chapters throughout the United States. Contact this office for the chapter nearest you.

Spirit and Breath Association
8210 Elmwood Avenue, Suite 209
Skokie, IL 60077
1-708-673-1384

This organization's goal is to assist those with lung cancer through a national telephone networking service (telephone counseling). The organization distributes the *Spirit and Breath Exercise Book*. For those individuals living in the Chicago area, support groups, a visitor program and newsletter is available.

Y-Me National Organization for Breast Cancer Information and Support, Inc.
18220 Harwood
Homewood, IL 60430
1-800-221-2141 (Patient Hot-Line, 9-5, CT, Weekdays)
1-708-799-8338 (General Information)
1-708-799-8228 (Patient 24 hour Hot-Line)

This organization provides information, telephone counseling, education, educational programs, and support groups for patients with breast cancer and their families and significant others. This organization maintains a "bank" of donated prosthesis and wigs for patients with limited financial resources.

United Ostomy Association
36 Executive Park, Suite 120
Irvine, CA 92714
1-714-660-8624

A nonprofit organization that provides speakers, literature, and monthly information meetings for people with ostomies. Volunteers, most of whom are ostomates, may visit patients with ostomies in the hospital or home with the consent of the patient's physician.

United Way of America
Mid-America Region
1400 East Touhy Avenue
Des Plaines, IL 60018-3305
1-708-707-6160

The staff of local offices of this organization are very knowledgeable of the support services available to cancer patients in the surrounding communities and can provide referrals to such resources.

PROFESSIONAL ORGANIZATIONS AND RESOURCES

American Association of Cancer Education
Sam Brown, EdD, Secretary
Educational Research and Development
University of Alabama at Birmingham
401 CHSD University Street
Birmingham, AL 35294

A multidisciplinary organization that provides education and training programs for professionals involved in cancer care. Annual meetings are held, and members receive the AACE Handbook upon joining.

American Pain Society
5700 Old Orchard Road, First Floor
Skokie, IL 60077
1-708-966-5595

A multidisciplinary organization, which is a national chapter of the International Association for the Study of Pain has members from many specialties in the fields of medicine, dentistry, psychology, nursing, other health professions and the basic sciences. Members include both investigators and clinicians in the field of pain and its treatment. One of the major goals of the Society is to promote education and training in the field of pain. Annual meetings are held.

Many states now have statewide Cancer Pain Initiatives, which is a multidisciplinary effort aimed at improving the management of cancer pain. It is a cooperative effort of clinical care facilities, higher education, government and many health care professionals including physicians, nurses, pharmacists, social workers, and others.

Call or write for more information.

American Society of Clinical Oncology
James B. Gantenberg, Executive Director
435 North Michigan Avenue
Suite 1717
Chicago, IL 60611
1-312-644-0828

Promotes and fosters the exchange of information relating to neoplastic diseases, with particular emphasis on human biology diagnosis, and treatment. The society publishes the *Journal of Clinical Oncology.*

Association of Community Cancer Centers
11600 Nebel Street
Suite 201
Rockville, MD 20852
1-301-984-9496

This organization provides a mechanism for the exchange of information among health professionals who believe high-quality cancer care should be available in the community. Publishes *Community Cancer Care Programs in the United States* and the *Oncology Issues: The Journal of Cancer Program Management.*

Association of Pediatric Oncology Nurses
6728 Old McLean Village Drive
McLean, VA 22101
1-703-556-9222

A professional organization open to all registered nurses with an interest in pediatric oncology. A quarterly journal, *JAPON,* an annual meeting, and local chapter activities are provided.

International Society of Nurses in Cancer Care
Carol Reed Ash, Secretary/Treasurer
Adelphi University School of Nursing
Box 516
Garden City, NY 11530
1-516-663-1001

The purpose of the International Society of Nurses in Cancer Care is to advance the knowledge and understanding of cancer nursing and to foster the dissemination of this knowledge and understanding. Nurses who are working in cancer care and who subscribe to the journal *Cancer Nursing* are eligible for membership.

Intravenous Nurses Society
2 Brighton Street
Belmont, MA 02178
1-617-489-5205

A professional organization open to all registered nurses with an interest in intravenous therapy. It publishes guidelines and standards for intravenous therapy and practice. The *Journal of Intravenous Therapy* and INS newsline are provided to members. A national meeting is held annually, and local chapters exist in more than 30 states.

Oncology Nursing Society
1016 Greentree Road
Pittsburgh, PA 15220-3125
1-412-912-7373

A professional nursing organization whose purpose is to promote the highest professional standards of oncology nursing. It provides support to oncology nurses; encourages study, research, and exchange of information; and publishes guidelines and standards for oncology nursing practice and education. A journal, *Oncology Nursing Forum,* and newsletter, *ONS News,* are provided to members. A national congress is held annually, and local chapters exist throughout the country. The ONS is also an ANA-accredited approver and provider of continuing education credits.

GENERAL PUBLIC INFORMATION

Center for Public Representation
121 S. Pinckney Street
Madison, Wisconsin 53703
1-800-369-0388

This organization is a non-profit law firm, training center and publishing house for the *unrepresented* that publishes easy-to-read practical self-help books on topics such as Guardianship, Senior Citizens and the Law, Health Care for Children with Chronic Illnesses, Power of Attorney, Planning for Long-Term Care, and the Uninsured. Call or write for catalog and ordering information.

Consumer Information Center
U.S. General Services Administration
Consumer Information Center-2D
P.O. Box 100
Pueblo, Colorado 81002

A governmental agency that provides free or low-cost federal publications of consumer interest including food and nutrition, health, drugs, health aids, medical problems, selecting a nursing home, and Federal Programs and Benefits. A catalog is available for $1.00.

Food and Drug Administration
Office of Consumer Affairs
HFE-885600
Fishers Lane
Rockville, MD 20857
1-301-443-3170

A consumer source on publication concerned with food-related subjects, FDA regulations, cosmetics, general medical drug information, medical devices, radiological health, and/or health fraud.

U.S. Department of Health and Human Services Public Health Service
Agency for Health Care Policy and Research
Suite 501
2101 East Jefferson Street
Rockville, MD 20852
1-800-952-7664

This governmental agency distributes health care literature for the general public, patients and their families and health care professionals.

U.S. Department of Labor Occupational Safety and Health Administration (OSHA)
Directorate of Technical Support
200 Constitution Avenue, N.W.
Washington, DC 20210
1-202-523-7047

The Occupational Safety and Health Administration (OSHA) is involved in the development and enforcement of occupational safety health standards and strives to ensure safe and healthful working conditions for every worker in the U.S. The directorate of technical support can provide information regarding work related hazards and occupational injuries and illnesses.

PERSONAL CARE RESOURCES

About Faces Permanent Cosmetics
1001 Bridgeway Blvd., Suite 432
Sausalito, CA 94965
1-415-331-0663

This company specializes in permanent cosmetic application, a tattoo process in which pigments are applied to the eyelids, eyebrows and lips to match skin tone. This process is used for alopecia areata (loss of facial and body hair), and loss of hair due to chemotherapy.

Airway
3960 Rosslyn Drive
Cincinnati, OH 45209
1-800-888-0458

This company manufactures a line of breast prosthesis called *The Portrait Group* along with fitting aids, brassieres and swimsuits. Call company to identify a dealer near you.

Alkin Hair Company
254 West 40th Street
New York, NY 10018
1-212-719-3070

This company matches hair samples that can then be braided, woven, or used for extensions. Call for information.

Caring Touch® Division International Hairgoods, Inc.
6811 Flying Cloud Drive
Eden Prairie, MN 55344
1-800-424-7567

This company manufactures and distributes cranial hair prostheses for men, women and children; eyebrow and moustache prostheses; and turbans and related supplies to a network of trained *Caring Touch* service centers. The company also offers patient educational materials on hair loss and the available appearance options. Call for information.

Designs for Comfort, Inc.
P.O. Box 8229
Northfield, IL 60093
1-800-443-9226

This company has developed a combination cap and hairpiece called the *Headliner* as an alternative to wigs. The *Headliner* is available in a variety of colors and fabrics. This product may be reimbursed by individual insurance companies as a hair prosthesis. Call to order by mail or locate a dealer near you.

Fairs' OPS, Inc.
P.O. Box 5760, Greenway Station
Glendale, AZ 85306
1-602-978-4435

This company distributes ostomy prosthesis support (OPS) undergarments. These undergarments are available for both men and women. Call for information.

Frends Beauty Supply
5270 Laurel Canyon
N. Hollywood, CA 91607
1-818-769-3834

This company offers cosmetics, camouflage makeup, eyelashes, and eyebrows. For mail order catalog, send $3.75. You will receive $3.00 credit toward your first purchase.

Holly Cosmetics/Medical Image Products
4947 Brownsboro Road
Louisville, KY 40220
1-800-222-3964

This company offers a line of corrective cosmetics. Information about the Holly Cosmetics line and a video are available by mail. Call to order information and a video, or to find a consultant near you. This company is involved in the *Look Good, Feel Better* program.

Intimacies by Alice
3 Hudson Watch Drive
Ossining, NY 10562
1-914-923-2010

This company manufactures a line of sleepwear and daywear, including loungewear, sportswear, and lingerie, for women who have had breast surgery. These are available in specialty boutiques or by mail order. Call for more information.

Jodee
5085 West Park Road
Hollywood, FL 33021
1-800-821-2767
1-305-987-7274

This company provides mastectomy products. Call to request a catalog, which includes bras, prostheses, and accessories.

Mary Catherine's
1914 N.E. 42nd Avenue
Portland, OR 97213
1-800-843-3215

A boutique for intimate apparel for women who have had breast surgery. Call or write for a catalog that includes bras, prostheses, and swimwear.

Nearly Me
316 W. Florence Avenue
Inglewood, CA 90301
1-310-330-7500 (Los Angeles)
1-800-421-2322

This company offers a line of breast prostheses, mastectomy swimwear, and accessories. Prostheses are available for all kinds of surgeries in a wide range of prices. Call for more information and a dealer near you.

Worldwide Home Health Center, Inc.
926 East Tallmadge Avenue
Akron, OH 44310
1-800-621-5938 (in Ohio)
1-800-223-5938

This company is a distributor for health care products and services. A free catalog is available that includes breast prosthesis, skin care products, and ostomy products.

EDUCATIONAL RESOURCES

ABLEDATA
Adaptive Equipment Center
Newington Children's Hospital
181 East Cedar Street
Newington, CT 06111
1-203-667-5405
1-800-344-5405

This is a continually updated product information database with entries for more than 1,700 commercially available products from over 2000 manufacturers. Detailed information is included on products for use in all aspects of independent living, including personal care, transportation, communication, and recreation. A printed copy of the database will be provided in response to an inquiry specifying the type of product desired or type of activity or function to be achieved. The database is also available through direct on-line searching or in a CD format for microcomputers. You can get up to 8 pages of information free.

American Cancer Society
1559 Clifton Road, N.E.
Atlanta, GA 30329
1-404-320-3333 (General Information)
1-404-329-7616 (Department of Nursing)

ACS offers printed and audiovisual materials as well as educational programs for nurses and other health care professionals. Scholarships are available for masters degree and doctoral students in cancer nursing.

American Pain Society
5700 Old Orchard Road, First Floor
Skokie, IL 60077
1-708-966-5595

The American Pain Society, a national chapter of the International Association for the Study of Pain is a not-for-profit educational and scientific organization. One of the Society's major goals is to promote education and training in the field of pain. The Society has developed a handbook, *Principles of Analgesic Use in the Treatment of Acute Pain and Chronic Cancer Pain: A Concise Guide to Medical Practice–2nd Edition*. For more information call or write to the American Pain Society.

CancerFax
NCI International Cancer Information Service
9030 Old Georgetown Road
Building 82, Room 219
Bethesda, MD 20892
1-301-402-5874 (on fax machine handset)
1-301-496-8880 (for technical assistance)

The National Cancer Institute has combined computer with fax technology and now offers a service to any health care professional with a fax machine current data on cancer treatment from NCI's comprehensive data base. Two types of summaries are available: (1) written to meet the informational needs of the health care provider and (2) written in language geared toward the general public. There is no charge for the service, you only pay for the cost of the telephone call. This service is available 24 hours a day, 7 days a week.

Cancer Information Service

1-800-4-CANCER

The Cancer Information Service is available to answer questions by telephone from the general public, patients and their families, and health professionals. Printed materials on many topics related to cancer are available to callers without charge.

Department of Health and Human Services

Public Health Service
Agency for Health Care Policy and Research
Executive Office Center
2101 East Jefferson Street, Suite 501
Rockville, MD 20852
1-800-952-7664

This governmental agency distributes health care literature for the public, patients and their families, and health care professionals. Call or write for more information.

National Cancer Institute

Bethesda, MD 20205
1-301-496-7403

Cancer Information Clearing House is an information service for organizations that use or develop materials for public and professional information and education. The Clearing House provides information exchange, either in form of bibliographic services or in custom searches of its collection of 7000 citations of cancer informational and educational materials and services.

International Cancer Information Center sponsors CANCERLINE, which includes (1) 400,000 citations and abstracts of articles published since 1963 on all aspects of cancer, (2) descriptions of 10,000 ongoing cancer research projects, and (3) 4,500 summaries of clinical investigations of new anticancer agents and treatment modalities.

Physician Data Query (PDQ) is a computer data base for retrieval of cancer treatment information. Providing easy access to state-of-the-art cancer information, the data base has three interlinked files, organized and internally arranged to allow interactive searching and retrieval of information.

National Rehabilitation Information Center

8455 Colesville Road, Suite 935
Silver Spring, MD 20910-3319
1-800-346-2742

This organization distributes a bibliographic database, **REHABDATA,** covering disability and rehabilitation research literature including citations to research reports from the National Institute on Disability and Rehabilitation Research sponsored centers and other sources such as scholarly papers, selected journal articles, audiovisual materials and other reference documents.

Office of Cancer Communications

NCI Building 31, Room 10A16
Bethesda, MD 20892
1-301-496-5583

This office, a branch of the National Cancer Institute, provides services for both the public and health care professionals, including information and publications on a wide variety of cancer topics.

University of Texas
M.D. Anderson Cancer Center

Patient Education Office
1515 Holcombe–Box 21
Houston, TX 77030
ATTN: Patient Education Clearinghouse
1-713-792-7128

M.D. Anderson Cancer Center Patient Education Office staff work with multidisciplinary committees to assess, implement, and evaluate educational activities for patients and their families. Teaching plans, printed materials, and audiovisual aids are available at a nominal cost to reinforce the instructions and information provided by individual members of the health care team.

The Patient Education Materials Clearinghouse serves as a distribution center for printed patient education materials. Call or write to obtain ordering information.

RECOMMENDED BOOKS/PAMPHLETS

Cetus Oncology Resource Guide

Cetus Corporation
500 W. 8th Street
Suite 100A
Vancouver, WA 98660
1-800-466-0701

The Cetus Oncology Resource Guide was created in support to the oncology team and their patients. The guide is intended to be used as an informational directory on adjunctive support services available locally, regionally, and nationally.

Domiciliary Terminal Care
A Handbook for Doctors and Nurses

by Derek Doyle
Churchill Livingstone
New York, NY

This handbook, published in 1987, is a useful guide for health care professionals providing terminal care in the home setting.

Dying at Home: A Family Guide for Caregiving

by Andrea Sankar
The Johns Hopkins University Press
Baltimore and London

This book, published in 1991, is a helpful guide for families wishing to care for their loved one at home during the terminal stages of illness.

Palliative Care of the Terminally Ill
by J. F. Hanratty
Radcliffe Medical Press
Oxford

This handbook, published in 1989, is also a handy reference for health care professionals providing terminal care in the home.

Mastering the Medicare Maze
Center for Public Representation
121 S. Pinckney Street
Madison, Wisconsin 53703
1-800-369-0388

This book provides easy-to-read information about just what Medicare is and how to appeal its decisions. The book contains considerable practical advice.

Regional Resource Guide
Center for Consumer Healthcare Information
P.O. Box 16067
Irvine, CA 92713-9950
1-800-627-2244

This 4-volume community resource guide is very comprehensive and contains information on available resources for a wide variety of health care needs, including home care, rehabilitation, support agencies, counseling, medical equipment and supplies as well as others. Call or write for more information.

The Role of the Oncology Nurse in the Office Setting
Susan B. Baird, RN, MPH
Editor-in-Chief
Kristine Hartigan, RN, OCN
Debra Holton-Smith, RN, BSN
Associate Editors
Presented as a professional service by Adria Laboratories
Division of Erbamont Inc.
Columbus, OH 43215

This publication is a useful guide for nurses working in the ambulatory setting. Professional and patient care issues are discussed in this publication.

Please Note: Literature is also available through the Support Service Organizations and the Professional Organizations listed in this Appendix.

CHAPTER 27

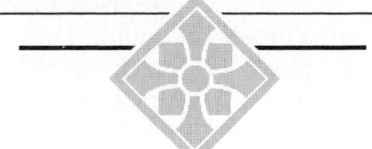

Nutrition

Lisa Schulmeister

Cancer and its treatment may affect the nutritional status of the patient in a variety of ways. Besides being subject to metabolic effects, patients are emotionally stressed when nutritional intake is impaired. Because eating is a basic bodily function and often a social activity, inability to eat or difficulty in eating may have a profound physical and psychologic impact on the individual with cancer.

EFFECTS OF CANCER ON NUTRITIONAL STATUS
Nutritional Components and Their Functions

Cancer may affect the metabolization of the nutritional components necessary to sustain life: carbohydrates, proteins, fatty acids, vitamins, minerals, and electrolytes. An alteration in the metabolization of these components affects the nutritional status of an individual, that is, the degree to which an individual's need for nutrition is met by his or her intake.

Carbohydrates are the sugars that provide energy for immediate use. They are converted to glycogen or fat for long-term storage or are converted to other molecules in the body. Carbohydrates can be divided into three classes: monosaccharides, disaccharides, and polysaccharides.

Monosaccharides are simple one-molecule sugars. Examples are fructose and dextrose (glucose). Disaccharides are two-molecule sugars. An example is sucrose (table sugar). Polysaccharides are complex sugars characterized by many molecules. Examples are starch and dextran.

Glucose is the fuel for most of the cells of the body. It is metabolized rapidly in the presence or absence of oxygen. Each gram of glucose provides 3.4 kcal. Carbohydrates are also a long-term source of energy. When glucose intake exceeds demand, it is converted into glycogen or fat. Both sources of energy are stored in the body and used when a glucose shortage occurs. When metabolized by certain processes, the glucose molecule can be used as the basis for other molecules, including amino acids and fatty acids.

Amino acids are the building blocks of the body. Proteins are many amino acids joined into one molecule. Amino acids are divided into two categories: essential and nonessential. Essential amino acids must be supplied from the diet because the body is unable to synthesize them from glucose or other amino acids. Nonessential amino acids need not be supplied from the diet because the body is able to synthesize them.

Functions of amino acids include maintenance and growth. When tissue breakdown exceeds synthesis or when glucose for energy is lacking, the result is wasting of protein from muscles and loss of mass. Amino acids assist in the regulation of body processes and make up many enzymes found throughout the body. Enzymes are the chemical regulators of many of the synthetic processes in the body. During starvation the body uses proteins as a source of energy. Each gram provides 4 kcal.

Lipids and fatty acids serve many roles in the body. Fatty acids are basic molecules, and lipids are long chains of fatty acids. Lipids may be saturated or unsaturated, depending on the number of double-bonded carbons in their structure. Lipids are an excellent source of energy, supplying 9 kcal per gram. They are also the long-term storage form of glucose. Fat-soluble vitamins are transported by lipids. Many fat-soluble vitamins (A, D, E, and K) are transported throughout the body bound to fatty acids. The fat content of food is responsible for the taste of many foods and the feeling of fullness that results from eating. Lipids also provide insulation and padding.

The fatty acids are precursors to many hormones, including testosterone and estrogen. They are also the basis for cholesterol.

Vitamins are compounds used in a number of enzymatic steps that regulate many processes. Normal amounts of the adult daily requirements (ADR) of vitamins are obtained by consuming a balanced diet. Vitamins can be divided into two groups: fat-soluble and water-soluble. Fat-soluble vitamins are stored by the body in fat. Deficiencies take a long time to develop because these vitamins are stored. Vitamin A is important in maintaining vision and in tooth and skeletal development, and it acts as a precursor to cholesterol. Vitamin D acts to regulate protein and calcium metabolism. Vitamin E is an antioxidant; that is, it prevents or lessens damage to body tissue caused by atmospheric oxygen. Vitamin K helps maintain the clotting ability of blood.

Water-soluble vitamins are not stored in the body and are readily eliminated in the urine. Deficiencies may develop quickly if inadequate quantities are consumed. Vitamin C is used in the formation of collagen, enhances iron absorption, and serves as an antioxidant. B-complex vitamins are cofactors in many enzymatic reactions.

Macroelements, or electrolytes, maintain osmotic pressure and water balance, facilitate nerve conduction and muscle contraction, and perform other functions. The macroelements are sodium, potassium, chloride, calcium, magnesium, phosphorus, and sulfur.

Trace elements are so named because they are needed by the body in small quantities. Deficiencies can develop quickly, but clinical signs of deficiency may not be apparent for a long time. Trace elements include zinc, manganese, copper, chromium, selenium, iron, and cobalt, among others.

Systemic Effects

Alterations in the normal metabolism of carbohydrates, proteins, and fats result in increased energy expenditures. The body of the person with cancer responds to the increased demand for glucose required by cancer cells and normal body cells with a high rate of gluconeogenesis. Gluconeogenesis is the synthesis of glucose by the liver and renal cortex from noncarbohydrate sources such as lactate and amino acids. When protein is broken down to provide amino acids for this process, muscle wasting results. Progressive wasting is called cachexia.[6,48,77] The anorexia-cachexia syndrome of advanced cancer is poorly understood. Psychological causes often reflect anxiety about cancer, its possible progression, depression, anticipatory phenomena, and learned food aversions.[46]

Fat metabolization is affected in individuals with cancer. Stored fat in the form of fatty acids is mobilized from adipose tissues and released in the bloodstream for use as fuel for energy production. This process is controlled by the inhibitory effects of insulin. These inhibitory effects are compromised in individuals with cancer. Body stores of fat are depleted as the disease progresses.[8,67]

Vitamin deficiencies observed in persons with cancer include a deficiency of vitamin A in many individuals with cancer of the lung and alimentary tract. Thiamine and vitamin C deficiencies have also been reported in various malignancies. Iron deficiency may result from the unavailability of iron in the diet or from malabsorption.

Fluid and electrolyte imbalances may result from direct and indirect effects of tumors. Parathyroid, lung, kidney, and colon tumors may produce an ectopic parathyroid-like hormone that deposits calcium in the renal tubules and may result in renal failure. Hypercalcemia may also cause a concentrating effect that leads to polyuria and water depletion. Leukemias and lymphomas may induce hyperuricemia, hyperphosphatemia, and hyperkalemia as a result of electrolytes released by cellular breakdown. A common presentation of bronchiogenic carcinomas, such as small cell, is the syndrome of inappropriate secretion of antidiuretic hormone (SIADH). This syndrome is characterized by urinary loss of sodium and excessive retention of water by the renal tubules. Renal tumors may secrete renin and in turn cause increased secretion of aldosterone, resulting in hypokalemia.[74]

Patients who are nutritionally depleted can have decreased immunocompetence, which becomes more severe as the disease progresses. Malnutrition decreases the size of the lymphoid tissues. Lymphatic structures such as the spleen, lymph nodes, and thymus participate directly in the immune response, and a decrease in their size contributes to immunosuppression. Decreased function of B-cell and T-cell lymphocytes will also result from malnutrition. Fewer T cells, especially helper T cells, and phagocyte dysfunction are common. The greater the malnutrition, the greater the deficiency of T lymphocytes. This produces delayed hypersensitivity response. The immune system works with cancer treatment to destroy tumor cells. Preservation of both nutritional status and the function of the immune system are thus important considerations in cancer therapy.[14,45]

Local Effects

Several local effects of cancer may alter the nutritional intake of the affected individual. Impaired ingestion may be caused by mechanical and anatomic alterations. Patients with cancer of the head and neck area, esophageal cancers, and brain tumors may have trouble with opening the mouth, chewing, and swallowing as well as with peristalsis. Obstruction of the esophagus can inhibit the passage of food. Gastric tumors often cause pain and distention. Cancers along the alimentary tract may cause obstructions, and they often inhibit the absorption of nutrients.

Cancer of the small intestine affects the digestion and absorption of food. A fistula of the bowel may develop as a result of tissue necrosis from a gastrointestinal (GI) tract tumor and induce electrolyte imbalance and malabsorption because of a lack of nutrients.

NUTRITIONAL CONSEQUENCES OF CANCER TREATMENT
Effects of Various Modes of Treatment

Surgical alterations in any area of the alimentary tract from the mouth to the anus may cause temporary or occasionally permanent alterations in nutritional intake or absorptive capabilities. Surgical procedures that alter the patient's ability to chew or swallow may prompt the need for soft or blenderized foods, and tube feedings may be required. Assessment and correction of malnutrition has led to improvements in the preoperative and postoperative management of patients with head and neck cancers over the past 20 years.[76] Partial or total gastrectomy can cause severe nutritional problems. When the greater portion of the stomach is removed, the intrinsic factor is not produced in quantities sufficient for the absorption of Vitamin B_{12}, and pernicious amemia develops. With resection of the stomach, the quantity of food that can be consumed at one time is limited, and frequent, small feedings are necessary. Dumping syndrome may also appear after gastrectomy; a few minutes after ingestion, food is dumped into the jejunum, and nausea, cramping, and diarrhea follow. Malabsorption of fat occurs in patients who have undergone a gastrojejunostomy. The duodenum is bypassed and pancreatic insufficiency results. Malabsorption of fat impairs absorption of fat-soluble vitamins and calcium. Iron absorption is also decreased, and anemia occurs.[36]

Radiation therapy may affect the normal tissues surrounding the treatment areas. Patients with cancer of the head and neck have both acute and chronic symptoms. Specifically, the normal tissues of the salivary gland, oral mucosa, muscle, and occasionally bone may be affected. In the acute phase, inflammation and swelling of tissues with resulting discomfort may affect nutritional intake. Taste changes, such as a diminished sense of taste or metallic taste when eating red meats, may cause aversion to food and decreased intake. Xerostomia, or diminished production of saliva, is a long-term side effect of radiation therapy. Pain and difficulty swallowing often occur. Saliva substitutes and topical anesthetics for oral use may be helpful, and eating moist foods is recommended.[41,60]

Irradiation of the small intestine produces vomiting, anorexia, diarrhea, and gastric distention. Antiemetics taken 30 minutes before treatment, low-residue diet, and adequate hydration may alleviate or minimize these side effects. Generally, these acute effects resolve with the completion of therapy.[70]

Chemotherapy may produce side effects that impair the patient's nutritional status. Chemotherapy causes nutritional deficiencies by promoting anorexia, stomatitis, taste alterations, and alimentary tract disturbances. Deficiencies of vitamins B_1, B_2, and K, and of niacin, folic acid, and thymine may also result from chemotherapy. Taste alterations, such as an aversion to red meat, are common with platinum based products. Cool foods with little aroma as well as bland foods are often tolerated well. Topical application of analgesics often minimizes the discomfort of stomatitis.[25]

Other common side effects of chemotherapy are nausea and vomiting. The severity of symptoms and their effect on nutritional status varies from patient to patient. Use of antiemetics and dietary measures may help.[61] Nausea and vomiting may have a psychogenic component; anticipatory nausea and vomiting before a chemotherapy treatment are not uncommon. Odor, sight, and even thought of food may produce emesis in some patients. Relaxation and diversion therapy is sometimes indicated. Aversions to specific foods may occur as a result of the association of those foods with nausea and vomiting. The most promising intervention is the use of "scapegoat" foods; foods or beverages intentionally introduced before the treatment period to block formation of a food aversion.[59]

The side effects of biotherapy are generally less severe than those of chemotherapy. Anorexia is a common complaint, and nausea and vomiting occur infrequently. Diarrhea may occur, depending on the agent used.

Nutritional Assessment

A nutritional assessment can screen for potential or existing problems in nutritional status, provide a data base for individuals at high risk, and determine response to treatment or dietary interventions. Although all patients should be assessed, particular attention should be given to the elderly patient. Older adults experience physiologic effects of aging that impair their nutritional status. For instance, one in five older adults experience xerostomia. Assessment of the patient's eating patterns, nutrient intake, and supplement use, and influences on eating habits should be completed prior to initiation of cancer treatment.[24,38,66]

Several methods can be used to estimate or quantify the nutritional status of the patient. See box sum-

---

COMPONENTS OF NUTRITIONAL ASSESSMENT

Nursing history
Date diagnosed
Type of cancer
Type and duration of therapy
Concurrent medications
Concomitant medical conditions
Surgical procedures
Side effects of therapy
Allergies

Psychosocial assessment
Home environment
Family support
Coping abilities
Self-image
Perceptions of role of nutrition
Cultural, religious considerations

Physical assessment
General overall appearance
Hair texture
Skin turgor and integrity
Condition of mouth and gums
Performance status
Alterations in elimination, comfort, etc.

Dietary evaluation
24-hour recall of intake
Food perferences
Food allergies
Use of vitamin supplements
Changes in diet or eating on life-style patterns
Observation of intake
Evaluation of nutrient composition

Biochemical measurements
Serum albumin
Hemoglobin, hematocrit
Serum transferrin
Total lymphocyte count
Creatinine
Urine urea nitrogen
Creatinine-height index
Skin testing

Anthropometric data
Height
Weight
Weight change over time (actual weight compared with ideal body weight)
Triceps skin fold thickness
Midarm muscle circumference
Subscapular skin fold thickness

---

marizing nutritional assessment above. A simple method is clinical observation. A thorough nursing history will identify concurrent health problems such as diabetes, hypertension, and malabsorption, which may affect nutrition. Psychosocial factors, including the home environment, food preparation methods, and the patient's body image should be noted. A physical assessment will reflect the overall nutritional status of the patient. Specifically, examination of the hair, teeth, gums, and general muscle tone may provide an early indication of nutritional deficiencies.[40] A functional assessment will determine the patient's ability to prepare meals and feed self.

Dietary evaluation is also a simple and effective tool for assessing nutritional status. A 24-hour food diary, a complete dietary history with notations of food allergies and preferences, and direct observation of intake coupled with evaluation of nutrient composition are methods for dietary evaluation. Much of this information can be collected from the patient; however, the patient may not report accurately. Direct observation of the patient's intake by a consistent nurse or dietitian is more precise but has limitations for patients who are not hospitalized.[36]

Biochemical measurements include lab values such as serum albumin, which is used to estimate visceral protein levels; serum transferrin, which reflects the body's ability to make serum proteins; and total lymphocyte count, which tests immunocompetence. Skin testing can reveal T cell–mediated immunocompetence, and urine urea nitrogen may be measured to estimate skeletal muscle mass.

Anthropometric measurements are the patient's midarm muscle circumference (MAMC), triceps skin fold thickness (TSF), subscapular skin fold thickness (SST), and weight for height as compared with reference standards. The measurements estimate subcutaneous fat stores, energy reserves, and skeletal muscle protein mass. Moreover, measuring weight and comparing it with the patient's ideal body weight and monitoring changes in weight over time will assist in identifying any downward trend in nutritional status.

Nutritional Intervention

Nutritional therapy for individuals with cancer has been shown to decrease the morbidity and mortality of cancer by preventing weight loss, increasing response to treatment, minimizing the side effects of therapy, and improving quality of life. The extent of nutritional support provided depends on the overall goals of the patient and health care team, and it may be palliative or quite aggressive.[34]

The individual patient's needs determine the type of nutritional support required. Factors include the patient's functional abilities and limitations, severity of the nutritional deficiency, potential for complications, duration of therapy, psychologic effect, and cost.

NUTRITIONAL SUPPORT
Oral Nutrition

After the need for nutritional support has been established, the next step is to determine the method of delivery. The oral route is most desirable. Supplemental oral nutrition may range from simple measures such as adding gravies and sauces to more complex interventions. The degree of intervention is based on the severity of the nutritional deficiency.

For individuals who have a mild weight loss, the first step is to determine the cause. In older adults, anorexia may be a contributing factor to weight loss. Possible etiologies include social, psychological, medical, and age related factors.[53] Individuals who are eating slightly less may benefit from frequent small meals and snacks. Foods high in protein such as cheese, fish, and poultry and foods high in calories are recommended. Family members and caregivers should offer a variety of foods; foods not appealing at one time may be favorites at another. Milkshakes, peanut butter on crackers, and prepackaged puddings are snacks that are not only nutritious but also easy to prepare.

Individuals who have a mild weight loss because of alterations in skin integrity of the oral mucosa (stomatitis) or taste alterations may benefit from a high-calorie bland diet. Avoidance of seasoning and experimentation with alternative flavorings such as vanilla may be beneficial. Use of a topical analgesic for stomatitis may reduce discomfort. Good mouth care cannot be overlooked; slight modifications may be needed. Substitution of baking soda or use of a toothpaste specifically for sensitive mouths may be indicated. Patients should avoid commercial mouthwashes, as they contain additives and flavorings that are often painful for those with altered oral mucosal integrity. Cold foods, particularly popsicles, ice cream, and frozen yogurt, often have a numbing effect and may be tolerated. Liquids that are known to have high acidity such as orange and lemon juice should be avoided.[65] Patients experiencing xerostomia may encounter difficulties maintaining adequate nutritional intake. The addition of liquids, particularly sauces and gravies, may be helpful.[63]

Although weight loss may be mild, early nutritional guidance decreases the incidence of severe deficiencies that may occur later on. In addition to dietary interventions, psychosocial support is indicated. Ineffective individual and family coping often occurs when the patient begins to lose weight. Efforts by family members to encourage a better intake are sometimes met with resistance. Frustration for both patient and family results as the patient perceives the relatives to be unsympathetic and lacking in understanding. Family members often perceive a lack of effort on the part of the patient and become frustrated at their inability to do more for the patient. Nurses should listen to problems with nutrition and provide guidance and instruction when indicated.

Nondietary interventions for patients with a mild weight loss include varying surroundings, eating at the table with family and friends, and arriving at the table immediately before meals to minimize the effect of food odor on appetite. Using small plates and eating more often may be helpful.

Patients with a moderate to severe weight loss require more intensive nutritional intervention. Unless prohibited, the oral route is the most advantageous. As with any weight loss, an examination of causes is a beginning point. Specific deficits can be determined and an individual plan of interventions can be designed. In addition to small, frequent meals and snacks, use of additives such as gravies and sauces will boost caloric intake. Medications may assist in controlling the side effects of the disease or treatment that may be affecting intake. Antiemetics given 30 minutes before meals and use of artificial saliva to control the symptoms of stomatitis are examples of pharmacologic interventions. Several randomized, controlled studies have also suggested that use of megestrol acetate with a dose range of 320 to 1600 mg per day improves appetite and food intake in patients with anorexia and advanced cancer.[71]

If indicated, provide high-calorie, high-protein supplements such as Isocal (Mead Johnson), Polycose (Ross), and Vivonex (Norwich Eaton). Monitor for alterations in elimination when using lactose-based products; some patients experience diarrhea and do not tolerate these formulas.

Psychosocial support and other measures such as varying surroundings for mealtimes, being well rested before meals, and participation in meal planning may help some patients.

Enteral Nutrition

Although oral nutrition is preferred, adequate intake may not be possible for patients who are anorexic, hypermetabolic or unconscious or who have a mechanical impairment. For these patients, it may be necessary to use a feeding tube. The enteral route is preferable because it uses the GI tract. Using the gut for feeding maintains the GI tract's digestive and absorptive capabilities and assists in maintaining GI motility. Metabolic comparisons show a more nearly normal usage of some nutrients with the enteral than with the parenteral route. Parenteral feeding is indicated for patients who have totally nonfunctioning GI tracts, who require bowel rest, or who are intolerant of enteral nutritional support.[54]

Assessment of nutritional status is essential for determining which patients are candidates for tube feedings. Generally, patients with functioning GI tracts who are unable to ingest adequate nutrients to meet their metabolic demands are candidates for tube feedings. Indications include numerous cancer diagnoses and related disorders (see box on p. 646).

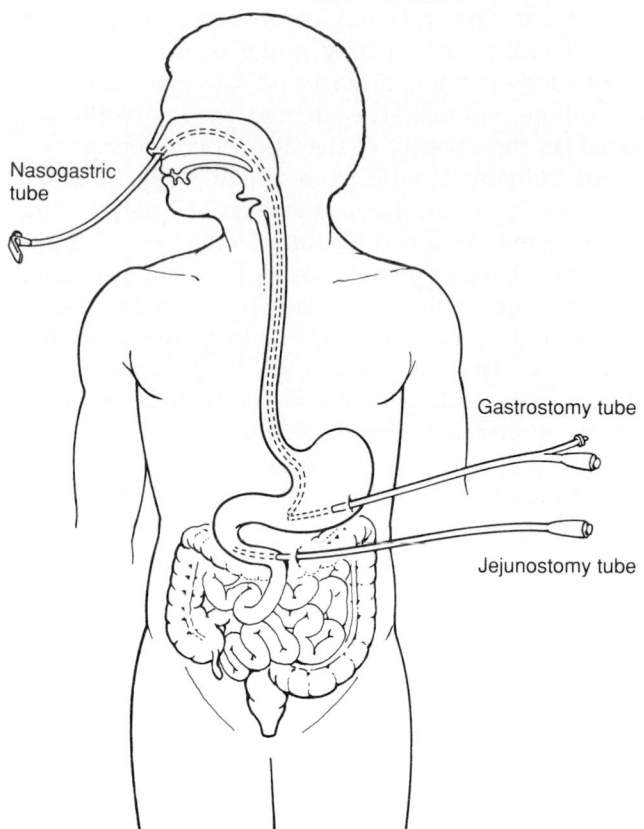

Figure 27–1 Three routes for tube feeding.

Tube feedings can be administered by the nasogastric, nasoduodenal, nasojejunal, esophagostomy, gastrostomy, and jejunostomy routes (Figure 27-1). Passage of the feeding tube through the nose into the stomach or intestine is most common. It is best tolerated when a small, flexible feeding tube is used. Larger, stiffer tubes may damage the mucosa of the GI tract and irritate the nose. Feeding ostomies generally require surgical percutaneous insertion. A feeding ostomy is indicated for long-term therapy, whenever obstruction makes insertion through the nose impossible, or after gastrointestinal surgery. Ostomy tubes eliminate nasal irritation and are more cosmetically acceptable to the patient. Possible complications include infection or skin irritation around the feeding-tube site; however, this risk is lessened with appropriate skin care.[50]

Nasogastric, esophagostomy, and gastrostomy feedings allow the digestive process to begin in the stomach. Aspiration may occur more easily with gastric feedings than with intestinal feedings because only the gastroesophageal sphincter is functioning to prevent gastric reflux. Nasoduodenal, nasojejunal, and jejunostomy feedings, which are delivered directly into the small intestine, use both the gastroesophageal and pyloric sphincters to prevent reflux. Tube selection is based on several factors, including the duration of therapy, history of abdominal procedures, gastrointestinal function, level of debilitation, and the discharge plan. Adequate digestion and absorption occur in the small intestine; however, when feedings are improperly selected or administered, nausea, diarrhea, and cramps can result.[29,30,52,62]

A cervical esophagostomy is a surgically created skin-lined canal extending from the border of the neck to the area below the cervical esophagus. The feeding tube is passed through this opening to the stomach for each feeding and removed after the feeding is finished.

ADMINISTRATION OF TUBE FEEDING.   The size of the tube selected for enteral feedings should be the smallest through which the food will flow. A variety of tubes are available. Most are made of soft, flexible material such as polyurethane or silicone rubber. These tubes do not stiffen when exposed to gastric juices and are more comfortable for the patient than are stiff tubes. The tubes are available in different French sizes and lengths, and most are radiopaque.[78]

The volume and concentration of nutriment delivered by tube feeding should meet the individual's specific needs. A patient who has been without adequate food intake before tube feeding requires a period of adaptation before full volume and strength can be tolerated. Isotonic formulas are more easily tolerated than hypertonic formulas and do not require the same degree of dilution. The duodenum and jejunum are more sensitive than the stomach to both volume and osmolality. Therefore, duodenal or jejunal feeding should be low in osmolality and delivered by continuous drip or pump.[51]

Bolus feedings of enteral formulas are administered usually at 250 to 400 ml over a few minutes five to eight times daily. Patients who are intolerant of bolus feedings may have nausea, diarrhea, aspiration, abdominal distention, and cramps.[51,56]

Gravity feedings may be intermittent or continuous. Gravity flow rates may be inconsistent and so must be assessed frequently. Even if checks are made as frequently as every half hour, accidental bolus delivery is possible. Ideally, the tube position should be checked two to three times daily and gastric residual should be checked every 2 to 4 hours. Feedings to the distal duodenum or jejunum should be given by continuous pump infusion to prevent dumping syndrome.

Continuous feedings may be given during the night over 10 to 12 hours or around the clock. They should be started at 50 ml or less and advanced only if the patient shows no diarrhea, cramping, or other signs of intolerance. When the desired rate has been reached, the strength can be increased as tolerated. Generally, an isotonic or nearly isotonic formula can be started at full strength; hypertonic or concentrated formulas are usually started at half strength (half formula, half water).

Various feeding sets, containers, and pumps are available for tube feeding. Selection of equipment and supplies is based on the formula to be given, rate and frequency of feedings, tube site, and other considerations, including the care giver's preference. Most feeding bags and administration sets are large enough to accommodate 500 to 1000 ml of formula. To prevent bacterial contamination when a large container is used, the amount of formula in the bag should approximate that which can be given over 8 hours. In warm environments, a feeding bag with a pouch for an ice bag is desirable to prevent curdling of the formula and bacterial contamination. New formula should not be added to formula that has already been hanging for 8 hours at room temperature. The container and tubing should be rinsed well before adding formula. With very careful cleaning, a feeding bag may be used for two days; however, discarding the bag after 24 hours is recommended.[21,51]

Some formulas are available in screw-top prefilled bottles, which decrease the chance for bacterial contamination. If a dilute formula is required, some formula must be wasted to allow for the addition of water, adding to the overall cost of the formula.

There are several enteral pumps that can provide a controlled rate of administration. Most have internal batteries to allow limited mobility and have alarm systems that indicate problems or completion of feeding. Most pumps have occlusion and low battery alarms and are simply designed to allow easy troubleshooting. An enteral pump is usually indicated if the patient is being fed by the small intestine, if the feedings are given continually around the clock, or if the desired rate is less than 200 ml per hour.

PSYCHOLOGIC IMPACT OF TUBE FEEDINGS. Recognition of the psychologic and social needs of the patient receiving (tube feedings) is an important component of nursing care. Patients facing long-term feedings must adapt to the loss of control over food selection and consumption. Since eating is a social, cultural, and sometimes religious activity, adaptation may be difficult. In addition, alterations of body image related to the presence of a nasogastric or percutaneously inserted feeding tube may cause distress.[42]

Thirst, taste deprivation, and inability to satisfy the appetite are common complaints of tube-fed patients. Patients may feel self-conscious surrounded by the equipment and supplies needed for formula administration and may find mobility limited by the feeding pump and pole. Limiting tube feedings to night hours or using gravity administration may enhance adaptation.

An assessment of the patient's life-style, home environment, body image, and motivation for tube feeding is critical before implementing therapy. Exploration of the patient's perceptions of the importance of food and eating will assist in identifying areas of concern and provide a good starting point for teaching. Involvement of the patient and family in the tube feedings is helpful. The rationale for all procedures should be described, and the patient and family should be encouraged to assist in the feeding.

Occasionally, patients are allowed some oral intake, usually fluids and soft, bland foods. Patients receiving all their nutrition from tube feedings may be permitted to chew gum or suck on hard candies, thus satisfying their sense of taste and their desire to chew.

Patients requiring long-term enteral therapy may benefit from meeting with other tube-fed patients. The support and role models provided often ease the transition to tube feeding.

MONITORING THE PATIENT.   The patient's weight is a simple test for assessing whether caloric and fluid needs are met. Weighing the patient daily or every other day will alert the care giver of a deviance from the anticipated weight gain or maintenance. If the patient loses weight during tube feeding, adjustments of the rate, formula, or calorie content may be made quickly.

Serum proteins may also be monitored, usually every 7 to 10 days. In the presence of malnutrition, there is decreased albumin synthesis. With optimal enteral nutritional support, there will be a rise in serum albumin and protein levels as the patient receives adequate calories and protein. A more sophisticated monitoring tool is a study to assess the balance between nitrogen intake and output. A 24-hour urine collection for urine urea nitrogen is obtained and analyzed. Nitrogen balance results when the output from the urine, skin, and stools approximates the intake.[42]

Table 27-1   Common Complications of Enteral Nutrition

Complication	Etiology
MECHANICAL	
Nasal irritation and erosion	Use of rigid, large-bore tubes
Esophagitis, pharyngitis	
Tube dislocation	Coughing or pulling on tube, tube migration
Tube occlusion	Kinked tube, inadequate irrigation, formula incompletely crushed, or incompatible medications
GASTROINTESTINAL	
Abdominal distention	Rapid infusion rate, delayed gastric emptying, formula intolerance
Nausea, vomiting	Rapid infusion rate, delayed emptying, formula intolerance, malabsorption, electrolyte imbalance, contaminated formula
Diarrhea	Rapid infusion rate, formula intolerance, malabsorption, contaminated formula
Constipation	Long-term use of low-residue solutions, inadequate fluid intake
RESPIRATORY	
Aspiration pneumonia	Gastric reflux of aspiration (especially with large-bore tubes), improper tube placement, large gastric residuals, patient positioned lower than 30° head elevation
METABOLIC	
Hyperglycemia	Underlying diabetes, sepsis, stress, intolerance to infusion rate
Hypokalemia	Concurrent diuretic, insulin, or antibiotic therapy
Hyperkalemia	Metabolic acidosis, renal insufficiency, excessive potassium in formula
Hypernatremia, dehydration	Insufficient water (especially if hyperosmolar, high-protein formulas are used)

Complications of Tube Feeding

Many of the complications of tube feedings are preventable through appropriate selection of formula and tubes, proper administration, and frequent monitoring. Complications may be mechanical and metabolic and may affect the gastrointestinal and respiratory systems (Table 27-1).[5,9,18,43,55]

A common complication is tube clogging as a result of inadequate flushing or improper administration of medication. Several commonly administered medications may occlude tubes if administered improperly (Table 27-2).[1] Patency of clogged tubes can often be restored by irrigating the tube with carbonated beverages, such as colas and ginger ale.

Home Enteral Therapy

An estimated 52,000 patients per year receive enteral nutrition at home.[20] Patients with advanced head and neck cancer are frequently candidates for home enteral support. In one study, home enteral nutrition was given for a median of 94 days, resulting in stable nutritional indices for the patients studied.[10]

Once it is determined that a patient needs enteral therapy and discharge is anticipated, the patient is assessed. A caregiver is selected if the patient is unable to perform self-care. The capabilities of the caregiver are assessed, the home environment is discussed, and the caregiver is trained until he or she can independently care for the tube-fed patient. Home supervised visits may also be conducted, and occasionally tube feedings are initiated in the home. General care of the tube-fed patient at home includes tube care, feeding, and assessment of complications and goal achievement (see box on p. 651).[79]

Parenteral Nutrition

Parenteral nutrition therapy supplies all of the essential nutrients by means of the intravenous route. Parenteral therapy may be called hyperalimentation and may be partial or total. Many patients receive partial parenteral nutrition in the form of dextrose solutions as part of their usual care. Total parenteral nutrition (TPN) supplies all of the daily requirements for protein and calories directly into the bloodstream. Parenteral nutrition is indicated for patients who have totally nonfunctioning gastrointestinal tracts, require bowel rest, or are intolerant of enteral therapy. Cancers of the GI tract and related obstructions are often indications for TPN. Because absorption of nutrients is impaired in such cases, TPN is often the only option available. The effects of cancer therapy, including radiation enteritis and intractable diarrhea, are also indications for TPN, as are other diagnoses.[19,23,35] See box on p. 651.

The delivery routes for TPN are peripheral and central veins. Peripheral administration of TPN solutions is accomplished by using the veins of the arm. The external jugular vein in the neck may also be used. With the peripheral route, the following should be considered[26,72]:

Table 27–2 Compatibility of Tube Feeding Products with Commonly Employed Drug Additives

Product Name, Manufacturer, Dose	pH of Product	pH of Mixtures	Compatibility of Mixtures	Comments
GASTROINTESTINAL AGENTS				
Donnatal Elixir, A.H. Robins, 10 ml	4.8-4.9	6.2-6.7	C	
Docusate Sodium (DDS), Lederle, 15 ml	6.2	6.4-6.7	C	
Lomotil Liquid, Searle, 5 ml	3.3-3.4	6.1-6.5	C	
Phenobarbital Elixir, Parke-Davis, 5 ml	6.5	6.5-6.7	C	
COUGH AND COLD PREPARATIONS				
Actifed Syrup, Burroughs Wellcome, 5 ml	5.6	6.2-6.4	C	
Benadryl Elixir, Parke-Davis, 10 ml	5.2	6.4-6.5	C	
Benylin DM Syrup, Parke-Davis, 10 ml	4.8-4.9	5.7-5.9	C	
Dimetane Elixir, A.H. Robins, 10 ml	2.7-2.8	5.2-5.4	Id Ce	Adhesive gelatinous material forms that clogs feeding tubes.
Dimetapp Elixir, A.H. Robins, 10 ml	2.6-2.7	5.1-5.3	I Ce	Enteral foods show some breakdown. Problem can be minimized by slow addition of elixir with stirring.
Phenergan Syrup, Wyeth, 10 ml	5.1-5.3	5.4-6.0	C	
Robitussin Expectorant, A.H. Robins, 10 ml	2.6	3.8-4.2	I Ce	Viscous flocculent precipitate forms capable of clogging feeding tubes.
Sudafed Syrup, Burroughs Wellcome, 10 ml	2.5	4.5-4.8	I Ce	Viscous, somewhat gelatinous mass forms instantly upon mixing.
Terpin Hydrate Elixir, Barre Lab, 10 ml	6.4-6.6	6.5-6.8	C	
Tylenol Elixir, McNeil, 10 ml	4.7	6.0-6.3	C	
ANTIPSYCHOTIC AGENTS				
Haldol Drops, McNeil, 1 ml	3.2-3.4	5.5-5.7	C	
Mellaril Oral Solution, Sandoz, 5 ml	3.8	5.5-5.9	I Ce	2-ml (200-mg) dose causes granulation of four enteral products studied at mixing interface. These granules clog feeding tubes.
Sinequan Concentrate, Pfizer, 2 ml	5.7	6.2-6.3	C	Although contrast light shows some particle growth, it is generally compatible with four enteral products studied.
Thorazine Concentrate, Smith, Kline & French, 1 ml	3.0	5.5-6.0	I Ce	Some particle growth and granulation at point of mixing may clog feeding tubes.

C, compatible; *Ce,* compatible with vital; *I,* incompatible; *Id,* physically incompatible.   *Continued.*

- Peripheral administration provides limited calories, generally fewer than 2500 kcal/day, as well as a limited amount of protein, less than 100 grams per day.
- Solutions administered peripherally can be very irritating to the vein, especially if dextrose is more than 10%.
- Solutions may be stopped quickly; tapering and weaning are not needed.

- Peripheral administration is useful for short-term nutritional support.

Administration of TPN via the central route is done using a central venous access device placed into a major vein such as the superior vena cava. Central venous access devices used for TPN include ports; triple lumen catheters; Broviac, Hickman, and Groshong catheters; and occasionally Swan-Ganz lines.[7,73] With the central route, the following should be considered:

Table 27–2 Compatibility of Tube Feeding Products with Commonly Employed Drug Additives—cont'd

Product Name, Manufacturer, Dose	pH of Product	pH of Mixtures	Compatibility of Mixtures	Comments
ANTIBACTERIAL AGENTS				
Bactrim DS Suspension, Roche, 10 ml	5.6-5.7	6.0-6.2	C	Slight increase in viscosity occurs when mixed with small volumes of enteral products.
Gantrisin Suspension, Roche, 10 ml	5.1	5.5-5.8	C	Some viscous drag is noted when mixed with small volumes of four enteral products studied.
Mandelamine Suspension, Forte, Parke-Davis, 1 ml	Oil base	Oil base	I	Mixtures become tacky and somewhat gelatinous (obvious signs of oil synuresis).
Pen-Vee K, Wyeth, 5 ml	6.5	6.5-6.6	C	pH of enteral product and penicillin VK are identical, favoring both chemical and physical stability.
E.E.S. Granules, Abbott, 5 ml	7.6	6.7-6.8	C	Slight increase in viscosity occurs when mixed with a small volume of enteral product.
Keflex Suspension, Dista, 5 ml	4.0-4.2	6.2-6.3	C	Vigorous stirring and slow addition of suspension are suggested.
Polymox Suspension, Bristol, 5 ml	5.6-5.7	6.3-6.4	C	Distributes uniformly with no phase separation or granulation.
MISCELLANEOUS AGENTS				
Feosol Elixir, Menley & James, 5 ml	2.2	3.3-3.7	I Ce	Completely jelling and clogging of feeding tubes results. Crushed iron tablets also present some problems unless well diluted.
KayCiel Elixir, Berlex, 15 ml	6.2	6.2-6.6	C	Product mixes readily with enteral products studied.
KCL Liquid, Barre	4.1 (10%) 3.6 (20%)	6.2 5.5	I I	Products found to be incompatible at mixing interface. Extent of incompatibility can be minimized by adding slowly and mixing vigorously.
Dilantin Suspension, Parke-Davis, 5 ml	4.9	5.5-6.0	C	Slight increase in viscosity occurs when mixed with small volumes of enteral products studied.
Lanoxin Elixir, Burroughs Wellcome, 2 ml	7.0	6.5-6.8	C	Product is compatible upon mixing. If permitted to remain 24-48 hours, rubbery mass results.

C, compatible; Ce, compatible with vital; I, incompatible; Id, physically incompatible.

- Central administration can provide a large amount of calories and protein.
- Final dextrose concentrations can be as high as 35% and final amino acid concentrations can be more than 5%.
- These solutions cannot be discontinued suddenly. Abrupt cessation may induce profound hypoglycemia. Tapering down the rate and concentration is the most effective method for discontinuation.

COMPONENTS OF PARENTERAL NUTRITION. The three main components of total parenteral nutrition (TPN) are glucose, amino acids, and fats. The glucose content of TPN, usually in the form of dextrose 50%, provides both immediate and long-term energy. Amino acids or proteins are provided with or without electrolytes and are usually ordered in concentrations of 5.5% or 8.5%. The lower concentration is indicated for patients with hepatic or renal dysfunction or failure. Administration of fats with TPN is required because the TPN solution stimulates the production of insulin, which in turn prevents fat from being metabolized. A fatty acid deficiency may result. Fat is provided through intralipids, usually in a concentration of 10% or 20%, and may be piggybacked or added to the TPN solution. Exact formulations are specific to the patient; they depend on individual requirements, tolerances, body chemistry, and disease processes (Table 27-3).

A TPN formula that combines the dextrose, amino acids, and fat emulsion in one container is often called a three-in-one or total nutrient admixture. Eliminating the need for piggybacking lipids allows for a closed system that reduces the risk of infection, minimizes

central venous catheter inserted. The additional lumens provide access for drug administration and blood sampling. Patients with single-lumen catheters who require medications must either have the line flushed before and after administration of medication or have the medication added to the TPN bag.[7,75] Several drugs have been tested to be compatible with TPN formulas for at least 12 hours.[28,31,32] See box on p. 653.

Administration of Parenteral Nutrition

Total parenteral solutions may be given continuously or by cycling. Cycling is most often used for patients receiving TPN at home during the night because it allows them to be mobile during the day. The disadvantage of cycling TPN is that patients must be able to tolerate a high-volume load. Cyclic TPN may be increased slowly at the start and then tapered at the end of the cycle. Programmable pumps are widely used to prevent or minimize hyperglycemia and hypoglycemia as blood sugars rise and fall. Compact, portable TPN pumps are also available with programmable functions. The portable pump, worn in a backpack-type carrying bag, is best suited for the ambulatory patient.

Patients requiring long-term parenteral nutrition face different challenges than those needing TPN for only a short time. Long-term therapy is most often accomplished in the home; the patient or designated caregiver performs many of the procedures.[64] Patients must be motivated to receive TPN at home and must be able to provide competent self-care. Assessment of capabilities before implementing home TPN is critical, because many patients are extremely anxious about performing highly technical procedures. Usually anxiety resolves with education and time.

Many patients note an altered self-image with long-term TPN. Their self-perceptions are undermined by being underweight or even cachexic, and this is compounded by the presence of a central venous access device connected to the TPN formula and equipment. Sleep disturbance may be induced by depressive illness, anxiety, nocturnal urination, and occasionally pump alarms.

When TPN is given to those requiring complete bowel rest, the absence of food intake may be traumatic. Eating is a major social and cultural event, and prohibiting food for several weeks disrupts the patient's life.

Patients may voice concerns about the cost of total parenteral therapy. Although usually covered by insurance and Medicare, home TPN may cost $400 or more per day. In the hospital TPN is a third more costly, and long-term inpatient TPN is financially prohibitive. Often the patient is facing loss of income because of cancer and its treatment and may incur

manipulations, and cuts waste. Often three-in-one solutions are ordered for patients receiving TPN at home because they are convenient and easy to administer. If lipids are piggybacked, TPN is generally given two to three times per week.[11,28]

Many patients receiving TPN have a multilumen

Table 27–3   Adult and Pediatric Parenteral Solution Formulas

ADULT

Base solution

40%-50% dextrose in water	500 ml
8.5%-10% crystalline amino acids	500 ml

Additives to each unit

Sodium chloride, acetate, or lactate	40-50 ml
Potassium chloride	20-30 mEq
Potassium acid phosphate (10-20 mM phosphorus)	15-30 mEq
Magnesium sulfate	15-18 mEq
Multivitamin infusion	10 ml
A	3,300 IU
D	200 IU
E	10 IU
Ascorbic acid	100 mg
Folic acid	400 μg
Niacin	40 mg
Riboflavin	3.6 mg
Thiamine	3 mg
B_6 (pyridoxine)	4 mg
B_{12} (cyanocobalamin)	5 μg
Pantothenic acid	15 mg
Biotin	60 μg

Additive to any one unit twice weekly

Vitamin K	10 mg

Intravenous fat emulsion 10% or 20%

500 ml 2-7 times weekly	50-100 gm
Carbohydrate calories	850 kcal
Protein calories	150 kcal
Fat calories	1000-2000 kcal
Nitrogen	6.5-8 gm
Amino acids	40-50 gm

PEDIATRIC

Base solution

40% dextrose in water	500 ml
8.5% crystalline amino acids	500 ml

Additives to each unit

Sodium chloride	25-30 mEq
Potassium acid phosphate	30-40 mEq
Magnesium sulfate	12-15 mEq
Calcium gluconate	25-35 mEq
Multivitamin infusion	
A	0.07 mg
D	10 μg
E	7 mg
K	200 μg
Ascorbic acid	80 mg
Folic acid	140 μg
Niacinamide	17 mg
Riboflavin	1.4 mg
Thiamine	1.2 mg
B_6 (pyridoxine)	1 mg
B_{12} (cyanocobalamin)	1 μg
Dexpanthenol	7 mg
Biotin	20 μg
Intravenous fat emulsion 10%, 3-7 times weekly	50-75 ml/kg

INFUSION RATE

	115 ml/kg/day
	115 kcal/kg/day
	3 g protein/kg/day

DRUGS TESTED TO BE COMPATIBLE WITH TOTAL PARENTERAL NUTRITION FORMULAS FOR AT LEAST 12 HOURS

Aminophylline
Antibiotics
  Cephalothin
  Clindamycin
  Erythromycin
  Gentamicin
  Methicillin
  Oxacillin
  Penicillin G
  Tetracycline
  Tobramycin
Antineoplastics
  Cyclophosphamide
  Cytarabine
  Fluorouracil
  Methotrexate
Corticosteroids
H_2 Receptor antagonists
  Cimetidine
  Ranitidine
Heparin
Insulin
Iron dextran
Metoclopramide hydrochloride
Narcotic analgesics
  Hydromorphone
  Meperidine
  Morphine

---

large medical bills. Patients with limited financial resources may find that anxiety related to the cost of care compounds the adjustment process.

An assessment of the patient's life-style, home environment, family and support systems, body image, and perceptions about TPN should be conducted when it is started. During hospitalization frequent assessments are needed to assist in identifying patients who are candidates for TPN at home.[44]

MONITORING THE PATIENT AND COMPLICATIONS OF THERAPY.   Patients beginning TPN must be monitored frequently to assess side effects and complications of the treatment. Daily monitoring of vital signs, weight, and lab values may indicate metabolic changes requiring the adjustment of TPN formula or its rate of administration. The metabolic and technical problems sometimes associated with TPN are numerous. Some are related to the insertion of the central venous access device. Other problems include electrolyte imbalance, infection, and volume overload (Table 27-4). With frequent monitoring by an experienced staff or well-educated patient performing self-care, the risk of complications is greatly reduced.

HOME PARENTERAL NUTRITION.   Since the late 1960s total parenteral nutrition has been administered successfully in patients' homes. It is estimated that 3000 patients currently receive home TPN, and increased growth is predicted as technologic advances continue.[27] Even in rural areas, home parenteral nutrition has become commonplace.[58] Home TPN has been particularly beneficial for pediatric oncology patients.[4]

Screening patients for home TPN includes assessment of the home environment, availability of a caregiver, learning abilities or disabilities, physical limitations, and motivation to learn procedures. Ideally,

education of the caregiver is begun before discharge. Teaching sessions over several days are best for teaching the complex procedures of administration of home TPN. See box on p. 654. Provision of a take-home booklet is recommended and return demonstrations performed by the caregiver are often beneficial. One key aspect of at-home care is assessment of the central venous access device and dressing change procedure.[62]

Infectious complications of long-term central venous catheters include infections of the tunnel and exit site, catheter related bacteremia, and septic thrombophlebitis.[17] There is currently lack of standardization of dressing change procedures in the home setting. One recent study suggests that transparent dressings on central venous catheters were associated with an increased risk of catheter tip infection.[37] Astute assessment and meticulous dressing change technique by the care giver minimize this complication.[12,68]

Follow-up visits in the home are essential. Although many patients may appear quite competent in the hospital, a home visit assures that procedures are followed appropriately. A home assessment also provides the opportunity to determine whether TPN formulas and supplies are stored correctly and whether infection control measures are observed. See Chapter 26.

Patients vary in the number of teaching sessions and follow-up visits required to assess compliance. Many need a visiting nurse for blood sampling and monitoring on a schedule. The frequency of clinic visits for evaluation by the physician varies according to the patient's needs; it ranges from once a week to every 6 months.

ETHICAL CONSIDERATIONS

Recently, increased attention has been given to evaluating the use of supportive nutritional therapies. The widespread use of home parenteral therapy has raised several ethical issues, including potential overutilization and inequitable access since it is the well-insured patient that primarily receives TPN.[33,49] The use of inpatient TPN has also come under scrutiny. Preoperative TPN in well nourished patients appears to be unwarranted at this time; however, efficacy of preoperative TPN in malnourished surgical patients has been established.[15] Further research is needed to determine how nutritional support influences nutritional status, abnormal host metabolism, gastrointestinal symptoms, and/or tumor growth.[16]

Nutritional support of the terminally ill patient with cancer remains controversial. Frequently, family members insist on feeding their loved one. Nurses should advocate for the patient by teaching that loss of appetite often occurs.[3,69] Nursing interventions

Table 27–4 Common Complications of Parenteral Nutrition

Complication	Etiology
NONMETABOLIC	
Allergy or sensitivity	Sensitivity to either the amino acid solution or the lipid emulsion
Infection	Catheter-related sepsis
Volume overload	Improper pump rate
Catheter placement	Puncture of or injury to nearby organs or vessels
Pneumothorax	
Arterial puncture	
Hematoma	
Thoracic duct puncture	
Brachial plexus injury	
Pulmonary embolism	
METABOLIC	
Hyperglycemia/Hyperosmolarity	Inability to metabolize high glucose concentration of formula
Hypoglycemia	When TPN is abruptly discontinued, high insulin levels cause rebound drop in blood sugar
Vitamin or mineral deficiencies	Administration of formulas lacking sufficient vitamins or micronutrients
Fatty acid deficiencies or overload	Insufficient or excessive administration of lipids
Hyponatremia	Formulas without sufficient sodium content
Hypokalemia, hyperkalemia	Insufficient or excessive potassium content
Hypocalcemia, hypercalcemia	Insufficient or excessive calcium content
Hypomagnesemia	Insufficient magnesium or increased metabolism of magnesium

---

CARE OF THE PATIENT RECEIVING PARENTERAL NUTRITION AT HOME

Catheter care
1. Change dressing and assess venous access device per frequency ordered by physician or institution or agency policy.
2. Flush with saline or heparin if cyclic schedule.

Preparation of medication
1. Inject additives (that is, vitamins) into pre-mixed bags.
2. Assemble bag and connect tubing.

Operation of equipment
1. Connect and disconnect pump.
2. Program pump if cyclic schedule or enter rate, volume, and other data.
3. Perform equipment troubleshooting.

Assessment of complications
1. Assess for electrolyte imbalance and presence of hyperglycemia.
2. Observe feet and fingers for edema.
3. Monitor temperature and urine for sugar and acetone.

Assessment of goal achievement
1. Weigh daily or every other day.

---

should be directed at structural or functional deficits, such as stomatitis, nausea and vomiting, and then managing concurrent but exacerbating symptoms like fatigue and dyspnea.[22] The use of intravenous hydration may be helpful in loosening pulmonary secretions, decreasing gastric secretions, and correcting fluid and electrolyte imbalances in select patients. However, the potential benefits of intravenous hydration must be carefully weighed against the potential risk of infection, the effect of the therapy on the patient's quality of life, and the cost of intravenous therapy.

Termination of nutritional support should occur when the patient, family, physician, and nurse judge that the patient no longer benefits from the nutritional support.[2,39,47] The decision must be made in accordance with accepted community standards of care and in compliance with applicable law.[2]

More than half of all patients with malignant disease eventually try unorthodox treatment. Nutritional therapies are often used, particularly by patients with advanced disease.[13] On-going communication with patients and their families about nutritional concerns is essential.

CONCLUSION

Cancer and its treatment affect nutritional status to varying degrees. Patients with local and systemic effects require ongoing assessment and prompt intervention. Nutritional support ranges in complexity depending on needs, and those needs change over time. Oral supplementation, the simplest type of support, is most effective when the patient is highly motivated, has manageable or temporary side effects, and can ingest and digest nutrients. Enteral and parenteral nutrition may be required for individuals with more severe symptoms and for those with demonstrated physical impairments of the gastrointestinal tract. In

Nursing Management

The additional nursing interventions listed below can be made depending on the specific alteration in intake or digestive abilities.

NURSING DIAGNOSES AND SUGGESTIONS FOR DIETARY MODIFICATIONS FOR COMMON PROBLEMS THAT MAY AFFECT INTAKE
- Nutrition, alterations in: less than body requirements related to:

Taste/olfactory changes
Use tart food to stimulate taste buds.
Use extra seasoning.
Try sauces and flavor additives.
Substitute fish and chicken for red meat.

Dysphagia
Eat soft or liquid foods.
Use sauces and gravies.
Eat small meals frequently.
If eating is painful, eat bland foods.

Dyspepsia
Avoid fatty and spicy foods.
Avoid gas-producing foods.
Use antacids.
Avoid lying down after meals.

Anorexia
Vary surroundings.
Eat with family and friends.
Try new foods and recipes.
Use smaller plates.
Eat high-calorie snacks.
Drink high-protein shakes.
Try hard candy.
Use distraction: radio, TV, etc.

Gastrointestinal mucositis
Avoid acidic fruits and juices.
Eat cool foods.
Use a topical analgesic before eating.

Nausea and vomiting
Drink clear liquids and advance diet as tolerated.
Drink flat beverages.
Avoid sweet, rich, and fatty foods.
Try dry foods (toast, crackers).
Try easily digested foods (rice).
Avoid food odors.
Eat cool foods.
Eat small, frequent meals.
Use antiemetics 30 minutes before meals.

- Elimination, alterations in: related to:

Dumping syndrome
Avoid fatty foods.
Avoid concentrated foods.
Eat small, frequent meals.
Drink liquids 30 minutes before and after meals.

Constipation
Drink adequate fluids.
Eat high-fiber foods.
Exercise regularly.
Avoid cheese and concentrated foods.

Diarrhea
Drink adequate amounts of fluid.
Drink fluids providing electrolytes.
Avoid milk products.
Avoid fatty, gas-producing foods.
Avoid high-fiber foods.
Eat high-potassium foods.

spite of their complexity, enteral and parenteral nutrition are commonly administered in the home, with family members as care givers. Advances in home therapies and nutritional support have enabled individuals with cancer and nutritional deficiencies to remain at home and have promoted an improved quality of life.

BIBLIOGRAPHY
1. Altman E and Cutie AJ: Compatibility of enteral products with commonly employed drug additives, Nutr Supp Serv 4:8, 1984.
2. American Society for Parenteral and Enteral Nutrition: Standards for home nutrition support, Nutr Clin Pract 7(2):65, 1992.
3. Barnie DC: Percutaneous endoscopic gastrostomy tubes: the nurse's role in a moral, ethical, and legal dilemma, Gastroenterol Nurse 12:250, 1990.
4. Bendorf K and Meehan J: Home parenteral nutrition for the child with cancer, Issues Compr Pediatr Nurs 12:171, 1989.
5. Benya R and Mobarhan S: Enteral alimentation: administration and complications, J Am Coll Nutr 10:209, 1991.
6. Beutler B: Cachexia: a basic biochemical mechanism, Nutrition 5:129, 1989.

7. Brendel V: Catheters utilized in delivering total parenteral nutrition, NITA 7:488, 1984.

8. Brennan MF: Nutritional support. In DeVita VT, Hellman S, and Rosenberg SA, editors: Cancer: principles and practice of oncology, Philadelphia, 1985, JB Lippincott Co.

9. Campbell SM: Adult enteral nutrition. In Young LY and Koda-Kimble MA, editors: Applied therapeutics: the clinical use of drugs, Vancouver, Washington, 1988, Applied Therapeutics, Inc.

10. Campos AC, Butters M, and Meguid MM: Home enteral nutrition via gastrostomy in advanced head and neck cancer patients, Head Neck 12(2):137, 1990.

11. Campos AC, Paluzzi M, and Meguid MM: Clinical use of total nutrient admixtures, Nutrition 6:347, 1990.

12. Capka MB and others: Nursing observations of central venous catheters. The effect on patient outcome, J Intrav Nurs 14:243, 1991.

13. Cassileth BR and Berlyne D: Counseling the cancer patient who wants to try unorthodox or questionable therapies, Oncology 3(4):29, 1989.

14. Chandra RK: Protein-energy malnutrition and immunological responses, J Nutr 122(3 suppl):597, 1992.

15. Chen MK, Souba WW, and Copeland EM: Nutritional support of the surgical oncology patient, Hematol Oncol Clin North Am 5:125, 1991.

16. Chlebowski RT: Nutritional support of the medical oncology patient, Hematol Oncol Clin North Am 5:147, 1991.

17. Clarke DE and Raffin TA: Infectious complications of indwelling long-term central venous catheters, Chest 97:966, 1990.

18. Cogen R and Weinryb J: Aspiration pneumonia in nursing home patients fed via gastrostomy tubes, Am J Gastroenterol 84:1509, 1989.

19. Copeland EM: Total parenteral nutrition in the cancer patient: the present as viewed from the past, Nutrition 6(4 suppl):2, 1990.

20. Crocker KS: Planning for home parenteral and enteral nutrition, Continuing Care 8:18, 1989.

21. Curtas S and others: Bacteriological safety of closed enteral nutrition delivery systems, Nutrition 7:340, 1991.

22. D'Agostino NS: Managing nutritional problems in advanced cancer, Am J Nurs 89(1):50, 1989.

23. Daly JM and others: Nutritional support of patients with cancer of the gastrointestinal tract, Surg Clin North Am 71:523, 1991.

24. Davies L and Knutson KC: Warning signals for malnutrition in the elderly, J Am Diet Assoc 91:1413, 1991.

25. Dreizen S and others: Nutritional deficiencies in patients receiving cancer chemotherapy, Postgrad Med 87:163, 1990.

26. Drescher M: Advances in peripheral vein nutrition, NITA 6:533, 1985.

27. Dudrick SJ and others: 100 patient years of ambulatory home total parenteral nutrition, Ann Surg 199:770, 1984.

28. Ebbert-Sauer ML: Adult parenteral nutrition. In Young LY and Koda-Kimble MA, editors: Applied therapeutics: the clinical use of drugs, Vancouver, Washington, 1988, Applied Therapeutics, Inc.

29. Eisenberg PG: Pulmonary complications from enteral nutrition, Crit Care Nurse Clin North Am 3:641, 1991.

30. Fay DE and others: Long-term enteral feeding: a retrospective comparison of delivery via percutaneous endoscopic gastrostomy and nasoenteric tubes, Am J Gastroenterol 86:1604, 1991.

31. Filibeck D: A review of the stability and compatibility problems associated with total parenteral nutrition solutions, Nutr Supp Serv 5:67, 1985.

32. Frey AM: Taking the confusion out of multiple infusion: IV medications and TPN, NITA 6:460, 1986.

33. Fry ST: Ethical issues in total parenteral nutrition, Nutrition 6:329, 1990.

34. Fry ST: Ethical aspects of decision-making in the feeding of cancer patients, Semin Oncol Nurs 2:59, 1986.

35. Grant JP: Proper use and recognized role of TPN in the cancer patient, Nutrition 6(4 suppl):6, 1990.

36. Groenwald S: Nutritional disorders. In Groenwald S, editor: Cancer nursing: principles and practice, Boston, ed 2, 1990, Jones & Bartlett, Inc.

37. Hoffman KK and others: Transparent polyurethane film as an intravenous catheter dressing. A meta-analysis of the infection risks, JAMA 267:2072, 1992.

38. Horwath CC: Nutrition goals for older adults: a review, Gerontologist 31:811, 1991.

39. Jansson L and Norberg A: Ethical reasoning concerning the feeding of terminally ill cancer patients. Interviews with registered nurses experienced in the care of cancer patients, Cancer Nurs 12:352, 1989.

40. Jeejeebhoy KN, Detsky AS, and Baker JP: Assessment of nutritional status, J Parenter Enteral Nutr 14(5 suppl):193, 1990.

41. Johnson J and others: Reducing the negative impact of radiation therapy on functional status, Cancer 61:46, 1988.

42. Kittelberger-Bockus SB, Cataldo CB, and Steinbaugh ML: Tube feedings: clinical application, Columbus, 1986, Ross Laboratories.

43. Kohn CL and Keithley JK: Enteral nutrition. Potential complications and patient monitoring, Nurs Clin North Am 24:339, 1989.

44. Koithan M: Home total parenteral nutrition complications, NITA 8:231, 1985.

45. Lehmann S: Immune function and nutrition. The clinical role of the intravenous nurse, J Intraven Nurs 14:406, 1991.

46. Lesko LM: Psychosocial issues in the diagnosis and management of cancer cachexia and anorexia, Nutrition 5:114, 1989.

47. Lin EM: Nutrition support. Making the difficult decisions, Cancer Nurs 14:261, 1991.

48. Lindsey AM: Cancer cachexia: effects of the disease and its treatment, Semin Oncol Nurs 2:19, 1986.

49. Mahmood T and Rubin AD: Home-based intravenous therapy for oncology patients, N J Med 89(1):43, 1992.

50. Meguid MM, Eldar S, and Wahba A: The delivery of nutritional support: a potpourri of new devices and methods, Cancer 55:279, 1985.

51. Metheny NM: Twenty ways to prevent tube-feeding complications, Nursing 85(15):47, 1985.

52. Monturo CA: Enteral access device and selection, Nutr Clin Pract 5(5):207, 1990.

53. Morley JE: Anorexia in older patients: its meaning and management, Geriatrics 45(12):59, 1990.

54. Muggia-Sullam M and others: Postoperative enteral versus parenteral nutrition support in gastrointestinal surgery, Am J Surg 49:106, 1985.

55. Mullan H, Roubenoff RA, and Roubenoff R: Risk of pulmonary aspiration among patients receiving enteral nutrition support, J Parenter Enteral Nutr 16:160, 1992.

56. Murphy JI: Tube feeding problems and solutions, Adv Clin Care 5(2):7, 1990.

57. Murphy LM and Lipman TO: Central venous catheter care in parenteral nutrition: a review, J Parenter Enteral Nutr 11:190, 1987.

58. Murray ND and Vanderhoof JA: Home TPN in sparsely populated areas, Nutr Clin Pract 4(2):62, 1989.

59. Nahikian-Nelms ML: General feeding problems. In Bloch AS, editor: Nutrition management of the cancer patient, Rockville, Maryland, 1990, Aspen Publishers, Inc.

60. Padilla GV: Gastrointestinal side effects and quality of life in patients receiving radiation therapy, Nutrition 6:367, 1990.

61. Pisters KM and Kris MG: Management of nausea and vomiting caused by anticancer drugs: state of the art, Oncology 6(2 suppl):99, 1992.

62. Ponsksy JL and others: Percutaneous approaches to enteral alimentation, Am J Surg 149:102, 1985.

63. Rhodus NL and Brown J: The association of xerostomia and inadequate intake in older adults, J Am Diet Assoc 90:1688, 1990.

64. Ricour C: Home TPN, Nutrition 5:345, 1989.

65. Robuck JT and Fleetwood JB: Nutritional support of the patient with cancer, Focus on Crit Care 19(2):129, 1992.

66. Roe DA: Geriatric nutrition, Clin Geriatr Med 6:319, 1990.

67. Ropka ME: Nutrition. In Johnson BL and Gross J, editors: Handbook of oncology nursing, New York, 1985, John Wiley & Sons.

68. Segura M and Sitges-Serra A: Clinical predictors of infection of central venous catheters used for parenteral nutrition, Infect Control Hosp Epidemiol 12:407, 1991.

69. Stephany TM: Nutrition for the terminally ill, Home Healthc Nurse 9(3):48, 1991.

70. Strohl RA: The nursing role in radiation oncology: symptom management of acute and chronic reactions, Oncol Nurs Forum 15:429, 1988.

71. Tchekmedyian NS, Hickman M, and Heber D: Treatment of anorexia and weight loss with megestrol acetate in patients with cancer or acquired immunodeficiency syndrome, Semin Oncol 18(1 suppl 2):35, 1991.

72. Timmer JG: Use of peripheral veins for TPN, Nutrition 5:346, 1989.

73. Viall CD: Daily access of implanted venous ports. Implications for patient education, J Intrav Nurs 13:294, 1990.

74. Vokes TJ and Robertson GL: Disorders of antidiuretic hormone, Endocrinol Metab Clin North Am 17:281, 1988.

75. Watson D: Piggyback compatibility of antibiotics with pediatric parenteral nutrition solutions, J Parenter Enteral Nutr 9:220, 1985.

76. Williams EF and Meguid MM: Nutritional concepts and considerations in head and neck surgery, Head Neck 11:393, 1989.

77. Wilmore DW: Catabolic illness. Strategies for enhancing recovery, N Engl J Med 325:695, 1991.

78. Wright B and Robinson L: Enteral feeding tubes as drug delivery systems, Nutr Supp Serv 6:33, 1986.

79. Young CK and White S: Preparing patients for tube feeding at home, Am J Nurs 92(4):46, 1992.

CHAPTER 28

Pain Management

Carol J. Swenson

Pain has an element of blank;
It cannot recollect
When it began, or if there were
A day when it was not.

"Pain Has an Element of Blank"
Emily Dickinson

Nurses play a major role in the successful management of the person who is experiencing cancer pain by preventing the situation of pain that Emily Dickinson describes — to not be able to remember when the pain was not there. One of the Oncology Nursing Society's Position Statements on Cancer Pain is that **"NURSES ARE RESPONSIBLE AND ACCOUNTABLE FOR IMPLEMENTATION AND COORDINATION OF THE PLAN FOR MANAGEMENT OF CANCER PAIN."**[70] In all health care settings this is important, because the nurse is the professional person who most often conducts the assessment on an on-going basis and therefore can determine whether the pain has increased, whether side effects are being managed effectively and, most importantly, whether the patient and family are satisfied with the pain relief provided. Nurses must accept the responsibility and accountability for the plan of care in the management of cancer pain.

With the pharmacologic agents and technology currently available, it is unfortunate when untreated cancer pain causes patients to suffer unnecessarily. Levy[41] states that 90% to 99% of pain can be relieved in the highly-controlled settings of hospices or palliative care units, yet the question remains whether medications and technology are being adequately used to control cancer pain. Pain affects a person's sleeping pattern, family, work, and social relation-ships. Ultimately, it affects a patient's quality of life and possibly the will to live.

DEFINITIONS

Pain—"Whatever the experiencing person says it is, existing whenever the experiencing person says it does"[45] is the most global and client-centered pain description. The American Pain Society[5] and the ONS Position Paper on Pain[69] both use Merskey's definition of pain as "an unpleasant sensory and emotional experience associated with actual or potential tissue damage, or described in terms of such damage.[54] From these two descriptions of pain, it becomes apparent that pain is multidimensional and subjective. Because pain is a subjective experience, *the patient is the only authority* on its existence — not the health professional.

Other definitions that assist in the understanding of the pain experience are suffering, tolerance, addiction, and dependence.

Suffering—an experience, either physical or mental, that the person dislikes (e.g., adversity, agony, anguish, torment, trouble). Suffering is more global than pain, because pain implies only the physical sphere whereas suffering may be spiritual, emotional, or social as well as physical. Suffering is distinct from pain and can occur with or without the presence of pain.

Drug tolerance—the involuntary need for increasing doses of analgesic to achieve the same level of pain relief. The actual incidence of tolerance is not known and many people will never develop it. When an increase of medication is required, it is most often an event of disease progression,[29] but tolerance must be considered. The use of non-opioids together with opioids will help to delay the possible onset of tolerance. Weissman and colleagues[82] state that "tolerance will develop more rapidly following IV or intraspinal administration than after oral or rectal administration." When drug tolerance develops, first there is a decreased duration of relief, then decreased level of pain relief. If tolerance is suspected, the person can be switched to another opioid. When switching to another opioid, use one third to one half of the equianalgesic dose because cross-tolerance between narcotics is incomplete and the person may otherwise be overmedicated.[5]

Addiction—the use of narcotics for the psychological euphoric effect and *not* for the analgesic effect; there is overwhelming involvement with obtaining and using drugs for other than approved medical reasons. Addiction as a result of medically prescribed narcotics is rare (<1:1000). Porter and Jick[62] report that of 11,882 hospitalized patients who had received at least one opioid injection during hospitalization there were only four cases of documented addiction in patients with no previous history of addiction.

Most often health care professionals overestimate the incidence of addiction following prescribed opioids for medical purposes. Keep in mind that the lay public are often also frightened of potential addiction and need education of the appropriate use of opioids and assurance that addiction is a nonissue in cancer pain management.

Physical dependence—the body's adaptation to the use of opioids without which abstinence syndrome (or withdrawal symptoms) will occur based on physiologic changes.

The person with cancer who is on opioids for longer than 3 to 4 weeks will be physically dependent, but is not addicted.[5,78] The physically dependent person will not have the craving for the euphoric effect and will not be engaging in drug-seeking behaviors. (See "Decreasing Doses", p. 667 for directions on "weaning" the physically dependent person from opioids.)

According to McCaffery's definition, nurses must believe every patient who says that he or she has pain in order not to inadvertently miss treatment of pain. Lack of observable pain does not mean lack of pain.

THEORIES OF PAIN

In the past, theories of pain were developed due to the lack of the capability to determine precisely what occurs physiologically during the pain experience. Some of the past theories were:

- *Specificity*—The intensity of nociceptive stimulus and perception of pain are directly correlated and travel along specific pathways from the pain receptors to the spinal cord.
- *Gate control theory*—Nociceptive impulses are transmitted via the spinothalamic tract but can be modulated in the spinal cord, brainstem, or cerebral cortex. Two types of afferent fibers have been identified: thinly myelinated A-delta fibers and unmyelinated C fibers. The substantia gelatinosa in the dorsal horn of the spinal cord is the proposed site of the "gating" mechanism. McGuire and Sheidler[51] state that "activity in the large fibers can 'open' the gate, while activity in the small fibers can 'close' it." Melzack and Wall, as well as others, have modified their theory over the past 25 years.[51]
- *Endorphins and enkephalins*—in the mid-1970s these "morphine within" opioid-like in the brain and spinal cord were discovered.

Today, studies are involved with the exact physiology of pain and people are researching the neurodynamics of pain. Paice[59] writes of "unraveling the mystery of pain" and describes the primary afferent fibers, dorsal horn of the spinal cord, spinothalamic tract, cortex, and modulatory systems and their interactions in the transmission and interpretation of pain.

Science may have progressed beyond the theory stage, but much is yet to be learned of this complex phenomenon called pain.

TYPES OF PAIN

Some of the ways that pain can be categorized are (Table 28–1):

Acute pain—This pain is brief in duration (less than 3 to 6 months), the cause is usually known, the intensity may range from mild to severe, and the treatment is aimed at elimination of the cause.

Table 28–1 Characteristics of Acute and Chronic Pain

Acute Pain	Chronic Pain	Chronic Cancer Pain
Identifiable cause	Cause hard to find	Usually identifiable cause
Short duration	Lasts longer than several months	Duration varies
Sudden onset	Begins gradually and persists	Onset varies
Well defined	May or may not be well defined	May or may not be well defined
Limited	Unlimited	Unlimited
Decreases with healing	Persists beyond healing time	May persist beyond healing
Reversible	Exhausting and useless	Exhausting and useless
Objective signs and symptoms	Objective signs absent	Objective signs absent
Anxiety	Depression and fatigue	Depression, fatigue, and anxiety

Chronic pain—Chronic pain extends beyond 3 to 6 months, the cause may or may not be known, it has not responded to treatment and/or does not subside after the injury heals. The intensity may range from mild to severe and treatment varies.

Chronic cancer pain—Cancer pain may be both *acute and chronic*. There is the time element of chronic pain, the intensity may be severe, the pain can be described as "intractable" (i.e., not able to be relieved), and may be due to several etiologies.

INCIDENCE OF CANCER PAIN

Not all people with cancer experience pain. The incidence of cancer pain is difficult to determine, but several experts agree that the figure is 40% to 80% when considering all types and stages of cancer.[8,9,28,61,82] Foley[29] states that 60% to 90% of patients with advanced cancer experience moderate to severe pain. In 1993 the American Cancer Society (ACS) estimated cancer deaths at 526,000, which means that between 316,000 and 473,000 people in the United States experienced pain related to their diagnosis of cancer during 1993.

Whether pain occurs in cancer is dependent upon several factors. The major factors include:

- *Location* of the primary or metastatic site of cancer. If there is bony involvement (as occurs with spinal metastases) or neural involvement (by direct tumor invasion or compression of any nerve tissue) the pain will be more severe than pressure due to organ involvement.
- *Stage* of the tumor activity.
  A client in a later stage of cancer experiences pain more often and at a more severe intensity than a person who is in an early stage of disease. Spross[71] states that 79% to 90% of people with advanced disease report pain.

ETIOLOGIES OF CANCER PAIN

There may be many causes for pain in the person with cancer.

Direct Tumor Involvement

Direct tumor involvement (e.g., proliferation of malignant cells within bone, nerves, viscera, or soft tissue) is a cause for pain. The site of the pain produces different sensations and intensities. Also the location of the site impacts on the type of analgesic indicated. The types of pain produced by direct tumor involvement may include:

- *Somatic pain* (nociceptive) — results from stimulation of afferent nerves in the skin, connective tissue, muscles, joints, or bones. It is usually described as *"dull, sharp or aching"* and is localized. The response to analgesics is usually good.
- *Visceral pain* —involves organs in the thoracic or abdominal area. It can be caused by infiltration, pressure, or distention. The pain is described as *"constant, aching, or deep."* This type of pain may be referred to surface areas. Visceral pain may be seen in advanced pancreatic or liver cancer.
- *Neuropathic pain* (deafferentation) — results from peripheral or central nerve injury and is usually described as *"burning, shooting, or tingling."* Response to analgesics is usually poor.
- *Cancer Pain Syndromes* — By definition, a syndrome is a number of different types of pain, different etiologies of pain, and different methods of treatment. Some of the known pain syndromes due to direct tumor involvement are:
- *Bone involvement* —"Multiple bony metastases are by far the most common cause of generalized bone pain," according to Portenoy.[61] In the case of vertebral involvement, it is imperative that the nurse report this occurrence, since pain alone will precede nerve compression and prompt intervention may prevent neurologic deficit formation.
- *Peripheral nerves* — Sites where this may occur include the chest wall and retroperitoneal space, which may produce pain in the back, abdomen, or legs.
- *Brachial plexus* — This is usually a result of a primary lung tumor (Pancoast's syndrome) and there is aching in the shoulder and upper back. According to Portenoy[61] up to 50% of clients with Pancoast syndrome will go on to develop cord compression if left untreated. Again, it is imperative that pain is assessed thoroughly, reported accurately, and treated promptly.
- *Epidural spinal cord compression* — "Over 95% of patients with epidural spinal cord compression report pain, which may be focal or referred."[61] The pain will precede any sensory or motor deficit and again it is mandatory that any new back pain be communicated immediately.

Cancer Treatment

Surgery, radiation therapy, or chemotherapy may exacerbate pain. Some of the syndromes that may follow cancer treatment include:

- *Postthoracotomy pain syndrome*—The intercostal nerve may be damaged at the time of surgery. This will usually be described as a "burning" pain (neuropathic).
- *Postmastectomy pain syndrome*—The intercostobrachial nerve may be damaged at the time of surgery. This is usually described as a "burning" pain (neuropathic) and may occur soon after surgery or months later.
- *Postamputation syndrome*—This may be due to the formation of a neuroma which has both lancin-

ating (shooting) and "burning" components or it may be a phantom sensation that exhibits both continuous dysesthesias and "shooting" pain.[61]

- *Multiple neural involvement*—There may be several neural areas affected by chemotherapy (principly the vinca alkaloids [e. g., vincristine] or cisplatinum). This paraesthesia or dysesthesia tends to be dose-related and will generally improve over 6 to 12 months.
- *Mucositis*—The inflammation of the oral mucosa as a side effect of some of the chemotherapeutic agents (especially the antimetabolities) can produce intensely painful ulcerations. It is not uncommon for patients to require opioids to relieve pain during this period of time.
- *Postradiation pain*—There may be inadvertent damage to the spinal cord, mucosa, or bone.

The pain associated with cancer therapies may occur immediately or long after the therapy is started, making it more difficult to determine whether the pain is due to a complication of therapy or recurrent disease.

Pain Unrelated to Cancer

Conditions unrelated to cancer (e.g., arthritis, decubitus, tension headache, diabetic neuropathy, etc.) can cause pain for the cancer patient.

If someone is immunocompromised it is not unusual for the person to develop herpes zoster (shingles). Following the treatment and healing phase, there can remain a post-therpetic neuralgia that can be difficult to manage and needs to be addressed as a neuropathic pain in origin.

Remember that *any* pain usually has special significance for the client with cancer. Whether it is a "routine" headache or gastritis, the fear is that the pain represents an extension of the cancer. *All reports of pain must be evaluated.*

When there is obvious trauma to a body part, the source of one's pain is evident, but with cancer it is often difficult to determine the anatomic injury that may be occurring and full assessment and evaluation is warranted.

FACTORS AFFECTING ONE'S RESPONSE TO PAIN

An individual's response to pain is influenced by several factors, which helps explain why pain is such a complex experience.

Anxiety

Anxiety is considered to be the most important factor affecting an individual's response to pain because it affects a person's ability to tolerate and cope with pain. Because increased anxiety increases pain, any strategy nurses can use to decrease a patient's anxiety will help to control pain.

Measures to decrease anxiety (distraction, relaxation, and so on) will be covered in a later section of this chapter. It is important to ask the patient and family members what has helped control the patient's anxiety in the past. Many of these measures can be incorporated into the patient's individual plan of care.

Past Experience of Pain

In general, the more experience of pain one has in childhood, the greater the perceptions of pain in adulthood. It is important for the nurse to discuss past pain with the patient. The nurse should also determine what measures have helped relieve pain in the past. Even though some measures may seem unlikely to help, if they are not harmful or contraindicated, they may aid the patient's pain treatment plan. The nurse should also find out what measures have not helped relieve pain in the past.

Culture and Religion

Acceptable responses to pain are learned at a very early age. Cultural and religious practices in one's family play an important role in the pain experience. Some cultures may view the expression of pain or suffering as a weakness, so they tend to minimize pain. Other cultures expect expression of pain so they may have greater overt manifestations of pain.

It is important to realize that not all people manifest pain in the same way and that there is no right or wrong way. The nurse should accept all patients' expressions of pain, regardless of their cultural or religious backgrounds.

BARRIERS TO ADEQUATE CANCER PAIN MANAGEMENT
Lack of Education

It has been well documented that there has been a lack of professional health care education regarding pain management that has resulted in less than optimal pain management for the person with cancer.[15,26,42,81] When 28 nursing text books were reviewed,[26] it was found that only one book accurately described the differences between physical dependence and addiction. McCaffery and Beebe[44] describe health professionals as often unaware of their lack of knowledge about pain control despite the fact that 81% of bacculaureate nursing programs accredited by the National League for Nursing includes some class content on pain.[46]

Whether in basic or continuing educational opportunities, nurses traditionally have not been taught how to assess pain or to use different treatment modalities, especially medications, appropriately. Many nurses are not familiar with the pharmacokinetics of analgesics, the types of analgesics available, equianalgesic dosages, novel routes of delivery, or principles of scheduling administration. McCaffery and Ferrell[47] report that although the percentage of nurses knowing that the risk of addiction is less than 1% has increased (i.e., an improvement), during a 1988 to 1989 survey of 2459 nurses, there were 21.6% who still thought that at least 25% of patients receiving opioids for pain relief would become addicted.

There is a call for reeducation of all health team members so that adequate pain control can be achieved. Positive advances have been made in recent years and nurses have been instrumental in the development of the hospice movement, oncology nursing's focus on symptom management (i.e., pain), and individual state cancer pain initiatives.

With today's knowledge and technology, nurses can assist the patient and family to achieve better pain management outcomes.

Regulatory Issues

Misconceptions also exist about narcotic regulations both nationally and within many states that promote the limitation of narcotics from being prescribed even when needed for successful pain management.

Myths and Misconceptions

The lay public and some health professionals have held many myths and misconceptions about cancer pain management that are now beginning to be addressed. Some of these myths and misconceptions include:

- The person taking pain medications will *easily* become addicted
- Cancer pain cannot really be relieved; it's part of the disease
- The "strong stuff" must be saved for later when the pain gets "really bad" or else nothing will be available
- "Shots" are stronger than pills
- If opiates are administered routinely, death will be hastened due to respiratory depression

Denying the existence of pain may function as a coping mechanism as any presence of pain may be viewed as disease progression. This must be evaluated in light of other factors: personality trait of stoicism, cultural beliefs, attitudes, and so on. Myths and misconceptions must be addressed by the health care professional in the initial assessment of pain and in subsequent reassessments.

RECENT DEVELOPMENTS IN CANCER PAIN MANAGEMENT

During the 1970s the hospice movement established itself in the United States. Throughout the country in large and small communities, home-care, free-standing, hospital-based, or agency-affiliated programs started serving the specific population who had a life-expectancy of 6 months or less. With this focus of care delivery, pain became one of the central symptom management issues. Hospice nurses were leading the way in recognizing the uniqueness of cancer pain and became the nursing profession's experts through hands-on practice.

The International Association for the Study of Pain (IASP) was formed in 1974. The American Pain Society (APS) is a national chapter of IASP.

In 1982 the World Health Organization (WHO) established a program in the cancer unit to study the incidence of cancer pain and to provide guidelines for cancer pain management. A 1984 meeting resulted in the publication of the booklet *Cancer Pain Relief* in 1986. The international WHO three-step analgesic ladder has been implemented in a number of countries (Figure 28–1). This ladder provides logical steps of progression of analgesics to treat the needs of the person who has pain. A revised edition, *Cancer Pain Relief and Palliative Care,* was published by the WHO in 1990.

In 1986 the World Health Organization established the Wisconsin Cancer Pain Initiative as the demonstration project site of the United States to "develop a comprehensive program to reduce cancer pain in the state of Wisconsin."[72] In 1991, there were 21 states with Cancer Pain Initiative Programs[74] and by 1993 there were 32 states with cancer pain initiative programs and five other states that were trying to organize programs. All of the established programs have nurse involvement and some state programs are led by a nurse. Activities of state cancer pain initiatives address the issues of: government regulations, myths and misconceptions of lay people and professionals, and professional education of pain management strategies. (See Figure 28-2 for a map and Appendix C, which lists contact persons as of June 1993.)

In 1990 the American Pain Society published its Standards on Acute and Cancer Pain. This interdisciplinary professional pain organization recognized that there was a means of setting criteria against which quality of practice could be measured. (See Section on Quality Assessment and Improvement.)

In 1990 the Oncology Nursing Society published its detailed document, "Oncology Nursing Society Position Paper on Cancer Pain,"[68,70] which includes:

- Introductory Material
- Scope of Nursing Practice Regarding Cancer Pain
- Ethics
- Practice (problem identification, assessment, planning, implementation and coordination, evaluation)
- Education (basic, graduate, continuing, patient and public)
- Research

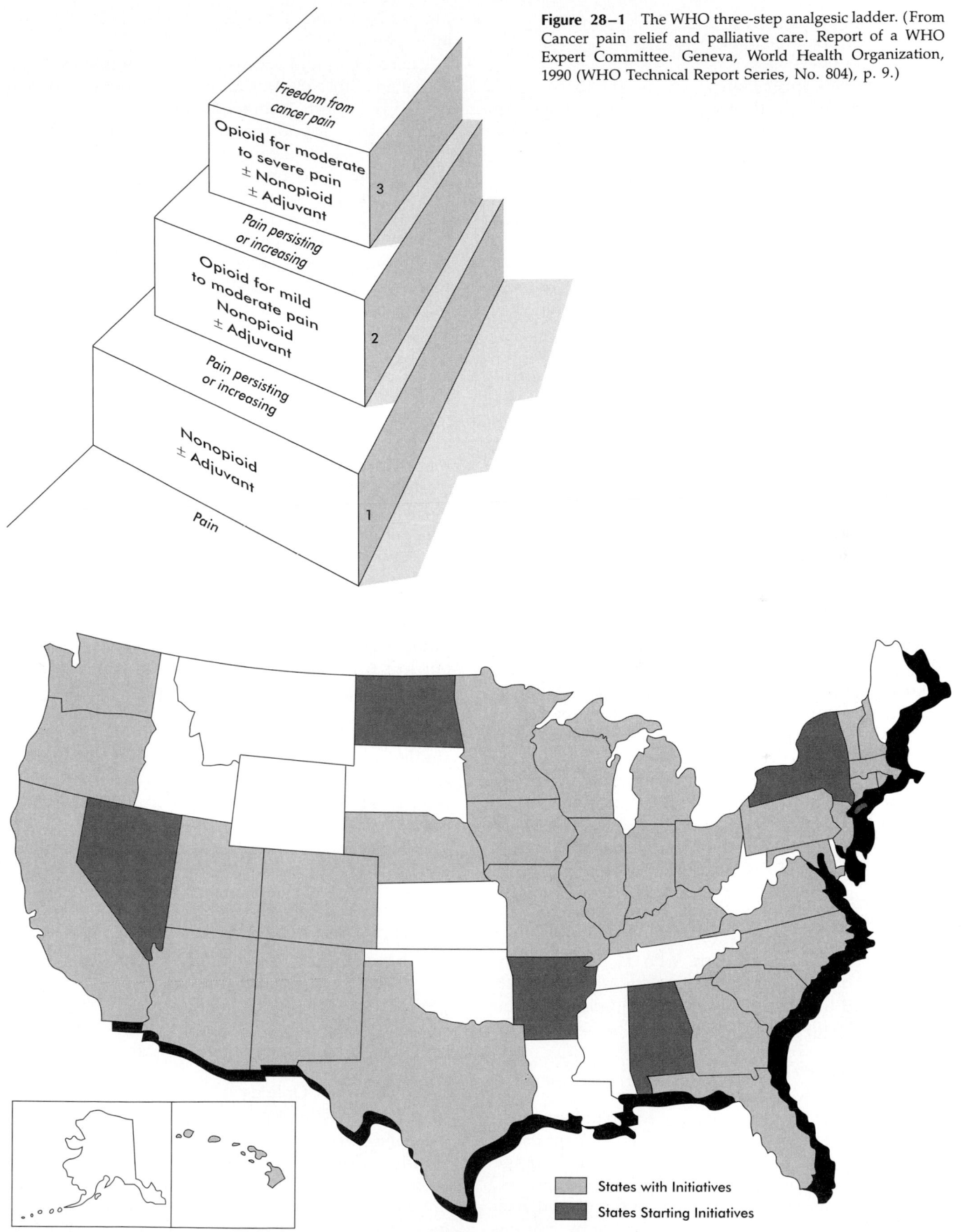

Figure 28–1   The WHO three-step analgesic ladder. (From Cancer pain relief and palliative care. Report of a WHO Expert Committee. Geneva, World Health Organization, 1990 (WHO Technical Report Series, No. 804), p. 9.)

Freedom from
cancer pain

Opioid for moderate
to severe pain
± Nonopioid
± Adjuvant

3

Pain persisting
or increasing

Opioid for mild
to moderate pain
Nonopioid
± Adjuvant

2

Pain persisting
or increasing

Nonopioid
± Adjuvant

1

Pain

☐ States with Initiatives

■ States Starting Initiatives

Figure 28–2   State cancer pain initiatives (March 1993).

- Resources
- Nursing Administration
- Social Policy
- Pediatric Cancer Pain

This document is a thorough and concise paper on quality pain management and nursing's role in providing this management.

In 1991, the governmental Agency on Health Care Policy and Research (AHCPR) formed an expert panel to develop guidelines on pain management. It was decided that there would indeed be the need for two separate documents, one on acute operative and trauma pain and one on cancer pain. In 1992 the acute pain guideline was published and the cancer pain guideline followed in 1993.

In 1992 the Joint Commission on Accreditation for Healthcare Organizations included pain management as one of its standards. (See Section on Quality Assessment and Improvement.)

There have been a vast amount of time and effort in studying the problem of cancer pain, identifying barriers, and establishing practice guidelines and standards. The time has now arrived to implement what we already know and make an impact on our patients who experience cancer pain.

PHARMACOLOGIC INTERVENTIONS
Non-Opioid Analgesics

The non-opioids work primarily at the peripheral nervous system level and are used for mild to moderate pain especially of bone metastases, soft-tissue infiltration, or arthritis. The categories of non-opioids include aspirin, acetaminophen, and the Nonsteroidal Antiinflammatory Drugs (NSAIDs).

Most nonsteroidal anti-inflammatory drugs (NSAIDs) block the production of prostaglandins, which are chemicals that are produced when cells are damaged.[83] NSAIDs have potential gastrointestinal (GI) side effects and this may limit their use over time. Inturrisi[35] and Wilke[83] note that all NSAIDs except choline magnesium trisalicylate (Trilisate) will interfere with platelet aggregation and, therefore, may not be appropriate for someone who is thrombocytopenic. Non-opioids are often given together with opioids and therefore a lower dose of opioid may be effective[65] (Table 28–2).

Opioid Analgesics

The opiates work primarily at the central nervous system (CNS) level. Those opioids used for mild to moderate pain often have acetaminophen or aspirin together with the opiate. Be aware of the total dosage of aspirin/acetaminophen consumed per 24 hours. The maximum dose of either should not exceed 6000 mg per 24 hours. If two tablets containing 500 mg each are taken every 3 hours, the total would be 8000 mg per 24 hours. (Table 28–3, see Table 28–6 for relative potency.)

There are opioid agonists used for moderate to severe pain (Table 28–4). Cancer pain management may indeed require these opioids over time.

It has been found that there is no ceiling effect of morphine, which means that the dose can continue to be escalated to provide analgesia with increased pain levels. For some drugs there is a ceiling and beyond that ceiling dose there is no added analgesic benefit. There are exceptional instances where clients may require 1000 to 2000 mg of morphine, or even more, per 24 hours and the person will be alert, ambulatory, and participating in activities of daily living.

After many years of experience with meperidine (Demerol), caution is now being expressed in two areas. First, it should never be used on a continuous basis for cancer pain treatment as the metabolite (normeperidine) is a central nervous system stimulator[38] and this can lead to tremors or seizure activity with repeated dosing. Second, the AHCPR *Clinical Practice Guidelines* include the warning against the use of meperidine for people who are taking monoamine oxidase inhibitors. "Severe adverse reactions, including death through mechanisms that mimic malignant hyperthermia have been reported when these drugs are used together."[1]

The question as to the efficacy of heroin over morphine has been studied with the conclusion that heroin does *not* offer any advantage over morphine when an equianalgesic conversion is done.[39,78] Heroin (diamorphine) is metabolized to morphine before it reaches the opiate receptors of the brain. Prior to the studies being done, heroin was most often the narcotic of choice in the Brompton's Cocktail in hospice programs in England; now oral morphine is routinely used.

Mixed agonist-antagonists may also be used for moderate to severe pain. Be cautious in using mixed agonist-antagonists to manage cancer pain for the following reasons:

- After using agonists (e.g., morphine), withdrawal-like symptoms can be precipitated when a mixed agonist-antagonist is given.
- If given with an agonist, the mixed form will antagonize and give poor pain relief with possible increase in psychomimetic effects.

Special Issues of Opioids

TITRATION/ESCALATING DOSES. Most often an increasing need for medication is indicative of progressive disease or a developing complication and thorough assessment is warranted. When it is determined that more medication is needed to manage an individual's pain, the safe plan of increasing the dose is: *increase 25-50% of the previous dose.*

Table 28–2 Nonopioid Analgesics

Drug	Recommended Dose and Interval	Comments
PARA-AMINOPHENOL DERIVATIVE		
Acetaminophen (Tylenol, Panadol, Anacin-3, Excedrin, Midol, Sine-Aid)	500-1000 mg q4-6 hr	Similar to aspirin in analgesic and antipyretic effects, but only slight anti-inflammatory effects. May not have effect on platelet aggregation. May cause liver toxicity.
ACETYLSALICYLICS		
Acetylsalicylic acid (aspirin)	50-1000 mg q4-6 hr	First choice analgesic if able to tolerate; standard anti-inflammatory; increased bleeding time due to inhibition of platelet aggregation
NONACETYLATED SALICYLATES		
Choline magnesium trisalicyte (Trilisate)	1000-1500 mg q8-12 hr	Minimal effect on platelet aggregation (platelet-sparing); available in liquid.
Diflunisal (Dolobid)	500-1000 mg q8-12 hr	Longer action; minimal antipyretic effect; minimal GI side effects.
Salsalate (Disalcid; Salsitab)	750-1000 mg q8-12 hr	May have minimal effect on platelet aggregation; minimal GI side effects
NSAIDs (NONSTEROIDAL ANTI-INFLAMMATORY DRUGS)		
Propionic acid derivatives:		
Ibuprofen (Motrin, Nuprin, Advil, Medipren)	200-400 mg q4-8 hr	Available as oral suspension.
Fenoprofen (Nalfon)	200 mg q4-6 hr	
Naproxen (Naprosyn)	250-500 mg q6-8 hr	Available as oral liquid.
Naproxen sodium (Anaprox)	275-550 mg q6-8 hr	Faster onset than naproxen.
Ketoprofen (Orudis)	25-50 mg q6-8 hr	
Indole acetic acid derivatives:		
Indomethacin (Indocin)	25-50 mg q8-12 hr	Available as oral suspension and rectal suppository; high incidence of side effects: GI symptoms.
Sulindac (Clinoril)	150-200 mg q8-12 hr	Lower incidence of renal toxicity; GI side effects common
Tolmetin (Tolectin)	200 mg q6-8 hr	Weak analgesic effect.
Anthranilics:		
Mefenamic acid (Ponstel)	250 mg q6 hr	Not recommended for use longer than 7 days.
Meclofenamate (Meclomen)	50-100 mg q6-8 hr	Diarrhea may occur as well as other GI side effects
Oxicam:		
Piroxicam (Feldene)	10-30 mg q6 hr or 20 mg qd	Not recommended for patients with renal or liver dysfunction; effect may not be seen for 7-12 days.
Pyrrololacetic acid:		
ketorolac (Toradol)	30 mg q6 hr	Only injectable NSAID; not recommended for use longer than 7 days; equivalent to 10 mg parenteral morphine; oral form also available.

Note: It is important to remember that all of the NSAIDs have similar side effects, especially GI irritation. All of these drugs should be administered on a full stomach and with milk. In addition to GI irritation, GI bleeding can be a serious problem related to the inhibition of platelet aggregation and NSAIDs should be used with caution in thrombocytopenic patients. See note on choline magnesium trisalicyte.[35,83]

Example:
Current dose: 60 mg PO morphine q4h
Add: 15-30 mg PO morphine q4h, thus
NEW PRESCRIPTION: 75 to 90 mg PO morphine q4h
Continue assessment to determine whether additional increases are needed.

RESCUE DOSES.   Obtain an order for an immediate release analgesic to use for breakthrough pain. The "rescue" medication should be the same drug (e.g., morphine) as the scheduled analgesic; a liquid immediate-release formula will act more rapidly than a tablet form. This dose should equal 33% to 50% of the regularly scheduled every 4 hour dose or calculate 10% of the total 24 hour requirement.

Example:
If 180 mg oral morphine are required per 24

Table 28–3 Opioids for Mild to Moderate Pain

Drug	Starting Oral Dose Range	Comments
Codeine	30–60 mg q4 hr	Usually combined with a NSAID; use cautiously with impaired ventilation, bronchial asthma, increased intracranial pressure and liver.
Hydrocodone bitartrate 5 mg + acetaminophen 500 mg (Vicodin, Lortab)	i-ii tablets q4 hr	Only available with acetaminophen.
Oxycodone hydrochloride 5 mg (Roxicodone)	5-10 mg q4 hr	Available alone or with aspirin or acetaminophen; elixir = 5 mg/ml, also available 20 mg/ml. Caution with impaired ventilation, bronchial asthma, increased intracranial pressure, and liver failure.
Oxycodone 5 mg + acetaminophen 325 mg (Roxicet, Percocet)	i-ii tablets q4 hr	
Oxycodone 5 mg + acetaminophen 500 mg (Tylox)	i-ii tablets q4 hr	
Oxycodone 5 mg + aspirin 325 mg (Perdocan)	i-ii tablets q4 hr	
Propoxyphene hydrochloride 65 mg (Darvon)	i-ii tablets q4 hr	Toxic metabolite, norpropoxyphene, accumulates with repeated dosing and overdose is complicated by convulsions; often combined with NSAID.
Propoxyphene napsylate 65 mg (Darvocet N)	i-ii tablets q4 hr	

Note: Be aware of the total dosage of aspirin or acetaminophen consumed per 24 hours. The maximum dose should not exceed 6000 mg per 24 hours. If two tabs containing 500 mg each are taken q 3 hr, the total would be 8000 mg per 24 hr.

Table 28–4 Opioids for Moderate to Severe Pain

Drug	Equianalgesic Parenteral Dose	Oral Morphine Equivalent	Comments
MORPHINE-LIKE AGONISTS			
Morphine	10 mg	30 mg	Standard of comparison for narcotic analgesics; 3-4 hr duration; 8-12 hr sustained-release tablets are available
Hydromorphone (Dilaudid)	1.5 mg	7.5 mg	High concentration is available for parenteral use; also available PO and R
Methadone (Dolophine)	10 mg	20 mg	Good oral potency; long plasma half-life (24-36 hr); accumulates with repetitive dosing
Levorphanol	2 mg	4 mg	Long plasma half-life (12-16 hr)
Oxymorphone (Numorphan)	1 mg	—	Not available orally; 5 mg rectal suppository = 5 mg parenteral morphine
Meperidine	75-100 mg	300 mg	Shorter-acting than morphine (2.5-3.5 hr); Toxic metabolite (normeperidine accumulates with repeated dosing, causing CNS excitation which can lead to seizures; avoid use in patients on monoamine oxidase inhibitors due to potential adverse reaction that mimics malignant hyperthermia and may lead to cardiovascular collapse.
Fentanyl (Sublimaze)	0.1 mg	—	Transdermal fentanyl patch (Durogesic) 25-50 mcg/hr roughly equivalent to 90 mg sustained-release morphine per 24 hr; there is a 12-hr delay in onset and offset of patch; fever increases dose rate.
MIXED AGONIST-ANTAGONISTS			
Pentazocine	60 mg q3-4 hr	150 mg q3-4 hr	May cause psychotomimetic effects; may precipitate withdrawal in narcotic-dependent patients; not recommended for cancer patients.
Nalbuphine (Nubain)	10 mg q3-4 hr	—	Not available orally; incidence of psychotomimetic effects lower than pentazocine.
Butorphanol (Stadol)	2 mg q3-4 hr	—	Not available orally; incidence of psychotomimetic effects lower than pentazocine.
PARTIAL AGONIST			
Buprenorphine (Buprenex)	0.3-0.4 mg q6-8 hr	—	Not available orally; may precipitate withdrawal in narcotic-dependent patients; not readily reversed by naloxone.

These doses are recommended starting doses from which the optimal dose for each patient is determined by titration. Although single-dose studies established the relative potency of PO/IM morphine as 6:1, in practice, repetitive dosing is the rule, and a ratio of 3:1 is more commonly used. For IM doses, the time to peak analgesia ranges from 30-60 minutes; after oral administration, the peak analgesic effect is about 2 hours.

Tables based on: Acute pain management: Operative or medical procedures and trauma. (1992). Agency for Health Care Policy and Research (AHCPR). Publication No. 92-0032; American Pain Society: Principles of analgesic use in the treatment of acute pain and chronic cancer pain, ed 3, 1992; Inturrisi CE: Management of cancer pain—Pharmacology and principles of management, Cancer 63(11):2310-2311, 1989; McCaffery M and Beebe A: Pain—A clinical manual for nursing practice. St. Louis, 1989, Mosby, pp. 78-79; and Weissman DE, Burchman SL, Dinndorf PA, and Dahl JL: Handbook of cancer pain management, Wisconsin, 1992, Cancer pain initiative.

hours, at 10% the rescue dose would be 18 mg. If 30 mg oral morphine are scheduled q4h, at 50% the rescue dose would be 15 mg.

If greater than or equal to 3 rescue doses are required per 24 hours, then obtain an order that includes that amount in the ATC (Around the Clock) dosing. Do maintain the order for rescue dosing. (See General Principles of Analgesic Administration, #4.) DECREASING DOSES.   If a person's pain decreases (e.g., following palliative radiation to bone metastases, or a nerve block being done), the opioid requirements may indeed decrease dramatically. According to the American Hospital Formulary Service,[3] abstinance syndrome (withdrawal) will occur if someone has required 240 mg or more of morphine per day for 30 days.

S & S Withdrawl during 1st 24 hours:
- Restlessness
- Lacrimation
- Rhinnorrhea
- Yawning
- Perspiration
- Gooseflesh
- Restless sleep
- Mydriasis

S & S Withdrawl during 24 - 72 hours:
- Twitching/muscular spasms
- Kicking movements
- Severe aches in back, abdomen, and legs
- Nausea, vomiting, diarrhea
- Coryza and severe sneezing
- Increase in all vital signs (T, P, BP, and R)

To safely "wean" the person from the opioids and prevent abstinence syndrome from occurring the following formula is used:
Give 50% of the previous order for 48 hours and then reduce by 25% q48h until <10 to 15 mg (parenteral morphine equivalent) per 24 hours.
Example: Client has been receiving 180 mg morphine sulfate PO/24 hours (at a 3:1 ratio this is 60 mg parenteral morphine per 24 hours)
Day 1 & 2–90 mg PO morphine sulfate/24 hours
Day 3 & 4–70 mg PO morphine sulfate/24 hours
Day 5 & 6–50 mg PO morphine sulfate/24 hours
Day 7 & 8–40 mg PO morphine sulfate/24 hours
Day 9 & 10–30 mg PO morphine sulfate/24 hours
    (this is 10 mg parenteral morphine equivalents)
Day 11–nothing

DURATION OF OPIOIDS.   Be aware that not all opioids have the same duration of effectiveness; some opioids are short-acting, some are long-acting, and some are in the middle. Scheduling must be according to how long the medication is actually lasting or pain will occur.

Short-acting opioids
  fentanyl (Sublimaze)   ½ hr

Intermediate-acting opioids
  meperidine (Demerol)   2-3 hr
  morphine   3-4 hr
  hydromorphone (Dilaudid)   3-4 hr
  codeine   3-4 hr
  oxycodone   3-4 hr
  propoxyphene (Darvon)   3-4 hr
Long-acting opioids
  methodone (Dolophine)   6-8 hr
  levorphanol (Levodromoran)   6-8 hr

Equianalgesia is the conversion of one route to another or from one opioid to another in an equivalent amount. When converting from one route of administration to another or from one opioid to another, it must be done in such a manner as to not undermedicate or overmedicate the client. This concept is just beginning to be realized and nurses can do much to educate other health care professionals in the process of equianalgesic conversion.

Example:
Mr. Payne received the following analgesics yesterday. Calculate the total 24-hour parenteral morphine equivalents that he received. (See Morphine Equianalgesic List Table 28-5 and Narcotic Oral Equivalent Chart Table 28-6.)

Morphine 5 mg IV × 8 (5 mg × 8) = 40 mg
Tylenol #3 × 6 (2.3 mg × 6) = 13.8 mg
Tylox × 4 (2.8 mg × 4) = 11.2 mg
Parenteral morphine equivalents/24 hrs = 65.0 mg
Oral morphine equivalents/24 hrs = 195.0 mg
    (oral : parenteral = 3:1)
SR morphine (q 12 hour) would be = 90.0 mg
    (sustained release morphine)
For breakthrough pain he would require = 30.0 mg
    (1/3 of 12-hr dose)

OPIOID SIDE EFFECT MANAGEMENT.   With the administration of opioids, side effects may often occur. The questions then become: Are expected side effects being managed effectively? Are there any unexpected side effects?

The expected side effects are:
Constipation.   Constipation does *not* diminish over time. All patients on opioids should be given stool softeners and agents to increase bowel motility to prevent constipation as opioids inhibit peristalsis in the GI tract.[5,41,80] Glare and Lickiss[30] describe 90% of patients in a palliative care program as experiencing constipation. Preventing severe constipation requires treating consistently and prophylactically. Often the discomfort of constipation is more distressing to the patient than other pain. If there are not orders for a bowel regimen, obtain them immediately (Table 28-7).

Walsh[80] offers the *SOS* plan:
  I. *S*tool softener (docusate sodium—Colace)

Table 28–5 Morphine Equianalgesic List

	IM	P.O.	Morphine Equivalent IM
NARCOTIC AGONISTS:			
Morphine	10 mg	30 mg	10.0 mg
Dilaudid (hydromor- phone)	0.5 mg		3.5 mg
	1.0 mg		7.0 mg
	1.5 mg	7.5 mg	10.0 mg
	2.0 mg		14.0 mg
		1.0 mg	1.3 mg
		2.0 mg	2.6 mg
		4.0 mg	5.3 mg
Numorphan (oxy- morphone)	1.0 mg		10.0 mg
Levo-Dromoran (levorphanol)	2 mg	4.0 mg	10.0 mg
Fentanyl (sublimaze)	0.1 mg (100 mcg)		10.0 mg
Dolophine (metha- done)	10 mg	20 mg	10.0 mg
Demerol (meperi- dine)	25 mg		4.0 mg
	50 mg		7.0 mg
	75 mg	300 mg	10.0 mg
	100 mg		14.0 mg
NARCOTIC MIXED AGONIST/ANTAGONISTS:			
Stadol (butorphanol tartrate)	2 mg		10.0 mg
Buprenex (buprenor- phine)	0.3 mg		7.5 mg
	0.4 mg		10.0 mg
Nubain (malbuphine)	10 mg		10.0 mg
NSAID:			
Toradol (ketorolac)	30-90 mg		6-12.0 mg
repeated doses	30 mg	30 mg	12.0 mg

Data from Inturrisi CE: Pharmacology of narcotic analgesics. Symposium on management of cancer pain, New York, 1984, H.P. Publishing Co, Inc., p. 23; Inturrisi CE: Management of cancer pain—Pharmacology and principles of management, Cancer 63 (11):2310-2311, 1989; McCaffery M and Beebe A: Pain—Clinical manual for nursing practice, St. Louis, 1989, Mosby, pp. 78-79.

II. *O*smotic laxative (Milk of Magnesia) if stool softener does not work

III. *S*timulant laxative (bisacodyl—Dulcolax)

Nausea/vomiting. In a study conducted by Campora, Merlini, and Pace,[13] 18% of patients on morphine had moderate to severe nausea and 28% experienced emesis; Levy[41] states that approximately 40% of patients receiving narcotics will develop mild to moderate nausea. The intensity of nausea and/or vomiting in patients receiving opioids varies from patient to patient and from opioid to opioid. The etiology of the nausea/vomiting appears to be the result of the effect of opioids on the chemoreceptor trigger zone. This side effect generally decreases after 2 to 3 days of repeated dosing[45,80] as tolerance to the side effect develops. Treat the side effect aggressively; it may require ATC (around the clock) management for 1 to 2 weeks. An-

Table 28–6 Narcotic Oral Equivalent Chart

NARCOTIC ORAL EQUIVALENTS

The importance of pain management for patients with cancer is recognized by oncology nurses, and "alteration in comfort" is a frequent nursing diagnosis with this patient population.

The Narcotic Oral Equivalent Chart was developed to visually display whether a shift from morphine to a morphine equivalent has resulted in an increase or decrease in potency.

Determining the "true" potency of a drug can be especially difficult when patients receive medication that combines a narcotic with a nonsteroidal anti-inflammatory drug such as aspirin or acetaminophen.

The chart ranks medications from the lowest potency of morphine equivalence to the highest. When choosing between different medications, this tool can assist nurses in identifying dosages and making decisions that will prove more beneficial to patients.

Oral Narcotic	IM Morphine Equivalent
Tylenol® #1 (7.5 mg codeine + 300 mg acetaminophen)	1.1 mg
Dilaudid® (hydromorphone 1 mg)	1.3 mg
Codeine 30 mg	1.5 mg
Tylenol® #2 (15 mg codeine + 300 mg acetaminophen)	1.5 mg
Darvon® (propoxyphene hydrochloride 65 mg)	1.6 mg
Darvocet-N® 50 (proyxphene napsylate 50 mg + acetaminophen 325 mg)	1.6 mg
Demerol® (meperidine 50 mg)	1.6 mg
Tylenol #3 (30 mg codeine + 300 mg acetaminophen)	2.3 mg
Percocet® (oxycodone 5 mg + acetaminophen 325 mg)	2.4 mg
Percodan® (oxycodone 5 mg + aspirin 325 mg)	2.4 mg
Vicodin® (hydrocodone bitartrate 5 mg + acetaminophen 500 mg)	2.9 mg
Tylox® (oxycodone 5 mg + acetaminophen 500 mg)	2.8 mg
Darvocet-N 100 (propoxyphene napsylate 100 mg + acetaminophen 600 mg)	3.1 mg
Morphine 10 mg	3.3 mg
Tylenol #4 (60 mg codeine + 300 mg acetaminophen)	3.8 mg

From Swenson CJ, Sikorski K, DeWaters T, and Bucknell Ryan S: Narcotic oral equivalents, Oncol Nurs Forum, 18(5):942, 1991.

tiemetic trials are warranted if nausea/vomiting is a problem. (See Table 28-7 for nursing management of side effects.)

Sedation. Because opioids have a depressant effect on the central nervous system, some drowsiness can be anticipated. Once pain management is achieved, do not confuse normal extended sleep patterns with sedation. Be aware that the person may have been exhausted from interrupted sleep patterns due to previous pain and may, in fact, sleep for extended pe-

Table 28–7   Nursing Management of Side Effects

Nursing Dx.	Interventions	Rationale

Alteration in bowel elimination: constipation	Assessment at regular intervals:
	  Are bowel sounds present?
	  What is the normal elimination pattern?
	  Is there an established bowel elimination pattern of every ≤3 days?
	  Number of stools per day
	  Character of stool
	  Absence of stool elimination
	Action: Treat prophylactically
	  General nursing measures
	    Promote adequate fluid intake of 2-3 L/day
	
	    Encourage high fiber diet
	    Promote exercise/activity as tolerated
	  Obtain orders for medications and administer as needed:
	    Docusate sodium (e.g., Colace, Modane Soft)
	      range: 1-2 tablets TID
	    Senna (e.g., Senokot)
	      range: 2-4 tablets BID
	    Docusate sodium + senna (e.g., Senokot-S)
	      range: 2-4 tablets BID
	    Bisacodyl (e.g., Dulcolax; a bisacodyl enema = Fleet)
	      range: 2-3 tablets HS
	
	    Colyte
	      range: 8 oz QD or BID
		The opiate side effect of diminished neural stimulation resulting in constipation will *not* diminish over time
		
		Provide hydration to bowel contents
		
		Increase bulk
		Improve general tone and stimulation
		
		Stool softener that lowers surface tension, permitting water and fats to penetrate and soften stools
		Mild natural laxative derivative from the cassia plant; it induces peristalsis
		Stool softener plus mild laxative (see above)
		
		A contact laxative that stimulates sensory nerves to produce parasympathetic reflexes resulting in increased peristaltic contractions of the colon
		An electrolyte lavage; a glycol acts as an osmotic agent and there is virtually no net ion absorption or loss

Alteration in nutrition: less than body requirements (nausea and/or vomiting)	Monitor and record I & O
	Weigh every 3-5 days, if appropriate
	Record number of episodes of emesis per 24 hours
	Teach patient/family techniques to improve nutritional intake:
	  Small, frequent meals
	  Reduce odors
	  Eat in pleasant surroundings
	  Do not lie flat immediately after a meal
	Administer antiemetics as needed:
	  Hydroxyzine (e.g., Vistaril, Atarax)
	    range: 25-50 mg q 4-6 hours
	
	  Prochlorperazine (e.g., Compazine)
	    range: 10 mg q 4-6 hours
	  Thiethylperazine (Torecan, Norzine)
	    range: 10 mg q 8 hours
	  Chlorpromazine (e.g., Thorazine)
	    range: 10-25 mg q 4 hours
	  Metoclopramide (e.g., Reglan)
	    range: 10-20 mg q 6 hours
	  Haloperidol (Haldol)
	    range: 0.5-1.0 mg q 4-8 hours
		The side effect of nausea/vomiting is usually transitory and will subside within 7-14 days
		
		Has antiemetic, analgesic, and mild sedative activity (APS, 1992, p. 29) as well as being an antihistamine
		Antiemetic
		
		Antiemetic
		
		Antiemetic; use if sedation is desired
		
		Promote gastric emptying
		
		Antiemetic; use if patient is too sedated

Continued.

Table 28–7   Nursing Management of Side Effects—cont'd

Nursing Dx.	Interventions	Rationale
Potential for sleep pattern disturbance (sedation) or alteration in thought processes (confusion)	Assess and document: Patient's ability to communicate and comprehend Patient's disorientation/confusion, agitation, or impaired memory Interview patient/family: Are they comfortable with the level of alertness or is it troublesome in any way? Discuss other possible causes with other members of the health care team. Administer stimulants as needed: Caffeine 65 mg (to 200 mg/day) Methylphenidate (e.g., Ritalin) range: 10-15 mg (divide between early A.M. and noon) Dextroamphetamine (e.g., Dexedrine) range: 5-10 mg A.M.[82]; 2.5-10 mg[5] Orient to person, place, and time prn	Sedation and/or confusion due to opiates will decrease with repeated dosing. The individuality of each person is to be respected. Impaired renal function, hypercalcemia, or brain metastases can be the cause of confusion/sedation rather than the opiates. Stimulant; has been shown to increase analgesia when given with aspirin-like drugs[5] Stimulant; has analgesic properties; low toxicity (4%) includes hallucinations and paranoia; tolerance may develop within 1 month and dose require escalation.[10] Stimulant; side effects may include anxiety, anorexia, or nervousness. Confirm reality
Potential for ineffective breathing pattern (respiratory depression related to use of opiates)	Assess rate, depth, and quality, especially after dose escalation. Respiratory rate ≥10 Breathing pattern is even and unlabored If respiratory depression is questioned, assess for hypoxia: Labored respirations Tachypnea Tachycardia Cyanosis Position is semi- or high-Fowler's Distinguish between respiratory depression due to opiates and a natural change if patient is terminal. Administer naloxone (Narcan) *only after determination of true respiratory depression.* Discuss rare occurrence of true respiratory depression with patient/family.	True respiratory depression related to opiates is rare in the person who is not opiate-naive as the body develops a tolerance to the side effects. Physiologic changes that occur with hypoxia. A natural change in respiratory pattern (Cheyne-Stokes) occurs as death approaches. Opiate antagonist; use with caution to avoid profound withdrawal, seizures, and severe pain. The APS[5] recommends a dilute solution (0.4 mg in 10 ml saline) administered as 0.5 ml IV push every 2 minutes. Provide education and support to reduce fears of causing death rather than providing pain relief.

riods initially just to "catch up." The questions to ask are:

- Is the person alert and oriented when awake?
- Has the person established a good nighttime sleep pattern?
- Is the person arousable from sleep?

If sedation persists for more than 3 to 5 days, possible added stimulation might be required. (See Table 28-7 for nursing management of side effects.)

Confusion and/or hallucinations.   These are most often temporary. Be aware of impaired renal function (as it will have an impact on the clearance of the narcotics) and other possible causes of confusion to be ruled out: cerebral metastases, hypercalcemia, sepsis, and so on. Tolerance to these side effects usually develops within 48 to 72 hours. (See Table 28-7 for nursing management of side effects.)

Pruritis.   This intense itching is more often observed with the administration of intraspinal narcotics, and is not frequently seen with the other routes of administration. The person will exhibit this first on the face and may be unconsciously rubbing or scratching at the nose or cheeks. This can be managed with an antihistamine or with even a dilute infusion of a mixed agonist/antagonist or naloxone. Pruritis is not life-threatening, but is certainly bothersome. Rapid nursing intervention will enhance the comfort level of the client.

Respiratory depression. Tolerance to this potential side effect develops rapidly (see box at right). The Texas Cancer Plan states that we have an inordinate fear of respiratory depression.[32] Pain is a natural antagonist to the respiratory depressant effects of opiates and therefore pain provides a natural stimulant. A sleeping rate of six to eight respirations per minute may be perfectly normal in the totally relaxed person. The "arousable factor" is a satisfactory guide: Can the person be aroused rather quickly from sleep? This will stimulate respirations. "New respiratory symptoms are virtually never a primary drug effect in those receiving stable doses of narcotics."[60] When doses are escalated, respirations should be monitored for any drastic change even though it is unlikely. Make certain that the patient/family understand that respiratory depression is a *rare* occurrence with continued use of opioids and that death is not being promoted.

Naloxone (Narcan) is an opiate antagonist, but must be used with caution to avoid profound withdrawal, seizures, and severe pain. The APS[5] recommends diluting 0.4 mg in 10 ml of saline and giving 0.5 ml IV push every 2 minutes. (See Table 28-7 for nursing management of side effects.)

Potentiators

By definition to potentiate is to endow with power or make potent. A word of caution is required regarding what is referred to as the use of "potentiators" to increase the effectiveness of an analgesic. Medicine and nursing have long taught that when the phenothiazine promethazine (Phenergan) is added to a narcotic, it will intensify (or potentiate) the analgesic effect of the narcotic. Studies by McGee and Alexander[48] and Dundee and Moore[21] show that, in fact, promethazine may only increase the intensity of one's pain. Margo McCaffery calls this an *antianalgesic* effect. What is observed in the client is more a potentiation of the side effects: increased sedation, hypotention, and respiratory depression. The American Pain Society[5] states that "except for methotrimeprazine [Levoprome 10-20 mg. available in parenteral formulation only], *phenothiazines neither relieve pain nor potentiate opioid analgesia*" (p. 30). Hydroxyzine (Vistaril, Atarax) does have analgesic properties and may be a useful adjunct for the client who is also anxious or nauseated.[5]

GENERAL PRINCIPLES OF ANALGESIC
ADMINISTRATION

1. *Choose the analgesic appropriate to the type and level of pain.* The choice of a non-opioid or weak, moderate, or strong opioid should be based on pain

---

GUIDELINES FOR RESPIRATORY DEPRESSION

1. Always have a baseline respiratory rate.
2. Respiratory depression is usually slow in onset and preceded by sedation.
3. Respiratory depression usually occurs
   7 minutes after IV
   30 minutes after IM
   90 minutes after SC
4. Use a flow sheet to record respiratory rate and pain relief.
5. Dilute Narcan 0.1 to 0.4 mg in 10 ml saline and administer intravenously over 2 to 4 minutes.

From McGuire L: Pain. In Beare PG and Myers JL: Principles and practice of adult health nursing, St. Louis, 1990, Mosby.

---

intensity which is determined through careful assessment (see Figure 28-1).

The concept of an orderly progression from the occurrence of pain to its successful management can be visualized as the rungs of a ladder in the following sequence:

A. Pain exists
B. Use a non-opioid with or without an adjuvant drug
C. If pain persists or increases . . .
D. Use an opioid for weak to moderate pain, with or without a non-opioid, and with or without an adjuvant drug
E. If pain persists or increases. . .
F. Use an opioid for moderate to strong pain, with or without a non-opioid, and with or without an adjuvant drug

The top rung of this ladder is freedom from cancer pain. This orderly progression allows for trials of various medications at all levels and assures that everything is being attempted to control the pain across the spectrum.

2. *Choose the easiest and most cost-effective route of administration.* Based on the KISSING principle (Keep it Sanely Simple in Narcotic Giving)—*Use the oral route whenever possible!* If nausea and/or vomiting prohibit this route, try the rectal route. Consider the following progression of routes:
   • Oral
   • Rectal
   • Transdermal
   • Subcutaneous
   • Intramuscular
   • Intravenous
   • Intraspinal (epidural or intrathecal)

3. *Schedule administration.* Around the Clock (ATC) dosing is mandatory to achieve a steady-state of analgesia and avoid the peaks and valleys that produce cycles of pain periods alternating with sedation. Never use a PRN schedule as the pain level

Table 28–8   Adjuvant Coanalgesics

Drug	Dose	Indications	Comments
TRICYCLIC ANTIDEPRESSANTS			
Nortriptyline (Pamelor, Aventyl)			Less orthostatic hypotension; available in liquid form.
Desipramine (Norpramin, Pertofranc)			Less sedation and anticholinergic effects
Imipramine (Tofranil)			
Doxepin (Sinequan)			
Amitriptyline (Elavil)	25-150 mg daily (hs); start at low dose and titrate upward to effect	Neuropathies and postherpetic neuralgia (especially burning pain)	Side effects include: dry mouth, urinary retention, sedation, orthostatic hypotension, delirium. May potentiate narcotics by blocking reuptake of serotonin (a neurotransmitter)

The analgesic therapeutic dose of antidepressants is ⅛-⅙ of dose required to treat clinical depression.

Drug	Dose	Indications	Comments
ANTIHISTAMINES			
Hydroxizine (Vistaril, Atarax)	25-50 mg PO or IM q4-6 hr	Pain together with nausea, anxiety	Has analgesic effects (50 mg IM = 5 mg morphine), as well as antianxiety, antiemetic, and antihistamine effects; very irritating to tissue.
ANTICONVULSANTS			
Carbamazepine (Tegretol)	100 mg q6-8 hr	Neuropathic lancinating pain (shooting/stabbing)(e.g., postherpetic sedation, and neuralgia, tic-like pain due to nerve injury)	Side effects include: vertigo, sedation, confusion, and bone marrow suppression
Clonazepam (Klonopin)	0.25 mg q12 hr		
Phenytoin (Dilantin)	3-5 mg/kg/day		Ataxia, skin rash, liver function abnormalities. Plasma levels should be monitored.
Sodium valproate Baclofen (Lioresal)	150 mg q8 hr	Tic-like pain	

then escalates and the patient must spend time just to "catch up" to prior levels of analgesia. The important feature here is to stay ahead of the pain and this principle requires teaching and reinforcement by nurses as it differs from usual pain management to which patients are accustomed.

4. *Be prepared for breakthrough pain.* Whatever the medication, route, or frequency of administration, always make certain that there is an order available for "breakthrough" pain. This is a sudden, and sometimes brief, increase in pain that may be due to increased activity or a particular motion. This "rescue dose" is administered over and above the regularly scheduled ATC medication. If three to four analgesic doses are required each 24 hours, the ATC regularly scheduled doses should be in-

creased to include the amount used for previous breakthrough pain while still maintaining a PRN dose for future breakthrough pain.

5. *Plan treatment of side effects.* Management of side effects must be done aggressively and often should be prophylactic. Be aware that the following side effects may occur with the repeated administration of opioids:
   - Constipation (does *not* decrease over time)
   - Nausea/Vomiting (usually temporary lasting about 1 week)
   - Sedation (usually temporary)
   - Respiratory Depression (rarely occurs)
   - Other: Confusion/hallucinations, dizziness, urinary retention

6. *Never use placebos* Placebos have no place in the

Table 28–8 Adjuvant Coanalgesics—Cont'd

Drug	Dose	Indications	Comments
STEROIDS			
Dexamethasone (Decadron)	10-20 mg ×1 then 4 mg q6 hr (16-96 mg) if spinal cord compression	Neural pain due to infiltration or compression (e.g., brachial or lumbosacral plexus); increased intracranial pressure; spinal cord compression	Less mineralcorticoid effect; reduces edema in tumor and nerve tissue. Chronic use: weight gain, Cushing's syndrome, increased risk of GI bleed with NSAIDs.
Methylprednisolone (Prednisone)	16 mg TID		
Prednisone	20-80 mg/day		
BENZODIAZEPINES			
Diazepam (Valium)	5-10 mg PO or IV TID	Acute anxiety or muscle spasm associated with acute pain	Side effects: sedation, respiratory depression (also used in the treatment of terminal dyspnea); *not* effective analgesic except for muscle spasm.
Lorazepam (Ativan)	1-2 mg PO or IV TID		
STIMULANTS			
Caffeine	65 mg	Lethargy; counteract sedative effect of opioids	Side effects: insomnia, tachycardia, palpitations, anorexia; may produce additive analgesia.
Dextramphetamine (Dexedrine)	2.5-7.5 mg AM & noon	Same	Same
Methylphenidate (Ritalin)	5-15 mg/day	Same	Same; tolerance may develop over 1 month and the dose may need to be escalated[10]

Data from Acute pain management: Operative or medical procedures and trauma, 1992. Agency for Health Care Policy and Research (AHCPR). Publication No. 92-0032; American Pain Society: Principles of analgesic use in the treatment of acute pain and chronic cancer pain, ed. 3, 1992; Inturrisi CE: Management of cancer pain—Pharmacology and principles of management, Cancer, 63 (11):2310-2311, 1989; McCaffery M and Beebe A: Pain—A clinical manual for nursing practice. St. Louis, 1989, Mosby, p. 78-79; and Weissman DE, Burchman SL, Dinndorf PA, and Dahl JL: Handbook of cancer pain management, Wisconsin, 1992, Cancer Pain Initiative.

oncology client population. As McCaffrey states, "Pain is whatever the client says it is, whenever he says it does."

Adjuvant (Coanalgesic Drugs)

Several medications have been found to be analgesic for particular types of pain. These drugs may be ordered for other than their usual indications (Table 28-8).

ANTIDEPRESSANTS. These can produce analgesia in particular circumstances and are appropriate despite a lack of emotional depression; they seem to act by increasing the serotonin level.[14] Indications are neuropathic pain (especially burning), depression, or insomnia. Gonzales[31] describes the use of amitriptyline for posttherpetic neuralgia.

The analgesic therapeutic dose of antidepressants is only one eighth to one sixth of the dose required to treat clinical depression.

ANTICONVULSANTS. Indications are for neuro-pathic pain (especially shooting or stabbing), lancinating pains (e.g., post herpetic pain), tics, or myoclonic jerks.

STIMULANTS. Indications are to increase analgesic effect of other medications, or to reduce the sedative effect of opioids.

CORTICOSTEROIDS. Indications are for nerve infiltration or compression, bone pain, increased intracranial pressure, anorexia, or mood disorders.

Routes of Administration

ORAL. See box on p. 674. This is the route of choice for economy, safety, and ease in pain management. Even severe pain requiring high doses of narcotics can be managed orally as long as the client is able to swallow medication without difficulty. It is very important to convert the parenteral to oral doses correctly as they are different and the amounts cannot be interchanged (see Table 28-5). Education may be required to convince the client/family that they do

---

ROUTES OF ADMINISTRATION

Oral
- Preferred route for analgesics; patients maintain control
- Allows greater mobility
- Drug levels peak in 1 to 2 hours
- Ease in administration
- Cost efficient

Rectal
- Good for patients who are NPO, nauseated, or unable to swallow
- May be more expensive than oral route and more difficult to obtain
- Most often a 1:1 ratio with oral

Transdermal
- Good for patients who are NPO, nauseated, or unable to swallow
- Takes 14-24 hours to peak initially; lasts approximately 17 hours after removal
- Each patch lasts 2-3 days
- Ease in administration
- Difficult to titrate

Subcutaneous infusion
- Provides prolonged parenteral administration of narcotics and/or intermittent bolus
- Avoids repetitive injections
- Avoids peaks and valleys in bloodstream
- Avoids need for intravenous access
- Readily managed at home
- Recommended for cancer patients who cannot take anything by mouth
- Requires use of infusion pump with alarms

Patient-controlled analgesia (PCA)
- Allows patient to receive a predetermined intravenous bolus of a narcotic by a pump mechanism
- Gives patient sense of control, less anxiety
- Provides quick pain relief
- Patient may require less narcotic
- Eliminates the need for repeated injections

IV continuous infusion
- Provides constant narcotic intravenous infusion to maintain constant blood levels
- No peaks and valleys in blood levels
- Recommended when unable to achieve pain control through oral or rectal routes with high dosages of narcotics or unable to use oral/rectal route
- Requires use of infusion pump with alarms

IV bolus
- Good for acute pain and/or procedures
- Provides most rapid onset but shortest duration
- Not recommended for constant pain due to peaks and valleys in bloodstream

IM injection
- Should be used mainly for acute short-term pain
- Painful administration; rotate sites
- Not recommended for chronic long-term pain especially cancer pain
- Not recommended for use with children, emaciated patients, or patients with a decrease in muscle mass

Spinal administration
Epidural
Dose: 5-10 mg morphine
Pain relief: 12-24 hours
Intrathecal (subarachnoid)
Dose: 0.5-1.0 mg morphine
Pain relief: up to 36 hours
- Narcotic (usually morphine) administered through catheter into epidural or intrathecal space
- May be intermittent bolus or by continuous infusion pump
- Careful selection of the patient necessary as procedure is expensive and may be risky
- Side effects include nausea, vomiting, pruritus, sedation, urinary retention, respiratory depression
- Possible complication of infection and/or meningitis

---

not need "shots" to control the pain and that parenteral administration does not mean stronger medication. As long as the equianalgesic amount is the same, the analgesic effect will be the same. Sustained release morphine is now available, which makes 12-hour dosing effective.[40]

The buccal or sublingual surface may be used for absorption of liquid analgesics in small quantities. Data from controlled clinical studies are not available, but anecdotes from practice support the idea.[44]

Buccal: The space between the cheek and gum of the upper molars; this does not stimulate salivation

Sublingual: Beneath the tongue; administration guidelines are 1 cc every 3 min. According to Stanley and Ashburn,[73] the highest permeability occurs sublingually.

RECTAL. If oral administration is not possible due to the presence of nausea/vomiting, if the person is unable to swallow, or if there is dysphagia present, the same dose of oral medication administered rectally can also achieve pain relief. Controlled studies are not available to support the practice fully, but it appears that the rectal mucous membrane absorbs equally to the oral cavity (thus a 1:1 ratio) and may prevent the necessity of changing to a parenteral route. The limitations for this route include the presence of diarrhea, anal/rectal fissures, or thrombocytopenia.

Available Prepared Suppositories include:[16,44]
Morphine [Upsher-Smith]   (5, 10, 20, or 30 mg)
Hydromorphone (Dilaudid) [Knoll]   (3 mg)
Oxymorphone (Numorphan) [DuPont Pharmaceuticals]   (5 mg)

TRANSDERMAL.   A new form of administration is now on the market in the form of a controlled-release "patch." Durogesic (Janssen) is fentanyl, a short-acting narcotic, which is available as a 72-hour continuous release product and clients/families can manage these with ease. Be aware that there will be a delay of approximately 14-24 hours[37] until the peak level of analgesia is reached and supplemental medications will be required. It may require a trial period to make certain that the dose is correct and that the product does indeed provide analgesia for a 72-hour duration for the client.

SUBCUTANEOUS.   This is an often overlooked route since intravenous administration has become customary. The ratio of dosing for subcutaneous versus IM/IV is 1:1. A small gauge (25 or 27 gauge) butterfly needle can be placed anywhere there is adequate subcutaneous tissue (e.g., abdomen or even thigh if the individual is not ambulatory) and the line may be used continuously or intermittently. The site should be inspected every 8 hours for redness, edema, and tenderness, but the butterfly needle can be left in place for 5 to 7 days without changing sites if there are no complications. Ideally, the medication should be concentrated so that there is ≤1 cc infused per hour, but it is possible to administer even larger amounts if absorption is adequate. Bruera et al[11] describe the successful subcutaneous infusion of narcotics and fluids at the rate of 20 to 100 cc/hr with the addition of hyaluronidase and KCl. Any medication with a parenteral formulation can be used for subcutaneous infusion.

Moulin et al[56] compared the efficacy of subcutaneous and intravenous routes and found no statistically significant differences in pain intensity, pain relief, mood, or sedation between the two routes. Johanson[36] reports a cost savings of $350 per week with subcutaneous administration rather than intravenous.

INTRAVENOUS.   For home use, a permanent central venous access device would probably be required. Unless the client requires the access for other purposes (e.g., hydration, nutrition, antibiotics), it adds considerable cost (the device, surgeon's fee, surgical suite costs, and maintenance) without additional benefit over other routes for pain management. If the client cannot swallow, has diarrhea, and has inadequate subcutaneous tissue, this may be the route of choice. It can be used intermittently (with a flushing schedule) or continuously via a Patient Controlled Analgesic (PCA) system.

PATIENT CONTROLLED ANALGESIA (PCA).   This method of pain control involves a machine-delivery system that is programmed by the nurse and can deliver a basal (continuous) amount with an incremental/bolus (intermittent) amount or a combination of both. Ideally, a PCA system will be programmed to have a continuous (Basal) infusion that covers the usual analgesic requirements and a bolus option available to treat breakthrough pain incidences. This type of technology can be used either subcutaneously or intravenously and allows the patient to have control over this area of life, namely pain management.

INTRAMUSCULAR.   Although this route has been used over time for pain management, it is least preferred for the person with cancer who may require medications for an extended period of time. Sites may become limited, absorption may become erratic, and, more importantly, it requires the *added pain* of an injection when the intent is to *relieve pain.*

DIRECT CENTRAL NERVOUS SYSTEM (CNS) ADMINISTRATION.   When a person has been trialled on the other methods of analgesic administration and they are not effective (e.g., intolerable side effects, high dose levels), a route that may indeed provide relief is via the opiate receptors of the spinal column. The analgesia is produced by the direct effect on the opiate receptors in the dorsal horn of the spinal column. The sites may be:

> *Epidural*—a catheter is placed between the vertebral column and the dura. The patient will require about one tenth the amount of narcotic as required parenterally.
>
> *Intrathecal*—a catheter is placed in the subarachnoid region. The patient will require about 1/100 of the narcotic as required parenterally.

The placement of the catheter requires strict aseptic technique by a skilled physician. The epidural or intrathecal catheter may be tunneled to the exterior for intermittent injection or a port/pump may be implanted for continuous infusion with a bolus option. There is extended pain relief (12 to 24 hours) following a single injection, but for some individuals a continuous infusion may be more efficacious.

Direct CNS analgesia is a relatively new area in nursing practice, and it requires that each state determine what its Nursing Practice Act allows in regard to an intraspinal catheter (e.g., inject [and if nurses may inject, which medications may be injected?]). Nurses working with spinal administration of narcotics must have documentation of adequate educational preparation for care. The agency/institution must have policies and procedures to govern practice.

Wilke[83] advocates the use of preservative-free solutions until current research determines whether preservatives are harmful or not. One other area of question is whether to use alcohol or provodone-ioidine in cleansing the injection port. Most of the guidelines specify provodone-ioidine due to the known toxic effect of alcohol to the spinal cord.[4]

As this pain management modality is costly, it is

usually not considered unless there is a life expectancy of 3 months or more. It falls into the category of "high-tech" and the other modalities warrant trials first.

See the box on p. 674 for a summary of the routes of administration.

NONPHARMACOLOGIC PAIN RELIEF TECHNIQUES

There are many activities that nurses can teach the client/family to do that aid in the reduction of pain. These interventions are most effective when the pain level is low, but can also be used as an adjunct to medications when the pain is moderate. Currently there is a lack of research to support many of these mechanical or psychosocial interventions, but in many instances they have merit and warrant a trial basis.

Most of the interventions are inexpensive and easy to perform. Most have low risks and few side effects, and, very importantly, they provide the ability for the patient to have some control over this aspect of their pain management.

Noninvasive pain relief techniques can be useful alone or as adjuncts to the management of pain. The mechanical techniques consist of cutaneous stimulation (therapeutic touch, pressure, heat, cold, massage, and transcutaneous electrical nerve stimulation [TENS]). Behavioral pain relief techniques include distraction, imagery/visualization, music, humor, prayer, education, play therapy, biofeedback, and hypnosis.

Mechanical Interventions	Behavioral Interventions
Cutaneous stimulation	Relaxation
Therapeutic touch	Distraction
Pressure	Imagery/Visualization
Massage	Music
Heat/cold	Humor
TENS	Prayer
	Education
	Play therapy
	Biofeedback
	Hypnosis

Noninvasive Mechanical Interventions

CUTANEOUS STIMULATION.   Cutaneous stimulation is any activity that stimulates the skin for the purpose of relieving pain. According to the Gate Control Theory of pain, this stimulates the large nerve fibers, which "closes" the gate to pain-conducting small nerve fibers.

HEAT AND COLD.   Because applications of heat and cold are so common and because they have been used for so long, nurses may underestimate their value in pain control. Both heat and cold decrease pain and muscle spasm. Deciding which therapy to use should

Table 28–9 Effects of Heat and Cold

	Heat	*Cold*
Pain	Decreased	Decreased
Muscle spasm	Decreased	Decreased
Inflammation	Increased	Decreased
Blood flow	Increased	Decreased
Hemorrhage	Increased	Decreased
Edema	Increased	Decreased

From McGuire L: Pain. Beare PG and Myers JL: Principles and practices of adult health nursing, St. Louis, 1990, Mosby.

be based on the physiologic effects desired (Table 28-9).

There are important factors that the nurse should keep in mind whenever using heat or cold therapy: the age of the patient, medical history, condition of the skin, and any discomfort. Some patients may benefit from alternating heat and cold therapy. However, if the patient cannot tolerate heat or cold therapy, it should be discontinued.

TRANSCUTANEOUS ELECTRICAL NERVE STIMULATION (TENS).   TENS consists of a pocket-sized battery-operated device that provides a continuous mild electrical current to the skin via electrodes. The electrodes are generally placed on or near the painful site. The stimulation is again of the large nerve fibers, which will "close" the gate.

TENS units have different dials so that the patient can adjust the intensity, rate, and pulse width (duration) to achieve a soothing, pleasant sensation.

The nurse plays an important role in teaching these techniques, in assessing whether they are being done correctly, and in evaluating whether they are indeed effective.[45]

Behavioral Interventions

Behavioral interventions focus the person's mind on something other than the pain sensation. They may be effective because they assist to decrease the person's anxiety. These techniques are very individual as to the person's preference and will be effective only when the person believes that they will work.

In order for behavioral interventions to be effective, the nurse must explore the interest areas of the client, determine which areas may have meaning for the client, and determine if the client believes the approach will make a difference in relieving pain. Each technique requires time to teach and practice in order to become effective. Briefly, the techniques are described below:

RELAXATION.   State of relative freedom from both anxiety and skeletal tension. Some examples include distracting thoughts, rhythmic breathing, peaceful images, quiet environment, and repetition.[45]

DISTRACTION. Distraction is focusing on stimuli other than the pain sensation. This is often done without realizing that it is a form of analgesia and is reducing the sensation of pain. Distraction helps alter the patient's ability to tolerate pain. Some examples include music (auditory distraction), tapping (tactile distraction), TV or flowers (visual distraction), people, and humor. Each of these activities may easily be employed with little or no cost and used as an adjunct to medications, but be aware that distraction has a short duration and does not replace pharmacologic analgesics.[45]

IMAGERY/VISUALIZATION. Mentally creating a picture is the use of one's imagination. This may be a focus on a close person, a place of enjoyment, a past event, or anything that is thought to bring pleasure. Examples of imagery include: emptying the sandbag, breathing out pain, and a ball of healing energy. The mind is occupied and therefore the pain is reduced in focus.[45]

MUSIC. Music (tapes, records, CDs, live performances) is used to take the thoughts away from the painful sensation. This is very individual as to the person's preference, and the client's choice must be explored. A teenager's choice of music would probably not be the choice of the person over 70, and the person trained in classical music may not be a country/western fan.[45]

HUMOR. Laughter is used as a distraction. Humor can provide immediate distraction, but it also can provide prolonged pain relief even up to 2 hours. Does the person have a favorite comedian? Are there audio or visual recordings available of that person performing? Is there a joke book that would match the person's sense of humor? Encourage the use of humor as many people who experience an ongoing pain find that they have little to laugh about.[45]

PRAYER. The use of communication with a higher power. Obviously the client's religious beliefs need to be explored. Is the person a Christian and accustomed to talking with God? Is the person a Hindu for whom there are many gods? Is the person a Moslem who prays to Allah? Is the person an atheist for whom there is no god or higher power and for whom this would not be an option?

PLAY THERAPY. Play therapy is the use of games or toys. This can be especially useful for children, but also for adults. To play is to involve the person physically and mentally in an activity and thus provide distraction. To a child, dolls can become the object taking on the pain. To an adult, a board game may provide a scene of competition and focus from which they are not otherwise involved.

BIOFEEDBACK. Biofeedback is the ability to alter the body functions (e.g., heart rate, blood pressure, muscle relaxation) by intentional mental focusing. This requires the skill of a professional person who is trained in the technique and may be more difficult in the home setting, but the person may have utilized this approach in the past and it is worth exploring as an adjunct during this time of pain.

HYPNOSIS. Hypnosis is the use of psychotherapy to alter the affective component as well as the sensory component of pain; the patient's perception of pain is modified. Hypnosis has been used to decrease stress, but studies on its efficacy in pain control are lacking. Hypnosis requires a professional who is skilled in teaching hypnosis and again may not be feasible for the home setting. Ahles[2] questions how effective this technique might be for patients with other than mild to moderate pain. More research is required in this area.[45]

Invasive Techniques

NERVE BLOCKS. The nerve block is an injection of an anesthetic agent into or near a nerve to numb pain pathways. The nerve block can be performed with either a local temporary anesthetic agent or a permanent neurolytic agent. Local anesthetic agents provide pain relief for several hours to days.

NEUROSURGICAL PROCEDURES. Neurosurgical procedures for pain relief are surgical or chemical (alcohol) interruption of pain pathways. It is essential that patients be carefully selected for these procedures and that they completely understand the potential risks and benefits.

ACUPUNCTURE. Acupuncture, the insertion of needles at various points into the body to relieve pain, comes from the Latin words acus, needle, and pungere, puncture. This invasive technique is based on an ancient Chinese theory of two opposing forces, yin and yang, the Chinese theory says that pain and illness are caused by an imbalance of yin and yang.

It is theorized that acupuncture works because it stimulates large nerve fibers to close the gate in the spinal cord to pain impulses. It is also postulated that acupuncture causes the release of endorphins.

QUALITY ASSESSMENT AND IMPROVEMENT

Pain, as well as other aspects of health care, must be assessed for quality management. Accurate evaluation of improvement must incorporate measurement of outcomes, which for pain includes patient satisfaction. Several groups have addressed this issue and have set standards that can be applied to an individual healthcare agency.

1. The Oncology Nursing Society (ONS) together with the American Nurses' Association (ANA) in 1987 published the "Standards of Oncology Nursing Practice." The "standards are primarily in-

tended to help nurse generalists provide effective care and pursue professional development", ANA and ONS, p. 4.

2. The Joint Commission on Accreditation of Healthcare Organizations (JCAHO) has included in their 1992 Manual for Hospitals the following section under Patient Rights:

   R1.1 The organization supports the rights of each patient.

   R1.1.1 Organizational policies and procedures describe the mechanism by which the following rights are protected and exercised:

   R1.1.1.2.2 The care of the dying patient optimizes the comfort and dignity of the patient through

   R1.1.2.2.2 *effectively managing pain*

   This is the first time that pain has been included in JCAHO standards and signifies the importance of addressing pain management as an individual patient's right.

3. The American Pain Society has developed "Standards for Monitoring Quality of Analgesic Treatment of Acute Pain and Cancer Pain." (See Appendix A) Each of the standards is identified as structure, process, or outcome and can be utilized in an agency's Quality Assessment and Improvement program. The document includes a patient interview tool to measure patient satisfaction.

4. The Agency for Health Care Policy and Research (AHCPR), an interdisciplinary federal panel of health care experts, in 1993 released the Guidelines on Acute Pain Management: Operative or Medical Procedures and Trauma.

5. In 1993 the Agency for Health Care Policy and Research (AHCPR) published Cancer Pain Management (With Applications to Selected Nonmalignant Conditions).

Thus, there are now a national accrediting body, national professional organizations, and the federal government that have developed and published information that asks the basic questions:

- Is pain being addressed as a symptom?
- How well is pain being managed?
  . . . from the client's point of view?
  . . . from the professional's point of view?
- Is there adequate documentation? Siehl[66] states "only when our documentation of specific pain interventions is complete, then so is the application of our knowledge in relieving pain for our patients."
- What education is needed (professional and lay)? Max[43] proposes that education alone may not be sufficient to change behaviors and that guidelines and tools need to be developed to ease assessment and communication between and among patients and health care professionals.

The issue of the effectiveness (or the lack of effectiveness) of pain management has also become a legal issue. Angarola and Donato[7] report that a jury awarded $15 million in damages to a family as a result of nursing actions that caused increased pain and suffering through withholding narcotics during terminal illness. Cushing[17] states that the jury award was later set aside and an undisclosed settlement figure was substituted. Yes, pain management is becoming a quality of care issue.

Text continued on p. 684.

Nursing Management

Although the care of patients with pain is multidisciplinary, in most cases *nursing care is the cornerstone.*[45] Pain management is a challenge that every nurse must face when caring for a patient with cancer. Regardless of the setting, the nurse has a vital role in pain management because the nurse has the ongoing contact with the patients in pain. Nurses must be vocal in the area of cancer pain. A nurse who is an advocate for cancer pain management need not be a pain expert, but rather one who is dedicated to the problem of cancer pain relief.

ASSESSMENT

Nursing is involved in obtaining a detailed quantitative and qualitative assessment of the client's pain experience. Pain is a subjective experience and it is only the person who has the pain who is able to legitimately describe the event in detail. As early as 1987, the National Institute of Health (NIH) Consensus Development Conference stated that "nurses have well-established pivotal roles in the assessment and management of pain".[57] Nursing's qualitative assessment includes observations of behavior and appearance and the client's description of sensations and personal impact of the pain. The quantitative assessment includes the client's description of the intensity of the pain and the analgesic requirements over time.

Qualitative assessment includes:

- Reported Symptoms Associated with Moderate to Severe Pain Spross et al[68] identify the following symptoms:

Mood disturbances: Anxiety, depression, anger, and irritability

Decreased ability to concentrate/communicate

Loss of appetite, nausea, and vomiting

Sleep disturbances/sleep deprivation

Sexual dysfunction/lack of interest

Splinting, limited mobility, disuse syndromes

Fatigue

Behavioral changes

- Classification of Pain

  Acute—less than 3-6 months

  Chronic—longer than 3-6 months

- Location

  Is it confined to one area or does it radiate?

  Has it changed from a previous location or extended beyond a previous site?

- Quality—Because the source of pain can vary, it is imperative that the nurse elicit a description that describes the pain most accurately. Use the client's own words for what the pain feels like. Keep in mind that the following descriptors may indicate a particular type of pain:

  Burning—Possibly neuropathic pain

  Stabbing—Possibly neuropathic pain

  Dull or sharp—Possibly somatic pain

  Constant or deep—Possibly visceral pain

- Duration

  Onset—When did it start?

  Intermittent—Does it last briefly after movement?

  Constant—Does it never go away?

- Aggravating and Relieving Factors

  What makes the pain worse? . . . better?

  Does it help to lie down, stand, sit up?

  What has person tried?

  Analgesics?

  Type?

  Dose?

  Frequency?

  Positioning

  Heat/Cold

  Massage

  Does the pain interfere with Activities of Daily Living (ADLs)? Is sleep affected (awakens due to pain)? Is sociability limited?

  What is the expectation for pain relief?

  An acceptable level that is tolerable

  No pain

Quantitative assessment includes:

- Intensity

  0 to 10 with "0" being no pain and "10" the worst pain imaginable. The intensity may be a verbal or visual identification. (See Figure 28-3 for a form of visual analog scale.) A conversion of

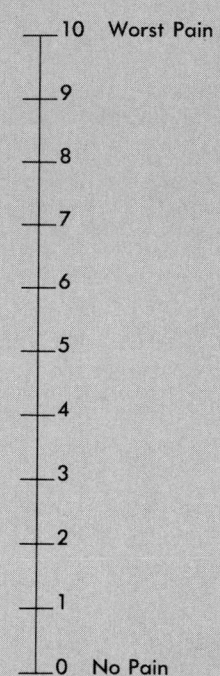

Figure 28–3 Vertical visual analog scale. This scale may be duplicated for use in clinical practice. (From McCaffery M and Beebe A: Pain: Clinical manual for nursing practice, St. Louis, 1989, Mosby.)

numbers into word descriptors for the levels may include:

0 = None

2 = Mild—pain unnoticed with activity

4 = Discomforting—sometimes interferes with activities or sleep

6 = Distressing—usually interferes with activities or sleep

8 = Severe—severely "restricts" person

10 = Excruciating—unable to tolerate

- Equianalgesic amounts per 24 hours

  It is important for the nurse to calculate what the total amount of analgesics required per 24 hours has been and convert this into the common language of morphine equivalents. (See Equianalgesia, p. 667, for details.)

Figure 28-4 is an example of a pain assessment chart that contains both qualitative and quantitative elements. The continuing assessment portion allows for a graphic display of pain intensity over time, which is valuable information for all members of the health care team.

Continued.

NURSING DIAGNOSES

Once the assessment of pain is completed, appropriate Nursing Diagnoses may include:
- Alterations in:
     Comfort (pain, sleep, and/or pruritis)
     Mobility
     Coping
     Elimination (constipation or diarrhea)
     Protective mechanisms (e.g., risk of spinal cord compression)
- Knowledge deficit (specify) (e.g., action of analgesics, schedule of administration, potential side effects)
- Anxiety
- Fear
- Fatigue
- Spiritual distress
- Social isolation/changes in relationships
- Hopelessness[68]

PLANNING

- Where is the client on the World Health Organization (WHO) stepladder of pain management? (See Figure 28-1.)
- Is current treatment adequate?
- Does physician need to be contacted for additional orders?
- Do the client and family understand (and agree with) the current treatment plan?
- Is the client satisfied with pain relief or is more pain relief desired?

NURSING INTERVENTIONS

See Table 28-10 for nursing management of cancer pain for nursing interventions. Appendix B contains a sample protocol that depicts the flow of assessment, the nursing interventions, and reassessment until pain management is achieved.

EVALUATION

Once assessment, planning, and interventions have been implemented, evaluation then proceeds to determine effectiveness of pain management. Evaluation includes:
- *Daily Pain Diary*
   The client/family record this on an ongoing basis.
       Intensity — Is the pain rating score lower than it was before?
       Analgesic intake (per 24 hours)
- *Satisfaction* — Is the client/family pleased with the effect of the analgesic therapy? What more can be done?

- *Quality of Life* — Is the client doing what she/he wants to do? Is pain interfering in any way with activities or personal interactions?

PATIENT TEACHING

Nurses play a major role in the teaching process. It may be spontaneous and informal or a lengthy session with resources (see Appendix C for available printed materials.) Some of the areas of client education include:
- Cause of pain
- Anticipated outcome (pain relief)
     Is the Client expecting no pain or manageable pain?
- What to report to MD/RN
     Unmanaged side effects
     Uncontrolled pain
- Medication information (schedule, dose, refills, and drug interactions)
- Side effects of medications and what to do to prevent or treat them (e.g., patient may be drowsy the first few days of narcotic use, but this effect will pass)
- Information to restructure attitudes and beliefs regarding addiction, medications, etc.
- Plan for follow-up and who to call for emergency assistance
- Client's and providers' responsibilities for pain management plan

GERIATRIC PAIN ISSUES

A segment of our population that has been often overlooked in the management of pain is the elderly. With the increase in longevity and the resultant "aging population" we must, as health professionals, develop a more acceptable attitude toward administering pain medications and controlling pain in the elderly.

McCaffrey and Beebe[44] have a chapter devoted to this topic with explanations and recommendations. Some of the *myths* that impede health care professionals in adequately managing pain in the elderly are:

1. Pain is a natural outcome of growing old.
2. Pain perception, or sensitivity, decreases with age.
3. The potential side effects of narcotics make them too dangerous to use to relieve pain in the elderly.
4. If the elderly patient appears to be occupied, sleeps, or can be otherwise distracted from pain, then he or she does not have much pain.
5. If the older person is depressed, especially if there is no known cause for the pain, then

Continu

Pain Assessment Chart (For Admission and/or Follow-up)

1. Patient _____   2. DX _____

Assessment on Admission

Date _____ / ____ / _____   Pain ☐   No Pain ☐   Date of Pain Onset _____ / ____ / _____

1. Location of Pain (indicate on drawing)

2. Description of Predominant Pain (in patient's words) _____

   _____

   _____

3. Intensity [Scale 0 (no pain) – 10 (most intense)] _____

4. Duration & when occurs _____

5. Precipitating Factors _____

6. Alleviating Factors _____

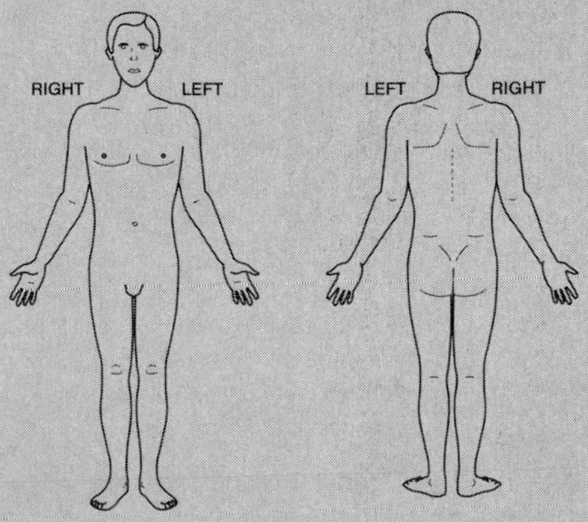

   _____

7. Accompanying Symptoms
   GI: Nausea ☐   Emesis ☐   Constipation ☐   Anorexia ☐
   CNS: Drowsiness ☐   Confusion ☐   Hallucinations ☐

   Psychosocial: Mood _____   Anger _____

   Anxiety _____   Depression _____

   Relationships _____

   _____

8. Other Symptoms

   Sleep _____   Fatigue _____

   Activity _____   Other _____

9. Present Medications _____

   _____

   _____

   Doses and times medicated last 48 hours _____

   _____

10. Breakthrough Pain _____

    _____

Signature: _____

Figure 28–4   Pain assessment chart.   *Continued.*

Continuing Pain Assessment and Interventions

Date/Time													
Med(s)/Dose													

Most Intense Pain

10													
9													
8													
7													
6													
5													
4													
3													
2													
1													
0													

No Pain Sensation 0

Blood Pressure													
Respiration													
Nausea													
Emesis													
Constipation													
Anorexia													
Drowsiness													
Confusion													
Hallucination													
Sleep													
Activity													
Mood													

INSTRUCTIONS: Ask patient to rate the intensity of his/her pain.
Plot this rating on the graph and connect the dots.

Figure 28–4, cont'd.   For legend see p. 681.

Table 28–10   Nursing Management of Cancer Pain—Cont'd

Nursing Dx.	Interventions	Rationale

Alteration in comfort, pain due to . . .	**Assessment:**
	Conduct on a systematic, ongoing basis
	Utilize a tool that addresses:
	  Qualitative components:
	    Reported symptoms
	    Mood disturbances (anxiety, depression, anger, irritability)
	    Decreased ability to concentrate/communicate
	    Loss of appetite, nausea, and vomiting
	    Sleep disturbances/sleep deprivation
	    Sexual dysfunction/lack of interest
	    Splinting, limited mobility, disuse syndromes
	    Fatigue
	    Behavioral changes
	    Interference with Activities of Daily Living (ADLs)[68]
	  Location (one or more sites)
		For accurate knowledge of patient's pain status and outcome of previous analgesic interventions.
		
		A change in location may be a new pain or a referred pain.

	Quality:
	    Burning (neuropathic)
	    Stabbing (neuropathic)
	    Dull or sharp (somatic)
	    Constant or deep (viseral)
	  Duration:
	    Onset
	    Intermittent or constant
	  Aggravating and relieving factors:
	    Standing, sitting, lying down
	    What has the person tried? (analgesics, heat/cold, massage, positioning)
	  Expectation for pain relief (an acceptable level or no pain?)
		Particular descriptor may indicate a specific type of pain. Use the patient's own words for what the pain feels like.
		
		Incorporating previously effective methodologies into the plan of care recognizes the past involvement of patient and family strengthening a sense of personal control.
		If the patient's expectations are not realistic (i.e., total pain relief and no side effects), disappointment in the health care system could arise.

	Quantitative components:
	    Intensity (0-10 scale)
	
	    Equianalgesic amount required per 24 hours
	
	Planning:
	  Determine whether current treatment is adequate and whether patient is satisfied with the pain relief
	Interventions:
	  Administer analgesics according to pain requirements and based on the principles of cancer pain management
	  Investigate the possible use of behavioral interventions in addition to analgesics
	  Instruct patient on behavioral pain management interventions
	  Collaborate with other health care professionals (e.g., physician, pharmacist, social worker) to use team approach to care
		Consistency in measurement gives a measurable means to determine an increase or decrease in severity.
		A common base of amounts (i.e., morphine) provides a consistent measurement of analgesic requirements.
		
		See analgesic tables (28-2 to 28-4) for specific medication information.
		
		Active participation in pain relief measures will increase the sense of personal control.
		
		An interdisciplinary team approach will address the total spectrum of pain.

Continued.

Table 28–10 Nursing Management of Cancer Pain—Cont'd

Nursing Dx.	Interventions	Rationale
Alteration in comfort, pain due to . . . —Cont'd	Evaluation and documentation:	

	Utilize tools to measure
	  Intensity
	  Satisfaction
	  Quality of life
		Written information is available to the interdisciplinary team.

	Conduct evaluation at intervals appropriate for severity of pain as a problem	The evaluation frequency is dependent upon whether pain is an active patient problem.

depression is causing the pain. Pain is a symptom of depression and would subside if the depression were effectively treated.

6. Narcotics are totally inappropriate for all patients with chronic nonmalignant pain.

With so many myths regarding pain in the elderly, what physiologic realities does the nurse need to keep in mind when addressing pain in the elderly?

• Distribution of Drugs:

There are changes in the body composition (an increase of fat and decrease in heart, kidney, and muscle mass) as aging occurs, therefore, usual adult doses may need to be decreased to avoid toxic drug levels in the blood and tissue. Decreased circulating proteins due to serum proteins, malnutrition, or chronic disease potentially result in greater drug effect from higher concentrations of unbound drug, with a greater risk of toxic effect.

• Metabolism of Drugs:

There is limited research in the area of hepatic metabolic rates in relation to aging, but it may be safer to allow for longer intervals between doses in the elderly.

• Excretion of Drugs:

A decrease in renal mass, renal blood flow, glomerular filtration rate, and tubular secretion can all occur in the kidney due to aging. With reduced function the drugs or their active metabolites may remain in the body longer.

General Conclusions

When working with an elderly population, analgesics are appropriate for pain management with the following considerations

1. The dose may need to be *decreased*
2. The interval between doses may need to be *lengthened*
3. The frequency of assessment and evaluation is *increased*

CONCLUSION

Nurses *are* central to the successful management of cancer pain. As Spross[67] stated in her ONS/Schering Clinical Lecture, "pain is an emergency for the person with cancer and, because of the distress it causes, nurses should respond with the same sense of urgency that exists when nurses respond to spinal cord compression or hypercalcemia."

NOT ONLY *CAN* YOU MAKE A DIFFERENCE IN SUCCESSFUL CANCER PAIN MANAGEMENT FOR THE PATIENT WHO IS EXPERIENCING PAIN, YOU *DO* MAKE THE DIFFERENCE.

BIBLIOGRAPHY

1. Agency for Health Care Policy and Research (AHCPR) "Acute Pain Management: Operative or Medical Procedures and Trauma. Clinical Practice Guideline." Rockville, MD: U.S. Department of Health and Human Services, Publication No. 920032, 1992.
2. Ahles T: Psychological techniques for the management of cancer-related pain. In McGuire DB and Yarbro CH, editors: Cancer Pain Management. Orlando, FL, 1987, Grune & Stratton, Inc.
3. American Hospital Formulary Service: Opiate Agonists. Bethesda, MD: American Society of Hospital Pharmacists, 1991, p 1148.
4. American Nurses' Association Position Statement on the Role of the Registered Nurse in the Management of Analgesia by Catheter Techniques, Am Nurse, February:7, 1992.
5. American Pain Society. Principles of analgesic use in the treatment of acute pain and chronic cancer pain—a concise guide to medical practice, ed 3.

(Copies available through the American Pain Society, PO Box 186, Skokie, IL 60076-0186).

6. American Pain Society Subcommittee on Quality Assurance Standards. Standards for monitoring quality of analgesic treatment of acute pain and cancer pain. Oncol Nurs Forum 17(6):952, 1990.

7. Angarola RT and Donato BJ: Inappropriate pain management results in high jury award. (letter), J Pain Sympt Manage 6(7):407, 1991.

8. Bonica JJ: Preface—A short course on the management of cancer pain, J Pain Sympt Manage (Suppl) 2(2):S3-S4, 1987.

9. Brescia FJ: Introduction: A short course on the management of cancer pain, J Pain Sympt Manage (Suppl) 2(2):S5, 1987.

10. Bruera E, Brenneis C, Paterson AH, and MacDonald RN: Use of methylphenidate as an adjuvant to narcotic analgesics in patients with advanced cancer, J Pain Sympt Manage 4(1):3, 1989.

11. Bruera E, Legris MA, Kuehn N, and Miller MJ: Hypodermoclysis for the administration of fluids and narcotic analgesics in patients with advanced cancer, J Pain Sympt Manage 5(4):218, 1990.

12. Cahill C, Panzaulla C, and Spross JA: Pediatric cancer pain. In Oncology Nursing Society Position Paper on Cancer Pain—Part III). Oncol Nurs Forum 17(6):948-951, 1990.

13. Campora E and others: The incidence of narcotic-induced emesis. J Pain Sympt Manage 6(7):428, 1991.

14. Cleeland C, Foley KM, and Levy MH: Stepped management of cancer pain, Patient Care 15:170, 1989.

15. Cohen FL: Postsurgical pain relief: Patients' status and nurses' medication choices, Pain 9:265, 1980.

16. Cole L and Hanning CD: Review of the rectal use of opioids, J Pain Sympt Manage 5(2):118, 1990.

17. Cushing M: The legal side: Pain management on trial, Am J Nurs 92(2):21, 1992.

18. Dalton JA: Nurses' perceptions of their pain assessment skills, pain management practices, and attitudes toward pain, Oncol Nurs Forum 16(2):225, 1989.

19. Diekmann JM, Engber D, and Wassam R: Cancer pain control: One state's experience, Oncol Nurs Forum 16(2):219, 1989.

20. Donovan MI: An historical view of pain management: how we got to where we are! Cancer Nurs 12(4):257, 1989.

21. Dundee JW and Moore J: The myth of phenothiazine potentiation, Anesthesiology 16:95, 1961.

22. Eland JM: The child who is hurting, Semin Oncol Nurs 1(2):116, 1985.

23. Enck RE: Parenteral narcotics for pain control in the home care environment, Caring 9(5):38, 1990.

24. Ferrell BR and Schneider C: Experience and management of cancer pain at home, Cancer Nurs 11(2):84, 1988.

25. Ferrell BR and Ferrell BA: Easing the pain, Geriatr Nurs July/August:175, 1990.

26. Ferrell BR, McCaffery M, and Rhiner M: Pain and addiction: An urgent need for change in nursing education, J Pain Sympt Manage 7(2):117, 1992.

27. Ferrell BR, Wisdon C, Rhiner M, and Alletto J: Pain management as a quality of care outcome, J Nurs Qual Assur 5(2):50, 1991.

28. Foley KM: Cancer pain syndromes, J Pain Sympt Manage (Suppl) 2(2):S13, 1987.

29. Foley KM and Arbit E: Management of cancer pain. In DeVita VT, Hellman S, and Rosenberg SA, editors: Cancer: Principles & Practice of Oncology, ed 3, Philadelphia, 1989, JB Lippincott Co.

30. Glare P and Lickiss JN: Unrecognized constipation in patients with advanced cancer: A recipe for the therapeutic disaster, J Pain Sympt Manage 7(6):369, 1992.

31. Gonzales GR: Postherpes simplex type 1 neuralgia simulating postherpetic neuralgia, J Pain Sympt Manage 7(2):320, 1992.

32. Guidelines for Treatment of Cancer Pain. Final Report of the Texas Cancer Council's Workgroup on Pain Control in Cancer Patients. Texas Cancer Council, 1991.

33. Hill CS and Fields WS: Advances in pain research and therapy, Vol 11, New York, 1989, Raven Press.

34. Inturrisi CE: Pharmacology of narcotic analgesics. Symposium on the management of cancer pain, New York: HP Publishing Co.

35. Inturrisi CE: Management of cancer pain—Pharmacology and principles of management, Cancer 63(11):2308, 1989.

36. Johanson GA: IV versus SQ opioid infusions for cancer pain, Am Hospice Palliative Care July/August:6, 1991.

37. Johanson GA: New routes of opiate administration, Am Hospice Palliative Care, July/August:4, 1992.

38. Kaiko RF and others: Central nervous system excitatory effects of meperidine in cancer patients, Ann Neurol 13:180, 1983.

39. Kaiko RF: Heroin: Facts and comparisons, PRN Forum 4:1, 1985.

40. Lapin J and others: Cancer pain management with a controlled-release oral morphine preparation, J Pain Sympt Manage 4(3):146, 1989.

41. Levy MH: Pain management in advanced cancer, Semin Oncol 12(4):394, 1985.

42. Marks R and Sachar E: Undertreatment of medical inpatients with narcotic analgesics, Ann Intern Med 78:173, 1973.

43. Max MB: Improving outcomes of analgesic treatment: Is education enough? Ann Intern Med 114(4):342, 1991.

44. McCaffery M and Beebe A: Pain: A Clinical Manual for Nursing Practice, St. Louis, 1989, Mosby.

45. McCaffery M: Managing your patients' adverse reactions to narcotics, Am J Nurs 89(10):166, 1989.

46. McCaffery M: Pain management: Nurses lead the way to new priorities, Am J Nurs 90(10):45, 1990.

47. McCaffery M and Ferrell BR: Opioid analgesics: Nurses' knowledge of doses and psychological dependence, J Nurs Staff Develop 8(2):77, 1992.

48. McGee JL and Alexander MR: Phenothiazine analgesia—fact or fantasy? Am J Hosp Pharm 36:633, 1979.

49. McGuire DB and Yarbro CH: Cancer Pain Management. New York: Grune & Stratton, Inc.

50. McGuire DB: Cancer pain: Pathophysiology of pain in cancer, Cancer Nursing 12(5):310, 1989.

51. McGuire DB and Sheidler VR: Pain. In Groenwald SL and others, editors: Cancer Nursing—Principles and Practice, ed 2, Boston, 1990, Jones and Bartlett Publishers.

52. McGuire L: Administering analgesics. Which drugs are right for your patients? Nursing 90:34, 1990.

53. McLaughlin-Hagan M: Continuous subcutaneous infusion of narcotics, J Intrav Nurs 13(2):119, 1990.

54. Mersky H: Classification of chronic pain: Description of chronic pain syndrome and definitions of pain terms, Pain 3:217, 1986.

55. Miaskowski C and Donovan M: Implementation of the American Pain Society quality assurance standards for relief of acute pain and cancer pain in oncology nursing practice, Oncol Nurs Forum 19(3):411, 1992.

56. Moulin DE, Kreeft JH, Murray-Parsons N, and Bouquillon AI: Comparison of continuous subcutaneous and intravenous hydromorphone infusions for management of cancer pain, Lancet 337:465, 1991.

57. NIH Consensus Development Conference: The integrated approach to the management of pain, J Pain Sympt Manage 2(1):35, 1987.

58. Paice JA: The phenomenon of analgesic tolerance in cancer pain management, Oncol Nurs Forum 15(4):455, 1988.

59. Paice JA: Unraveling the mystery of pain, Oncol Nurs Forum 18(5):843, 1991.

60. Portenoy RK and Coyle N: Controversies in the long-term management of analgesic therapy in patients with advanced cancer, J Pain Sympt Manage 5(5):307, 1990.

61. Portenoy RK: Cancer pain—Epidemiology and syndromes, Cancer 63(11):2298, 1989.

62. Porter J and Jick H: Addiction rate in patients treated with narcotics (letter), New Engl J Med 302(2):123, 1980.

63. Relieving Pain: An analgesic guide. Principles of analgesic use in the treatment of acute pain and chronic cancer pain. American Cancer Society. Am Nurs 88(6):815, 1988.

64. Rogers AG: The successful use of controlled-release morphine, J Pain Sympt Manage 5(5):331, 1990.

65. Schug SA and others: A long-term survey of morphine in cancer pain patients, J Pain Sympt Manage 7(5):259, 1992.

66. Siehl S: The need for quality assurance in pain management, J Pain Sympt Manage 5(4):215, 1990.

67. Spross JA: Cancer pain and suffering: Clinical lessons from life, literature and legend, Oncol Nurs Forum 12(4):23, 1985.

68. Spross JA, McGuire DB, and Schmitt RM: Oncology Nursing Society Position Paper on Cancer Pain—Part I (Scope of Nursing Practice Regarding Cancer Pain, Ethics and Practice), Oncol Nurs Forum 17(4):595, 1990.

69. Spross JA, McGuire DB, and Schmitt RN: Oncology Nursing Society Position Paper on Cancer Pain—Part II (Education, Research and list of cancer pain management resources), Oncol Nurs Forum 17(5):751, 1990.

70. Spross JA, McGuire DB, and Schmitt RN: Oncology Nursing Society Position Paper on Cancer Pain—Part III (Nursing Administration, Pediatric Cancer Pain and Appendices), Oncol Nurs Forum 17(6):943, 1990.

71. Spross JA: Pain management: Issues in the hospital setting. In Pain Management Issues in Research and Practice. American Cancer Society publication, 1992.

72. Spross JA: Cancer pain relief: An international perspective, Oncol Nurs Forum 19(7 supplement):5, 1992.

73. Stanley TH and Ashburn MA: Novel delivery systems: Oral transmucosal and intranasal transmucosal, J Pain Sympt Manage 7(13):163, 1992.

74. Steele JA: Twenty-one states operate cancer pain initiatives, J Nation Cancer Inst 83(22):1613, 1991.

75. Swenson CJ, Sikorski K, DeWaters T, and Bucknell Ryan S: Narcotic oral equivalents, Oncol Nurs Forum 18(5):942, 1991.

76. Thorpe DM: Comprehensive pain care: The relief of pain and suffering, Dimens Oncol Nurs 4(1):27, 1990.

77. Twycross RG and Lack SA: Oral morphine: Information for patients, friends and families, Beaconsfield, Bucks, England: Beaconsfield Publishers, Ltd. (Available through Roxane Laboratories, Inc.)

78. Twycross RG and Lack SA: Oral morphine in advanced cancer, ed 2, Beaconsfield, Bucks, England: Beaconsfield Publishers Ltd. (Available through Roxane Laboratories, Inc.)

79. Vetter TR: Pediatric patient-controlled analgesia with morphine versus meperidine, J Pain Sympt Manage 7(4):204, 1992.

80. Walsh TD: Prevention of opioid side effects, J Pain Sympt Manage 5(6):362, 1990.

81. Watt-Watson JH: Nurses' knowledge of pain issues: A survey, J Pain Sympt Manage 2(4):207, 1987.

82. Weissman DE, Burchman SL, Dinndorf PA, and Dahl JL: Handbook of cancer pain management, ed 3, From the Medical College of Wisconsin and the University of Wisconsin Medical School in conjunction with The Wisconsin Pain Initiative.

83. Wilke DJ: Cancer pain management: State-of-the-art nursing care, Nurs Clin North Am 25(2):331, 1990.

84. World Health Organization (WHO). Cancer pain relief and palliative care, Geneva, Switzerland: World Health Organization, 1990.

Appendix A

STANDARDS FOR MONITORING QUALITY OF ANALGESIC TREATMENT OF ACUTE PAIN AND CANCER PAIN*

AMERICAN PAIN SOCIETY SUBCOMMITTEE ON QUALITY ASSURANCE STANDARDS†

[From American Pain Society Subcommittee on Quality Assurance Standards. Standards for monitoring quality of analgesic treatment of acute pain and cancer pain. Oncol Nurs Forum 17(6):952-954, 1990.]

Summary

Hospital and chronic care facilities in the United States have active "quality assurance committees" that monitor selected outcomes of care, working toward steady improvement in results. In order to harness these existing mechanisms to improve pain treatment, the American Pain Society has drafted a set of standards that embody five key elements for favorably influencing behaviors of patients and clinicians: 1) ensuring that a report of unrelieved pain raises a "red flag" that clinicians cannot ignore; 2) putting information about analgesics conveniently at hand where orders are written; 3) promising patients responsive analgesic care and urging them to communicate pain; 4) providing policies and safeguards for the use of modern analgesic technologies; and 5) monitoring the facility's success in implementing these measures.

Introduction

Undertreatment of acute pain and chronic cancer pain persists despite decades of efforts to provide clinicians with information about analgesics (NIH Consensus Conference, 1986; Donovan, 1987; Hill, 1989). Traditional educational approaches, we believe, must be complemented by interventions that more directly influence the routine behaviors of clinicians and patients to ensure that pain is communicated and that treatment is rapidly adjusted to provide relief (Soumerai, 1984; Morgan, 1986; Hodes, 1989; Edwards, 1990; Max, 1990).

In the United States, virtually all healthcare facilities have "quality assurance committees" composed of physicians, nurses, pharmacists, other clinicians, and administrators. Each committee chooses a number of clinical objectives that it considers important to monitor. They examine *process*, that is, whether the appropriate personnel follow the proper procedures in dealing with the clinical problem, and *outcome*, the result for the patient. Outside organizations, most notably the Joint Commission on Accreditation of Healthcare Organizations (JCAHO) (O'Leary, 1987), make regular inspections of facilities to assess how well they are monitoring care. Because the economic viability of facilities often depends on successful accreditation, administrators provide strong incentives for professionals to comply.

To support individual clinicians who wish to make pain relief a targeted outcome in their facilities (as recommended by a recent NIH Consensus Conference [1986]), the American Pain Society has developed the following draft standards with the informal advice of JCAHO staff. The standards will be disseminated through publication in medical and nursing journals and through mailings to hospitals. Some facilities also may wish to examine treatment of chronic pain not due to cancer or nonpharmacological treatments. We have focused, however, on the drug treatment of acute pain and cancer pain because there is already a consensus regarding treatment methods.

To facilitate their use, a number of other materials will be distributed along with these standards, such

---

*For publication in Proceedings of the VI World Congress on Pain, Elsevier, 1990.

†Subcommittee members: Mitchell B. Max, National Institute of Dental Research, Bethesda, MD (chair); Marilee Donovan, Rush-Presbyterian-St. Luke's Medical Center, Chicago, IL; Russell K. Portenoy, Memorial Sloan-Kettering Cancer Center, New York, NY; Charles S. Cleeland, University of Wisconsin, Madison, WI; L. Brian Ready, University of Washington, Seattle, WA; Daniel B. Carr, Massachusetts General Hospital, Boston, MA; W. Thomas Edwards, University of Massachusetts Medical Center, Worcester, MA; Mary A. Simmonds, Pennsylvania State College of Medicine, Hershey, PA; and Wayne O. Evans, Rehabilitation Center for Pain, Indianapolis, IN. Send correspondence to: Mitchell B. Max, MD, National Institutes of Health, Building 10, Room 3C-405, Bethesda, MD 20912.

as the American Pain Society's pamphlet, *Principles of Analgesic Use for the Treatment of Acute Pain and Chronic Cancer Pain* (American Pain Society, 1990, Standard II); a brief questionnaire, included in the appendix, to assess patient satisfaction with analgesic care (Standard IC); and a patient education brochure, still in preparation, that declares the facility's commitment to responsive analgesic care.

American Pain Society Quality Assurance Standards for Treatment of Acute Pain and Cancer Pain in Hospitals and Chronic Care Facilities

PREFACE (TO BE INCLUDED WITH STANDARDS). In the majority of patients with acute pain and chronic cancer pain, comfort can be achieved with the attentive use of analgesic medications. Historically, however, the outcomes of analgesic treatment often have not been satisfactory, largely because clinical care units have had no systems in place to ensure that the occurrence of pain is recognized and that when pain persists, there is rapid feedback to modify treatment. These suggested standards are offered as one approach to developing such a system. Individual facilities may wish to modify these standards to suit their particular needs.

The guidelines are intended both for clinical facilities in which only conventional analgesic methods are used (e.g., intermittent parenteral or oral analgesics) as well as in those using the most modern technology for pain management. In either case, the quality of pain control will be enhanced by a dedicated pain management team whose personnel acquire special training in pain relief. Newer, more aggressive methods of pain control, such as patient-controlled analgesic infusion, epidural opiate administration, and regional anesthetic techniques, may provide better pain relief than intermittent parenteral analgesics in many patients, but they carry their own risks. Should institutions choose to use these methods, they must be delivered by an organized team with frequent follow-up and titration and with adequate briefing of the primary caregivers. Such teams should be organized under one of the recognized medical departments of the facility. Specific standards for such methods, monitored by that department, might well augment the general guidelines articulated here.

I. ACUTE PAIN AND CHRONIC CANCER PAIN ARE RECOGNIZED AND EFFECTIVELY TREATED
Required Characteristics (Process)

IA. A measure of pain intensity and a measure of pain relief are recorded on the bedside vital sign chart or on a similar record that facilitates regular review by members of the healthcare team and is incorporated in the patient's permanent record.

IA1. The intensity of pain/discomfort is assessed and documented on admission, after any known pain-producing procedure, with each new report of pain, and routinely, at regular intervals that depend upon the severity of pain. A simple, valid measure of intensity will be selected by each clinical unit. For children, age-appropriate pain intensity measures will be used.

IA2. The degree of pain relief is determined after each pain management intervention, once sufficient time has elapsed for the treatment to reach peak effect (e.g., one hour for parenteral analgesics, two hours for oral analgesics). A simple, valid measure of pain relief will be selected by each clinical unit.

IB. Each clinical unit will identify values for pain intensity rating (e.g., greater than the midpoint on the pain intensity scale) and pain relief rating (e.g., < 50% at its maximum) that will elicit a review of the current pain therapy, documentation of the proposed modifications in treatment, and subsequent review of their efficacy. This process of treatment review and follow-up should include participation by physicians and nurses involved in the patient's care. As the general quality of treatment improves, the clinical unit will upgrade this standard to encourage a continuous process of improvement.

Required Characteristics (Outcome)

IC. At regular intervals (to be defined by the clinical unit and the quality assurance committee), each clinical unit will assess a randomly selected sample of patients who have had surgery within the past 72 hours, have another acute pain condition, and/or have a diagnosis of cancer. Patients will be asked whether they have had pain during the current admission. Those who have experienced pain will then be asked about:

1. current pain intensity.
2. intensity of the worst pain experienced within the past 24 hours (or other interval selected by the clinical unit).
3. degree of relief obtained from pain management interventions.
4. satisfaction with responsiveness of the staff to reports of pain.
5. satisfaction with relief provided.

II. INFORMATION ABOUT ANALGESICS IS READILY AVAILABLE (PROCESS).   Information about analgesics and other methods of pain management, including charts of relative potencies of analgesics, is situated on the unit in a way that aids writing and interpreting orders. Nurses and physicians can demonstrate the use of this material. Appropriate training to treat patients' pain is available to health professionals and included in continuing education activities.

III. PATIENTS ARE PROMISED ATTENTIVE ANALGESIC CARE (PROCESS).   Patients are informed on admission, verbally and in a printed format, that effective pain relief is an important part of their treatment, that their communication of unrelieved pain is essential, and that health professionals will respond quickly to their reports of pain. Pediatric patients and their parents will receive materials appropriate to the age of the patient.

IV. EXPLICIT POLICIES FOR USE OF ADVANCED ANALGESIC TECHNOLOGIES ARE DEFINED (PROCESS).   Advanced pain control techniques, including intraspinal opioids, systemic or intraspinal patient-controlled opioid infusion (PCA) or continuous opioid infusion, local anesthetic infusion, and inhalational analgesia, must be governed by policy and standard procedures that define the acceptable level of patient monitoring and the appropriate roles and limits of practice for all groups of healthcare providers involved. Such policy should include definitions of physician accountability, nurse responsibility to patient and physician, and the role of pharmacy.

V. ADHERENCE TO STANDARDS IS MONITORED (PROCESS)

Required Characteristics (Structure and Process)

VA. An interdisciplinary committee, including representation from physicians, nurses, and other appropriate disciplines (e.g., pharmacy), monitors compliance with the above standards, considers issues relevant to improving pain treatment, and makes recommendations to improve outcomes and their monitoring. Where a comprehensive pain management team exists, its activities are monitored through the parent department's quality assurance body, which also may serve as the facility's quality assurance committee for pain relief. In a nursing home or very small hospital where an interdisciplinary pain management committee is not feasible, one or several individuals may fulfill this role.

VB. At least the chair of the committee has experience working with issues related to effective pain management.

VC. The committee meets at least every three months to review process and outcomes related to pain management.

VD. The committee interacts with clinical units to establish procedures for improving pain management where necessary and reviews the results of these changes within three months of implementation.

VE. The committee provides regular reports to ad-

ministration and to the medical, nursing, and pharmacy staffs.

Example of Patient Outcome Questionnaire (Standard IC) (To be filled out by interviewer)

1. At any time during your care, have you needed treatment for pain?
   _____Yes _____No

2. Have you experienced any pain in the past 24 hours?
   _____Yes _____No

3. On this scale, how much discomfort or pain are you having right now? (Category, numerical, or VAS scales may be used for questions 3-5.)
   _____ (record rating)

4. On this scale, please indicate the worst pain you have had in the past 24 hours.
   _____ (record rating)

5. On this scale, please indicate how much relief you generally obtained from the medication or other treatment you were given for pain.
   _____ (record rating)

6. Select the phrase that indicates how satisfied you are with the way your nurses treated your pain. Very satisfied, satisfied, slightly satisfied, slightly dissatisfied, dissatisfied, very dissatisfied

7. Select the phrase that indicates how satisfied you are with the way your doctor treated your pain. Very satisfied, satisfied, slightly satisfied, slightly dissatisfied, dissatisfied, very dissatisfied

8. When you asked for pain medication, what was the longest time you had to wait to get it?
   _____ Record answer or choose from: 15 minutes or less, 15-30 minutes, 30-60 minutes, more than one hour, never asked for pain medication

9. Was there a time that the medication you were given for pain didn't help and you asked for something more or different to relieve the pain?
   _____Yes _____No
   If your answer is "yes," how long did it take before your doctor or nurse changed your treatment to a stronger or different medication and gave it to you?
   _____Record answer or choose from: 1 hour or less, 1-2 hours, 2-4 hours, 4-8 hours, 8-24 hours, more than 24 hours

10. Early in your care, did your doctors or nurses discuss with you that we consider treatment of pain very important, and did they ask you to be sure to tell them when you have pain?
    _____Yes _____No

11. Do you have any suggestions for how your pain management could be improved?

APPENDIX B
Sample Pain Management Protocol*

I. According to pain assessment, the following analgesics will be used:

PAIN	ANALGESIC	ROUTE	INITIAL DOSE/FREQ.
A. Mild (1-2)	Acetaminophen or aspirin or ibuprofen	PO	650 mg q4h ATC 400 mg q4h ATC
B. Moderate/discomfort (3-4)	Acetaminophen/codeine (Tylenol #3)	PO	2 tablets q4h ATC
	Acetaminophen/hydroco-done (Vicodin or equiva-lent)	PO	2 tablets q6h ATC
C. Severe/distressing (5-7)	Acetaminophen/aspirin/ox-ycodone (Percodan, Perco-cet, Tylox)	PO	2 tablets q4h ATC
D. Very severe/(8-10)	Roxanol concentrate (20 mg/cc) Morphine Sulfate Immediate Release (MSIR) or	PO	10-30 mg q4h ATC
	Hydromorphone (Dilaudid)	PO	4 mg q4h ATC

After 48 h of successful analgesia with MSIR or hydromorphone, or if the patient is already taking strong opioids, may convert to sustained-release morphine (MS Contin or Oromorph). ATC = Around the clock.

II. Constipation Management

DRUG	DOSE/FREQUENCY	PURPOSE
A. Docusate sodium + senna (Senokot-S)	1-2 tablets TID Range: 1 daily to 4 tablets TID	Stool softener
B. If no bowel movement in 48 hours: Dulcolax	2-3 tabs qHS to TID	Stimulant

Rule: one Senokot-S for every 15 mg morphine or its equivalent

III. Nausea Control

DRUG	DOSE/FREQUENCY	PURPOSE
Prochlorperazine (Compazine)	10 mg PO, R, q4-6h 10 mg spansule q12h 25 mg R supp. q12h 10 mg IM q6h prn	Antiemetic
or Triethylperazine (Torecan)	10 mg PO, IM daily to TID, 1-3 times daily	Antiemetic
If gastric stasis, Metaclopramide (Reglan)	10 mg PO q6h (Range: 10 mg q8h to 20 mg q6h)	Promote gastric motility

IV. *Additional Medications*

DRUG	DOSE/FREQUENCY	PURPOSE
Choline Magnesium Trisalicylate (Trilisate)	1500 mg PO q8-12h 600 mg PO q6h	Non-narcotic Salicylate Prostaglandin inhibitor
Ibuprofen (Advil, Motrin)		NSAID NSAID
Naproxen (Naprosyn)	250-500 mg PO BID	Neuropathic pain (shooting)
Carbamazepine (Tegretol)	200 mg PO BID-QID	Neuropathic (burning)

*Adapted from Northern Illinois Hospice Association, Rockford, IL. From Hackman E: Pain management for the terminally ill. Unpublished Master's degree project, Northern Illinois University, 1990.

Desipramine (Norpramine)	25 mg HS (10 for elderly) (Increase by 1 tab q2-3 days until 100-300 mg at HS)	
Dexamethasone (Decadron) or Prednisone	Variable	Antiinflammatory
Lorazepam (Ativan)	1 mg PO HS, or tritrate from 0.5 to 2 mg. BID or TID	Antianxiety

V. *Route*

A. *Oral* if possible!

B. If dysphagia is present:

1. Sublingual/buccal morphine, although not FDA approved, is found to be effective when rectal route is contraindicated; use 1:1 ratio.

2. Rectal forms of aspirin/acetaminophen/ morphine and most antiemetics are available. Although not approved, sustained-release, oral morphine may be given rectally. Use 1:1 ratio.

3. Morphine may be administered by subcutaneous infusion. Caregivers must be instructed about management of the pump. Oral to subcutaneous ratio = 3:1.

4. Intrathecal, epidural, or central venous access infusions will be considered only if all other routes fail to achieve adequate control.

VI. *Guidelines for "rescue doses"*

1. If on sustained-release morphine q12h, supplement with ⅓ of the dose q4h prn.

2. If 3 more "rescue doses" are required per 24 hours for breakthrough pain, total the dose of analgesics per 24 hours and divide into the new ATC dosing schedule.

APPENDIX C
Resources

ORGANIZATIONS

American Cancer Society, National Office (ACS)
1599 Clifton Road
Atlanta, GA 30329
404-320-3333

American Pain Society (APS)
A national chapter of the International Association for the Study of Pain.
5700 Old Orchard Road, First Floor
Skokie, IL 60076-0157
708-966-5595

International Association for the Study of Pain (IASP)
A multidisciplinary professional organization
909 NE 43rd Street, Suite 306
Seattle, WA 98105-6020
206-547-6409

National Cancer Institute (NCI)
Office of Cancer Communications
NCI/NIH
Bethesda, MD 20892
1-800-4-CANCER

National Hospice Organization (NHO)
Publishes *Hospice* magazine (professional orientation) and *The Hospice Journal* (research orientation)
1901 North Moore Drive, Suite 901
Arlington, VA 22209
703-243-5900

Oncology Nursing Society (ONS)
501 Holiday Drive
Pittsburgh, PA 15220-2749
412-921-7373

WHO Cancer Pain Relief Program
American Association for World Health
1129 20th Street N.W. Suite 400
Washington, DC 20036
202-466-5883

Wisconsin Cancer Pain Initiative
3675 Medical Science Center
University of Wisconsin Medical School
1300 University Avenue
Madison, WI 53706
608-262-0978

STATE CONTACTS

An asterisk indicates that the state has an initiative.

ALABAMA
John J. Marsella, MD
1504 Tacoma St.
Dothan, AL 36303
(205)793-8105

ARIZONA*
Eugenie A. Obbens, MD
222 West Thomas Road, Suite 415
Phoenix, AZ 85013
(602)650-6306
(602)650-7161 fax

Cheryl Lewis
1225 W. Atlantic Dr.
Gilbert, AZ 85234
(602)835-0711
(602)835-9716 fax

ARKANSAS
A. Reed Thompson, MD
4301 W. Markham, Slot 543
Little Rock, AR 72205-7199
(501)686-5140
(501)664-4381 (private ofc.)

CALIFORNIA*
Pamela J. Haylock, RN
220 Ware Road
Woodside, CA 94062
(415)851-5620 phone & fax

Theresa Ferrer-Brechner, MD
6001A Truxtun Ave. Ext., Suite 180
Bakersfield, CA 93309
(805)861-9542
(805)631-7160 voice mail
(805)861-9548 fax

COLORADO*
Carol Balmer, PharmD (President)
Box C-238
School of Pharmacy
University of Colorado
4200 E. 9th Ave.
Denver, CO 80262
(303)270-7709
(303)266-5795 pager
(303)270-6281 fax

CONNECTICUT*
Didi Loseth, RN, MSN
705 Sport Hill Rd.
Easton, CT 06612
(203)261-6630 home
(212)639-8708 (Mem. Sloan-Kettering)
(212)717-3081 fax

Rich Gannon, RPh
41 Sunset Ave.
Meriden, CT 06450
(203)237-7849 (home)
(203)524-2003
(203)524-7066 fax

DELAWARE
Gretchen W. Jones, RN, MS, OCN
P.O. Box 581
Hockessin, DE 19707
(302)658-7468

FLORIDA*
Lisa O. Sienon, RN, OCN
Lee Moffitt Cancer Center
Pain Service
P.O. Box 280179
Tampa, FL 33682-0179
(813)972-8456
(813)972-8495 fax

GEORGIA
Anne Marie Mckenzie, MD
1719 Pine Ridge Dr. NE
Atlanta, GA 30324
(404)686-2320
(404)686-4889

HAWAII*
Hob Osterlund, RN, MS
The Queen's Medical Center
1301 Punchbowl Street
Honolulu, HI 96813
(808)547-4726
(808)547-4032 fax

Linda Person, RN (Chair)
Oncology Unit
Kaiser Medical Center
3288 Moanalua
Honolulu, HI 96819
(808)834-3869
(808)834-3990 fax

ILLINOIS*
Michael E. Frederich, MD (President)
Medical Director
Hospice of Southern Illinois, Inc.
305 South Illinois
Belleville, Illinois 62220
(618)235-1703
1-800-233-1708
(618)235-2828 fax

Mary Cooper, RN
Chair Region I (Central and Southern Illinois)
441 Hay Street, Suite 203
Decatur, IL 62526
(217)875-3913
(217)428-1243 fax

Carol J. Swenson, RN, MS, OCN
Chair Region II (Northwestern Illinois)
Swedish American Hospital
1400 Charles Street
Rockford, IL 61104
(815)968-4400 pager 128
(815)968-3713

Martha Twaddle, MD
Hospice of the North Shore
2821 Central Street
Evanston, IL 60201
(708)866-4601
(708)866-6023 fax

INDIANA*
Neil Irick, MD (Chair)
Pain Resource Center
2020 West 86th Street
Suite 310
Indianapolis, IN 46260
(317)872-2332
(317)872-2889 fax

Julie Painter, RN, OCN
Oncology Clinical Nurse Specialist
Regional Cancer Center
1500 North Ritter Avenue
Indianapolis, IN 46219
(317)355-4848
(317)351-7739 fax

IOWA*
Peggy Christ, RN (Co-chair)
Jennie Edmundson Hospital
933 E. Pierce Street
Council Bluffs, IA 51502

Eric Goldsmith, D.O. (Co-chair)
1440 E. Grand
Des Moines, IA 50314

KENTUCKY
Lin Edwards, RN, MS
Director of Program Development
Hospice of Louisville
3532 Ephraim McDowell Drive
Louisville, KY 40205-3224
(502)456-6200
(502)456-6655 fax

MAINE
Beth Place
Visiting Nurse Svc.
RR 2, Box 921
Wells, Maine 04090
(207)985-8085 home
(207)284-4566 work

MARYLAND*
Rebecca Finley, PharmD
University of Maryland Cancer Center
22 South Greene Street
Baltimore, MD 21201
(410)328-7683
(410)328-6896 fax

Beth Gregory, PharmD (Co-chair)
John's Hopkins Oncology Center
Carnegie 180
600 N. Wolfe St.
Baltimore, MD 21205
(410)955-6591
(410)955-0125 fax

Julie A. Steele, MPH, CHES (Co-chair)
National Cancer Institute
Office of Cancer Communications
9000 Rockville Pike
Building 31, Room 4B43
Bethesda, MD 20892
(301)496-6792
(301)402-0894 fax

MASSACHUSETTS*
Margaret Barton Burke, RN, MS, OCN
c/o American Cancer Society, Mass. Division
247 Commonwealth Avenue
Boston, MA 02114
(617)267-2650
(617)469-9549 (home)

MICHIGAN*
Josefina Magno, MD
International Hospice Institute
Henry Ford Hospital
2799 West Grand Boulevard
Detroit, MI 48202
(313)876-9234
(313)874-4044 fax

Stuart Weiner, MD
Academy of Hospice Physicians
3371 Beecher Road
Flint, MI 48532
(313)733-7270
(313)733-0250 fax

MINNESOTA*
Thomas E. Elliott, MD (Chair)
The Duluth Clinic, Ltd.
400 East Third Street
Duluth, MN 55805
(218)722-8364
(218)725-3030 fax

Paula Sallmen, RN, OCN, BAN
Virginia L. Piper Cancer Institute
Abbott Northwestern Hospital
800 E. 28th St. at Chicago
Minneapolis, MN 55407-3799
(612)863-4633
(612)863-4689 fax

MISSOURI*
Marianne Nalley, RN
Professional Education Director
3322 American Ave.
Jefferson City, MO 63131
(314)893-4800
(314)893-2017 fax

NEBRASKA
Elaine J. Pohren, MSN, RN
Pain Center
University of Nebraska Medical Center
600 S. 42nd Street
Omaha, NE 68198-5640
(402)559-4364

NEVADA
Carl R. Noback, MD
Noback Pain Center
630 S. Rancho Drive, Suite A
Las Vegas, NV 89106
(702)870-1111
(702)870-7121 fax

NEW HAMPSHIRE*
Marion B. Dolan
Heritage Home Health
169 Daniel Webster Hwy., Suite 7
Meredith, NH 03253
(603)279-4700
(603)279-1370 fax

NEW JERSEY*
Alice Duigon, MSN, RN, CS, OCN
798 Michigan Avenue
Toms River, NJ 08753-4507
(908)929-4281 (phone and fax)
(for fax, call beforehand so machine is set)

Donna Bocco (Chair)
2600 U.S. Hwy. 1
P.O. Box 2201
New Brunswick, New Jersey 08902-0803
(908)297-8000

NEW MEXICO*
Walter B. Forman, MD (Chair)
Department of Veteran's Affairs Medical Center
2100 Ridgecrest Drive
Albuquerque, NM 87108
(505)256-2795
(505)256-2882 fax

Carol Dolan, RN, MSN
University of New Mexico Cancer Center
900 Camino de Salud NE
Albuquerque, NM 87131
(505)277-2858
(505)277-2841 fax

Mark T. Holdsworth, PharmD
Assistant Professor
College of Pharmacy
Nursing/Pharmacy Building
University of New Mexico
Albuquerque, NM 87131
(505)277-2858
(505)277-6749 fax

Antonio Goncalves, PhD
Director, Behavioral Oncology
University of New Mexico Cancer Center
900 Camino de Salud NE
Albuquerque, NM 87131
(505)277-2858
(505)277-2841 fax

NEW YORK
Kimberly Calder, MPS
Cancer Care, Inc.
1180 Ave. of Americas
New York, NY 10036
(212)302-2400
(212)719-0263 fax

Terry Altilio
Memorial Sloan Kettering Cancer Center
Social Work Department
1275 York Avenue
New York, NY 10021

Bruce Kaplan, MD
Dept. of Anaesthesia
Booth Memorial Medical Center
5645 Main St.
Flushing, NY 11355
(718)670-1080
(718)445-8597 fax

NORTH CAROLINA*
Faye W. McNaull, RN, OCN
Durham VA Medical Center
508 Fulton Street
Durham, NC 27705
(919)286-0411 (beeper 416)
(919)286-6896 fax

Jo Ann Dalton, RN, EdD
Associate Professor
School of Nursing
7460 Carrington Hall
University of North Carolina
Chapel Hill, NC 27599
(919)966-1582
(919)966-7298 fax

NORTH DAKOTA
LaRae Palmer, RN
Hospice of the Red River Valley
702 28th Avenue North
Fargo, ND 58102
(701)237-4629
(701)280-9069 fax

OHIO*
Warren Wheeler, MD (Chair)
Belinda Reed
Ohio Cancer Pain Initiative
3732 C Olentangy River Road
Columbus, OH 43214
(614)442-0608

OKLAHOMA
Barbara Bilderback, RN, MS
Department of Education
St. Francis Hospital
6161 S. Yale Avenue
Tulsa, OK 74136
(918)494-1193

OREGON*
Kelly Scott, PharmD (Chair)
Oregon Cancer Pain Initiative
P.O. Box 6313
Portland, OR 97228-6313
(503)229-7760
(503)790-1208 fax

PENNSYLVANIA*
Georgia Trostle, RN (Executive Director)
Hershey Medical Center
P.O. Box 850 C1710
Hershey, PA 17033
(717)531-6849
(717)531-6916 fax

Mary A. Simmonds, MD (Chair)
Cowley Associates
Plaza 21, Suite 2-1
425 N. 21st Street
Camp Hill, PA 17011
(717)761-7400
(717)761-1796 fax

RHODE ISLAND*
Phoebe Fernald, RN, MS, OCN
Rhode Island Hospital
Dept. Medical Oncology
593 Eddy St.
Providence, RI 02903
(401)444-5013
(401)444-4184 fax

SOUTH CAROLINA*
Francine R. Margolius, EdD, RN
Medical University of South Carolina
College of Nursing
171 Ashley Avenue
Charleston, SC 29425-2402
(803)792-4612
(803)792-2969 fax

TENNESSEE
John A. Campa III, MD
Chief, Neuro-Oncology Pain Service
Centennial Medical Center
2702 Hillmeade Drive
Nashville, TN 37221
(615)342-4520
(615)342-4577 fax

TEXAS*
C. Stratton Hill, Jr., MD
Director, Pain Service
UTMD Anderson Cancer Center
1515 Holcombe Blvd. Box 8
Houston, TX 77030
(713)792-2824
(713)794-4999 fax

Deborah Thorpe, RN, MS
UTMD Anderson Cancer Center
1515 Holcombe Blvd. Box 82
Houston, TX 77030
(713)792-7318
(713)794-4999 fax

UTAH*
Perry G. Fine, MD
Associate Professor
Department of Anesthesiology
University of Utah Health Sciences Center
50 North Medical Drive
Salt Lake City, UT 84132
(801)581-6393
(801)581-4367 fax

Arthur G. Lipman, PharmD
Professor of Clinical Pharmacy
The University of Utah
Department of Pharmacy Practice
College of Pharmacy
Salt Lake City, UT 84112
(801)581-5986
(801)581-3716 fax

VERMONT*
Amy Becker, PharmD
Department of Pharmacy
Medical Center Hospital of Vermont
111 Colchester Ave.
Burlington, VT 05401
(802)656-5083
(802)656-4832 fax

VIRGINIA*
Thomas J. Smith, MD (Chair)
Medical Director
Dalton Oncology Clinic
Box 230 MCV Station
Richmond, VA 23298-0230
(804)786-0450
(804)371-8453 fax

Susan Robinson, RN
Massey Cancer Center
Box 37
Richmond, VA 23298-0037
(804)786-0450
(804)371-8453 fax

WASHINGTON*
Nigel Bush, PhD
Fred Hutchinson Cancer Research Center
1124 Columbia Street - FB600E
Seattle, WA 98104
(206)667-PAIN
(206)667-3531 fax

Judy Kornell, RN, MN, OCN
Fred Hutchinson Cancer Research Center
1124 Columbia Street FB600E
Seattle, WA 98104
(206)667-5021
(206)667-3531 fax

WISCONSIN*
June L. Dahl, PhD
3675 Medical Sciences Center
1300 University Avenue
Madison, WI 53706
(608)262-0978
(608)262-1257 fax

PROFESSIONAL PUBLICATIONS

"Acute Pain Management: Operative or Medical Procedures and Trauma. Clinical Practice Guideline". Agency for Health Care Policy and Research (AHCPR) Publication No. 92-0032.

"Acute Pain Management in Adults: Operative Procedures (Quick Reference Guide for Clinicians)". AHCPR Publication No. 92-0019.

"Acute Pain Management in Infants, Children and Adolescents: Operative and Medical Procedures (Quick Reference Guide for Clinicians)". AHCPR Publication No. 92-0020.

Center for Research Dissemination and Liaison AHCPR
  Publication Clearinghouse
P.O. Box 8547
Silver Spring, MD 20907
800-358-9295 or 301-495-3453

APS Journal
  Official Journal of the American Pain Society
  Churchill Livingstone Inc.
  5 S. 250 Frontenac Road
  Naperville, IL 60563
  800-553-5426

Journal of Pain and Symptom Management
  A multidisciplinary publication that supports research
  and education in all areas of palliative care.
  Elsevier Publishing Co., Inc.
  Subscription Customer Service
  655 Avenue of the Americas
  New York, NY 10010
  212-633-3950

"Cancer Pain Management (With Application to Selected
  Nonmalignant Conditions)". Agency for Health Care Policy and Research (AHCPR).
  See Acute Pain Management publication for address and
  telephone number.

"Cancer Pain Release"
  A publication of the World Health Organization Collab-
  orating Center for Symptom Evaluation
  634 WARF
  610 Walnut Street
  Madison, WI 53705
  608-262-0727

"Cancer Pain Relief and Palliative Care" (1990)
  76-page handbook for pain management compiled by international experts.
  WHO Publications Center—USA
  49 Sheridan Avenue
  Albany, NY 12210
  518-436-9686

"Effective Pain Management for Cancer Patients" (1992)
  A monograph on the latest in cancer pain education and
  treatment.
  Bonica, J. J.
  Distributed by Pharmacia-Deltec, Inc.
  1265 Grey Fox Road
  St. Paul, MN 55112
  1-800-426-2448 or 612-633-2556

"Handbook of Cancer Pain Management"
  Weissman DE, Burchman SL, Dinndorf PA, and Dahl JL:
  (3rd ed., 1992)
  Wisconsin Pain Initiative
  3675 Medical Sciences Center
  1300 University Avenue
  Madison, WI 53706
  608-262-0978
  ($3.00 per copy, plus postage)

"Innovations in Cancer Pain Management" (1992)
  40-page booklet written by national experts
  Janssen Pharmaceutica Inc.
  40 Kingsbridge Road
  Piscataway, NJ 08855
  1-908-524-9378

"Oncology Nursing Society Position Paper on Cancer Pain
  Monograph"
  Oncology Nursing Society (1990)
  501 Holiday Drive
  Pittsburgh, PA 15220-2749
  412-921-7373
  ($7.00 per copy for non-member; $6.00 for member)

"Oral Morphine in Advanced Cancer" (2nd ed., 1989)
  Twycross, R. & Lack, S.
  Bath, England: Bath Press
  (Available through Roxane Laboratories)
  P.O. Box 16532
  Columbus, OH 43216
  1-800-848-0120

"Principles of Analgesic Use in the Treatment of Acute Pain
  and Chronic Cancer Pain: A Concise Guide to Medical
  Practice" (3rd ed., 1992)
  29-page booklet
  American Pain Society
  5700 Old Orchard Road, First Floor
  Skokie, IL 60077-5595
  708-966-5595

"Pain: Clinical Manual for Nursing Practice" (1989)
  McCaffery M and Beebe A
  C.V. Mosby Company
  11830 Westline Industrial Drive
  St. Louis, MO 63146

"3-Step Analgesic Ladder for Management of Cancer Pain"
  (1991)
  A summary pocket guide of pharmaceutical review.
  Portenoy, R.K.
  (Available through Roxanne Laboratories)
  P.O. Box 16532
  Columbus, OH 43216
  800-848-0120

PATIENT INFORMATION
Booklets

*"Cancer Pain Can Be Relieved" (1988)
*"Children's Cancer Pain Can Be Relieved" (1989)
*"Jeff Asks About Cancer Pain" (1990)
  (Addresses the adolescent with cancer pain.)
  Wisconsin Cancer Pain Initiative
  3675 Medical Sciences Center
  University of Wisconsin Medical School
  1300 University Avenue
  Madison, WI 53706
  608-262-0978
  ($0.50 plus postage each for non-Wisconsin residents)

"How to Talk to Your Doctor About Acute Pain"
  Ronald Melzak, Paul Paris, and Ada Rogers (1987)
  DuPont Pharmaceuticals Biomedical Department
  E.I. DuPont de Nemours & Co., Inc.
  Wilmington, DE 19898
  1-800-543-8693

"Oral Morphine: Information for Patients, Families and
  Friends"
  Robert G. Twycross and Sylvia Lack (1987)
  Roxanne Laboratories
  P.O. 16532
  Columbus, OH 43216
  1-800-848-0120

"Questions and Answers About Pain Control: A Guide for
  People with Cancer and Their Families"
  National Cancer Institute (1986)
  Printed and distributed by the American Cancer Society
  (Available through local ACS offices)
"Relieving Pain"
  Ronald Dubner and Mitchell B. Max
  National Institutes of Health, 1988
  Produced by the Office of Clinical Center Communica-
    tions
  National Institutes of Health
  Building 10, Room IC255
  9000 Rockville Pike
  Bethesda, MD 20892
  301-496-2563
"Up-to-Date Answers to Questions About Measuring Pain"
  (to help patients living with cancer)
  Purdue Frederick Company, 1991
  Norwalk, CT 06850-3590
  203-853-0123

Groups

International Pain Foundation
  Supports public education about pain disorders and their
    treatment through literature and information.
  909 N.E. 43rd Street, Room 306
  Seattle, WA 98105-6020
  1-206-547-2157

VIDEOTAPES

"Cancer Pain Control: Winning the Battle"
"Cancer Pain Control: Controlling Your Cancer Pain"
  (both are client-oriented with "Controlling Your Cancer
  Pain" being more specific on the "how-to")
  Marshfield Video Network
  Marshfield Clinic
  1000 North Oak Avenue
  Marshfield, WI 54449
"No Fears . . . No Tears: Children with Cancer Coping with
  Pain"
  Canadian Cancer Society
  (professionally oriented)
  available through local ACS offices

CHAPTER 29

Protective Mechanisms

Suzanne Shaffer

Numerous mechanisms protect the human being from foreign substances and invading organisms. It is the purpose of this chapter to look at these mechanisms and their importance to the person with cancer, the nursing process, related nursing diagnoses, and nursing interventions.

IMMUNITY

Immunity is a protective mechanism that serves to maintain the integrity of the body against foreign substances or agents. The study of immunity was based on the study of infectious diseases but cannot be limited to such and now encompasses the areas of organ transplantation, blood transfusion, cancer, and autoimmunity.

Three main functions of the immune system include: defense against invading organisms, homeostasis—removal of dead "self" cells, and surveillance—removal of mutant cells.

The major purpose of a fully functional immune system is to distinguish self from not-self. The ability of the body to develop tolerance of self-produced antigens is a part of this function. There are two basic types of immunity: innate and acquired. Innate immunity is a nonspecific immune system function. Acquired immunity is specific and dependent upon the recognition of self and not-self.[35,45]

Innate Immunity

Innate immunity is a nonspecific response to any breach of the skin and mucous membranes. This type of immunity is present at birth and is species specific. Innate immunity provides initial protection against foreign substances and invading organisms. There are four mechanisms of innate immunity: mechanical barriers, chemical barriers, fever, and inflammation.[1,10,32,35]

MECHANICAL BARRIERS. Mechanical barriers include epithelial surfaces such as skin and mucous membranes, and their projections along the gastrointestinal, respiratory, and genitourinary tracts. Intact skin and mucous membranes present an effective physical barrier to the entrance of organisms and toxins. Epithelial surfaces carry receptors for specific antigens on the cell surfaces. These receptors are essential for maintaining the skin and mucous membranes' normal microorganism flora. Secretory IgA, an antibody, prevents the attachment of pathogenic organisms to epithelial cells. Routine exfoliation of epithelial cells, with loss of adherent organisms, also serve to limit invasion by organisms.[1,17,32]

CHEMICAL BARRIERS. Chemical barriers include such substances as saliva, mucus, tears, sweat, gastric juices, sebum, cerumen, lysozyme products, and numerous other substances secreted by the body. These prevent entry of potentially harmful substances and organisms by various mechanisms such as pH, viscosity, and the presence of other substances with antimicrobial activity that physically inhibits attachment and invasion by organisms.[1,35]

FEVER. Fever (elevated body temperature) is a protective mechanism directed against temperature-sensitive organisms such as bacteria and viruses. These organisms secrete substances that act as pyrogens, elevating body temperature in response to their presence. Temperature-sensitive organisms such as these rarely survive sustained body temperature elevations in excess of 39° C (103° F). Warm-blooded animals elevate body temperature by internal means in response to pyrogens such as bacterial toxins and leukocyte products (cytokines) when inflammation and/or immune response occurs.[10] Fevers of 38.2° to 39.5° C are generally well tolerated.

Fever is a defense mechanism that has a positive

effect on the survival of patients with life-threatening infections. Recent investigations have identified the immune enhancing effect of fever on antigen recognition and sensitization.[59] There appears to be increasing support for the positive effects of fever and that aggressive antipyresis for low-grade temperature elevations may be detrimental.*

INFLAMMATORY RESPONSE.   The inflammatory response is a local reaction initiated when mechanical or chemical barriers of the body are invaded by organisms. This limited, nonspecific response is initiated and mediated by phagocytic white blood cells such as neutrophils, eosinophils, basophils, monocytes, and macrophages. It does not require recognition of self. The process of inflammation is not complete until all invading organisms, dead and dying phagocytic cells, and necrotic cellular debris are removed by macrophages (histiocytes) and tissue damage is repaired by fibroblasts.[35,44]

Acquired Immunity

Acquired immunity is the body's specific neutralizing response to foreign invaders and their products. This type of immunity is not fully functional at birth. It may take 6 to 7 years for the immune system to mature, and as a person reaches late middle age, its level of functioning begins to decline,[35,52,62] as evidenced by increased autoimmune disorders and cancers.

There are two main mechanisms of acquired immunity: cell-mediated immunity and humoral immunity. Both employ lymphocytes as effector cells.[35,62]

LYMPHOCYTES.   Lymphocytes are small, round, mononuclear cells, which make up approximately 30% of the peripheral circulating leukocyte population. Lymphocytes are derived from pleuripotential stem cells found in the bone marrow. Two major subtypes of lymphocytes have been identified: thymus-derived or thymus-dependent lymphocytes (T cells) and bursa-derived or bursa-dependent lymphocytes (B cells).[35,62]

CELL-MEDIATED IMMUNITY.   Cell-mediated immunity (CMI) uses T cells as the primary effector cell. T cells function as immunoregulatory and cytotoxic cells. CMI provides defense against intracellular bacteria such as *Mycobacterium tuberculosis* and *Listeria monocytogenes*, fungi, viruses, and protozoa (see box, top right). Delayed hypersensitivity reactions are a type of CMI. Transplantation rejection, by both graft and host, is caused in part by the T cell and its ability to distinguish self from not-self. Immune surveillance, or the body's inherent ability to prevent cancers, is also thought to be a function of CMI with the natural killer cell (NK cell or large granular lympho-

---

*References 10, 18, 34, 37, 47, 59, 63.

> ### INFECTING ORGANISMS ASSOCIATED WITH CELLULAR IMMUNE DEFICIENCY
>
> | *Intracellular bacteria* | *Viruses* |
> |---|---|
> | Mycobacterium tuberculosis | Herpes simplex |
> | Atypical mycobacterium | Herpes zoster |
> | | Cytomegalovirus |
> | | Epstein-Barr |
> | *Listeria monocytogenes* | Hepatitis B |
>
> | *Fungi* | *Protozoa* |
> |---|---|
> | Candida albicans | Pneumocystis carinii |
> | Cryptococcus neoformans | Cryptosporidium |
> | Aspergillus species | Toxoplasma gondii |
> | Histoplasma capsulatum | Giardia lamblia |
> | | Isospora belli |

> ### CELL-MEDIATED IMMUNE DEFICIENCIES
>
> *Primary immune deficiencies*
> *Predominantly T-cell*
> Chronic mucocutaneous candidiasis
> Nezelof syndrome
> DiGeorge syndrome (thymic aplasia)
> *Combined T-cell and B-cell*
> Ataxia-telangectasia
> Severe combined immune deficiency
> Severe combined immune deficiency with adenosine deaminase deficiency
> Short-limbed dwarfism
> Wiscott-Aldrich syndrome
>
> *Secondary immune deficiencies*
> *Malignant disease*
> Acute lymphoblastic leukemia
> Chronic lymphocytic leukemia
> Hairy cell leukemia
> Hodgkin's disease
> Mycoses fungoides and Sézary syndrome
> Non-Hodgkin's lymphoma
> Advanced carcinomas
> *Therapeutic*
> Cytotoxic drugs
> Immunosuppressive agents
> Radiation therapy
> *Infections*
> Human immune deficiency virus
> Cytomegalovirus
> Epstein-Barr virus
> Non-A/Non-B hepatitis
> Leprosy
> Tuberculosis
> Histoplasmosis
> Cryptococcosis
> Toxoplasmosis

cyte) being the primary effector cell of surveillance.[30]

Cell-mediated immune deficiencies may be congenital or acquired (see box above). Congenital anomalies include children born without thymus glands or those with poorly functioning thymus glands. Death usually occurs in the first years of life caused by infection. Secondary or acquired causes of diminished T cell function are more common and include acquired immune deficiency syndrome (AIDS), Hodgkin's disease, organ transplantation immunosuppression, and some autoimmune disorders. Persons who have defects in their cell-mediated immunity, regardless of cause, are susceptible to opportunistic infections from a host of bacteria, viruses, fungi, and protozoa and to the development of cancers, particularly those arising from lymphoid tissue.[35,62]

HUMORAL IMMUNITY. Humoral immunity is the part of acquired immunity that involves the production of antibodies. Antibodies are substances produced by plasma cells (sensitized B cells) in response to specific recognition of an antigen (foreign substance). They are serum proteins called immunoglobulins. There are five major categories of immunoglobulins: IgG, IgM, IgA, IgD, and IgE. The body has an unlimited ability to produce different antibodies against specific antigens. Antibodies function by neutralizing toxins, agglutinating and lysing microorganisms and other cells, and serving as opsonins (coating organisms and making them more palatable to phagocytic cells).

Defects in humoral immunity, like those of cell-mediated immunity, may be congenital or acquired (see box, top right). Agammaglobulinemia and some types of hypogammaglobulinemia may be congenital. These produce lifelong susceptibility to severe bacterial infections. Secondary humoral immune deficiencies, most commonly hypogammaglobulinemias, are often related to lymphoproliferative disorders such as chronic lymphocytic leukemia, non-Hodgkin's lymphomas, and plasma cell dyscrasias such as multiple myeloma and Waldenstrom's macroglobulinemia. Acquired idiopathic hypogammaglobulinemias occur without known cause. Regardless of cause, the person with a defective humoral immune system is susceptible to infection by high-grade (nonopportunistic) encapsulated bacteria, both gram-positive and gram-negative. These infections are often life-threatening and recurrent.[34]

INTERACTIONS. The specific immune response requires complex interaction between cell-mediated and humoral immunity. The macrophage (a phagocytic WBC) is necessary for the proper functioning of this response. The macrophage processes and presents the antigen to the T cell for recognition and elicitation of response. The primary responsibility of the T cells is recognition of self. In the presence of not-self antigens, a number of processes are elicited. Among these is the production of lymphokines. Lymphokines, part of a larger group called cytokines, are soluble chemical mediators that facilitate intracellular communication among T cells, B cells, macrophages,

---

HUMORAL IMMUNE DEFICIENCIES[44,62]

Primary antibody deficiencies
X-linked hypogammaglobulinemia
X-linked hypogammaglobulinemia with growth hormone deficiency
Transient hypogammaglobulinemia of infancy
Common variable unclassifiable hypogammaglobulinemia
Selective immunoglobulin deficiencies (IgA, IgG-subclass)
Autosomal recessive hypogammaglobulinemia

Primary mixed T- and B-cell deficiencies
(See cell-mediated immune deficiencies listed in box on p. 699)

Secondary antibody deficiencies
Chronic lymphocytic leukemia
Acute lymphoblastic leukemia
Non-Hodgkin's lymphoma—B-cell origin
Multiple myeloma
Heavy chain disease
Waldenstrom's macroglobulinemia
Thymoma
Nephrotic syndrome
Protein losing enteropathies
Burns
Splenectomy

EXAMPLES OF CYTOKINES

Monokines
Interleukin-1 (IL-1) or endogenous pyrogen (EP)
Tumor necrosis factor (TNF)
Interferon, alfa (leukocyte) (IF)
Granulocyte-colony stimulating factor (G-CSF)
Granulocyte/macrophage-colony stimulating factor (GM-CSF)
Interleukin-6 (IL-6)

Lymphokines
Macrophage activating factor (MAF)
Macrophage inhibition factor (MIF)
Interferon, gamma (immune) (IF)
Interleukin-2, T-cell growth factor (IL-2)
Interleukin-3, Multi-CSF growth factor (IL-3)
Interleukin-6, B-cell differentiation factor (IL-6)
Chemotactic factor (CF)
B-cell growth factor (BCGF)
Tumor necrosis factor (TNF)
Lymphotoxin (LT)

---

and other phagocytic cells. Particular lymphokines (see box above) may cause activation of macrophages, sensitization of other T cells, and conversion of B cells to plasma cells with resultant production of antibodies. T cells are also regulatory cells of the immune system. Helper/inducer T cells (T4 or CD4 lymphocytes) stimulate and promote immune system function, while suppressor T cells (T8 or CD8 lymphocytes) inhibit or prevent immune system functioning. T8 or CD8 lymphocytes may also become T cells capable of "cell-to-cell" combat.[35,62]

SKIN
Anatomy and Physiology

The skin is one of several mechanical barriers that can prevent the entrance of invading organisms and toxins and maintain homeostasis. The skin is composed of the epidermis, dermis, and assorted derivatives of epidermal/dermal origin, which include hair, nails, cutaneous glands, and teeth.[17]

The epidermis, or topmost epithelial layer, primarily functions to conserve water. Pigment-forming cells called melanocytes reside within this layer. Constant mitotic activity replaces dead cells. Repair and replacement occur from the bottom up; old cells are lost through wear and tear of daily living and are replaced by new cells developing underneath.[17]

The dermis, or inner layer of skin, determines skin thickness. It is thickest on dorsal surfaces of the body, palms of hands, and soles of feet and thinnest on ventral surfaces including the abdomen and genitalia. The dermis contains blood vessels, lymphatics, and sensory nerve endings.[17]

The skin is a multifunctional organ. Its recognized functions include the following[1,17]:

- Distinguishes between pain, temperature, and touch
- Regulates loss of water and electrolytes
- Regulates body temperature by vasoconstriction and vasodilation
- Absorbs substances applied directly to the skin
- Excretes excess water and electrolytes
- Prevents entrance of external gases, liquids, and pathogens as long as intact and so protects the internal body
- Provides nutrition to underlying structures through abundant blood supply

Pathophysiology

A person with cancer may experience multiple disruptions of skin integrity.

DISEASE-RELATED CAUSES.   Disease-related causes of skin integrity disruption include primary skin malignancies such as malignant melanoma, basal cell carcinoma, squamous cell carcinoma, Kaposi's sarcoma, and mycoses fungoides. Metastatic tumors of the skin, such as chest wall recurrence in breast cancer, and leukemic and lymphomatous infiltrates (leukemia cutis and lymphoma cutis respectively) may also disrupt skin integrity. Cutaneous manifestations associated with remote effects of malignancy, such as acanthosis nigricans, acquired icthyosis, dermatomyositis, and exfoliative dermatitis, may cause disruption of skin integrity secondary to scratching and

cracking of skin. Thrombocytopenia with resultant petechiae, purpura, and ecchymoses may lead to increased fragility of the skin.[17]

TREATMENT-RELATED   CAUSES.   Treatment-related causes of skin impairment include those associated with chemotherapy such as drug extravasation, alopecia, hyperpigmentation, hyperkeratosis, photosensitivity, ulceration, and radiation recall reactions.[17] Skin reactions associated with nonantineoplastic agents include allergic skin eruptions, Stevens-Johnson reactions, and erythema multiforme. Radiation therapy skin reactions may progress to wet or dry desquamation. Surgical incisions and other invasive procedures such as needle biopsies and vascular access devices also disrupt skin integrity.[17]

COMPLICATING   FACTORS.   Complicating factors that may interfere with the maintenance of skin integrity include immobility, malnutrition, obstruction, infection, and pruritus.

ASSESSMENT.   Skin assessment should include a thorough inspection of all skin surfaces with attention focused upon the following: color, vascularity, bleeding (location, type and amount), lesions (appearance, number, location, distribution, and ulceration), edema, moist areas, and general condition of hair and nails. If lesions are present, assess for general characteristics, morphologic structure (nodularity, scaling, crusting, erosions, and fissures), size (measure), drainage (color, character, amount, and odor), associated pain and tenderness, depth of lesions (measure) and presence of vital structures within the lesion (i.e., carotid artery). Palpate high risk areas (chest, abdomen, neck, and scalp) with palms of hands for presence of "silent" lesions. Metastatic lesions are generally hard and immovable. Assessment should also include attention to any history of allergies, medications, and past and present skin disorders. Risk assessment is an integral part of the nursing process.

Medical Management

Treatment of skin complications may include antibiotics, antifungals, and antivirals for infection, surgical procedures for incision and drainage, debridement, skin grafting, radiation therapy for obstructive phenomena, chemotherapy to treat the underlying disease for relief of pruritus, and management of disfiguring, non-healing or ulcerating malignant skin lesions.

MUCOUS MEMBRANES
Anatomy and Physiology

The oral mucosa provides a mechanical barrier to inhibit the invasion of microorganisms. The oral mucosa is composed of three layers: an outer layer of stratified, squamous epithelium; a middle layer, the lamina propria, consisting of fibrous fingerlike projections that extend into the epithelium and contain blood vessels, nerves, and glandular tissue; and an inner submucosal layer that varies in thickness with the function at specific anatomical locations. The lamina propria and epithelium are separated by basement membrane. Stem cells of the basement membrane divide and differentiate into the various cells of the surface epithelium. These cells have an estimated life span of 3 to 5 days. It is estimated that the surface epithelial layer of the oral mucosa is replaced every 7 to 14 days. When loss exceeds the rate of replacement, shallow ulcerative lesions occur. Repair continues at a fixed rate, which may leave large areas of mucous membrane denuded of surface epithelium. Intact mucous membranes provide an effective mechanical barrier against harmful exogenous and endogenous organisms. The normal oral flora, mainly consisting of gram-positive bacteria, gram-negative bacteria, and fungi, serve to inhibit the growth of pathogenic organisms. Other mucous membrane-covered surfaces exhibit similar function and growth and replacement patterns.[9,20]

Pathophysiology

The following terms are defined for the purpose of this discussion:

- *Stomatitis*—a general term referring to the inflammatory reaction and shallow ulcerative lesions occurring on the mucosal surfaces of the mouth and oropharynx 7 to 14 days after the administration of certain chemotherapeutic agents and following radiation therapy to the head and neck.[9,25]
- *Mucositis*—a general term referring to the inflammatory reaction and shallow ulcerative lesions occurring on mucosal surfaces, not limited to the mouth and oropharynx, frequently associated with the administration of certain chemotherapeutic agents and following radiation therapy to mucous membrane-bearing sites. Stomatitis, esophagitis, gastritis, enteritis, colitis, proctitis, and vaginitis are examples of treatment-related mucositis.[16,31]

DISEASE-RELATED CAUSES.   Disease-related causes of the disruption of mucous membranes include primary tumors of the head, neck, gastrointestinal tract, respiratory tract, and genitourinary tract; agranulocytic oral ulcers; gingival hypertrophy and infiltration associated with acute leukemia; non-Hodgkin's lymphoma or acute leukemia involving Waldeyer's ring; and Kaposi's sarcoma among others. Disease-related immunosuppression may lead to superinfection with *herpes simplex* (HSV), *Candida albicans,* and other opportunistic agents.[9,20]

TREATMENT-RELATED   CAUSES.   Treatment-related causes of mucous membrane disruption include

---

ANTINEOPLASTIC AGENTS TOXIC TO MUCOUS MEMBRANES	
Antimetabolites	***Antibiotics***
Cytosine arabinoside	Actinomycin
5-Fluorouracil	Adriamycin
6-Mercaptopurine	Bleomycin
6-Thioguanine	Daunomycin
Methotrexate	Mithramycin
	Mitomycin C
Plant alkaloids	
Vincristine sulfate	***Miscellaneous***
Vinblastine sulfate	Hydroxyurea
Etoposide (VP-16)	Procarbazine hydrochloride

---

chemotherapy-induced mucositis (see box above), radiation-associated mucositis, xerostomia (dry mouth), parotitis (inflamed and swollen salivary glands), osteoradionecrosis of the bone (late destruction of irradiated bone and subsequent loss of teeth), and surgical procedures. Chemotherapy effects are systemic and may be wide-spread. Radiation-associated effects are site specific and involve only the areas within the treatment port.

COMPLICATING   FACTORS.   Complicating factors include infections, which may become systemic; bleeding from nonintact mucosal surfaces; poor nutritional status; and pain secondary to the lesions. Preexisting periodontal disease predisposes to more severe complications of disease- and treatment-related mucositis as well as chronic exposure to chemical and physical irritants.[9,20]

ASSESSMENT.   Numerous oral assessment tools are available in the nursing literature. Most assess the lips, tongue, mucous membranes, gingiva, teeth, saliva, voice, and ability to swallow. The use of an oral assessment tool provides the ability to assign numerical (objective and comparative) scores to the examination. It also provides a common base (language) for ongoing physical assessment and evaluation of patient outcomes.[9,20,22,26]

Oral assessment requires the use of readily available tools including a pair of exam gloves, gauze sponges, flashlight, and tongue depressor. Oral assessment should be done at least twice daily and the findings documented in the patient record. The patient and family should be taught the techniques of assessment so that they can follow the progress when the patient is sent home. The patient and family should also be instructed to report any changes in oral sensation or taste and the appearance of lesions.[26,53]

Rectal and vaginal mucosal assessment in the neutropenic patient should be limited to visual inspection only. This prevents trauma to ulcerated mucosa and decreases the potential for dissemination of infection through manipulation of the rectal and vaginal tissue. The patient should be questioned about the presence or absence of rectal or vaginal bleeding, pain, itching, discharge, drainage, and other discomfort or changes in sensation.[16,67]

Medical Management

Treatment of complications involving nonintact mucous membranes includes antibiotics, antifungals, and antivirals for superinfections; platelet transfusion and antifibrinolytic agents for bleeding from mucous membranes; topical and systemic analgesics for pain; and dilation of strictures involving the esophagus and vagina.

BONE MARROW SUPPRESSION
Anatomy and Physiology

The bone marrow is the production site for all formed blood elements: erythrocytes, granulocytes, monocytes, lymphocytes, and megakaryocytes. During early fetal development, hematopoiesis (production of blood) occurs in the liver and yolk sac. By the 20th week of gestation, the bone marrow begins to produce blood cells and by the 30th week, the bone marrow has achieved normal cellularity. At birth, active bone marrow is found in all bones of the body. With age, the functional marrow space contracts, so that by adulthood active marrow is found primarily in the axial skeleton, sternum, ribs, vertebral bodies, pelvis, skull, and in the proximal ends of the long bones.[32,35]

Bone marrow is a spongy organ made up of a fibrous network of connective tissue called stroma. The stroma is supported within the marrow cavity by spicules of bone radiating to the center of the bone marrow cavity from cortical bone. The bone marrow is a highly vascular organ with numerous nutrient arteries and interconnecting venous sinusoids. Poorly understood regulatory mechanisms prevent immature blood cells from entering the venous sinusoids and circulating blood until they reach maturity.[32,35]

All blood cells arise from a common progenitor cell called the stem cell.[35] The stem cell probably resembles and cannot be distinguished by sight from the small mature lymphocyte. The stem cell pool is self-renewing; for every stem cell that enters the differentiation and maturation pool, another cell returns to the stem cell pool. Conditions causing destruction of the stem cell pool lead to the development of marrow aplasia. Stem cells may be either pleuripotential (uncommitted) or unipotential (committed) (Figure 29-1).

Stem cells, having entered a designated cell line, mature under the influence of specific hematopoietic growth factors. The first to be identified and the best known of these growth factors is erythropoietin

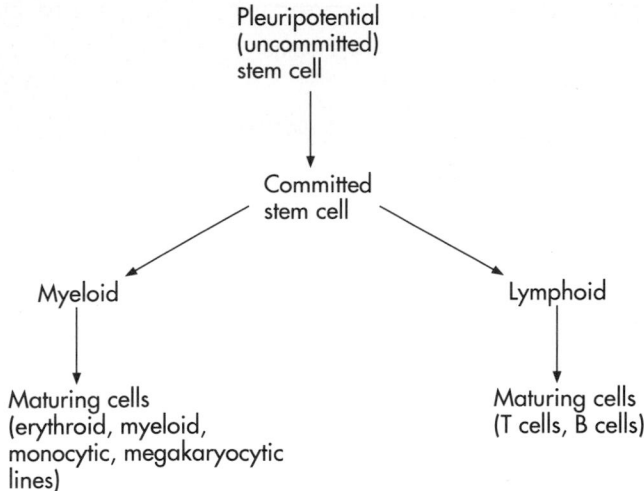

Figure 29-1 Stem cell differentiation and maturation.

(EPO), a glycoprotein hormone produced by the kidney. EPO is necessary for proper differentiation and maturation of erythrocytes (RBCs). EPO levels are regulated by tissue oxygen levels. EPO production reflects need for oxygen carrying capacity via hemoglobin. Current research has led to the identification of several other hematopoietic growth factors. Recombinant DNA technology has made it possible to produce large quantities of these growth factors, allowing increased clinical trials. Those growth factors undergoing trials include recombinant granulocyte/macrophage-colony stimulating factor (rGM-CSF), granulocyte-colony stimulating factor (rG-CSF), interleukin-3 (rIL-3) or multi-CSF, and macrophage-colony stimulating factor (rM-CSF). The target cells of the growth factors both vary and overlap. rGM-CSF and IL-3 are multilineage in that they stimulate and regulate most of the cell lines of the myeloid series (i.e., granulocytes, monocytes, macrophages, erythrocytes, and/or megakaryocytes), while rG-CSF and rM-CSF are lineage restricted (affecting only the neutrophil or monocyte/macrophage lines respectively). rGM-CSF and rG-CSF have received limited approval from the Food and Drug Administration. rGM-CSF has been released for use in accelerating recovery following autologous bone marrow transplantation for nonmyeloid malignancies and rG-CSF has received approval for the prevention of febrile neutropenia following myelosuppressive chemotherapy for nonmyeloid malignancies. Neither CSF stimulates platelet production to any great extent. It is hoped that through the development of other growth factors or combinations of growth factors that prolonged myelosuppression will be a thing of the past.[38,50,60]

Once a stem cell has entered a particular cell line, differentiation and maturation occur in a manner characteristic of erythroid, myeloid, lymphoid, or

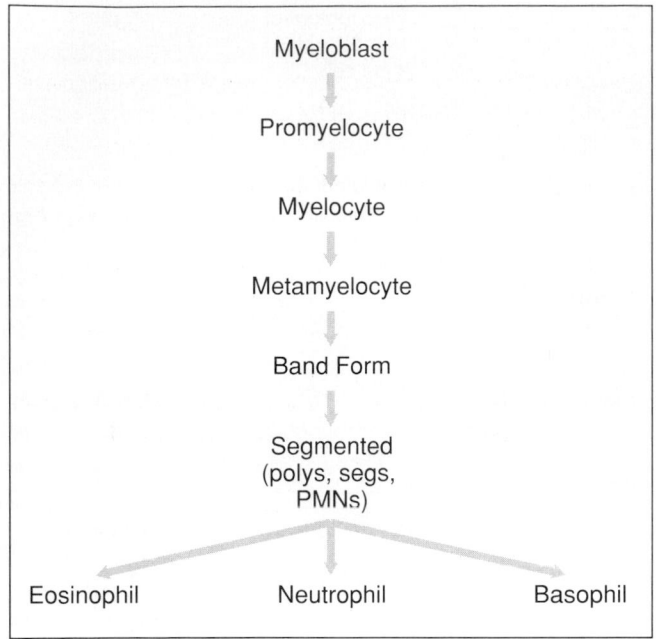

Myeloblast

↓

Promyelocyte

↓

Myelocyte

↓

Metamyelocyte

↓

Band Form

↓

Segmented
(polys, segs,
PMNs)

Eosinophil   Neutrophil   Basophil

Figure 29–2   Myeloid maturation.

megakaryocytic cells (Figure 29-2). Residence (maturation) time within the marrow varies from cell line to cell line and with the body's need for the cell type. Some cell lines have storage pools. Once released into circulation, life span ranges from 6 to 8 hours for the neutrophil to 120 days for the erythrocyte. The marrow is able to respond to increased need for particular cells by permitting early release from the maturation and storage pools.[35,44]

Pathophysiology

Pathologic bone marrow conditions arise from a defect in the stem cell or the marrow microenvironment. The stem cell defect may be intrinsic, as in the leukemias, or extrinsic, as in exposure to stem cell toxins such as benzene or chloramphenicol. Microenvironment problems may occur intrinsically, as in myelofibrosis, a myeloproliferative disorder characterized by replacement of the marrow cavity with fibrous tissue, or extrinsically, as when a nonhematologic malignancy metastasizes to the marrow. Replacement followed by marrow failure may occur. Treatment of malignant disorders by chemotherapy or radiation therapy may alter the stem cell pool and its environment permanently.[35]

DEFINITION OF TERMS.   The following terms are defined for the purpose of this discussion:

- *Leukopenia*—a condition said to occur when the total leukocyte complement is reduced. Leukopenia is a nonspecific finding and usually reflects a decrease in all WBCs (Table 29-1).
- *Granulocytopenia*—a condition said to occur when

the absolute granulocyte complement is reduced. When granulocytopenia occurs, there is a decrease in neutrophils, eosinophils, and basophils.

- *Neutropenia*—a condition that exists when there is an absolute decrease in the number of circulating neutrophils, usually less than 1000/mm³. The absolute neutrophil count (ANC) is calculated as follows:

$$\underset{0.10}{\text{Segs (\%)}} + \underset{0.10}{\text{Bands (\%)}} \times \underset{2000}{\text{White blood cell count}} = \underset{= 400/mm^3}{\text{ANC}}$$

Neutropenia is associated with a profound impairment in the inflammatory response, leading to lack or minimization of the usual signs and symptoms of infection such as erythema, swelling, heat, and pain.[11,12,27] Purulence is not present. Neutropenia is the single most important predisposing factor to infection in the person with cancer:

ANC > 1,500/mm³ = normal risk
ANC < 1,000/mm³ = moderate risk
ANC < 500/mm³ = severe risk
ANC < 100/mm³ = extreme risk

Neutropenia may be related to basic disease processes such as acute nonlymphocytic leukemia or aplastic anemia. Neutropenia may also occur as a result of myelosuppressive treatment for malignant disease such as chemotherapy or radiation therapy.

- *Immunosuppression*—a condition that exists when lymphocyte function or interaction is suppressed. Immunosuppression may result from either disease process or treatment. Selective immunosuppression may inhibit either cell-mediated or humoral immunity. Immunosuppression may be primary or secondary, secondary immunosuppression being the most common. Immunosuppression secondary to corticosteroid therapy is the most common secondary or acquired suppression. Acquired immunodeficiency syndrome (AIDS) resulting from depletion of immunoregulatory T cells occurs following infection with the human immunodeficiency virus (HIV). Primary lymphoid malignancies such as chronic lymphocytic leukemia and non-Hodgkin's lymphoma may also cause immunosuppression.[35]
- *Anemia*— a condition characterized by a decrease in circulating hemoglobin levels or circulating erythrocytes. Anemia occurs when loss or destruction exceeds production of RBCs. This may occur from acute hemorrhage, replacement of normal marrow elements with abnormal cells, loss of the stem cell pool, decreased or ineffective production of RBCs, and accelerated destruction

Table 29–1 Types of Circulating Leukocytes

Type of WBC	% of WBC	Function
Neutrophil	50-70	Phagocytosis, inflammation
Eosinophil	1-4	Chemotaxis, allergies
Basophil	0-4	Anaphylaxis, allergies
Monocyte	2-9	Phagocytosis, inflammation, differentiation into macrophages
Macrophage	—	Circulating and fixed, phagocytosis, antigen processing and presenting cell for the T-cell
Lymphocyte	20-40	Specific immune response, cell-mediated immunity and humoral immunity

of RBCs. Anemia may result from both basic disease process and treatment.[35]

- *Thrombocytopenia*—a condition characterized by decreased numbers of circulating platelets or thrombocytes.[8,33] Thrombocytopenia may result from decreased or ineffective production of platelets secondary to marrow replacement by tumor, exposure to marrow toxins or infectious agents, and ionizing radiation. Thrombocytopenia may also result from increased destruction secondary to immune mediated conditions such as immune thrombocytopenia purpura (ITP) or coagulopathies such as disseminated intravascular coagulation (DIC). In some instances platelet numbers may be normal or increased and a bleeding tendency still exist. This abnormal bleeding may result from a qualitative platelet defect.[33] The most common causes of qualitative platelet defects are ingestion of aspirin or similar drugs that interfere with normal platelet function, and the presence of abnormal platelets secondary to myeloproliferative disorders.[35]
- *Pancytopenia*—a term used when there is a deficiency of all the cell elements of the blood (erythrocytes, platelets, and all the white blood cells [neutrophils, eosinophils, basophils, monocytes, macrophages, and lymphocytes]).

COMPLICATING FACTORS. Complications associated with bone marrow suppression include increased susceptibility to infection secondary to neutropenia, fatigue associated with anemia, and increased risk of bleeding secondary to low platelet counts.

ASSESSMENT

Infection. Daily assessment of the cancer patient should include identification of risk factors for the development of infection, such as neutropenia, lymphopenia, and immunosuppressive therapy. Close observation for the usual signs and symptoms of infection is necessary because neutropenic patients may exhibit little or no inflammatory response[11] (see box on this page). Fever and, occasionally, hypothermia represent serious infection in the immunocompromised.[40]

SIGNS AND SYMPTOMS OF INFECTION
Temperature > 38° C (100° F)
Flushed skin, diaphoresis
Shaking chills
White, cream-colored lesions in mouth
Erythema, swelling, or pain in skin, throat, eyes, joints, perineal or rectal areas
Cough, chest pain, tachypnea, or dyspnea
Changes in character or color of sputum, urine, or stools
Dysuria or frequency of urination
Malaise, lethargy, myalgias, or arthralgias
Skin rash
Confusion, mental status change

Changes in usual respiratory pattern (rate, depth, breath sounds, sputum production), in gastrointestinal tract functioning (nausea, vomiting, dysphagia, hiccoughs, abdominal pain, cramping, diarrhea, rectal pain or itching), and in the genitourinary system (dysuria, oliguria, anuria, pelvic pain, vaginal or urethral discharge) are frequently associated with infection.[12,13,15] Breaks in the integrity of the skin (head and neck, axillae, intertriginous areas, buttocks, and perineum) and mucous membranes (oral, anal, vaginal) represent portals of entry for infectious organisms and should be duly noted. Sepsis, or blood-borne systemic infection, produces significant morbidity and mortality. Assessment for and early detection of sepsis is important in caring for the severely neutropenic patient[48,58] (see left-hand box on p. 706).

Bleeding. Assessment for bleeding should include the following: a check of daily laboratory values for hemoglobin and platelet count; a check of medications that may alter platelet production or function; assessment for the presence of petechiae and ecchymoses, prolonged bleeding from venipunctures, minor cuts, or scratches, frank bleeding from any body orifice, and occult blood in excreta and vomitus.[33,35]

Anemia. Assessment for anemia and its resultant fatigue should include the following: a check of daily laboratory values for hemoglobin and platelet count, a check for presence of occult blood in the excreta of

---

**SIGNS OF IMPENDING SEPTIC SHOCK
(HYPERDYNAMIC OR WARM SHOCK)**

Mental confusion
Chills and fever
Skin flushed and dry
Blood pressure normal or slightly low
Widened pulse pressure
Tachycardia
Tachypnea
Hypoxemia
Urine output normal to slightly increased

**INFECTING ORGANISMS ASSOCIATED WITH
NEUTROPENIA**

Gram-negative bacteria
Pseudomonas aeruginosa
Klebsiella and *Enterobacter* species
Escherichia coli

Gram-positive bacteria
Staphylococcus aureus
Streptococcus pyogenes

Fungi
Candida albicans
Aspergillus species
Mucorales species

Long-term vascular access devices
Staphylococcus epidermidis
Corynebacterium JK

---

the thrombocytopenic patient, a check for the presence of frank bleeding from any body orifice, and assessment of the pattern of fatigue and its impact upon life-style.[35]

Medical Management

INFECTION. The medical management of suspected infection in the neutropenic or otherwise immunocompromised patient includes its prompt recognition with a workup including cultures, radiologic studies, a thorough physical assessment, and the immediate institution of broad-spectrum, empiric, intravenous antibiotics. Blood cultures should be obtained from both peripheral and central venous access sites, if present, for aerobic and anaerobic bacteria, fungi, and viruses if indicated. Cultures from body orifices, other body substances, and any suspicious lesions should be obtained before initiating antibiotic therapy.[12,13,57] Sites of infection in the neutropenic patient are the following:

- Lungs
- Skin
- Oral cavity
- Gastrointestinal tract
- Genitourinary tract
- Blood

The choice of antibiotics will be based on the prevalence and sensitivities of organisms commonly cultured at the health care facility[57] (see box above, right). The usual combination is that of an aminoglycoside and a semisynthetic penicillin with good antipseudomonal effect. Antibiotic coverage may be narrowed when the culture results are available. Antibiotic therapy usually continues for a minimum of 10 to 14 days or until the patient's neutrophil count recovers to over 1,500/mm³. If the patient continues febrile for greater than 72 hours it is advisable to reculture, and depending upon previous culture results, change antibiotic therapy. If the patient has a vascular access device and the current antibiotics do not have good coagulase-negative Staphylococcus coverage, therapy

may need to be changed to include a drug such as vancomycin. If the patient's clinical course deteriorates or there is reason to suspect the infecting agent may be either fungal or viral, amphotericin B (an antifungal) or acyclovir (an antiviral) or both may be added empirically.[57]

BLEEDING. Bleeding related to thrombocytopenia may be manifested as petechiae, purpura, ecchymoses, bleeding from a hollow viscus (GI tract, lungs, or GU tract), intracranial hemorrhage, or occult bleeding identified through the routine testing of excreta.[33] Workup of a suspected bleed should include a thorough physical examination, radiologic examination as indicated by the clinical presentation, and laboratory evaluation, including a complete blood count (CBC), prothrombin time (PT) and partial thromboplastin time (PTT), and fibrinogen and fibrin degradation products (FDPs) if indicated.[2] Treatment depends upon the cause of the bleeding. If the bleeding is secondary to thrombocytopenia or a qualitative platelet defect, platelet transfusions will be of value. If the bleeding results from a coagulopathy such as DIC, platelets and coagulation factors may be replaced, using concentrates, cryoprecipitate, or fresh frozen plasma. Epsilon aminocaproic acid (Amicar) may be added to inhibit lysis of the clot by the fibrinolytic system.[8,33,35,46]

ANEMIA. Symptoms of anemia may occur at variable levels of hemoglobin, depending upon the rapidity with which it has occurred, the age of the patient, and status of the cardiorespiratory system.[29] Findings may include the following: palpitations, shortness of breath, orthopnea, congestive heart failure with pulmonary edema, angina, fatigue, weakness, intolerance of cold, tinnitus, digestive complaints, difficulty in concentration, and numerous other nonspecific findings.[29,62] The workup should include a thorough physical assessment looking for the site of bleeding and the level of cardiorespiratory compensation. Laboratory examination should include complete blood count, reticulocyte count, lactic dehydrogenase, bilirubin, and a hemolysis screen if indicated.[62] Transfusion of red blood cells is indicated if there is evidence of cardiac decompensation or if low hemoglobin levels are combined with low platelet counts. Transfusion of whole blood is not indicated unless there is massive bleeding and volume replacement cannot be accomplished by other means. Replacement of circulating red cell mass to improve oxygen carrying capacity should be accomplished by transfusion of packed red blood cells. This provides for more efficient use of blood components and less risk of volume overload.[49]

TRANSFUSION THERAPY

The use of blood component therapy is one of the more common supportive therapies employed in the care of the person with myelosuppression. Even so, transfusion therapy must be used with care. While major mismatch transfusion reactions are rare and usually result from clerical error (the patient received the wrong unit of blood), febrile transfusion reactions are quite common. Febrile reactions are caused by the recipient reacting to donor leukocyte antigens. This can be discomforting for the patient and may accelerate alloimmunization or sensitization to transfused blood. Historically, febrile reactions have been dealt with by using premedications that may suppress the response or through the administration of leukocyte-poor blood products. Saline-washed RBCs provided significantly reduced numbers of leukocytes although this is costly in time, money, and loss of RBCs. Early leukodepletion filter required extra processing and cooling of the RBCs. Leukocyte-poor platelets were rarely provided. Recent technologic advances have produced more efficient filters that are both user friendly and are available for platelets. The provision of leukocyte-poor blood components is more important for those persons who are expected to require transfusion support for prolonged periods and alloimmunization prevention.[6] Other potential benefits from leukodepletion include (1) decreased risk of bloodborne pathogens that reside in leukocytes, such as cytomegalovirus (CMV), and (2) possible decreased risk of transfusion-associated graft-versus-host disease.[3,6,42]

CMV infection, especially CMV pneumonitis, carries a significant risk for morbidity and mortality in patients who are severely immunosuppressed. CMV transmission may occur when a CMV negative (CMV −) recipient is transfused with blood from a CMV positive (CMV +) donor. The virus may remain dormant in lymphocyte for years following active infection. CMV + persons with normal immune system functioning are unaffected by the virus since their immune system keeps the virus in check. Interest is great regarding methods of reducing risk for the CMV − person. Leukodepletion of blood components may help decrease the risk by removing potentially infectious leukocytes.[6] Another method that is showing promise is the development/identification of a CMV − blood donor pool. This necessitates screening and designation of CMV − donors. Not in widespread use, this method is costly, time-consuming, and removes potential donors from the general blood donor pool.

Since the mid-1980s when HIV transmission via blood transfusion was confirmed, there has been a great interest by potential blood transfusion recipients in directed donations (the personal selection of one's blood donors). It has been assumed that directed donors would be safer than donors from the volunteer pools, when in fact it has been shown that the incidence of infectious disease markers is higher in directed donor population. A more recent problem with directed donations is transfusion-associated graft-versus-host disease (TA-GvHD).[6] While exeedingly rare, TA-GvHD carries a mortality rate approximating 100%. The high mortality rate is associated with bone marrow failure. TA-GvHD has been associated most frequently with directed donations from first degree relatives such as parents or siblings. TA-GvHD occurs when the transfusion recipient has two nonidentical HLA haplotypes and the transfusion (lymphocyte) donor is homozygous for either of the HLA haplotypes of the recipient. The recipient is unable to recognize the donor lymphocytes as "not-self" while the donor (transfused) lymphocytes are able to recognize the recipient as "not-self." The lymphocyte reaction is essentially the same as that seen following allogeneic marrow transplantation. The exception is that the recipient marrow stem cells are a target organ for the GvH reaction, while in BMT associated GvHD, the marrow stem cells are of donor origin and therefore "self" and are not reacted against. The potential for TA-GvHD following directed donation is such that it is recommended that all blood components from first degree relatives be irradiated prior to transfusion. Irradiation of blood components prior to transfusion is standard procedure for marrow transplant recipients and premature or other immunocompromised neonates. It is possible that leukodepletion filtration may decrease the risk of TA-GvHD but is not as effective as ionizing radiation.[3,6,42]

Text continued on p. 717.

Nursing Management

NURSING DIAGNOSES FOR THE PERSON WITH CANCER AND POTENTIAL DISRUPTION OF SKIN INTEGRITY[13,41,43,56]

- Skin integrity, impaired, potential/actual, related to immobility, malignant skin lesions, infectious skin lesions, nonspecific rashes, irritation from urinary and/or fecal incontinence, abrasions resulting from scratching and shearing forces, invasive therapeutic procedures, radiation skin reactions, "recall" skin reactions, chemotherapy extravasations, lymphatic and/or vascular obstruction, decubiti, and/or malnutrition
- Infection, potential for, related to impairment of skin integrity secondary to any of the above contributing factors, related to surgical incision; related to presence of long-term venous access device
- Pain related to any of the above contributing factors; pruritus related to basic disease process and/or adverse drug reaction; pain related to postherpetic neuralgia
- Body image disturbance related to malignant skin lesions, extremity edema, and alopecia

INTERVENTIONS

Assessment

- Inspect high risk skin areas for color, vascularity, edema, injuries, scars, lesions, nodules.
- Document assessment at least once a shift.

Preventive measures to maintain intact skin

- Use draw sheet for turning and positioning.
- Elevate head of bed to maximum of 30 degrees except for mealtimes.
- Use footboard to prevent sliding.
- Provide over-bed trapeze to assist in position change.
- Lift patient to change position rather than pulling or sliding.
- Use devices to decrease pressure areas, such as alternating pressure mattresses, Clinitron or Kin-aire types of beds.
- Use heel and elbow protectors.
- Provide meticulous skin hygiene — mild soap, thorough rinsing, patting dry (not rubbing), air dry when feasible, apply lotions to skin over bony prominences.

Malnourishment

- Follow general preventive measures.
- Provide adequate nutritional support.
- Assess risk daily.

Incontinence

- Follow general preventive measures.
- Offer bedpan and urinal every 2 hours.
- Wash buttocks and perineum after each incontinence, pat or air dry.
- Place waterproof pads between draw sheets rather than next to patient's skin.
- Evaluate need for bowel and bladder retraining program.

Immobility

- Follow general preventive measures.
- Use splints and braces to prevent contractures.
- Use dietetic and nutrition consultants.
- Initiate referrals to rehabilitation medicine, social services, and vocational rehabilitation.
- Institute bowel program with stool softeners and laxatives to prevent constipation.
- Provide diversionary activities to prevent boredom.

Pruritus

- Follow general preventive measures.
- Maintain hydration of the skin by increasing fluid intake, applying water-soluble emollients to damp skin, and providing a humidified environment.
- Keep fingernails short and smooth.
- Wash hands frequently.
- Use alternative methods of skin stimulation such as pressure, massage, vibration, and cold compresses.
- Avoid inciting agents and tight, irritating, nonabsorbable clothing.
- Prevent vasodilation by providing a cool environment and cool baths and showers, avoiding alcohol- and caffeine-containing foods and beverages, and decreasing anxiety level through use of distraction.
- Institute medical treatment as prescribed, which may include treatment of the underlying malignancy, antihistamines, corticosteroids, tranquilizers, and topical agents.

Maintenance of normal skin integrity should be a major emphasis of nursing management. This includes continued assessment, evaluation of risk, prevention of skin breakdown, and specific interventions should impaired skin integrity occur. Systematic protocols or care plans should be implemented to ensure continuity of care.

PATIENT AND FAMILY EDUCATION

Patients and families need to be taught the importance of maintaining intact skin, the fundamentals of assessing skin, and how to prevent breakdown by proper positioning and padding to prevent pressure points. Patients and families should be taught the signs and symptoms of infection and when and whom to notify on the health care team.

INTERVENTIONS FOR NONINTACT SKIN

Assessment

- Inspect skin lesions and document: general character, location and distribution, configuration, size (measure), morphologic structure (nodularity, scaling, crusting, erosions, fissures), drainage (color, amount, character, odor), depth of lesion, presence of vital structure in lesion (carotid artery).
- Monitor for signs and symptoms of infection (elevated temperature, tachycardia, tachypnea, change in color and odor of drainage, erythema).
- Evaluate for associated signs and symptoms (pain and tenderness).
- Evaluate patient's physical and psychologic responses to lesions.
- Assess patient and family's ability to care for problem in the home.

General maintenance interventions

- Follow general preventive measures.
- Implement infection measures.
- Implement measures to prevent bleeding and trauma.
- Provide adequate pain control.
- Obtain Enterostomal Therapy/Skin Care Specialist consult.
- Obtain Home Health referral well in advance of discharge.

Nonulcerating lesions

- Follow general preventive measures.
- Use dry dressings to protect against irritation and trauma.
- Use occlusive dressings with topical medications for increased penetration.

Ulcerating lesions

- Cleanse area with antibacterial soap using gentle motion. Rinse well. Prevent cross-contamination if local infection is present. May use half-strength hydrogen peroxide and normal saline for effervescent cleansing. Do not use on healing tissue.
- Follow recommended protocol for debridement (i.e. cotton swabs, wet-to-dry soaks, continuous soaks, or proteolytic enzymes).

Prevention and management of local infection

- Irrigate with antibacterial agent as prescribed.
- Use sterile technique.

- Administer systemic antibiotics as prescribed.
- Obtain specimens for culture as prescribed or if fever is present.
- Apply dry, sterile, non-adherent dressing. Change and cleanse every eight hours or more often as needed.

Hemostasis

- Use silver nitrate sticks or styptic pencils as prescribed for mild oozing.
- Apply 1:1000 epinephrine or topical thrombin to areas with moderate oozing as prescribed. Local radiation or application of hemostatic dressings may be used.

Drainage

- Change dressing as frequently as necessary (as soon as it is wet).
- Use absorbent dressings for small/moderate amounts of drainage or on areas too large to pouch.
- Apply drainage bag or ostomy pouch for copious amounts of drainage. Apply skin protectant to surrounding skin to prevent irritation and breakdown.
- Secure sterile dressings with Montgomery straps, stretchable gauze, or Stomahesive.

Odor

- Cleanse wound and change dressing as frequently as necessary.
- Obtain culture and sensitivities of wound.
- Apply commercial anti-odor agents to outside of dressings.
- Administer agents such as metronidazole (orally or topically) to control odor caused by anaerobes.
- Place shallow tray of activated charcoal in patient's room.
- Place commercial room deodorizer in room. Is room deodorizer more offensive than wound odor?

PATIENT AND FAMILY EDUCATION

In addition to teaching general preventive measures to maintain intact skin, it is a given that the patient/family unit is to be taught the signs and symptoms of infection and who and when to notify when they occur. Treatments and procedures should be discussed: clean or sterile technique, handwashing technique, disposal of used/soiled materials and dressings, environmental and personal hygiene practices, measures to prevent cross-contamination, application and expected effects of medications, measures to maintain hydration and nutrition, and measures to control bleeding. The primary caregiver must be instructed in the performance of the dressing procedures in the home.

Nursing Management

NURSING DIAGNOSES FOR THE PERSON WITH CANCER AND POTENTIAL DISRUPTION OF ORAL MUCOUS MEMBRANES[4,13,19,52]

- Oral mucous membranes, altered, related to: side effects of chemotherapy or radiation therapy, local infection or tumor
- Infection, potential for, related to: side effects of systemic chemotherapy and/or radiation therapy to the head and neck
- Knowledge deficit regarding good oral hygiene techniques; side effects of cancer therapy and radiation therapy
- Pain related to oral/esophageal mucositis as evidenced by patient's complaints of discomfort; excess or viscous oral secretions and/or oral lesions leading to discomfort and/or stimulation of the gag reflex
- Nutrition, altered, less than body requirements related to oral discomfort: as evidenced by decreased caloric intake, weight loss of more than 10% of preillness weight, and weakness
- Communication, impaired verbal, related to oral discomfort, increased or decreased salivation

INTERVENTIONS

Measures to decrease inflammation of mucous membranes

- Avoid exposure to chemical or physical irritants such as commercial mouthwashes, alcohol, tobacco, and hot and spicy or coarse foods.
- Encourage adequate fluid intake (>3 l/D).
- Use a systematic oral care protocol, which includes oral hygiene measures before and after each meal and at bedtime as a minimum and every 2 hours around the clock when oral mucositis is present.

Measures to increase comfort

- Use topical protectant and analgesic agents.
- Use systemic analgesics when pain is uncontrolled by topical agents.
- Safe, effective agents for oral care include normal saline (1 tsp/1 L of water) and sodium bicarbonate (1 tsp/1 L of water) alone or in combination (1:1).
- Brushing and flossing are the best defense against plaque build-up, but should be discontinued when the ANC is less than 1000 mm^3 and/or the platelet count is less than 50,000 mm^3 or mucositis is present. Toothettes or a gauze wrapped finger may be used instead.
- Low pressure irrigation set-ups such as a gavage bag, IV solution bag with tubing (500 ml normal saline), bulb syringe may be used to soften and remove debris. Suction equipment should be available for those patients at risk for aspiration.
- Water soluble lubricants may be used for dry, cracked lips.
- Dentures should be cleaned with a denture brush and an antimicrobial detergent such as chlorhexidine gluconate when oral care is done. Rinse with normal saline or water.
- Dentures should be removed while sleeping and as often as possible to give mucosa a rest. Soak dentures in commercial denture cleanser/soak when not in use. Solution should be changed daily.
- Dentures should not be worn except for meals when mucositis is present or ANC is less than 1000 mm^3 and/or platelet count is less than 50,000 mm^3 even when no oral pathology is present.
- For mild to moderate mucositis, implement oral care protocol every 2 hours while awake and every 4 hours during night.
- For severe mucositis, implement oral care protocol every 1 to 2 (not to exceed 2) hours during day and every 2 to 4 (not to exceed 4) hours during night.

Measures to minimize complications

- Modify dietary intake to include bland, soft, or liquid food (avoiding acidic foods and liquids) high in calories and protein, served at room temperature or cool, *not* hot or cold.
- Encourage use of oral hygiene measures before eating.
- Administer topical or systemic analgesics before meals.
- Provide calorie-containing liquids of choice for patient to sip frequently.
- For xerostomia (dry mouth), provide artificial saliva at bedside for patient use. Encourage patient to rinse mouth with water at least every 2 hours while awake. Provide beverages and sauces with meals to help alleviate difficulty swallowing.
- Identify alternative means of communication such as magic slates, notes, cards, and direct, short-response questions.

Medical treatment

- Administer antibiotics, antifungals, and antivirals as prescribed.
- Administer analgesics as needed. Patient may require around the clock systemic analgesia.
- Administer dietary supplements, enteral, or parenteral nutrition as prescribed.

- For bleeding from oral mucosa, administer antifibrinolytics and platelets as prescribed, and/or apply topical thrombin and gelfoam.
- Obtain swabs (specimens) for bacterial, fungal, and viral cultures and sensitivities.

Nursing management or oral and esophageal mucositis includes systematic assessment and documentation of condition of oral cavity at least once a day, informing the physician of any abnormalities, and utilizing a consistent and safe systematic oral care plan around-the-clock.[9,20,21,22] Promote comfort through the use of topical anesthetics and systemic analgesics, maintain optimal nutritional status, teach patient/family to utilize interventions to prevent/minimize oral mucositis, and use precautions when caring for the unresponsive patient to prevent aspiration while administering oral care.

PATIENT AND FAMILY EDUCATION

Teaching should include emphasis on the following:
- Importance and technique of daily oral assessment
- Signs and symptoms of mucositis and infection
- Importance of continuing use of a systematic oral care protocol at home
- Importance of fluids and adequate nutrition
- Necessity of dietary changes secondary to the presence or absence of oral and esophageal lesions
- Avoidance of trauma to mucous membranes secondary to smoking, smokeless tobacco, alcohol, extremes of temperature, chemical irritants such as commercial mouthwashes, and physical irritants such as highly seasoned or hard- or sharp-textured foods and poorly fitting dentures.

NURSING DIAGNOSES FOR THE PERSON WITH CANCER AND THE POTENTIAL FOR VAGINAL/RECTAL MUCOSITIS

- Tissue integrity, impaired, related to: side effects of chemotherapy and/or radiation therapy as evidenced by signs and symptoms of mucositis
- Infection, potential for, related to nonintact vaginal and/or rectal mucosa
- Knowledge deficit regarding safe sexual practices, good personal hygiene; side effects of mucositis related to cancer therapy
- Pain related to mucositis evidenced by the patient's complaints of painful urination, defecation, and/or sexual intercourse
- Diarrhea related to gastrointestinal mucositis; painful defecation related to rectal mucosa
- Sexuality patterns, altered, related to decreased energy and potential fear of trauma and/or infection

INTERVENTIONS

Measures to decrease inflammation of mucous membranes
- Avoid exposure to chemical and physical irritants such as tampons, deodorant-containing vaginal pads or liners, deodorant-containing "personal hygiene" sprays, douches, rectal thermometers and suppositories, and vaginal and anal intercourse.
- Encourage adequate fluid intake.
- Wash perineum with soap and water following each urination and defecation; pat or air dry.

Measures to increase comfort
- Use sitz baths.
- Avoid standing or sitting for long periods of time.
- Avoid irritating, constricting, nonabsorbent underclothing.

Measures to minimize complications
- Modify dietary intake to minimize diarrhea and constipation.
- Encourage frequent perineal hygiene measures.
- Instruct female patients to wipe from front to back following urination and defecation.
- Avoid trauma to either vaginal or rectal mucosa.
- Monitor patient for signs and symptoms of vaginal infection and/or rectal cellulitis/abcess. Culture as needed. Notify physician.

PATIENT AND FAMILY EDUCATION

- Teach personal risk factors for development of mucositis—chemotherapy, radiation therapy.
- Teach signs and symptoms of mucositis, such as pain, itching, and discharge or drainage, which should be reported.
- Use measures to prevent complications.
- Identify situations that require professional interventions, such as fever, diarrhea, and uncontrolled pain.

Nursing management of vaginal and rectal mucositis includes frequent, indirect assessment of signs and symptoms of mucositis, prevention of diarrhea and constipation, encouragement of bathing of perineal and rectal areas after each urination and defecation, teaching female patients to wipe front to back to prevent contaminating vaginal and urethral areas with fecal organisms, and teaching sexual practices that minimize trauma and risk of infection.

Teaching should include the signs and symptoms of mucositis and infection, whom and when to call, and sexual and elimination practices that prevent or minimize the risk of trauma and infection. Vaginal intercourse should be avoided while platelet and neutrophil counts are low and if mucosal ulcerations are present. Intercourse should be permitted and encouraged after recovery of blood counts and mucosa.

This may help prevent development of vaginal strictures and webbing, which may occur after pelvic irradiation. Women who are not sexually active may need to use vaginal dilators to maintain vaginal patency following pelvic irradiation. Condoms should be worn by the male partner to prevent transmission of organisms through nonintact mucosa. Adequate lubrication should be obtained using a water-soluble, not a petroleum-based, product. Anal intercourse should be avoided.[13,16]

Nursing Management

NURSING DIAGNOSES FOR THE PERSON WITH CANCER AND INCREASED SUSCEPTIBILITY TO INFECTION[2,13,52]

- Infection, potential for, related to:
    Disease entity
    Side-effects of treatment
    Neutropenia, immune suppression, etc.
    Disruption of mucous membranes and/or skin
    Presence of long-term venous access device
- Body temperature, altered, potential for, related to infection secondary to neutropenia, immunosuppression, non-intact skin and/or mucous membranes.
- Knowledge deficit regarding basic disease process, treatment, signs and symptoms of infection, neutropenic precautions
- Sexuality patterns, altered, related to decreased energy and potential fear of trauma and/or infection.
- Social isolation related to therapeutic environment or fear of acquiring an infection.
- Anxiety related to knowledge of diagnosis, treatment, and prognosis
- Fear related to discharge concerning home management and self-care, and uncertainty about long-term outcome.

PREVENTIVE MEASURES

Prevention of infection in susceptible individuals is an important nursing measure. *Hand-washing is the single most important action for the health care professional, the patient, the patient's family, and visitors.* The importance of adequate hand-washing using running water, soap, and friction cannot be overstated. The health care professional must use good hand-washing technique before and after any direct patient contact. Gloves are not to be used as a substitute for good hand-washing.[12,15]

Protective isolation techniques vary from institution to institution. The Centers for Disease Control no longer recognizes or recommends protective isolation for persons who are immunosuppressed or neutropenic. Protective isolation can be thought of more as a "mind set" than an actual category of isolation.[24,55] It must become second nature for the nurse caring for the neutropenic or immunosuppressed patient to be aware of the patient's increased risk and the risk the nurse represents to the patient.[12,27,28] Most institutions advocate the use of a private room, good hand-washing practices, and an infection-free staff to care for the patient. Dietary restrictions for the neutropenic patient may include an order for "cooked diet" only. Raw fruits and uncooked vegetables are often excluded because of soil contact and multiple personnel handling during storage and preparation.[12,14,27]

INTERVENTIONS

General preventive measures

- Wash hands with soap, water, and friction before and after all direct patient contact.
- Provide private room if possible. If unavailable, ensure uninfected roommate.
- Provide infection-free staff to care for patient.
- Give nursing care to neutropenic patient first to decrease risk of cross-contamination.
- Provide meticulous skin and oral hygiene for patient.
- Provide cooked diet only—no raw fruits or uncooked vegetables.
- Do not allow live plants or cut flowers in standing water in room.
- Avoid all sources of stagnant water in room such as water pitchers, denture cups, humidifiers, and respiratory therapy equipment. Change daily.
- Screen visitors for illnesses.
- Avoid overcrowded areas such as waiting rooms.
- Utilize Universal Precautions/OSHA requirements when caring for all patients.

Prompt recognition of suspected infection

- Assume that any change from the ordinary is infection until proven otherwise.
- Assess patient's risk of infection by calculating ANC and reviewing patient history for predisposing factors such as basic disease process, myelosuppressive therapies, immunosuppressive therapies, and antibiotic therapy.
- Assess skin and mucous membranes each shift and document in patient record.

- Assess vital signs including temperature at least every 4 hours and document in patient record.
- Notify physician of temperature elevation greater than 38.2° C (101° F), changes in skin and mucous membrane integrity, lesions, or rashes and any altered level of consciousness.
- Facilitate workup of suspected infection by obtaining ordered cultures, blood specimens, and radiologic studies in a timely manner.
- Initiate and administer antibiotics as prescribed in a timely manner.
- Observe and assess patient for adverse effects of antibiotic administration.

Nursing management of the infected cancer patient is a complex and challenging task. Infection is the most common cause of death for the person with cancer. Nurses represent a crucial and constant part of the care team—and frequently the difference between life and death for the patient.[28]

Nursing management of infection demands its prompt recognition, which requires the health care professional to maintain a high index of suspicion. Literally anything out of the ordinary could be infection. The nurse's intuitive feelings are frequently helpful in the absence of objective findings of infection. Physician notification and documentation of the nursing assessment in the patient record are essential parts of the nursing process.[12,15,27,36]

The nurse's assistance in the workup of suspected infection will include timely retrieval of specimens for culture, coordination of radiologic studies, and facilitation of physical assessment by the physician and nurse.[13,18]

Empiric antibiotic therapy should be instituted within 4 hours of an initial temperature spike and the obtaining of cultures. It is the nurse's responsibility to provide for timely and safe administration of antibiotics. Scheduling, timing of infusions, and knowledge of drug toxicities and interactions are also the responsibility of the nurse (Table 29-2).[43,46,51,57]

Frequent assessment of the patient with suspected infection is essential. Vital signs including temperature should be measured no less frequently than every 4 hours. Other key points of assessment should include auscultation of breath sounds, auscultation and palpation of abdomen, observation of skin and mucous membranes, and assessment of level of consciousness.[12]

Fever management includes administration of antipyretics and the use of tepid baths, cooling blankets, ice packs, and other nonpharmacologic methods of reducing elevated body temperature. Once antipyretics have been instituted and fever recurs, it is often less physiologically stressful to administer them on an around-the-clock schedule to avoid the see-saw

pattern of hyper- and hypothermia. It is important to prevent shivering, which increases body temperature. Parenteral meperidine and morphine or both may be administered to alleviate rigors.[18,34,37]

Early recognition of septic shock is essential to patient survival. Impending sepsis is frequently suggested by the findings of tachycardia, tachypnea, widened pulse pressure, elevated body temperature, hot dry skin, and altered mental status. Survival is improved if sepsis is recognized before circulatory collapse occurs.*

Patient and family education

Educational efforts should center upon teaching the patient and family the signs and symptoms of infection, which may include any of the following: fever, cough, dysuria, shortness of breath, oral ulcers, diarrhea, nausea, and vomiting. Because of the risk of septic shock associated with neutropenia, it is imperative that the patient and family take any fever seriously and notify the appropriate health care professional. Teaching should be explicit about when and whom to call and include a list of telephone numbers giving the patient and family 24-hour access to the health care setting.[23]

"Survival teaching" should be individualized to each patient, taking into consideration readiness to learn and ability to take charge of their lives and illness. Content may include laboratory test interpretation; calculation of an absolute neutrophil count; keeping a journal of dates, drugs, dosages, blood counts, and side effects; neutropenic precautions; hand-washing technique; personal hygiene practices; activity; diet; and sexual practices.[23]

NURSING DIAGNOSES FOR THE PERSON WITH CANCER AND INCREASED RISK OF BLEEDING[2,13]

- Injury, potential for, bleeding related to decreased platelet count/basic disease process/cancer treatment
- Knowledge deficit regarding thrombocytopenia and increased risk of bleeding; signs and symptoms of bleeding
- Sexuality patterns, alteration in, related to decreased energy and potential fear of trauma and/or infection
- Anxiety related to knowledge of diagnosis, treatment, and prognosis
- Fear related to discharge concerning home management and self-care, and uncertainty about long-term outcome

*References 7, 15, 36, 39, 48, 58.

Table 29–2   Nursing Implications of Antibiotic Administration

Drug	Side Effects	Implications
AMINOGLYCOSIDES		
Amikacin Gentamicin Tobramycin Vancomycin	Nephrotoxicity and ototoxicity	Monitor renal function carefully. Monitor for signs of hearing loss, tinnitus, and vertigo. Observe for signs of superinfection. Follow infusion guidelines carefully.
PENICILLINS		
Carbenicillin Ticarcillin Piperacillin Mezlocillin	Skin rashes, drug fever, anaphylaxis, hypokalemia, and abnormal platelet function	Monitor renal function carefully. Elicit allergy history. Be prepared for possible allergic reaction. Monitor CBC and liver function tests carefully. Monitor serum electrolytes (K and Na). Observe for signs of superinfection.
CEPHALOSPORINS		
First, second, and third generation drugs	Skin rashes and drug fever	Monitor renal function carefully. Observe for phlebitis if given peripherally. Observe for signs of superinfection.
MONOBACTAMS		
Aztreonam	Seizures, altered taste, diarrhea, nausea, vomiting, skin rash, superinfection, anaphylaxis	Elicit history of allergies. Monitor liver function. Monitor renal function. Monitor coagulation. Monitor neurotoxicity. Observe for signs of superinfection.
CARBAPENEM		
Imipenem/cilastin	Seizures, somnolence, hypotension, nausea, diarrhea, vomiting, rash, phlebitis, anaphylaxis	Elicit allergy history. Monitor renal function. Monitor liver function. Monitor CBC and Coombs' test. Observe for signs of superinfection.
ANTIFUNGAL AGENTS		
Amphotericin B	Hypokalemia, fever, rigors, phlebitis, nausea, vomiting, headache, nephrotoxicity, ototoxicity, and elevated liver enzymes	Monitor renal function carefully. Monitor serum electrolytes carefully. Monitor liver function tests carefully. Premedicate with diphenhydramine, acetaminophen, and meperidine. Administer additional meperidine IV as ordered for relief of rigors. Monitor patient's temperature at baseline and during infusion. Infuse slowly, preferably with infusion pump. Drug is a colloid. Administer with nonfiltered tubing. Agitate bag frequently to maintain in suspension. Keep out of direct sunlight.

PREVENTIVE MEASURES

Care should be taken to prevent bleeding in the thrombocytopenic patient. Measures should include those that maintain skin and mucous membrane integrity.[2,8,29,35]

Provision of a safe environment falls within the confines of nursing practice. In severely thrombocytopenic patients, bed rails should be up at all times, the patient should be up with assistance only, and the patient who is weak or showing signs of bleeding should be on complete bed rest.

All excreta and vomitus should be tested for the presence of occult blood. The results of each test should be entered in the patient record and the physician notified if the results vary significantly from previous testing.

Obtain laboratory tests as ordered. Know results and how they are related to the patient's risk for bleeding. Be able to interpret lab results in terms of platelet disorder, coagulation factor deficiency, mixed coagulopathy, and lack of vascular integrity.[33]

INTERVENTIONS

General preventive measures

- Limit invasive procedures.
- Provide safe environment (e.g., side rails up, assistance with ambulation).
- Avoid intramuscular injections.
- Avoid aspirin-containing medications or nonsteroidal anti-inflammatories.
- Suppress menses in premenopausal female patients by hormonal manipulation as ordered by the physician.
- Avoid hard toothbrushes or tooth flossing.
- Avoid use of rectal thermometers, suppositories, enemas, or rectal examinations.
- No alcohol-containing beverages.

Assessment of bleeding

- Check laboratory values for platelet count, hemoglobin and hematocrit, and any other coagulation studies, such as prothrombin time (PT), partial thromboplastin time (PTT), fibrinogen, and fibrin degradation products (FDP) to assess patient's risk of bleeding.
- Assess skin and mucous membranes for presence of petechiae, purpura, and ecchymoses, document in patient record, and notify physician of any evidence of bleeding.
- Assess for any evidence of frank bleeding (e.g., epistaxis, hemoptysis, hematemesis, hematochezia, melena, hematuria, or vaginal bleeding), document in patient record, and notify physician if present.
- Quantitate amount of frank bleeding as accurately as possible, document, and report.

- Hemetest all stools, urine, and emesis for the presence of occult blood whenever the platelet count is less than 50,000/mm³.
- Apply pressure and/or pressure dressings to venipunctures, bone marrow aspiration and biopsy sites, and other sites of invasive procedures until hemostasis occurs.
- Observe sites of invasive procedures, such as vascular access device placement, for continued hemostasis and notify physician if bleeding is present or recurs.
- Administer appropriate medications to prevent activities that raise intracranial pressure such as vomiting, coughing, sneezing, and straining in stool.
- Report any complaints of headache with or without change in level of consciousness or vital signs.
- Administer platelet transfusions and other blood component therapy as ordered.
- Obtain physician order and administer premedications of diphenhydramine, acetaminophen, and/or corticosteroids to patient with history of transfusion reaction.
- Monitor patient for signs and symptoms of transfusion and take appropriate measures (see Table 29-3).

Patient and family education

- Assess skin and mucous membranes daily for evidence of bleeding.
- Assess personal risk of bleeding by knowing current platelet count and other pertinent lab values.
- Assess for and report any evidence of frank bleeding including petechiae, purpura, and ecchymoses.
- Avoid all aspirin-containing compounds. Read the label. Don't take any medications unless prescribed by your physician.
- Report any feelings of increased weakness, change in stool color and consistency, emesis, headache, and change in level of consciousness.
- For nosebleed, apply ice pack across bridge of nose and pressure to nostrils below bridge of nose. If bleeding does not stop within 5 minutes or bleeding is profuse, notify physician. Anterior or posterior nasal packs may be required.

Nursing management of the bleeding patient depends upon prompt recognition of the problem so that definitive therapy can be undertaken. Bleeding precautions should be initiated when the platelet count drops below 50,000/mm³. Frequent assessment should be made of vital signs, mental status, skin and mucous membranes, sites of invasive procedures, and all excreta and vomitus for occult blood. Signs of intracranial hemorrhage include decreased level of consciousness, headache, seizures, unequal pupil size and reaction, hypertension, and bradycardia. Administration of antiemetics, cough suppressants, and stool softeners and laxatives when indicated may help lower the risk of intracranial hemorrhage by preventing the sudden raising of intracranial pressure while retching, coughing, and straining at stool.[29,35]

Platelet transfusion is generally the treatment of choice for bleeding secondary to thrombocytopenia. Indications for platelet transfusion are not always clear. Some physicians may prefer to wait for signs of bleeding before transfusing platelets; others may opt to transfuse with platelets prophylactically when the platelet count drops below 20,000/mm^3. Platelet transfusions may be random donor (obtained from multiple units of fresh whole blood), single donor (obtained by platelet pheresis), or single donor, HLA matched (obtained by platelet pheresis from a related, matched donor). Transfusion reactions occur most frequently with random donor platelets and usually consist of febrile reactions, urticaria, or both. This type of transfusion reaction is most likely to be related to leukoagglutinins and may be alleviated by premedication or leukocyte-poor platelets. Alloimmunization (development of antiplatelet antibodies) occurs after exposure to platelet transfusions. When this occurs, optimal response to platelet transfusions fails to occur and the platelet count remains the same or drops lower. With alloimmunization it may be necessary to reserve platelet transfusions for times of active bleeding.[2,46,49]

PATIENT AND FAMILY EDUCATION

The educational process for the patient and family should include practical guidelines for the prevention of bleeding, such as using acetaminophen instead of aspirin, always checking the ingredients of over-the-counter medications, not taking any medications unless prescribed by the physician, avoiding trauma, what to do for ecchymoses, when to call the physician if bleeding occurs or is suspected, what is serious bleeding, and how to recognize intracranial hemorrhage.[23]

NURSING DIAGNOSES FOR THE PERSON WITH CANCER AND FATIGUE ASSOCIATED WITH ANEMIA

- Activity intolerance, potential/actual related to anemia secondary to bone marrow suppression; related to decreased tissue perfusion secondary to anemia as evidenced by fatigue, motor weakness, and inability to perform activities of daily living
- Gas exchange, impaired, related to decreased oxygenation secondary to anemia (decreased hemoglobin)

- Sexuality patterns, alteration in, related to decreased energy secondary to anemia
- Mobility, impaired physical, related to decreased strength and endurance
- Knowledge deficit related to basic disease process; signs and symptoms of anemia

PREVENTIVE MEASURES

Preventive measures include the following: frequent assessment of skin and mucous membranes for pallor; cardiovascular system for signs of decompensation such as irregular rhythms, murmurs, changes in blood pressure and pulse rate, peripheral edema, and dyspnea; pulmonary exam for changes in rate and depth of respirations and rales; and neurologic exam for altered levels of consciousness and inability to concentrate. Nurses should be aware of current laboratory values for hemoglobin, hematocrit, reticulocyte count, and platelet count. Persons known to be anemic should be encouraged to monitor their activity closely to prevent overtiring.

INTERVENTIONS

Nursing management of the patient with fatigue associated with anemia should include teaching energy conservation techniques, helping the patient cope with the changes in life-style that severe fatigue may dictate, providing the time and opportunity for the patient to ventilate anger, frustration, and feelings of depression, monitoring patient activity, planning activities to prevent overtiring, and transfusing packed red blood cells as ordered by the physician. The nurse must be aware of safe transfusion practices, signs and symptoms of transfusion reactions, and indications for premedication and administration of leukocyte-poor blood[49] (Table 29-3).

PATIENT AND FAMILY EDUCATION

Teaching plans should include the following instructions:

- Rest when tired—anemia and fatigue are expected and temporary side effects of treatment for cancer.
- Develop a progressive ambulation plan—don't try too much at one time.
- Pace your activities—try to maintain as normal a life-style as possible; plan periods of exercise and rest.
- Seek assistance with such things as child care, meal planning and preparation, laundry, and housecleaning.
- Eat a nutritionally balanced diet.
- Maintain usual patterns of sleep.[6,13]

Table 29–3   Transfusion Reactions

Type of Reaction	Signs and Symptoms	Interventions
Hemolytic	Fever, chills, back pain, substernal tightness, dyspnea, circulatory collapse, urticaria, vomiting, diarrhea, hemoglobinuria, renal shutdown, bleeding diathesis	Prevent by proper identification of patient and blood for transfusion. Discontinue the transfusion. Send to blood bank and obtain urine and blood specimens per hospital policy for transfusion reaction workup. Administer saline diuresis, furosemide, and mannitol to prevent acute tubular necrosis.
Allergic	Urticaria, itching, bronchospasm, anaphylactoid reactions	Elicit history of prior allergic reactions. Premedicate with diphenhydramine and/or corticosteroids. If reaction occurs, stop the transfusion. Follow hospital policy for suspected transfusion reaction. For anaphylactoid reaction, administer epinephrine, maintain airway and perfusion. Administer additional emergency measures as needed.
Febrile (leukocyte antigens)	Fever with or without rigors, tachycardia, tachypnea, hypotension, cyanosis, fibrinolysis, leukopenia	Elicit history of febrile reactions. Premedicate with acetaminophen. If reaction occurs, stop the transfusion and follow hospital policy for suspected febrile reaction. Administer saline washed or leukocyte-poor red blood cells.
Bacterial (gram-negative organisms and endotoxin release)	Fever, rigors, circulatory collapse, mental confusion, septic shock	Maintain proper blood storage and administration conditions. Stop the transfusion immediately. Obtain blood for cultures, return blood to lab for culturing. Administer emergency treatment as needed. Administer antibiotics as ordered.

CONCLUSION

Protective mechanisms such as skin, mucous membrane, and bone marrow protect the body from foreign substances and invading organisms. The patient with cancer undergoing the various treatment modalities becomes at risk for breakdown of one or all of these protective mechanisms. Nursing management requires prompt recognition of the signs and symptoms of infection, bleeding, and skin breakdown so that definitive therapy can be implemented. Nurses caring for these patients are key members of the health care team at this crucial time.

BIBLIOGRAPHY

1. Adams A: External barriers to infection, Nurs Clin North Am 20(1):145, 1985.
2. Alexander EJ: Injury, potential for, related to thrombocytopenia. In McNally JC and others, editors: Guidelines for oncology nursing practice, ed 2, Philadelphia, 1991, WB Saunders Co.
3. Anderson KC and Weinstein HJ: Transfusion-associated graft-versus-host disease, N Engl J Med 323:315, 1990.
4. Baird SB, McCorkle R, and Grant M: Cancer nursing, Philadelphia, 1991, WB Saunders Co.
5. Baird SB: Decision making in oncology nursing, Toronto, 1988, BC Decker, Inc.
6. Baranowski L: Filtering out the confusion about leukocyte-poor blood components, J Intrav Nurs 14:298, 1991.
7. Barry SA: Septic shock: special needs of the patient with cancer, Oncol Nurs Forum 16(1):31, 1989.
8. Bavier AR: Alterations in hemostasis. In Johnson BL and Gross J, editors: Handbook of oncology nursing, New York, 1985, John Wiley & Sons.
9. Beck S: Impact of the systematic oral care protocol on stomatitis after chemotherapy, Cancer Nurs 2:185, 1979.
10. Bernheim HA, Block LH, and Atkins E: Fever:

pathogenesis, pathophysiology, and purpose, Ann Intern Med 91:261, 1979.

11. Bodey GP: Quantitative relationship between circulating leukocytes and infection in patients with acute leukemia, Ann Intern Med 64:328, 1966.

12. Brandt B: Nursing protocol for the patient with neutropenia, Oncol Nurs Forum 17(1s):9, 1990.

13. Brown MH and others: Standards of oncology nursing practice, New York, 1986, John Wiley & Sons.

14. Carlson AC: Infection prophylaxis in the patient with cancer, Oncol Nurs Forum 12(3):56, 1985.

15. Chernecky CC and Ramsey PW: Critical care of the client with cancer, Norwalk, CN, 1984, Appleton-Century-Crofts.

16. Clark JC: Mucous membrane integrity, impairment of, related to vaginal changes. In McNally JC and others, editors: Guidelines for oncology nursing practice, ed 2, Philadelphia, 1991, WB Saunders Co.

17. Couillard-Getreuer DL: Skin. In Johnson BL and Gross J, editors: Handbook of oncology nursing, New York, 1985, John Wiley & Sons.

18. Cuhna BA, Digamon-Beltran M, and Gobbo PN: Implications of fever in the critical care setting, Heart Lung 13(5):460, 1984.

19. Cunningham M: Dental prosthetics: physiologic and microbial insults, Oncol Nurs Forum 11:78, 1984.

20. Daeffler RJ: Oral hygiene measures for patients with cancer, I, Cancer Nurs 3:347, 1980.

21. Daeffler RJ: Oral hygiene measures for patients with cancer, II, Cancer Nurs 3:427, 1980.

22. Daeffler RJ: Oral hygiene measures for patients with cancer, III, Cancer Nurs 4:29, 1981.

23. Derdiarian A: Informational needs of recently diagnosed cancer patients, Nurs Res 35(5):276, 1986.

24. Donovan C: Protective isolation, Oncol Nurs Forum 9(3):50, 1982.

25. Dudjak LA: Mouth care for mucositis due to radiation therapy, Cancer Nurs 10:131, 1987.

26. Eilers J, Berger AM, and Peterson MC: Development, testing and application of the oral assessment guide, Oncol Nurs Forum 15:325, 1989.

27. Ellerhorst-Ryan JM: Complications of the myeloproliferative system: infection and sepsis, Semin Oncol Nurs 1:244, 1985.

28. Eperson S: Nursing support of host defenses, Crit Care Nurs Q 9(1):51, 1986.

29. Fisher SG: Bleeding. In Johnson BL and Gross J, editors: Handbook of oncology nursing, New York, 1985, John Wiley & Sons.

30. Gallucci BB: The immune system and cancer, Oncol Nurs Forum 14(6s):3, 1987.

31. Goodman M and Stoner C: Mucous membrane integrity, impairment of, related to stomatitis. In McNally JC and others, editors: Guidelines for oncology nursing practice, ed 2, Philadelphia, 1991, WB Saunders Co.

32. Grady C: Host defense mechanisms: an overview, Semin Oncol Nurs 4(2):86, 1988.

33. Griffin JP: Be prepared for the bleeding patient, Nursing 16(6):34, 1986.

34. Griffin JP: Fever, when to leave it alone, Nursing 16(2):57, 1986.

35. Griffin JP: Hematology and immunology: concepts for nursing, Norwalk, CN, 1986, Appleton-Century-Crofts.

36. Griffin JP: Nursing care of the critically ill immunocompromised patient, Crit Care Nurs Q 9(1):25, 1986.

37. Gurevich I: Fever: when to worry about it, RN Dec:14, 1985.

38. Haeuber D: Future strategies in the control of myelosuppression: the use of colony-stimulating factors, Oncol Nurs Forum 18(2S):16, 1991.

39. Hall KV: Detecting septic shock before it's too late, RN Sept:29, 1981.

40. Henschel L: Fever patterns in the neutropenic patient, Cancer Nurs 8(6):301, 1985.

41. Herberth L and Gosnell DJ: Nursing diagnoses for oncology nursing practice, Cancer Nurs 10(1):41, 1987.

42. Holland PV: Prevention of transfusion-associated graft-versus-host disease, Arch Pathol Lab Med 113:285, 1989.

43. Hughes WT: Empiric antimicrobial therapy in the febrile granulocytopenic patient, Infect Control Hosp Epidemiol 11:151, 1990.

44. Jett MF and Lancaster LE: The inflammatory-immune response: the body's defense against invasion, Crit Care Nurs Sept/Oct:63, 1983.

45. Kemp D: Development of the immune system, Crit Care Nurs Q 9(1):1, 1986.

46. King NH: Controlling bleeding when the platelet count drops, RN, Aug:25, 1984.

47. Kluger MJ: Fever: role of pyrogens and cryogens, Physiol Rev 71:93, 1991.

48. Lamb LS: Think you know septic shock? Nursing 12(1):34, 1982.

49. Lichtiger B and Huh YO: Transfusion therapy for patients with cancer, CA 35(5):1, 1985.

50. Lieschke GJ and Burgess AW: Granulocyte colony-stimulating factor and granulocyte-macrophage colony factor, N Engl J Med 327:28, 1992.

51. Link DL: Antibiotic therapy for the cancer patient: focus on third generation cephalosporins, Oncol Nurs Forum 14(5):35, 1987.

52. McNally JC and Stair J: Potential for infection. In

McNally JC and others, editors: Guidelines for oncology nursing practice, ed 2, Philadelphia, 1991, WB Saunders Co.

53. Malkiewicz J: What assessing the mouth can tell you, RN May:65, 1982.

54. Montrose PA: Extravasation management, Semin Oncol Nurs 3(2):128, 1987.

55. Nauseef WM and Maki DG: A study of the value of simple protective isolation in patients with granulocytopenia, N Engl J Med 304:448, 1981.

56. Owen P: Skin integrity, impairment of, related to malignant skin lesions. In McNally JC and others, editors: Guidelines for oncology nursing practice, ed 2, Philadelphia, 1991, WB Saunders Co.

57. Pizzo PA: Management of fever and infection in the patient with cancer, Mediguide Infect Dis 2(4):1, 1983.

58. Rice V: The clinical continuum of septic shock, Crit Care Nurs Sept/Oct:86, 1984.

59. Roberts NJ: Impact of temperature elevation on immunologic defenses, Rev Infect Dis 13:462, 1991.

60. Rostad M: Current strategies for managing myelosuppression in patient with cancer, Oncol Nurs Forum 18(2s):7, 1991.

61. Rostad M: Injury, potential for, related to anemia. In McNally JC and others, editors: Guidelines for oncology nursing practice, ed 2, Philadelphia, 1991, WB Saunders Co.

62. Smith SL: Physiology of the immune system, Crit Care Nurs Q 9(1):7, 1986.

63. Styrt B: Antipyresis and fever, Arch Intern Med 150:1589, 1990.

64. Walsh TJ and others: Empiric therapy with amphotericin B in febrile granulocytic patients, Rev Infect Dis 13:496, 1991.

65. Williams LT, Peterson DE, and Overholser CD: Acute periodontal infection in myelosuppressed oncology patients: evaluation and nursing care, Cancer Nurs 5(6):465, 1982.

66. Workman ML: Immunological late effects in children and adults, Semin Oncol Nurs 5(1):36, 1989.

67. Yeomans AC: Rectal infections in acute leukemia, Cancer Nurs 9(6):295, 1986.

CHAPTER 30

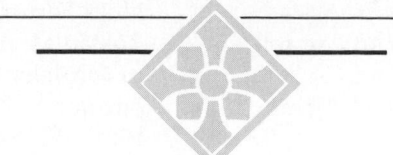

Psychosocial Issues

Noella Devolder McCray

I wanted a perfect ending so I sat down to write the book with the ending in place before there even was an ending. Now I've learned the hard way that some poems don't rhyme, and some stories do not have a clear beginning, middle and end. Like my life, this book has ambiguity. Like my life, this book is about not knowing, having to change, taking the moment and making the best of it without knowing what is going to happen next.[59]

INTRINSIC FACTORS
The Personal Meaning of Cancer

INDIVIDUAL RESPONSE.   Living with uncertainty, as poignantly described by the late comedienne Gilda Radner, is the major challenge that faces every individual diagnosed with cancer, as well as those with whom significant relationships are shared. The future, which once may have seemed to hold unlimited potential, immediately becomes limited when viewed within the context of a cancer diagnosis. As noted by Weisman, "cancer is not just another chronic disease, it evokes many of the deepest fears of mankind."[77] The meaning a cancer diagnosis holds for a particular individual is highly personal and is derived from numerous sources, including past experiences with cancer, cultural biases, and information gained from the lay press. Each of these sources may or may not be accurate, may or may not be helpful, and may or may not lead to positive coping and adaptation. The individual, and those with whom significant relationships are shared, have all had different experiences, which influence their interpretation and expectations. Thus, while similar behaviors or response patterns may emerge and be observed by the nurse, it is crucial to remember that each individual diagnosed with cancer experiences a unique situation framed by highly personal life experiences.

The specific kind of cancer and necessary treatment influences the unique challenges to be faced and the potential responses. Visible physical changes can accentuate or minimize the personal and social impact. Crucial differences in response also arise from the extent of altered daily functioning. With time and experience the meaning and implications of the diagnosis evolve but adaptation and uncertainty remain as haunting challenges.

The initial diagnosis may have been preceded by varying levels of concern, ranging from a low level of suspicion associated with routine examinations to the steadily increasing anxiety and suspicion associated with sequential diagnostic procedures. The individual and family initially experience the shock of an unexpected diagnosis or the pain of having their worst fears confirmed. The personal meaning of cancer evolves over time.

TIMING AND ROLE STRAIN.   The timing of a cancer diagnosis in terms of the developmental level of the individual and the individual's family may exacerbate or mitigate the feelings produced by the diagnosis.[24] Age and stage of life affect perceptions, understanding, and acceptance. The diagnosis of a malignancy in a child, young adult, or a person experiencing a productive middle age is often viewed as more devastating than in the elderly individual who has seemingly completed significant life events.

Timing is significant not only in terms of development but also in relation to other stressors. Periods of life transitions, such as marriage, childbirth, retirement, or death in the family can intensify responses. The point in time influences the degree of role strain incurred by each individual involved. The perceived burdens of care can lead family members to struggle with feelings of guilt, resentment, or anger. Roles may change dramatically. Partial or full unemployment can drain financial resources as well as change roles. These changes can be accompanied by altered communications in relationships.

Nurses are cautioned not to consider an initial response as permanent or representative of the way the individual and family will cope in the future. Weisman and Worden have described the initial response as that of the existential plight.[78] During approximately the first 100 days following diagnosis, the individual attempts to address some of the existential issues related to the diagnosis, including those related to dying, the future, and the meaning life has had. During this same time, the individual is presented with a treatment plan and therefore must simultaneously begin to learn to cope with recovery from surgical procedures and side effects of cancer therapies.

The significance of the initial diagnosis period cannot be overemphasized. A wide range of responses are observed as the individual and family attempt to adapt to an overwhelming situation. It is particularly important to refrain from labeling a particular response as abnormal or maladaptive. There is nothing normal about being diagnosed with a life-threatening disease, nor is there a right way to face the threatened loss of a loved one. Because all individuals have the potential to learn, to grow, and to change, the foundations of their psychosocial care are respect and a nonjudgmental attitude. A major determinant of their coping success can be a nurse's ability to "coach" them through this tumultuous time.

SPIRITUAL DISTRESS.   The person with cancer and those with whom significant relationships are shared may experience some degree of spiritual distress as they struggle with the effects of the diagnosis and its meaning. The perceived misfortune or tragedy uncovers concerns about the unfair distribution of suffering in the world. This often begs a confrontation with the concept of a kind and loving God. Attempts to explain or transform bad into good and pain into privilege are often used to defend God.[38]

Questions may outnumber answers. "Why Me?" may never be satisfactorily answered. While some feel enriched by their faith at this time others may feel robbed by it.

The nurse can be supportive by being aware of and showing respect for differing religious beliefs. More importantly, the nurse provides support through nonjudgemental listening and providing an opportunity for telling the individual's story. Through such listening the appropriateness of a referral to clergy can be ascertained. While some are comforted by displays of faith others are best served by supportive listening. An assessment of spiritual distress can guide the nurse but such an assessment can be effectively done only after the nurse has reconciled a personal spirituality that accepts ambiguity and differences.

Providing Support for Psychosocial Adjustment

Complex psychological and social issues are interwoven aspects of the response to a diagnosis of a chronic disease process. Recognition of this fact has led professional caregivers to establish concurrent care goals—disease control and quality of life. As the medical understanding and management of cancer have progressed steadily, so have the understanding and management of psychosocial issues. Psychosocial oncology has become a distinct field of study and practice. An emerging theoretical base provides the pathways for intervention.

INTERDISCIPLINARY TEAM APPROACH.   As the aspects of care are interwoven so are the roles of professional caregivers. Interdisciplinary team care is the standard in quality care delivery. Some aspects of psychosocial care are best suited to the psychologist, psychiatrist, clergy, social worker, or counselor. Another potential team member is the lay volunteer or another cancer survivor who is trained and matched with a patient to provide special support. Each team member can contribute to altering perceptions of the situation, improving coping abilities, and altering the overall response to the situation. Nurses in various settings contribute to psychosocial care, either directly or indirectly through referrals and coordination of care. Each interdisciplinary team member serves the patient and family best when working together in an interdisciplinary manner.

STRUCTURED ASSESSMENT.   Nurses and all health care professionals benefit from a structured assessment or data base from which they can determine the capacity of the patient and family to manage the situation.[23] Symptom and well-being inventories can be used to measure anxiety, depression, hostility, somatization, and general distress or well being.[68] This assessment requires time and is best accomplished after the establishment of a trusting relationship.

Data can be collected over a period of time and should be recorded in a systematic way. Published guides are available for conducting a psychosocial assessment.[23] The system adopted should be one that is workable within the constraints of the setting yet complete enough to form an objective base for establishing priorities and reasonable care goals.

As a result of nursing and other team members' assessments, numerous nursing diagnoses related to psychosocial care can be made[53] (see box on p. 722). Each diagnosis must be substantiated by a data base and then followed with a plan of care. The plan of care should document nursing goals and the patient's goals as stated by the patient.

ADAPTATION PROCESS.   The goals of cancer therapy range from disease cure to palliation of symptoms. Thus the degree of personal threat experienced

---

NURSING DIAGNOSES RELATED TO PSYCHOSOCIAL CARE*

Adjustment, impaired	Impaired problem-solving
Anxiety	Ineffective management of therapeutic regimen
Body image disturbance	Knowledge deficit (specify)
Caregiver role strain	Noncompliance (specify)
Coping, defensive	Parenting, altered
Coping, family: potential for growth	Parenting, altered, potential
Coping, ineffective family: compromised	Powerlessness related to illness and hospitalization
Coping, ineffective family: disabling	Relocation stress syndrome
Coping, ineffective individual	Self-esteem, disturbance
Decisional conflict (specify)	Self-esteem, chronic low
Denial, ineffective	Self-esteem, situational low
Family processes, altered	Sleep disturbance related to anxiety and/or depression
Fear	
Grieving, anticipatory	Social interaction, impaired
Grieving, dysfunctional	Social isolation
High risk for caregiver role strain	Spiritual distress (distress of the human spirit)
Impaired communication (decreased attention and concentration)	Violence, potential for: self-directed or directed at others

*NANDA approved—1992

---

by the individual and the subsequent ability to adapt or cope will vary over time. The process of adapting is characterized by a series of transitions in terms of knowledge of the disease process, emotional responses on the part of the individual and significant others, and the need to negotiate changes in life-style patterns to adjust to the demands of treatment. While individuals diagnosed with cancer share many issues of common concern, these issues may vary according to the position the individual occupies on the cancer care continuum.

Adaptation to cancer can be addressed from several time frames: initial diagnosis, treatment, recurrence, advanced disease, and death, or long-term survival. The needs of the individual differ at each point on the continuum. Artificially dividing the cancer experience into such phases can be helpful in describing human responses. However, the potential then exists of failing to recognize that human emotional responses do not have artificial boundaries.

Initial Diagnosis and Treatment. The common experience is that of being told the diagnosis. Immediately after the disclosure of a cancer diagnosis, each person sets out upon a unique path characterized by highly individual physical and psychosocial responses to a situation marked by uncertainty. The primary concern of the newly diagnosed person is life versus death.[77] Family and friends also share these initial concerns. They experience an acute grief reaction to the diagnosis itself and the uncertainty of the outcome. Grief reaction as a response to chronic illness can be viewed from the framework of attachment theory.[82] Attachment theory is based on the premise that the level of distress experienced is directly related to the significance the individual places upon the body function

or part that is threatened.[82] This theoretical framework can serve as a basis for a nursing assessment. When treatment is initiated, the individual who values physical appearance may find coping with threatened alopecia most difficult, and the individual who is career-focused may be highly distressed by therapy-related fatigue and subsequent loss of function. The nurse must therefore also consider the impact the potential loss will have upon the individual's body image (see Chapter 31).

During the initial diagnostic and treatment stage, the individual and family are often overwhelmed and have trouble comprehending all that is said. A study of newly diagnosed cancer patients provided valuable information regarding the process of informing the patient of the diagnosis.[40] Half of the individuals studied were initially told of their diagnosis when they were alone or with only other medical personnel present. Greater distress was reported by those told in a recovery room or by telephone. Many individuals reported feeling numb or shocked and particularly vulnerable in instances when they were alone. They reported a need to have their sense of personal tragedy acknowledged.[40]

Although further study is needed of ways to minimize the trauma of presenting the diagnosis, this preliminary study has implications for nurses in recovery rooms, physicians' offices, and all settings where a diagnosis is confirmed. The physician who makes treatment recommendations, often a consulted oncologist, is in the position of reexplaining the diagnosis a second or third time. Thus, by the time the individual is presented with a specific treatment plan, he or she may be overwhelmed with the information given and not understand the diagnosis or treatment plan. The nurse who is present at this time is in the best position to assess the response and level of understanding. The nurse who anticipates this situation may recommend that the patient come accompanied by a friend or family member and use a tape recorder to enhance understanding and retention of information. The nurse can repeat information, validate understanding, and gently encourage participation in treatment decisions and goal setting.

The process of clarifying information and reducing confusion can be facilitated by various nursing interventions.[18,73] Paper and pencil can be provided to encourage the individual to write down questions that come to mind and record answers received. Questions and concerns may then be prioritized and can serve as the basis of further discussion with physicians and other care providers. Information can then be reviewed by the patient or family at their convenience. These suggestions illustrate the coaching function of the nurse who helps individuals move from the confusion of the unfamiliar to a sense of mastery of their situation.[4]

Recurrence. While an ever-increasing number of individuals diagnosed with cancer achieve long-term control and are eventually considered cured of their disease, a significant proportion of individuals do not achieve such a goal. When cure is not feasible, the goal of therapy is control, or the longest possible disease-free period. This goal presents the patient and family with the doubled-edged sword of hope and fear. The hope of defying the odds is bound by the fear of recurrence. Statistics may predict life expectancy based on diagnosis, pathology, and stage of disease, but do not consider the individual's response. Each individual's experience is physically and psychosocially unique and somewhat unpredictable.

The fear of recurrence and lack of predictability have been cited as the source of a decreased personal sense of control.[25,55] This sense of uncertainty can be manifested in a variety of behaviors. The patient and family may blame health care providers or each other as they review the events leading to diagnosis, treatment, and recurrence. The nurse can show support by allowing the individual to retell their story, thus acknowledging their pain and grief.

When initial therapy is completed, the individual may experience a fear of abandonment by health care providers. Less frequent appointments and examinations can become a source of anxiety. A study of men with testicular cancer who were nearing the completion of therapy revealed an increase in the number of phone calls and outpatient visits to health care providers to validate the significance of minor physical changes.[25] This time period is also anxiety-provoking for family members. While the individual may be making every attempt to get back to normal, family members and friends may be constantly monitoring for symptoms of recurrence. They may manifest their concern through frequent phone calls to review symptoms or paradoxically encouraging nonreporting or minimizing concerns.

Family members may find themselves emotionally drained. The immediate need to support the loved one diminishes and they are left with their own anxieties. The patient's complaints of fatigue, a cough, or gastrointestinal disturbances may all be interpreted by the family as proof that the cancer is recurring. Nurses can assist the individual and family by acknowledging their concerns as real and assessing physical findings to determine the need for further evaluation.

When recurrence is documented the nurse can assist the patient and family by providing an understanding of its significance. The recurrence signifies an increased tumor cell burden occurring at an interval of time related to the growth rate of the specific cancer cell line. The return of clinically evident disease indicates an inadequate response to initial therapy. The recurrence does not necessarily mean there is no chance for cure. In some instances reinstitution of the same therapy or a second line therapy can achieve a second remission or a cure.

The psychosocial response to a recurrence is dependent on several variables. A study of a large number of patients with a wide variety of malignancies revealed surprising findings.[79] Thirty percent of the population studied found the experience of recurrence less traumatic than the initial diagnosis. This group reported their initial treatment experience as smooth or uneventful. Individuals who experienced greater emotional distress were most often physically debilitated and experiencing a decrease in function. The study also noted that individuals who lived with a realistic expectation of recurrence were much less distressed than those who believed the disease was completely eradicated. Individuals who had completed therapy but were in remission less than 1 year were the most concerned about relapse. Those who experienced longer periods of remission began to allow themselves the hope of a cure, so recurrence was more emotionally distressing to this group. It is important to note that the individuals who lived with the realistic possibility of recurrence were not, as a group, pessimistic about their future. Rather, they were hopeful that they would experience another remission. While the concerns of individuals experiencing recurrent cancer deserve greater study, the nurse is cautioned not to assume that patients who experience a recurrence are universally overwhelmed or depressed. Current symptoms, functional status, previous experience with cancer therapy, and ongoing expectations since initial diagnosis are important variables in determining how one copes with recurrence. The nurse remains in a central supportive role at this time.

Long-term Survival. When the individual's disease-free period extends, the fear of recurrence seems to decrease.[13] Professionals must note that the publicly regarded milestone of a 5-year disease-free survival period may no longer be considered appropriate in certain diseases.[27] A vital component of the care of people experiencing disease-free status is to provide them with current, appropriate information regarding the significance of the length of the disease-free interval in relation to their particular situation and the important role of follow up. When disease control is not an attainable goal, and palliative care is given, the challenge of creating a vision of hope still exists.[19] The caregiver's provision of measures to relieve physical and psychosocial distress can foster the hope for comfort and peace.

Patient and Family Coping Strategies

ALTERATIONS IN COPING. The personal meaning a cancer diagnosis holds for individuals and their loved ones and possible outcomes of cancer therapies are the source of multiple and complex issues faced by the individual and family for the balance of life. Nurses are cautioned to avoid labeling any behavioral responses as permanent or ineffective. The nursing diagnosis accepted by NANDA (see box on p. 722) for this process is "Ineffective coping related to." The determination of ineffective or effective coping is more often the nurse's judgment call than the patient's own determination.[14,69]

Measurement of effectiveness relies upon patient self report. Studies of such reports by large numbers of cancer patients have formed the basis of lists that identify coping strategies as ineffective, effective, or positive.

The goal of coping is problem resolution. Coping may be simplistically viewed as what one does about any problem in order to feel better. This involves recognition of a problem and some degree of action followed by a personal evaluation of the efficacy of the action. The person diagnosed with cancer brings to this new situation a coping history.

Positive coping strategies have been characterized by several different types of behaviors. The following list provides examples of some strategies, identified by specific behaviors.[77]

- Avoidance behaviors are minimal: denial of the potential problem is minimized by gaining appropriate information, including referrals to appropriate health care providers.
- Realities are confronted: the possible outcomes of cancer therapies are realistically acknowledged and addressed.

- Problems are redefined into a solvable form such as: scheduling therapy to minimize disruptions in work and family activities.
- Alternatives are considered such as: having a backup plan for needed child care arrangements.
- Open and mutual communication with significant others is maintained: the feelings, concerns, and anxieties of the individual and significant others are addressed with honesty by both parties.
- Constructive help, including adequate medical care, is sought. The individual seeks a second opinion or actively searches for health care providers with whom he or she feels comfortable.
- Support is accepted when offered and assertive behavior is used when necessary. The individual accepts support that is helpful and recognizes behaviors that are not helpful.
- Morale is enhanced through self-reliance or the use of available resources. The individual pursues activities that are personally meaningful and in addition recognizes that compromises may need to be made, such as working part-time or reducing the amount of time spent in volunteer activities.
- Self-concept is as important as symptom relief and the individual who, while living with compromise, maintains a sense of control and does not behave as if powerless, continues to value self as a functioning being.
- Hope is self-pride, not self-deception. The ability to hope for a cure, increased life expectancy, or for an inevitable peaceful death does not indicate a lack of knowledge or understanding of the situation. Hope may include time-focused activities, such as the desire to witness the birth of a first grandchild.

Weisman also reports behaviors described by patients as not helpful when used consistently.[77] Ineffective coping strategies include withdrawal, suppression, the excessive use of alcohol or other drugs, passive acceptance, and reckless impulsive behaviors. It is important to note that the individual or family may use an ineffective style in an isolated situation, usually in response to extreme stress. Some of these behaviors are understandable in the context of an individual's background. Withdrawal to prepare one's questions or explanations to family members may be quite effective for the normally quiet, self-reliant individual. Passive acceptance may be culturally related or based on a fear of being labeled a "bad" patient or a "difficult" family. The length of time such behaviors are used is more important than their use in an individual situation. Individuals and their families who choose to consistently engage in impulsive behaviors, substance abuse, or suppression of symptoms may require the assistance of a clinical nurse specialist, social worker, or physician.

The nurse's role in fostering coping begins with an assessment of previous stressors and coping responses. Many individuals clearly assert that no matter how successfully they have coped with previous experiences they are now overwhelmed by the cancer diagnosis.

The needs of the individual, family, and friends change over time and all coping strategies are not needed simultaneously. A flexible and resourceful style can emerge in response to change.

Nonjudgmental Support

In aiding the patient and family through the adaptation process the nurse contributes the most when offering nonjudgmental support. The nursing focus can be to assist the individual in building upon past successes and learning from those experiences in which the individual's self-assessment of coping was that of needing improvement.

By focusing on learning from experiences, the nurse conveys nonjudgmental support and teaches the patient a reframing technique that supports positive change.

It may be helpful for the individual and family to engage in education programs that teach coping skills. The American Cancer Society's program "I Can Cope" encourages the development and mastery of skills that facilitate an understanding of cancer as a chronic disease, self-care management of common therapy-related side effects, and the recognition and acceptance of emotional concerns. Family members and friends are also encouraged to attend "I Can Cope" sessions to recognize and cope with their own concerns. The success of such programs has been well documented.[32]

EXTRINSIC FACTORS
The Nurse's Self-Assessment

PERSONAL MEANING.   In order to render quality psychosocial care to the individual with cancer and the family, the impact of the disease must also be viewed from the perspective of the nurse. The nurse and other caregivers can experience a wide range of emotional responses. The meaning a cancer diagnosis holds for a particular nurse is framed within the nurse's own life experience.

PROFESSIONAL EXPERIENCE.   The care brought to each situation builds upon previous experiences and influences expectations. An individual newly diagnosed with cancer may remind the nurse of other similar patients or the nurse may be reminded of personal experiences with family or close friends who have faced cancer.

Such memories may be positive or negative, help-ful or unhelpful. Patients' families may also serve as a reminder of positive or negative experiences. The challenge for the nurse is to realize that similarities, unless consciously recognized, may hinder an accurate assessment of the actual needs of an individual and family.

Cancer patients' and nurses' perceptions of caring behaviors have been identified and compared.[39,43] In two different studies, the patient's initial perception of the most important nurse-caring behaviors were the technical components of good physical care delivery. Patients initially did not report valuing aspects of a trusting relationship as highly as did the nurse. This discordance should be viewed carefully by nurses. Nurses can appreciate that through the provision of quality physical care they can establish a trusting relationship for psychosocial care. The nurse can also appreciate that the strain of facing never-ending physical and psychosocial needs can lead to exhaustion. The literature well supports the fact that constant caregiving demands can lead to such exhaustion.[8] Nurses then must reevaluate strategies for self-care.

Theoretical Psychosocial Models

CRISIS THEORY.   Crisis is a state provoked when a person faces an important obstacle in relation to life goals and for a time finds it insurmountable through the use of customary problem-solving methods.[7] Not every untoward event results in crisis or illness, but it does present an upset in the steady state.[31] Crisis occurs as an emotional response to a threatening situation.

Crisis theory describes three phases of response. In the precrisis phase the individual seeks to maintain equilibrium by adapting to physical and psychosocial changes within the context of normal life events. Problems arise. The problem itself is not the crisis. Crisis occurs as a response to a problem. Within the context of cancer, the perceived degree of threat associated with the discovery of a breast lump, for example, may initiate a crisis response in a woman with a strong family history of breast cancer. The important factor is the individual's perception of threat. The expectations and fears are derived from the family history of cancer. The crisis response is initiated not by a confirmed diagnosis but by the perceived threat.

The crisis phase is characterized by disorganization. Attempts are made to solve the problem, which may or may not be successful. In the example of a woman with a newly discovered breast lump, several possibilities emerge. The woman may respond by attempting to ignore the lump yet be haunted by an anxiety about progressive disease because of her delayed action in seeking care. She may minimize her findings and delay seeking attention while busying herself with other activities. Or she may alleviate her distress by seeking immediate medical evaluation and becoming proactively involved in her treatment planning.

In the postcrisis phase, again several possibilities can emerge. Successful problem resolution reduces the crisis and can influence the individual's functioning in future crisis situations. If the postcrisis period is marked by deterioration in physical and emotional function, the individual may function at a level lower than in the precrisis state. If new skills are learned and personal growth occurs, future functioning may be at a higher level of coping.

Oncology nurses can use the crisis intervention model to foster personal growth. The nurse can assist the individual through the initial difficulty by teaching problem-solving skills that aid in regaining personal control. Such teaching and support can assist individuals and families to achieve a higher level of postcrisis functioning.[61]

AREAS OF PREDOMINANT CONCERN. Studies of large numbers of cancer patients have yielded data regarding psychosocial impact. The issues patients and families reported they "frequently worried about" have been clustered and identified by Weisman and Worden as seven areas of predominant concern[79]:

- *Health concerns*—level of worry is related to the individual's interpretation of disease spread and significance of therapy-associated symptoms.
- *Self-appraisal*—changes in physical appearance or employment status influence self-esteem and body image.
- *Work and finances*—physical disability, temporary or permanent job changes, questions of insurance coverage, or any change in financial status can be a great source of emotional distress.
- *Family and significant others*—general mood swings or specific sexual concerns can strain relationships.
- *Religion*—the regularity of church attendance does not always indicate the depth of a belief system. Some feel comfort from a religious belief while other feel abandonment.
- *Friends and associates*—the kindness of friends and associates is appreciated, but the limitations of such relationships are acknowledged. Specific expectations may be absent.
- *Existential concerns*—regardless of the prognosis given, the individual struggles with finite existence and the possibility of early death.

PSYCHOSOCIAL STAGING. As goals of therapy are adjusted to the stage of disease progression, likewise supportive care is adjusted to various psychosocial stages of response to the disease process. Weisman and Worden have described four psychosocial stages that can be considered in conjunction with the physical stage of disease[78]:

- *Stage I: Existential Plight*—the first 100 days following diagnosis have been described as the period of existential plight. The initial period, when the diagnosis has been confirmed, is described as that of impact distress. As time progresses, the initial shock becomes focused on coping with treatment plans and therapy side effects. Regardless of prognosis, the fear of death during this time is recurrent. In general, emotional distress parallels the degree of physical change.
- *Stage II: Mitigation and Accommodation*—this stage encompasses the issues faced during remission or the time after which cure is designated. Adjustments are related to long-term side effects and the fear of recurrence. Successful adjustment includes living with minimal emphasis on disease-related changes and achieving preillness function and autonomy. Reinvestment in life occurs as plans for the future are again made.
- *Stage III: Decline and Deterioration*—recurrence signals a time-limited prognosis. The realization of disease return may be related to the degree of symptoms experienced. The actual life expectancy may remain unclear. This stage may last for a long time or progress rapidly to preterminality.
- *Stage IV: Preterminality and Terminality*—this stage acknowledges the beginning of the dying process. Symptom control and personal choices should guide care. From preterminality to death, caregivers can provide safe conduct or passage for the dying.

DEATH AND DYING. The landmark work that facilitated much of our understanding of the dynamics of dying was done by Kubler-Ross. She identified five stages associated with the dying process: denial, anger, bargaining, depression, and acceptance.[37] Some professionals later misinterpreted these data and believed it was important to progress through the stages in an orderly series from diagnosis until death. Some felt it important to help the individual move from stage to stage. Professionals sometimes reported feelings of inadequacy when their patients did not die in a stage of acceptance. In reality, the stages are to be understood as fluid and changing. The fluid nature of individual responses can make the assessment difficult.

Kavanaugh built upon the research of Kubler-Ross and described two major tasks to be accomplished in the dying process.[34] The first task is for the dying person to receive permission to die from every important person that will be left behind. This task may be accomplished for some, all, or none of the family or friends of the dying. When accomplished, it may be in an open, direct manner or very subtly. The second task is for the dying person to voluntarily let go of every important person and possession held dear. This task is also very highly individualized. At any given time the dying person, family, and friends (including professionals) may be struggling with different stages or tasks. Nurses have a supportive role in the midst of these individual responses.

Professional rewards come from recognition of efforts in this process. Nurses can recognize that family members who do not abandon the dying, in the face of their own discomfort, may silently be granting permission for the death. The individual who acknowledges the joy and difficulties experienced in life may be able to picture the world without his or her presence and voluntarily let go of life.

Common Misconceptions

DENIAL AND HOPE.   Denial and hope are often misunderstood and can therefore lead to inaccurate assessments. The term *denial* is sometimes used by health care providers to describe individuals who do not verbalize or display an understanding of the severity of their situation. Denial may also be described as minimization of physical or psychosocial distress, withdrawal, or distortion of information. Denial is a process rather than a fixed style.[67] Specific aspects of the disease situation, such as the prognosis, may be denied. Prognosis may be acknowledged only to certain individuals and then not consistently. Selection of limited situations or relationships for open disclosure is often based on the perceived safety of the situation or relationship. Caregivers can feel shut out and therefore misconstrue the response as denial.

Denial can be an extremely helpful mechanism. Staying consistently in touch with all of the emotional aspects of a life-threatening situation is neither realistic nor helpful. In the midst of apparent denial, the individual may be struggling with a competing increased awareness. This process can therefore be adaptive rather than maladaptive. Concern over a maladaptive response may be appropriate when an individual consistently engages in self-destructive behaviors or refuses therapy that offers long-term control or cure.

There may be a confusing period in the patient's adjustment and response that is also confusing to the witness. It is seen when the emotional distress of advanced disease or impending death is so painful that escape routes are sought. Individuals who have previously articulated knowledge of their prognosis suddenly embark on a course of behaviors or statements that seem to reflect little knowledge or acceptance of reality. Patients or families may say "when I

am better" or "we are planning a trip to Europe in a couple of months when he is stronger." Or there may be a sudden avoidance of questions about their condition. This phenomenon has been described as a period of middle knowledge.[77] During this period caregivers may best respond by gently refocusing the individual toward reality. Statements such as "I hope you are able to go, but it may not be possible" do not support unrealistic expectations but rather support the concept of hope.

The concept of hope is quite elusive. It is a highly personal experience that represents one's imagined future. Hope has been defined as an emotion, an expectation, an illusion, and a disposition.[49] It has been characterized as having two distinct subsets: generalized hope, which is a positive view of life or the world, and particularized hope, which is directed toward a specific outcome with a personal meaning.[17] A study addressing the relationship between hope and coping in individuals diagnosed with cancer found a positive correlation between hope and effective coping.[28] In this study, subjects still receiving therapy were more hopeful than those to whom only supportive care was given. The ability to perform self-care or carry out family responsibilities was also noted as significant to the degree of hope. A strong religious faith showed a positive correlation. Another study noted that being hopeful requires energy.[57] The latter study identified as hopeful those individuals who described meaningful lives and were peaceful regarding their situation.

Nursing assessment of psychosocial adjustment can be hampered by misconceptions of denial and hope. Hopeful attitudes can initially appear to be a denial of a grave situation. Strong religious beliefs can also be misinterpreted as false hope or maladaptive denial. The ability to differentiate comes from a strong nurse-patient-family relationship and a systematic assessment. The relationships and assessment evolve over time and are characterized by openness and a nonjudgmental approach that enables hope to exist.

SADNESS AND DEPRESSION.   Another challenging psychosocial assessment involves the distinction between sadness and depression. Sadness is a normal human response to a potential or real loss. Depression is a severe expression of normal sadness.[67] Sadness is uncomfortable for both the cared for and the caregiver.

When confronted with the diagnosis or recurrence of cancer, a grief reaction normally ensues. The grief reaction may be manifested in numerous ways: anger, inability to concentrate, lapses in short-term memory, withdrawal, or tearfulness. Individual and cultural variances are also noted. When such responses lead to an inability to carry out self-care or a prolonged state of diminished self-esteem, supportive intervention is needed. An assessment of preillness relationships and crisis response patterns is necessary. A history of family discord, substance abuse, or depression should be evaluated.

A complete assessment of emotional states includes a search for potential physical causes. The fatigue associated with cancer therapies, electrolyte abnormalities, or side effects of drugs may precipitate or aggravate depressive symptoms. When depressive symptoms persist, psychiatric consultation may be indicated.[44] Psychotherapy and pharmacologic intervention can help a subset of patients. Nursing interventions should focus on fostering a supportive environment that accepts a variety of emotional responses as appropriate and valid. Caution should be observed with individuals who internalize rather than verbalize feelings. Although catharses may be helpful for some, it must be recognized that a safe environment for catharsis demands a skillful therapeutic relationship. When individuals feel forced to verbalize feelings, they will subsequently feel awkward in the presense of the individual perceived to be responsible.[67] A team approach may be most helpful in assessing and managing sadness and depression.

MAXIMIZING QUALITY OF LIFE FOR PATIENT AND FAMILY

The myriad psychosocial issues that are a part of cancer nursing care stem from the individual response of the patient, family, friends, and society to a diagnosis and prognosis. Maximizing quality of life is the goal regardless of disease outcome. Both supportive care and survivorship involve specific issues that must be successfully addressed to maximize quality of life. A structured assessment can uncover misconceptions that may impede healthy coping and adjustment. Specific models of care and intervention techniques can be employed to influence the adjustment process and outcome.

Survivorship

From the time of its discovery and for the balance of life, an individual diagnosed with cancer is considered a survivor. During the experience the individual first fights to beat the disease and then to sustain disease-free survival.[52] Survivorship brings with it many aspects of rehabilitation. The physical, psychosocial, vocational, and financial effects of cancer are receiving more attention than ever.[41,64]

A new group of survivor has emerged to address these concerns. These individuals come together through various forums to search, explore, and learn together. They attend meetings, share newsletters, and write books. They exchange "war" stories and work together to achieve quality time. They have found meaning and usefulness in the concept of survival rather than cure.[71] The organization called the National Coalition for Cancer Survivorship (NCCS) was thus formed.

There are an estimated 8 million Americans with a history of cancer who share survivorship concerns. In an attempt to call public attention to the survivor's needs, the American Cancer Society put forth "The Cancer Survivor's Bill of Rights."[71] These rights address medical care, personal life adjustment, job opportunities, and insurance coverage. The aim is to have society foster a truly normal life span for cancer survivors.

In spite of progress in treatment, cancer continues to be associated with negative outcomes. With such a prevailing attitude, often too little thought is given to aggressive rehabilitation. The growing survivorship movement has refocused concern on life after treatment and the rehabilitation needs of cancer patients.

Cancer rehabilitation may be defined as the process of minimizing the physical, psychologic, social, and vocational dysfunction that may result from the disease or its treatment. Rehabilitation measures are aimed at restoration of function and prevention of further complications and include compensatory and supportive measures. When disabilities cannot be corrected, coping or adaptation must occur. Adaptation is an attempt to maintain sameness with a focus on altering to conform to demands and maintain the system.[6] The system may be the family, school, work, or community. Adaptation is not always achievable, and the broader concept of coping must then be explored. The goal of coping is problem resolution, which necessitates a change in both the person and the situation. With coping as a goal, the person uses a variety of resources to regain personal control. The problem may not be permanently solved, but the process can begin again.

Rehabilitation is dynamic, since abilities and goals are continually changing.[16] Confrontation is an integral part of the strategies employed.[6,77] Such rehabilitation involves measures that enable individuals to feel at home with their bodies, self-image, emotional status, social setting, and work.

PHYSICAL REHABILITATION. Physical rehabilitation should begin as soon as the likelihood of disability is recognized. Loss or dysfunction of a body part requires various approaches to physical rehabilitation. Surgical amputation of a body part or limb may lead to the need for a prosthesis and techniques to aid in maintaining function and prevent further complications, such as lymphedema after breast surgery. Other examples of physical consequences include loss of voluntary bowel or bladder control, loss of energy, loss of appetite, inability to speak or swallow, deterioration in muscle strength, inability to ambulate, or unstable gait.[16] Functional restoration will be dependent on the degree of impairment, disability, or handicap experienced. Other physical changes, such as impaired fertility, may be the source of distress requiring psychosocial rehabilitation.

Nurses and physical therapists can work together with the patient and family employing techniques, such as upper extremity range of motion, arm and hand strength or endurance, coordination, splinting, and compensatory techniques for sensory loss. In aiding with the adjustment to a physical loss, there is no substitute for the support and role modeling that can come from a peer, someone who has experienced the same loss. Referrals to such groups as Reach to Recovery or laryngectomy clubs can complement the efforts of nurses and therapists and bolster the self-esteem of the patient.

PSYCHOSOCIAL REHABILITATION. Because of their complexity, psychosocial needs are best assessed in a systematic manner.[62] The history should include information about the family makeup and relationships, work history, religious and community involvements, educational status, financial resources, and, when possible, clues to prior coping mechanisms. Emotional distress scales or similar types of measurements may be helpful in objectifying information.

Cancer survivors frequently perceive themselves as being treated differently by family, friends, and business associates. Myths, misconceptions, fear of recurrence, and poor communication may all contribute to the newfound disease of such relationships. Patients soon decide with whom they can talk about their illness. They may seek those less likely to be frightened or overwhelmed with anxiety.

Conflicting data exist regarding the long-term impact of a cancer diagnosis on marital relationships. Changes in body image, impaired fertility, degree of unresolved conflicts, and preillness maturity within a relationship must all be considered.[9,41] The cancer survivor who is single also has special concerns. Anxieties over developing intimate relationships center on explaining the cancer history, potential infertility, and body image changes.[9,80] These concerns should be clinically addressed proactively. A psychosocial data base can uncover such concerns and guide the caregiver in strengthening the adjustment process. A psychosocial plan of care should involve a team approach and consider developmental needs, realities of treatment, prognosis, and all aspects of rehabilitation.

When disease or treatment leaves the individual with residual impairment, specific rehabilitation goals aimed at restoration may be needed. Participation in activities of daily living can be the joint goal of patient, family, nurse, physical and occupational therapist, social worker, and psychologist. Techniques employed may include a life-style interview or checklist and information on energy conservation, pacing, work simplification, home adaptation, and adaptive equipment. Adaptive living techniques can foster the maintenance of self-esteem. The rehabilitation team can employ such techniques as stress management, relaxation, dealing with depression through activity, and making life-style changes to maximize independence.

EMPLOYMENT/VOCATIONAL REHABILITATION. Employment often means more than a source of income. A job or career may be a major part of feelings of identity and self-worth. Most successfully treated cancer patients are able to resume previous occupations with minor or no alteration in circumstances. Those who do face problems when returning to work cite the attitudes of employers and coworkers as a major concern.[48] Nurses should prepare patients for the possibility of such reactions.[51] Some patients recognize their own attitudes as the obstacle. Fear of recurrence and fatalism about the disease may be at the root of the problem. Some cancer survivors describe a sense of being locked into a current position or employer.[81] They are hesitant to change positions because of specific concerns about obtaining insurance benefits. Actual discrimination may be difficult to prove since it can be subtle.

The Americans With Disabilities Act (ADA) of 1990 requires equal opportunity in selection, testing, and hiring of qualified applicants with disabilities, including individuals with cancer or a history of cancer. This law prohibits discrimination against workers with disabilities and is similar to the Civil Rights Act of 1964 and Title V of the Rehabilitation Act of 1973. The individual who is familiar with these laws can protect themselves from discrimination through preventive strategies. Unless the effects of disease or treatment directly affect the individual's ability to perform the essential functions of a job there is no obligation to disclose information. It is important not to lie, but also not necessary to volunteer information. The employee should be prepared to educate the employer and to stress specific job qualifications and abilities.

Any person with a history of cancer, who meets specified job qualifications and can perform the essential functions of the employment position is protected under the Americans with Disabilities Act of 1990. The employer is required to provide reasonable accommodation. The Equal Employment Opportunity Commission (EEOC) assumes the federal government role of enforcing the standard. Local government offices can assist in investigations or claims.

When residual effects of disease or treatment alter the individual's ability to continue in the pre-illness job, vocational rehabilitation interventions may be necessary. Retraining, partial disability, or full disability may be the only alternative for some. In these situations a rehabilitation team is needed to establish specific and realistic goals.[16,26] Oncology nurses, along with rehabilitation specialists, can assist in successful reentry.[62] The rehabilitation team can also assist in educating employers to dispel cancer myths.

Finances, Insurance, and the Law

An individual's insurance coverage and financial resources greatly influence access to care and quality of care. The uninsured and underinsured are at the mercy of indigent care providers or limited state and federal programs. Limited services and limits on coverage place individuals in the compromised position of under reporting of health problems. This situation fosters delayed diagnosis and treatment, increased acuity, and spiraling of health care cost.

The cost of care adds to the individual and family's burden of living with cancer. They may be faced with the dilemma of forced choices: limited job mobility, paying medical bills vs. living expenses, not reporting symptoms, seeking financial assistance, changing relationships, and insurance limitations as a subtle form of discrimination.[58]

Insurance companies can decide the type of insurance contract they will sell and to whom. Contracts are negotiated with employers and with individuals. The contract cost is determined by the coverage limits. The individual with evidence of persistent or recurrent disease may be considered a high risk to the insurance industry. The concept of excess mortality (observed death rates vs. standard expected rates) is used in calculating premiums. Private insurance companies can establish waiting periods, deny coverage, and cancel policies based on the provision of each policy.

Currently no federal law guarantees a right to adequate health insurance. Cancer survivors do have the opportunity of keeping the health insurance obtained through their employer even after they are no longer employed. This opportunity is provided through The Comprehensive Omnibus Budget Reconciliation Act (COBRA) and The Employee Retirement and Income Security Act (ERISA). The COBRA plan can provide short term coverage while seeking new employment or a new group plan. The ERISA law entitles the individual to file a claim when benefits are denied through discrimination. The ERISA law is enforced by the Pension and Welfare Benefits Administration of the United States Department of Labor. Nurses and other interdisciplinary team members can support the individual with financial concerns by sensitively assessing their situation and educating them about rights and resources.

Providing Comfort in Terminal Care

When cure or disease control are no longer attainable goals, there is a shift to palliative care in what is commonly referred to as the terminal phase of illness. The transition into this phase may be gradual and the shift in care needs are not always recognized and acknowledged. As caregiving needs change, role strain may increase. The distinct needs of the patient and the caregiver must be recognized. The literature provides a systematic description and distinction between the needs of patient and primary caregiver.[83]

Nurses who recognize differing levels of need and need awareness in the patient and family can respond sensitively with supportive care. The nurse must be able to focus attention on the patient's goals, as stated by the patient, without neglecting the needs of the family. By asking questions and listening, the nurse can distinguish facts from feelings and ethical concerns. Clinical judgment suffices when dealing with the facts of disease progression and symptoms, but a more ethical decision-making process is required to deal with value-laden concerns. When values come in conflict ethical dilemmas can arise.

ADVANCED DIRECTIVES. When addressing quality of life issues and clarifying values, the health care team approaches the subjects of no code, living wills, and hospice care. The cornerstone belief is that when death is inevitable, dignity is essential. Though not universally accepted, it is a common belief that it is not detrimental to tell a patient death is near. Honest communication should be tempered with sensitivity. In the context of such open communication, the wise physician may suggest that the patient prepare for the possibility of becoming unable to communicate and participate in treatment decisions.

A Supreme Court ruling has affirmed the constitutional right of liberty to refuse any medical treatment, including life-prolonging procedures and the right to name an agent to be a surrogate decision-maker for health care issues when the individual loses the personal capacity to do so. These rights are proclaimed by enacting an advance directive that is a signed, dated, and witnessed document. Some states require notarization of the document. The individual who signs such a document must provide copies to their family, physician, and other appropriate individuals and discuss the specific details with these individuals.

HOSPICE CARE. Discussion of care goals will lead to planning for a method of care delivery. When the focus of care is on the needs of the patient and family, attempts are made to leave as much control as possible in their hands. This approach serves to reaffirm life.[6] The setting and use of available health care agencies are determined by the individual situation. Regardless of the setting or agencies involved, the hospice approach or philosophy can serve the spectrum of needs. Hospice involves physical care, counseling services, volunteer assistance, respite care, support at the time of death, and bereavement follow-up. The coordination of care is based on stringent assessment of the resources, both internal and external, of the individual and family.[76]

Changes in health care reimbursement reward early discharge and home care. Home care and palliative needs require nursing assistance. The availability of a constant care provider is essential. Nurses coordinate the multidisciplinary care delivery. While delivering skilled care directly, they also teach family and friends how to deliver personal care. Hospice has therefore been described as primarily a nursing intervention.[50] Physical comfort is the priority. When physical symptoms are well managed, the dying may have the emotional energy to prepare themselves for death.

The dying individual has the right to choose which decisions to be involved in and which are of less concern.[42] Some individuals may wish to plan their own funeral and tell others of the plan, either verbally or in writing. Some may wish to make concrete arrangements for the family's financial and legal stability while avoiding conversation about feelings related to the dying process. During the dying process, less fear may be described than earlier in the disease process, yet a sense of disbelief may still be maintained.[74] The hospice nurse assesses the emotional position and lends gentle support without pressure to influence the response.

The needs of family members are unique to each member. Nursing assessment should identify the type of support family members are seeking.[84] The challenge of nursing is to prioritize the needs of patient and family members, noting the degree of congruence or discordance. The nurse can then more readily distinguish between reasonable and ideal psychosocial care.

BEREAVEMENT.   The nurse who cares for the dying knows that grief does not begin with death or end with the funeral. With long-term illness, there is an opportunity to prepare for the actual loss by anticipating it. Anticipatory grief may or may not ease or shorten the bereavement process. The degree of emotional attachment and quality of communication within relationships influence the impact and outcome of grief. Constant pain, suffering, and a protracted death can increase the emotional pain. During the period of anticipation, the family may rehearse the impending death and feel depressed but also attempt to readjust their lives. At the time of death, there may be little display of emotion. Nurses and other caregivers may perceive a premature detachment. Therapeutic assessment throughout the illness and dying process can lessen the chance of misinterpreting the grieving process.

Grief and mourning have many faces. Descriptions of normal grief come from reports of common symptoms. Crying, depressed mood, and sleep and eating disturbances are commonly reported. The sequence of events is reported as phases of shock and disbelief, developing awareness, and resolution.[67]

The time necessary for grief resolution is highly variable. Behavioral adaptation may be a response to societal expectation and not a barometer of emotional healing. Clear evidence of grief resolution may be the ability to speak of the lost relationship comfortably and realistically, recounting pleasures and disappointments of the relationship.

Psychosocial management of the bereaved ideally begins with assessment of coping resources before the death. Helping the family know what to expect may ease the impact. Practical information and helpful acts convey compassionate support. The nurses' composure can create an atmosphere of control. When nurses' genuine feelings and emotional responses are controlled rather than denied, the bereaved are most therapeutically served. Extended care for the bereaved can take many forms: presence at funeral services, notes of sympathy, phone calls at specific intervals, support group offerings, or social gatherings. Such extension of care by professionals can be preventive medicine for the bereaved.

There are no timetables for grief and bereavement. The extent of follow-up must be individualized to the bereaved's needs and the constraints of the professional and institutional resources. Focus on high-risk needs and further referrals may be the priority.

Support for the Caregiver

PRIORITY-SETTING.   During the entire course of coping with cancer, there are psychologic and social effects on family functioning. The process can become destructive or turn in a positive direction toward personal growth. The direction taken at each crisis point may differ for each family member based on their unique perceptions of crises as threat or opportunity. Varied perceptions and expectations can lead to communication barriers. Such barriers can impede effective coping and personal growth. Nurturing can remove such barriers. Therapeutic interventions by a nurse or other caregiver are critical at these susceptible times. Interventions can become therapeutic when preceded by careful assessment and mutual goal-setting. Each individual's goals or priorities must be considered.

In distinguishing between ideal and reasonable goals, priority-setting becomes of paramount importance. Priority-setting often parallels a hierarchy of needs. Physical needs must be met first. Emotional and social needs are more complex. The individual who successfully meets these needs may experience the personal growth that permits addressing spiritual needs. Care demands must be assessed in light of the priorities.[56] The clarification of goals and priorities fosters shared responsibilities. The level of communication needed to establish priorities can also aid in minimizing demands, making problems manageable, and preventing burnout.

Burnout is a syndrome of physical and personal exhaustion accompanied by negative attitudes and loss of concern for self and others. Family members and professional caregivers alike risk such a response when giving highly specialized care in emotionally charged situations. A cycle of frustration, helplessness, and cynicism can develop. The risk of burnout can be reduced by voicing frustration appropriately, developing a support system, setting priorities, and establishing reasonable expectations.[69]

LIFE ENHANCEMENT SKILLS. High-quality care and avoidance of burnout can be achieved when life enhancement skills are developed. Life enhancement begins with self-care. Attending to the needs of others must be balanced with attending to one's own needs. A nutritious diet, adequate sleep, and physical exercise aid in physical self-care. Psychic and social comfort can be achieved through a variety of activities that provide a form of decompression. Prodromal signs of distress or inappropriate coping must be recognized and confronted. Life enhancement skills are developed from a philosophy of being true to self, a personal spirituality and commitment to caring for self and others. These skills can include such things as exercise, reading, writing, crafts, hobbies, music, dance, drama, and humor. Such skill development fosters resilience. With resilience, crisis can eventually be perceived as an opportunity for growth.

The crisis of cancer begins as a psychosocial response to a biologic growth but can become a psychosocial and spiritual growth process of life enhancement. This response is supported by nurses who have chosen a profession of life enhancement.

Nursing Management

FACILITATING POSITIVE COPING
The Nurse's Role as Coach

Nursing interventions for psychosocial care are aimed at facilitating positive coping. The coach or teacher of positive coping skills must possess a number of competencies.[4] First is the competency of *timing*. Timing is the art of capturing readiness to learn. Cancer nurses' competency is challenged here when information about disease, side effects of therapy, and self-care measures is to be taught at a time of high stress and overwhelming emotional responses. Teaching must be done progressively and repeatedly. Initial goals are to obtain informed consent, advise of immediate side effects, and assure safe self-care behaviors. The second competency is *integration*. Early rehabilitation is achieved when the nurse teaches self-care strategies that emphasize the healthy aspects of the individual and integration of the implications of illness and recovery into their life-style. The third competency is *understanding*. The nurse who skillfully listens to the patient's interpretation of information can mobilize appropriate psychologic and spiritual resources. Fourth is the competency of *interpretation*. Interpretation provides the patient with a rationale for treatments, procedures, and self-care measures. Skillful interpretation will reduce the sense of being overwhelmed. The fifth competency is *coaching*. The nurse coach assists the patient through difficult events such as bone marrow aspirations, venipunctures, nausea and vomiting, and alopecia. The nurse who gently coaches the patient through stressful and unfamiliar situations, one step at a time, can provide maximum support and facilitate successful coping.

Promoting Self-Care

Whether the goal be cure, control, or palliation, coping is most often facilitated when self-care is fostered. Situations and times will dictate the need for caregivers to assume aspects of care. Self-determination may then be more important than actual self-care. The skills needed for self-care and self-determination do not always come naturally. In many chronic diseases, model patient education programs have been developed to foster self-care and effective coping.

The "I Can Cope" program, developed by Johnson and Norby and offered through the American Cancer Society, is a model cancer education program that teaches self-care and coping skills. The series of classes addresses learning about the disease and treatment, managing side effects, dealing with emotions, maintaining physical fitness, enhancing sexuality, and identifying and using resources. The class learning is enhanced by audiovisuals and printed materials that can later be used as reference guides for self-care. The self-help strategies taught in the classes are also described in a book of the same title, *I Can Cope*.[32]

The Patient's Sense of Maintaining Control

Studies suggest that cognitive information — that is, specific facts about the disease or treatment — is preferred by individuals during the initial phase of therapy. As treatment progresses, behavioral information is more readily assimilated. Determining individual learning needs is an important component of fostering self-care. The work of the "I Can Cope" program originators suggests that many individuals also respond to information that focuses on sensory experiences such as relaxation or massage.[33] Although research is needed to determine the type of information most beneficial to groups and individuals, the nurse can best meet any need by using professional experience and individualized assessment as a guide. The ultimate goal is to foster self-care and aid the patient in maintaining a sense of control in the situation.

Assisting the Patient with Goal-Setting

When the patient or family experiences episodes of feeling overwhelmed either physically or emotionally, goal-setting can be a helpful intervention. This process begins by asking the patient what outcome is desired. The nurse can help determine what goals are attainable within specific time frames. The nurse can provide assistance in establishing attainable goals within specific time frames. For example, this technique can be used to coach the individual through periods of inadequate fluid intake. Another attainable goal may be to come to the dinner table at least once a day rather than eating in one's room. Such small and attainable goals can build feelings of success. Periodic review of attained goals can be a morale booster for even the most withdrawn individual. Such coaching functions by the nurse aid in reaching the goal of positive coping.

Referral for Counseling

Cancer patients rarely employ a maladaptive coping style in a consistent manner. However, there are occasions when particular behavioral patterns are a manifestation of an inability to cope effectively and require the intervention of an individual with advanced skills in psychosocial assessment. The experienced nurse is frequently in a position to recognize these patterns and to make a referral for further assessment. First it is important to observe for consistency, especially when dealing with a new diagnosis or recurrence. Some assessment techniques require advanced practice skills to determine the extent of maladaptive coping.[86] Maladaptive coping may manifest itself as three or more of the following behaviors:

- Poor eye contact and little facial expression, slow speech
- Nonfluctuating, generally negative mood
- Appetite significantly depressed, refusing adequate nutrition
- Sleep pattern characterized by early morning awakening, insomnia, or excessive daytime sleeping
- Lack of attention to hygiene and activities of daily living

The initial diagnosis or recurrence of cancer may initiate or exacerbate several of these behaviors. A complete assessment includes noting the persistence of such behaviors. Even in the absence of the symptomatology described, there may be indications for referral to specially skilled psychosocial caregivers.

Coping can be ineffective without being maladaptive. Many individuals are at risk of developing further problems if appropriate psychosocial assessment and intervention do not take place. Nurses may ask the patient or family to keep a log of feelings or responses during treatment or at critical times of change. Such a technique may aid in documenting negative thought or behavior patterns and confirm the need for a skilled counseling referral.[36]

Noncompliance can be a manifestation of ineffective coping and indicate the need for referral or a psychosocial consultation. Lack of compliance usually represents unmet needs or signifies a lack of understanding. Noncompliant behavior may also be a manifestation of anger, anxiety, or depression. Failure of an individual to follow a recommended treatment regimen may stem from other concerns, such as economics, a desire to avoid side effects, or a genuine lack of comprehension regarding the treatment regimen. To ensure continuity of care, patient compliance should be continuously monitored. Complex information should be tailored to meet individual needs, and specific behaviors that enhance compliance should be identified and reinforced.[3] Caregivers often perceive noncompliant behavior as a conscious decision to annoy the caregiver. Adequate assessment can deter such a perception.

BEHAVIORAL TECHNIQUES
Rationale

Specific behavioral interventions may be useful adjuncts in facilitating positive coping. Such interventions are particularly helpful in the management of anxiety, nausea and vomiting, and chronic pain. Behavioral techniques are most effective when combined with standard management approaches to specific problems. The comfort of patients receiving emetogenic chemotherapy may be enhanced by using relaxation therapy along with effective antiemetics. Distraction or the use of imagery along with appropriate analgesics may reduce pain perception. The use of rhythmic breathing during acutely painful procedures can reduce anxiety.

Behavioral techniques are to be taught, not imposed. Some individuals may resist behavioral approaches out of a fear of losing control or behaving in an embarrassing manner. An association with stage hypnosis may underlie such fear or reluctance. It is important to clarify concepts that are often misunderstood.[85] When presenting behavioral techniques as an option, it is important to point out that such techniques are successful because the person does remain in control of thoughts and functions.

Types of Behavioral Techniques

Relaxation, imagery, and hypnosis are three behavioral techniques that may be used individually or in combination. Relaxation is described as the absence of tension. Benson's relaxation response uses progressive muscle relaxation.[5] Reduction in tension can be physiologic or psychologic. Imagery has been described as the internal experience of an event without external stimuli.[85] A common imagery experience is that of a daydream. Imagery uses the imagination to visualize and sense an experience. Hypnosis is the induction of a trancelike state.[70] The trance is described as a wakeful dissociative state characterized by an increased receptivity to suggestion. These techniques require varying degrees of training. After successful training, nurses can teach patients to do progressive relaxation alone or with the use of music or directed audio tapes. These techniques can be used as an adjunct in the management of chemotherapy-induced nausea.[10,22] Numerous scripts are available to assist nurses in implementing relaxation and imagery techniques.[46] Biofeedback is a technique that requires the use of monitoring instruments to assess muscle tension or thermoregulation. Some individuals are more attracted to such an approach than others and may benefit by a referral to someone qualified to implement such techniques. While the goals of relaxation and hypnosis may be similar, the approaches and techniques are quite different. Hypnosis is dependent upon the achievement of a trance state. Supervised training is necessary for the safe use of hypnotic techniques. After individualized assessment and mutual goal-setting have been completed by the nurse and patient, an appropriate technique may be selected.

CONCLUSION

The biologic disease process is unique for each individual, and the psychosocial response is equally individual. The psychosocial response extends to the family, friends, and professional caregivers. Meaningful support and therapeutic interventions can be difficult to deliver. A structured assessment and team approach can foster objective and complete data collection, support uniqueness, and aid in priority-setting. With such an approach, an open evolving system is established, and the potential arises for adaptation, positive coping, and holistic growth in the person with cancer and in family, friends, and caregivers.

BIBLIOGRAPHY

1. Anderson BI: Sexual functioning morbidity among cancer survivors, Cancer 55(1):1835-42, 1985.
2. Anderson J: Insurability of cancer patients: a rehabilitation barrier, Oncol Nurs Forum 11:42, 1984.
3. Barofsky I: Therapeutic compliance and the cancer patient, Health Educ Q 10(suppl):43, 1984.
4. Benner P: From novice to expert: excellence and power in clinical nursing practice, Menlo Park, CA, 1984, Addison Wesley.
5. Benson H: The relaxation response, New York, 1975, William Morrow Co.
6. Burns N: Nursing and cancer, Philadelphia, 1982, WB Saunders Co.
7. Caplan G: Principles of preventative psychiatry, New York, 1969, Basic Books.
8. Carpenter P and Morrow G: Clinical care of cancer patients: close personal interpersonal encounters of the difficult kind, J Psychosoc Oncol 3(4):67, 1986.
9. Cella DF and Tross S: Psychological adjustment to survival from Hodgkin's disease, J Consult Clin Psychol 54(5):616, 1986.
10. Cotanch PH and Strum S: Progressive muscle relaxation as antiemetic therapy for cancer patients, Oncol Nurs Forum 14(4):33, 1987.
11. Crothers HM: Employment problems of cancer survivors: local problems and local solutions. In Proceedings of the workshop on employment, insurance and the patient with cancer, New Orleans, 1986, American Cancer Society.
12. DePastino EP: The nurse as counselor, Oncol Nurs Forum 11(4):93, 1984.
13. Derogatis LR: Psychology in cancer medicine: a perspective and overview, J Consult Clin Psychol 54(5):632, 1986.
14. Devolder-McCray Noella: Ratings by health professionals of effective coping strategies for cancer patients. Master's thesis, University of Kansas, 1979.
15. Dodd M and Ahmed N: Preference for type of

information in cancer patients receiving radiation therapy, Cancer Nurs 10(5):244, 1987.

16. Dudas S and Carlson C: Cancer rehabilitation, Oncol Nurs Forum 15:183, 1988.

17. Dufault K and Martocchio B: Hope: its spheres and dimensions, Nurs Clin North Am 20(2):379, 1985.

18. Dyck S and Wright K: Family perceptions: the role of the nurse throughout an adult's cancer experience, Oncol Nurs Forum 12(5):53, 1985.

19. Einhorn LH, Crawford ED, and Shipley WU: Cancer of the testes. In DeVita V, Hellman S, and Rosenberg S, editors: Cancer principles and practice of oncology, ed 3, Philadelphia, 1989, JB Lippincott Co.

20. Fernsler J: A comparison of patient and nurse perceptions of patients' self-care deficits associated with cancer chemotherapy, Cancer Nurs 9(2):50, 1986.

21. Fobair P and others: Psychological problems among survivors of Hodgkin's disease, J Clin Oncol 4(5):805, 1986.

22. Frank JM: The effects of music therapy and guided visual imagery on chemotherapy-induced nausea and vomiting, Oncol Nurs Forum 12(5):47, 1985.

23. Freidenberg I and others: Assessment and treatment of psychosocial problems of the cancer patient: a case study, Cancer Nurs 3:111, 1980.

24. Germino B: The impact of cancer on the patient, the family and the nurse. In Living with cancer: fifth national conference on cancer nursing, New York, 1987, American Cancer Society.

25. Gorzynski JG and Holland JC: Psychological aspects of testicular cancer, Semin Oncol 6(1):125, 1979.

26. Gunn AE: Cancer rehabilitation, New York, 1984, Raven Press.

27. Henderson IC and others: Cancer of the breast. In DeVita V, Hellman S, and Rosenberg S, editors: Cancer principles and practice of oncology, ed 3, Philadelphia, 1989, JB Lippincott Co.

28. Herth K: The relationship between level of hope and level of coping, response and other variables in patients with cancer, Oncol Nurs Forum 16(1):67, 1989.

29. Hoffman B: Cancer survivors at work: job problems and illegal discrimination, Oncol Nurs Forum 16(1):39, 1989.

30. Hopkins MB: Information-seeking and adaptional outcomes in women receiving chemotherapy for breast cancer, Cancer Nurs 9(5):256, 1986.

31. Infante MS: Crisis theory, a framework for nursing practice, Reston, Va, 1982, Reston Publishing Co.

32. Johnson J and Klein L: I can cope: staying healthy with cancer, Minneapolis, 1988, DCI Publishing.

33. Johnson J and others: Sensory information instruction as a coping strategy in recovery from surgery, Res Nurs Health 1:4, 1978.

34. Kavanaugh R: Facing death, Baltimore, 1974, Penguin Books.

35. Killilea M: Social and community support systems. In Living with cancer: fifth national conference on cancer nursing, New York, 1987, American Cancer Society.

36. Kline PM: Reactive depression in the client with cancer. In Chernecky CC and Ramsey PW, editors: Critical nursing care of the client with cancer, Norwalk, Conn, 1984, Appleton-Century-Crofts.

37. Kubler-Ross E: On death and dying, New York, 1969, Macmillan.

38. Kushner H: When bad things happen to good people, New York, 1981, Schocken Books.

39. Larson P: Important nurse caring behaviors perceived by patients with cancer, Oncol Nurs Forum 11(6):46, 1984.

40. Lind S and others: Telling the diagnosis of cancer, J Clin Oncol 7(5):583, 1989.

41. Loescher LJ and others: Surviving adult cancers. Part 1. Physiologic effects, Ann Intern Med 111(5):411, 1989.

42. Martocchio B: Authenticity, belonging, emotional closeness and self-representation, Oncol Nurs Forum 14(4):3, 1987.

43. Massie M: The cancer patient: psychiatric complications and their management, current concepts in psycho-oncology and AIDS, Memorial Sloan-Kettering Cancer Center Syllabus, 1987.

44. Massie M and Holland J: Assessment and management of the cancer patient with depression, Advances in Psychosomatic Medicine 18:1, 1988.

45. Mayer D: Oncology nurses' versus cancer patients' perceptions of nurse caring behaviors: a replication study, Oncol Nurs Forum 14(3):48, 1987.

46. McCaffrey M and Beebe A: Pain clinical manual for nursing practice, St Louis, 1989, Mosby.

47. McCorkle R: Development of a symptom distress scale, Cancer Nurs 1:373, 1978.

48. Mellette S: The cancer patient at work, CA 35(6):360, 1985.

49. Miller JF: Inspiring hope, Am J Nurs 85(1):22, 1985.

50. Mor V and Masterson-Allen S: The hospice model of care for the terminally ill, Adv Psychosom Med 18:119, 1988.

51. Mullen F: Re-entry: the educational needs of the cancer survivor, Health Educ Q 10(suppl):88, 1984.

52. Mullen F and Hoffman B: An almanac of practical

resources for cancer survivors charting the journey, New York, Consumers Union, 1990.

53. North American Nursing Diagnoses Association: Conference Proceedings, St Louis, 1992, The Association.

54. Northouse L: Mastectomy patients and the fear of cancer recurrence, Cancer Nurs 4(3):213, 1981.

55. Northouse L: Family issues in cancer care, Adv Psychosom Med 18:82, 1988.

56. Oberst M and others: Caregiving demands and appraisal of stress among family caregivers, Cancer Nurs 12(4):209, 1989.

57. Owen D: Nurses' perspective on the meaning of hope in patients with cancer: a qualitative study, Oncol Nurs Forum 16(1):75, 1989.

58. Quigley K: The adult cancer survivor: psychosocial consequences of cure, Semin Oncol Nurs 5(1):63, 1989.

59. Radner G: It's always something, New York, 1989, Simon & Schuster.

60. Reiker PP, Edbril SD, and Garnick MB: Curative testes therapy: psychosocial sequence, J Clin Oncol 3(8):1117, 1985.

61. Rickel LM: Making mountains manageable: maximizing quality of life through crisis intervention, Oncol Nurs Forum 14(4):29, 1987.

62. Romasaas E and others: A method for assessing the rehabilitation needs for oncology outpatients, Oncol Nurs Forum 10(3):17, 1983.

63. Scanlon C: Creating a vision of hope: the challenge of palliative care, Oncol Nurs Forum 16(4):491, 1989.

64. Schmale AH and others: Wellbeing of cancer survivors, Psychosom Med 45(2):163, 1983.

65. Schover LR and Fife M: Sexual counseling of patients undergoing radical surgery, J Psychosoc Oncol 54(5):616, 1986.

66. Schwalb E and Crosson K: Helping you help your patients: the patient education program of the National Cancer Institute, Oncol Nurs Forum 15(5):651, 1985.

67. Simko LO: Psychosocial dimensions of cancer. In Groenwald SL, editor: Cancer nursing principles and practice, Boston, 1987, Jones & Bartlett Publishers, Inc.

68. Sneed N and others: Adjustment of gynecological and breast cancer patients to the cancer diagnosis: Comparisons with males and females having other cancer sites, Health Care for Women Int 13:11, 1992.

69. Snyder C: Oncology nursing, Boston, 1986, Little Brown & Co.

70. Spiegel H and Spiegel D: Trance and treatment, New York, 1978, Basic Books.

71. Springarn N: The new breed of survivors, Cancer News, American Cancer Society, 1988.

72. Stephens L: NANDA diagnosis questioned, ONS News 7(7):8, 1992.

73. Thorne SE: Helpful and unhelpful communications in cancer care: the patient perspective, Oncol Nurs Forum 15(2):167, 1988.

74. Vachon M: Psychotherapy and the person with cancer: an analysis of one nurse's experience, Oncol Nurs Forum 12(4):33, 1985.

75. Watzlawick P and others: Change: principles of problem formation and problem resolution, New York, 1974, WW Norton.

76. Wegman J: Hospice home death, hospital death, and coping abilities of widows, Cancer Nurs 10(3):153, 1987.

77. Weisman AD: Coping with cancer, New York, 1979, McGraw-Hill.

78. Weisman AD and Worden WJ: The emotional plight of cancer: significance of the first 100 days, Int J Psychiatry Med 7(1):145, 1976-77.

79. Weisman AD and Worden WJ: The emotional impact of recurrent cancer, J Psychosoc Oncol 3(4):5, 1986.

80. Welch-McCaffrey D: Oncology nurses as cancer patients: an investigative questionnaire, Oncol Nurs Forum 11(2):48, 1984.

81. Welch-McCaffrey D and others: Surviving adult cancers. Part 2. Psychological implications, Ann Intern Med 11(6):517, 1989.

82. Werner-Beland JA: Grief responses to long-term illness and disability, Reston, Va, 1980, Reston Publishing Co.

83. Wingate A and Lackey N: A description of the needs of noninstitutionalized cancer patients and their primary caregivers, Cancer Nurs 12(4):216, 1989.

84. Woods N, Yates B, and Primomo J: Suporting families during chronic illness, Image 21(1):46, 1989.

85. Zahourek RP: Relaxation and imagery: tools for therapeutic communication and intervention, Philadelphia, 1988, WB Saunders Co.

86. Zimberg M: Psychosocial isolation. In Brown MH and others, editors: Standards of oncology nursing practice, New York, 1986, John Wiley & Sons.

CHAPTER 31

Impact of Cancer on Sexuality

Judith A. Shell

Human beings are sexual from the time of birth until their death, and being sexual is a primary part of being human. If this factor is dismissed by the nurse or physician, the patient often perceives him- or herself as less than human. Until recently, health care professionals have been inclined to focus on the physical and emotional aspects of the human being while overlooking the psychosexual. This has been especially true with patients who are disabled, chronically ill, or over the age of 62.

Williams and colleagues reported in the late 1980s that "sexuality remains a sensitive, infrequently addressed issue in our society for health professionals as well as for the lay population."[72] Presently, however, attitudes are changing and sexual rehabilitation is beginning to be an integral part of cancer treatment. Reasons for this change in attitude may include: (1) better education concerning human sexuality; (2) a more receptive attitude by society; and (3) an increased demand for open discussion of sexuality issues.[1] *Sexuality* is a term that can mean different things to different people. In a broad sense, it may simply mean "acting or feeling like a male or female."[14] Often, the focus is on sexual "performance," when the definition should be more comprehensive. Thorn-Grey and Kern offer this explanation for sexuality: "The verbal, visual, tactual and olfactory communication which expresses love and intimacy between two people."[63]

Although nurses often feel a responsibility to address their patients' sexual concerns, many experience discomfort with this role. This discomfort may be due to: (1) personal feelings of anxiety regarding

sexual topics; (2) embarrassment about obtaining a sexual history; and (3) negative societal stereotypes about sexuality and chronic illness/disability.[17]

Even with expanded general knowledge of human sexuality, some studies have shown that the nurse's attitude concerning sexuality and illness has not altered.[18] However, increased confidence in sexual assessment and intervention may be attained if specific information and "how-to's" are made available. The Oncology Nursing Society and American Nurses Association Outcome Standards for Cancer Nursing Practice have provided guidelines for the nurse, which include the area of sexuality, and this chapter will expand on those guidelines with details with details of site-specific concerns.

PSYCHOSOCIAL DEVELOPMENT THROUGH THE LIFE CYCLE

Of the many patients faced with a diagnosis of cancer, most experience a life crisis. Although death is often the first fear, the potential for other stressors exists.[48] Surgery, adjuvant therapy (chemotherapy and radiation), the possible spread of malignancy, and an uncertain prognosis are all factors that necessitate lifestyle adjustments. Changes in role function and an altered body image or self esteem often threaten the patient with loss of feelings of femininity or masculinity, as well as sexual functioning. Masters and Johnson state that almost half of all couples who are physically and psychologically "healthy" have had sexual problems at some time during their relationship.[39] It is reasonable to assume, then, that many cancer patients will have sexual concerns given the added stressors of their disease.

A person's sexual expression will vary throughout the life cycle. Although personal beliefs and values

The author gratefully acknowledges Cathy Downer for typing and re-typing this manuscript.

737

Table 31–1 Psychosexual Stages of Development

Stage	Basic Psychosocial Task	Sexual Tasks
Infancy (0-2 years)	Acquiring basic trust, learning to walk, talk	Gender identity
Childhood (2-12 years)	Acquiring a sense of autonomy vs. shame and doubt; entering and adjusting to school	Pleasure-pain associated with sexual organs and eliminative functions; masturbation takes place with resulting shame and acceptance; secondary sex characteristics become evident
Adolescence (13-20 years)	Acquiring sense of identity vs. role confusion	Mastery over impulse control, acceptance of conflict between moral proscription and sexual urges, handling new physiologic functions (menses for girls and ejaculate for boys)
Young adulthood (20-45 years)	Acquiring a sense of intimacy vs. isolation; vocational effectiveness; interpersonal security, "sexual adequacy"	Sexual adequacy and performance plus fertility concerns and questions related to parenting
Middle adulthood (50-70 years)	Acquiring a sense of self-esteem vs. despair; adjusting to diminution of one's energy and competence; "empty nest syndrome" plus care of aging parents or their death; adjusting to change in physique and evidence of aging	For the female, menopause and resulting vasomotor changes, atrophy of breasts, clitoral size, and vaginal lubrication; for the male, delay on attaining an erection, a reduced compulsion to ejaculate, episodic impotence, possible prostatitis
Old age	Adjusting to loss of friends, family, confrontations with old age and dying, painful joint conditions, reduced hearing and visual acuity; adjustment to social stigmatization of being "old"	Reduced vitality, fear of incompetence or injury (coital coronary); fear of being viewed as "dirty old person"; unavailability of a partner (widowhood); limited physical capacity and reduced options

Reprinted with permission from Schain W: Sexual problems of patients with cancer. In DeVita VT, Hellman S, and Rosenberg SA, editors: Cancer: principles and practice of oncology, 1985, JB Lippincott Co.

are influential, interference with the psychosexual stages of development by an event like disease may cause sexual dysfunction (Table 31-1).[48] For the cancer patient, passage from one stage to the next may be precluded by the disease and its treatment or prognosis. Awareness of these stages will help the caregiver recognize patients at risk for possible sexual dysfunction.

In addition to these stages, there are various other factors of importance to keep in mind. The patient's personal reaction to his or her illness and previous experience with the disease should be explored. Where are they in the continuum between denial and acceptance? What are their expectations and fears? If the patient has a significant other or spouse, consideration should be given to the couple's prior strengths and the stability of the relationship. What were their feelings toward sexuality before the disease? If the partners were supportive before diagnosis, they tend to be supportive after diagnosis.[3,45,46] Marriage stability after cancer diagnosis and treatment is generally based on the precancer situation.

ANTICIPATION OF AND ADAPTATION TO THE EFFECTS OF CANCER

Once patients are assured of survival beyond the initial diagnosis, the quality of their life becomes a concern. Will they be able to function as "normal" people do? Taken-for-granted activities like work, recreation, travel, parenting, and sex take on a new importance. While undergoing treatment or in the recovery period, patients will experience fluctuating degrees of fatigue, anorexia and nausea, and discomfort and debilitation. These will affect their level of sexual interest and ability and their sense of adequacy and self-esteem. Depending on the type of cancer and therapy employed, specific physiologic and psychologic changes can impair normal sexual functioning and feelings of femininity or masculinity.

Sense of Adequacy

For some people, the mere process of being ill may cast doubt on their sexual identity and response, which, in turn, will reflect on their sense of adequacy. Because of the seriousness of their illness, cancer patients are often too embarrassed to raise questions about their sexual concerns. They may feel that worrying about such a relatively unimportant matter as sex is unjustified. It must be emphasized, however, that sexuality is physically and emotionally a source of satisfaction and great pleasure and also the most intimate way we share ourselves with others.

Male and female sexual response is normally integrated into the sexual response cycle (excitement, plateau, orgasm, and resolution). The *male sexual response* (desire, subjective arousal, erection, emission, ejaculation, and orgasm) has separate mechanisms of control and can therefore be affected independently.[67] Although cancer therapy may destroy the capability for an erection, the pleasure of sexual arousal and orgasm often remain intact. This factor is important because men are often worried about whether they can function as they did before. For an in-depth explanation of male and female sexual response, see von Eschenbach and Schover.[67]

Female sexual response (desire, subjective arousal, vaginal expansion and lubrication, and orgasm) is less well understood. Women with cancer may lose sexual desire during debilitating treatment, especially if the therapy affects the structure or innervation of the clitoris or vagina. This, along with painful intercourse, are factors that tend to interfere with orgasm. Emphasis here is on perceived damage resulting from therapy, which women feel will lead to rejection from their partner.[1]

Since the capability of relating sexually is extremely important in our culture, some patients may declare a lost interest in sex just to protect themselves from the embarrassment of lost orgasmic function or erectile failure.

Sexual dysfunction apart from the disability may also be present. This can be due to "special problems such as alcohol, drug abuse, a history of physical and sexual abuse, or a history of irresponsible sexual behavior."[14] Sexual inadequacy that is the result of a potentially fatal disease or other problems then predictably leads to a threatened self-image.

Sense of Self-Esteem

Even when there is no organic illness, feelings of unworthiness and incompetence lead to a negative body image. Cancer patients are at much greater risk of having a negative body image because of mutilating surgery and devastating side effects of therapy. Cancer and its treatment can produce considerable loss of economic independence, alter role behavior and significant relationships, and reduce sexual responsiveness. What follows is fear of abandonment, withdrawal, and sexual dysfunction. To enhance sexual self-esteem, resumption of the ability to function sexually one way or another becomes of paramount importance. This allows the patient to feel more desirable and retain the ability to relate intimately with others.[58]

Gratification and Performance

The feelings of belonging and receiving approval is closely associated with the process of giving and receiving sexual pleasure. Cancer patients often feel undesirable and unattractive and, because they are now typecast as "ill," feel they are not supposed to be

---

MOTIVES FOR SEXUAL INTERCOURSE
Desire for closeness
Wish to conceive
Attempt to control or manipulate one's partner
Nonverbal expression of affection
Defense against depression or anxiety
Bid for attention
Confirmation of worth
Defense against intimacy

Reprinted with permission from Schain W: Sexual problems of patients with cancer. In DeVita VT, Hellman S, and Rosenberg SA, editors: Cancer: principles and practice of oncology, 1985, JB Lippincott Co.

---

sexual. It has been reported that these patients desire touch more than overt sexual activity.[33] The reason for this is unclear but may be related to side effects, fatigue, weakness, and pain, which all cause diminished libido. However, it is also postulated that they feel sexual desires but take it for granted that their partner does not desire them. The partner, in turn, worries that the patient may be too sick to want sexual activity and feels guilty about having a sexual interest in someone who is sick and under treatment. Unfortunately, if these misconceptions persist, patients and their partners are likely to avoid the intimate and/or sexual contact that might be possible.

Schain explains that sexual functioning is part of the reflection of an individual's coping mechanisms and that sexual activity may reflect different motives at different times during the health-illness continuum (see box above). The cancer diagnosis may change the motive for sexual acts, and the couple may need to change their focus from one of performance and orgasm to one of touching and general pleasuring.

Nurses must not fail to see alternatives to stereotypical sexual behavior and acknowledge each patient's unique sexual identity. It is the nurse's responsibility to be free of fixed ideas and to continue to discuss sexual concerns at all stages of cancer and its treatment, regardless of the patient's circumstances or age. It must never be supposed that the patient who has raised no question has no concerns. Concentrated attention must be given to the issue of sexuality just as it is given to other aspects of cancer care because sexuality is one of the most fundamental aspects of humanity.

SITE-SPECIFIC ISSUES AFFECTING SEXUALITY

The following nursing diagnoses apply to the nursing interventions that will be discussed.[10]

Principal Nursing Diagnoses

- Sexual dysfunction related to impotence, ineffective coping, lack of knowledge, change or loss of body part, and physiologic limitations.

- Disturbance in self-esteem related to change in body image, self-concept, role performance, and personal identity

Secondary Nursing Diagnoses

- Activity intolerance related to fatigue
- Alteration in comfort related to acute/chronic pain, which decreases sexual desire
- Impaired verbal communication related to tracheostomy
- Social isolation related to cancer (incontinence, disfiguring surgery, superstitions of others)

Most discussions in the literature related to sexual problems of cancer patients begin with malignancies of the genital organs because cancer in this area is most likely to cause sexual dysfunction. Consequently, head and neck cancers, sarcomas that result in amputation, hematologic malignancies, and lung cancers are frequently overlooked or barely mentioned. Therefore, a nursing approach to these concerns will be addressed first.

Head and Neck Cancer

PHYSIOLOGIC AND BODY IMAGE ALTERATIONS. The social significance of youth and facial beauty continues to be profound and is exemplified through movies, television, and magazines. The few older people portrayed by the mass media are usually very attractive. Therefore the impact of head and neck cancer and its treatment can be particularly devastating since the defects caused by the disease are immediately recognizable. The patient feels grossly unattractive and frequently has difficulty with life's most basic needs such as talking, eating, and even breathing. Given these fundamental problems, it is not surprising that little or no attention is given to the need for closeness, touching, and genital sexual pleasures.

Sexual relationships may be influenced by the patient's age, smoking and drinking habits, and the general emotional impact of treatment. Many patients are more than 60 years of age at the time of diagnosis and may be entering a period of adjustment to a diminished sexual drive.[14] The patient may also be an alcoholic, which will influence treatment and the rehabilitation process. Metcalfe and Fischman explain that intimacy, trust, and open communication are frequently nonexistent in alcoholic relationships because intimacy is too threatening to the alcoholic individual.[42] Since alcoholic men and women are known to have a low sense of self-esteem, the nurse may have to focus on this issue first before moving on to the patient's feelings of masculinity or femininity.[64]

Patients with head and neck cancer often require rehabilitation, which may be accomplished with reconstructive surgery or prostheses or both. It is important to keep in mind that the expectations of the patient may differ from actual treatment results. Consequently, the patient may suffer one or more disappointments, as illustrated by the following anecdote:

A woman had an oral prosthesis made. The match and the appearance were excellent, and she regained confidence and employment and she delighted in sociability. Her praise and gratitude were profuse. However, once when we had lunch together she said, "I have so much to be thankful for and yet . . . ," and she turned away and she touched the prosthesis. "When I laugh, this never laughs, and when I take it off I sometimes wonder if I can go on."[14]

Head and neck cancer patients will necessarily face lingering cosmetic and functional impairments, which will impact on their body image and sexuality. Often, presurgical levels of function and esthetics cannot be restored.[71] Although attempts at prosthetic rehabilitation are noble, never forget that the patient's concept is often quite different from the medical concept. Rehabilitation will change the patient's practices and habits. Remember, to this patient, a kiss and a hug may be worth a thousand words.

Nursing Management

HEAD AND NECK CANCER
INTERVENTIONS FOR THE PATIENT WITH HEAD OR NECK CANCER

- A gastrostomy tube may be placed to rid the patient of nasogastric feeding tube, which interferes with kissing and facial petting.
- Sugarless mints and artificial saliva help to freshen stale breath caused by a dry mouth (from radiation therapy).[31] Artificial saliva (Moi-Stir, Xerolube) also helps prevent tooth decay.
- The patient may have a decreased sense of smell so that perfumes cannot be appreciated. Candles, scented or not, can provide a relaxed ambience for both patient and partner, though the fragrance is not appreciated by the patient.
- Tracheostomies should be cleaned of mucus and

covered lightly during sexual activity. (To obtain tracheostomy covers, see Resources at the end of this chapter.)
- Partners should be made aware that the patient's heavy breathing may sound different. If the larynx is removed, a sexy voice, whispered love talk, and other eroticisms will be eliminated.[26]

- Various positions may need to be tried for sexual activity because the partner may be fearful of cutting off the patient's air supply.
- Patients, especially females, may wish to wear fancy nightgowns with high necks or other erotic neckwear. Males may wish to wear a dickie.

Sarcomas of Bone and Soft Tissue and Limb Amputation

PHYSIOLOGIC AND BODY IMAGE ALTERATIONS.   Little information is available regarding the sexual adjustment of upper or lower extremity amputees. Commonly, concentration is placed on the patient's functional problems during and after prosthetic rehabilitation and any reference to sexuality is omitted.

Major limb amputation creates emotional hurdles for patients' perception of themselves, as well as acceptance by their partners (Figure 31–1). A decrease in self-esteem and a negative body image are common because of the presence of a gross defect that is obvious even when covered with clothes. The male may equate the loss of a limb to the loss of manhood. Some patients may view the surgery as a punishment for past transgressions.[27]

Cummings has discussed several potential sexual problems, which include the simple mechanics of body positioning during intercourse, immobility because of physical isolation, amputee fetishism, associated disease states that can alter sexual function, and phantom pain sensations.[13] Phantom limb pain can be quite disturbing and can in itself impair sexual functioning.

Amputees are admittedly apprehensive about their physical capabilities, but this fear often subsides once they begin prosthetic training, ambulation, or articulation. As patients become more independent, confidence in their sexuality usually returns.[44] Some patient fail to gain satisfaction from a prosthesis. Those patients then resort to using crutches rather than be restricted by the somewhat awkward movement of artificial limbs. They forfeit a better cosmetic appearance, however.

The life-style of amputees may be profoundly affected, especially if they have been independent and physically active. The range of problems usually depends on the extensiveness of the amputation. For example, a female with a shoulder disarticulation may find that simple tasks like styling hair and getting clothing to look good are difficult. Less dramatic upper extremity amputations allow for easier manipulation of a conventional hand prosthesis, a hook prosthesis, or a newer myoelectric powered hand (Figure 31–2).

Lower extremity amputees, especially those with hip disarticulations and hemipelvectomies, have a different set of uncertainties with prosthetics.[44] Most prevalent worries are socket discomfort, mobility, and energy expenditure. With an exoskeletal device, the socket area envelops the entire pelvis and adds to hip and waist measurements (Figure 31–3). One female patient stated that she couldn't tuck her blouses in

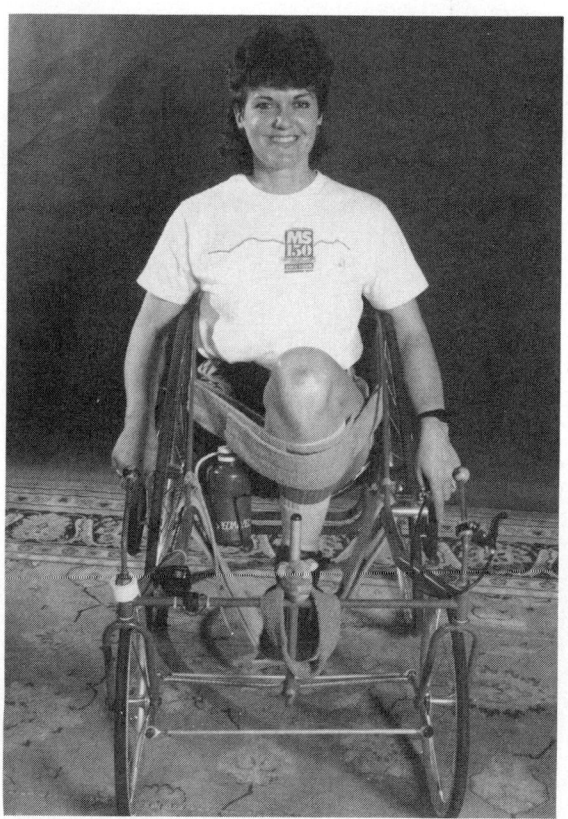

Figure 31–1 Lou Keyes, hemipelvectomy patient, in her racing wheelchair. Lou also uses a prosthetic device proficiently and crutches when she is in a hurry.

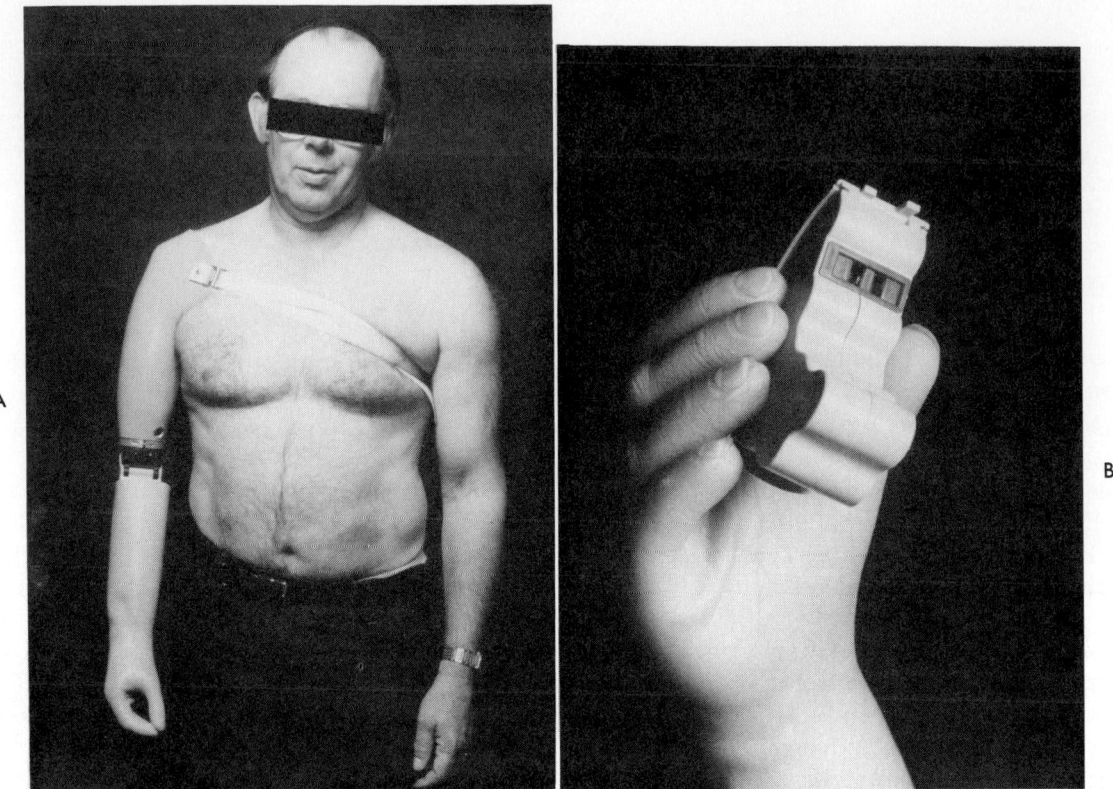

Figure 31–2 **A,** Above the elbow, myoelectric prosthesis. **B,** Myoelectric hand grasping object. (Courtesy of American Medical Systems, Minnetonka, Minnesota.)

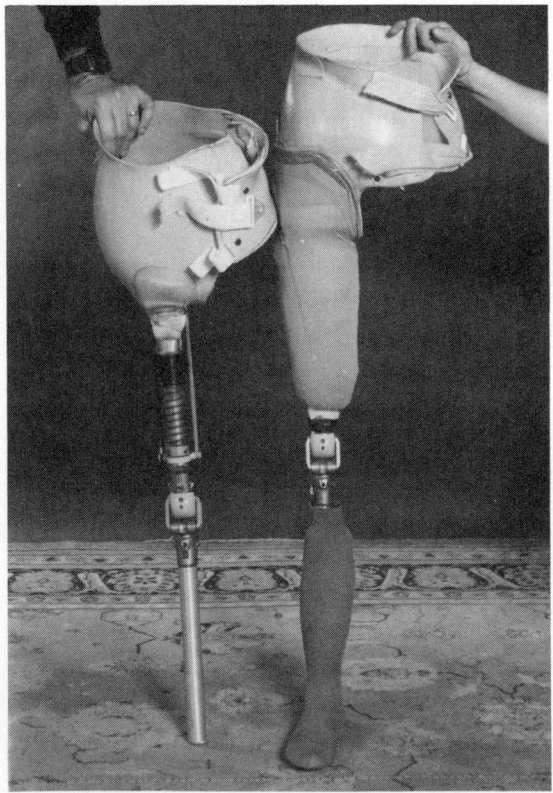

Figure 31–3 Prosthesis on left is a hip flexion bias system without a rotator knee and no flexibility in the socket—cost $11,000. Prosthesis on the right is a hip flexion bias system with a rotator knee and partially flexible socket—cost $13,000.

and thought her clothes looked too big. Females often have difficulty wearing sanitary pads during menses and may wish to use double tampons. All amputees must deal with undesirable noises produced by prosthetic joints, and even buying a pair of shoes can be disconcerting.

For those patients without partners, there may be a support group or sporting activities to become involved in—like wheelchair racing. These are great opportunities to meet people and share like experiences. The more the patient gets out and about and regains self-confidence, the easier it will be to meet and interact with all kinds of people. (For more information, see Support Groups at the end of this chapter.)

For those patients with partners, feelings of maleness or femaleness can be regained with the partner's love, support, and understanding. A loving and intimate relationship can help restore self-confidence and determination to adapt to their disability.

Nursing Management

LIMB AMPUTATION

Not only is the amputee's body image and self-concept threatened, but often many taken-for-granted activities are either eliminated or severely hampered. Some suggestions that may be helpful to amputees in resuming an intimate relationship with their partners follow:

- After some experimenting, some amputees find that intercourse can be maintained without any modification or adjustment of positions.
- Some patients may expend slightly more energy, which may result in mild fatigue, but this rarely hampers sexual function.
- If balance and movement are a problem, pillows or other forms of cushions may be used to maintain a level pelvis.[48]
- Lovemaking does not always have to occur in the bedroom. A sofa or large chair can be used to balance on, or the female can lean against a chair while her partner makes love from behind.
- The female may need to assume the superior position during coitus.
- An upper extremity amputee may wish to use a side-lying position with the existing arm free to balance themselves.
- Hemipelvectomy patients may have extra folds of skin used to make their flaps. Since these patients may be uncomfortable exposing themselves to their partners, these skin folds can be held in place by a "compression sock." This sock compresses the folds into a hiplike shape, and the sock can then be modified with an opening in the crotch to provide for intercourse.

HEMATOLOGIC MALIGNANCIES
Impact of Therapy Side Effects on Body Image

Although the diagnosis of lymphoma/leukemia or multiple myeloma can be terrifying, treatment does not comprise surgery or amputation, which can cause disfigurement. What the individual may not realize, however, is that chemotherapy and/or radiation therapy can be just as devastating to sexuality. Except for multiple myeloma, these diagnoses are often made in young, active people who see themselves as infallible, and they often do not comprehend the impact of the illness until well into their therapy.

Most men and women experience reduced desire for sexual intercourse during chemotherapy treatments, particularly during the first few days after receiving their drugs. This is usually due to increased weakness, fatigue, and intermittent nausea and vomiting. Also, whether the patient is young or old, male or female, defacement due to hair loss can destroy self-confidence. Another problem for acute myelocytic leukemia patients is the prolonged hospitalization during chemotherapy with consequent lack of privacy.

Lack of sexual eagerness can also be induced by an effect on the testes or ovaries. Hormone levels can decrease resulting in difficulty with erections and vaginal dryness.[5] Fortunately, these problems are often temporary, and hormone levels and sexual desires return to normal after chemotherapy or radiation therapy ends.

Myelosuppression and its consequences can cause fatigue and shortness of breath, which decrease sexual desire. Concern about bleeding and infection will be present due to low platelet and white blood cell/absolute neutrophil counts. A perfect environment for a vaginal yeast infection may be created, which inflames the lining of the vagina and causes itching and burning during intercourse. The male patient's ability to have an erection may also be affected. Creativity will be necessary to promote sexual intimacy.

Many patients will experience moments of anxiety and depression throughout their treatment, and therapy can last for up to 3 years. The nurse should stress the importance of maintaining involvement in activities and relationships with their friends when they feel good. Advise patients on ways to ask for assistance with activities of daily living and remind them not to be ashamed to ask for help, as they have most likely often helped others.

A discussion may be needed to assess the feelings of the spouse or significant other. It is helpful to identify ways they can support the client's feelings of self-worth and masculinity or femininity. Encourage them to reassure the client that sexuality and lovability are not affected by appearance only.

One of the most stressful events for any patient is alopecia. Some patients may feel that hair loss is even worse than amputation, and because of its effect on body image, sexual inadequacy can ensue. Be sensitive when explaining this side effect to any client, male or female, and provide them with the information in the box on this page.

SUGGESTIONS FOR PATIENTS WHO EXPERIENCE ALOPECIA

- Use a mild protein-based shampoo, cream rinse, and conditioner. Rinse the hair well and pat dry, *not* vigorously. Shampoo every 4 to 7 days.
- Avoid excessive brushing and use a wide-toothed comb/brush.
- Avoid hair spray and hair dye. Permanents are OK, but if hair loss is expected, it is best to wait until regrowth to perm the hair.
- Avoid electric hair dryers and curling irons, clips, bobby pins, barrettes, and pony tails.
- Many types of hats and caps are available. Purchase some kind of head wrap or turban, whether it is winter or summer, because the hair helps to keep the head warm. Even in warm weather, the head can get very cold if left uncovered in an air-conditioned environment.
- Use sunscreen on scalp when outside.

Nursing Management

HEMATOLOGIC MALIGNANCIES

INTERVENTIONS

- The patient who is neutropenic should be advised against oral and anal sexual manipulation. Remind the client and partner that gratification may be derived from simply touching and holding. The couple may bathe together. Bubbles, a little candlelight, and some wine (in plastic glasses) make for an intimate experience. The couple can share each other intimately, and the warm water may help ease some of the general aches and pains.
- Intercourse can be planned for after antiemetics are given and when the medications will be most effective.
- Advise patients to avoid the stress of heavy meals and liquor before intercourse.

- To avoid fatigue, a nap before intercourse may be helpful. The supine position or a side-lying position uses less energy. Also, avoid temperature extremes if possible.
- The importance of contraceptive measures during chemotherapy and radiation must be emphasized to all patients. Although chemotherapy will affect sperm count and ovulation, the patient cannot depend on this alone for contraception.[43] Teratogenic effects are seen during the first trimester of pregnancy, especially if the female is under treatment.[11,15] Studies are currently under way to determine possible effects on future generations.[23,36]
- Encourage sperm banking before initiation of chemotherapy.
- If the patient's complexion is pale due to decreased RBCs, encourage bright colors and the use of make-up to enhance appearance.

Breast Cancer

PHYSIOLOGIC AND BODY IMAGE ALTERATIONS. Today's society has idealized the female breast to such an extent that it has become a "sociosexual" symbol of sexuality and femininity.[48] Physiologically, removal of a breast should not decrease sexual desire or activity, but in reality many studies have demonstrated high levels of stress in regard to sexual functioning among mastectomy patients.[3,46] Mastectomy makes an obvious change in the body's contour, which can lead to fears about loss of identity as a woman and a desirable sexual being. The partner's perceived importance of a breast can also impact the female's perspective should she choose mastectomy.

Anxiety is also present regarding the cancer diagnosis.

The patient who is treated with lumpectomy and radiation therapy has concerns about her sexuality as well. Although this patient's breast is preserved, she may experience a skin reaction and increased fatigue while receiving radiation treatment. This can last for several weeks and also lead to decreased desire for sexual activity. Long-term depression and maladjustment are not as likely in this population, but it is just as important to assist these patients with their doubts and anxieties.

A woman's response to treatment for breast cancer and its corresponding threat to sexuality will depend on several conditions[48]:

- Her feelings about her femininity
- The value she bestows on her missing breast
- Her physical discomfort
- The response of her significant other
- The reinforcement she receives from the nurse regarding her sexual identity
- Her sense of self-worth

The status of the patient's preoperative sexual relationships and her interpretation of sexual satisfaction must also be ascertained. Cultural and religious attitudes will also influence "acceptable" sexual practices.

Rarely addressed are the single, divorced, widowed, and lesbian population (to be discussed later). Lewis and Bloom, years ago, made the assumption that these women may have a more difficult time adjusting to their new situation and resuming sexual relations.[35] An excellent resource for this population, as well as for married women, is the Reach to Recovery program (see Support Groups at the end of this chapter). This program tries to pair the patient with a volunteer mastectomy patient of the same race, side of mastectomy, social status (married, widowed, divorced), etc.[21] The volunteer explains exercises for the affected side's arm, tells where to get prostheses and clothing, and gives emotional support.

Rehabilitation may consist of reconstructive surgery, which is often done several months after treatment. Occasionally surgical repair must be done before good reconstruction can be accomplished. Although the reconstructed breast will never look like the original breast, some women exercise this option because they feel it looks more natural. A multitude of breast prostheses are also available; some of them are listed in the Resources at the end of this chapter.

Breast cancer and its treatment can be an overwhelming blow to a woman's femininity, and it is the nurse's responsibility to assist her not only with treatment but also with the preservation of her sexuality.

Nursing Management

BREAST CANCER

Many articles in the literature quote Mildred H. Witkin and her personal and professional experience with mastectomy.[48] One of her recommendations is for the couple to experience the loss of the breast together in the hospital. The partner may wish to assist with dressing changes and caring for the mastectomy wound. For example, a few years ago, one of my lumpectomy and radiation patients had a skin reaction on her breast and had to have daily dressing changes. Her husband was a willing participant and even created a "cross your heart" bandage for his wife. My patient expressed to me several months later how much it meant to her to experience his care and interest during her treatment.

Another behavioral prescription from Witkin is that the couple stand nude in front of a mirror and express the thoughts and feelings this elicits.[47] In this circumstance the patient is likely to feel less vulnerable since she and her partner are both nude. Of course, not all couples will be able to accept or handle this type of exercise, and they should be encouraged to use their own coping strategies. Since coping mechanisms will vary from person to person and couple to couple,

numerous behaviors will be exhibited. These will range from allowing the partner to participate in care and view the mastectomy scar immediately to not allowing anyone but the physician to see the wound. Support is continually needed to promote healthy adjustment by the patient.

When making love, these suggestions may be incorporated.

- Until the woman is ready to disrobe or let her partner touch the wound area, she can wear a fancy camisole or short nightgown. This camouflages the area but is still sexually stimulating for the couple.
- To minimize a direct view of the woman's missing breast, the partner may assume the superior position (missionary position) or use a rear-entry position. *Joy of Sex*, edited by Dr. Alex Comfort, is an excellent reference for positions a couple may use to increase sexual pleasure.
- The couple may make love by candlelight to decrease the impact of the change in body contour.
- Concentration on a certain sexual task (sensate focus) may increase stimulation and reduce appearance concerns. One suggestion is a touching exercise, explained in depth in the American Cancer

Society's book *Sexuality and Cancer: For the Woman Who Has Cancer, and Her Partner*. The focus is initially on massaging the extremities and back and ignoring the genital sexual organs, and the result is relaxation and sensual pleasure.[50]

• Since many women derive great pleasure from stroking, sucking and manipulation of the breast during foreplay, the remaining breast can continue to be stimulated if the woman so desires. Reassure the patient that manipulation will not cause another breast cancer.

Female Pelvic and Genital Cancer

PHYSIOLOGIC AND BODY IMAGE ALTERATIONS.   As in breast cancer, the surgery needed to cure female patients from cancers of the genital organs can be very threatening to a woman's sexuality.[3]

A threat to a woman's capability of being physically sexual can lead to a lost sense of femininity.[57] As the patient progresses through treatment, McDonald and colleagues report that fluctuations in self-esteem and body image occur.[40] The female sexual response cycle will most likely be affected if treatment affects the structure and innervation of the clitoris and/or the vagina.

Surgical resection and/or radiation therapy for cancer of the cervix, uterus, ovary, vulva, diethylstilbestrol (DES) exposure, and bladder can be either simple or quite extensive. Women faced with this type of treatment have many apprehensions:

• Threat to life
• Feelings of lost femininity
• Concern about what their external region will look like
• Ability to have intercourse and, if so, whether it will be painful
• Fear that long with the loss of fertility will come loss of vitality and orgasmic potential
• Fear of physical aging, diminished libido, loss of vaginal lubrication, and dyspareunia

To prevent extensive morbidity and sexual dysfunction from the previously stated concerns, early intervention with counseling is imperative for the gynecologic cancer patient.

Nursing Management

FEMALE PELVIC AND GENITAL CANCER

The following nursing interventions apply to radical hysterectomy, partial or total pelvic exenteration, radical vulvectomy, cystectomy, and radiation therapy.

Radical Hysterectomy

As discussed in Chapter 11, in radical hysterectomy, the vaginal canal is shortened somewhat (up to one half) but is not believed to be sexually appreciable in all cases. Penile thrusting may be uncomfortable since the trigone of the bladder and sigmoid colon may be closely associated with the new vaginal apex.

Donahue and Knapp suggest alternate methods of intercourse that can be most helpful (see box on p. 747).[16] Delayed resumption of bladder function introduces an embarrassing problem. If a long-term indwelling catheter is present, vaginal sexual relations can be impeded. Partners may change positions, and rear entry intercourse can be practiced.[62] To prevent dislodgement, the catheter can be placed up over the lower abdomen and taped into place. Alternate ways of expressing physical love can also be fulfilling and can include oral, anal, and digital expressions.

Pelvic Exenteration

There may be several factors of adjustment that this particular surgery generates.[2] These can include adaptation to a urinary conduit, bowel conduit, or both, and this can cause worry about appearance and appliance fit, possible leakage, and odor. The vulva will be extensively denervated, which results in decreased erotic sensations. Creation of a neovagina may also be necessary. Clitoral swelling and pain may occur, requiring a clitoridectomy for relief.[65] It is understandable that many patients report decreased frequency of sexual activity and satisfaction and a loss of sexual self-confidence.

To assure the most beneficial adjustment psychologically and sexually for the patient and her partner, it is necessary to provide specific alternatives and realistic information *before* surgery. Unfortunately, some women have been told that sexual intercourse will feel the same and be as good as before the surgery. Many women complain of the inability to voluntarily constrict the vaginal introitus, and for those women with a neovagina, some allege that it is too short or too large or associate it with an increased chronic discharge.[48] Some women maintain orgasm ability,

---

ALTERNATIVE COITAL POSITIONS AND COITAL EQUIVALENTS

- Angle of penile thrust can be altered by elevating the woman's hips on 1 to 2 pillows.
- Deeper vaginal barrel can be mimicked by enclosing the penis within one or both palms.
- Some patients find that vaginal penetration from behind between closely adducted thighs will increase pleasure.
- If coitus is not possible, the basic mechanics of cunnilingus (application of tongue or mouth to the vulva) and fellatio (sexual gratification by intromission of the penis into another individual's mouth) should be explained.

From Donahue V and Knapp R: Sexual rehabilitation of gynecologic cancer patients, Obstet Gynecol 49:118, Jan 1977; with permission.

but others lose it or achieve orgasm only with extra effort. Also, after reconstruction there is usually decreased vaginal sensation. To promote total healing and the ability to detect early recurrence, a waiting period of 12 to 18 months is advised before resumption of sexual intercourse.[16]

Young women exposed to DES during gestation with consequent vaginal cancer are treated in another way. This group also requires vaginal reconstruction and presurgical counseling and education. Once reconstruction has taken place, coitus is encouraged immediately, if possible and appropriate.[6,43] Since these women are often in their teens when diagnosed, intercourse is not always possible for moral or religious reasons or simply for lack of a partner. In this case, silastic stents are placed to maintain a patent vaginal canal. These young women understandably become easily discouraged because of the discomfort and peculiar stretching sensation caused by the stents.

Another alternative to the stents is the use of a small-to-medium sized dildo. Young women have few objections to use of a dildo, since it is flesh colored, soft plastic, more pliable, and more comfortable than a dilator.[57]

Positive encouragement and support are vital if these women are to feel as normal as possible. This support will be especially meaningful if it comes from other women who have experienced the same kind of reconstruction.

Alternatives to sexual intercourse available to women who have had vaginal reconstruction and to those not interested in such surgery may include nudity, cuddling, and general pleasuring; autoeroticism and mutual masturbation with a partner; oral-genital relations and anal love play; and fantasy.

Radical Vulvectomy and Cystectomy

Cancer of the vulva usually occurs in women who are well past menopause, and these elderly women are often reluctant to come forward for treatment until the disease has progressed. As a result, the therapy can have a particularly frightful impact on body image and sexual identity.[4]

For early stage disease, patients are usually treated with skinning vulvectomy, laser treatment, and/or wide local excision rather than simple vulvectomy. Skinning vulvectomy is a technique used by Rutledge, which "excises vulva skin and conserves fat, muscle and glandular structures below the skin."[43] A split thickness graft from the inner thigh is then applied to cover the denuded area.[43] This procedure gives an optimal cosmetic and functional result. Laser treatment involves destruction of the lesion by vaporizing the tissue. There is excellent healing with this procedure, but there is not a thorough pathologic review of the diseased specimen.[43] Patients have few complaints of dyspareunia or decreased sexual responsiveness with laser therapy. Topical 5% fluorouracil cream used over a 2 to 3 month period of time is another treatment choice. It is advocated by some clinicians, but most find it impractical since the cream must be applied until desquamation occurs.[43] This produces a significant degree of local discomfort, and intercourse can be painful until healing takes place. In radical vulvectomy, the fine sensory perception experienced during foreplay is destroyed and must be compensated for by excitement of other erogenous zones such as the earlobe, breasts, fingers, toes, and inner thighs.[30]

It is imperative that the patient's partner be included in all education and counseling because of the radical nature of the treatment and long recuperative period after therapy. Patients comment that adequate information is rarely given so they can begin to alter their sexual expectations, and others state that the treatment is embarrassing and creates an isolated feeling.[1,4]

Little is mentioned in the literature concerning female patients undergoing cystectomy and the sexual problems that arise from excision of the bladder and more than one third of the vagina. Problems identified are vaginal tightness and dryness and self-conscious anxiety because of the ostomy. Scarring can develop as well as numbness and lost sensation due to impaired innervation of the perineum. Recommended remedies may include a vaginal estrogen cream and vaginal dilators to help decrease dyspareunia. Most women like to cover their ostomy appliance with a fabric cover, and feminine lingerie may also be worn during sexual activity. Kegel exercises are helpful to relieve tension and decrease dyspareunia.[55] Positive reinforcement and specific suggestions can make an important difference in the woman's achievement of a satisfying sexual adjustment.

Radiation Therapy

Both external therapy and internal radiation insertion can cause irritating side effects, which are disruptive to sexual activity. Diarrhea, skin reaction of the external genitalia, and especially vaginal irritation, stenosis, and dryness are the most troublesome.[28] To prevent a diminished sense of femininity, a discussion with pertinent facts and proposals should precede radiation therapy.

The vagina will react to radiation by becoming shorter and narrower, having adhesions and problems with lubrication. The nurse may suggest the following:

- Continued sexual intercourse during treatment is usually encouraged to decrease possible adhesions and prevent shortening. Sometimes tissues may become tender, or an external skin reaction may necessitate stopping sexual intercourse. It can be resumed when healing and comfort allow.
- A good water-soluble lubricating jelly is always needed to decrease vaginal discomfort and can be applied privately or as part of foreplay.[57]

- During sexual activity, the hips may be elevated or the adducted thighs lubricated to emulate a deeper vaginal barrel and improve sexual stimulation for a male partner. The female superior position allows her more control but is usually not as comfortable. Rear entry is another alternative.[28]
- Vaginal dilators can be used if a woman does not have a sexual partner or is not sexually active. Sexually active women may also use dilators during treatment if intercourse is too exhausting. Normal sexual activity is preferred because some women hesitate to place foreign objects into their vaginas, and some are concerned about implications of masturbation. Sometimes dilators are indeed necessary, and the patient's compliance will increase if she is made aware that complete vaginal stenosis will occur, obstructing the physician's view in follow-up, if not used.[43]

It is important to be sensitive to both the patient and her partner when explaining dilator use.

Male Pelvic Cancer

PHYSIOLOGIC AND BODY IMAGE ALTERATIONS.   Men as well as women have stereotypical roles that society expects them to live by. They are supposed to be heroes and good providers, to hide their emotions and be strong, not to touch each other unless engaging in sports, never to relate on an emotional level or be dependent on another.[60] Masculinity is also equated with activity and productivity; a man must never admit to possible physical problems and

Table 31–2   Effects of Surgery on Male Sexual Functioning

Surgery	Direct Effect	Indirect Effect
AP resection	Damage to sympathetic and parasympathetic nervous systems resulting in: 1. Varying degrees of impotence (erectile difficulties) 2. Ejaculatory problems 2.1. Retrograde ejaculation 2.2. Decreased amount ejaculate 2.3. Decreased ejaculatory force	Altered sexual expression as a result of: 1. Physical impairment 2. Body image change 3. Altered self-esteem 4. Fears 5. Pain
Radical cystectomy	As above but to a greater extent 1. May be 100% impotent 2. Retrograde or no ejaculation	As above
Pelvic exenteration	As with AP resection and radical cystectomy	As above
Radical prostatectomy	Stress incontinence (temporary) Varying degrees of impotence	As above
Orchiectomy	Loss of gonads and testosterone resulting in: 1. Sterility 2. Decreased libido	As above
Cord surgeries Paraplegia; Quadriplegia; (tumor removal, pain control)	As with AP resection	As above

From Shipes E and Lehr S: Sexuality and the male cancer patient, Cancer Nurs 5:375, Oct 1982; with permission.

must always be in control.[60] Pertaining to sexuality, the state of a man's penis is always of utmost importance. Consequently, when the male patient experiences a malignancy in the pelvis or genital area, his entire self-image may be threatened. After diagnosis and treatment are complete and the fear of death is no longer uppermost in the patient's mind, he concentrates on the sequelae.[25] The impact on self-image will be even greater if his sexuality is threatened.

When the malignancy involves the prostate, testicle, or penis, there is a temporary or permanent disturbance in relation to erection, emission, and ejaculation. Orgasm is not as frequently affected and can actually be achieved even when genital function is lost. See Table 31–2 for an in-depth description of common cancer surgeries of the male pelvis and their effect on sexual functioning.[60] To promote adjustment and sexual rehabilitation, support and assistance for the patient and his partner are essential through knowledge and specific interventions.

Nursing Management

MALE PELVIC CANCER
Prostate

Surgery for prostate cancer has a definite impact on male sexual potency, depending on how extensive it is. When transurethral resection (TUR) is employed in early stage disease, approximately 80% of these patients experience scanty or absent ejaculation, although they are still able to have an erection. Until recently, if the cancer had progressed and radical prostatectomy was the treatment of choice, 85% to 90% of these patients experienced erectile impotence. Now with nerve-sparing surgical techniques, one study reported that 86% of a group of men could achieve erections 1 year after surgery although others have not had this much success.[49] Problems can occur when radiation is used in lieu of surgery, because of probable fibrosis of the pelvic arteries.[56] Incidental reports of erectile impotence vary from 14% to 46% after treatment with external radiation. Interstitial treatment may be used if the tumor burden is small and incidence of impotence is reported between 7% and 13%.[73]

Endocrine treatment (castration, estrogen, and/or an LH/RH antagonist [Lupron]) commonly causes difficult and embarrassing problems such as gynecomastia, phallic atrophy, loss of libido, and erectile impotence.[25] Many men experience physical debilitation, depression, anxiety, and pain, all of which may decrease sexual desire.

One of the most important issues in the area of male pelvic cancers may be to help the patient and his partner develop a change in attitude toward sexual intercourse if erection is no longer possible or if it is impaired. As Schain so aptly put it, it might "be necessary to learn alternative responses to the notion that intercourse (with an erect penis in the vagina) is the point at which all sexual encounters should be finalized."[48] Even if frequency drops, the potential for sexual arousal remains with the correct stimulus:

- Many men become sexually aroused with erotic books, pictures, and/or movies.
- Long periods of foreplay, including romantic dinners, showering or bathing together, and using different rooms for lovemaking, may be stimulating. A changed or strange environment such as a local motel may bring new excitement.
- If a full erection is not possible, mutual masturbation may allow the patient to reach orgasm and ejaculation. The partner should massage the penis by pushing down with pressure at the base of the penis. The penis should not be pulled up toward the abdomen or it can lose blood. A female partner can assist erection by inserting a partially erect penis into the vagina and flexing her perineal muscles.[59]
- During ejaculation, semen may be propelled into the bladder, which may threaten the male's sense of masculinity. The partner, however, may enjoy oral stimulation more since she no longer has to taste or swallow semen.[51]
- If the patient has problems with urinary incontinence, he should empty his bladder before intercourse and perhaps wear a condom if this becomes worrisome to his partner. Remind the couple that urine is sterile and will not harm the partner.
- The risks and benefits of penile implants should be explained to the couple. Schover recommends waiting 6 months after surgery before installing a prosthesis.[51] The patient and partner may choose from several different types of prosthesis. A comparison of two of the types (Figure 31-4) is given in Table 31-3. An excellent resource is *Bio-Potency: A Medical Guide to Sexual Success* by Richard and Deborah Berg.
- Intracavernous injections into the penis using papaverine to stimulate erections is becoming a common treatment.[61]
- Finally, like other cancer patients, a male pelvic cancer patient may simply need physical closeness and intimacy. Sexual activity is not always what is needed to promote feelings of love and belonging.

Testicle

Not surprisingly, men with cancer of the testicle not only have problems with fertility, but also with their intimate relationships.[22] This population is generally

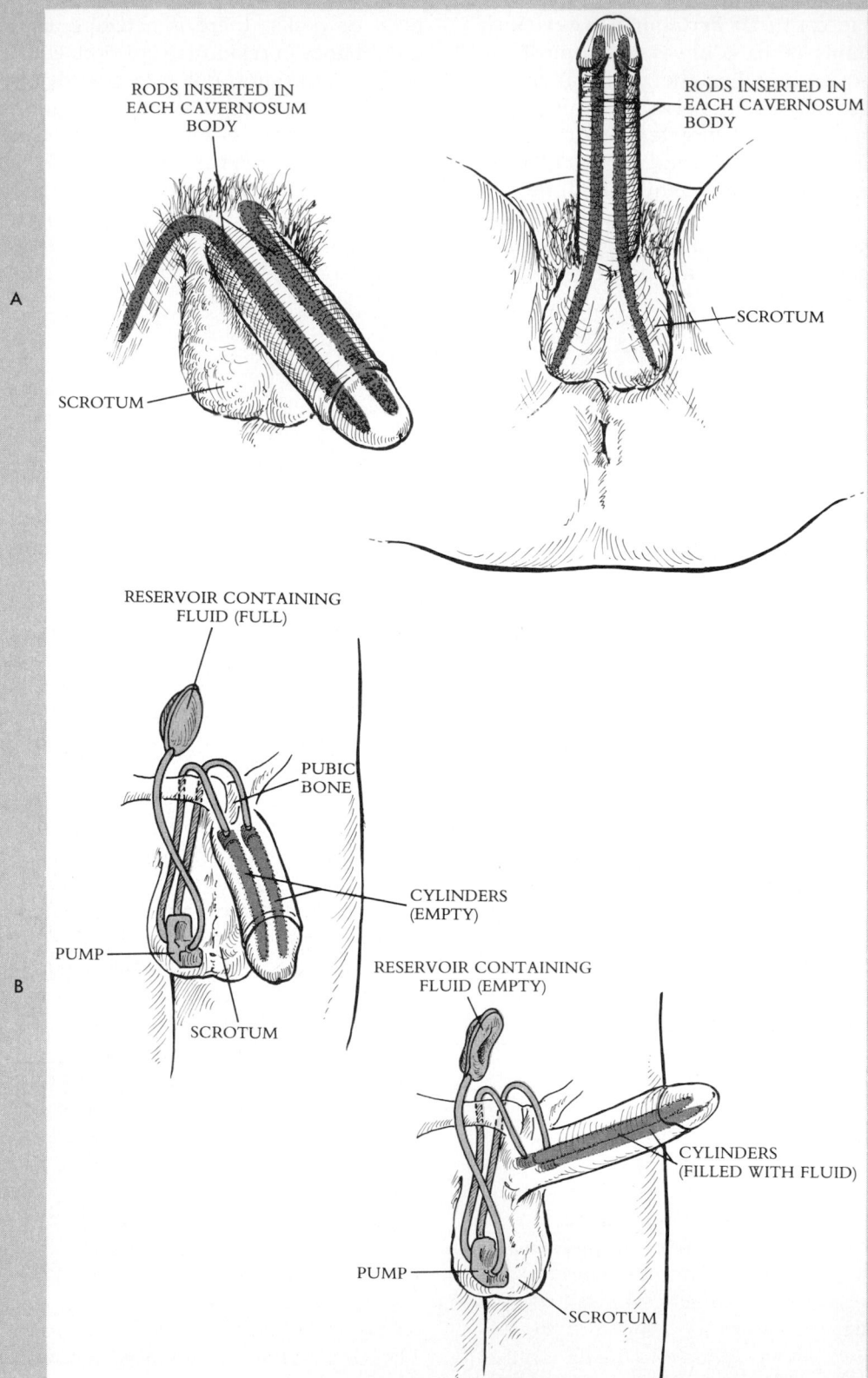

RODS INSERTED IN
EACH CAVERNOSUM
BODY

RODS INSERTED IN
EACH CAVERNOSUM
BODY

A

SCROTUM

SCROTUM

RESERVOIR CONTAINING
FLUID (FULL)

PUBIC
BONE

CYLINDERS
(EMPTY)

PUMP

B

SCROTUM

RESERVOIR CONTAINING
FLUID (EMPTY)

CYLINDERS
(FILLED WITH FLUID)

PUMP

SCROTUM

Figure 31—4   Penile prostheses can be of two types, **A,** In one type two semirigid silicone rods are implanted into the penis. **B,** In the second type two expandable cylinders are inserted into the penis and are connected by a tubing system to a fluid-filled bulb. (From Denney N and Quadagno D: Human sexuality, 1988, the CV Mosby Co.)

Table 31–3   A Comparison of Inflatable and Semirigid Penile Prostheses

Factor	Type of Prosthesis	
	Semirigid	*Inflatable*
Ease of concealment	May need special briefs; noticeable in locker room or at public urinal	No problem, although self-contained version may not lie down completely
Size of erection	Some loss of length and thickness	Normal thickness, some loss of length (self-contained version cannot add thickness)
Function during sexual intercourse	80% to 90% of patients satisfied	80% to 90% of patients satisfied
Infection during healing	Occurs in 1% to 2% of patients	Occurs in 1% to 2% of patients
Prosthesis erodes through spongy tissue inside penis	In less than 5% of patients	No problems
Prolonged pain after healing	Rare	Rare
Need to repair prosthesis	Rare	5% to 15% reoperation rates
Usual hospital stay*	2 to 4 days	2 to 5 days
Total costs*	$6,000 to $10,000	$10,000 to $12,000

*Based on our experience in 1987 with surgery performed under a general anesthetic.
From Schover L: Sexuality and cancer: for the man who has cancer, and his partner, New York, 1988, American Cancer Society; with permission.

young (15 to 34 years old) and in a crucial stage in life, and cancer treatment produces organic problems and sexual anxieties leading to dysfunction. When more treatment than unilateral orchiectomy is necessary, sexual dysfunction increases. Extensive surgery (retroperitoneal lymph node dissection [RLND]), radiation, and chemotherapy may cause erectile and orgasmic dysfunction.[34] To prevent sexual dissatisfaction, the couple should be educated and encouraged with the following information (this does not include fertility information):

- Stress the fact that normal sexual desire and pleasurable sensations, erection, and orgasm will probably continue. If sexual desire is lost, serum testosterone should be checked; replacement therapy may be needed.
- Alpha-adrenergic stimulating drugs can increase ejaculation and occasionally the intensity of orgasm for some patients who have had retroperitoneal lymph node dissection.[34]
- Loss of a testicle can cause embarrassment, and this can be remedied by a silicone testicular prosthesis to replace the lost testicle.
- Reinforce the fact that the cancer is not contagious through sexual activity and that radiation therapy will not contaminate the partner.
- For those patients with permanent erectile difficulties, see the suggestions under prostate cancer and penile implants.
- Encourage both partners to ask directly for the type of caressing and touching he or she prefers.[59]
- Remind the patient that often people feel awkward and anxious when resuming sexual activity, but sex-

ual relations, if physiologically possible, may resume about 6 weeks after pelvic surgery.
- If retrograde ejaculation is a problem because of RLND and cannot be reversed, Schover and Fife describe a technique to harvest sperm after orgasm. "Postorgasmic urine is immediately voided into a sterile container. Viable sperm cells are centrifuged out and placed in a nutrient solution preparatory to use in artificial insemination."[52]
- Sperm banking may be an option worth exploring if the number and motility of the sperm is adequate. This is costly and there is no guarantee that future artificial insemination will be successful. If the patient is interested, however, sperm banking must be done before chemotherapy begins.

Penis

Penile cancer, although very rare, results in the greatest risk of sexual dysfunction. Partial or total penectomy is usually needed to control the cancer. If partial penectomy is done, the penile stump usually becomes erect with stimulation and is long enough for intercourse with antegrade ejaculation.[51] If the entire glans penis is removed, a perineal urethrostomy is created behind the scrotum.[56] When it is stimulated to orgasm, ejaculation takes place through the perineal urethrostomy. Counseling for this man and his partner must include reassurance that both can be satisfied in several different ways:

- Some couples may wish to use a phallic-shaped vibrator as a substitute penis for partner satisfaction.
- If total penectomy has occurred, stimulation of the mons pubis, perineum, and scrotum can produce

orgasms with pleasurable contractions in the remaining cavernous musculature.[56]
- If partial penectomy has occurred, men report erections and orgasms of normal or near normal intensity with the phallic stump.[51]
- Female partners must be advised (without instilling avoidance of sexual contact) to have a yearly Pap smear since they may be at increased risk for cervical cancer from exposure to the human papilloma virus.[51]

Cystectomy

Sexual dysfunction after cystectomy is similar to that after radical prostatectomy. The surgery is similar except that with radical cystectomy, urethrectomy may be included, which further damages penile innervation or blood flow. The other major difference is that a urinary diversion must be done, which can result in the need for an ostomy appliance. Many patients choose to have a continent internal urinary reservoir or ileocolonic neobladder, and those men are reported to remain more sexually active than men with appliances.[51]

In addition to the interventions mentioned previously, following are a few ways to decrease anxiety from a urostomy:
- Before intercourse, the appliance should be emptied. Some patients secure the bag with a supportive belt.
- Like females, males may choose to wear a cover over their ostomy bag. Men may also wish to wear provocative underwear (silk boxer shorts) and expose only their genitalia during intercourse.
- To avoid friction on the stoma and pouch, other positions besides the missionary position may be tried.
- Some patients like to have their stomas touched during lovemaking, but they must be reminded that the stoma is fragile and too much rubbing may cause tearing. Objects should not be placed into the stoma.

Male pelvic cancer patients, like their female counterparts, must be treated with tenderness and understanding during the time of diagnosis, treatment, and long-term adjustment. Although many suggestions for mechanical aids and alternatives have been forthcoming, it is also important to remember the common expressions of affection and sexuality.

Colorectal Cancer

PHYSIOLOGIC AND BODY IMAGE ALTERATIONS.   Surgery for colorectal cancer often has a profound effect on body image and sexual responsiveness. Because of the societal taboos centered around eliminative functions, many men and women feel disgusted that their feces now come from the front of their bodies.[27] Women undergo feelings of having been violated, whereas men experience the surgery as castration or mutilation.[27,48] Some patients report embarrassment because they equate the cleaning of their stomas with masturbation. Others are distressed because they have no "vacation" from stoma maintenance. They must always make sure that there are adequate facilities for cleaning themselves in private; consequently, leisure activities may be compromised.[48]

Regardless of the type of surgical diversion performed (colostomy, ileostomy, or urinary diversion), patients express many common reactions. These reactions may include: (1) greater-than-expected fatigue and weakness; (2) feelings of fragility and vulnerability to harm; (3) despair at the initial viewing of the stoma; (4) feelings of invalidism and depression; (5) fear of accidents, odor, leakage, and staining; (6) excessive emotional investment in the stoma; and (7) feelings of lost personal control.[58] Understanding and support from the nurse are important for healthy recovery. If the nurse is not an ostomate herself, the patient may receive great reassurance from a fellow ostomate. Members of an ostomy organization usually visit the patient both before and after surgery and substantially reduce anxiety and depression. Rehabilitation is of utmost importance to these patients since they will probably have many productive years with an ostomy appliance.

Nursing Management

COLORECTAL CANCER

Many patients with colon cancer are not ready to talk about their sexuality and sexual activity immediately after surgery. Many say that sex is one of the farthest things from their minds. The subject should at least be broached so patients will feel more comfortable thinking about their sexuality and will feel freer to ask questions at a later date.

Sexuality education is more readily available for ostomates and their partners than for many cancers (see Resources at the end of this chapter). The following methods may be useful:

- Prepare the pouch before sexual activity by emptying and assuring the seal. If the ostomy is dry or controllable with irrigation, a small cover or patch may be sufficient cover.
- Deodorize the pouch (1 or 2 drops of Banish is helpful) and avoid foods that cause gas.
- Test out comfortable positions (e.g., lateral scissors position or rear entry).
- Wear attractive camouflage like a cummerbund or cloth cover for the pouch.
- To protect from leakage, a rubber sheet may be placed under the sheet and a towel on top of the sheet.
- Underwear with an opening up the center is provocative and also provides a cover.
- Males may experience retrograde ejaculation after surgery and should be warned of this to prevent thoughts that "things aren't working quite right."
- As previously mentioned, penile implants are an option for men unable to have an erection.
- Most important, a good sense of humor is necessary, because accidents will happen. The couple may even consider rehearsing for when the time comes.

LUNG CANCER
Physiologic and Body Image Alterations

Unlike many other malignancies discussed in this chapter, lung cancer has a dismal prognosis even when surgery has been performed, unless diagnosed in the very early stages. Little is realized in the literature in relation to psychosocial issues and the person with lung cancer, and no studies specific to sexuality and lung cancer are found. Reasons for this may be because these patients are often diagnosed with advanced disease that progresses rapidly and their performance status is often very poor.[7] Quality of life is always an important factor in relation to the person with cancer and should be especially important to those with a shortened life expectancy. Since treatment for these people is often palliative rather than curative, it is important to consider their feelings of masculinity, femininity, and self-esteem, along with the basic aspects of care such as pain control. Due to the often rapidly fatal nature of lung cancer, the patient and partner must make significant decisions and adjustments, which often affects the patient's sense of self-esteem and worthiness: (1) if the patient has been a smoker, he or she will probably have tremendous feelings of guilt to overcome or deal with; (2) if the patient's performance status is poor and remains so due to fatigue and weakness, they will be unable to continue as a productive member of the family; (3) if the patient/partner decide to take treatment (chemotherapy, radiation therapy), energy must be expended to cope with the side effects; and (4) if the patient/partner decide not to take treatment, there will be issues to resolve such as coping with an early death and caregiving. In regard to treatment decisions, Bernhard and others explain that, to the person with lung cancer, treatment is often associated with hope. "This allows active efforts in dealing with the course of disease and helps cancer patients manage free-floating anxiety."[8] Given all of the aforementioned anxiety-producing symptoms, side effects, and treatment regimens to deal with, it is not surprising that Bernhard and others report that lung cancer patients tend to withdraw socially.[8] All of these factors will have an effect on the relationship the patient has with his or her partner, and it is no wonder that there may be little time, energy, or desire for intimacy.

Nursing Management

LUNG CANCER
NURSING INTERVENTIONS

The nurse should encourage lung cancer patients and their partners to experience sexual closeness that does not necessarily lead to intercourse, which can exacerbate excessive fatigue and dyspnea. Along with the other interventions mentioned in this chapter, the following suggestions may be helpful:

- When experiencing sexual closeness, the significant other should continue to treat the patient as a partner rather than an invalid. These are the few moments when the patient can feel like a real person again.
- Make sure the significant other can be near to the patient when in an office setting or in a hospital bed.
- Being physically close, hand holding, sharing an intimate moment will enhance feelings of maleness and femaleness especially when the patient is getting treatment or is hospitalized.
- Soft caressing or light massage with oils or creams is sensual and can help reduce pain/discomfort.
- Mutual masturbation while watching adult movies promotes intimacy and conserves energy.
- Use strategies for managing dyspnea (see Chapter 15).

SPECIAL ISSUES INFLUENCING SEXUALITY
The Gerontologic Patient

Gendel reports an informal survey of one of her college psychology classes in which 75% of the class did not believe their parents were sexually active and 95% did not believe their grandparents could possibly be sexually active.[20] This small survey supports previous studies and documents beliefs that many hold, including health professionals. Older people face a double bias about their sexuality: it is assumed that "old" people are (1) too ill to be thinking sexually, and (2) incapable of sexual activity.[20] If attitudes such as these prevail, chances are few that sexual issues will be considered in these patients' general health care.

We must reflect on our own attitudes about sexuality and the aging population and ask ourselves some questions. How do I feel about my elderly parents or grandparents having sex? If I see two elderly people kissing and fondling each other, how do I react?[62] (See Figure 31–5.) Frank-Stromborg tells us that there is "a misunderstanding of the normal physiologic changes in sexual capacities and functioning that occur with advancing age. These changes alter sexual performance; they do not destroy it."[19] One interesting note in Gendel's article points this out: "An 82-year-old male patient who was to have his left testicle removed, but who had already undergone other pelvic surgery resulting in loss of erectile function, was requesting a testicular prosthesis. His current sexual style with his partner was mutual genital stimulation to orgasm without erection, but he did not want her to fondle an 'empty sac'."[20]

When providing sexual counseling for the elderly, be aware that all couples will not be interested in sexual activity. Respect for this option is necessary. However, the nurse should make sure that the couple is not abstaining because that is what is expected of them.

Various methods of sexual relating besides vaginal intercourse should be discussed with an elderly couple. For those patients who still have the desire for sexual involvement, the nurse may wish to encourage the following:

- A weak back and/or muscles can be helped by exercising those muscles. This will also make the person feel more sexually attractive.
- A nutritional diet from the basic four food groups can prevent depression and apathy, which may decrease sexual performance and interest.
- For the partners to achieve lubrication and erection, longer precoital stimulation may be needed to compensate for slowed physical response.
- Because of musculoskeletal changes, various positions for intercourse should be tried to promote comfort and save energy.[19,49,50]
- Both partners may not achieve orgasm; however,

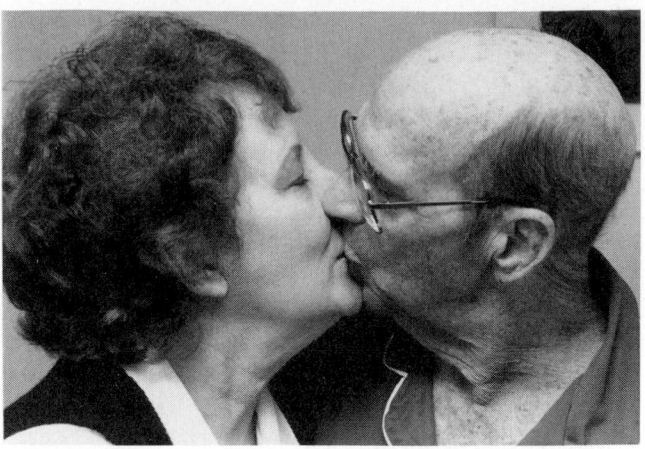

Figure 31–5 Henry and Margie sharing a tender moment.

sexual pleasuring can still be enjoyed. Also the male may have little or no ejaculate.
- During prolonged hospitalization or nursing home confinement, privacy should be provided for couples to hold, touch, fondle, and have intercourse if desired. This holds true for couples of any age.
- Warm baths, gentle massage, caressing and touching, masturbation, and fantasy all provide a sense of satisfaction and reassurance.
- Cleanliness, skin care (makeup, perfume, after shave), hair care, mouth care, and attractive clothing can enhance feelings of masculinity and femininity.

The Homosexual Patient

It must never be assumed that all patients have or wish to have a partner *or* that all partners are of the opposite sex. It is the nurse's responsibility to be knowledgeable about the entire patient population and not to be judgmental. All patients are entitled to competence and a caring attitude. This is not always easy, however, because the literature is not overflowing with knowledge concerning the homosexual cancer population, and it is not always clear that the patient is homosexual.

The sociocultural structure of male homosexual relationships differs from that of female homosexuals. Six types of sociosexual relationships have been identified for the male, ranging from one-night stands to stable cohabitation or "marriage."[27] Less is known about lesbian relationships, but there is less promiscuity and more of them marry.[27] The gay/lesbian sexual repertoire and erotic positions are similar to those of heterosexuals except when limited by identical anatomy. Hogan explains that "the number of different sex roles and activities the homosexual is willing to engage in is directly related to age, length of homosexuality, the degree of acceptance of sexual impulses, and homosexual orientation."[27]

As with heterosexuals, the precancer sexual relationship has an important effect on the stability of the postcancer relationship. Those homosexuals involved in a permanent sexual relationship usually have fewer problems. If the patient has been diagnosed with cancer and still has to "cruise" (look for a sexual partner), it will be as difficult to deal with their new body image as it is for the heterosexual patient. Successful "scoring" may be substantially decreased.[27]

Due to inexperience in the area of sensitivity to behavioral cues, obtaining information about sexual orientation may be missed because staff do not ask the right questions. Rather than asking about a spouse, husband, or wife, the nurse can ask the client if he or she is sexually active or whether they have a significant other.[38] Questions about sexual activity may deal with sexual preference such as "Do you prefer sexual activity with women, men, or both?"[38] Mapou tells us that " . . . most clients are not offended by such questions and those who are gay or lesbian are likely to appreciate the candor." The nurse should treat the significant other as a spouse and involve them in the treatment process. This is likely to promote self-confidence and self-esteem in both members of the couple.[38]

In a group of testicular patients who were gay, one man expressed worry that his homosexuality caused his testicular cancer. Others were embarrassed at the lack of semen at ejaculation and didn't know how to explain this to their partner.[54] Male homosexual ostomates often wish to use their stomas as receptacles for intercourse, and they must be emphatically cautioned against this practice. The stoma is fragile and can tear and bleed.

The Patient Experiencing Spinal Cord Compression

All cancers have the propensity to metastasize to other areas of the body including the spinal cord, and most of the cancers dealt with in this chapter can cause problems of this nature. Since the literature of rehabilitative medicine and nursing has dealt extensively with the issue of sexuality and the paralyzed patient, this chapter will not address the topic. The reader is referred to the Resources at the end of this chapter for information.

STERILITY, INFERTILITY, AND PREGNANCY

It has been reported that 5% of new cancer cases occur in patients aged 34 years or younger, and this means that approximately 5000 or more patients will be treated for cancer during their reproductive years.[5] The patient's age and sex, stage of development, the type, dose, and duration of therapy are all integral factors in relation to reproductive tissue damage.

Heiny reports several concerns in relation to reproductive damage and future capacity and they include: (1) abnormal sexual development, impaired sexual performance, and infertility; (2) potential damage to germ cells producing chromosomal changes; (3) transmission of the cancer-bearing gene to offspring; (4) problems with childbearing capabilities; and (5) likelihood for marriage.[24] Heiny found no conclusive evidence of congenital abnormality or cancer transmission except for genetic forms of cancer. She did find an increase in spontaneous abortion with combination (radiation and chemotherapy) therapy. The young cancer survivor tends to be less likely to marry than the average person.[24]

Generally speaking, male fertility is more susceptible to damage than the female's because of the constant mitotic cycles needed for spermatogenesis versus the relative inactivity of the female oocyte. Testes are more susceptible to injury than are ovaries because rapidly dividing cells are most often affected by cancer therapies. Consequently, many chemotherapeutic agents alone, and especially in combination, can cause azospermia, oligospermia, or permanent sterility. Alkylating agents such as nitrogen mustard, cyclophosphamide, and chlorambucil cause sterility in the majority of treated males. However, depending on the drugs used, drug dose, and length of treatment, fertility may return, and the time frame can vary from 15 to 49 months after completion of therapy.[5] Comparisons of different chemotherapy combinations are reported by Averett and others and one study showed that 3 of 21 patients in a MOPP regimen had return of spermatogenesis whereas all patients in an ABVD group showed recovery.[5] "Several reports suggest decreased sensitivity to chemotherapy-induced gonadol toxicity in the prepubertal testes compared with the adult testes."[5] Successful pregnancy is often limited due to abnormalities of the pretreatment sperm specimen. Frequently, the sperm have poor motility, and there are a growing number of patients who have attempted in vitro fertilization as treatment for male infertility with reported successes.[5]

Once again, age plays a role for the female concerning possible ovarian dysfunction after treatment with chemotherapy because there are progressively fewer germ cells in the aging ovary. Averett and others reported on several studies that used multiagent chemotherapy such as MOPP. " . . . 49 percent of patients experienced ovarian failure, and 34 percent had irregular ovarian activity, some of which progressed to complete ovarian failure. An age-dependent effect was noted since 89 percent of the patients with amenorrhea received treatment after age 25."[5] As with boys, the ovarian function of prepubertal girls seems less susceptible to damage from chemotherapy. One other major concern for women is cancer and pregnancy. Harris reports that one in 1800 pregnant women will have cancer, and all forms of neoplasms are found during pregnancy with breast, cervical, ovarian, lymphoma, and colorectal occurring most frequently.[23] Making a decision whether or not to treat the patient during pregnancy should take into consideration several factors: (1) "gestation age of the fetus; (2) maternal and fetal health at the time of diagnosis; (3) mother's prognosis and likelihood of future pregnancies after treatment; and (4) the known teratogenic effects of the drugs to be used."[70] If the administration of chemotherapy is initiated after the first trimester, there are surprisingly few complications associated with treatment. Also, pregnancy after chemotherapy is not usually discouraged although some oncologists are concerned about recurrence facilitated by hormonal and immunologic changes. Since there is little scientific data to support these worries, women should consider ultimate prognosis and the desire for children.

Finally, the children of patients treated with chemotherapy must be considered. Currently, there are no known studies available that show an increase in congenital anomalies or other diseases in these children. One study did a chromosomal analysis of 24 children whose parents had been treated with chemotherapy and found 23 with normal karyotypes.[5] In addition, one other study that followed another subset of children up to 12 years (median follow-up 2.5 years) showed growth, development, and school performance to be normal. If the parent is treated with a combination of chemotherapy and radiation therapy, there appears to be more complications of pregnancy. Wives of male patients have more spontaneous abortions and female patients have more offspring with a variety of problems. Many scientists feel that prolonged observation must be done to better define the possible mutagenic nature of chemotherapy and radiation therapy in these children.

ASSESSING AND PRESERVING THE SEXUAL HEALTH OF THE CANCER PATIENT

Nursing Assessment Techniques

When performing a sexual health assessment, several elements can enhance both the nurse's and the patient's comfort during the discussion[37]: Key elements that will promote optimal patient teaching can be found in the box on this page.

There are several different approaches to sexual history-taking. Three sets of questions are presented here:

McPhetridge includes assessment of the effects of the illness on sexuality as a part of the nursing history.[41] For our purposes, these questions might read as follows:

- Has having cancer (or its treatment) interfered

SEXUAL HEALTH ASSESSMENT

- Privacy is essential when doing the assessment. If the patient is not in a private room, move to another area if possible. An office, conference room, or a vacant patient room is preferable.
- Assure the patient of confidentiality. This tends to decrease the level of anxiety markedly. Usually it is good to include the partner, but it may be necessary to meet privately with the client at first to establish rapport.
- Try to obtain a sexual history early in your association with the patient (see the approaches that follow). This implies that sexuality is an important and natural part of good health. Fatigue and how it can affect the patient's sexual activity may be included during an explanation of chemotherapy side effects. In this way one can introduce the concept, talk about it somewhat, and come back to it without making the patient uncomfortable.
- Avoid overreaction in your verbal and nonverbal communication. Wide eyes and an open mouth are not conducive to trust. Also try not to be bored. Listening with genuine interest helps to convey acceptance.
- Move from less sensitive to more sensitive issues.
- Determine the patient's goals for treatment.
- Realize when a problem is too complex to handle or when you do not know enough to be therapeutic and refer the problem on, e.g., clinical nurse specialist, psychologist, or sexual rehabilitation counselor.

---

with your being a mother (wife, husband, father)?
- Has your cancer (or its treatment) changed the way you see yourself as a man (woman)?
- Has your cancer (or its treatment) caused any change in your sexual functioning (sex life)?
- Do you expect your sexual functioning (sex life) to be changed in any way after you leave the hospital?[41]

Kolodny and others recommend general basic questions in the original contacts with patients when it is known that sexuality is likely to be affected by treatment.[29] The focus in this brief sexual history is on sexual functions.

1. Are you sexually active? (If "yes," then 2)
2. What is the approximate frequency of your sexual activity?
3. Are you satisfied with your sex life? (If "no," then proceed.) Why not?

For men:
4. Do you have difficulty obtaining or maintaining an erection?
5. Do you have difficulty with control of ejaculation?

For women:

6. Do you have difficulty becoming aroused?

7. Do you have any difficulty having orgasm?

For both men and women:

8. Do you have pain with intercourse?

9. Do you have any questions or problems?[29]

VerSteeg describes an early assessment approach that is more comprehensive and addresses the following areas[66]:

- *Couple's relationship.* What kind of relationship is it? What are its strengths, resources, coping abilities, degree of closeness, and importance of sexual aspects?
- *Understanding of cancer and its treatments.* What do they understand about the disease and its treatments? What is their understanding of the anatomy and physiology involved? What do they know about changes from therapy, its side effects, and their duration?
- *Impact on sexuality.* What do they understand about the impacts of cancer and its treatment—physically, psychologically, and socially? What do they understand about effects on sexuality and fertility?
- *Preparation for changes.* How do they want to prepare for expected changes? What kind of anticipatory guidance will help them be ready for common initial responses (anxiety and depression)? How can they explore alternatives, plan new responses, and communicate ideas and feelings?
- *Planning and participation in care.* How does the person being treated want to participate in planning for hospital care? What are the mutual expectations between patient and staff for self-care in the hospital and later at home? How will the partner be involved? What is his/her investment in various facets of care? What is the nature of support needed and how can the partner respond to that need?
- *Control and optimism will help.* What kinds of support will help the patient have a sense of control and optimism or hope regarding self, body, environment, and the unknowns involved in the situation?
- *Expansion of sexuality.* How does the couple want to expand their perceptions of sexuality and potential sexual activities? What are the best avenues of new learning for them, and in what order? Do they want information in printed form? Discussion with the nurse or with others who have had similar therapy? Do they want exercises to explore new behaviors together?[65]

The PLISSIT is a model frequently used for sexuality counseling or a nursing intervention.[12] Each step is taken depending on the nurse's knowledge and comfort level.

- *P = permission.* This promotes discussion and encourages the couple to continue in their present pattern of sexual activity plus suggests some risk taking.
- *LI = limited information.* Includes the permission already given plus some new information specific to their sexuality concerns.
- *SS = specific suggestions.* May include new activities for the couple, which may entail "homework."
- *IT = intensive therapy.* This is when the couple is referred on to a therapist for more intense treatment.[12]

A more complete model has been created by Schain.[46] Her model uses eight letters—PLEASURE—to cue the nurse to the topic area and to represent a good feeling. For a more in-depth explanation of this method, see Schain's article.

- *P = partner.* Is there one, how many, what kind of relationship? Problems identified and recommendations will depend on whether there is a partner or not.
- *L = lovemaking.* What are the motives for being sexually active? Permission to engage in autoerotic behavior may be helpful.
- *E = emotions.* What is the patient's attitude about the illness and sexual problems? If underlying psychologic problems surface, referral may be appropriate.
- *A = attitude.* What is the "norm" of sexual activity for this patient and what are your own values?
- *S = symptoms.* An explicit explanation of the problems in regard to the three phases of the sexual response cycle is needed here.
- *U = understanding.* What are the etiologic factors (intrapsychic, physiologic, relationship) contributing to the problem?
- *R = reproduction.* What is the desire to have children, and if this ability is eliminated, how does that affect the patient's life goals?
- *E = energy.* How does the problem interfere with the individual's overall psychologic and sexual comfort, and do they want formalized sexual counseling?[46]

PRESERVING INTIMACY

Today our patients survive longer after their treatment for cancer. Survivorship means that the nurse must look with the patient to rehabilitation. In sexual rehabilitation, the nurse's goal of helping to restore the patient's sexual function is followed closely by the goals of restoring self-image and self-esteem. Each patient's sexuality is unique and is reflected in touching, smelling, hearing, tasting, and visual stimulation. These create for the patient and partner their own special intimacy, sense of affection, and physical gratification. Many references have been made and suggestions given in this chapter, but when there are *no* acceptable alternatives within a relationship it is the nurse's duty to help the couple use their own coping strategies and strengths. The values and beliefs of the couple are important to the use and success of various alternatives. What may be an acceptable expression for some may not be for others. Sometimes all they need is to be given permission to try something different. Encourage them to take the risk, and be there to support them.

CONCLUSION

As health care professionals continue to struggle to understand and be comfortable with their own sexuality, cancer patients continue to ask for help in dealing with disease and treatment related to sexual issues. In this situation it is important to extend our efforts beyond the disease and focus on the whole patient. For all of us, receiving sexual pleasure and closeness is linked to a sense of belonging and worthiness. Being accepted is intimately bound to self-esteem. As one author put it, "self-esteem is the sum total of all our feelings about ourselves . . . it is the reputation we share of ourselves with ourself."[9]

Resources

- Tracheostomy covers may be obtained from Byram Health Care Center, Inc., Tracheo-stoma Bibs, 2 Armonk Street, Greenwich, CT 06380, 1-800-354-4054.
- Available breast prostheses include the following:
  - Tri-Hawk Corp., Silima addition bound silicone, 1-213-622-0143.
  - Amoena Corp., A thin, soft silicone gel, 2150 Newmarket Place #116, Marietta, GA, 1-800-995-9559.
  - Nearly Me, cloth, poly/foam, or silicone; 1-312-478-7701 or 1-800-421-2322
  - Bosom Buddy, thin glass beads cushioned by cotton, covered with nylon; 1-208-343-9696
- Information on vaginal dilator is available from Syracuse Medical Devices, Inc., 608 Demong Drive, Syracuse, NY 13214. Cost of dilator: small–$4.50, medium—$5.50, large—$6.50.
- Literature on sexuality education for ostomates is available for a small charge from the United Ostomy Association, Inc., 36 Executive Park, Suite 120, Irvine, CA 92714, 1-714-660-8624.
- Options for men and women experiencing alopecia are as follows:
  - Great American Options, International Hairgoods, Inc., 6811 Flying Cloud Drive, Eden Prairie, MN
  - Headliner, Designs for Comfort, Inc., P.O. Box 8229, Northfield, IL 60093, 1-800-443-9226.
  - Sweetie Cap, Lan Care, Inc., 2747 17th Avenue Court, Moline, IL 61265, 1-309-762-4800

- Literature on rehabilitation for the patient with spinal cord compression is as follows:
  - Christina Mumma, editor: *Rehabilitation Nursing: Concepts and Practice,* ed 2, is available from Rehabilitation Nursing Foundation, 2506 Gross Point Road, Evanston, IL 60201.
  - Kolodny R and others: *Textbook of Human Sexuality for Nurses,* Boston, 1979, Little, Brown & Co.
- Literature with reference to sexuality issues:
  - Johnson J and Klein L: I Can Cope: Staying healthy with cancer, DCI Publishing, Minneapolis, MN, 1988.
  - Noyes D and Mellody P: Beauty and cancer, AC Press, Los Angeles, 1988.
  - Schouer L: Sexuality and cancer: For the woman who has cancer, and her partner, American Cancer Society, Inc., Atlanta, GA, 1988.
  - Schouer L: Sexuality and cancer: For the man who has cancer, and his partner, American Cancer Society, Inc., Atlanta, GA, 1988.

Support Groups

- Support groups for head and neck cancer patients are often sponsored by the American Cancer Society, such as The Lost Chord for laryngectomies.
- One of the first support groups in the country for amputees was founded in the Kansas City area by Lou Keyes and is called LEAPS. This stands for Lower Extremity Amputees Providing Support, and the telephone number is 1-816-361-3206. This group also has access to information about support groups nationwide.
- Reach to Recovery is a voluntary group of mastectomy patients sponsored and trained by the American Cancer Society (ACS). The ACS is located in most cities in the United States.
- Prostate cancer support groups (ACS).

BIBLIOGRAPHY

1. Anderson B: Sexual functioning complications in women with gynecologic cancer: outcomes and direction for prevention, Cancer 60:1987.
2. Anderson B and Hacker N: Treatment for gynecological cancer: a review of the effects on female sexuality, Health Psychol 2:203, 1983.
3. Anderson B and Jochimsen P: Sexual functioning among breast cancer, gynecologic cancer, and healthy women, J Consult Clin Psychology 53:25, 1985.
4. Anderson B and others: Sexual functioning after treatment of in situ vulvar cancer: a preliminary report, Obst Gynecol 71:13, 1988.
5. Averette H, Boike G, and Jerrel M: Effects of cancer chemotherapy on gonadal function and reproductive capacity, CA-A 4:4, 1990.
6. Baxley K and others: Alopecia: effect on cancer patients body image, Cancer Nurs 7:499, 1984.

7. Bernhard J and Ganz P: Psychosocial issues in lung cancer patients (Part 1), Chest 99:1, 1991.

8. Bernhard J and Ganz P: Psychosocial issues in lung cancer patients (Part 2), Chest 99:2, 1991.

9. Cantor R: Self-esteem, sexuality and cancer-related stress, Front Radiat Ther Oncol 14:51, 1980.

10. Carpenito L: Nursing diagnosis: application to clinical practice, Philadelphia, Vol 4, 1992, JB Lippincott Co.

11. Cooley M and Cobb S: Sexual and reproductive issues for women with Hodgkin's disease: overview of issues, Cancer Nurs 9:188, 1986.

12. Cooley M, Yeomans A, Cobb S: Sexual and reproductive issues for women with Hodgkin's disease: application of PLISSIT model, Cancer Nurs 9:248, 1986.

13. Cummings V: Amputees and sexual dysfunction, Arch Phys Med Rehabil 56:12, Jan 1975.

14. Curtis T and Zlotglow I: Sexuality and head and neck cancer, Front Radiat Ther Oncol 14:26, 1980.

15. Doll D, Ringenberg Q, and Yarbro Y: Management of cancer during pregnancy, Arch Intern Med 148, 1988.

16. Donahue V and Knapp R: Sexual rehabilitation of gynecologic cancer patients, Obstet Gynecol 49:118, Jan 1977.

17. Ducharma S and Gill K: Sexual values, training and professional roles, J Head Trauma Rehab 5:2, 1990.

18. Fisher S: The sexual knowledge and attitudes of oncology nurses: implications for nursing education, Semin Oncol Nurs 1:63, Feb 1985.

19. Frank-Stromborg M: Sexuality and the elderly cancer patient, Semin Oncol Nurs 1:49, Feb 1985.

20. Gendel E: Self-esteem and sexuality in older patients with cancer, Front Radiat Ther Oncol 20:166, 1986.

21. Glasgow M and others: Sexual response and cancer, CA-A 37:322, 1987.

22. Gritz E and others: Long term effects of testicular cancer on sexual functioning in married couples, Cancer 64:1989.

23. Harris B: Issues in nursing care of pregnant patients with cancer. In Lowdermilk D, editor: NAACOGs clinical issues in perinatal and womens health nursing, 1:4, 1990.

24. Heiney S: Adolescents with cancer: sexual and reproductive issues, Cancer Nursing 12:2, 1989.

25. Heinrich-Rynning T: Prostatic cancer treatments and their effects on sexual functioning, Oncol Nurs Forum 14:6, 1987.

26. Hoehm P and McCorkle R: Understanding sexuality in progressive cancer, Semin Oncol Nursing 1:56, Feb 1985.

27. Hogan R: Human sexuality: a nursing perspective, Norwalk, Conn, 1985, Appleton-Century-Crofts.

28. Jenkins B: Sexual healing after pelvis irradiation, Am J Nurs 86:920, 1986.

29. Kolodny R and others: Textbook of human sexuality, Boston, 1979, Little, Brown & Co.

30. Lamb M: Sexual dysfunction in the gynecologic oncology patient, Semin Oncol Nurs 1:9, Feb 1985.

31. Larsen G: Rehabilitation for the patient with head and neck cancer, Am J Nurs 82:119, Jan 1982.

32. Lefebure K: Sexual assessment planning, J Head Trauma Rehabil 5:2, 1990.

33. Leiber L and others: The communication of affection between cancer patients and their spouses, Psychosom Med 38:379, 1976.

34. Levison V: The effect on fertility, libido, and sexual function of post-operative radiotherapy and chemotherapy for cancer of the testicle, Clin Radiol 37:161, 1986.

35. Lewis F and Bloom J: Psychosocial adjustment to breast cancer: a review of selected literature, Int J Psychiatry Med 9:1, 1978–79.

36. Li F: Genetic studies of survivors of childhood cancer, Am J Pediatr Hematol Oncol 9, 1987.

37. MacElveen-Hoehn P: Sexual assessment and counseling, Semin Oncol Nurs 1:69, 1985.

38. Mapou R: Traumatic brain injury rehabilitation with gay and lesbian individuals, J Head Trauma Rehab 5:2, 1990.

39. Masters W and Johnson V: Human sexual response, Boston 1966, Little, Brown, & Co.

40. McDonald T and others: Impact of cervical intraepithelial neoplasia diagnosis and treatment on self-esteem and body image, Gynecol Oncol 34, 1989.

41. McPhetridge L: Nursing history: one means to personalize care, Am J Nurs 68:73, 1968.

42. Metcalfe M and Fischman S: Factors affecting the sexuality of patients with head and neck cancer, Oncol Nurs Forum 12:21, 1985.

43. Perez C, Hoskins W, and Young R: Gynecologic tumors. In DeVita VT, Hellman S, and Rosenberg SA, editors: Cancer: principles and practices of oncology, ed 3, Philadelphia, 1989, JB Lippincott Co.

44. Reinstein L, Ashley J, and Miller K: Sexual adjustment after lower extremity amputation, Arch Phys Med Rehabil 59:501, Nov 1978.

45. Renshaw D: Sexual and emotional needs of cancer patients, Clin Ther 8:242, 1986.

46. Schain W: A sexual interview is a sexual intervention, Innovations Oncol Nurs 4:2, 1988.

47. Schain W: Sexual and reproductive issues in breast cancer, Workshop on Psychosexual and Reproductive Issues Affecting Patients with Cancer, San Antonio, Texas, American Cancer Society, Jan 1987.

48. Schain W: Sexual problems of patients with can-

cer. In DeVita VT, Hellman S, and Rosenberg SA, editors: Cancer: principles and practice of oncology, ed 2, Philadelphia, 1985, JB Lippincott Co.

49. Schover L: Sexuality and cancer: for the man who has cancer, and his partner, New York, 1988, American Cancer Society.

50. Schover L: Sexuality and cancer: for the woman who has cancer, and her partner, New York, 1988, American Cancer Society.

51. Schover L: Sexual problems in men with pelvic or genital malignancies, Workshop on Psychosexual and Reproductive Issues Affecting Patients with Cancer, San Antonio, Texas, American Cancer Society, Jan 1987.

52. Schover L and Fife M: Sexual counseling of patients undergoing radical surgery for pelvic or genital cancer, J Psychosocial Oncol 3:15, 1986.

53. Schover L, Schain W, and Montague D: Psychologic aspects of patients with cancer: sexual problems of patients with cancer. In DeVita V, Hellman S, and Rosenberg S, editors. Cancer principles and practices of oncology, ed 3, Philadelphia, 1989, JB Lippincott Co.

54. Schover L and von Eschenbach A: Sexual and marital counseling with men treated for testicular cancer, J Sex Marital Ther 10:29, 1984.

55. Schover L and von Eschenbach A: Sexual function and female radical cystectomy: a case series. J Urol 465:465, Sept 1985.

56. Schover L: Sexual rehabilitation of urologic cancer patients: a practical approach, CA-A 34:66, 1984.

57. Shell J: Sexuality for patients with gynecologic cancer. In Lowdermilk D, editors: NAACOGs clinical issues in perinatal and women's health nursing, Philadelphia, 1990, JB Lippincott Co.

58. Shell J: The psychosexual impact of ostomy surgery. In Progressions: developments in ostomy and wound care, St Louis, 1992, Mosby.

59. Shell J: Sexual function and activity in the person with genitourinary cancer. In Berry D, editor: Urologic oncology nursing manual, Philadelphia, CoMed Communications, 1993.

60. Shipes E and Lehr S: Sexuality and the male cancer patient, Cancer Nurs 5:375, Oct 1982.

61. Sidi A and others: Intracavernous drug-induced erections in the management of male erectile dysfunction: experience with 100 patients, J Urol 135:704, 1986.

62. Steinke E and Bergen B: Sexuality and aging, J Gerontol Nurs 12:6, 1986.

63. Thern-Gray B and Kern L: Sexual dysfunction associated with physical disability: a treatment guide for the rehabilitation practitioner, Rehabil Lit 44:5, 1983.

64. Vanderpool J: Alcoholism and the self-concept, QI Stud Alcohol 30:59, 1969.

65. Vera M: Quality of life following pelvic exenteration, Gynecol Oncol 12:355, 1981.

66. VerSteeg M: Options for sexual expression. In von Eschenbach P and Rodriguez D, editors: Sexual rehabilitation of the urological cancer patient, Boston, 1981, Hall.

67. von Eschenbach A and Schover L: The role of sexual rehabilitation in the treatment of patients with cancer, Cancer 54:2662, 1984.

68. Wallace L: Sexual adjustment after radical genital surgery. Nurs Times 83:51, 1987.

69. Weaver S, Lange L, and Vogts V: Comparison of myoelectric and conventional prosthesis for adolescent amputees, AJ Occupat Ther 42:87, 1988.

70. Weeks D: Acute leukemia and pregnancy. In Lowdermilk D, editor. NAACOGs clinical issues in perinatal and womens health nursing. Philadelphia, 1990, JB Lippincott Co.

71. Welty M and others: The patient with maxillofacial cancer: surgical treatment and nursing care, Nurs Clin North Am 8:137, 1973.

72. Williams H and others: Nurses' attitudes toward sexuality in cancer patients, Oncol Nurs Forum 13:37, 1986.

73. Zinreich E and others: Pre- and post-treatment evaluation of sexual function in patients with adenocarcinoma of the prostate, Int J Radia Oncol Biol Phys 19:3, 1990.

APPENDIXES

APPENDIXES

APPENDIX A

Glossary

absolute risk—the number of specific cancer cases (breast) in a given population divided by the number of people (women) in the population—may be expressed as an average risk for every women in that group.

acquired immunity—specific and dependent upon the recognition of self and non-self.

active immunotherapy—the administration of biologic or chemical products that stimulate the immune system of the host.

adoptive immunotherapy (passive immunotherapy)—the direct transfer of cells or products of the immune system to a host.

allogenic—having cell types that are antigenically distinct.

allograft—a graft of tissue between individuals of the same species but of different genotype, called also allogenic graft.

aneuploid—having more or less than the normal diploid number of chromosomes.

antibody—an immunoglobulin protein produced by plasma cells and B cells in response to antigen, which has the ability to combine with the antigen that stimulated its production.

antigen—a molecule that is specifically recognized by antibody and by cells of the adaptive immune system.

attributable risk—the number of cancer cases in a population that are associated with a given risk factor and that could potentially be prevented by alteration or removal of those factors.

autologous—related to self, designating products or components of the same individual organism.

azotemia—an excess of urea or other nitrogenous bodies in the blood.

B-cells (B-lymphocytes)—cells derived from bone marrow stem cell in humans, capable of responding to antigen by the production of antibody.

biological response modifier (BRM)—an agent that can modify host reactions against disease, with resul-

tant potential to prevent progression of cancer or metastatic spread; includes, but not limited to immunotherapy.

biotherapy—treatment with agents derived from biologic sources and/or affecting biologic response.

capillary leak syndrome—shift of fluid from the intravascular space resulting in accumulation of fluid in the extravascular space; symptoms include hypotension, tachycardia, and weight gain.

CD4 cell—cell expressing the CD4 protein on its surface, primarily cells of the immune system, particularly T helper cells (T_4 cells) and monocytes/macrophages.

CD8 cell—cell expressing the CD8 protein on its surface, primarily a subpopulation of T cells, particularly cytotoxic T cells (T_8 cells) and suppressor T cells.

cellularity—the ratio of hematopoietic (blood forming) tissue to adipose tissue in the marrow.

cell mediated immunity—involving specifically immune T cells and cells of the natural immune system (natural killer [NK] cells and monocytes/macrophages), particularly important to the body's defense against viral-infected cells and malignant cells.

colony stimulating factor (hemopoietic growth factor)—a group of hormone-like glycoproteins that are secreted by a wide range of cells in the body and upon which the processes of hemopoieses are dependent. Substances that stimulates growth and/or orderly maturation of cells of the hematopoietic system.

commitment—process by which components of the hemopoietic hierarchy increasingly lose the potential to differentiate into alternative cell lines.

chemotactic—the movement of an organism or an individual cell, such as a leukocyte, in response to a chemical concentration gradient

cytokine—a protein hormone of the immune system that is responsible for communication with other cells of the immune system or with cells outside of this system

cytostatic—suppresses cell proliferation

cytotoxic—able to kill cells

deafferentation—the elimination or interruption of afferent nerve impulses, as by destruction of the afferent pathways

diaphanoscopy—examination with the diaphanoscope; transillumination.

diploid—an individual or cell having two full sets of homologous chromosomes

effector cell—cells of the immune system that mediate an immune response.

ELISA (enzyme-linked immunosorbent assay)—capable of detecting either antibody or antigen by the binding of an enzyme coupled to either anti-1g or antibody specific to the antigen; used to detect HIV antibodies.

epidemiologic approach—examines the frequency of the disease among relatives.

hemopoiesis—the process by which the various components of the blood are formed and mature.

gene therapy—insertion of a functioning gene into a human cell to direct the natural antiviral human cell response. Provide a new function to the cell.

genetic approach—studies the pattern of disease expression among relatives.

genome—the complete set of hereditary factors, as contained in the haploid assortment of chromosomes.

genotype—the entire set of genes one inherits from both parents.

glycoprotein—any of a class of conjugated proteins consisting of a compound of protein with a carbohydrate group.

haplotype—the group of alleles of linked genes contributed by either parent.

heterogeneous—derived from a different source or species; xenograft.

hematopoiesis—the process by which blood cells are produced in the bone marrow.

homogeneous—consisting of or composed of similar elements or ingredients; of a uniform quality throughout.

humoral immunity—specific immunity activated by antibody found in blood and lymph; particularly important in trapping viral and bacterial organisms that have not yet invaded cells of the body.

hybridoma technology—process by which fusion cells, produced by myeloma plasma cells, are introduced into an immunized mouse. The substance produced is a monoclonal antibody specific for a particular antigen that can be collected as a large quantity of a monoclonal antibody.

hyperbaric—characterized by greater than normal pressure or weight; applied to gases under greater than atmospheric pressure; as hyperbaric oxygen.

hypoguesic—abnormally diminished acuteness of the sense of taste.

idiotype—an antigenic determinant present on and characteristic of a certain antibody molecule, usually located in the variable region.

immunity—a protective mechanism that serves to maintain the integrity of the body against foreign substances or agents.

immunogenic—capable of stimulating an immune response.

immunoglobulin—a glycoprotein composed of heavy and light chains that functions as antibody; in humans, the five classes are designated as IgG, IgA, IgM, IgD, and IgE.

immunomodulation—alteration of the immune response to induce up-regulation, suppression, or tolerance.

immunosuppression—blocking or diminishing the functioning of the immune system.

immunosurveillance—a theory that postulates that the immune system plays an important role in the prevention of development of detectable cancer.

immunotherapy—treatment of disease by active or passive immunization or by the use of agents designed to modulate (stimulate or suppress) the immune response.

incidence—the number of newly diagnosed cases of cancer in a specified period of time (calendar year) in a defined population.

indolent—slow growing tumor

lymphokine—activated killer cell—effector cell capable of killing tumor cells: activated by cytokines derived from lymphocytes (lymphokine), particularly interleukin-2; has broad activity.

interferon (IFN)—a class of cytokines originally identified for their ability to inhibit growth of viruses within cells; selectively inhibit the synethesis of viral RNA in infected cells; immunoregulatory functions, including enhancing the activities of macrophages and natural killer cells.

interleukin (IL)—a class of cytokines produced by lymphocytes and/or macrophages in response to antigenic or mitogenic stimulation, which mediate communication between cells of the immune system.

in vitro—within a glass, observable in a test tube, in an artificial environment.

in vivo—within the living body.

karotype—the chromosomal constitution of the nucleus of a cell.

lentivirus—any of a group of retroviruses, including those that cause maedi and visna in sheep.

leukoagglutinin—an agglutinin directed against leukocytes.

leukocytosis—a transient increase in the number of

leukocytes in the blood, resulting from various causes as hemorrhage, fever, infection.

lymphocytapheresis—the selective removal of lymphocytes from withdrawn blood, which is then retransfused into the donor.

lymphokines—soluble factors released by stimulated lymphocytes.

lymphotoxin—a product of lymphocytes; lymphotoxin is toxic for certain tumor cells and shares several properties with tumor necrosis factor.

morbidity—the condition of being diseased or morbid; the sick rate; the ratio of sick to well persons in a community.

monoclonal antibody (MAB)—an antibody produced from a single clone of cells; MABs recognize a specific antigen.

monocytosis—increase in the proportion of monocytes in the blood.

monokines—cytokines such as tumor necrosis factor released by mononuclear phagocytes.

morphology—the science of the forms and structures of organisms.

mortality—the number of deaths attributed to cancer in a specified time period in a defined population.

multipotent progenitor cell—an early component of the hemopoietic hierarchy that has undergone some degree of differentiation, but still has the potential to develop into any of several of the cell lines and has limited self-replicative ability.

murine—pertaining to or affecting mice or rats.

myeloproliferative—pertaining to or characterized by medullary and extramedullary proliferation of bone marrow constituents.

myelopthisis—invasion of the bone marrow by neoplastic elements.

neuropathic—functional disturbances and/or pathologic changes in the peripheral nervous system.

oncogene—a gene involved in the transformation of a normal cell into a malignant cell, or a gene that increases neoplastic properties of a cell.

osteoradionecrosis—necrosis of the bone following irradiation.

outcome—the result of service delivery including patient, staff, and organizational performances.

nociceptive—receiving injury.

passive immunotherapy—the direct transfer of cells or products of the immune system to a host.

pleiotropic—the quality of a gene to manifest itself in a multiplicity of ways.

plexopathy—any disorder of a plexus, especially of nerves.

phenotype—the entire physical, biochemical, and physiologic makeup of an individual as determined both genetically and environmentally as opposed to genotype.

ploidy—the aggressiveness of a neoplasm by analyzing the cellular DNA content.

pluripotent stem cell—the most primitive of the blood cells in the hemopoietic hierarchy. These cells, as yet unidentified in humans, are the forerunners of all of the cell lineages. The pluripotent stem cell is characterized by infrequent cell cycling and the ability to self-replicate.

precursor cell—a nucleated cell that is morphologically recognizable as belonging to a specific lineage and that gives rise immediately to the mature components of the circulating blood.

prevalence—measurement of all the cancer cases both old and new, at a designated point in time.

primary prevention—measures taken to ensure that cancer never develops (decreasing the number of new smokers).

process—the manner in which service will be delivered. Procedures, practice guidelines/protocols, action plans, and documentation systems describe process.

progenitor cells—an early ancestor of the mature components of the blood. The pluripotent stem cells also is called a "common progenitor cell."

provirus—the genome of an animal virus integrated into the genetic material of a host cell.

radiobiology—that branch of science that is concerned with the effect of light and ultraviolet and ionizing radiations upon living tissue or organisms.

randomized—to make random for scientific experimentation.

recombinant DNA technology—process by which there is identification of a gene for a specific substance. The gene is then cloned and inserted into a bacterium that then serves as a factory to produce the desired substances (IL-2, TNF, IL-1).

refractory—not readily yielding to treatment.

relative risk—the incidence of cancer (breast) in a population (women) with a known or suspected risk factor (genetic) divided by the incidence rate of cancer (breast) in a population (women) without that risk factor (genetic).

reticuloendothelial—pertaining to tissues having both reticular and endothelial attributes.

retinoid—any derivative of retinal, whether naturally occurring or synthetic.

retrovirus—a large group of RNA viruses that carry reverse transcriptase.

reverse transcriptase—an enzyme that catalyzes RNA-directed polymerization of DNA.

secondary prevention—measures used for detecting and treating early diagnosed cancer while in its most curable stage.

sequestration—isolation of a patient; the net increase in the quantity of blood within a limited vascular area.

seroconversion—the change of a serologic test from negative to positive, indicating the production of detectable, circulating antibodies.

simian—pertaining to, characteristic of, or resembling an ape or monkey.

standard—a written value defining the rules, actions, results, or analyses that are related to the patient, staff, or system and are sanctioned by an authority.

standard of practice—a written value statement that defines the rules, actions, or conditions that direct patient care.

structure—the circumstances under which a service will be delivered. The organization's mission, philosophy, goals, and policies define its structure.

somatic growth factors—substance regulates growth of non-blood cells in the body. This is a more diverse and less well-understood system, with positive and negative regulation (insulin-like, epidermal, and platelet-derived growth factors).

stereotactic—pertaining to or characterized by precise positioning in space, said especially of discrete areas of the brain that control specific functions.

stratification—the art or process of stratifying; develop different levels.

suppressor T cells—a subset of T-lymphocytes that reduces the activity of other T and B cells.

syngeneic—having identical matched cell type.

T-cells (T lymphocytes)—thymus-dependent cells that are involved in a variety of cell-mediated immune responses.

tachyphylaxis—a rapidly decreasing response to a drug or physiologically active agent after administration of a few doses.

telangiectasis—the spot formed most commonly on the skin by a dilated capillary or terminal artery.

tenesmus—straining, especially ineffectual and painful straining at stool or in urination.

thermography—a technique wherein an infrared camera is used to photographically portray the surface temperatures of the body, based on the self-emanating infrared radiation.

threshold (for evaluation)—a pre-established level or pattern of performance related to an indicator at which further evaluation of the quality and appropriateness of an important aspect of care is initiated.

translocation—an interchange in which one segment of a chromosome is transferred to another chromosome, generally the result of breakage and abnormal reattachment.

trending—analyzing the results of numerous studies on the same indicator to identify patterns that may influence the quality of outcomes related to the important aspect of care or service being monitored.

tumor marker—a product produced by a cancer cell, or in response to the presence of cancer, that may be released into the circulation or may remain associated with the cancer cell.

tumor necrosis factor (TNF)—produced primarily by activated macrophages. TNF is cytostatic or cytotoxic for some neoplastic cells, induces hemorrhagic necrosis of some tumors, has a range of activities similar to lymphotoxin.

unipotent progenitor cell—early component of the hemopoietic hierarchy that has undergone further differentiation and is committed to one or two cells lines.

western blot—an immunoassay used for measuring antiviral antibody responses, useful for distinguishing antibody responses to specific viral proteins. Frequently used as a confirmatory test for HIV status.

window phase—the time between the dates of actual exposure leading to infection and development of detectable serum antibodies.

Outcome Standards for Cancer Nursing Practice

1. Prevention and Early Detection
2. Information
3. Coping
4. Comfort
5. Nutrition
6. Protective Mechanisms
7. Mobility
8. Elimination
9. Sexuality
10. Ventilation
11. Circulation

APPENDIX B   LABORATORY VALUES

Test	Purpose	Normal Values (Adult)	Nursing Action
Arterial blood gases	Assess respiratory status, acid-base balance.	pH 7.35-7, 45 P_{CO_2}, 35-45 P_{O_2}, > 70 HCO_3, 23-28 BE, 0 + 3 O_2 saturation, > 93% F_{IO_2}	Mark lab slip as for any O_2 therapy at time sample collected. Send specimen on ice to lab immediately. Apply pressure on puncture site for 5 min. Include respiratory rate and O_2 therapy status when reporting ABG's results to physician.
CHEMISTRY			
Electrolytes			
Calcium (Ca^{++})	Assess renal, neuromuscular bone status; parathyroid, thyroid function; increased levels with bone mets.	8.5-10.5 mg/100 ml	Observe for increased or decreased neuromuscular activity with Ca^{++} level < 7 mg or > 13 mg/dl.
Chloride (Cl^-)	Assess renal status, acid-base balance.	95-100 mEq/L	Potassium replacement therapy should be accompanied by a 1:1 ratio of potassium to chloride.
Magnesium (Mg^{++})	Assess renal, metabolic, neuromuscular status.	1.4-2.3 mEq/L	Assess antacid ingestion. Increased levels observe and implement seizure precautions.
Phosphorus (P)	Assess renal, parathyroid function, bone status.	2.5-4.5/100 ml	Assess dietary intake (e.g., starvation).
Potassium (K^+)	Assess renal status, endocrine, cardiac function, acid-base balance.	3.5-5.0 mEq/L	Monitor higher or lower level for potential cardiac toxicity; increased level metabolic acidosis.
Sodium (Na^+)	Assess renal status, endocrine function, acid-base balance.	135-145 mEq/L	Monitor fluid intake/output; implement precautionary safety measures if <120 mEq/L; decreased levels with metabolic alkalosis.
Albumin serum	Assess renal and nutritional status.	3.5-5.0 g/dl (20-day half-life)	
Prealbumin	Assess nutritional status.	17-42 mg/dl, short half-life	Provides an analysis of protein changes during previous 2 days.
Bilirubin	Assess hepatic, biliary tract, or hemolytic function; hemorrhage, drug toxicities, blood transfusion.	Total: 0.2-1.2 mg/100 ml Direct: 0.1-0.4 mg/100 ml Indirect: 0.1-0.8 mg/100 ml	
Calcitonin serum	Assess malignancy of thyroid.	50-500 pg/ml	
Cholesterol	Assess hepatic, pancreatic, biliary tract, thyroid function.	Age 40+: 150-300 mg/dl Age 30-39: 140-270 mg/dl Age 20-29: 120-240 mg/100 ml	High-fat, high-sugar diet may alter results.
Copper serum	Assess hepatic function.	70-165 µg/100 ml	
Creatinine serum	Assess renal urinary tract function bone status; ARF profile: Increased bun, creatinine, potassium; decreased sodium.	20-70 µg/24 hr 0.7-1.4 mg/100 ml	

Continued.

APPENDIX B LABORATORY VALUES — cont'd

Test	Purpose	Normal Values (Adult)	Nursing Action
Creatinine clearance serum	Assess renal status.	0.8-2 mg/100 ml	Serum level drawn to compare with urine sample.
Glucose serum	Assess pancreatic, liver or endocrine status, diabetes mellitus, hypoglycemia, malabsorption, Cushing's syndrome.	Fasting (FBS) 65-110 mg/100 ml	NPO past midnight before test. Report glucose levels of < 40 mg/dl to > 400 mg/dl immediately.
		2-hr postprandial (2-hrPP) glucose level should be within normal limits	Eating and specimen collection schedules must be coordinated.
Glycohemoglobulin	Assess pancreatic, liver or endocrine status, diabetes mellitus.	4.3-6.1%	Provides steady state of blood glucose level over 4 to 6 weeks.
Urea Nitrogen Blood (BUN)	Assess renal function, hydration status.	10-20 mg/100 ml	A ratio of BUN to serum creatinine of >10:1 may be suggestive of dehydration, GI bleeding, or decreased cardiac output
Uric acid serum	Assess renal function; hypercalcemia.	Female: 2.2-7.7 mg/100 mg Male: 3.9-9.0 mg/ml	Monitor intake and output; observe for elevations with rapidly dividing cell destruction; administer appropriate interventions.
Guaiac (fecal) or occult blood, Hemoccult	Determine presence of blood that is not visible.	Negative	Instruct patient to abstain from red meats for 48 to 72 hr before test.
HEMATOLOGY			
Complete blood count (CBC)	Assess clotting status, response to infection and inflammation.	RBC, WBC, platelets	
Red blood cells (RBC)	Assess anemias, hydration, oxygen transport; RBC fragmentation acute leukemia/myelodysplasia.	Female: 4.2-5.5 mil/mm^3 Male: 4.4-6.0 mil/mm^3 Older adult: 3.5 mil/mm^3	Do not draw blood sample from same extremity as IV infusion.
Hematocrit (Hct)	Assess blood loss, hydration, hematologic disorders.	Female: 37%-47% Male: 42%-52%	
Hemoglobin (Hgb)	Assess blood loss, anemias, dehydration.	Female: 12-16 g/100 ml Male: 14-18 g/100 ml	
RBC indices Mean corpuscular hemoglobin (MCH) [Normal color]	Assess anemias and polycythemia.	28-34 pg Older adult: 28-32 pg	
Mean corpuscular hemoglobin concentration (MCHC)	Assess chronic blood loss, lead poisoning.	30%-40% Older adult: 29-33%	
Mean corpuscular volume (MCV) [Size of RBC]		82-101 µg^3 Older adult: 90.5-105 µg^3	
Reticulocyte count	Assess anemia; bone marrow function.	Female: 0.5%-1.5% Male: 0.5%-2.5%	
White blood cell count (WBC)	Assess amount of infection, inflammation, and healing.	4,000-11,000/mm^3	Steroid drugs may suppress WBC's.

Test	Normal value	Purpose	Nursing implications
Differential neutrophils (polymorphonuclears [polys] or segmentals [segs])	42%-66% or 3,000-7,000 Older adult: 43%-79%	Determine presence of infection, inflammation, and stress.	Granulocytes include neutrophils, basophils, and eosinophils. Monitor for neutropenia; implement measures to prevent or minimize infectious process.
Band cells (stabs)	3%	Assess presence of recent infection.	
Basophils	0.4%-1.0% or 40-100/mm³	Assess status of polycythemia vera, leukemias, Hodgkin's disease, allergic reactions, and stress.	
Eosinophils	1%-3% or 50-400/mm³ Older adult: 0%-0.3%	Assess response to ACTH or epinephrine or status of allergy, leukemia, Hodgkin's disease.	
Lymphocytes	25%-33% or 1,000-4,000/mm³ Older adult: 11%-48%	Assess status of infection, especially viral, and stress.	
Monocytes	0%-9% or 100-600/mm³ Older adult: 1%-5%	Assess status of bacterial phagocytosis and healing.	
Erythrocyte sedimentation rate (ESR)	Female: 0-30 mm/hr Male: 0-20 mm/hr	Assess nonspecific inflammation and tissue injury; malignancy, rheumatic fever, and arthritis; acute and/or chronic infections.	
Platelets	150,000-450,000/mm³	Assess bone marrow, clotting status; increases in advanced malignancy.	Monitor for thrombocytopenia. Implement measures to prevent or minimize bleeding. Moderate risk < 50,000 Severe risk < 20,000; potential for CNS hemorrhage.
Platelet adhesion	5,000-18,000/mm³	Assess platelet function.	
Platelet aggregation	Visible < 5 min	Assess platelet function.	
Platelet volume	8-10 fl	Determine platelet size; assess purpura, DIC, anemias.	
	2.5 µm in diameter	Assess hematopoietic status; increased levels with neuroblastoma.	
Ferritin serum	Female: 5-100 ng/ml Male: 10-270 ng/ml	Assess anemias.	
Folic acid serum	4-16 ng/ml	Assess anemias.	
Iron serum	87-279	Assess amount of iron that could be carried if transferrin were completely saturated: Anemias, chronic blood loss, and liver disease.	
Total iron binding capacity (TIBC)	250-400		
Coagulation factors			
Factor I: fibrinogen	60-100 mg/ml	Assess clotting status, hemophilia.	Report abnormal results.
Factor II: prothrombin	10%-15% concentration	Assess vitamin K deficiency.	
Factor V: proaccelerin	5%-10% concentration		
Factor VII: proconvertin	5%-20% concentration	Assess von Willebrand hemophilia A.	
Factor VIII: antihemophilic globin	30%-35% concentration		
Factor IX: thromboplastin	30% concentration	Assess hemophilia B (Christmas disease).	
Factor X: Stuart-Power	8%-10% concentration		
Factor XI: morphilic	20%-30% concentration		
Factor XII: Hageman	0%	Assess for DIC.	
Factor XIII: fibrin stabilizing	1% concentration	Assess for bleeding tendency.	

Continued.

APPENDIX B   LABORATORY VALUES—cont'd

Test	Purpose	Normal Values (Adult)	Nursing Action
Coagulation time (Lee-White, clotting time)	Assess coagulation; monitor heparin therapy.	5-15 min	Assess for potential bleeding. Pressure may be required on puncture site for 5 min.
Fibrin split products (FSPs)	Assess degree of coagulation.	< 4 µg/ml	Monitor/Report elevated levels of FSP.
Fibrin degradation products (FDPs)	Assess disorders (e.g., DIC).	< 10	Monitor/Report elevated levels of FDP.
Fibrinogen	Assess ability to form clots; to assess for leukemia, liver damage, DIC.	160-300 mg/100 ml Older adult: 470-485 mg/100 ml	DIC profile: decreased platelets, fibrinogen, plasminogen; increased PT, PTT, FDP'S; report results STAT.
Prothrombin time (protime PT)	Assess coagulant activity of the "extrinsic" system including factors V, VII, X, fibrinogen, and prothrombin.	100%; also reported in seconds, approximately 11-15; varies with lab	Assess for potential bleeding. Pressure may be required on puncture site for 5 min. Report results as ratio of patient to control rather than seconds.
Plasminogen	Assess DIC.	73-122%	
Protamine sulfate	Assess coagulation, DIC.	Negative	
Activated partial thromboplastin time (APPT) or partial thromboplastin time (PTT)	Assess all plasma coagulation factors except VII and XII (e.g., stage II clotting disorders such as hemophilia).	APPT: 30-45 sec PPT: 16-25 sec	
Thrombin clotting time (thrombin time; TT)	Assess III clotting.	10-20 sec or within 3 sec of control	
Immunoglobulins	Assess immune system status.	Levels vary with age.	Report abnormal results.
IgA	Assess for autoimmune disease.	65-650 mg/100 ml	
IgD	Assess for multiple myeloma.	0-30 mg/dl	
IgE	Assess for potential allergies.	0-200 ng/ml	
IgG	Assess for multiple myeloma.	600-1,700 mg/100 ml	
IgM	Assess for hepatitis.	50-300 mg/100 ml	
ISOENZYMES			
Acid phosphatase serum	Assess prostate status, multiple myeloma, parathyroid or renal function.	< 4 ng/ml	Usually done on a serial basis for 3 days. Elevated in 75% of patients with bone metastases.
Alkaline phosphatase (ALP) serum	Assess status of bone and of renal, hepatic, intestinal, and biliary tract; indicator for GVHD, osteogenic sarcoma.	30-115 mU/ml	NPO 8 hours before test. Food can raise levels up to 25%.
Amylase serum	Assess pancreatic, renal, or salivary gland.	20-110 mU/ml	
CPK serum	Assess myocardial, muscle, and brain damage; infectious disease: HIV, hepatitis.	CPK: total Female: < 51 mU/ml Male: < 82 mU/ml CPK-MB bands 3% indicate cardiac damage. CPK-MM bands 97%-100% indicate muscle damage. CPK-BB bands 0% indicate brain damage.	Elevation of MB bands 3-6 hr after onset of acute myocardial infarction; peaks in 24 hr.

Test	Normal values	Use	Nursing considerations
Lactic acid dehydrogenase (LDH) serum	100-205 mU/ml	Assess hepatic, cardiac, renal, muscular, or RBC status.	Elevation seen 12-24 hr after onset of acute myocardial infarction; peaks in 2-6 days; elevation may indicate high-risk leukemia and lymphoma and/or relapse of these diseases.
Lipase serum	0-190 U	Assess pancreas.	
Serum glutamic-oxaloacetic transaminase (SGOT)	10-55 nU/ml	Assess status of many organs (e.g., liver, heart); cellular death (chemotherapy and radiotherapy).	Elevation seen 8-12 hr after onset of acute myocardial infarction; peaks in 48 hr.
Serum glutamic-pyruvic transaminase (SGPT)	4-28 mU/ml	Assess status of many organs (e.g., liver); cellular death (chemotherapy and radiotherapy); hepatitis, cirrhosis, mononucleosis.	

Other tests

Test	Normal values	Use	Nursing considerations

Cerebrospinal fluid values	Albumin mean: 29.5 mg/100 ml + 112 SD: 11-48 mg/100 ml
	Bilirubin: O
	Cell count: 0-5 mononuclear cell per mm³
	Chloride: 120-130 mEq/L
	Glucose: 50-75 mg/100 ml
	IgG mean: 4.3 mg/100 ml + 112 SD: 0-8.6 mg/100 ml
	Protein
	  Lumbar: 15-45 mg/100 ml
	  Cisternal: 15-25 mg/100 ml
	  Ventricular: 5-15 mg/100 ml
		Assess cerebrospinal system; brain tumor, CVA, meningitis.	Sterile procedure for specimen collection; send specimen to lab immediately. DO NOT refrigerate specimen, because refrigeration may inhibit growth of meningococus organisms and alter test accuracy.

Gastric analysis	Basal
	  Female: 2.0 + 1.8 mEq/hr
	  Male: 3.0 + 2.0 mEq/hr
	Maximal (after histalog or gastrin)
	  Female: 16 + 5 mEq/hr
	  Male: 23 + 5 mEq/hr
		Assess gastric function; carcinoma of stomach, pernicious anemia, and gastric atrophy.	NPO 8 hr before. Requires nasogastric tube insertion to collect specimen. Assess gag reflex after procedure.

Duodenal drainage	pH: 5.5-7.5 Amylase: over 1,200 U total Trypsin: 35-160% Viscosity: 3 min or less	Assess for duodenal ulcer status.	
Blood cultures	Negative: usually drawn from different site to coincide with temperature elevation	Determine presence of pathogens.	Implement precaution measures for potential infection. Administer prescribed antibiotics.
Papanicolaou smear (Pap)	Negative	Assess cervical tissue for presence of disease.	Collect three separate slide specimens.
Urinalysis	Color, turbidity: clear Negative for glucose, ketones, blood, bile, protein, bilirubin, crystals, RBC, WBC. Casts: not waxy; few hyaline, epithelial or granular	Screening tool; assess renal, endocrine status, infection.	Urine sample must be fresh for accurate results.

Continued.

APPENDIX B   LABORATORY VALUES — cont'd

Test	Purpose	Normal Values (Adult)	Nursing Action
Specific gravity		1.010-1.025 (urine osmolarity should always be higher than blood serum osmolarity)	
pH	Levels are affected by vegetarian, fruit, meat in dist.	5.0-7.5	
Acetone		Negative	
Amylase		24-76 μg/ml	
Bence-Jones protein	Assess oncologic status; multiple myeloma.	Negative	Keep urine container on ice.
Calcium	Assess parathyroid.	Negative	
Catecholamine	Assess renal system, Cushing's syndrome.	Epinephrine: < 20 μg Norepinephrine: < 100 μg Metanephrine: < 1.3 mg Vanillylmandelic acid: < 6 mg	
Creatinine clearance	Assess renal status.	75-125 ml/min Female: 0.8-1.8 g/24 hr Male: 1.0-2.0 g/24 hr	Collection container is kept on ice. Collect all urine for 24 hr.
Culture	Determine presence of pathogens.	Negative or < 10,000 organisms/ml	Usually drawn serially from different sites to coincide with temperature elevation.
Urobilinogen urine	Assess GI malfunction.	Up to 1 mg in a 2-4-hr specimen	Collection container is kept on ice.
24-hour urine	Assess renal status.	Same as creatinine clearance	
Viruses	Determine presence of virus.		Implement infection precautions for positive virus results; report positive results for all viruses.
HTLV I	Detect T-cell leukemia.	Negative	HIV: 1 — Seroconversion
HTLV II	Detect hairy cell leukemia.	Negative	2 — Lymph node involvement
HTLV III	Detect retrovirus (HIV) AIDS.	Negative	3 — Progressive lymphadenopathy
			4 — a — ARC fever; weight loss
			b — Neuropathy changes
			c — Infectious disease
			d — Malignancy
Herpes simplex	Detect herpes simplex virus I or II.	Negative	
Varicella zoster	Detect chicken pox, shingles	Negative	
Cytomegalovirus	Detect pneumonia.	Negative	
Epstein-Barr	Detect infectious mononucleosis.	Negative	
Rubella	Detect measles.	Negative	
Tumor markers are listed in Chapter 4.			
Hepatitis			
A — Anti-HAV, IgM	Infectious hepatitis.	Negative	
B — HBsAg, HBeAg	Serum hepatitis	Negative	
C — Anti-HCV	Posttransfusion non-A, non-B hepatitis	Negative	
D — Anti-HDV	Delta virus	Negative	
E — No test available	Enteric non-A, non-B hepatitis	Negative	

APPENDIX C   SELECTED DIAGNOSTIC TESTS

Diagnostic Test	Purpose	Procedure/Preparation	Postprocedure
Angiography	Used in various segments of the arterial system to determine vessel patency or the presence of an aneurysm, embolism, or arterial/venous malformations.	Assess for allergy to iodine preparation; NPO past midnight, sedation before procedure, local anesthesia before catheter insertion via fluoroscopy; contrast medium is infused via catheter; serial-timed radiographs are obtained.	A pressure dressing or sandbag may be applied to the entry site; monitor vital signs as ordered.
Barium studies	Assess for evidence of disease, anatomic abnormalities, malabsorption syndrome.	NPO status before test varies; 300-600 ml of contrast medium swallowed by patient for upper GI; lower GI preparation may include clear liquids, bowel prep of laxatives, suppositories, or enemas.	Large fluid intake is encouraged to promote barium excretion and minimize fluid loss.
Bone marrow biopsy	To examine the bone marrow for number, size, and shape of RBCs, WBCs, and megakaryocytes, estimation of cellularity, and determination of the presence of fibrotic tissue.	Aspiration of the marrow from the sternum, iliac crest, anterior and/or posterior iliac spine; proximal tibia in children; local anesthesia.	Apply pressure to puncture site; observe site for bleeding.
Bronchoscopy	Assess strictures, inflammation, or bleeding. Examine or remove pooled secretions and foreign bodies. Perform biopsy for analysis; place radiation beads for unresectable lung tumors.	NPO past midnight, sedation and atropine before procedure; fiberoptic bronchoscope inserted through nares.	Monitor vital signs; NPO status maintained until return of gag reflex.
Chest X-ray	Provide visualization of heart, lung, mediastinum, pulmonary vessels, trachea, bronchi, pleura, and diaphragm; assess response to therapy, location of monitoring catheters, pacemaker wires, etc., pleural effusions, neoplasms.	Optimal visualization requires that patient take in and hold a deep breath.	
Cholangiogram IV	Visualization of the biliary ductal system; assess inflammation; presence of stones and/or obstruction.	NPO past midnight; bowel preparation; IV infusion of iodine dye.	Assess that bilirubin level is <3.5 mg/100 ml so visualization is possible; if bilirubin is elevated, procedure may be cancelled; observe for allergic reaction from dye.
Colonoscopy	Examine the left, transverse, and right colon and sigmoid.	Clear liquid diet 1-3 days before; sedation and cathartics before exam, NPO past midnight; colonoscope inserted through anus.	Observe for unexpected bleeding.
Colposcopy	Provide direct visualization of the vagina, vulva, and cervical epithelium; to biopsy cervical tissue.	Colposcope is inserted into the vagina and advanced toward the cervix.	Monitor vital signs; observe for vaginal bleeding.
Computerized axial tomography (CT scan)	Noninvasive procedure to analyze tissue for density, assess for evidence of disease, inflammation, displacement, or enlargement.	May require NPO status; may be performed with or without a dye injection; CT scanning provides a cross-sectional image.	

Continued.

APPENDIX C   SELECTED DIAGNOSTIC TESTS — cont'd

Diagnostic Test	Purpose	Procedure/Preparation	Postprocedure
Culdoscopy	Permit observation of the uterus, fallopian tubes, ovaries, broad ligaments, rectal wall, and sigmoid colon from inside the cul-de-sac.	NPO past midnight; local, regional, or general anesthesia; surgical incision is made in the posterior vaginal wall; culdoscope is inserted into the vagina and passed through the incision into the cul-de-sac.	Monitor vital signs; observe for vaginal bleeding.
Cystoscopy	Permit direct examination of the urethra and bladder for strictures or bleeding sites; remove biopsy specimens of the prostate, bladder, and urethra; place urethral catheters.	May require sedation or anesthesia before exam; cystoscope is inserted into the urethra and advanced into the bladder.	Monitor for urinary retention or bleeding and for vital signs.
Echocardiography	Assess congenital ischemic or acquired heart disease, presence of pericardial effusion, structure and mobility of heart.	Gel is applied to the skin and the transducer is moved along the skin with some pressure. Heart valves and pericardial sac are examined.	Assist with hair washing.
Electroencephalography (EEG)	Assess intracranial pathophysiology and organic brain syndrome and determine presence and type of epilepsy.	From 16 to 32 electrodes are applied to the head with electrode paste.	
Electrocardiography (12-lead ECG)	Record electrical activity within the heart.	Electrodes are attached to patient's chest and to each of the four extremities.	
Endoscopic retrograde cholangiopancreaticography (ERCP)	Assess suspected biliary duct pathology and pancreatic disease.	NPO, sedative before procedure; IV line for medication administration; fiberoptic scope inserted for visualization.	Monitor vital signs; observe for bleeding; NPO status maintained until return of gag reflex.
Esophagoscopy with gastroscopy	Permits direct visualization of esophagus and stomach. Biopsy specimens, brushings or washings may be obtained.	NPO, sedative before procedure; local anesthesia. Fiberoptic scope is inserted through the mouth. IV line for medication administration.	Monitor vital signs; NPO status maintained until return of gag reflex.
I-125 fibrinogen uptake	Noninvasive test to identify suspected thrombus formation in the deep veins.		
Intravenous pyelogram (IVP)	Provide visualization of the kidneys, ureters, and bladder to determine abnormalities, obstruction, and/or hematoma.	Assess for allergy to iodine preparation; contrast medium is injected IV and concentrates in the urine; NPO for 12 hours before exam; bowel prep may be required.	Monitor vital signs; encourage fluid intake.
Laparoscopy	To permit visualization of pelvis and intestines; ovarian biopsy or other surgical procedures may be performed as part of laparoscopy (e.g., lysis of adhesions, tubal ligation.)	NPO past midnight; general anesthesia; a surgical incision is made and a trocar is inserted and then aspirated to ensure that intestine or large vessels have not been perforated; nitrous oxide or carbon dioxide may be inserted to create a pneumoperitoneum.	Monitor vital signs; observe for abdominal discomfort and bleeding.

Procedure	Purpose	Preparation	Nursing considerations
Liver biopsy	Assess liver malfunction or disease.	NPO 6-8 hours before, sedative before procedure; local anesthetic; needle insertion to obtain specimen.	Apply pressure to biopsy site; turn patient on right side; observe for bleeding; give vitamin K injection; monitor vital signs.
Lumbar puncture	Assess diagnosis of brain or spinal cord neoplasm, hemorrhage, meningitis, encephalitis, autoimmune disorders of CNS, and/or degenerative brain disease.	Sterile procedure; place patient in lateral decubitus (fetal) position; local anesthetic; obtain 3 sterile specimens.	Explain to the patient that he or she MUST lie still during the procedure; rest in bed (flat position) for 1 hr post-procedure.
Lymphangiography	Performed for staging purposes with lymphoma or to detect metastasis; to examine lymph vessels for obstruction.	Assess for allergy to iodine preparation; dye injected intradermally; serial-timed radiographs obtained.	Monitor vital signs; observe for respiratory distress.
Magnetic resonance imaging (MRI)	Noninvasive method for assessing tissue function and chemical composition of the body.	May require NPO status; contraindicated for patients with aneurysm clips or pacemakers because of magnetic field.	
Mammography	Determine presence of benign or malignant breast disease and cysts and to guide needle biopsy.	Breast is placed between the camera and film and compressed for a clear image.	
Mediastinoscopy	Allow visualization of mediastinum; potential biopsy of lymph nodes; to permit diagnosis and staging of cancer, infection, and sarcoidosis	NPO past midnight; sedation before procedure; local or general anesthesia before insertion of mediastinoscope via incision at suprasternal notch.	Monitor vital signs; potential for bleeding and dyspnea; NPO status until return of gag reflex.
Myelography	Permit visualization of the subarachnoid space to detect abnormalities of the spinal cord and vertebrae and locate obstruction in the flow of CSF	NPO for 4 hours before procedure; local anesthetic; needle inserted into lumbar space; contrast medium inserted with timed serial radiographs.	Monitor vital signs and neurologic status; follow postprocedure body position orders.
Nuclear medicine scans			
Bone	Detect focal defects in the bone, infection, fractures; to assess disease process.	Assess for previous reaction to contrast media; requires IV line for insertion of dye; serial radiographs are obtained; NPO and sedation may be required.	Encourage fluid intake to aid in urinary excretion of radionuclide.
Brain	Delineate subdural hematoma, arteriovenous malformation, thrombosis, abscess, neoplasm, glioma, or other metastatic tumors.	Assess for previous reaction to contrast media; requires IV line for insertion of dye; serial radiographs are obtained; NPO and sedation may be required.	Encourage fluid intake to aid in urinary excretion of radionuclide.
Gallium	Determine presence of neoplasms, lymphoma, bronchogenic cancer, Hodgkin's disease, or inflammation.	Assess for previous reaction to contrast media; requires IV line for insertion of dye; serial radiographs are obtained; NPO and sedation may be required.	Encourage fluid intake to aid in urinary excretion of radionuclide.
Liver and spleen	Detect lesions (e.g., cysts, hematomas, abscesses, adenomas, lacerations, and metastasis).	Assess for previous reaction to contrast media; requires IV line for insertion of dye; serial radiographs are obtained; NPO and sedation may be required.	Encourage fluid intake to aid in urinary excretion of radionuclide.

Continued.

APPENDIX C   SELECTED DIAGNOSTIC TESTS — cont'd

Diagnostic Test	Purpose	Procedure / Preparation	Postprocedure
Lung	Examine pulmonary vascular circulation and to locate pulmonary emboli.	Assess for previous reaction to contrast media; requires IV line for insertion of dye; serial radiographs are obtained; NPO and sedation may be required.	Encourage fluid intake to aid in urinary excretion of radionuclide
MUGA	Assess indices of ventricular effectiveness, ejection fraction, and ventricular volume of heart.	Assess for previous reaction to contrast media; requires IV line for insertion of dye; serial radiographs are obtained; NPO and sedation may be required.	Encourage fluid intake to aid in urinary excretion of radionuclide.
Renal	Provide data on kidney size, shape, location, and perfusion.	Assess for previous reaction to contrast media; requires IV line for insertion of dye; serial radiographs are obtained; NPO and sedation may be required.	Encourage fluid intake to aid in urinary excretion of radionuclide.
Thallium	Identify myocardial fibrosis and ischemia; perfusion imaging.	Assess for previous reaction to contrast media; requires IV line for insertion of dye; serial radiographs are obtained; NPO and sedation may be required.	Encourage fluid intake to aid in urinary excretion of radionuclide.
Thyroid	Assess location, size, shape, and anatomical function of the substernal or enlarged thyroid glands.	Assess for previous reaction to contrast media; requires IV line for insertion of dye; serial radiographs are obtained; NPO and sedation may be required.	Encourage fluid intake to aid in urinary excretion of radionuclide.
Oximetry	Assess arterial oxygen saturation (SaO_2); shock lung, pneumonia, asthma, mechanical ventilation status.	Place monitoring probe or sensor on the earlobe/fingertip.	Assure patient that test is noninvasive.
Paracentesis	Confirm presence of ascites; specimen analyzed for protein amylase, RBC, WBC, fat, specific gravity, and cancer cells; fluid may be removed for palliative measures.	Local anesthetic; insertion of trocar, then catheter for drainage; may be continuous flow set-up.	Monitor vital signs; observe and record fluid loss.

Pericardiocentesis	Needle aspiration of fluid from pericardial sac used for diagnostic or therapeutic purposes; ECG monitoring for localization and position of needle tip.	IV line for keep vein open rate; patient in supine position with head of bed elevated 60 degrees.	Observe and monitor vital signs, potential bleeding, and dyspnea.
Proctoscopy	Explore anus, rectum, and sigmoid colon.	Clear liquid diet, laxatives, NPO, enemas till clear before exam.	Observe for unexpected bleeding or sharp pain.
Sigmoidoscopy (flexible)	Examine left, transverse, right, and sigmoid colon with a flexible fiberoptic endoscope; biopsy and removal of polyps may be performed at this time.	Clear liquid diet 1-3 days, NPO 6-8 hours before; cathartics before exam; fiberoptic endoscope inserted via anus.	Observe for unexpected bleeding or sharp pain.
Thoracentesis	Obtain pleural fluid for analysis; therapeutic is performed to relieve intrathoracic pressure associated with excess fluid in the lung.	Local anesthesia before insertion of trocar, then chest tubes; needle insertion for biopsy may be guided by fluoroscopy.	Monitor vital signs; observe for respiratory distress, bleeding at entry site and excessive blood in sputum.
Tomography	To assess nodules or calcification in pulmonary mass or infiltrate.	Radiographic imaging through a predetermined cross section of the body; optimal visualization requires that patient take in and hold a deep breath.	
Ultrasonography Doppler	Noninvasive procedure using sound waves to assess tissue function, abscess, trauma; determine blood flow velocity.	Gel is placed on the patient and the transducer is moved along the skin with some pressure.	
Venography	Demonstrate nonfilling of a vessel; assess for abnormal valves, thrombophlebitis, or hematoma.	Assess for allergy to contrast medium; inject contrast medium; serial-timed radiographs are obtained.	Monitor vital signs; observe for bleeding at entry site.
Ventriculography	Observes size, shape, and filling of ventricles; detect lesions and/or cerebral anomalies.	Serial x-ray of the skull after air or contrast material is injected via burr holes in the skull.	Requires general/local anesthesia, NPO status past midnight; monitor vital signs postprocedure every 15 to 30 min for the initial 24 hr; head of bed elevated 10 to 15 deg for 24 hr; observe scalp dressing; monitor pain and administer analgesics.

BIBLIOGRAPHY FOR APPENDIXES B AND C

Herberman RB: Tumor markers. American Association for Clinical Chemistry NCI, Triton Diagnostics Inc., 1401 Harbor Bay Parkway, Almeda, CA 94501.

Littrup PJ et al: Prostate cancer screening: current trends and future implications, CA Cancer J Clin 42(4):198, 1992.

Pagana KD and Pagana TJ: Diagnostic testing and nursing implications, 3rd ed, St. Louis, Mosby, 1990.

Pesce AJ and Kaplan LA: Methods in clinical chemistry, St. Louis, 1987, Mosby.

Phipps WL, Long BC, Woods NF, and Cassmeyer VL: Clinical handbook of medical surgical nursing, 4th ed, St. Louis, 1991, Mosby.

Tietz NW, Finley PR, and Pruder EL, editors: Clinical guide to laboratory tests, 2nd ed, Philadelphia, 1990, WB Saunders.

Tilkian SM, Conover MB, and Tilkian AG: Clinical implications of laboratory tests. St. Louis, 1987, Mosby.

Wallach J: Interpretation of diagnostic tests, 5th ed, Boston, Little, Brown and Company, 1992.

Index